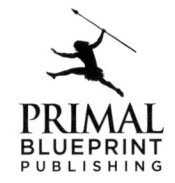

THE BORDEAUX KITCHEN

AN IMMERSION INTO
FRENCH FOOD AND WINE,
INSPIRED BY
ANCESTRAL TRADITIONS

TANIA TESCHKE   *Tania Teschke*

PRIMAL
BLUEPRINT
PUBLISHING

The Bordeaux Kitchen: An Immersion into French Food and Wine, Inspired by Ancestral Traditions

Copyright © 2018 Tania Teschke. All rights reserved.

Except as permitted under the United States Copyright Act of 1976, reproduction or utilization of this work in any form or by any electronic, mechanical, or other means, now known or hereafter invented, including xerography, photocopying, and recording, and in any information storage and retrieval system, is forbidden without written permission of the publisher.

Mention of specific companies, organizations, or authorities in this book does not imply endorsement by the author or publisher. Information in this book was accurate at the time researched.

Library of Congress Cataloging-in-Publication Data

Names: Teschke, Tania, 1971- author.
Title: The Bordeaux kitchen : an immersion into French food and wine :
  inspired by ancestral traditions / by Tania Teschke.
Description: Oxnard, CA : Primal Blueprint Publishing, [2018] | Includes
  bibliographical references and index.
Identifiers: LCCN 2017060470 (print) | LCCN 2018007138 (ebook) | ISBN
  9781939563408 (ebook) | ISBN 9781939563392 (hardcover)
Subjects: LCSH: Cooking, French. | Wine and wine pairing--France. | LCGFT:
  Cookbooks.
Classification: LCC TX637 (ebook) | LCC TX637 .T45 2018 (print) | DDC
  641.5944--dc23
LC record available at https://lccn.loc.gov/2017060470

Editor: Tracy Dunigan
Cover Design: Janée Meadows and Caroline De Vita
Interior Design and Layout: Caroline De Vita
Photography by Tania Teschke
Animal Illustrations by Arnaud Faugas
Copyediting, Proofreading, and Indexing: Tim Tate

Primal Blueprint Publishing, 1641 S. Rose Ave., Oxnard, CA 93033
Please contact the publisher with any questions, concerns, and feedback, or to obtain quantity discounts.
888-774-6259 or 310-317-4414
email: info@primalblueprintpublishing.com, or visit PrimalBlueprintPublishing.com.

DISCLAIMER: The ideas, concepts, and opinions expressed in this book are intended to be used for educational purposes only. This book is sold with the understanding that the author and publisher are not rendering medical advice of any kind, nor is this book intended to replace medical advice, nor to diagnose, prescribe, or treat any disease, condition, illness, or injury. It is imperative that before beginning any diet, exercise, recipes, or lifestyle program, including any aspect of the methodologies mentioned in *The Bordeaux Kitchen*, you receive full medical clearance from a licensed physician. If you are currently taking medication for health conditions, are pregnant or a growing youth, or have a current or past condition such as cardiovascular disease, cancer, diabetes, or other serious health condition, major dietary changes should be considered with extreme caution and the guidance of a trusted medical professional. The author and publisher claim no responsibility to any person or entity for any liability, loss, or damage caused or alleged to be caused directly or indirectly as a result of the use, application, or interpretation of the material in this book. If you object to this disclaimer, you may return the book to publisher for a full refund.

Printed in the U.S.A.

Foreword by Dr. Catherine "Cate" Shanahan v

1. Introducing *The Bordeaux Kitchen* 1

2. How I Came to Discover the Ancestral Lifestyle by Eating Like the French 7

3. The French Art and Tradition of Food and Wine 13

4. The Three Secrets to French Cooking: Farm Fats, Fresh Ingredients, and Cast-Iron Pots 29

5. Butchery Basics: Know Your Cuts and Hone Your Knives 71

6. Recipes, Stories, Cooking Tips, and Wine Pairings 93

   Beef – *Le Boeuf* 107

   Fish and Seafood – *Les Poissons et les Fruits de Mer* 159

   Lamb – *L'Agneau* 189

   Offal and Fats – *Les Abats et les Graisses* 217

   Pork – *Le Porc* 285

   Poultry, Eggs, and Rabbit – *La Volaille, les Oeufs, et le Lapin* 333

   Stocks and Sauces – *Les Fonds, Bouillons, et Sauces* 381

   Veal – *Le Veau* 419

   Vegetables – *Les Légumes* 431

   Desserts – *Les Desserts* 483

7. Know Your French Wines, How to Taste Them, and How to Pair Them with Food 513

8. Living with Intention, Family Food Organization, and Meal Planning 563

Appendixes 586

   My Roots 587

   Epilogue 591

   A Note on the Photography 592

   Acknowledgments 593

   Cooking Glossary 597

   Resources and Further Reading 603

   Endnotes 614

   Selected Bibliography 623

   Index 627

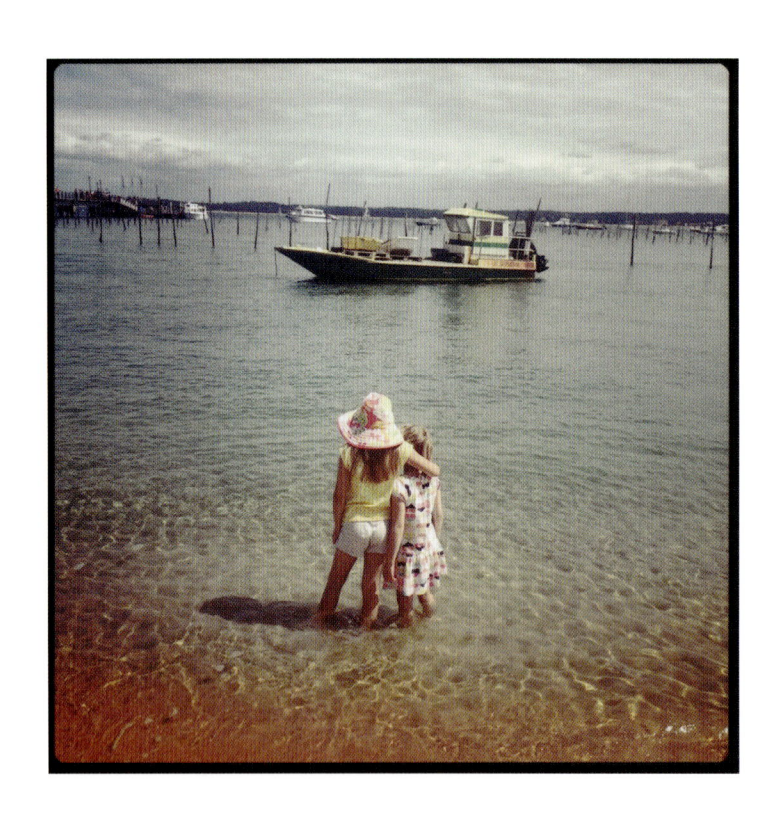

For my children, their children, grandchildren, and great-grandchildren,
lest their generations think they were forgotten before they even began.
For my family, near and far.
And for my husband, Toby.
I could not have done this without you.

FOREWORD

The French are perhaps one of the best examples of a culture that devotedly guards and celebrates its ancestral culinary traditions. But in recent decades, with the unfortunate worldwide trend toward low-fat diets and industrially processed food, many of the classic French recipes featuring fresh butcher cuts, organ meats, and hearty stocks have faded from memory. In *The Bordeaux Kitchen*, Tania Teschke reclaims the most nourishing and satisfying foods of ancestral French cuisine. With easy-to-follow recipes that deliver rich flavor and nutrient density, Tania shows that the French Paradox, eating rich foods that are high in fat while enjoying health and longevity, is actually not a paradox at all. And she does so at just the right moment. The growing food revolution has reawakened a passion for local, fresh, sustainably and humanely raised food. Athletes are experiencing tremendous performance benefits from a diet rich in natural, nutritious fats, even the long-disparaged saturated fats. Millions affected by chronic disease and autoimmune disorders are beginning to seek healing alternatives to a standard modern diet that is laden with sugar and vegetable oils. As many of our social interactions move into the virtual sphere, it is more important than ever to strengthen our real-time connections with family and friends. So, it is not surprising to see a renewed appreciation and celebration for the culinary traditions and whole food ingredients—often accompanied by a good wine—that are found in ancestral recipes.

When I first met Tania in 2016 at the Ancestral Health Symposium, I saw that her passion for food and wellness and her family's unique experiences living abroad could unite these elements together in an accessible book that would have broad appeal. Her years of cooking and studying in France and other European countries have rekindled her deep appreciation for ancestral traditions. She learned and tested her recipes alongside French chefs, as well as French grandmothers and friends. She visited farms throughout the Southwest of France and studied with some of the country's premier winemakers and oenologists.

Unlike the vast majority of French cookbooks, this is not a purely epicurean endeavor. *The Bordeaux Kitchen* answers the fundamental question driving Tania and so many of us: how can delicious traditional food heal our bodies and create conditions for optimal health? This book explains why eating an ancestral diet is healthier than a modern diet by drawing upon the work of leading nutrition researchers and authors. It brings what we've learned from the paleo/primal movement, the recently popular ketogenic diet, and carefully prescribed autoimmune protocols and shows us that through simple, traditional recipes we can nurture our health by procuring, preparing, and serving real food that is delicious and immensely satisfying.

I am particularly happy to see that *The Bordeaux Kitchen* is full of recipes with meat on the bone, organ meats, fermented foods, and raw foods—what I call the Four Pillars of the Human Diet. In *The Bordeaux Kitchen*, you'll find dozens of recipes made simple—from chops and steaks, to stews and stocks, to high omega-3-rich fish and seafood, to sauerkraut and sprouted nuts. You will also learn how to prepare calf's liver, sweetbreads, and, if you are daring enough, sheep's brains! You'll turn these raw ingredients into delicious, nutrient-dense meals that our bodies and our cells crave. Tania also shows us how cooking with animal fats, olive oil, and butter instead of toxic vegetable oils, adds not only beneficial fats and nutrients, but incomparable flavor to dishes. Finally, for those like me who enjoy a glass of wine now and then with a nourishing meal, Tania provides extensive education in the art of wine pairing—choosing the best wines, French or otherwise, to accompany each recipe. She explains how wine not only flavors a dish, but also accentuates the entire sensory experience of dining with family and friends.

Whether you come to *The Bordeaux Kitchen* as a foodie, Francophile, professional athlete, health-conscious parent, or all of the above, you'll find many French-inspired recipes to charm your palate and boost your and your family's health. You will also discover a new way of looking at food and your connection to culinary traditions. Get ready for an immensely satisfying journey to better health!

Catherine "Cate" Shanahan, M.D.
December 2017

Dr. Cate Shanahan is a board-certified family physician from Connecticut, author of the acclaimed *Deep Nutrition*, and former nutrition director for the Los Angeles Lakers. She specializes in medically supervised weight loss through ancestral-based eating, and is lauded for her passionate crusade against refined high polyunsaturated vegetable oils. Dr. Shanahan was trained in biochemistry and genetics at Cornell University's graduate school before attending Robert Wood Johnson Medical School. She practiced family medicine in Hawaii for 10 years, during which time she also studied ethnobotany. She became enlightened about the benefits of ancestral eating when she noticed the elderly patients eating traditional Hawaiian diets were healthier than younger patients who had adopted Western dietary habits. Her groundbreaking message, presented in the original edition of *Deep Nutrition* in 2009, was credited with helping to ignite the burgeoning ancestral health movement.

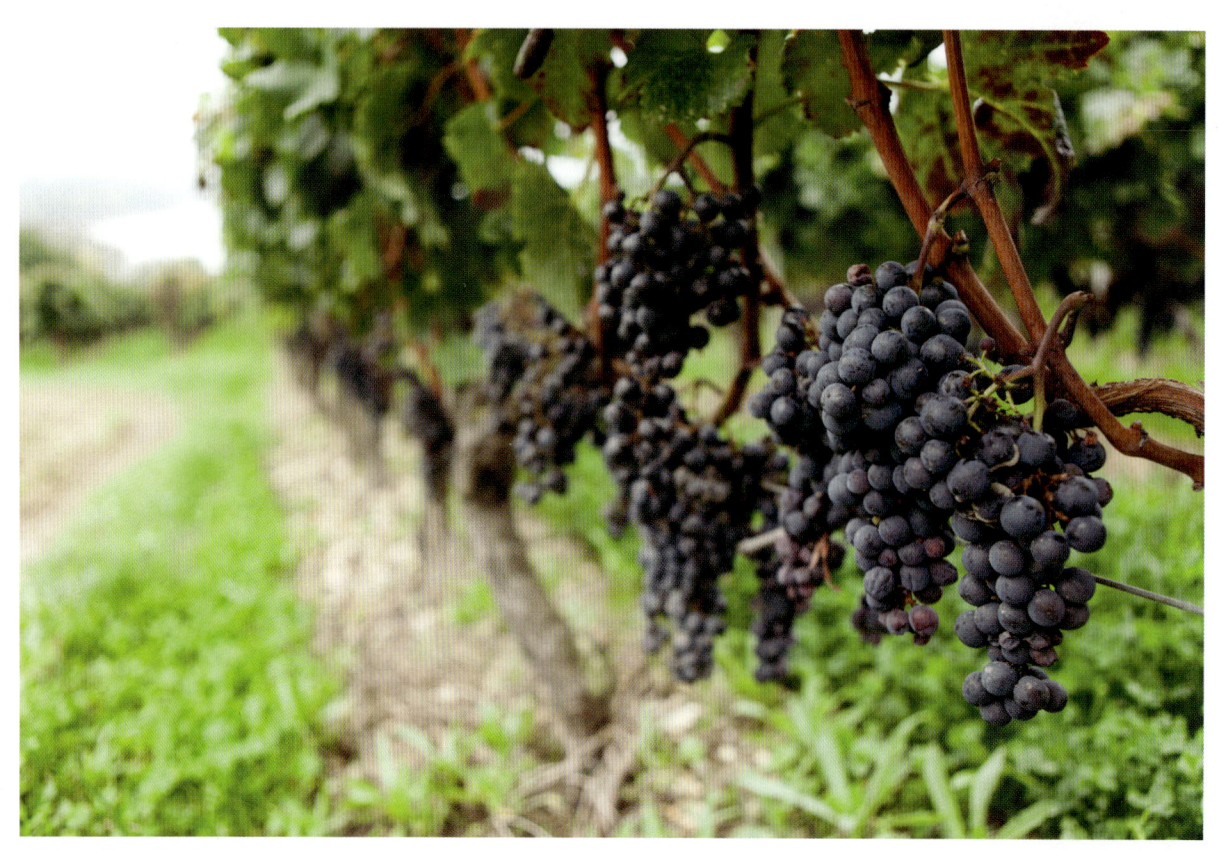

Château Biac, Bordeaux

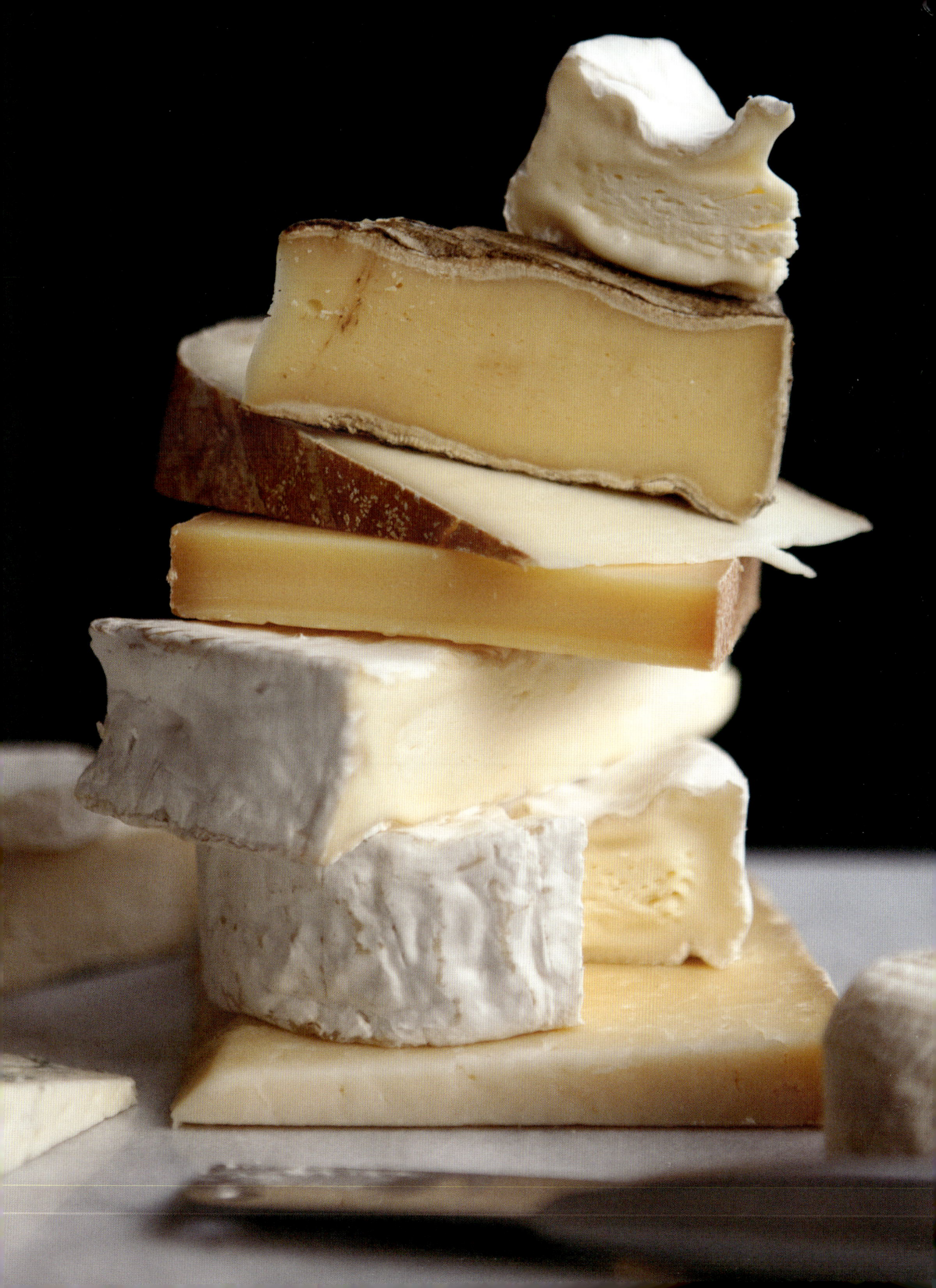

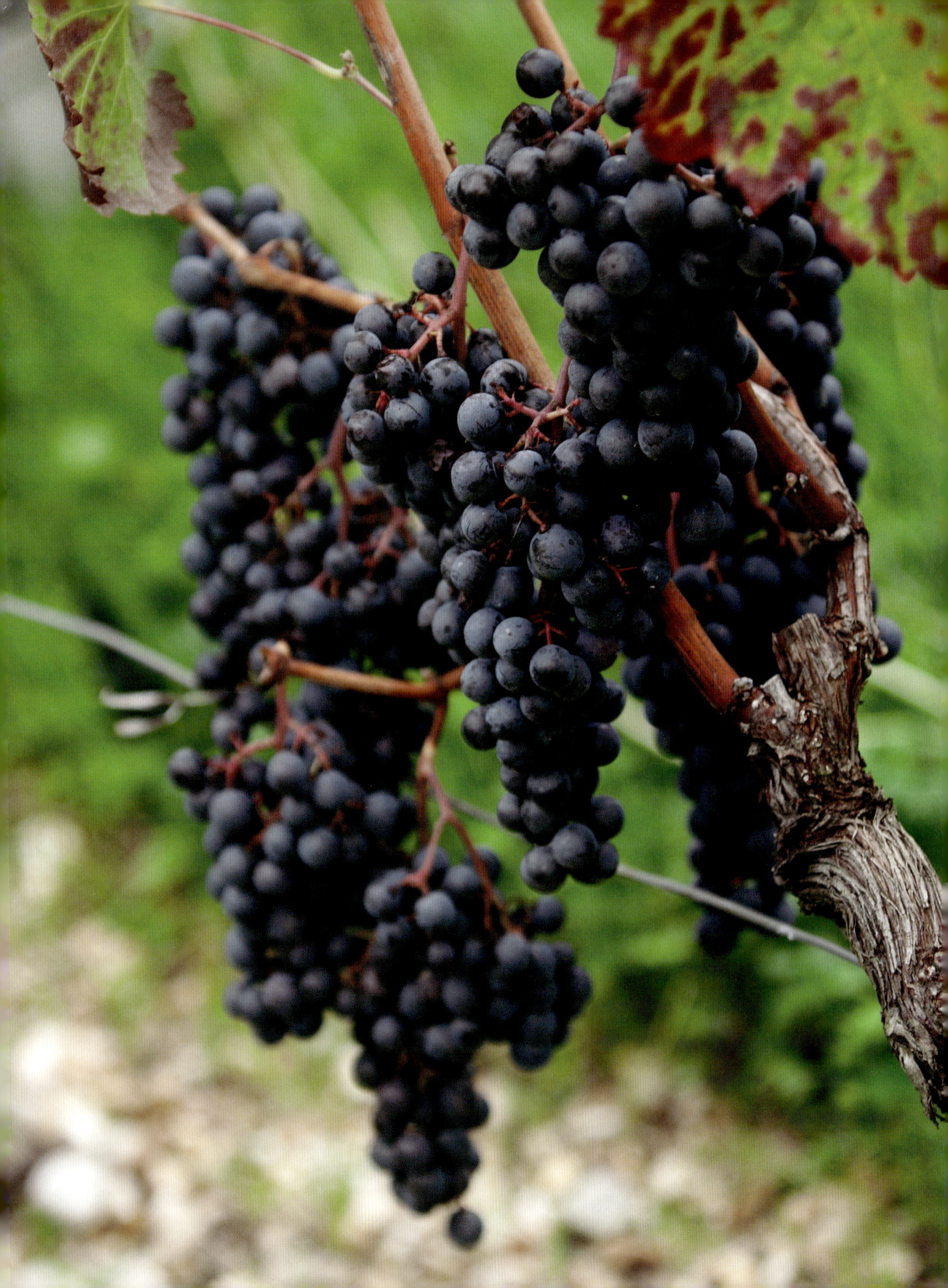

CHAPTER 1

INTRODUCING *THE BORDEAUX KITCHEN*

THE FRENCH PARADOX

People look at the French in bewilderment, wondering how they can eat such rich food, yet stay so slim. However, from an ancestral or primal/paleo perspective, there really is *no paradox* when you consider the time-honored traditions of French culture and cuisine. These traditions honor the use of natural and seasonal food, sourced locally when possible, and reflect a sensible approach (*une approche raisonnée*) to eating that enhances a healthy metabolism.

THE FRENCH ANCESTRAL APPROACH

The good news is that you, too, can live and eat as richly as the French, while enhancing your health through a primal/paleo lifestyle. As you will see in *The Bordeaux Kitchen*, traditional Southwestern French recipes in particular are beautifully and naturally suited to meet our primal nutritional needs. My wish is that these culinary traditions will inspire your family meal planning and nourish your sense of health, wellbeing, and community. I will also explain how to accompany these ideas and recipes with a glass of wine from time to time!

Primal, Paleo, and Ancestral— What's the Difference?

Throughout *The Bordeaux Kitchen*, you will frequently see the terms *primal*, *paleo*, and *ancestral*. Here's how I am using the terms in the text:

Primal/paleo diets consider the human diet dating back to the Paleolithic era (2.6 million years ago) to determine what to eat based on what food best served our evolution and survival as a species.

Ancestral diets focus on eating natural, whole food in the way it was traditionally prepared by our ancestors—unrefined, pesticide-free, non-GMO, using grassfed, full-fat, raw dairy, and organic ingredients when possible.

FRENCH CUISINE'S RICH TAPESTRY

Traditional French cooking has a common thread running throughout its cuisine. Regional culinary influences—from Alsace in the East to the Vendée in the West, and from Bordeaux in the Southwest to Burgundy, the medieval birthplace of "modern" French cooking—weave in their own rich color and texture by contributing their unique culinary treasures to the already resplendent cuisine of France. At its core, *The Bordeaux Kitchen* embraces an ancestral perspective to cooking by integrating traditional, time-honored recipes and wine pairings from all over France. Most of these nutrient-dense recipes originate from the French Southwest (*le Sud Ouest*), one of the richest culinary and agricultural epicenters of France.

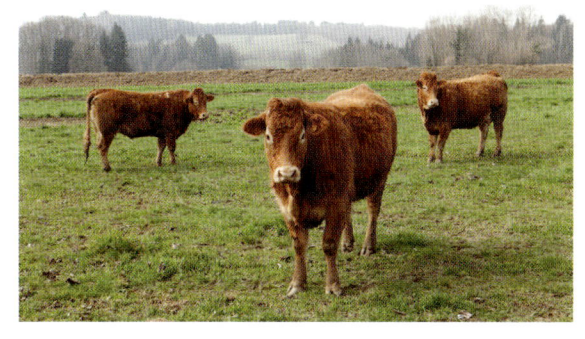

Grass-fed Limousine Cows of the French Southwest

INSPIRED BY THE FRENCH SOUTHWEST

From the French Basque region and the Pyrénées to coastal fishing towns, and from the Dordogne valley to world-class vineyards, my family and I discovered during three years of living in Bordeaux that the French Southwest has it all. It is a region where you can find everything from Basque lambs and black Pyrénées pigs to wild game, a wide array of local vegetables and cheeses, pastured duck and goose farms, oyster growers, and an assortment of fish along the Atlantic coast, not to mention some of the most-prized beef

‹ *Château Biac, Bordeaux Region*

breeds including *Bazas*, *Blonde d'Aquitaine*, *Charolaise*, and *Limousine*. The magic of the region's cuisine is in the preparation of these simple, local, fresh ingredients with flavorful herbs and healthy fats into some of the richest and most delicious French dishes. With such abundant resources, it is no wonder the French Southwest is known for its vast array of recipes that originate here and then flow out to influence the rest of France.

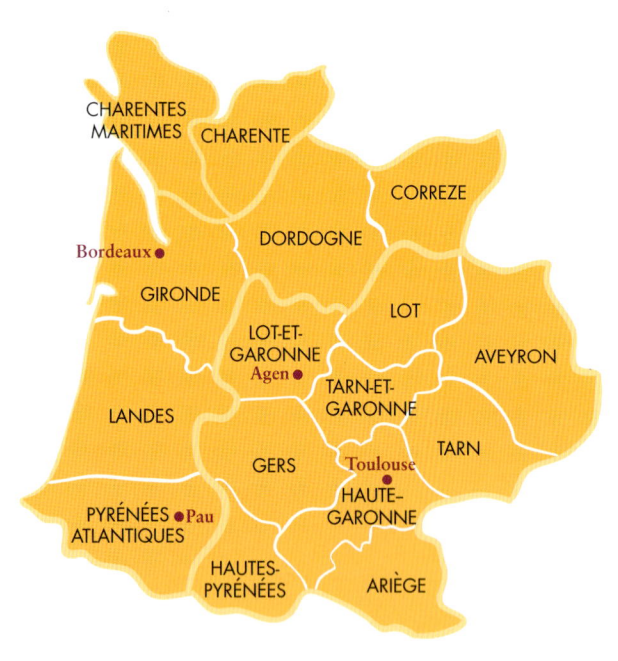

Departments of the Southwest Corner of France

And unlike the rest of France, many French Southwest sauces and dishes call for wine instead of cream in their preparation. This is because the Bordeaux wine region is known for its world-class wines that naturally complement the rich gastronomic history of the region, including delicious preparations of meats, seafood, and vegetables rounded off with nutritious and delectable fats.

Many people do not realize that some of their favorite French dishes originate from the Southwest of France—**Foie Gras** (page 244), **Duck Breast, *Magret de Canard*** (page 351), **Wine Trader's Rib Eye Steak, *Entrecôte Sauce Marchand de Vin*** (page 155)—yet they are apt to find them on French menus both in France and around the world. Yet, it is not only *what* the French eat, it's *how* they eat. I enjoyed making many of these recipes with energetic French grandmothers, passionate farmers, excitable butchers and chefs, devoted parents, and dedicated winemakers, who all showed me how preparing and enjoying ancestral recipes slowly and deliberately, in contrast with our hectic modern social and eating habits, can further enhance our health and the richness of our social connections.

THE FOUR FAT REGIONS OF FRANCE (AND THE FIFTH FAT)

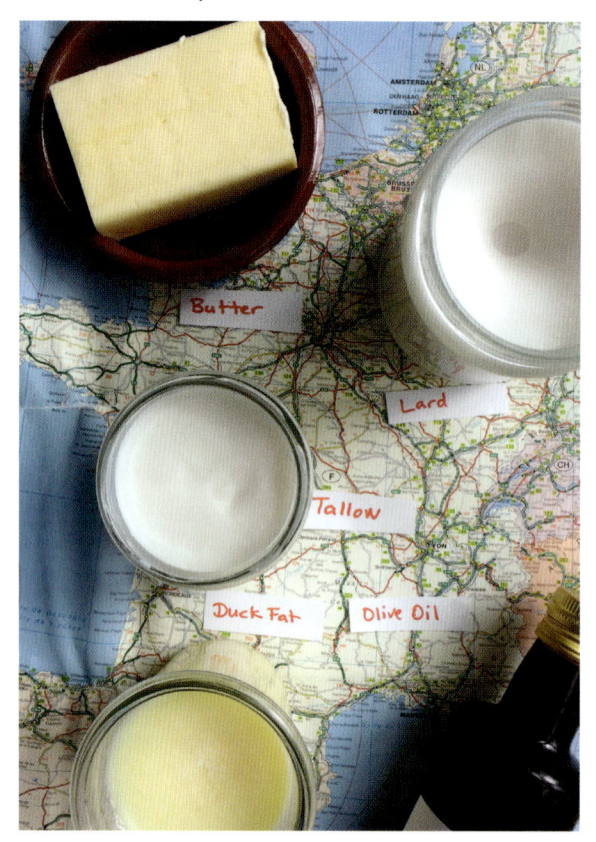

Fats of France

France can be divided into four regions with respect to its historical and regional use of fats for cooking, according to historian Waverley Root's book from 1958, *The Food of France*.[1] For the most part, this still holds true today, as the Northwest (Brittany and Normandy) predominantly uses butter, the Northeast (Alsace and Lorraine) primarily employs lard, the Southeast (Provence) most commonly uses olive oil, and the Southwest utilizes all of the above in addition to the venerable duck and goose fats, which in traditional Southwestern French cooking, outweigh the use of butter by a large margin. Paris, meanwhile, derives its influences from all around France, and each region likewise influences the others in what Root calls a "reciprocal culinary osmosis." I would add a fifth fat to these—the historically used tallow, a readily available, rich source of nutrients, now all but forgotten in modern kitchens. Add to this the fatty marrow of animal bones, rich in collagen and used to make restorative and flavorful stocks in French cooking, and there you have the foundations of a nutrient-dense, satiating cuisine!

MODERN QUANDARY

As I discuss in Chapter 3, "The French Art and Tradition of Food and Wine," French cooking methods have served as the foundation of modern cuisine around the world. And let us not forget that France still maintains among the lowest rates of coronary heart disease, though, like in most countries around the world, these rates are slowly increasing.[2,3] Despite its rich, interwoven cultural and gastronomic history and breadth of international appeal, France, like all "developed" nations, is not immune to an ever-increasing reliance on industrially refined "foods," nor to the associated health implications that accompany the modern "conveniences" of "fast food," supermarkets, and large-scale agricultural production.

A NECESSITY TO PRESERVE TRADITION

The Bordeaux Kitchen is a response to what I consider a necessity: not only to help preserve France's magnificent gastronomic legacy, but also to guide you past the health pitfalls of our modern diet toward the benefits of a rich French culinary tradition and a primal/paleo approach to living. This book presents some of the most nutrient-dense recipes in traditional French cuisine, a kind of French Ancestral Diet, the sheer opposite of its acronym, FAD. Not a new fad in any way, these are traditions to hand down to our children, lest they be lost amid the tide of trendy diets, consumed as modern fads and eventually cast aside. Rather, *The Bordeaux Kitchen* brings back an understanding of the vital role nutrient-dense foods have played in sustaining us for generations.

SHARED ANCESTRAL RECIPES

The Bordeaux Kitchen draws from a unique blend of what I learned while living in Bordeaux for three years, numerous cooking classes, and a year-long, scientifically oriented university course in wine tasting, in addition to the ancestral recipes shared by French chefs, butchers, grandmothers, mothers, and friends. Some are time-tested recipes, passed on to me directly from the cooks and chefs who have made them for their own families over the years, while others I have adapted to suit my own real food, home-cooking style. This cookbook also supplies you with unique diagrams in French and English depicting the cuts of meat for beef, lamb, pork, and veal to help guide your understanding of where these cuts of meat come from and why they are appropriate for a particular dish.

COMBINED WITH WINE

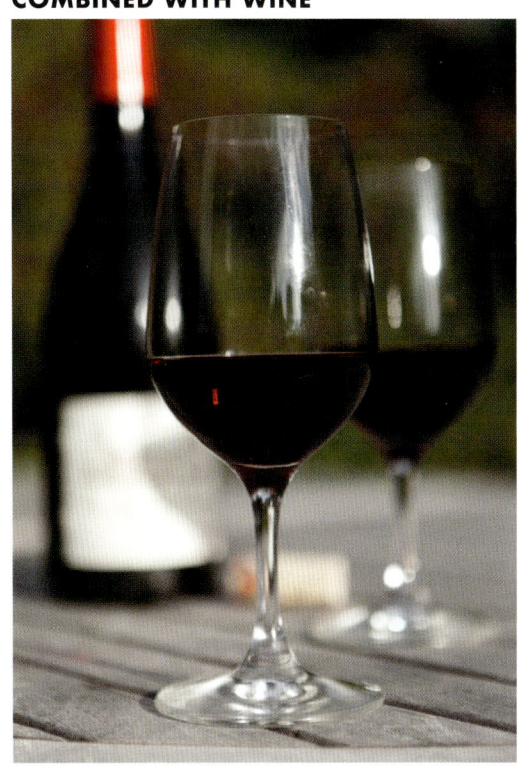

Many people like to enjoy a glass of wine now and then with their meal. Sips of wine, savored slowly, can add a memorable, sensual element to a meal. No one understands this like the French. Indeed, the Europeans have enjoyed wine over millennia. French dishes evolved with wine as a counterpart. Wine is often an ingredient, such as in **Chicken in Wine Sauce,** *Coq au Vin* (page 345), **Basque Chicken,** *Poulet Basque* (page 334), or **Beef Burgundy,** *Boeuf Bourgignon* (page 109). I am, therefore, delighted to share with you some wine-pairing suggestions along with the recipes, as well as some background on the wines of France and how to taste and enjoy them (see Chapter 7 – Know Your French Wines, How to Taste Them, and How to Pair Them with Food).

NUTRIENT-DENSE RECIPES FOR OUR MODERN DAY

The Bordeaux Kitchen describes certain French traditions, such as the importance of taking the time to procure, prepare, and enjoy real ingredients. This process adds up to something greater than its parts and embraces the value of bonding over home-cooked meals with family and friends. These "whole food" recipes, such as **Slow-Cooked Leg of Lamb,** *Gigot d'Agneau,* (page 209), **Pork Shoulder Cooked in Fat,** *Échine de Porc Confit* (page 311), **Pyrénées Country Pâté,** *Terrine de Compagne des Pyrénées* using pork liver, (page 314), and stocks made with chicken, fish, or veal, pages 417, 403, and 415), demonstrate the importance of the nutrient-dense animal fats, herbs, spices, and ingredients that have sustained families for generations, as evidenced by some of France's most famous original cookbooks dating back to the Renaissance, and in some cases, the Middle Ages. By welcoming the seasonality and freshness of locally grown food in all its flavor and nutrient-density, this book reflects the spirit of the way our ancestors ate. It is a call to reduce our modern-day reliance on industrially refined and processed "foods" and oils. Stripped of nutrients and authentic flavor, industrial "food" companies add sugar, high fructose corn syrup, and industrially-derived salts to processed "foods," replacing all the satisfying, naturally-occurring fats and mineral salts. The recipes in *The Bordeaux Kitchen* reflect a time when more attention and time were dedicated to nourishment (and thus, health) before the dawn of pesticides, mass food production, and the rapid degradation of our soil (thanks to modern agricultural practices), which has only escalated since the mid-20th century onward.

PAYING IT FORWARD

I have been deeply motivated to create this book as a guide for my family and for you, the reader. In learning about the undeniable link between health and food, I am learning how to nourish my family and to pass on, with each meal, this knowledge to my children. If I do not pay forward what I have learned, the knowledge is lost without reaching its full potential in subsequent generations. I am not formally trained as a chef, scientist, or nutritionist. But I found formal training not necessarily required in my search to understand how to properly nourish my family and to regain my health following a series of setbacks. *The Bordeaux Kitchen* is proof that with a bit of focus, anyone can learn to enjoy French cooking and reap the benefits of French ancestral wisdom.

MOTIVATION

After a decades-long journey of digestive and wellness issues, I am ready to share what I have learned about the importance of proper nutrition in overall health. Having explored diverse dietary paths—from vegetarianism back to meat eating, dabbling in ketosis (fat eating and fat burning), and letting go of refined sugar consumption and similar "refined food" addictions—I am now reclaiming the knowledge of our ancestors. Learning how to feed my family motivates me to get up in the morning and puts further distance between a near-death hospital experience in my mid-20s followed by years of lingering health problems. My improved state of health (not to mention the fact that this home-cooked food tastes delicious) motivated me to create *The Bordeaux Kitchen*!

SUPPORT

I would not be at this point, ready to give back, without the support of my husband and my two daughters who have shared in my suffering and triumphs all these years. I am profoundly grateful to them for sticking with me, putting up with my changes, ideas, and ups and downs. In return, I cook a variety of the most nutrient-dense meals their palates will tolerate. Nurturing a family toward truly healthful eating while surrounded by an industrialized "food" system is a slow process and challenge, but already after a few years of small steps and dietary tweaks, we have all experienced great improvements in mood, behavior, digestion, and energy. By embracing the culinary and cultural lessons of the French and the ancestral movement, I found an opportunity to teach sustainable, nurturing dietary habits to my family. May our journey inspire others to give this approach to *eating with intention*, focusing on relaxed family time spent around lovingly prepared meals, a chance to take root. Embracing the lessons of *The Bordeaux Kitchen* provides an opportunity for every family to learn sustainable, nurturing dietary habits, reduce their consumption of refined sugars and convenience "foods," and rely more on seasonal, nutrient-dense foods and satisfying, healthy fats.

INSPIRATION AND GRATITUDE

The healing and the learning are never really over; it is a lifelong journey for each of us. The creative outlets I have found through cooking, writing, and photography, combined with all I have learned from nutrition research, health podcasters, blogs, books, the primal/paleo and ancestral movements, and French cookbooks, among other sources, continue to inspire me on a daily basis. I am grateful for the interactions with people I have met throughout France, whether during my walks through the medieval streets of Bordeaux or in cooking classes, and of course the friends who have shared their love of cooking with me. I am endlessly impressed with their dedication to the crafts of cooking, butchery, wine making, and to the fine art of pairing food with wine. Not least of all, I am grateful for their patience in teaching me their beloved crafts and for the warmth they have shown me in the caring of their families, friends, and guests! I am grateful to have learned the secret behind the supposed French Paradox—which is that you can enjoy better health *by way of*, rather than *in spite of*, eating rich, delicious, traditional dishes. The ancestral traditions of French cuisine and the art of simply living in the moment, mindfully enjoying great food and loving company, is well worth celebrating and preserving. I invite you to join me, to immerse yourself in these traditions, and let *The Bordeaux Kitchen* be your guide.

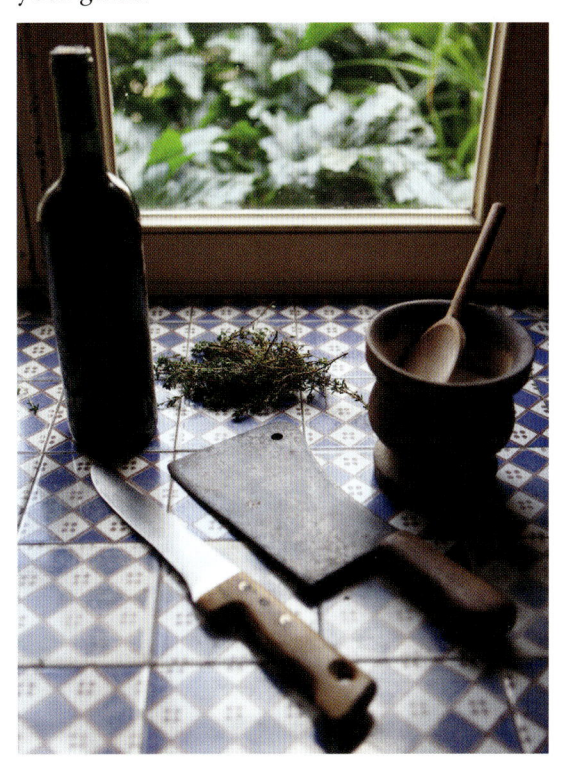

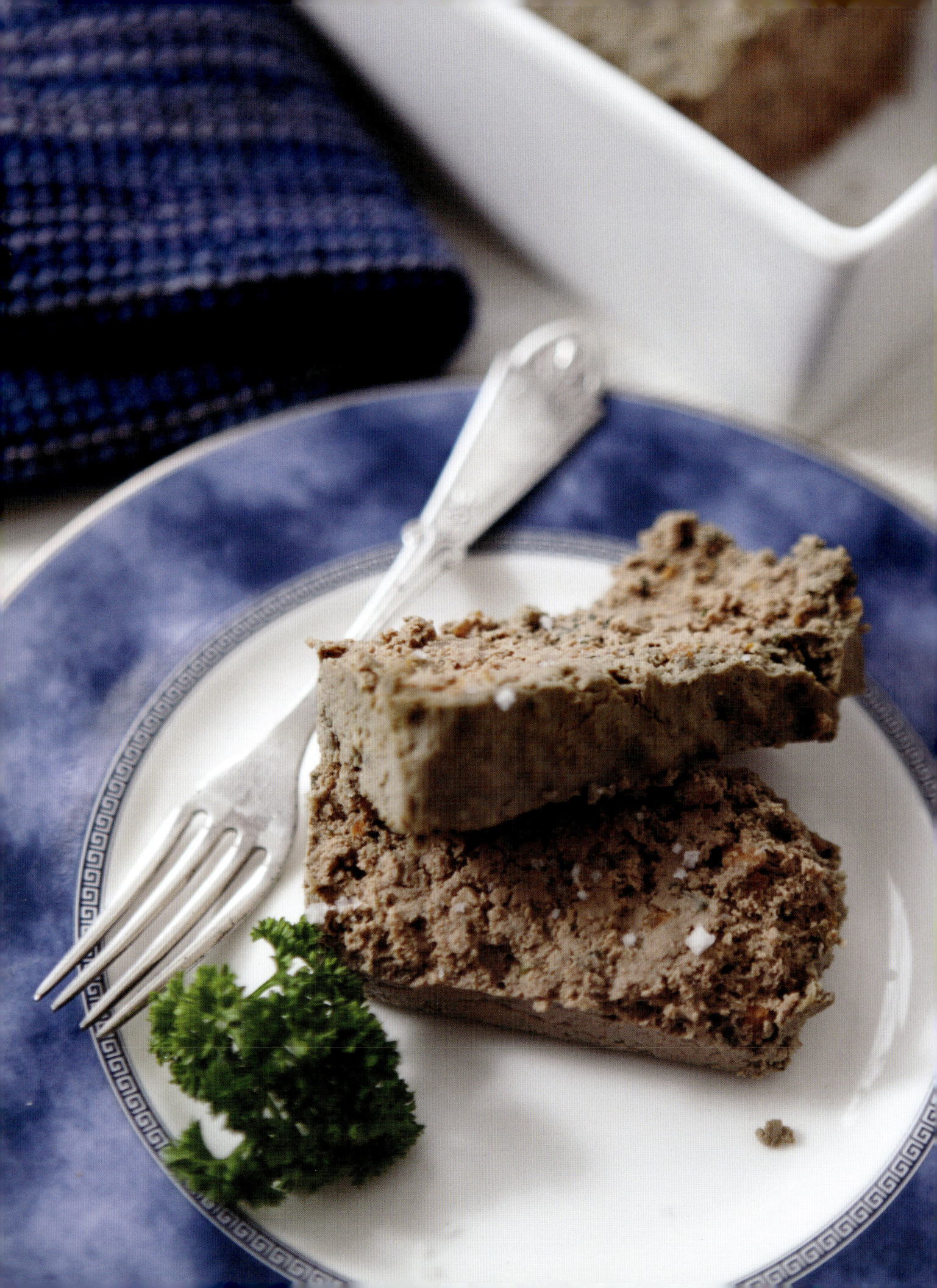

CHAPTER 2

HOW I CAME TO DISCOVER THE ANCESTRAL LIFESTYLE BY EATING LIKE THE FRENCH

"The greatest wealth is health."
—Virgil[1]

The Bordeaux Kitchen ties together what I have learned over the past two decades, about health, food, our environment, and other cultures, particularly during my three years studying food and wine in Bordeaux. This cookbook is also inspired by my deep connections to food that go back to my earliest childhood memories (see *My Roots* on page 587) and my love of France. Beginning in my teenage years, I was fortunate to study French and visit and live in France on several occasions.

I have always had an affinity for old world food, but it was an early brush with death at the age of 25 from a ruptured appendix and subsequent poor health that motivated me to search for better health. It was not until 2013, however, after two decades of poor digestion, unpredictable moods, and low energy, that I happened upon the ancestral lifestyle through a series of science, nutrition, and health podcasts and books while my family and I were living in Southwestern France. At the same time that I was learning about the key tenets of an ancestral lifestyle more in tune with our evolutionary past, I was also experiencing a traditional French lifestyle and learning how to cook like the French. I began to see the positive effects of the French diet and lifestyle on my symptoms and overall health.

And as it turned out, people in the ancestral movement were looking for precisely those things the French were already doing: cooking from scratch and *with intention*, using fresh, seasonal, nutrient-dense ingredients and animal fats. Instead of using industrially refined sugars, salts, and oils, the French used what I call "farm fats," such as butter, duck fat, and lard. In addition, the French tend to move more outdoors under their own power (on foot or bike) to procure many of these ingredients at local markets. Like their ancestors, the French still share meals regularly and convivially with family and friends, often pairing their food with wine and savoring it all slowly and mindfully for a total-sensory experience.

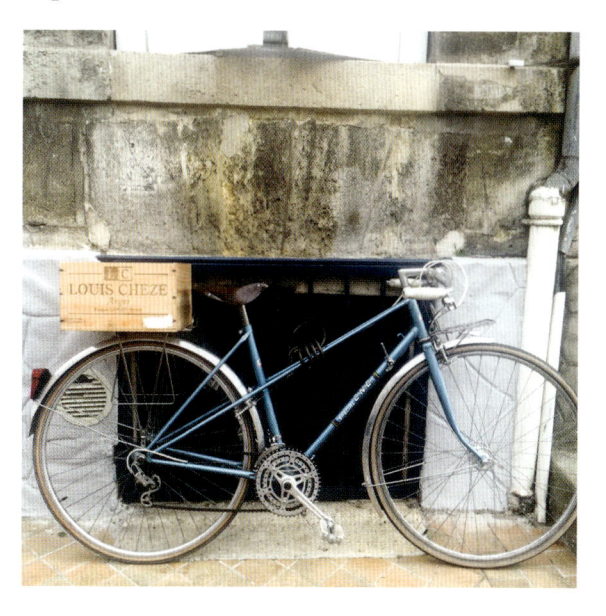

Mind you, my family and I were not exactly living off the land, cut off from civilization; we were living in Bordeaux, a city of over 240,000 people (and over 750,000 people in the greater Bordeaux area). Yet we were still able to integrate elements of the ancestral lifestyle into our modern lives, slowly but surely and without great difficulty, using the "French ancestral" lifestyle as a roadmap.

So, there I was in Southwestern France, learning about ancestral lifestyles through my research while experiencing firsthand how the French live, cook, and make wine. I seized the opportunity to learn from the French as much as possible about their cooking methods, real-food ingredients, fresh food preparation

‹ *Duck Liver Pâté (recipe on page 242)*

(including French butchery), and how to cook with traditional fats. I even learned how to prepare organ meats, and of course, how to taste and appreciate wine. Simultaneously, I was integrating all that I was learning from the ancestral health community on wellness and nutrition, such as prioritizing sleep and letting go of gut-disrupting and inflammatory sugar, refined "foods," and industrial oils.

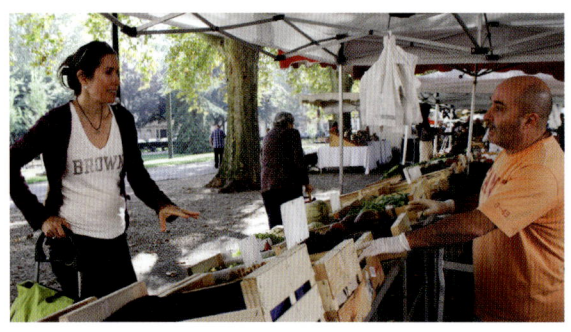

Tania at the Saint Seurin Market in Bordeaux talking with an organic produce vendor   Photo: Dr. Corinne Giesemann

I also saw digestive, hormonal, and energy benefits from the paleo and primal approaches by cutting out sugar and grains and lowering my consumption of carbohydrates in general. In their place, I increased the protein somewhat, but more so the animal fats in my diet. This strategy improved my health in numerous ways, as did avoiding restaurants, which was a challenge with so many nice French restaurants and cafés from which to choose. I really began to see results when I also focused on reducing stress and getting more sleep following the final exam of my intensive Bordeaux University year-long wine course. This meant no computer after dinnertime, going to bed right after (or even *before*) my children, and not going out in the evenings. It meant saying "no" to many social engagements for my children and me. It also meant being the "strange" mom at school who didn't send in candy and cookies for parties and who boycotted bake sales. Less was more. I was beginning to truly understand the extent to which nutrient-dense foods were the key to healing. The process of eliminating distractions also opened my eyes to the extent to which we depend on industrial "food" and energy systems to spoon-feed us during our rush-about modern-day lives.

Living in France gave me ample opportunity to seek out the wonderful flavors in natural foods that can be obscured when our tastes become accustomed to processed "foods." It also reintroduced me to the use and benefits of what I call the "farm fats:" butter, duck and goose fat, lard, olive oil, and tallow, the kinds of (primarily saturated and monounsaturated) fats that one could render or press by hand on one's own farm. I also learned how to cook and not be scared by offal, the most overlooked parts of animals that are actually the most nutritious. Learning to use and consume these fats and animal parts has been the key to sustainably satiating me between meals, thereby reducing by default my consumption of sugar and the resultant mood and energy swings. I even benefited from the loss of some abdominal "belly fat" that had stubbornly hung on for years after my second pregnancy.

THE TENETS OF *THE BORDEAUX KITCHEN*

In Bordeaux, I dedicated myself to learning the essential elements of French ancestral cuisine, combined with my discoveries from the primal and paleo community that can be incorporated into our modern lives to improve our health. I found seven key elements of the French ancestral approach that guide me today. These are the tenets of *The Bordeaux Kitchen*.

1. Cook your own food, and source it often, when possible, on foot or on bike.

2. Embrace animal fats from quality sources (such as your local butcher).

3. Focus on nutrient-density by rediscovering how to cook with organ meats from pasture-raised animals.

4. Do away with all industrially processed "foods," grains, and oils to break free from their toxicity and addictiveness.

5. Get in tune with the rhythms of nature, which means eating fresh, seasonal, and organic vegetables and herbs. Increase your movement and your access to sunlight in the day and more sleep at night.

6. Get over taboos about what constitutes "breakfast" or a "snack," and feed your family with intention.

7. Pair your meals with the right wine, and savor your food slowly with family and friends.

Throughout *The Bordeaux Kitchen* you will learn more about prioritizing these tenets You will learn how to prepare delicious and nutritious French-inspired meals for yourself, your family, and your friends, using techniques, utensils, and ingredients to ensure your success and delight. You will learn about French wine and how to pair wine with meals. You will learn about French butchery and why this is important to understanding the recipes. You will also learn some of the key principles of an ancestral lifestyle, including the value of consuming nutrient-dense foods, getting movement, sunlight, and sleep, the advantages of consuming organic produce and pasture-raised animals, and the benefits of letting go of sugars, grains, and industrially refined "foods."

THE BORDEAUX KITCHEN PERSPECTIVE ON ANCESTRAL DIETS

Our distant, pre-agricultural ancestors from tens of thousands of years ago had very basic cooking tools if any, and they were able to survive by eating animals almost entirely "nose-to-tail," deriving great nutritional benefit from the organs and fat in particular. This book respects and celebrates that ancestral ability to thrive on natural, whole food and animal sources by encouraging you to procure and enjoy local, seasonal, and pesticide-free produce, fish, and meat. At the same time, the recipes in *The Bordeaux Kitchen* demonstrate how our modern cooking methods and tools can help us to utilize every part of the animal in a practical and economically viable way, thanks to cast-iron pots, stainless steel pans, spatulas (for scraping every last bit of fat from a bowl), sharper knives, occasionally a food processor, and not least of all, the timeless knowledge of butchers, farmers, and cooks.

The recipes in The Bordeaux Kitchen focus on cooking with unprocessed and natural fats along with meats and vegetables, while relinquishing (except for a few sweetened desserts) the reliance on grains, breads, sugar, rice, and pastas that are now prevalent throughout Europe.

Our ancestors from the Middle Ages onward had iron pots and knives, but they were largely dependent on the agriculture and available products of the day. Also, by then, much of their diet consisted of grains and sweets (unlike our primitive ancestors). However, they did render animal fats, they hand-churned butter, and eventually hand-pressed olive oil (which was previously only used for self-anointment and religious purposes), and used all of these for cooking. The recipes in *The Bordeaux Kitchen* focus on cooking with these unprocessed and natural fats along with meats and vegetables, while relinquishing (except for a few sweetened desserts) the reliance on grains, breads, sugar, rice, and pastas that are now prevalent throughout

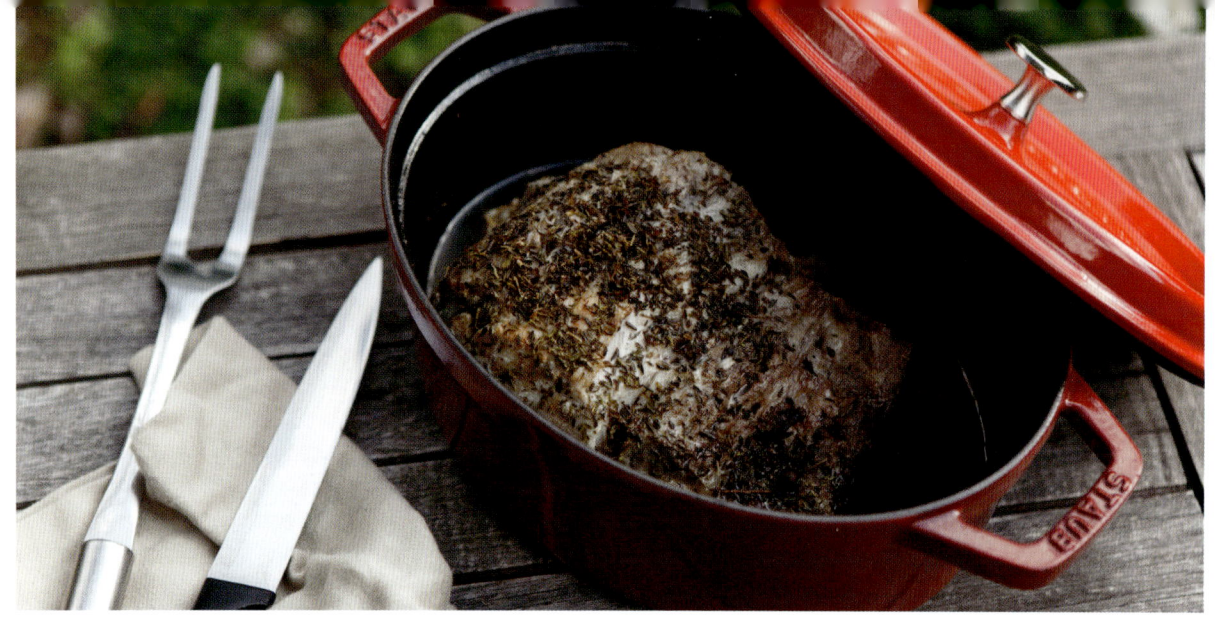

Pork Shoulder Confit (see page 311)

Europe. The spirit of cooking expressed through the recipes in The Bordeaux Kitchen reflects the French *joie de vivre*, the happiness and pleasure taken from communing with family and friends around a delicious, healthy meal and a good glass of wine. Thankfully, such French traditions have survived centuries of food modernization. They are part of the wisdom of the ages passed on to us from our ancestors.

What makes the recipes in The Bordeaux Kitchen different from our most recent ancestors' diets from about the late-1800s? Margarine came into use in the 1870s, pesticides were widely introduced following World War II, and animal fats in our diet were greatly reduced over the decades due to a widespread, though erroneous, belief that they were a major health risk. The public's resultant fear of dietary fat throughout the 20th century has only recently given way to a renewed understanding that animal fats are not only nutritious, but *essential* for many brain and hormonal functions. Rather than avoid animal fats, we should embrace them by cooking *all* parts of the animal. Unfortunately, some of today's modern French cuisine downplays cooking with animal fats, as the conventional wisdom to "eat light" has crowded out their use in favor of industrial oils, while only "moderate" quantities of olive oil and butter are called for in recipes, if at all.

My aim in The Bordeaux Kitchen is to reintroduce the most nutrient-dense, traditional French recipes and to reinvigorate our understanding and consumption of animal fats and hand-cultivated olive oils. Along with promoting a return to using these healthy fats in our diet, I encourage eating organic, sustainably grown foods and a return to the communal sharing of food with family and friends to foster a renewed sense of interest in and caring for one another. Using unrefined animal and saturated fats, combined with a return to more reasonably paced ancestral lifestyle patterns (such as seasonal eating and regular rhythms of rest and movement, and less use of artificial "blue" light) is critical for countering the ill-effects of toxic and nutrient-poor diets, as well as the sedentary, stressful habits of our unhealthy modern-day cultures.

The Bordeaux Kitchen, as a cookbook and blog, focuses on preparing traditional French recipes and includes the healthy fats that have sustained us nutritionally for generations, and indeed millennia, a sort of guide to the French ancestral diet and lifestyle. In addition to the recipes, I encourage you to slow down and enjoy the process of cooking and dining in the spirit of our shared ancestral history, a culture that, while not entirely forgotten, has been pushed aside in recent decades in the name of modern convenience. I am reclaiming this knowledge and wish to share it with you. I know *my* health depends on it. Perhaps yours does, too.

Bon appétit!

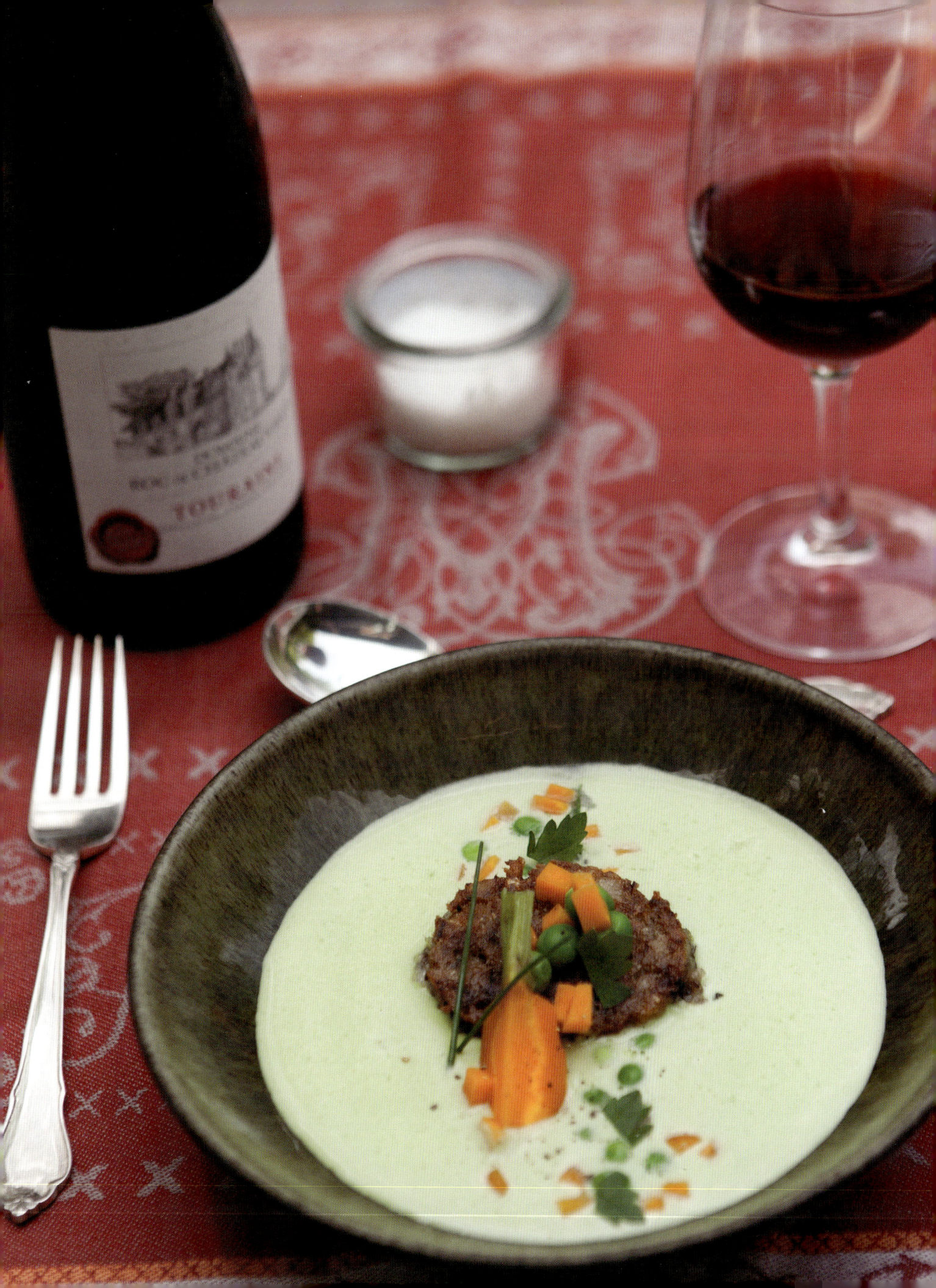

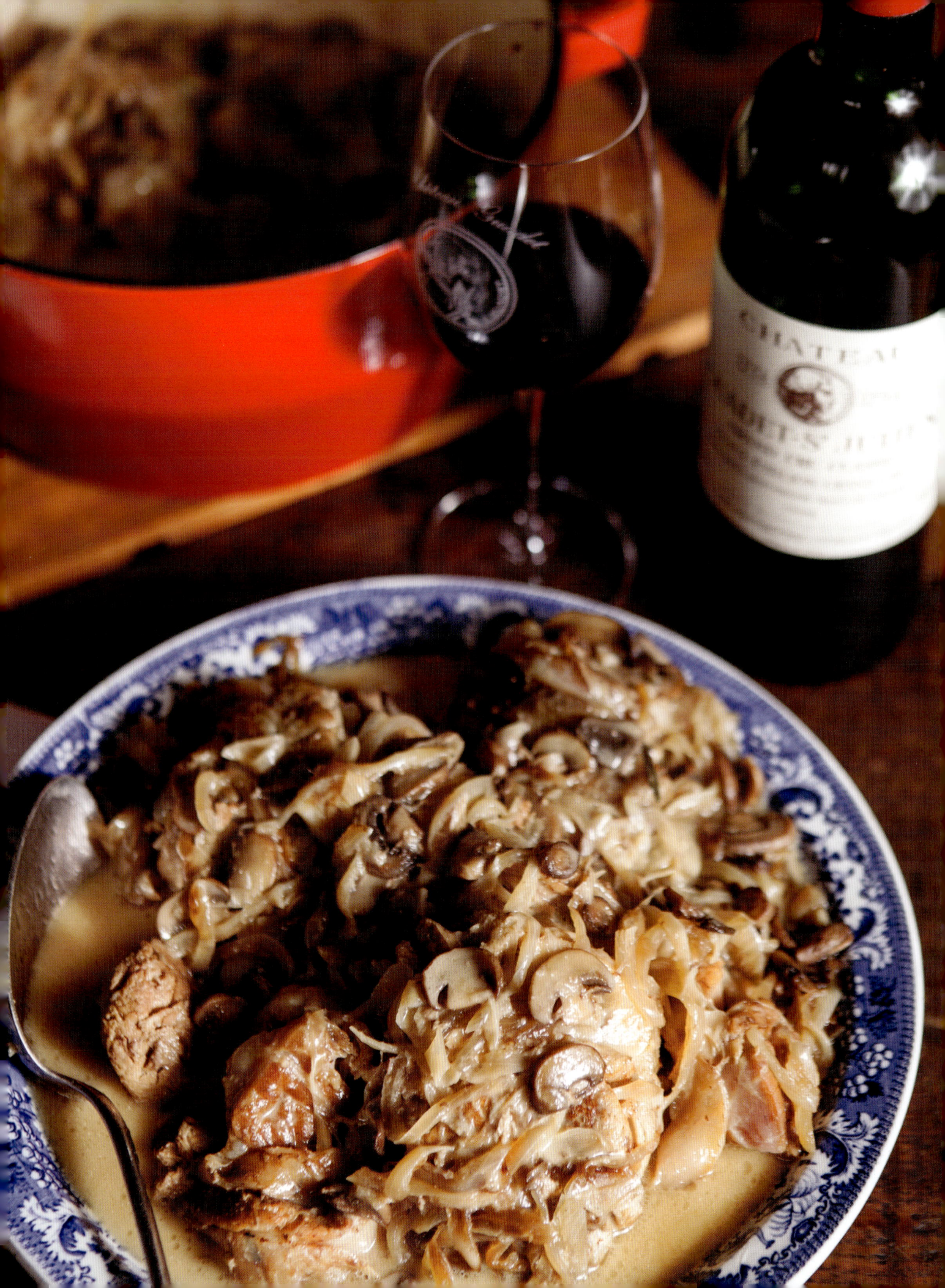

CHAPTER 3

THE FRENCH ART AND TRADITION OF FOOD AND WINE

"Recipes have to be studied in the double context of the techniques of the craft and the cultural circumstances of their time of origin."
—Barbara Ketcham Wheaton[1]

PRESERVATION OF TRADITION

I am hardly the first person to have discovered the wonders of French cooking. Traditional French cooking is often perceived around the world as the pinnacle of modern Western cuisine, if not its foundational bedrock. France's dual contribution of *haute cuisine*, the cuisine of royalty and fine restaurants, and *cuisine bourgeoise*, the everyday peasant cooking, together have formed and informed generations of chefs, culinary schools, and family cooks. Everyone from American bakers to Japanese chefs look to France to learn some of the finest, established methods of the culinary arts. *The Bordeaux Kitchen* focuses on recipes you might find in a typical three-course French meal of appetizer, main course, and dessert (*entrée, plat, et dessert*), cooked for family or friends. The multi-course French gastronomic meal (including the careful selection of ingredients and flavor combinations, the pairing of food with wine, and the sharing of the meal with family and friends) is so revered, it was even inscribed in the UNESCO Cultural Heritage List in 2010.[2]

La nouvelle cuisine, or "new cuisine," a term which has seen many iterations since the 1730s, transformed yet again in the 1960s.[3] With an emphasis on "lighter fare" (or less fat), *la nouvelle cuisine* also focused on artfully plating a dish so that you could "eat with your eyes," or admire the look and beauty of a dish. By contrast, the recipes appearing in *The Bordeaux Kitchen* are primarily meant to actually *satiate* you, rather than just look pretty or quell your hunger for an hour or two (though I have attempted to give each dish an appealing portrait nevertheless). The recipes employ what I call the "farm fats," those hand-churned, hand-pressed, or hand-rendered fats one could make on a farm: butter (or ghee), duck and goose fat, lard, olive oil, and tallow.

Selected Highlights of Food Culture in France and the United States

1306 *Traité de Cuisine écrit vers 1306* ("Treatise on Cooking written around 1306") is printed and published by Louis Douët d'Arcq in 1860. It is one of the earliest French texts on cooking and describes cooking by the seasons. "Medieval meals were influenced by the difficulties of supply and storage, by seasonal fluctuations in the availability of ingredients, by the dictates of the church calendar... The seasons determined to a large degree what was available for the cook to work with."[4]

Late 1300s *Le Viandier de Taillevent* ("Meat Cooking Manual by Taillevent") first appears and is attributed to Guillaume Tirel under the pseudonym Taillevent. It presents the way in which meats and vegetables are to be prepared for the upper classes and royalty. It becomes one of the most famous cookbooks, with multiple printings until 1604.[5]

1393 *Le Ménagier de Paris* ("The Goodman of Paris") manuscript is written by an elderly French townsman for his young wife as a guide to household maintenance and cooking, including the sourcing of seasonal foods and local meats.[6]

1400s (or Late Middle Ages) French cooking is still typified as the international fare of most western European countries, initiating from the courts, but does not yet include the recipes or cuisine of the French peasant class.[7]

1470 First printing presses come into use in Paris, France.

‹ *Blanquette de Veau (recipe on page 422)*

1500s The link between diet, ingredients, and health maintenance becomes the subject of discussion in the upper classes in France as they develop an increasing interest in the novel varieties of food from the New World such as corn, potatoes, sweet potatoes, sweet and hot peppers, and tomatoes. Sugar becomes more readily available, and the cultural focus on religious fasting begins to diminish. The seasons still "imposed strict limits on the kitchen."[8] Few cooks can read or write, thus their culinary and horticultural knowledge is passed down to apprentices and children through practice in the kitchen and garden.

1600s Cooking methods become standardized for efficiency and variety. "Writers use references to food to signal character traits, social class, and mood."[9] Still-life paintings of food begin to appear.

1650s The "garnished bouquet" (*bouquet garni*, a mix of herbs used in cooking), chocolate, coffee, and tea make their way into daily French life.

1651 "Classic French cuisine" is immortalized with the publication of *Le Cuisinier François* ("The French Cook"), published by La Varenne. The first great French cookbook, it is intended initially for the more prosperous classes and focuses on flavors, soups (*fond de cuisine*), and sauces, before trickling down to average French people.

1683–1679 Nicolas de Bonnefons publishes his culinary works emphasizing the seasonality and diversity of fruits, vegetables, animal meats and fats, as well as the use of "healthy" bouillons in French cooking.[10]

1700s Many of the recipes developed during this time remain "a part of the national French traditions: omelets, bouillon, soups, sauces, pastries."[11]

1765 The first "restaurant," from the word *restauration*, which means to become reinvigorated by the consumption of a soup (*bouillon*), opens in Paris by a man named Boulanger, a bouillon vendor who wants customers to be able to dine at tables to drink his restorative broths.

Late 1700s Cookbooks become sparsely published as food shortages increase levels of hunger and poverty among the population, leading up to the French Revolution.

1789–1799 The French Revolution topples the monarchical regime in France.

1800s France becomes known for its "lavish banquets" and for having the finest chefs and cuisine throughout Europe.[12]

1822 Sugar consumption in the U.S. is 6 pounds per person per year.[13]

1844-1846 French physician and retired military surgeon Dr. Jean-Francois Dancel conducts a seminar on obesity and excessive corpulence at the Academy of Sciences in Paris and subsequently publishes a book on this theme, promoting a dietary regime for humans that is low in carbohydrates and high in fat and protein content.

1863 The first public recommendation to eat a low-carb, high-fat diet comes in the form of a "Letter on Corpulence, addressed to the public," published in the U.K. by William Banting. The letter recommends eating animal meat, fats, and offal or fish (including at breakfast time), as well as reducing starches and sugars in the diet. Non-starchy vegetables, wine (and sherry or Madeira) are also encouraged as well as six to eight hours of sleep a night.

1869 An edible substance that is cheap, affordable and not likely to spoil (later known as "margarine") is invented by French chemist Hippolyte Mège-Mouriès, in response to the need for a butter substitute for Emperor Napoleon III's army and for the lower classes of French society.

1870-1880 Stone-grinding wheat mills begin to be replaced in Europe and the U.S. by roller mill technology which removes vitamins, minerals and fiber from wheat,[14] marking the beginning of industrially refined "foods."[15]

1880s Cotton seeds are subjected to a chemical process that produces polyunsaturated fatty-acids or PUFAs, known as vegetable oils, which are then introduced into the food supply as a substitute for the natural fats, lard, butter, and beef tallow.[16]

1895 Chocolate truffles are invented by French Patissier Louis Dufour.[17]

1900 Two grams of vegetable oils or PUFAs are consumed in the U.S. per person per day (while 99% of added fats in the American diet still consist of lard, butter, and beef tallow). By 2012, vegetable oil or PUFA consumption rises to 80 grams, for an average of 726 calories per person per day.[18]

1911 Trans fats are created when hydrogenation, a process by which hydrogen is chemically added to liquid oils to make them solid at room temperature, is invented in the U.S. Trans fats are later deemed unhealthy by the United States Department of Agriculture (USDA) due to the oxidation that occurs when heating these fats and which cause inflammation in the human body and cellular damage.[19, 20]

Early to mid-1900s "Economic necessity rather than traditional preferences dictate the use of margarines and vegetable oils" in France and Europe due to World Wars I and II.[21] Trans fat and margarine manufacturers in the U.S. market their products as healthier than butter, suggesting that animal fats are responsible for conditions such as heart disease.[22]

1916 First USDA dietary guidelines for children, "Food for Young Children," and for adults, "How to Select Foods," are presented.[23]

Post-World War II The post-war years see an increased availability and reliance on convenience and processed "foods." The search for a cure to heart disease leads to an interest in low-fat diets, thanks in part to studies cited by Ancel Keys, an American physiologist (1904-2004) who (many now think inaccurately) linked consumption of saturated fats to cardiovascular disease. American dietary food guidelines are changed to reflect Keys' (inaccurate and misrepresented) recommendations for low-fat diets, and much of the Western world follows suit.[24]

1962 *Silent Spring* is published by Rachel Carson, increasing awareness about indiscriminate industrial use of pesticides in the U.S.

1970s Mono-crop agricultural policies and the "energy crisis" in the U.S. dovetail to send food prices sky-high, when the energy-intensive cost of producing and transporting beef becomes prohibitively expensive.[25]

1971 Alice Waters opens *Chez Panisse* in Berkeley, California, one of the first restaurants to focus on sourcing local, organic food and ingredients. *Diet for a Small Planet* is published by Francis Moore Lappé about the wastefulness of meat production and its contribution to global food scarcity.

1980–1990s The emphasis on eating a low-fat diet to combat heart disease continues to be widely promoted around the world, leading to the popularity of vegetarian, Mediterranean, and low-fat diets.

1992 The USDA "Food Pyramid" is revised from the 1984 "Food Wheel" to guide Americans on their dietary intake. The U.S. Dietary Guidelines encounter some controversy due to the policies of farm subsidization and lobbying efforts of the agricultural industry, whose political influence, some believe, throws into question the scientific validity of the guidelines.[26, 27]

2000s–Present American sugar consumption increased by almost 40% between 1950 and 2000, including high fructose corn syrup, which increased from zero pounds per capita in the 1960s to almost 64 pounds per capita by 2000.[28, 29] Yearly increases in the consumption of refined grains, oils, and sugars in the U.S. and Europe correlates with increases in modern chronic diseases, including heart disease, diabetes, and obesity.[30] Worldwide, obesity has doubled since 1980,[31] while diabetes and obesity has quadrupled.[32] Cardiovascular disease is the number one cause of death worldwide.[33] Where is the world headed in the presence of these refined "foods" and in the absence of traditional foods and saturated animal fats?

Today The four processed foods—white flour, vegetable oils (PUFAs), trans fat (partially hydrogenated oil), and sugar—make up 63% of the U.S. diet (yet have virtually no micronutrients). According to Dr. Chris Knobbe, "This is the recipe for metabolic disaster."[34]

CULTURAL PRIDE AND HERITAGE

France is unique in that food and cooking have been revered there for centuries and are firmly rooted in the very fabric of French culture. This diverse culture varies from region to region, but collectively draws from a variegated, overlapping heritage from around Europe: Basque, Catalan, Celtic, Frankish, Gallic, Gascon, Nordic, and Roman, to name a few. Nevertheless, some traditions and habits can be said to be common among the French population. The French tend to eat seasonally, and they are proud of their locally grown produce and livestock. They might sometimes even be suspicious of food products from other regions. Shop owners share with pride the celebrated part of the country from which their food hails; for example, rosé wines from Provence match with a nice lunch of fire-roasted *Bresse* chicken (a breed of poultry from the controlled appellation of Bresse in Eastern France). Here Augustin Jallon shows off a Bresse chicken in front of his rotisserie shop *Le Poulailler d'Augustin* in Bordeaux, and we have a peek inside the shop.

Meals made of fresh, whole, natural food that is locally produced; homemade wines, cheeses, breads, and desserts; and hard work, rest, and integral relations within tightly-knit communities of small villages are some of the habitual and culinary threads that have traditionally held that cultural fabric together. Whether walking through town, visiting local markets and chatting with vendors, or communing with friends and neighbors over shared food, wine, cider, coffee, or tea, all of these activities encourage people to get outside, slow down, and live in the moment. These idyllic images and experiences are what make up an integral part of the traditional French experience.

REGIONAL PAIRING OF FOOD AND WINE

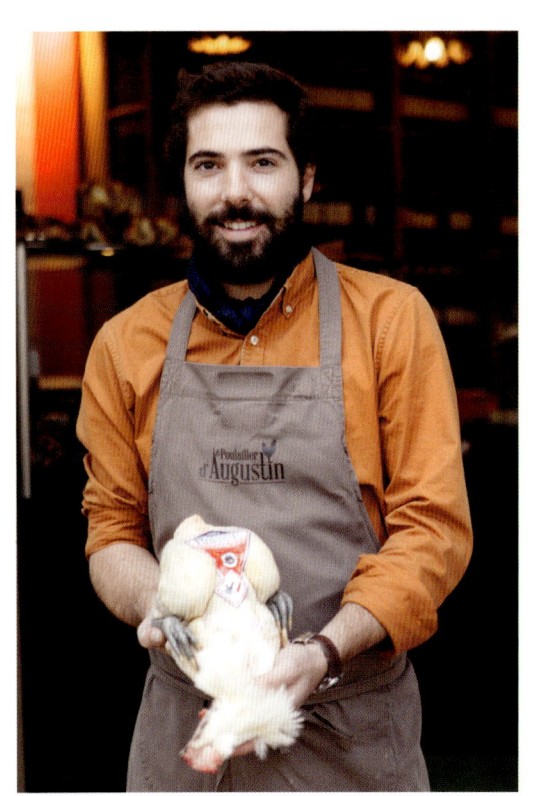

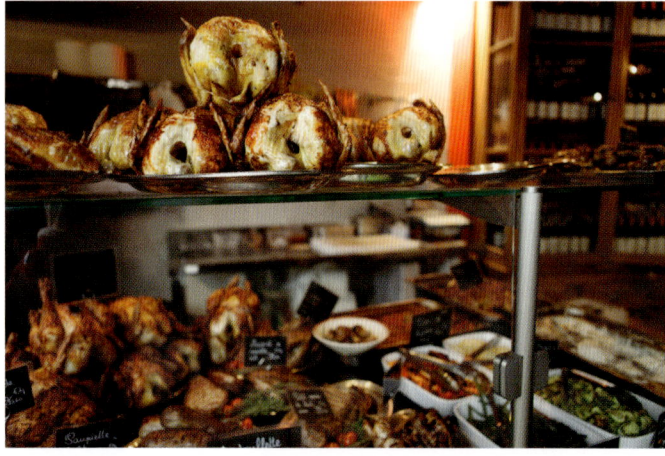

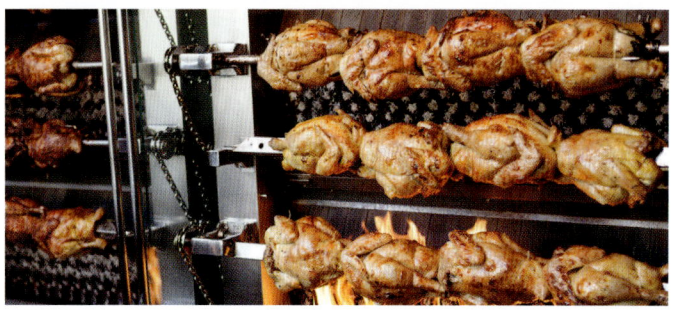

There is no room for processed "food" in the traditional French diet. On weekends, the French often gather with family, and since many urban French have relatives living in the countryside, it can still be said that they are inextricably linked to the land and the food it produces. Traditionally, French dishes produced from locally sourced, whole food are nutrient-dense and rich in saturated fat, with all the vitamins and minerals that entails. Locally grown wine is naturally endowed with polyphenols and healthful vitamins, albeit in small amounts. In fact, the most basic tenet of matching food and wine is to pair local dishes and foods, including cheeses, with local wines. Marrying these provides for a dense sensory experience. Whether it is cider with *galettes* (thin buckwheat pancakes) in Brittany (*Bretagne*), or lamb from Pauillac (a town North of Bordeaux in the Médoc region) paired with a Paulliac Cabernet Sauvignon blend, it turns out that local food goes best with locally-made beverages. *The simplest rule of thumb for matching a wine with a recipe in France is to choose a regional wine variety matching the regional origin of the dish.* This is part of what makes France and its authentic food and wine so unforgettable to those who visit.

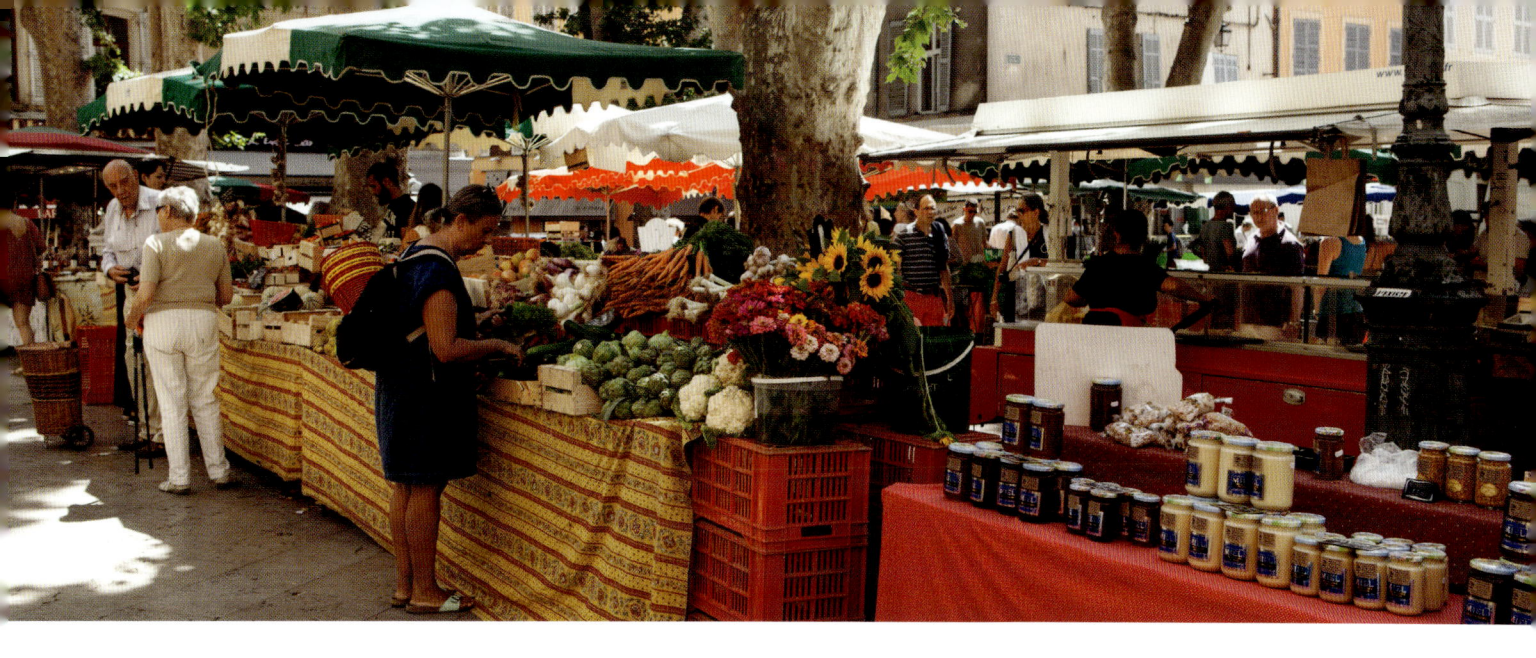

> The simplest rule of thumb for matching a wine with a recipe in France is to choose a regional wine variety matching the regional origin of the dish.

TASTE AND *TERROIR*

This idea of "regional pairings" essentially comes out of the idea of *terroir*, the concept that climate and geography, indeed the very soil itself (and by extension, the soil microbiome) along with the cultivator's hand, give the food and wine grown in a region its own distinctive taste and flavor. In her book, *The Improvisational Cook*, Sally Schneider quotes this principle as "what grows together goes together," in reference to this culinary tradition in France and other countries.[35] The words *terroir* and taste (*goût*) go together often: "The taste of the terroir" (*le goût du terroir*) and "cooking from the terroir" (*la cuisine du terroir*), as Paula Wolfert refers to the French Southwest culinary tradition in her 1983 and 2005 editions of *The Cooking of Southwest France*.[36]

Even French children's books celebrate the agronomic and regional diversities of their country. One colorful picture book, *Le Tour de France de la Famille Oukilé* by Béatrice Veillon, depicts illustrations of each region's treasures, from sightseeing and food to natural and architectural highlights. Another illustrated and compelling children's book series *Questions? Réponses!* covers French cultural and historical themes from Paris to pirates. "Point of interest" road signs dot the French highways, proudly drawing tourists' attention to local sights such as the prehistoric Lascaux caves in the Dordogne-Périgord region of the French Southwest. When not

CHAPTER 3

traveling long distances, the French are well known for walking or biking to get around town when conducting their daily business or meeting friends at a local café or bistro.

CULTURAL CONNECTION AND DISCONNECTION WITH FOOD

The French connection and appreciation of their food sources stems from a rich cultural tradition and pride in stewardship of the land. This is in stark contrast to America's relationship with its food and sources. This may stem from the culturally "ingrained" USDA dietary guidelines created for Americans in 1916 which transformed from simple lists of food into recommended "nutrient groups," then into "food groups" and "food pyramids," and eventually to "food plates."[37] What may have begun as a reasonable concern by the U.S. government regarding nutrient deficiencies, caused no doubt by an increased reliance on refined foods (see timeline on page 14), turned into a cultural food-disconnect.

The creation of the controversial "Food Pyramid" by the USDA in 1992 was heavily influenced by industrialized agricultural lobbyists. The resulting pyramid combined "fruits and vegetables" as if they were one and the same food group. All fats, oils, and sweets were to be consumed minimally (particularly saturated fats), while "healthy whole grains," (bread, cereal, rice and pasta— the very grains that are so pro-inflammatory and that often cause insulin-resistance in so many people) were recommended at a whopping 6 to 11 servings per day.[38] These guidelines not only advised Americans about nutrition, according to the so-called "experts" and industrial lobbyists, they also shaped programs affecting school children, veterans, and social welfare recipients across the nation. Currently, carbohydrates make up over 75% of the current recommended USDA "Food Plate," while saturated fats are limited, if not discouraged altogether by their absence in the discussion.[39]

In his 2012 book *Folks, This Ain't Normal*, Joel Salatin cites American consumers' complacent relationship to their food as a symptom of years of disconnect from its source—the land and the people who cultivate it. I agree with Salatin's premise that this complacency can be *changed* with improved education about how food is grown and sourced. Luckily, change is afoot in the U.S. The growing popularity of home gardens, local farmers' markets, and investments in projects like "cow shares" (in which multiple families buy a "share" in a cow) are some of the ways Americans are moving toward sustainable and healthier eating habits.

The French Use of Fats

In his 1958 publication, *The Food of France*, journalist and well-traveled Francophile and food historian Waverley Root wrote that France could be divided into four regional groups of French cooking, based on the type of *fats* they primarily use. "Though each area tends to adhere most faithfully to its own school," Root wrote, "none is unaware of the others. Thus at the outset, French cooking is gifted with the great asset of variety."[40] For the most part, these divisions still hold true today, though as I mentioned in Chapter 1 (page 2), traditionally (as evidenced by some of the first French cookbooks and other writings from the Middle Ages onward), tallow has also been a widely used fat in traditional French cooking and may be considered the fifth of the fats used in France.

Types of "farm fats" used regionally:
- Butter – Northwest (Brittany and Normandy), Central and Northeastern France
- Lard – Alsace, Lorraine, Auvergne
- Olive Oil – Provence, the Cote d'Azur and Corsica
- Animal Fats (primarily duck, goose and lard, but also butter) and Olive Oil – French Southwest (Aquitaine, Midi-Pyrénées including Gascony, Basque and Béarn region, and parts of Languedoc-Roussillon, Limousin and Poitou-Charentes)

CULINARY DIVERSITY

Records as far back as the late 1300s show an emphasis on the seasonality and diversity of fruits, vegetables, animal meats, and fats (including fish), as well as "healthy" bouillons, made from the bones of animals, widely employed in French cooking.[41] The diversity of fats used in Southwest French cuisine, including butter and olive oil, is a testament to the region's culinary diversity and is represented in the numerous surf and turf recipes represented in this book.

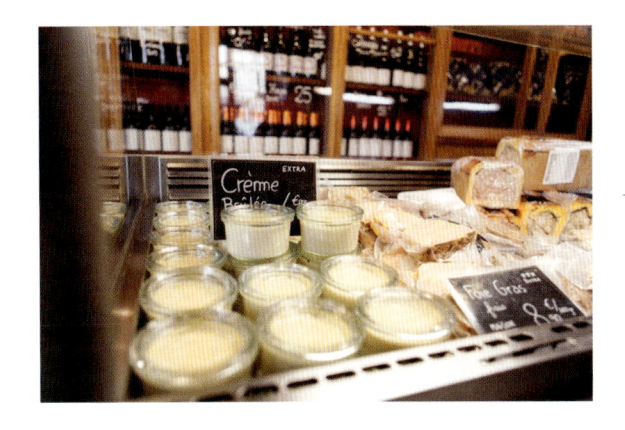

The regional divisions regarding the types of fat used in French cooking as defined by Waverley Root are still largely true today. The exception to this is the modern (since the late 1800s) introduction of industrially-refined oils (such as safflower, cottonseed, rapeseed/canola, and soybean), which are now used more ubiquitously than ever in restaurants and households and are recommended in cookbooks and on culinary websites. This reliance on industrially-refined oils rather than on "farm fats" has grown significantly over the past several decades in the modern world in an attempt to reduce the use of saturated fats and to make use of cheaper alternatives. Not surprisingly, the increased incidence of modern chronic diseases corresponds to this growing reliance on industrially-refined oils. It turns out that the French Paradox, coined in 1991 by Dr. Serge Renaud, a professor at the University of Bordeaux, to describe the seemingly contradictory idea that French people can eat duck fat and drink red wine while maintaining low rates of cardiovascular disease, is actually not a paradox at all. Instead, it is the very fats and nutrient-rich foods used in cooking, and indeed, the very essence of the traditional French way of life, that supports good health.[42]

It turns out that the French Paradox, coined in 1991 by Dr. Serge Renaud, a professor at the University of Bordeaux, to describe the seemingly contradictory idea that French people can eat duck fat and drink red wine while maintaining low rates of cardiovascular disease, is actually not a paradox at all. Instead, it is the very fats and nutrient-rich foods used in cooking, and indeed, the very essence of the traditional French way of life that supports good health.[42]

CHAPTER 3

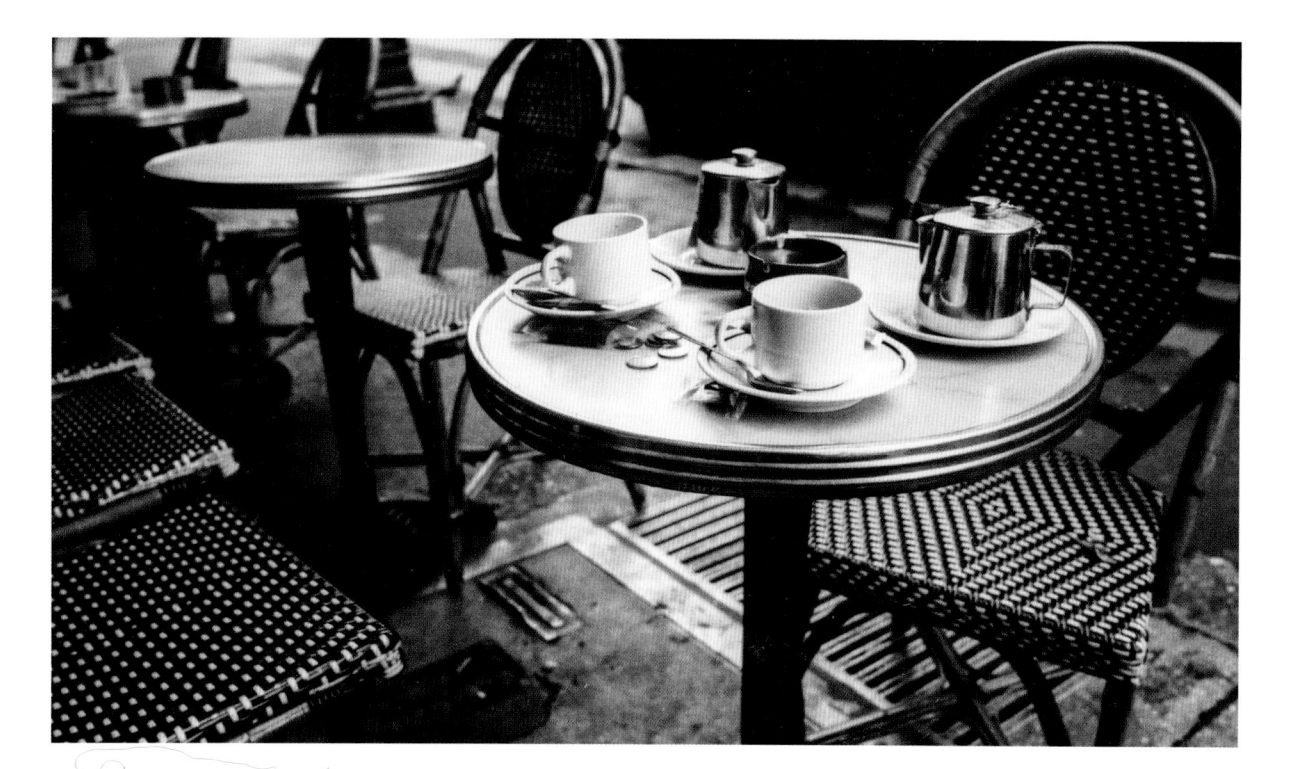

I am hardly the only proponent for using fats in French cooking. According to Kate Rhéaume-Bleue in her 2012 publication "Vitamin K2 and the Calcium Paradox," the K2 in the fats consumed by the French is the very lifesaving ingredient that protects them. "The French Paradox isn't a paradox at all," she writes. "The very same pâté de foie gras, Camembert, egg yolks and creamy, buttery sauces that we inaccurately labeled 'heart attack on a plate,' liberally supply the single most important nutrient (Vitamin K2) to protect heart health."[43] President and co-founder of the Weston A. Price Foundation Sally Fallon Morrel, who herself was inspired by French culinary traditions after studying in the South of France, encourages the use of nutrient-dense foods and cooking with animal fats in her books, among them *Nourishing Broths*, *Nourishing Fats*, and *Nourishing Traditions*. Dr. Catherine Shanahan also states that French cuisine stands firmly on what she calls the "Four Pillars of the Human Diet," in which the foods consumed are: meat on the bone, fermented and sprouted, organs and other "nasty bits," and fresh, unadulterated plant and animal products.[44]

Unfortunately, even for the French, particularly in bigger cities, the art of traditional cooking is disappearing, as busy people succumb to the modern conveniences and temptations of fast and packaged "foods," rushed lunches while working, and eating on the go. When I began taking cooking classes after moving to Bordeaux, I was surprised at how afraid some of the French participants were to use generous amounts of butter in certain recipes. While the chefs advocated using butter or olive oil, no mention was made about using other animal fats.

As far as taking the time to eat a good meal, fortunately, some French (and other Europeans) still do take lunch breaks, at times even over a glass of wine, with a friend, spouse, or colleague. Most people continue to value the Sunday family meal at grandmother's house, *chez mamie*. And most people will take the time at some point to stop in a café to meet with a friend or read the newspaper. Taking this time in *the French way* is culturally equated with wellness. After all, who doesn't dream of sitting in a French café watching the world go by for a few moments?

LEARNING FROM THE PAST
When we examine the anecdotal evidence of what people who are now octogenarians through centenarians typically ate when they were children, we are told breakfasts consisted of real food like seasonal garden vegetables, farm-fresh eggs, bacon and other home-cured meats, yogurts, cheeses, soups, homemade breads or porridges, and other farm-style foods to carry them through the day. Lunches were sufficient to sustain the energy required for labor, and dinners satiated families throughout the night. This is in complete contrast with today's French "continental breakfast" of coffee, croissant with jam and/or butter, and orange juice. Seeking anecdotal evidence, which often seems more reliable than scientifically conducted studies, I surveyed friends about what their parents and grandparents ate for breakfast.

My friend, Malika Faytout, a fellow wine course classmate, relayed stories about her great-grandfather's experience growing up in the French countryside in the late 1800s. Men would leave early in the morning for work, after a coffee, followed by a mid-morning break of soup, leftovers, meat or lard and bread, often washed down with some wine. Malika's parents, born in the 1940s, on the other hand, grew up eating a more modern breakfast of chocolate milk or milk with coffee and bread with jam. However, Malika's parents lived off the land and grew up eating local foods. They, along with her great-aunt, Tante Lucie, born in 1931, (whose Millas dessert recipe may be found on page 484) are all alive and well and continue to make meals at home using seasonal ingredients from the surrounding countryside. My husband fondly remembers dining on chocolate soup and bread for breakfast when he was a 10-year-old American exchange student living outside of Paris in the early 1980s. Luckily, his host family supplemented the baguettes and chocolate bars with eggs and yogurt for breakfast and served dinners of **Braised Veal Stew** (page 422). My own first experience in France was as a 14-year-old staying with American friends of our family who lived in Grenoble in the Southeast French Rhône-Alps region. My host mother, Jo, delighted in showing me markets and procuring local breads, butter, jams, cheeses, charcuterie, and honey, all of which I of course instantly fell in love with.

Born in 1903, Waverley Root, wrote in his book *The Food of France* that growing up in New England, he "thought nothing of starting the day with a breakfast of steak, potatoes, and mince pie, in the winter at least…" adding, he "would not do it now, and I doubt if anyone does, even those who, at today's prices, can afford a breakfast steak." By 1958, when his book was published, Root had begun to evidence the American culture shifting away from nutrient-dense fats and whole foods, at least for the breakfast meal. Similar shifts in diet occurred around the modern world as the decades progressed and modern societies transitioned to a reliance on refined "foods." As early as 1906, Will Keith Kellogg, an American industrialist, launched the Battle Creek Toasted Corn Flake Company and began to change the face of morning breakfasts in America. A superb account of this dietary shift and the origins of the fat-phobic craze that followed, in addition to an accounting of the correlating worldwide epidemics of diabetes and obesity, is presented by Nina Teicholz in *The Big Fat Surprise*. Though we must be careful to not confuse correlation with causation, there has been increasing evidence to suggest links between our modern diets and our modern chronic diseases.

SCHOOL LUNCHES IN FRANCE
In France today, school lunches, (often subsidized by the French government), are served in courses. Although not primal/paleo, they are balanced (*balancé*) and typically include a variety of dishes, such as traditionally prepared roasts, salads, and soups, accompanied by modern-style foods like pastas, breads, or pizza. A combination of raw or cooked vegetables and fruits, along with more "processed foods," such as plain

yogurt with sugar or a choice of fruit or sweet pudding, is often offered along with water to drink. Candy and cake are relegated to birthday and other celebrations, although to a mom on an anti-sugar kick like me, even these seem far too frequent. Some French children with whom my children played indicated that they actually *want* bacon and eggs for breakfast, but they are served these on the weekends only when their parents have more time, and probably because of the ubiquitous *fear of fats*. Instead, children are typically fed biscuits, cereal, and low-fat milk. Again, this is anecdotal evidence, but it speaks to the fact that even the French have changed their dietary habits, and, in my opinion at least, are losing out on the nutrients that only a nutrient-dense, higher-fat, ancestral-style breakfast or meal can provide.

TO MARKET—*AU MARCHÉ*
Whether by maintaining a small herb or vegetable garden, or by regularly shopping at local farmers' markets, the French still maintain the cultural practice of staying connected to the food they eat, as well as to those who produce it. Many French still walk with their wheeled caddies or bike with their baskets to their neighborhood markets. These markets are places for friendly connection, where time slows down. (You can sometimes even hear nostalgic Edith Piaf tunes from an accordion player at the market or outside a café.) Getting to know the local fishmonger, butcher, or organic farmer is one way of ensuring a high-quality product, and sometimes better prices. Gourmet grocery shops (*épiceries fines*) are another charming and specialized, if more expensive, option. Building community, it can be said, is part of our DNA; our species evolved living in tight-knit, socially cohesive units. This kind of community cohesiveness is enhanced in French towns and villages, where most people typically live in small apartments, with small refrigerators, compared to those in the U.S. This encourages getting outside frequently and walking, biking, or socializing in the open air, especially at outdoor cafés.

Of course, not even the French can escape the modern influences or impacts of the growing use of pesticides or the dominance of large supermarkets (*grandes surfaces*) and strip malls, which tend to define parts of the urban and suburban landscape in France as they do in other parts of the modernized world. The relatively new reliance on processed "foods," oils, and sweets (even in France), has led to nutrient deficiencies and metabolic disorders such as obesity, diabetes, cancer, autoimmune, degenerative, and chronic diseases like fibromyalgia, Alzheimer's, Parkinson's, and multiple sclerosis (MS).[45] Now, even the likes of cookbook author Paula Wolfert has turned to "food as medicine" to treat her own affliction of Alzheimer's disease.[46]

It is no wonder shopping separately at individual markets, be they a butcher, dairy, bakery or hardware store, seems inconvenient compared to the one-stop grocery store chains that abound in every community. In our rushed modern lives, making a supermarket run by car may *seem* more time and energy efficient, but it ends up robbing us of the slower, more humanly-scaled pace of procuring goods, not to mention the opportunity for exposure to sunlight and the outdoors, or the health benefits of walking or biking to a neighborhood market and the human connections maintained by chatting with a neighbor. Not surprisingly, I have driven home exhausted after trips to the large, one-stop supermarket, yet I feel energized from walking to the local farmers' market where I can chat and ask the vendors of the chicken, honey, and vegetables I like, how and where their products are grown and processed.

There is also the matter of food quality, as the difference in freshness of produce typically sold in local markets far surpasses the mass-produced, packaged "foods" available in the supermarket. In pre-refrigeration days, Saturday markets came about so that Sunday's roast could be bought the day before, rather than earlier in the week, risking spoilage. My French culinary teacher and friend, Chef Frédéric Schueller, admonishes his students to visit the local and street markets more frequently, lest they disappear into history. As a chef, teacher, and father, he understands the importance of maintaining the relationships and routines of the traditional market. He, of course, has an established relationship with the butcher, poultry, herb, and dairy vendors at the central market, *Capucins,* in Bordeaux, where he regularly takes his students.

Capucins Market, Bordeaux

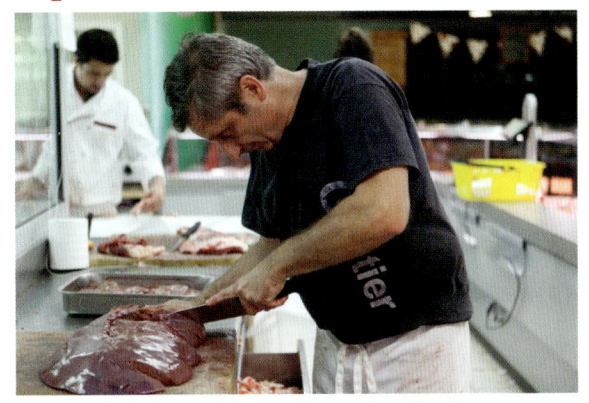

Yannick of the Gautier Butcher Shop Slicing Veal Liver

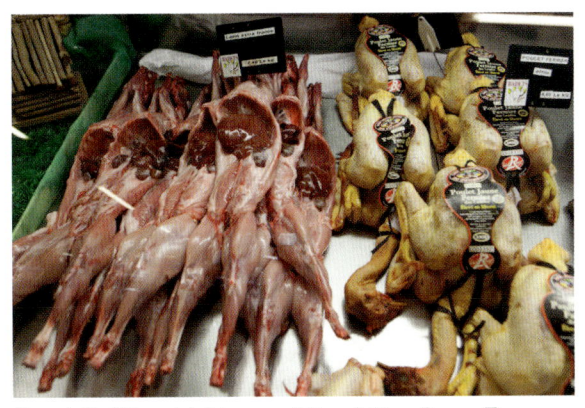

French Rabbits with Livers and French Free-Range Farm Hens for Sale

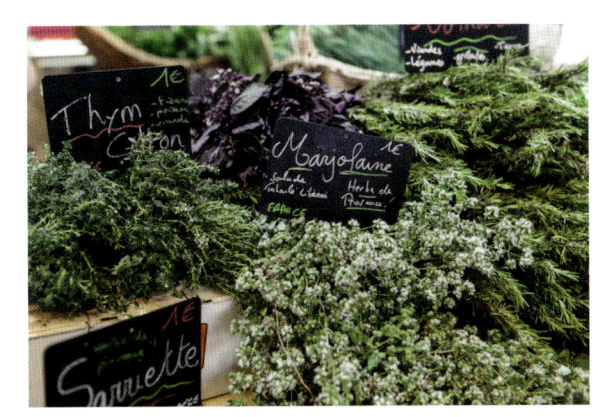

Fresh Herbs for Sale

Though the numbers of patrons at local French markets are now declining in favor of large grocery store chains that offer lower prices and convenience, many French are still willing to pay a premium for fresher foods from local sources and to support their local food producers and vendors.[47] Traditionally, a large percentage of French daily life and monthly income was dedicated to shopping at markets and small shops (*épiceries*), and to preparing and sharing food. In the U.S., patronage at farmers' markets has increased in recent years, though the trend seems to be rising relatively slowly.[48] The vibrant, communal aspect to shopping at local markets is evident from the socializing that occurs among vendors and neighbors and from the subsequent sharing of food and wine with family and friends. This kind of psychological wellbeing, borne of traditional, communal relationships, cannot be nurtured with a quick croissant, sandwich, soda, candy bar, or microwaved meal on-the-go. It is not surprising, then, that what is nutritionally deficient is also psychologically and sensory deficient as well. *Living with intention* by choosing healthy, locally grown or produced food and nurturing relationships with our local farmers simply mirrors how we evolved to eat.

In spite of the lure of modern conveniences, many of the French still do carry on some of their culinary traditions by taking the time to regularly procure, prepare, cook, eat, and share their food. We are not as disconnected as our modern lifestyles and media would have us believe. Many of our grandparents' lessons about food and nurturing community live on in us today. We just need to acknowledge this wisdom by living intentionally and making conscious choices when nourishing ourselves and our families, and by understanding that food really is our best medicine. Hippocrates is often attributed with having said: "Let food be thy medicine and medicine be thy food."

Traditionally, every French *grandmère* had her repertoire of recipes which she naturally passed down, along with her baking, butchering, canning, farming, or gardening knowledge, to the next generation. This transfer of horticultural and culinary knowledge, from one generation to the next, parent to child, cook to cook, farmer to son, just like master butcher to apprentice butcher, was necessary before the advent of literacy and the printing press and the appearance of cookbooks. Today the familial custom of handing down culinary and other traditions is disappearing. These legacies would disappear altogether if not for the chefs, cookbooks, and fine restaurants that focus on traditional French cooking. But, in spite of the support and interest in traditional French culinary traditions, the push to go "low-fat" has not escaped even the French. Traditional recipes that call for using animal fat, rather than industrially-processed oils, are often passed over in favor of the faster, packaged fare of the modern diet. I have yet to see a modern French recipe online or in a recent French cookbook where tallow, for example, is named as the preferred cooking fat. *The Bordeaux Kitchen* counters this trend.

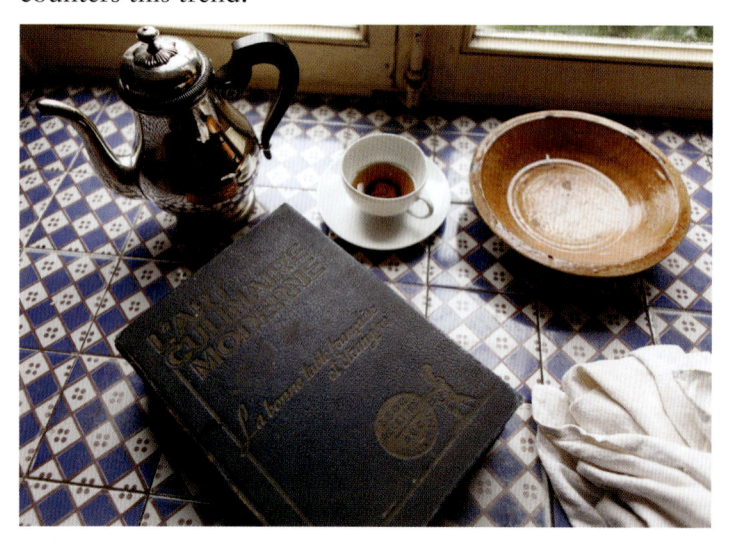

The Bordeaux Kitchen is my attempt to rekindle an interest in the traditional French recipes and cooking methods that are not only the bedrock of French cuisine, but that also reflect the wisdom of the primal/paleo and ancestral approaches. This cookbook demonstrates at-home, real cooking methods that everyone can master with some practice. I encourage you to eat in the French tradition with friends and family to help slow down the pace of eating so that you can properly digest and more thoroughly enjoy the flavors and textures of your meal, and yes, the wine. This is where the French *joie de vivre* comes from!

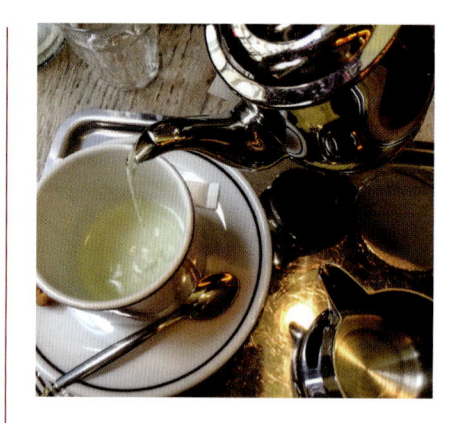

French Ancestral Secrets to Eating:

Take your time.

Know your source.

Walk outside and socialize.

Procure foods that are fresh, local and in-season.

Eat slowly.

Eat diversely.

Eat in good company.

Do not snack between meals.

An afternoon coffee or tea in good company is preferred.

Do not consume water with a meal.

Pair and share wine, slowly sipped.

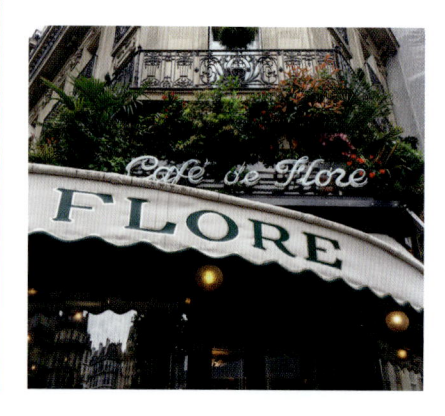

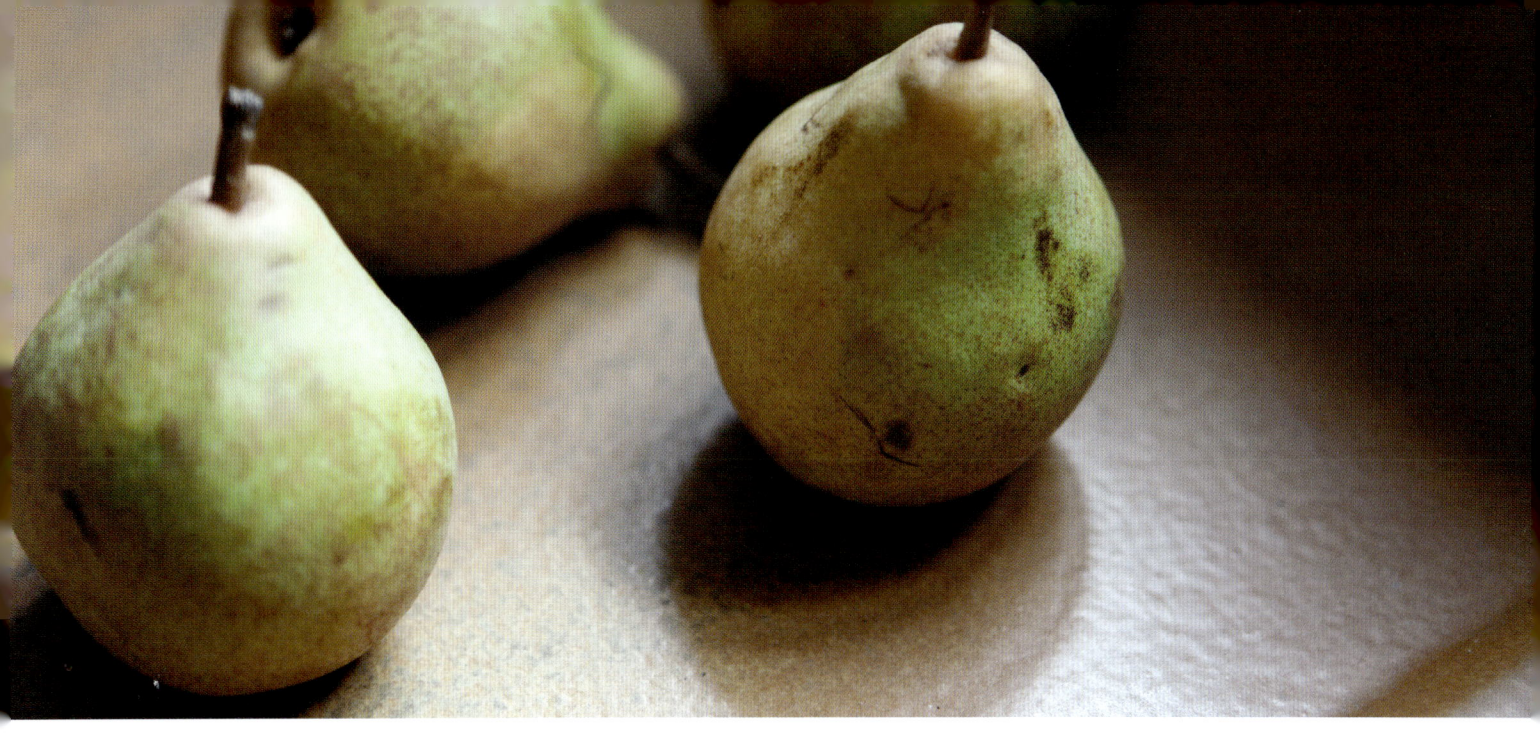

Seasonal Eating in France

The nutrients and flavor of fruits, nuts, and vegetables are of highest quality when grown locally, picked ripe, and consumed soon after. The following list shows some of the regional fruits and vegetables available throughout France (either from its mainland or its territories), neighboring Spain, or elsewhere in Europe that have worked their way into French culinary culture. Interestingly, many of the aromas of these fruits and a few vegetables can be found in French wines, as well. The list below provides a seasonal timeline that corresponds with the months of ripeness of these fruits and vegetables in the Northern Hemisphere. This seasonal time frame is, of course, stretched as long as possible thanks to the use of greenhouses and other technological developments that extend the growing season. This list serves as a basic guide, nonetheless, for determining the best time to consume these fruits and vegetables.[49]

The Seasons — *Les Saisons*

Spring: March–May

Summer: June–August

Autumn: September–November

Winter: December–February

Fruits — *Les Fruits*

Apple – *Pomme*: July-March
Apricot – *Abricot*: Summer
Blackberry – *Mûre*: April-October
Blueberry – *Myrtille*: July-October
Cherry – *Cerise*: May-August
Chestnut – *Marron* or *Châtaigne*: August-December
Currant – *Groseille*: July-August
Cranberry – *Airelle*: July-August
Fig – *Figue*: August-October
Grape – *Raisin*: September-October
Kiwi – *Kiwi*: November-March
Lemon – *Citron*: Summer
Melon – *Melon*: May-August
Mandarine – *Mandarine* (Clementines and Tangerines are varietals): November-February
Mirabelle plum – *Mirabelle*: July-September
Nectarine – *Nectarine*: July-August
Orange – *Orange*: September-April
Peach – *Pêche*: June-September
Pear – *Poire*: July-March
Plum – *Prune*: July-September
Quetsche plum – *Quetsche*: July-October
Quince – *Coing*: September-October
Prune – *Pruneau*: August-September
Raspberry – *Framboise*: June-October
Rhubarb – *Rhubarbe*: May
Strawberry – *Fraise*: April-August
Walnut – *Noix*: September-April

CHAPTER 3

Exotic Fruits and Year-Round Eating

I would add the pomegranate, *le grenade*, to the list of fruits. It is not native to France, but nevertheless, the pomegranate is in season between November and February. Rich in nutrients, pomegranate seeds serve as a great topping for salads. Also available in France year-round, thanks to importation, are the exotic fruits: avocado, banana, coconut, mango, and pineapple. Figuring out when to eat these during the year is difficult, because at the equator, they are always in season. Therefore, it is up to each individual to decide their comfort level with the carbon footprint and energy expenditure of importing food when considering how much or how little to include these fruits into one's diet and recipes. This is a tough call because avocado and coconut, in particular, are much loved by the primal/paleo community and contain healthy fats. If we argue that our ancestors originated at the equator anyway, then perhaps there is less of a moral dilemma about eating some imported food that is healthy for us. The French are certainly well accustomed to eating exotic fruits and relish their aromas in certain white wines. Bananas, mango, pineapple, and apples, along with stone fruits like pears, contain loads of phytonutrients and vitamins, but also fructose (sugar). In excess, even a natural sugar like fructose can upset the delicate balance required for microbiome and liver health. Therefore, I would recommend limiting consumption of these fruits, regardless of their availability during the year.

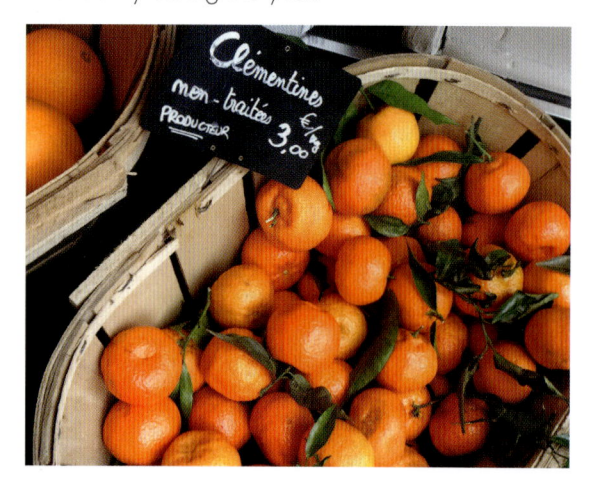

Vegetables — *Les Légumes*

- Artichoke – *Artichaut*: May–October
- Beet – *Betterave*: June–December
- Broccoli – *Brocoli*: July–November
- Brussel sprouts – *Chou de Bruxelles*: September–February
- Cauliflower – *Chou-Fleur*: May–August
- Chard – *Blette*: April–October
- Corn – *Maïs*: July–October
- Cucumber – *Conconbre*: April–October
- Eggplant – *Aubergine*: May–September
- Endive – *Endive*: November–April
- Fennel – *Fenouil*: Summer and Autumn
- Garlic – *Ail*: April–September
- Green bean – *Haricot Vert*: June–October
- Leek – *Poireau*: September–March
- Lettuce – *Laitue*: April–October
- Parsnip – *Panais*: October–February
- Pattypan squash – *Pâtisson*: July–September
- Pea – *Petit Pois*: June–July
- Pepper – *Poivron*: Summer
- Potato – *Pomme de Terre*: May–February
- Pumpkin – *Citrouille*: Autumn
- Radish – *Radis*: April–October
- Salad greens – *Salades*: April–November
- Salsify – *Salsifis*: October–March
- Spinach – *Épinard*: April–June and October–November
- Squash – *Courge*: August–October
- Tomato – *Tomate*: May–October
- Turnip – *Navet*: May–June
- Winter squash – *Potiron*: July–November
- Zucchini – *Courgette*: May–October

Carrots, celery, and onions fall into the "year-round" category, as do cabbage and some mushrooms, because various species are available throughout the year, depending on the region. My children eat cucumbers and tomatoes daily, except for the few winter months when they are not available in our local, organic produce store. Somehow, we manage without these family favorites, though it can make for a longer winter. Nevertheless, they make quite a colorful comeback when they reappear in the market in the spring!

Boeuf Carottes (recipe on page 116) ›

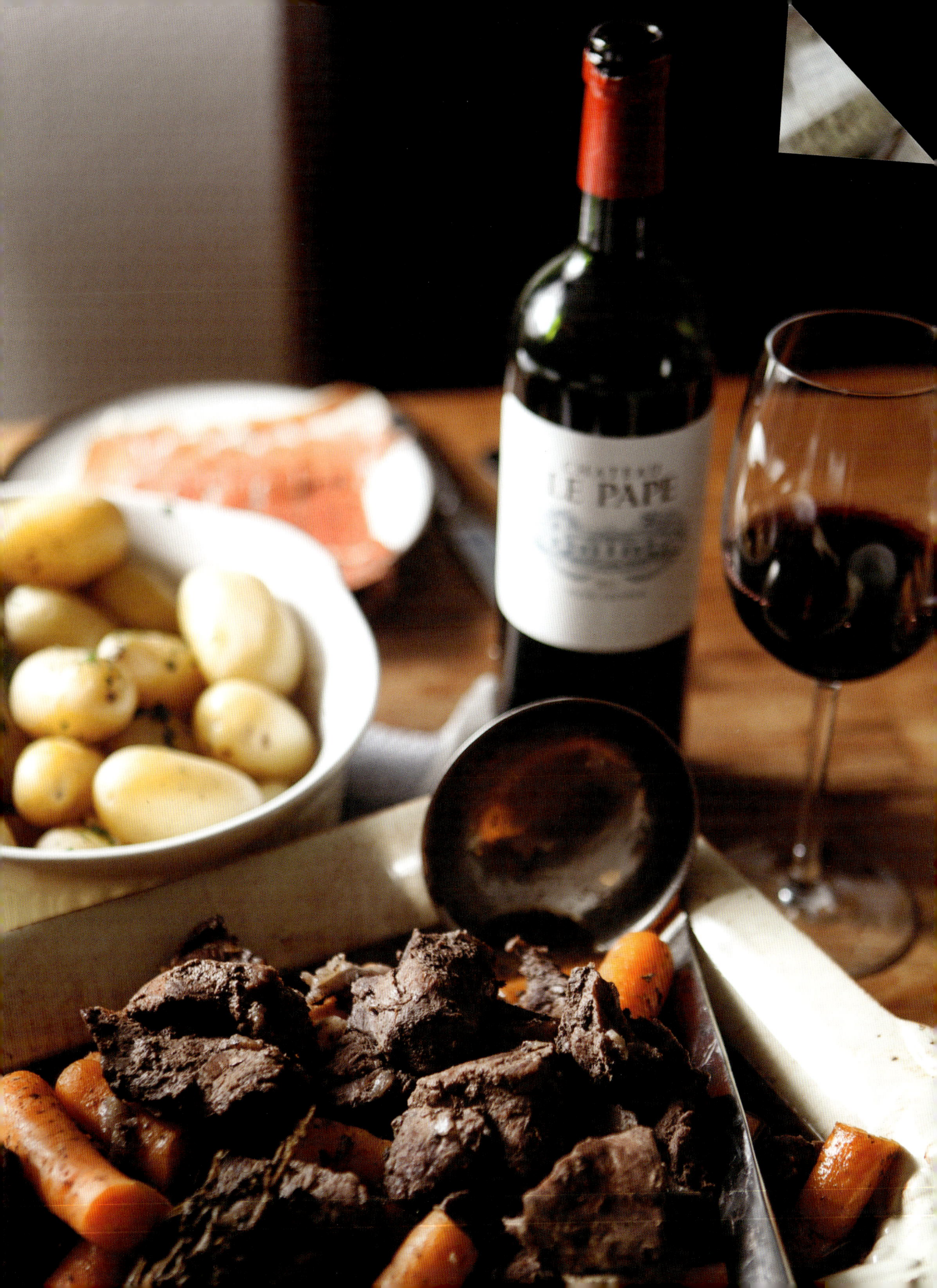

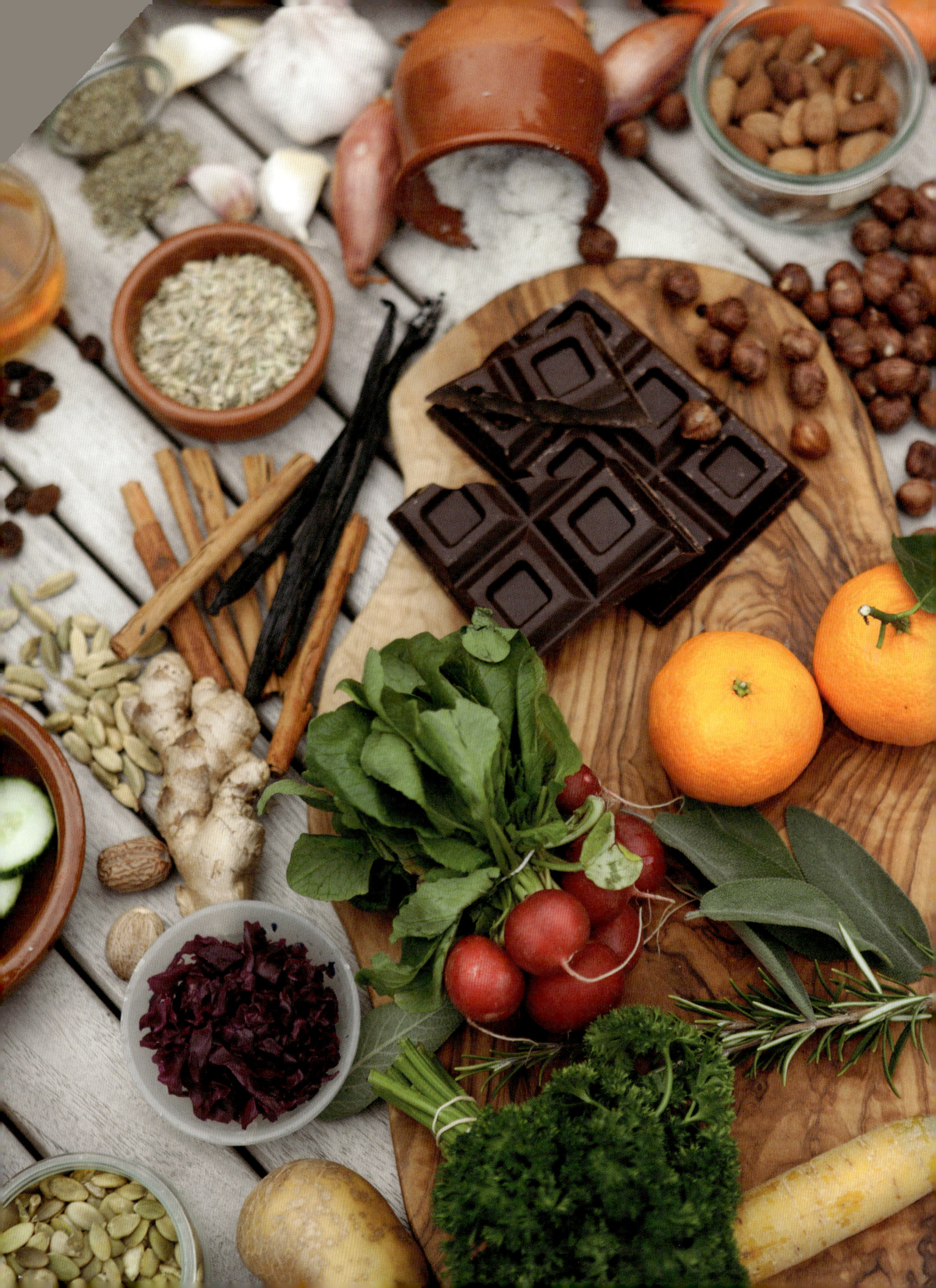

CHAPTER 4
THE THREE SECRETS TO FRENCH COOKING: FARM FATS, FRESH INGREDIENTS, AND CAST-IRON POTS

NOT JUST ANY OLD DUCK

Imagine this scenario: You have two duck breasts, one sautéed in canola oil in a cheap, Teflon-coated pan, salted with refined table salt, flavored with artificially flavored orange syrup, and served with a dipping sauce of high-fructose-corn-syrup plum jam, and a side of boxed scalloped potatoes flavored with mineral-deficient sodium chloride and corn syrup. The other duck breast is sautéed in its own fat in a cast-iron pot, salted with coarse grains of mineral-rich Celtic sea salt, flavored with fresh organic orange rind and juice, and served with a dipping sauce of homemade plum marmalade and a side of sautéed potatoes cooked in duck fat and flavored with fresh herbs and more sea salt. Which would you prefer? (See the recipe for **Orange Duck Breast** on page 351.)

You can almost taste the difference as you read about the amazing layering of flavors, isn't that right (*n'est-ce pas*)? The difference is not only in taste. The second duck breast is also more nutritious thanks to the ingredients and the right cooking implement. Expensive? I would argue that the cost of the fresh ingredients is lower than the industrially processed ones if you view the initial purchase of good ingredients like high-quality sea salt and fresh herbs (perhaps grown in your own herb garden) as a long-term investment in maintaining your good health. I would also argue that taking the time to chop herbs, slice potatoes, and relish that homemade jar of plum marmalade is time well spent. Nor does it take much more time than dumping the boxed, industrial ingredients together and calling it a meal. As I have mentioned before, the time spent in meal preparation can be considered a meditative process, preparing your body for receiving nutrient-dense, warm food. Ancestral eating is worth the time and investment. The nutrient-density of real, high-quality foods, in my experience, is an investment in your health.

In this chapter we explore the three elements or the "secrets to French cooking" that make this cuisine so delicious, nutritious, and immune to fads: the use of farm fats, fresh ingredients, and cast-iron pots!

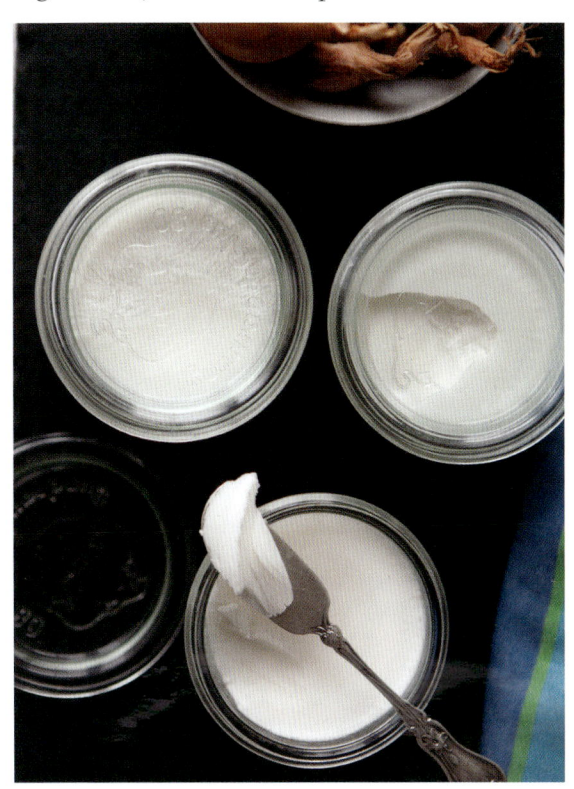

Rendered Lard

THE SECRET TO FRENCH COOKING #1: FARM FATS

From an ancestral perspective, our proverbial French great-grandmother rendered, pressed, and used a variety of what I call "farm fats": butter, beef and lamb tallow, lard and bacon fat, duck and goose fat, as well as hand-pressed olive oil, which turn out to be the most nutrient-dense fats for cooking. These are what people cooked with before margarine and vegetable oils. Indeed, industrial seed oils—polyunsaturated fats or PUFAs—were not invented until the 1880s. Our ancestors ate animal fats, butter, duck fat, lard, and tallow even before olive oil, which was primarily used in antiquity for anointing oneself (as Odysseus did before his voyage in *The Odyssey*) rather than for cooking. With the exception of olive oil, a predominantly monounsaturated fat, the traditional "farm fats" are primarily composed of saturated fats.

A FEW WORDS ABOUT SATURATED FAT
Contrary to current dietary advice, I contend that eating saturated fat is not, in itself, harmful,[1] and in fact, is what keeps us *healthy and satiated*. Moreover, if you follow the conventional advice and avoid saturated fat, you forego some of the most nutrient-dense foods that help our bodies thrive, such as organ meats, the animal-derived cooking fats, and whole, unpasteurized dairy products. Organ meats are rich in micronutrients (vitamins A, K2, B12, and zinc, for example) that are not found in such accessible doses in plants. These and many other micronutrients are fat-soluble and therefore *require* adequate fat to be digested and absorbed.

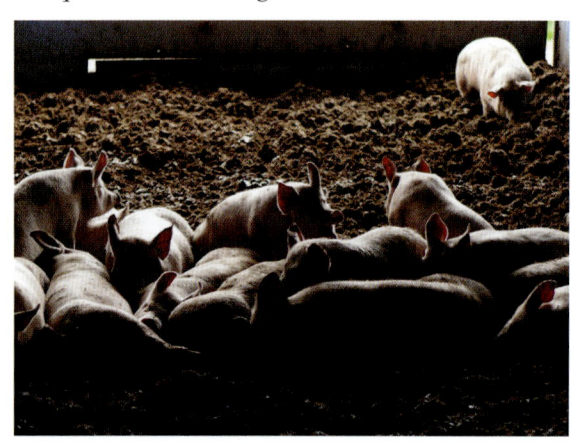

Organic, but Not Grass-fed

Just to be clear, when I talk about eating healthy saturated fats, I am talking about organic (free from synthetic pesticides) meat, organ meat, dairy, and eggs from *high-quality*, grass-fed, pasture-raised animal sources. (There is a difference between organically fed and grass fed, such as the photo of the pigs shown here who are fed organic feed in small numbers per lot, but are nevertheless not grass fed.) Grass-fed sources of animal fat contain the delicate omega-3 fatty acids necessary for good health, as well as the saturated fats which protect the omega-3s from oxidation, counter inflammation, and nourish our brains.[2] Meanwhile, animal fat and meat from factory farms generally contain far fewer nutrients than those from sustainably-raised sources because these products come from less-healthy animals raised on hormones, antibiotics, and grain-based feed in unhealthy, cramped, and often indoor Concentrated Animal Feeding Operations, or CAFOs.[3] Another critical factor to be aware of is that fat, otherwise known as adipose tissue, stores toxins. This is a measure taken by our bodies and animals' bodies for several reasons, one of which is to protect our vital organs and blood from toxins. Therefore, animal fats from organic (synthetic pesticide-free, herbicide-free, and fungicide-free) and pastured (grass-fed) sources are likely to contain fewer toxins and contribute to the cycle of regenerating the soil. Growing one's own vegetables or tending one's own sheep is of course an idyllic and worthy dream, but supporting one's local, organic farmers is another, more practical way for most of us to consume organic foods. This is why I believe choosing only *quality* animal fats is best—for our own health, the animals' welfare, and of course, the environment.

Saturated animal fats are essential for brain health and proper endocrine function. These fats do not spike insulin levels and help keep inflammation at bay. Author of *Primal Fat Burner,* Nora Gedgaudas, provides numerous studies and backup research to support her thesis that "fats from healthy animal sources and unrefined tropical oils are paramount to the functioning of our physiology and for robust health."[4] What's more, she explains how we gain a metabolic advantage by burning "ketones, the energy

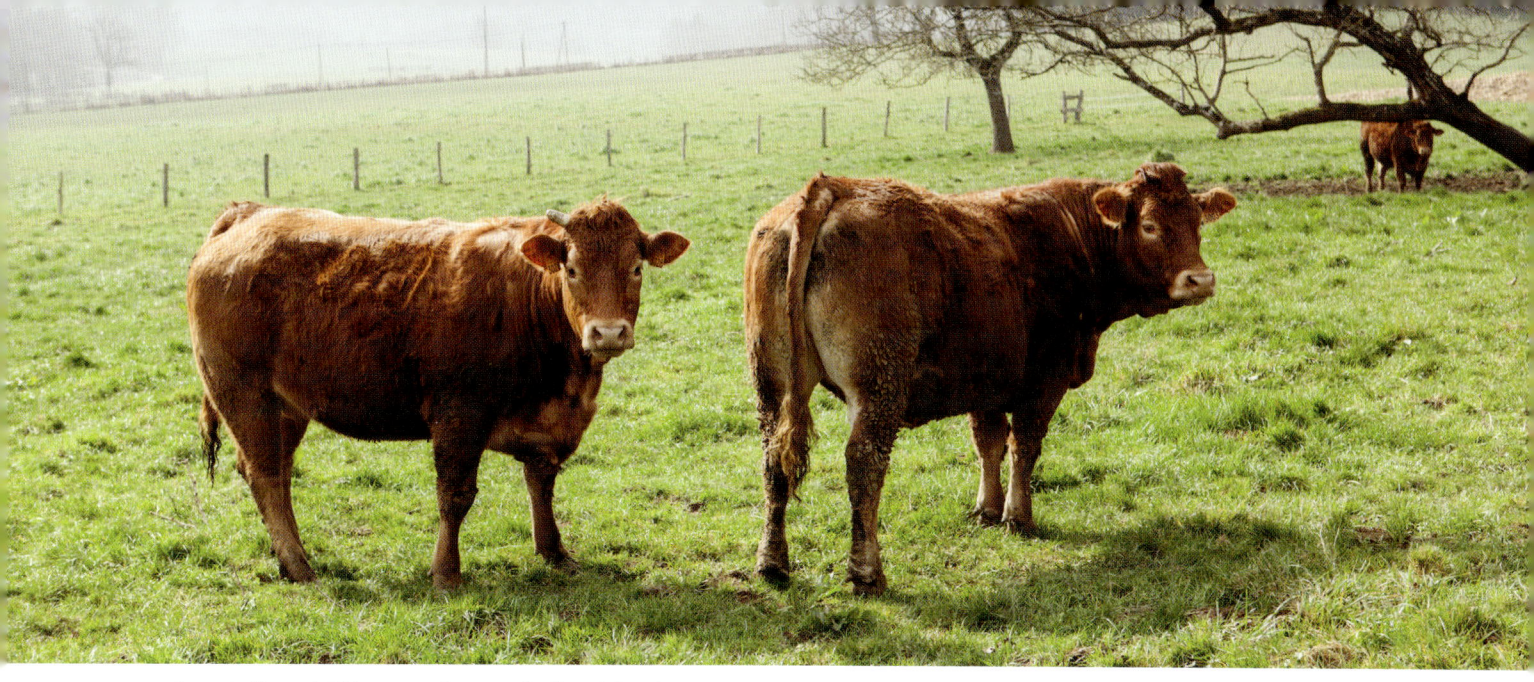

Organic Grass-fed Limousine Cows in the French Southwest

units of fat, instead of glucose, the energy from carbohydrates in the form of starches and sugars."[5] The effects of fat burning give us endurance while reducing cravings, protecting our mitochondria and organs, regulating our insulin levels, stabilizing our moods, and reducing our overall risk of disease.[6] It must be added here, that we are talking about eating saturated fats in the *absence* of sugars and starches.[7,8]

There are studies suggesting that diets rich in saturated fats (from natural sources) actually *protect* our arteries and nervous system from damage and disease. This may be in part because, quite simply, eating quality animal fats does not raise insulin levels like consuming carbs or too much protein. Looking broadly and longer-term, it is clear that disease rates for many modern diseases have *not* dropped since the low-fat craze began, but rather have *increased*. There are many studies, such as the eight-year long Women's Health Initiative study conducted beginning in 1993 on over 48,000 women, that show no decrease in risk of heart disease (nor weight loss or lower risk of breast or colorectal cancer) from diets low in dietary fat but high in vegetables, fruits, and grains.[9,10]

There are numerous multi-year studies that show no greater risk of heart disease mortality from diets high in saturated fats,[11] while replacing saturated fats with polyunsaturated fats (industrially refined vegetable oil) or carbohydrates (sugars and grains) have been shown to raise the risk of non-fatal heart attacks.[12] We now know that replacing saturated fats with carbs not only increases risk of heart disease, but it also causes increased oxidation (inflammation) and impaired glucose tolerance (weight gain, diabetes, obesity), debunking the decades-long, misleading "Diet-Heart Hypothesis."[13,14] The USDA even toned down its long-held admonition to limit dietary cholesterol in the 2015 dietary guidelines.[15] We now understand that cholesterol is an essential component of brain health and overall health, and that high *dietary* cholesterol is *not* the same as high *serum* cholesterol.[16] We also know that the body returns to homeostasis no matter how much cholesterol one consumes.[17] Without adequate cholesterol, we risk having problems with memory and brain function, including dementia, and the widely-used cholesterol-lowering statin drugs may make the situation worse.[18]

Studies suggest that diets rich in saturated fats from grass-fed animal sources, high in omega-3 fatty acids actually protect our brains from cognitive decline.[19,20] What's more, many experts agree that eating quality grass-fed animal fats (particularly as part of a low-carb, high-fat diet) does not raise insulin levels or contribute to diabetes and obesity, like consuming carbs or excessive protein does.[21] In my mind, these kinds of studies support my argument that the French enjoy good health *because* of their rich diet, not *in spite* of it.

As I added more saturated fat to my own diet and to that of my family's in preparing recipes for *The Bordeaux Kitchen*, I noticed *more immediate* positive changes. I was more satisfied after meals. I snacked less. I craved sugar less. I slept better. My kids' moods stabilized, and their focus improved. Eating more saturated fat, my already slim husband *lost* an excess 15 pounds he never knew he had. There were, and still are, fewer colds and flus, fewer outbursts and mood swings. I realize my family's experience is just one piece of anecdotal evidence. But if you look across the primal/paleo community, one thing is clear: as you increase quality fats in your diet, and consume fewer carbs and sugar, you naturally shed excess body fat and stabilize blood sugar.

Of course, most French who cook in ancestral ways know all this instinctively—that meals based on fresh, local, quality animal fats will bring satiety and nutrition and will encourage sharing with others. No one roasts a leg of lamb (page 209) and sautés potatoes in duck fat (page 468) just to eat alone in front of the television. When you prepare a meal with quality ingredients and natural fats, it is something to share with others. Why do this only for special occasions when this can be part of your daily routine? The recipes in *The Bordeaux Kitchen* will show you how to bring healthy saturated fat into your repertoire of meals. In the Butchery chapter, I explain how to choose quality sources and cuts of meat to maximize nutrient density.

FAT: THAT UNFORTUNATE HOMONYM
In *The Big Fat Surprise*, author Nina Teicholz discusses "the unfortunate homonym" of the word "fat" which refers both to the dietary fat that we eat and the adipose tissue or "fat" that collects in our bodies due to hormonal and blood lipid reactions to the food we eat. We need to separate the concept of farm fats from body fat and from the adjective that applies to being "unattractively" overweight. The unfortunate homonym confusion has only grown in severity in recent decades with the rapid rise in rates and prevalence of diabetes and obesity in modern cultures and the mistaken fear that eating fat makes us fat and gives us heart disease.

SATURATED FAT DOES NOT MAKE US FAT
Saturated fats from warm-blooded animals are solid at room temperature and become liquid when heated. When we consume these fats, they go through a process of assimilation in our gut and are passed on to the cells and organs, like the brain, as needed. Fat travels through the bloodstream in lipoproteins, nourishing the cells. Saturated fats are the robust, slow-burning log on our fire. Industrially refined oils (polyunsaturated fatty acids, or PUFAs, which I discuss later in the "A Few Words on Industrial Seed Oils" sidebar on page 41), however, "trick" our cells by posing as fuel, yet they do not provide the nutrients necessary for energy production in the cell mitochondria. Instead, these refined "trick fats" sap us of energy, accumulate in the body, and cause oxidative damage. The body is reluctant to burn the poor fuel from these PUFAs, which leads to stubborn fat storage.[22] It turns out that our adipose tissue (body fat) is actually an endocrine organ[23] that releases hormones[24] on which our body depends for regulation of brain function, reproduction, and metabolism.[25]

LOW-FAT DIETS AND HEART DISEASE
Meanwhile, excessive amounts of refined carbohydrates in the fat-fearing, low-fat, high-carb Standard American Diet (SAD diet) glycate, or stick to our cells, increasing our blood sugar levels.[26] These excessive sugars also stiffen up our cell walls and bind to hormone receptors, disrupting our hormonal function, causing insulin resistance, and

making our cells prone to oxidation.[27] They also glycate and therefore increase our LDL cholesterol particles and triglycerides in the blood,[28] blocking off our capillaries and blood vessels.[29] It is these refined carbohydrates (glucose and fructose) which, when consumed in excess, are quickly burned like kindling, or else are converted to "stored fat" (our adipose tissue) by the liver.[30] What's more, low-fat diets end up being high-carb diets because carbohydrates are substituted for the missing fats. These are generally processed carbs that attempt to satiate with added refined salts and sugars because they are lacking the satiating effect of fat, leading to numerous poor health conditions.

Dr. William Davis, author of *Wheat Belly*, has summed up "low-fat" diets as follows: "Cutting fat does not reduce the risk of heart disease, in fact, it causes incredible metabolic distortion … it causes high blood sugar, hyperglycemia, a rise in fasting glucose, insulin resistance, growth of belly fat, hypertension, metabolic syndrome, diabetes, pre-diabetes."[31]

DON'T CUT OUT THE FAT
Nutrient density turns out to be a much better factor to use when choosing your food than the lack of fat. Remember *The Bordeaux Kitchen* Tenets from Chapter 2 (page 8)? Eating nutrient-dense food is critical to our wellbeing. Animal fat is nutrient dense. Our brains are made up of 70%-80% fatty acids, and our hormones (comprised of sterols, including chole*sterol*) are fats. Many of the nutrients we need to survive and thrive can only be metabolized in the presence of fats such as the *fat-soluble* vitamins A, Bs, and C.[32] Nina Teicholz's book *The Big Fat Surprise* cites decades' worth of evidence showing that excessive carbohydrates are driving up rates of obesity and diabetes because of their spiking effect on insulin levels in the body. Even combining high-fat food with high-sugar intake, such as when eating cheesecake, creates a problem because excess sugar in the blood ends up getting stored as fat.[33]

"Saturated fat does a body good."[34] Unlike carbohydrates and even protein, fat does not affect insulin levels. Those of us who had been cutting out the saturated fats (butter, lard, tallow, fat from fowl) for the past several decades have been depriving ourselves of the very nutrients that we evolved to consume and thrive on as a species. The great experiment in recent decades with low-fat diets and the fear of consuming animal fats has contributed to increases in a range of modern diseases that have led to great suffering and untold premature deaths.

FATTY ACID RATIOS AND THE BRAIN
Our brains are made of 70-80% fatty acids. The quality fat that we eat helps nourish our brain and the rest of our body. However, as we have seen, not all fats have the same effect on the body. In general, the modern diet lacks omega-3 fatty acids and contains too many omega-6s. Our optimal ratios of omega-6 to omega-3 should be closer to 4 to 1, or 1 to 1, instead of 10 to 1 or higher.[35,36] (Omega-6 fatty acids compete with omega-3s for vitally important spots at the cellular membrane level and can squeeze out the presence of omega-3s. Omega-3s fight inflammation, while omega-6s are largely pro-inflammatory.[37]) Michael A. Schmidt, author of *Brain Building Nutrition* and *Beyond Antibiotics*, is one of many scientists who talks about the dangers of skewing our fatty acid ratio in the direction of omega-6s when we consume industrially adulterated "foods": "Fatty acids that we consume in the diet… form the membrane, the cell architecture throughout the body and actually the brain architecture, which then influences how we perceive, how we sense, our ability to move, our mood, our ability to recall and to think, and our cognition, if you will, our ability to associate our actions with an outcome. Fatty acids have an impact on all of that by virtue of their effect on brain architecture, so you could almost say fatty acids have the power to change who we are." If this isn't food for thought, then nothing is.

DEBUNKING THE ERA OF "FEAR AND DISGUST" OF FATS

There are many great books about fats. One in particular I must mention yet again: *The Big Fat Surprise* by Nina Teicholz. It recounts the history of the myths surrounding saturated fats and the rise of industrial seed oils and trans fats and their use in processed "foods." Romy Dollé's book *Good Fat, Bad Fat* goes into an in-depth study of the many fats. Another excellently organized reference admonishing us to avoid PUFAs and that contains a scientific look at fats at the molecular and cellular levels is Dr. Cate Shanahan's newly revised and reprinted *Deep Nutrition*. And if you're worried about eating too many calories, read either *Good Calories, Bad Calories* or *Why We Get Fat*, both by Gary Taubes, to understand the faulty foundation of the U.S. "food pyramid," upon which, unfortunately, so much of our modern nutrient-poor diet (even in U.S. public schools, tragically) is based. If you eat to satiation a good combination of what I call "farm fats" (see page 18), vegetables, eggs from pastured poultry, offal, and proteins, you will be less likely to overeat in the first place. We tend to overeat the things that are easy to eat and are dense in calories but nutrient-poor. (See titles by Robb Wolf and Mark Schatzker on the hyper-palatability of processed "foods" in the Resources and Further Reading section on page 603.) Another excellent recent reference volume on animal fats is *Nourishing Fats: Why We Need Animal Fats for Health and Happiness* by Sally Fallon, president of the Weston A. Price Foundation (WAPF).

CHOLESTEROL CONUNDRUM

With all this talk about fat, what about cholesterol? Just like the French Paradox, which, as we've seen, is not really a paradox, the cholesterol conundrum really is not a conundrum. It has been proven in many studies that dietary cholesterol does not affect cardiovascular disease as purported for decades by the Diet-Heart Hypothesis, in which saturated fat was linked to heart disease and fat became feared. There is no or very low association between dietary cholesterol and heart disease.[38] I refer you again to Nina Teicholz's book as well as to Denise Minger, who recounts the history of this epic fallacy and fear in her book *Death by Food Pyramid*. The book shows that it is actually *carbohydrate* consumption that increases triglycerides in the blood—one large factor connected to heart disease.

THE FATS OF FRANCE: A REVIEW

According to Waverley Root's 1958 book, *The Food of France*, one can divide France into four parts, based on which fat predominated in local cooking. This breakdown is still useful for the most part today: Dairy production is widespread in the northwest of France (Brittany and Normandy, but also in eastern France in Burgundy, Jura, and Savoie). Butter is used in many French dishes, and is sometimes clarified to remove the casein proteins, elevate the smoke point (discussed at the end of the following section), and create a creamier effect, such as in Hollandaise or Béarnaise sauces. The northeast (Alsace, Lorraine, Auvergne) is a region where lard and the venerable duck and goose provide the primary cooking fats. Olive oil is most commonly used in dishes from France's southeast (Provence and Corsica). And in the Southwest (into which I would place Bordeaux and its surrounding regions, in addition to Gascony and the Basque country and Béarn and even Languedoc-Rousillon, which borders on the southwest but also extends to the Mediterranean Sea), all of the above fats apply, making southwestern French food so very rich in so many ways!

FARM FATS ARE SATURATED FATS

The fat from pastured animals contains a combination of monounsaturated, polyunsaturated, and a majority (60 to 70%) of saturated fat. Saturated at the molecular level means that a fatty acid molecule is made up of a stable string of carbon atoms bonded with hydrogen atoms. No nicks or dents to put a chink in its armor (whereas industrially processed oils, as I discuss later, have many chinks in the armor and are highly toxic and susceptible to oxidation). Saturated fats like butter, lard, and tallow remain solid at room temperature. Olive oil is primarily made of monounsaturated fats and is liquid at room temperature. Consuming fat is what allows us to absorb many of the nutrients and vitamins in our food, including many of those in vegetables, which is where the term "fat-soluble vitamins" gets its meaning. Let us remember that an animal, such as a pig or cow, stores vitamin D in its fat. So, a vegetarian, as I was in my early twenties, misses out on the, dare I say, healing and necessary nutritional benefits of eating animal fat. The omega-3s we might think we are getting when we consume chia, flax, or other plant oils are poorly converted by our human bodies, unlike the cow or the chimpanzee. We can only assimilate up to 6% of these omega-3s from vegetable sources, and unfortunately, they oxidize easily, often before they are consumed.[39,40] Thus, the well-intentioned vegetarian (or vegan) sacrifices herself yet again, as I did, with a nutrient-poor, and dare I say, *damaging* diet. There's also the environmental degradation caused by farming all those GMO soy "foods" like soy burgers and nuggets to replace the real thing, meat,[41] to say nothing of the fact that soy and other GMO cereal grains and grasses like wheat and corn are heavily sprayed with glyphosate, whose increase in use over recent decades correlates with a rise in chronic modern diseases[42,43] and autism,[44,45] as well as mitochondrial malfunction and microbiome disruption.[46,47]

Saturated fat could be translated to mean "does not oxidize," that is to say, the molecule is saturated and does not attract free radical oxygen molecules to latch onto it, *unlike* the polyunsaturated fats (canola, corn or soy bean oil, for example). Lard and tallow, for this reason, do not turn rancid easily and can be cooked on high heat. Therefore, these two fats, along with duck fat, are usually what are recommended in the recipes for "browning" (caramelizing) meat in *The Bordeaux Kitchen*. The sugars in the meat are browned, but the saturated fats hold up to the heat.

The smoke point (*point de fumée*) of a fat or oil matters in the cooking process, because at the smoke point temperature, the enzymes and other helpful compounds break down and oxidation occurs. The smoke point of each fat or oil varies somewhat depending on its source,[48] therefore I have provided a range of temperatures in the following descriptions. If we cook with these fats and oils *below* the smoke point as much as possible, and avoid charring (blackening), we can maximize the health benefits of cooking with these fats and add tremendous flavor to our meals.

BUTTER

You could almost consider butter on its own among the Secrets to French Cooking, it is so flavorful and rich, giving cooked food, whether savory or sweet, that special *oomph*, that *je ne sais quoi*. Julia Child and butter are often referred to together. (Julia Child, the American diplomat's wife who became famous for translating French cuisine into a language and manner Americans could understand, remained true to the French tradition by using butter where called for in recipes. "And if you're afraid of butter, which many people are nowadays," she said while making mashed potatoes with French chef Jacques Pépin on public television in 1997, "you just put in cream!"[49]) In France, some butters are geographically certified, much like other French agricultural products. Butter can be made from cream or whey, with or without added salt. For the purposes of the recipes in this book, I use sweet cream butter, adding salt to the dish separately. Brittany is one region where they use local sea salt in making butter, *beurre de Breton*, and they are quite proud of this. Rightly so, it is delicious! Indeed, different milks and processes produce different butter. Some chefs add herbs to their butters. Butter is so versatile and in France can be used as a simple staple ingredient or served as a luxurious condiment.

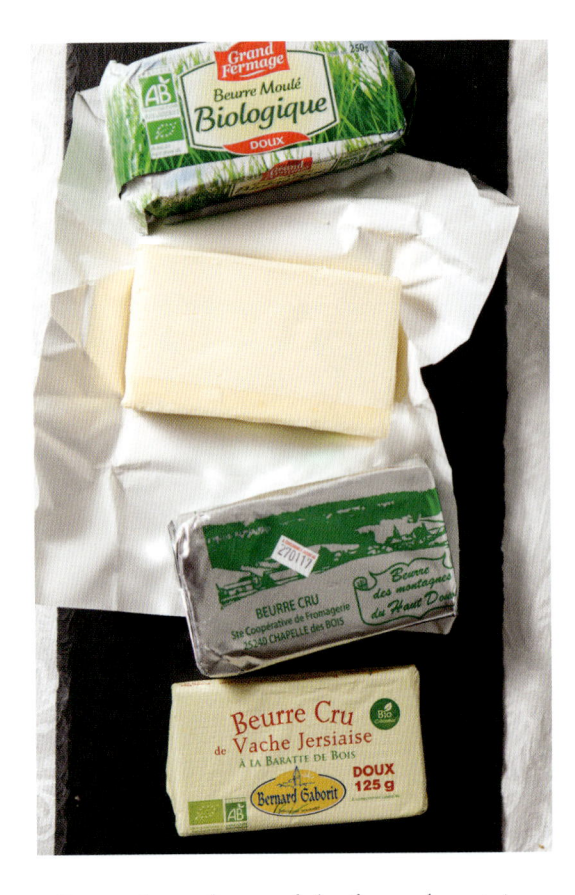

Butter is made up of the fat and protein from milk. Butter contains 12%-15% short and medium-chain fatty acids. If the animal (cow, goat, sheep, camel, buffalo) has grazed (as it evolved to) on pesticide-free grasses, the milk it provides is called "grass fed" or "pastured" (not to be confused with "pasteurized," which means heated until all bacteria and enzymes are killed). The healthful properties of butter from grass-fed cows are significant, providing vitamin K2 along with antioxidant and cancer-fighting omega-3 fatty acids and conjugated linoleic acids (CLAs) and other nutrients.[50,51,52,53] Some like to say that vegetables exist for the enjoyment of butter! As long as you do not have sensitivities to the protein casein in butter, or do not suffer from any estrogenic (hormonal) or immunogenic or inflammatory effects from dairy, then this is a powerfully healthful fat. Unpasteurized grass-fed butter contains many of the living bacteria and enzymes one would enjoy in raw milk. As this is an animal fat, organic *and* grass fed is best. Raw butter and cream can be a challenge to find, but are well worth the search. A small amount of high-quality organic grass-fed raw dairy goes a long way. (The Weston A. Price Foundation houses abundant literature on raw dairy. There is also a website to check out: rawmilk.org. See more on dairy in the Fresh Ingredients section later in this chapter.)

As for its cooking properties, butter, when heated, loses its moisture through evaporation, raising the temperature of the remaining milk proteins which then undergo the Maillard reaction: the proteins brown, and the sugars in the butter "caramelize." The resulting brown, tasty butter is called *noisette* in French, also the name for "hazelnut," probably for the resulting caramel color and nutty flavor. Beyond this point, butter will burn anywhere from 250°F to 300°F (121°C to 150°C). Clarified butter (*beurre clarifié*), which has been melted slowly and then separated from the casein protein (that floats to the top of the pan and is discarded), has a higher smoke point than butter. I have seen its estimate range from 356°F to 485°F (180°C to 252°C).

GHEE

A type of clarified butter often used in South Asian and Middle Eastern cooking, ghee has a smoke point of 450°F to 485°F (232°C to 252°C), or possibly a bit higher, and is an even more meticulously refined version of butter. It contains 25% or more short and medium-chain fatty acids, almost double that of butter.[54] The Ayurvedic practice (the primary health treatment system originating from India) of making ghee comes from the warmer, southern regions of India where butter would spoil if not transformed into ghee. Those with casein sensitivities can sometimes use ghee for cooking. Ghee can have a nutty flavor. When it is hand-processed in small batches, ghee can sometimes taste even more like it came from a cow than butter does.

BACON FAT

What's not to love about bacon? It is essentially caramelized meat in fat. Anything caramelized is delicious to us: butter, nuts, and yes, bacon. The Maillard reaction is at play here again, browning the sugar molecules in the fat to make it taste so good. Bacon fat in particular adds that smoked or salty flavor. Just be careful about what has been added to your bacon. You can cure your own pork bellies in salt, garlic, and vinegar (page 86), to be sure of no unwanted additives. Or find a butcher or online service (such as Pete's Paleo or U.S. Wellness Meats) for cured sugar-free and industrial preservative-free bacon. I use bacon fat to add fat and flavor to vegetables such as broccoli, squash, and sweet potatoes.

LARD – SAINDOUX

Lard is the general word for pork fat. Fatback, synonymous with lard (*saindoux*) comes mostly from the back and is the fat just beneath the skin of the pig. (Leaf lard, which comes from around the viscera, is the most prized and taste-free lard to render, used for baking for example, but fat-back lard is more plentiful and really just as good.) Lard is such a great source of dietary fat, especially from pastured hogs which have received sunlight on their backs and have converted this, as we do, through the skin into vitamin D. We absorb the vitamin D and other nutrients when we eat "fatback" or lard. Lard has a smoke point of 360°F to 374°F (182°C to 190°C), and is versatile and useable in all French cooking. See instructions for **Rendering Lard (Pork Fat)** on page 267. Pork caul (*crépine*) comes from the viscera, holding the organs of the pig in place. It has a web-like look to it and is not used as a cooking fat, but rather to wrap around meat dishes to hold them together or to tuck around pâtés in jars.

FAT FROM FOWL

Duck fat (*graisse de canard*) is at the heart of French cuisine from the southwest. It is what makes the dish **Sarlat Sautéed Potatoes** (page 468) so delicious, along with any vegetable or dish where you need fat to cook. Equally delicious and nutritious is goose fat, *graisse d'oie*. Duck and goose fats are high in oleic fatty acids and are 55% monounsaturated fatty acids (MUFAs), shown to lower triglycerides.[55] Duck fat, goose fat, and chicken fat have a high smoke point of about 375°F (190°C) and are flavorful and excellent for "browning" meats and vegetables. Rendering duck or goose fat is simple. See instructions for **Rendering Duck (or Goose) Fat** on page 266. The cracklings are delicious, like popcorn but with much more flavor! Added to vegetables, they are almost a meal in themselves. You can also use them to make **Duck Rinds** (page 359.)

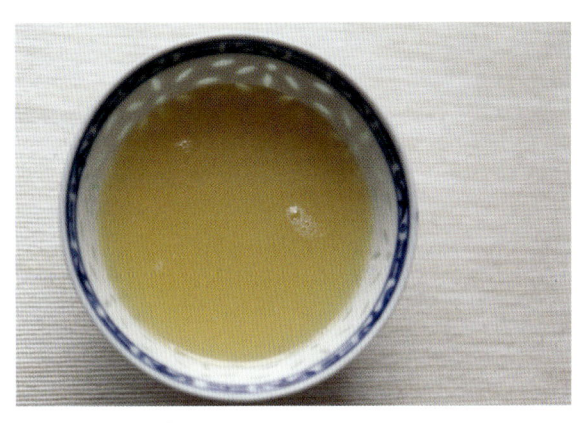

Rendered Duck Fat

TALLOW – LE SUIF

Beef and lamb fat when rendered is called tallow. (Suet is the visceral fat surrounding the kidneys and may be chopped or rendered for cooking.) These fats have distinct flavors and odors, lamb being much more aromatic, even too strong for some people. But if I am cooking lamb meatballs (*kefta*), for example, I will use lamb tallow for the frying, if I have any. Beef tallow was used to fry french fries in fast food restaurants until sometime in the 1970s, when the propaganda against animal fats and the use of cheaper industrial vegetable oils usurped this practice. When I cook with tallow, I smell that distinct french fry aroma from my childhood. Tallow's smoke point ranges from 400°F to 420°F (204°C to 215°C), which makes it excellent for higher heat sautéing, braising, or browning meats and vegetables. Rendering tallow is also easy. See instructions for **Rendering Tallow (Beef Fat)** on page 268. What is left over are beef cracklings, which you can freeze for later use or throw in with sautéed vegetables. I mix them with chopped leeks and a bit of duck fat and sea salt for extra flavor. In France, farm fats are available in grocery stores, spice shops (*épiceries*, from the word "spice," *épice*), butcher shops, and at the markets. I look for the organic versions to reduce the potential for toxins in the fats. If you do not want to render your own fats, you can buy rendered tallow, lard, and duck fat from Fatworks and U.S. Wellness Meats online.

OLIVE OIL – *L'HUILE D'OLIVE*

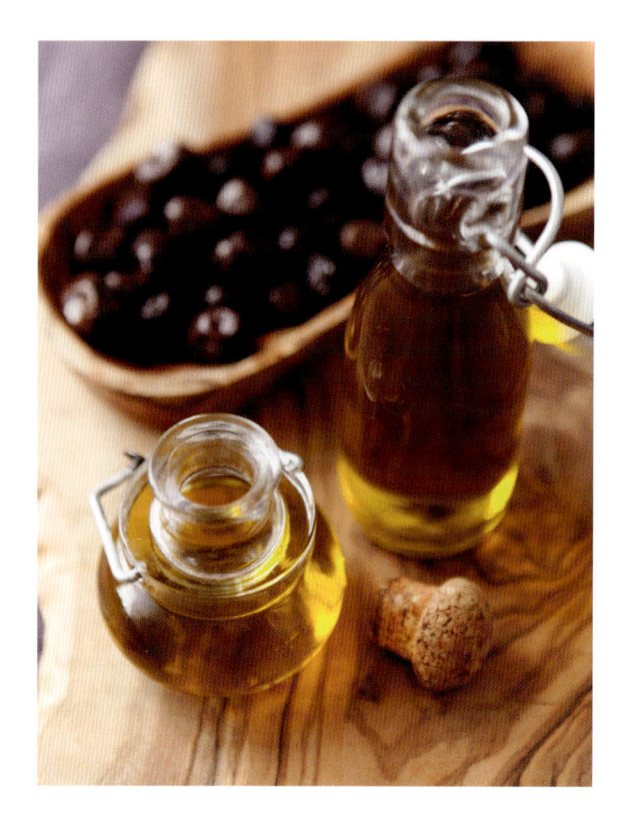

Oh, there is so much to say about olive oil! The Romans brought olives to France, along with their way of life, and indeed this fruit grows naturally in the Mediterranean region of France. This is one oil that has been harvested by hand and used in cooking for millennia. I consider olive oil among the great cooking fats to use in French recipes (usually not on high-heat settings), thanks to its rich flavors, monounsaturated fat profile, and ability to help us assimilate fat-soluble vitamins from vegetables.

Handmade batches of cold-processed, extra virgin, organic olives are the best, which is why, with olive oil, you get what you pay for.[56] The cheapest "olive" oils may not be 100% pure. In the U.S., only 60% to 70% of the oil is required to actually come from olives to be considered olive oil. The rest could be a hazardous mixture of other industrial oils, which adds to shelf life, but dilutes an otherwise good product and ruins the good omega fatty acid ratios. A monounsaturated fat, extra virgin olive oil that is cold pressed, especially if it looks cloudy (meaning it is unfiltered), has a varying smoke point between about 320°F and 375°F (160°C and 190°C). It is used for its flavor in many dishes, especially in the Mediterranean part of France. In my recipes, I keep the oven temperature at 365°F (185°C) so as not to burn the olive oil. As a monounsaturated fat, MUFA (which means only one spot along its fatty acid chain, called a double bond, can acquire an oxygen molecule and oxidize), olive oil is much more stable and less hazardous to our health than industrial vegetable seed oils. These refined seed oils are polyunsaturated fats and have numerous spots at which oxygen can bind and "oxidize" in storage, during the cooking process, and in our bodies. Three strikes—you're out!

But several properties of olive oil make it less suitable for high heat cooking. Olive oil's anthocyanins (pigmented flavonoids that contribute to flavor), polyphenols (with antioxidant properties like hydroxtyrosol), and other antioxidants (like beta-carotene and vitamin E) are temperature sensitive. Olive oil will oxidize (without its protective olive skin), if it sits by the stove, oven, or in the sun. Therefore, for most of my high-heat cooking, I opt for other cooking fats, particularly duck or goose fat, ghee, lard, tallow, or coconut oil, depending on the recipe. Refined, "light" olive oil has a higher smoke point of about 465°F (240°C), but it is just that: refined. With regard to the recipes in *The Bordeaux Kitchen*, when I list "olive oil" as an ingredient, I mean organic (where possible) extra virgin olive oil.

OLIVE OIL VS. ANIMAL FATS IN TODAY'S FRENCH COOKING

The most surprising thing about modern French chefs, is that many of them have abandoned cooking with traditional fats. Instead, they typically use olive oil when cooking at high temperatures to sear foods, rather than using tallow with beef, or lard with pork. These animal fats, being saturated, are more stable and resistant to oxidation and have similar or slightly higher smoke points than olive oil. Luckily, French chefs still also use butter or clarified butter (or even a combination of olive oil and butter) to maintain that traditional flavor and texture. My Bordeaux-based American friend Dewey Markham, Jr. says he was trained in French cooking school to use the combination of butter and olive oil so as to increase the smoke point while also retaining the flavor of olive oil in the finished food. At least the French chefs I have learned from are using olive oil and not industrial vegetable oils. I cannot say as much for what "lower end" restaurants and cafés are using. One would hope they are all using high-quality olive oil and butters.

Nevertheless, there are several points where French chefs and cooks might have strayed from their ancestral tradition. First, why not use lard, tallow, or duck fat? There is a dearth of these wonderful farm fats in modern recipes. I surmise that modern French chefs (and others around the world in culinary schools) are *trained* now to use either olive oil or butter and do not question their training. Second, the basis for this training may date back as far as 1869 in France, when alternative fats like margarine were first invented.[57] Over time, people began to avoid cooking with animal fats, which carried through society from one generation to the next. Now we have arrived at a place where the norm is cooking with refined oils and the exception is relying upon the "farm fats." It seems to me that chefs (and culinary schools) are just responding to demand. People are *afraid* of consuming tallow (it is also not generally sold in stores), so tallow is off the menu and replaced by the popular favorite olive oil, or worse, a low-quality refined seed oil. In addition to the risks of dilution and corruption by the refining process, olive oil oxidizes readily at higher temperatures, especially low-quality versions bought on the cheap. Oxidation causes free radicals in the body, which in turn cause tissue damage and inflammation. And who needs that? We already have enough cell damage from the stresses of modern life, including pollution, lack of sleep, pesticides, poor soils, overuse of medications, etc. By cooking with saturated fats like butter, duck and goose fat, lard and tallow—of high quality and ideally from grass-fed and pasture-raised sources—you will be rewarded with wholesome nutrients and flavor, while lowering the risks of oxidation and inflammation. Reserve the high-quality olive oil for when it is truly needed in cooking and for cooler temperatures while taking advantage of the other flavors available to you. And you will eat and cook with joy!

OTHER OILS

Organic virgin coconut oil is a very popular cooking oil in the primal/paleo world as it is tasty, versatile, has a relatively high smoke point (depending on how refined it is)—ranging from 350°F to 400°F (171° to 204°C)—and is made up partially of medium-chain triglycerides (MCTs), a form of fat that is easily metabolized by our brains. For this reason, consuming MCTs separately or in coconut oil is becoming more common for those wishing to increase their brain function, or even those with more advanced neurological diseases of the brain such as Alzheimer's or Parkinson's. However, these oils can be tough on the digestive system in that they can cause loose stools if consumed in large quantities. Sustainably harvested red palm oil has similar properties to coconut oil, but it is much harder to find a truly reliable, sustainable source. Industrially-run palm oil plantations have wreaked massive havoc on the local environment (deforestation, habitat destruction, air and water pollution to name a few) for the sake of producing hydrogenated palm oil, which is hazardous to our health, as all hydrogenated oils are. West African red palm oil is one that does not contribute to the destruction of orangutan habitats, as the palm oil from Indonesia does. Coconut and red palm oils are refined to varying degrees. Therefore, much like olive oil, you get what you pay for. A small-batch processed certified organic coconut oil without fillers will be more expensive but less industrially altered (in theory, with less environmental impact) than one that has gone through a more extensive refining process and been mixed with undisclosed additives. Regulations do not exist, in the U.S. at least, to label coconut oil for additives. Skinny Fat & Co is one responsibly-run, additive-free coconut oil I have tried, and it is indeed more expensive than the others as you are paying for their due diligence to quality and good stewardship.

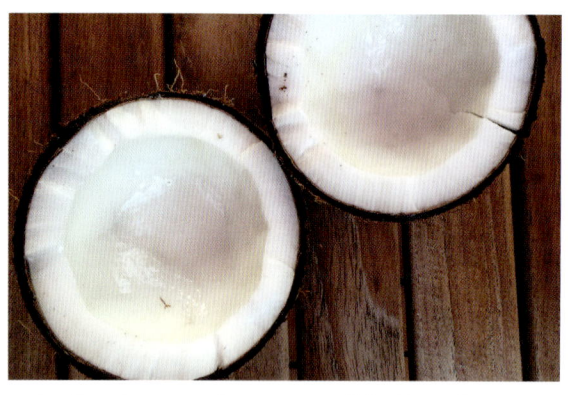

As for the use of coconut oil in French cooking, many recipes originate from France's overseas island territories of Guadeloupe and Martinique and in parts of Southeast Asia, known in colonial times as *Indochine* to the French. These tropical lands provided recipes and ingredients that have been woven into the fabric of French cuisine over time. Though coconut oil does not figure prominently in *The Bordeaux Kitchen*, it can easily replace other oils or fats in recipes depending on your taste and what is in your pantry.

Here are a few other oils that are not generally used for cooking in *The Bordeaux Kitchen* or in traditional French cuisine but can be used on occasion as substitutes for the farm fats.

Avocado Oil – *L'Huile d'Avocat* Though not common in French cooking, avocado oil is a versatile oil I have used for medium- to high-heat cooking as it has a high smoke point of 520°F (271°C). But it is also delicious on salads, and it is a key ingredient in Mark Sisson's Primal Kitchen Mayonnaise. Avocados are high in mono-unsaturated fats and make a flavorful and satisfying addition to salads.[58]

Grapeseed Oil – *L'Huile des Pépins de Raisin* This is a popular French choice as a salad topping for its delicate, nutty flavor. It has a good ratio of omega fatty acids if it has been cold-pressed, but it is very prone to oxidation and is not used as a cooking oil in France.

Walnut Oil – *L'Huile de Noix* Walnut oil is used in France, as the walnut has long been cultivated in the region of Périgord in France's southwest. Although walnut oil is less frequently used than olive oil in France overall, it has a favorable fatty acid ratio, and is used often in the French southwest on salads and even cheeses, particularly goat cheese.

Macadamia Nut Oil – *L'Huile de Macadamia* This is a delightfully nutty fat and good replacement option for higher-heat cooking, as it said to have a smoke point of about 413°F (212°C). It is also delicious on salads, but is not used in traditional French recipes.

Sesame Seed Oil – *L'Huile de Sésame* Roasted or unroasted, sesame seed oil provides a nice flavor and can have a smoke point of about 350°F to 410°F (177°C to 210°C), but should not be overused. Consider it, like grapeseed oil, more of a condiment.

As with all nuts and seeds, care should be taken when using nut and seed oil as these contain phytic acids, anti-nutrients that can cause adverse reactions in the body, and are to be avoided for those on autoimmune diets so as not to unnecessarily stress already taxed immune systems.

A Few Words on Industrial Seed Oils

Notice that industrially altered oils such as canola (rapeseed), corn, cottonseed, rice bran, safflower, soy, sunflower, and "vegetable," even expeller "cold" pressed, are not on the farm fats list. These oils are highly susceptible to oxidation, do not stand up well to industrial processing, and are therefore highly toxic.[59] In fact, thanks to their industrial processing, these vegetable oils are stripped of any of their original antioxidants and are, essentially, liquid oxidative stress in a bottle. Oxidative stress causes rapid aging as well as abnormal development and abnormal growth. Generations of children have been born into this experiment now, and we are seeing the effects."[60] If you do one thing only, cut out these oils from your diet. (This may mean bringing your own 100% olive oil to a restaurant, as they are likely to be using cheaper replacements or mixtures with industrial seed oils.)

These oils are cheap for industry to produce, but they do not nourish us. In fact, they harm us over time in a process of oxidation, chronic inflammation, neurological damage, and aging in the body. These altered, toxic, oxidized molecules end up everywhere in the body, disrupting cellular metabolic function[61] and causing alterations in tissues from the brain to the ovaries.[62] Moreover, they can be carcinogenic and cause DNA mutations which can be passed down to our children and affect fertility (in men and women).[63] It's downright tragic for our health that industrial seed oils are so ubiquitous in packaged, processed "foods" (like chips and many so-called "healthy" foods—just look at the labels), but also in restaurants across the United States.[64] And let us not kid ourselves, France's (and Europe's) lower-end restaurants are not immune to using these oils, either.

As Dr. Catherine Shanahan has said, "Nature does not make bad fats, factories do… It is the refining process that does all the damage."[65] Industrial seed oils are products usually made with hexane in a petrochemical process at high heats, pressurized, deodorized, bleached etc., in which any semblance of nutrition is lost and the omega-6 to omega-3 ratio is altered to produce an unhealthy ratio way beyond the normal one-to-one ratio for which our bodies are suited. In nature, soybeans and sunflower seeds contain antioxidants. When industrially processed, they are stripped of these and chemically altered. The resulting oils, called PUFAs because they are made up of molecular chains of polyunsaturated fatty acids, contain multiple ("poly") double carbon bonds in close proximity to one another. These double carbon bonds are unstable and attract oxygen molecules to bind with them, causing oxidative damage to the molecule. Once these molecules are altered, no amount of exogenous antioxidants can reverse the damage. These oxidized molecules build up in our bodies, worsening oxidative damage and inflammation and aging us over time.[66] Saturated fats, present in lard, butter, and tallow—the farm fats—do not oxidize. Fats that occur in nature are more easily metabolized and utilized in nature (i.e., by us). The less food is altered, the better off we are. Lard is much more of a whole food than any refined oil, and there's less risk of free radical damage. There are so many reasons for us to go back to the farm!

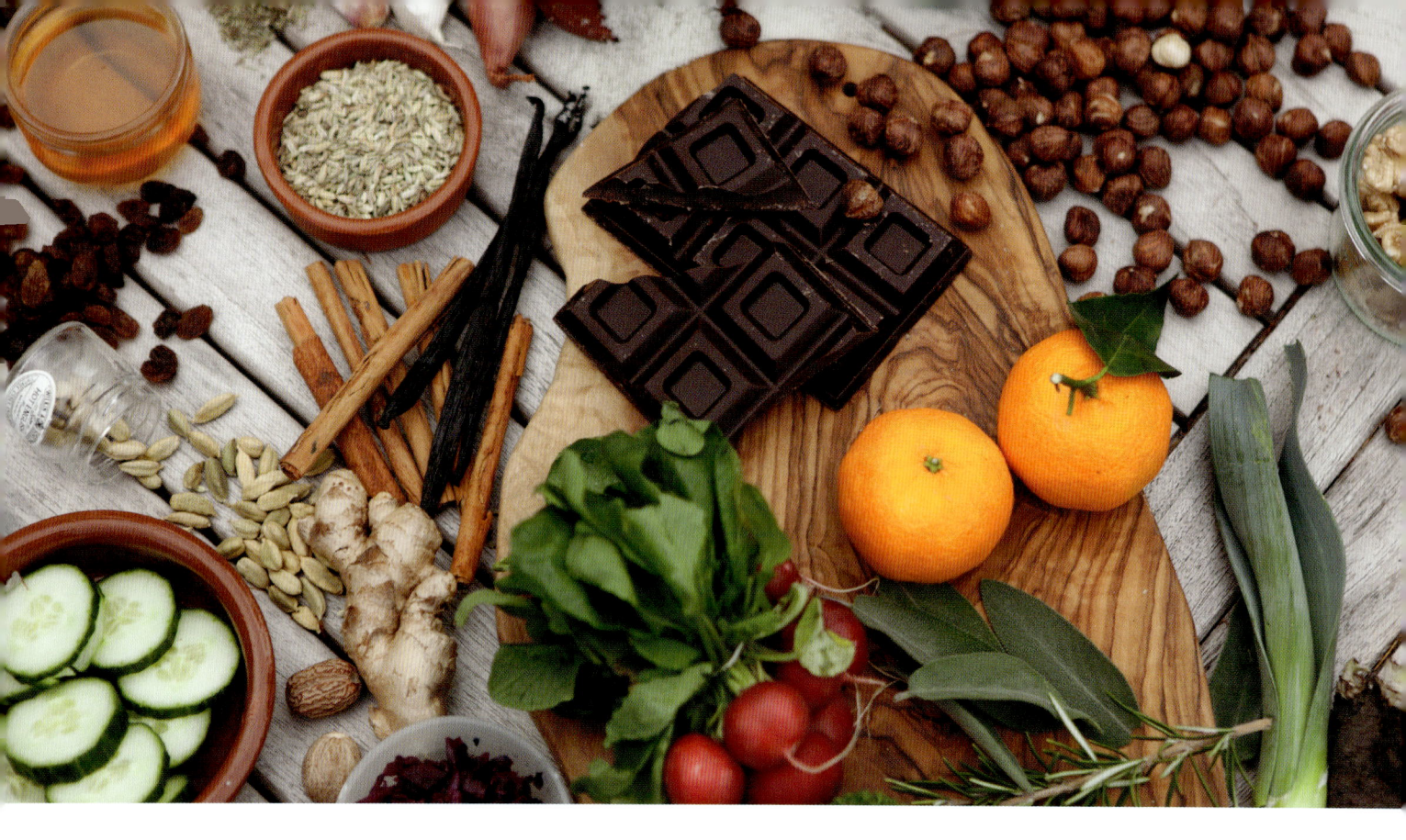

THE SECRET TO FRENCH COOKING #2: FRESH INGREDIENTS

Fresh ingredients are by definition in-season and, for the most part, locally-grown. Whatever was ready to be picked or harvested is what landed on our ancestors' proverbial plates. Although many ingredients, such as certain dried spices, cured meats, or pickled and preserved items, were available year-round for use in recipes. An ancestrally minded way of life means equating nutrient-dense meals with real, whole, fresh, and organic ingredients. Experimenting with seasonal food (while supplementing with dried, preserved, and fermented ones) is a key strategy in ensuring your diet is nutrient-dense, like that of our ancestors.

Following is a glossary-style collection of ingredients that a French great-grandmother might have used (and that I use today, as can you) when following the French ancestral recipes in The Bordeaux Kitchen.

AROMATIC HERBS

Fresh, aromatic herbs include things one can grow in one's own garden or indoor pot, such as basil, laurel (bay leaves), rosemary, thyme, sage, marjoram, peppermint, and savory. According to Dr. Stephen Masley, author of the *The Thirty-Day Heart Tune-Up* and a trained chef, herbs are anti-inflammatory. He encourages their use in cooking for that reason as well as their taste-enhancing qualities. What's more, herbs are less likely to have been tinkered with in terms of their genetic material over the ages and are nutrient-dense. Rosemary (*romarin*), for example, is soothing and invigorating to smell, has anti-microbial effects,[67,68] and grows plentifully in the South of France. Thyme (*thym*) is also native to southern Europe and is very common in French cooking. Marjoram (*marjolaine*) is a Mediterranean herb used sometimes in *herbes de Provence*, a combination of aromatic herbs commonly used to flavor dishes in the South of France. Garlic (*ail*) is used in a majority of recipes in this part of the world. Combining these creates an impact on the taste buds even my children like. The freshness of these ingredients and adequate sea salt make for a winning combination for lamb chops and pork ribs, as well as beef steaks, that never gets old!

SPICES

Spices such as cinnamon, curcuma (turmeric), ginger, fennel, nutmeg, pepper, and star anise can be found in many French recipes, depending on the regional cuisine and outside influences. When it comes to spices, France's colonial past and overseas territories touch French cuisine with spices that appear in traditional North African (*Afrique du nord*) dishes such as *tajines*, where ginger and turmeric feature prominently, or Southeast Asian (*Indochine*) curries, in which star anise, coriander, or cumin are used.

The term *quatre épices* refers to a grouping of four spices: black pepper, cinnamon, clove, and nutmeg, but could also include chili pepper or ginger. The "Quatre Épices" shrub from France's island of La Réunion in the Indian Ocean is similar to allspice. Allspice can be used in place of *quatre épices*. *Cinq épices* refers to a grouping of five spices: cinnamon, clove, fennel, black pepper, and star anise, but it could also include cardamom or ginger; it comes originally from Chinese traditional cuisine. It is used in some French dishes to modify the flavor profile. For many reasons, black pepper is one of the most common spices, and historically one of the most highly-valued spices, and it figures in most spice combinations. Besides enhancing flavor on its own, black pepper increases the absorbency of other herbs and spices, such as curcumin, and amplifies their health benefits, and it even helps reduce oxidative stress in the body and inflammation in the brain.[69]

A "garnished bouquet" (*bouquet garni*), a combination of bay leaves, thyme, leek, rosemary, parsley, or savory tied in a small bundle with string, forms the basis of many traditional, slow-cooked French recipes. Bay leaves are plentiful if you have a laurel tree. If you should be so lucky as to receive a branch of leaves from a friend or neighbor's tree, as I was in Bordeaux, you can leave them out to dry before storing them. They can also be used fresh, just like most herbs.

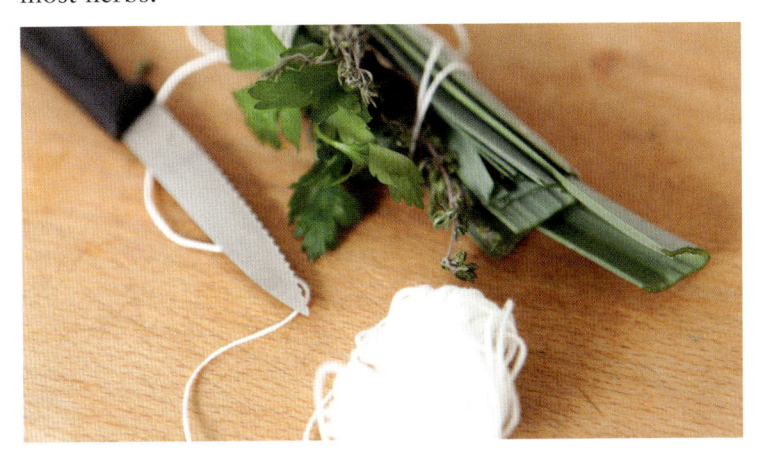

Herbs and spices are nutrient-dense and have a variety of properties helpful in supporting good health. Chop staple herbs like fresh rosemary in batches when you have time, and store in the freezer or refrigerator in a glass jar. They will liven up almost any meat dish in no time.

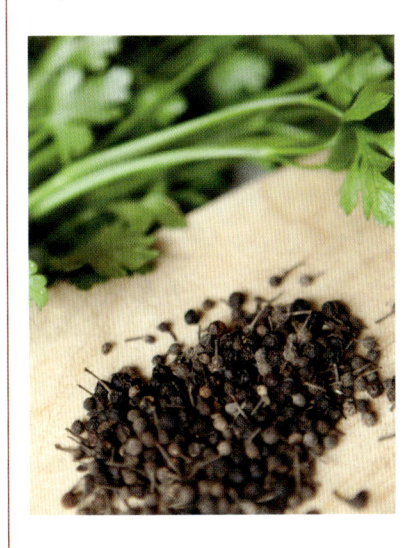

The combination of carrots, onion and celery (or celery root), often in a 1:2:1 ratio respectively, is called *mirepoix*, and is the basis for many stocks, broths, and soups.

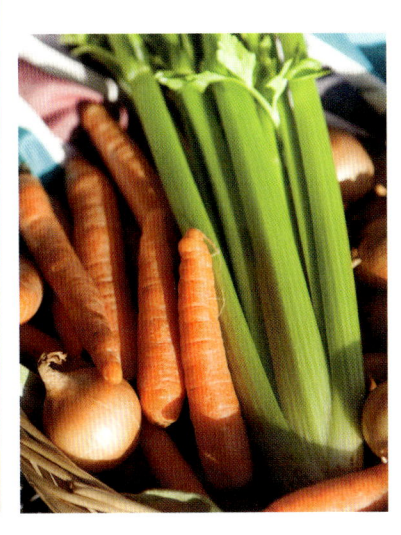

CHAPTER 4

GARLIC

Along with herbs and spices, garlic, shallots, onions, and carrots round out the flavor profile for many of the recipes in this book as well. It is always good to have these kinds of ingredients on hand, as any combination of these will almost guarantee great flavor in your food.

Garlic has both antifungal and antimicrobial properties (though it is also a FODMAP[70], making it more difficult for some to digest), and many healing remedies throughout history have included garlic. Since garlic figures so prominently in French recipes, it's helpful to keep garlic on hand. Garlic can be stored in a bowl or basket on the counter, but it can also be very helpful when you are in a pinch for time to have some peeled or even minced garlic on hand. I have found that crushing a clove of garlic beneath the wide, flat side of a knife makes it easier to peel off the skin. The age-old chef's trick of crushing garlic in this way allows the aromas to be released while keeping the garlic itself encased in its skin when used in dishes where the garlic flavor is desired but the garlic itself is not. (I just eat the garlic in the end, regardless.) Crushing garlic also has the effect of allowing the enzymes to work their medicinal magic in the garlic clove, making its antimicrobial and vitamin powers that much more potent. Garlic has even been shown to reduce ear pain.[71] Garlic has so many beneficial uses!

CRUSHING, PEELING AND CHOPPING GARLIC RAPIDLY

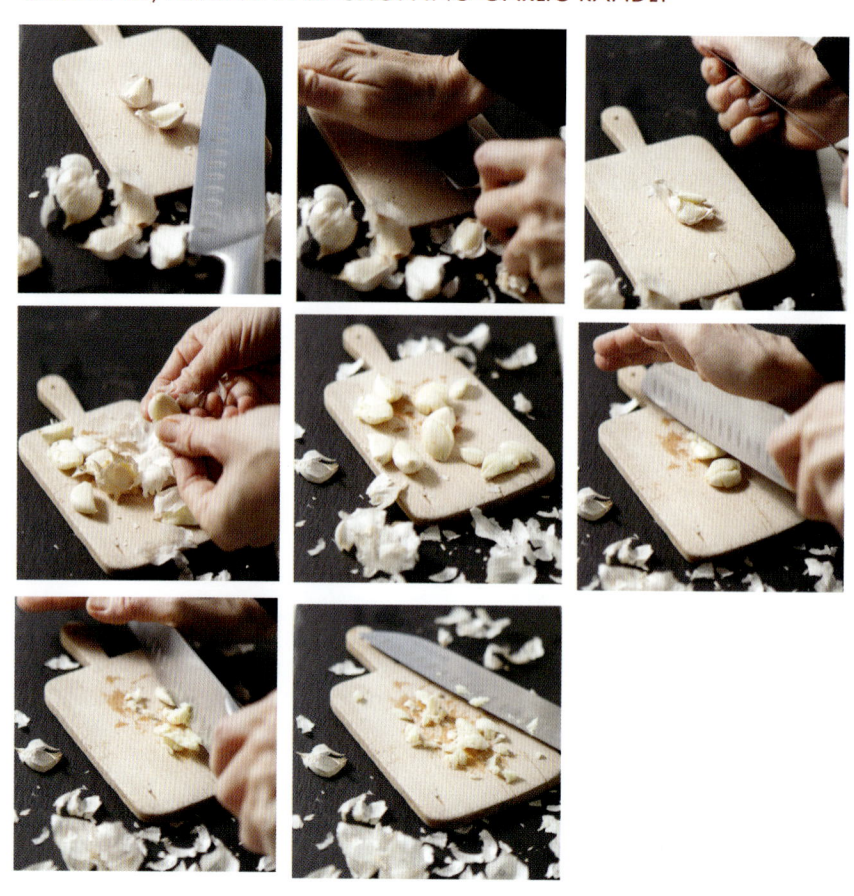

French chefs will usually remove the green germ or stem inside the garlic clove, especially when it begins to sprout while in storage, as they say it is difficult to digest this green germ. Cookbook author David Lebovitz has documented taste tests that show that garlic mayonnaise with the green germ tastes more bitter, but that garlic cooked with the green germ does not.[72] It's up to you. To remove the germ, slice the clove in half and pull it out from each half. I use a small paring knife to pry out the germ. It takes extra time but can be oddly satisfying.

MEET THE SHALLOTS

Where there is garlic, there are often also onions or shallots, other sulfurous, flavorful ingredients. The difference between the yellow or white onion and the shallot is that the shallot is sweeter and subtler, a more kid-friendly kind of onion, one could say. Shallots differ in color from pink to yellow and in size, but are usually more oblong than onions. The red onion is less potent and sweeter than the yellow or white onion but still different from the shallot.

SALT – NOT YOUR ORDINARY TABLE SALT

Another secret of French cooking is the use of mineral-rich, unrefined sea salt, or Celtic sea salt as it is often called in the U.S. In our modern food paradigm, there is a *fear of salt*. Iodized, refined "table salt" *should* be feared, as it is made up of only one compound: sodium chloride, plus some added iodine "for good measure," along with silicates and de-caking agents. This is not a healthful combination, and in fact requires many times more magnesium molecules from our own bodies to metabolize this industrial salt than it does to metabolize natural salts. Sodium chloride, "table salt," thus depletes our magnesium and calcium, while sea salt has 72 minerals in perfect proportion.[74] Salts harvested from the sea—Pacific, Atlantic, or Mediterranean—as well as mountain salts, such as European or Himalayan mountain salts, contain the trace minerals we need to survive in a form that is *readily absorbed* by our bodies.[75] To get around the lack of iodine in sea salt, add sea vegetables or shellfish, in particular oysters and clams, to your diet. Sea vegetables such as dulse, kombu, nori, and wakame can be easily added to bone broths or fish stock to increase the iodine content.

For those suffering from taxed adrenals (fatigue and low energy), a pinch of sea or mountain salt in a glass of water can help with the proper retention of salt in the body.[76] A pinch of this kind of salt in a glass of water every morning can also help our adrenal glands with their burden of daily stresses.[77] I begin and end my day with a pinch of sea salt in

Short Cut: Pre-chopped Garlic in Olive Oil

When I have time, I peel an entire bulb of garlic at a time, mince it either by hand or in a mini food processor (often sold as an "immersion blender" or "chopper"), place the minced garlic in a glass jar, and cover the garlic in olive oil, which serves to preserve the garlic for up to four or five days in the refrigerator. I have used minced garlic kept in the refrigerator for up to five days and it retains its flavor well. The garlic does begin to smell strongly after several days, however, as if it has begun to ferment a bit. At the very least, allow garlic to "aerate" a bit right after cutting it before using it in a recipe; this increases the potency of its antimicrobial characteristics.[73]

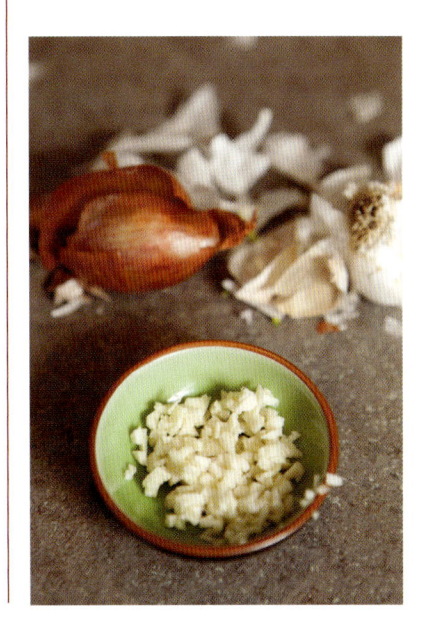

CHAPTER 4

Île de Ré Salt Harvesting

Just off the Southwestern French Atlantic coast on the island of Île de Ré, Thomas Citeaux and his wife Marie-Marie harvest sea salt in earthen pits, a practice followed since the Middle Ages. Thomas recommends one teaspoon (five grams) of sea salt per day to maintain good health. Some salt-o-philes, such as Dave Asprey, of Bulletproof Coffee fame, offer eight grams as a good amount of daily salt intake, however he warns against the pollution coming from the seas that may be present in sea salts. He recommends instead Himalayan salt, a salt formed from dried up ocean water from eons ago, untouched by humankind. Himalayan salt mining is a hazardous practice performed primarily in Pakistan, but the salt does have valuable properties and has an entrancing pink color, showing signs of the minerals it carries. Beautiful salt lamps are made using large pink salt crystals as a soothing source of light. Unrefined, natural mineral salts, whether from ancient seabeds or today's seas are essential to our existence and have all their minerals intact.

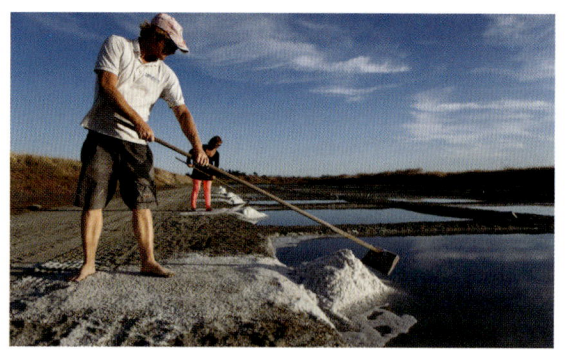

Thomas and Marie-Marie Citeaux work the salt beds in July at sunset, raking up the coarse sea salt after it has become concentrated into each bed from water evaporation. It is left in pyramids to dry overnight.

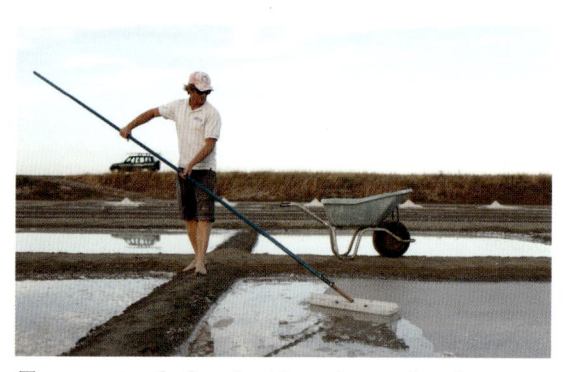

Thomas scrapes the fleur de sel from the water's surface.

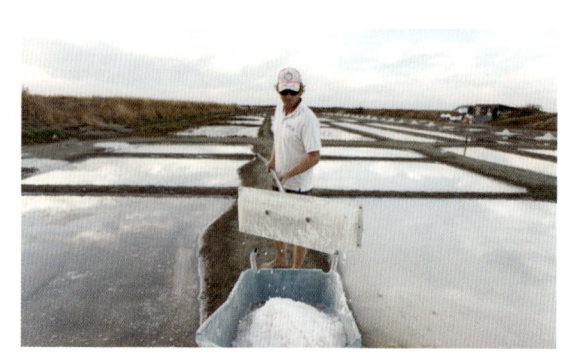

The pinkish-white fleur de sel is dropped into a wheel barrow...

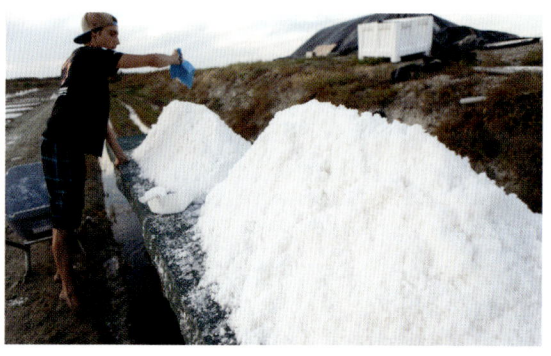

... and placed in a mound of salt to be packaged up.

my water glass. If you are salt-phobic, you may find my recipes saltier than your low-salt diet might have allowed. Just work your way up, feeling confident that the right kind of salt will nourish you and make your food taste delicious, requiring fewer spices, sauces, and tricks to get you to eat it!

Seawater is a rich source of magnesium, which is absorbed through the skin when we swim in the sea, an activity many seaside-living French do year-round. French or "Celtic" sea salt is harvested in two forms: large grain (*gros sel*), which is greyish or reddish in color due to the variety of minerals it contains, and flower salt (*fleur de sel*), the top layer of salt that dries in the sun. Salt harvesters compete to see who can harvest the whitest, purest grains of this finer, more expensive, delicate salt. The large grain sea salt can be ground into finer salt, *sel de mer fin*, for use in cooking but can also be left as larger grains especially for use in soups and stews. *Fleur de sel* is often used as a finishing touch, a chef's secret topping to a savory dish or dessert. The fine, white cubes are pleasing to the eye and delicate on the tongue, and add a subtle crunch. *Gros sel* offers a lovely crunch and a varied terrain on a dish with robust flavor for those who are not salt-phobic!

EGGS

Eggs are nutrient dense and are a rich source of saturated fat, fat-soluble vitamins, and water-soluble nutrients such as choline.[78] A chicken egg supplies everything a growing chick needs to become a chick and can provide us with powerful nutrients and fats as well. In France, the egg (from the chicken) is used in countless recipes. It is hard to avoid. It should be noted, however, that chicken eggs are often implicated in allergic reactions and are therefore not part of autoimmune dietary protocols (such as AIP). Duck eggs are sometimes more tolerable to some, but are harder to find. Duck, goose, and quail eggs are consumed in France, but much less frequently than chicken eggs. When I list an egg in a recipe, I mean a chicken egg. But I also mean organic and pasture-raised, where possible. Organic refers to the chicken feed being organic and non-GMO, and to the fact that no hormones or antibiotics are used on the chickens. Organic, pastured eggs are in a class of their own, compared to the eggs from conventionally-raised chickens.[79] As with grass-fed meats, "pastured" (or "grass-fed") eggs are from chickens who are free to roam around, pick and scratch in grass, dirt and dung for worms, maggots, and seeds. This goes way beyond the "free range" label, which may not be as "free" as our imaginations would like. Free range legally means that the hens are "free to roam," but usually only through a small door attached to their pen to an "open area." This does not mean they actually go out of their enclosure. "Pastured" or "pasture-raised" are the words to look for on an egg carton in the U.S.

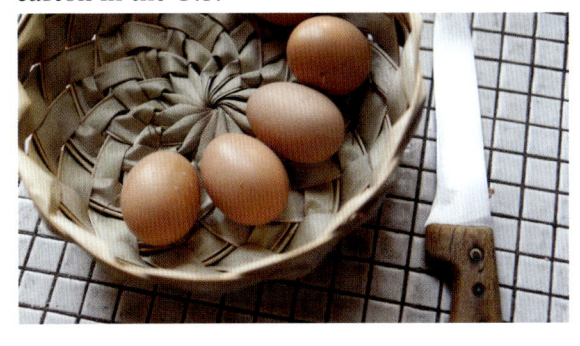

NUTS AND SEEDS

Nuts and seeds are nutrient dense, containing vitamins, minerals, and diverse fatty acid compositions, and they make great snacks. They can be used as flavorful garnishes in salads, as nut butters, or occasionally ground into flour. However, every living organism has a defense mechanism, whether we perceive it outwardly or not. The main objective genetically for organisms, including plants, is to pass on their seeds, their genetic material, to the next generation. To achieve this, legumes, nuts, and seeds have their own "poisons" and tools called phytates and lectins. Phytates bind with minerals like iron and zinc and therefore reduce their absorption in the blood. For these reasons, people with autoimmune or digestive problems might want to avoid nuts and seeds altogether. In their natural, whole, fresh state, however, sunflower seeds, for example, are surrounded by their own protective antioxidants, which protect the antioxidants in our bodies as well.[80] To disarm the anti-nutrients, we soak and sprout nuts and seeds and use them as garnish on salads, or we grind them into flour or nut butters.

SOAKING, SPROUTING, AND DEHYDRATING NUTS AND SEEDS

Most nuts and seeds can be soaked in water overnight, so as to encourage them to sprout, releasing enzymes and phytates that might otherwise interfere with our proper digestion and absorption. The soaking water should be discarded.

HOMEMADE ALMOND MILK

Homemade nut milks can be made while soaked nuts are still wet, skin on, with two parts fresh added water to one part nuts. Almond milk is made this way in a blender on a high setting for 30 seconds. Once the almonds are liquefied, the "milk" can be separated from the almond meal by wringing the solids in a cheesecloth. (See photo A.) The remaining solids can be spread on a baking pan and dried under a low temperature, between 130°F to 150°F (55°C to 65°C) for a couple of hours. This becomes your almond meal for a recipe, and the milk can be used immediately in a shake, sauce, or dessert (see **Aunt Lucie's Millas** on page 484), drunk straight up, or else frozen for future use. (See photo B.) After nuts have been soaked overnight, pour them in a colander, dry them off with a towel, and spread them out on a baking pan to be dried, also between 130°F to 150°F (55°C to 65°C) for 24 hours.

If you need "blanched almonds" (peel removed), this is the time to remove the skins, before you dehydrate them and while they are still wet. Once dehydrated, they can be used in cooking, baking as ground almond flour, or ground into blonde almond butter. (See the following section on making nut butters.) They can be roasted for 10 to 15 minutes at 325°F (160°C), but observe them carefully so that they do not over roast. How many batches of nuts have I burned, or over roasted because I walked away! Sadly, over-roasted nuts never get eaten.

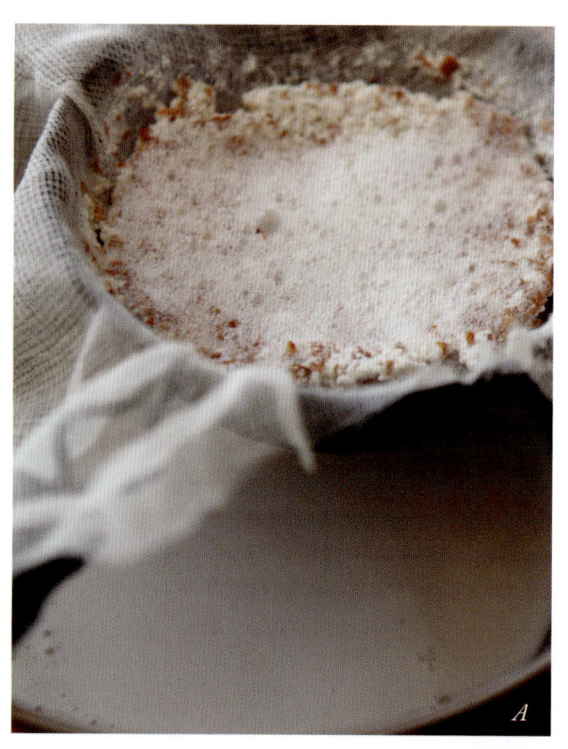

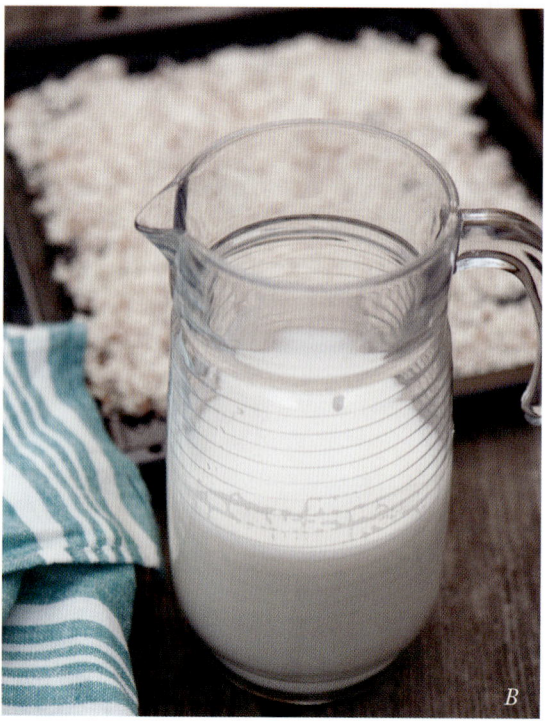

Homemade Almond Milk

48

THE BORDEAUX KITCHEN

NUT BUTTERS

Dried nuts and seeds, whether roasted or not, can be made into nut butters. I have made almond and Brazil nut butters with great success. I add coconut oil and sea salt to add flavor. I have even tried a hazelnut chocolate spread, which you achieve by adding cocoa powder. It's not for everyone, but there is lots of room for mixing according to your family's tastes. I have even roasted peanuts and made peanut butter, which my kids love. Peanuts, however, are a legume and even more so than other nuts, are particularly prone to mold. As legumes, they have a lower nutrient density value along with the usual phytates and lectins, however, peanut butter is really tasty and goes so well with chocolate!

NUT AND NON-GRAIN FLOURS

The most common nut flours found in French dishes include almond, chestnut, hazelnut, and walnut. Chestnut trees are very common in the French southwest and have been in use for food there since about the 11th century.[81] Chestnuts, ground into flour, have protected certain populations in southwestern France from famine through the centuries, as chestnut flour was often used to make bread. For recipes that require flours other than almond or hazelnut, which I grind myself, I generally purchase pre-ground chestnut or walnut, as they are consistent and finely ground. The warning here would be that being finely ground, these are still "refined" flours, with cellular walls broken down to a certain degree in the refining process. They are easy to gobble down, and can potentially be absorbed very quickly into the blood stream, spiking blood sugar and disrupting the gut microbiome, much like refined grain flours. Therefore, sparse use of any of these flours is recommended, as is the consumption of sugars, desserts, and baked goods in general for the same reasons.

Other non-grain flours derived from root vegetables that are used in ancestral cooking are arrowroot, cassava (or yucca) root flour, plantain flour (or smashed fresh green plantains), tapioca starch (derived from cassava), and tigernut (a tuber) flour, each of which can be substituted in certain recipes depending on your tastes, needs, and the availability of the ingredients in your pantry. Certain flours and grains can be sprouted, something recommended by the Weston A. Price Foundation (WAPF) on their website and in their publications. Guar gum, konjac root flour, and xantham gum are non-starchy thickeners popular among the ketogenic diet community, however, when it comes to the "gums," some people are sensitive to these. In the Desserts chapter, I have used mainly chestnut flour, almond meal (almond meal is ground almonds with the skin on, almond flour is from skinless

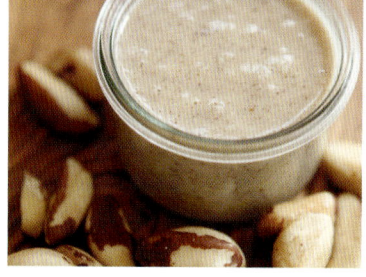

Noisy Brazil Nut Butter

Every time I announce that I am going to make a nut butter, my family members scatter. Turning hard nuts to a butter pretty much requires a food processor, and it is deafeningly noisy, especially when using Brazil nuts because of their large size. Nevertheless, Brazil nuts are famous for their selenium. Two Brazil nuts a day is said to be sufficient to replenish that mineral. I love the creamy flavor of Brazil nut butter and sometimes make a batch to dip into with a spoon now and then after a meal. Run two cups of Brazil nuts in the processor. After one minute, add two pinches of fine sea salt. While the machine is running, add one tablespoon of coconut oil and allow to blend for 15 more seconds, then turn off the processor. This process takes a total of about two minutes. Scrape the nut butter out of the processor into a sealable jar. Store in the refrigerator for up to ten days. (At room temperature it is runny, but it solidifies in the refrigerator.) It is so yummy it may not last ten days. Paired with dark chocolate, it's almost too good to be true. If you haven't been eating sugar for a while, you will notice that the Brazil nut butter tastes quite sweet. Balanced with the salt, it's delicious just by the spoon, but also yummy with carrots or celery for a snack. For almond butter (also unavoidably noisy in the food processor), use one cup of almonds (roasted or just sprouted and dehydrated), two tablespoons coconut oil, and two pinches of salt, which makes about 6 ounces.

Grilled Pine Nuts – Pignons de Pin Torrifiés

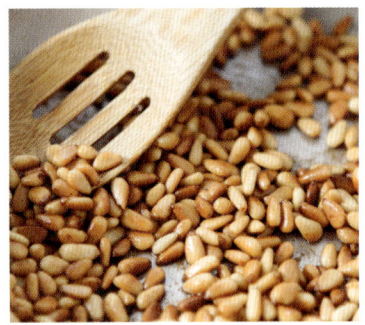

Something often used in French cooking to garnish dishes or in salads are pine nuts. They are usually grilled to add to their flavor. An easy way to grill them is to place the pine nuts along with some olive oil in a pan and a pinch of salt and allow them to cook on medium heat. (Try two tablespoons of olive oil for one cup of pine nuts.) Stirring (*rémuant*) frequently, the pine nuts will begin to brown. Remove them from the pan when they have reached their desired color or degree of grilling. (Grilling time takes about eight to ten minutes.)

or "blanched" almonds), coconut flour, or walnut flour, and in the Stocks and Sauces chapter, I have used primarily cassava flour in lieu of wheat flour.

SOAKING LEGUMES

In order to reduce the phytates present in legumes, such as lentils, they may be soaked for 24 hours and then allowed to sprout over the course of one to three days. It is not clear that this will make them any easier to digest for some people. I love hummus, but even if I soak, sprout, and pray to the legume gods, my digestive tract still cannot yet handle the rough and tumble of the legume (chick pea or lentil) to the system. My children like it, occasionally, with raw veggies. Remember that peanuts, and therefore peanut butter, fall into the legume category.

MUSHROOMS IN FRANCE

Mushrooms come in various forms and are used in countless French recipes, and they are indeed the stars in many dishes, especially when it comes to the prized French truffle, *la truffe*, black or white. I have included mushrooms or truffles in my selection of recipes only in **Beef Burgundy** (page 109), **Braised Veal Stew** (page 422), and **Chicken in Wine Sauce "Coq au Vin"** (page 345), an homage to Julia Child's *Coq au Vin*, because mushrooms (mold and fungus) can be an allergen to some people. However, they may be added to many a dish, as desired, such as stews, salads, and sautés. Indeed, the French adore cooking with mushrooms and truffles, and do so frequently.

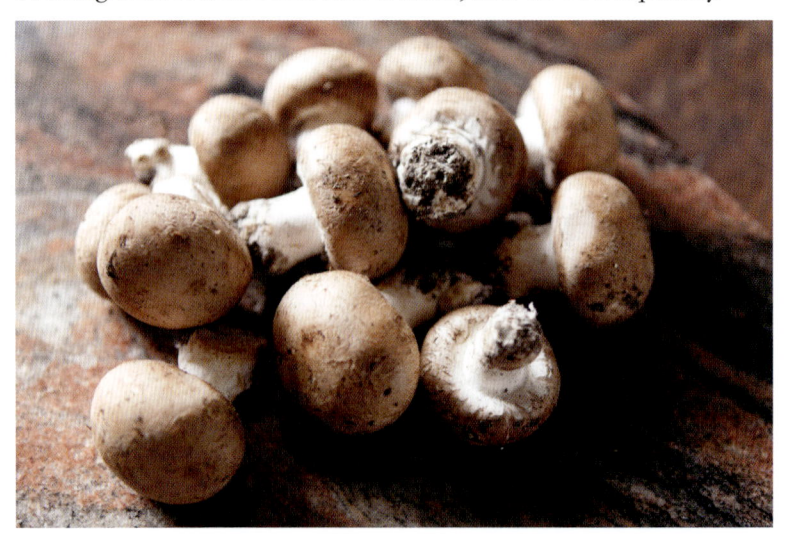

Mushrooms contain vitamins. The porcini mushroom (*cèpe*), the "king" of mushrooms which grows around Bordeaux, contains vitamins B, D, E, and K as well as the minerals iron, potassium, and phosphorus. Cèpes are in season from August to October and show up in many dishes in restaurants and homes around Bordeaux during that time. The only thing they don't show up in is ice cream, though some chef may come up with a recipe. The *Bordelais* will sauté porcini mushrooms in butter, garlic, and olive oil, or they might include them in a mushroom omelet, sautéed first in butter and garlic. Other commonly used mushrooms which you might add to an omelet (*une omelette*) or other dish in France include *chanterelles* or *girolles*, which are bright yellow-orange in color, black chanterelles or black trumpets (*trompettes de la mort*), sweet tooth or hedgehog mushrooms (*pieds-de-mouton*), which are light orange in color, or the elusive and highly-regarded truffle.

THE NOBLE TRUFFLE

Truffles are another one of those foods in France that, when in season, entire festivals celebrate. The celebrated black truffles of the Périgord region of France (*truffes noir* or *truffes Périgord*) are found in limestone soils growing around the roots of oak, hazelnut, and linden trees. There are also *truffes de Lorraine* and *truffes de Bourgogne*, named after their regions of origin. White truffles are primarily from the Piedmont region of northern Italy and they are very expensive. Harvested, carefully measured, and thinly sliced, tiny bits of the noble truffle may appear in almost any dish you can imagine and are even stuffed into cheeses. Sows are used to search out the truffles in the wild because they are so good at rooting them out. But the sows must be muzzled, lest they eat the prize!

NIGHTSHADE VEGETABLES

"Nightshades" are flowering plants in the *Solanaceae* family and include peppers, eggplants, white potatoes, and tomatoes. Nightshades produce substances called alkaloids which can have toxic or beneficial effects on people. Those sensitive or suffering from autoimmune problems should avoid eating these vegetables. While I have included a number of recipes in this book containing these nightshades, the majority of the recipes do not, as I cannot eat them myself and have therefore found ways around this issue.

ROOT VEGETABLES IN FRANCE

Celery Root (Celeriac) – *Céleri Rave*: Celeriac is a yellowish-brown tuber with a bumpy surface to its bulbous shape and is endowed with B vitamins and phosphorous. It can make for a good risotto substitute or boiled and mashed into something akin to mashed potatoes with less of the starch.

Ginger – *Gingimbre*: Ginger is a root vegetable known and used for its many healing and medicinal qualities but is also a beloved spice in French dishes originating from Asia and North Africa.

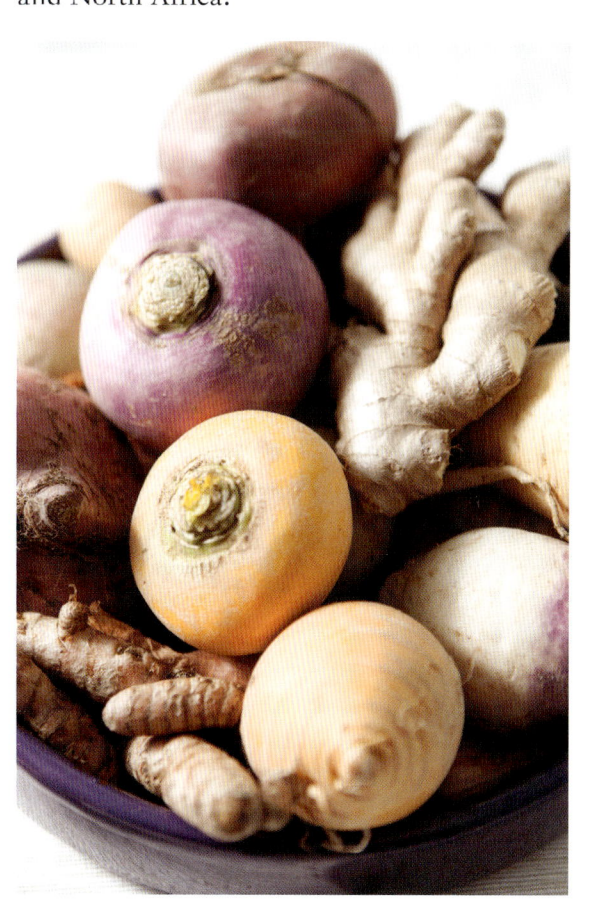

Jerusalem Artichoke – *Topinambour*: The Jerusalem artichoke is not native to Europe, but rather to North America, and is used by some French chefs as an alternative to mashed potatoes. It is rich in inulin, which is a prebiotic, feeding the gut microbiota in the colon, but can cause intestinal gas and should be consumed carefully for those with sensitive digestive tracts.

How to Make Sauerkraut

To make sauerkraut (either using red or white cabbage or a combination of both), I chop the cabbage into quarters, cut out the core, and then slice the quarters into fine strips (photo A). I then add one tablespoon of fine salt for about two pounds (900 grams) of cabbage (photo B), and rub the cabbage pieces together and break them apart with my hands for about 10 minutes to extract the juices. My hands need a rest after that! At this point, some caraway seeds (*graines de carvi*) may be mixed in if desired. I place the cabbage with all its juice into a clean glass jar, add a weight (I use a small jar of marbles), pressing down on the cabbage until it is submerged in its own liquid (photo C). I leave it on the counter covered with a cloth towel for five to seven days (the sauerkraut will probably have a rim of foamy bubbles, telling you the microbes are hard at work), then remove the weight, cover the jar, and refrigerate. It lasts for pretty much as long as it takes you to eat it. Homemade probiotics! Carrots and other vegetables may be pickled the same way in this process.

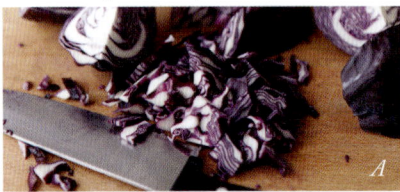

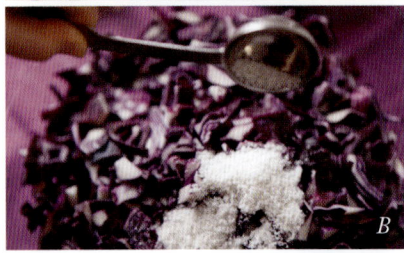

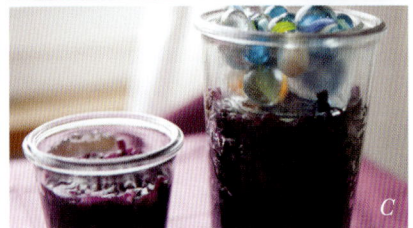

Kohlrabi (Turnip Cabbage) – *Chou-Rave:* Kohlrabi is a German turnip, turnip cabbage, in the Brassica family, and can be eaten raw or boiled/steamed.

Parsnip – *Panais:* Parsnip is a root vegetable that looks like a whitish carrot and is related to both the carrot and to parsley. It has a sweet, carroty taste with a slight bitterness. French chefs also use parsnips to replace potatoes or to add flavor to a mashed-potato dish.

Rutabaga: The rutabaga, or Swedish turnip, is in the Brassica family. Like the Jerusalem artichoke, rutabagas may also be used in dishes in place of potatoes.

Salsify – *Salsifis:* Salsify is a root vegetable in the dandelion family with a brownish-black exterior and a white interior.

Turmeric – *Curcuma:* Turmeric is an Asian root vegetable with properties that counter inflammation in the body. In tropical regions it can be grown year-round, otherwise it must be planted at the end of spring and harvested at the end of summer. This root, freshly grated or dried, can be used in many recipes. An ingredient in many East Asian recipes, turmeric has powerful anti-inflammatory properties, particularly when combined with black pepper for better absorption, and can be used in many recipes for those on a healing journey with nutrient-dense foods. Grate it fresh, or use the powder in ground beef dishes, such as **Ground Beef Parmentier** (page 137). It will add a golden yellow or orange color (beware, your children will notice this) and possibly a bit of its earthy aroma.

Turnip – *Navet:* Turnip is a white and lavender-colored root vegetable, boiled or baked, whose leaves are also edible. In France it is available for a short time in the spring and figures in the **Springtime Lamb Stew** recipe (page 213).

PICKLED CABBAGE, PICKLED CARROTS

Pickling is one of the earliest forms of preserving food. Using natural bacteria found on the vegetables, the vegetables' own juices, salt, and water, an enzymatic process of lacto-fermentation (lactic acid fermentation) occurs over several days in which the bacteria convert the sugars (carbohydrates) in the vegetable into the energy they need, called lactic acid. According to Sally Fallon of the WAPF, this kind of fermentation increases vitamin C. *Choucroute* in French, but known in the U.S. by its German equivalent "sauerkraut," is made from cabbage (red or white) and most commonly eaten with pork or pork sausage, fowl, and wild game. I mix my homemade white sauerkraut warmed with bacon bits (*lardons*).

PRESERVED LEMONS – *CITRONS CONFITS*

Another influence from North Africa is the use of pickled lemons in French cuisine. These add a flavorful combination of tartness and sweetness at the same time in recipes like salmon tartare (*tartare de saumon*), tagines, desserts, and a variety of other dishes. A similar process to making sauerkraut is used to pickle lemons. Slice the lemons into quarters or eighths, leaving the slices connected at one end, salt each lemon, squish them into a glass jar, adding salt between layers of lemons, and submerge them beneath their own liquid. Additional liquid (lemon juice) may be needed. Keep them covered and airtight for several weeks before use. Some chefs wait a year before breaking into their jars of *citrons confits*!

VINEGAR: THE ANSWER TO ALL OUR PROBLEMS?

Vinaigre (literally "soured wine"), especially apple cider vinegar, is useable in food preparation such as in sauces and bone broth (to extract minerals from the bones), natural hair products, to improve gut health, and in cleaning products that can remove calcium deposits. Chef Célia of the Michelin star St. James Restaurant in Floirac outside Bordeaux uses white vinegar to wipe plates clean that may have water spots on them. This sanitizes and creates a brilliant surface on the plate onto which she and Michelin star chef Nicolas Magie add their creations. The question is, what *can't* you do with vinegar?

Many French recipes call for white or red wine vinegar, balsamic vinegar, Xeres or Banyuls vinegar, or apple cider vinegar. Those sensitive to the yeasts in vinegar may want to stay clear of vinegar or test it before using it, but overall, vinegar adds flavor along with its many health benefits. Add baking soda to a basic white vinegar and you have yourself a powerful cleaning product. Even diluting one-part vinegar to three or four parts water in a spray bottle will give you an easy cleaner for bathrooms and kitchen.

NATURAL SUGARS: DATES, HONEY, RAW CANE SUGAR

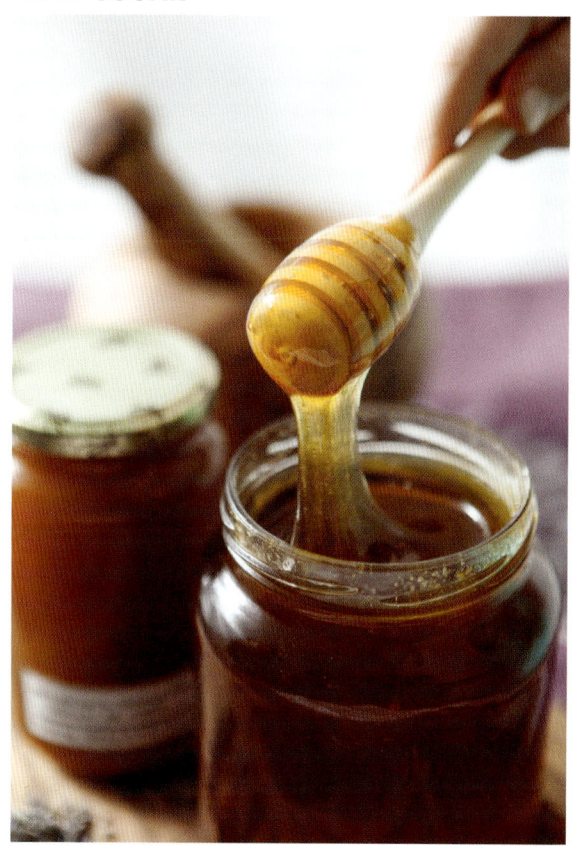

Raw Honey

Brown sugar from organic sugar cane still contains molasses and can be obtained from fair trade vendors (see *A Word on Fair Trade* on page 55). At the very least, this is a much better choice over the ubiquitous, refined white sugar, but it is still sugar, and therefore should be used with much discretion.

Thanks to France's historically close ties with Northern Africa, dates have become part of many dishes, being stuffed, chopped, or puréed into all manner of dishes, but particularly in sweet *tajines*, North African-style stews. Again, dates, especially the large "medjool" variety found in the U.S., are absolute sugar bombs and should be treated accordingly.

Like everything else in France, the best French honeys are from local producers. It is an easy sweetener to find around France, raw or pasteurized. The consumption of raw honey conveys the benefits of the enzymes

CHAPTER 4

and microbial richness found in honey, from which many cures, pastes, compresses, and medicaments are made. For cooking, honey is a lovely natural sweetener, though vulnerable to burning. I found French recipes calling for white or brown sugar could usually be modified to take honey or maple syrup instead. (Between the two, I would choose honey over maple syrup in most cases, because it is not already boiled like maple syrup and can be used in its raw state.) These sweeteners are still fructose, to which many people, including myself, are sensitive to in varying degrees. But the good thing is, one can reduce or eliminate these sweeteners as much as one likes. And if one is not dependent on sweetness for flavor, then the dishes will still satisfy, especially when adequate fat (such as dairy fat or lard) is used in their preparation.

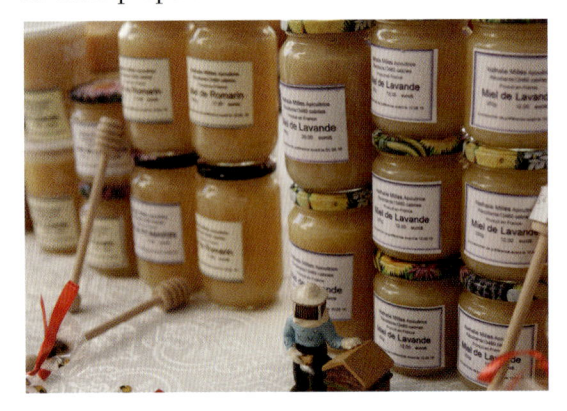

OTHER SWEETENERS

Like refined flours, standard white sugar is akin to, or in many cases more addictive than, cocaine and should be avoided. It also can be the product of GMO sugar beets.[82] One interesting factoid about sugar is that we need the help of 56 magnesium molecules to metabolize one molecule of sucrose. While magnesium is present in the molasses-containing raw cane sugar, white refined sugar is stripped of its magnesium-containing molasses.[83] Consuming refined sugars causes magnesium deficiency, which has numerous negative downstream effects on our health.[84,85,86]

Agave is a processed fructose, marketed as a natural alternative, but which actually has a similar glycemic effect as high fructose corn syrup and in general should also be avoided.

There are some sweeteners that are available to us today that were not available to our great-grandmothers, but this does not mean they cannot be useful to us at times. These sweeteners, such as monk fruit, stevia, and some sugar alcohols (erythritol, for example) can give us sweetness with a lower glycemic load.

Monk fruit sweetener comes from the monk fruit, an Asian fruit with antioxidants and sweetness that does not come from natural sugar, therefore it has little or no effect on blood sugar levels.[87] It comes in a white or golden powder form, appearing much like regular sugar.

Stevia is derived from a plant and is sold in liquid or powder formulations. It has caught on in the sugar industry but is often mixed with other artificial sweeteners and care must be taken in choosing a pure form. Stevia is favored for its lack of effect on blood glucose levels, but it should be avoided if autoimmunity is a factor in one's health journey.

Sugar alcohols such as xylitol, maltitol, and erythritol have varying effects on the gut, but low effect on blood glucose levels. Erythritol is generally derived from the fermentation of corn or sugar cane and is said to have no effect on blood sugar and can be found in powdered form like regular sugar. Researching these before consuming them and assessing their potential effects on your body is recommended. There are increasing numbers of studies suggesting that certain industrial artificial sweeteners, never available to our ancestors, must be avoided.[88] Watch out for them as added ingredients in processed yogurts and other packaged "foods."

FRUIT AND JUICES

Fruit comes up in many dishes, both sweet and savory, in French cooking. I have included a limited selection of recipes containing fruit in the Desserts section, as fruit is still "nature's candy." Fruit is made up of fructose sugars and fibrous cellulose. The fiber in fruit helps slow down the metabolizing of the fructose, whereas juice has this fiber stripped away. The glycemic load of fruit juice is very high, forcing the liver to turn it all to fat, raising blood sugar levels and contributing to insulin resistance.[89] Some people, like me, react to fructose, perhaps because of an overloaded liver (called non-alcoholic fatty liver disease) from years of fructose inundation. The good news is, you can lower your fatty liver score, as I have, by simply cutting down on or cutting out the fructose. As with any sweetener, fruit is probably something to be consumed more sparsely than say, vegetables. Of course, certain fruits contain vitamins and phytonutrients of great benefit to us, and each person should find his or her own threshold of happiness when it comes to fruit. Berries are particularly dense in phytonutrients and are popular ingredients in French dessert recipes, and they make for a great sweetener for desserts, salads, and shakes. For more on the effects of fruit on the body, check out Romy Dollé's book, *Fruit Belly*.

A WORD ON FAIR TRADE
Fortunately, the concept of Fair Trade, in which the producer is given a fair market price for his or her goods, is spreading not only into consumer decision-making but also into a wide variety of goods offered by food producers and marketers around the world beyond coffee, tea, and cocoa, the most common Fair Trade goods. A Fair Trade product, whether packaged, transformed, or still a raw material, gives the buyer some amount of assurance that the farmer who actually grew that food has been fairly compensated, and that the buyer is contributing with his or her choice to a positive cycle of agriculture. Fair Trade organic chocolate, for example, tends to have fewer random additives; look for the ones made with organic cane sugar. Together with the organic food principle of sustainably grown and harvested foods, Fair Trade makes a powerful vote for a healthful, sustainable, equitable lifestyle that will demonstrate high integrity, consciousness, and respect in ways that monoculture, industrial agriculture, does not.

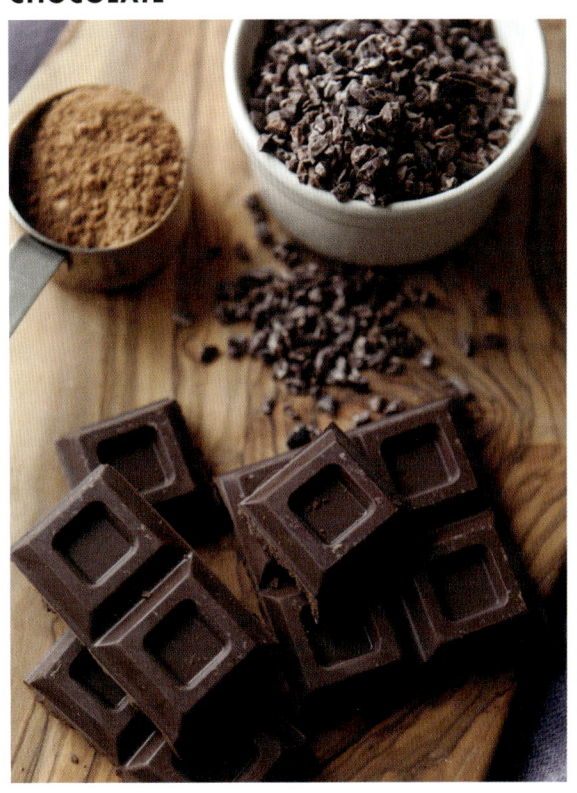

CHOCOLATE

Chocolate was the first of the foreign drinks to arrive in Europe, arriving in France in the mid-1600s and then showing up in a recipe as a thickener in Massialot's *Cuisinier roïal et bourgeois* in 1691.[90] Remember that your 70% or 80% chocolate still has some sweetener in it. This may be good old Fair Trade raw cane sugar or one or more of the sugar alcohols (which can also cause stomach upset in some people). Examine the labels. The cheap chocolates we grew up on in the U.S. are often not made from fair-trade cocoa beans. It's absolutely counter-intuitive to be giving this "chocolate" junk to our children on Halloween or for snacks, when the cocoa pods are often harvested by children in forced labor conditions and the candy contains sugar that often can lead to tooth decay, behavioral problems, diabetes, and obesity.

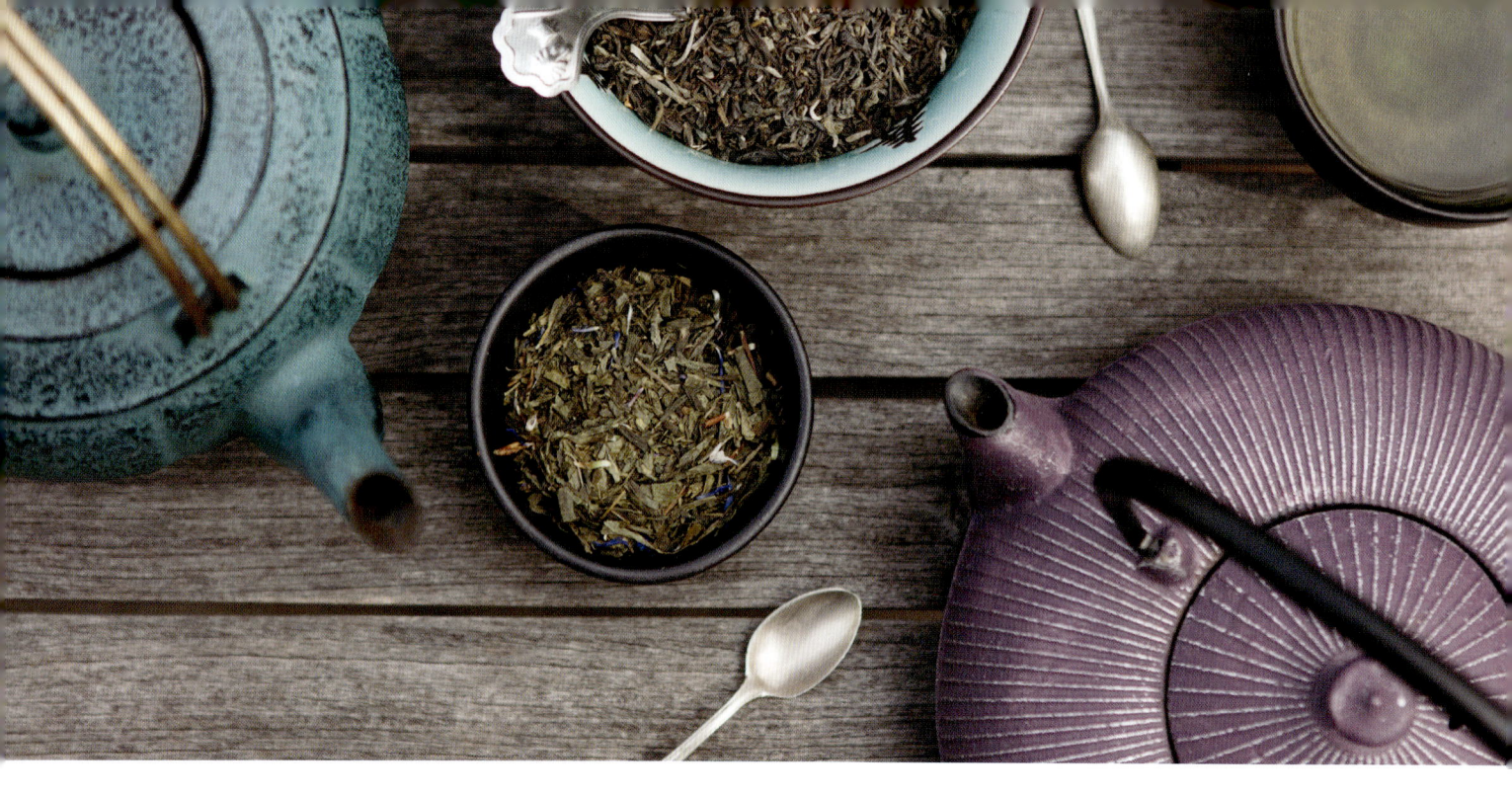

I go for 100% cacao when I can find it. In French organic stores, there is usually a 100% option. In the U.S., organic cacao nibs, unsweetened powder, and 100% bars are readily available online, but again, examine the ingredients and look for the Fair Trade label. No sugar, just cacao, or else a bit of organic raw cane sugar. When I'm looking for a quick dessert, one square with some sea salt and a spoonful of coconut oil is usually all I need.

COFFEE AND TEA

Trade in tea in France began in the mid-1600s, and coffee followed soon thereafter in 1660.[91] It seems as if no French person begins his or her day without coffee. In France, the coffee tends to be small in quantity and potent in flavor and caffeine. *Un café* is actually a small *espresso* (originally Italian) from which other drinks like *caffè latte* and *cappuccino* are made. *Café crème* in France is basically diluted espresso with added milk or cream. Even after living so many years in Europe, I have only recently begun to consume an occasional coffee. I enjoy the fact that coffee aromas elicit romantic visions of cafés in Paris. Tea (*thé*) is commonly served in a small pot with a tea bag. (Beware, some tea bags can be made with gluten.) As a bit of a tea snob, if I am out and about, I like to search out tea houses that serve Fair Trade, organic loose-leaf teas. It can be a challenge to find, but that is part of the fun! At home, I use fresh sage and rosemary from my garden, fresh or dried organic thyme, and organic loose-leaf teas and herbs, ranging from green tea to lavender to passionflower to verbena. I love to mix!

DAIRY OR NON? MORE ON THE TRADITION OF BUTTER IN FRENCH COOKING

Cooking without butter in France sounds like Italian food without the olive oil. But thanks to all the other farm fats, butter can be avoided if necessary. If butter, and any dairy product for that matter, brings about allergic reactions, cross-reactivity with other allergens like gluten, or insulin-inducing responses, these are best avoided. I haven't quite gotten myself to where I can eat butter, but I am hopeful for the future and use ghee instead for myself. I cook my children's eggs in unpasteurized butter and place a slab on their vegetables at dinner. Cheese can also elicit a cascade of reactions (as in my case, skin irritation, redness and dryness, and inflamed sinuses) that can last for weeks. Obviously in such cases, it is better to avoid cheese, yogurt, and all dairy from cow's milk until digestion, skin, and other reactions are no longer a problem. Some find that milk and cheese from goats or sheep cause fewer or no adverse reactions. Be patient, as I keep hearing about people who can once again tolerate dairy products from cow's milk. It can just take a while. There is always hope!

In general, raw, unpasteurized, full-fat dairy is the richest in nutrients and in the enzymes and "good" bacteria that battle the "bad guys" in our systems. Pasteurize the dairy, and you have a sterile white mass that may only serve to spike your insulin, especially if the dairy product has had its fat removed, such as in low-fat or skim milk.[92] If you have ever tasted full-fat, raw cream, it is heaven on earth. It is so rich and creamy, there is no need for sugar. Sadly, for some people like me, cream can cause skin flare ups. Hopefully not for long, though. Dairy can also cross-react with gluten or other potentially inflammatory foods, depending on the person and their state of health, therefore, it's best to see for yourself and your own family about what is the best quantity and kind of dairy, if any, to consume. As for my own children, they love drinking raw milk, spooning organic sour cream onto their meats, and eating raw fresh goat cheese with honey.

CHEESE – LE FROMAGE

France is almost synonymous with the word "cheese," *fromage*. In France there are 45 AOP (appellations of protected origin—*Appellations d'Origine Protégées*) located around the country. If the name of the origin is in the name of the cheese, you can trust that it comes from that place, where the producers have followed specific guidelines for the harvesting and maturation of the cheese. The name of the cheese often indicates from which animal milk (or combined milks) it was made. Generic bries and camemberts exist, and might be less expensive but also perhaps not of the rigorous quality expected of an AOP cheese. The longer or more precise the name, the higher the chance that that cheese comes from some place interesting! Rocamadour cheese comes from the Rocamadour goats, who live on the steep hillsides around the medieval town of Rocamadour, a town itself hewn into the rocky hillside. Roquefort, if authentic, comes from the moist, cool caves in Roquefort in southern France, where the cheese is allowed to grow moldy and age. The taste is powerful, but sadly so are the adverse effects of this cheese on the immune-compromised.

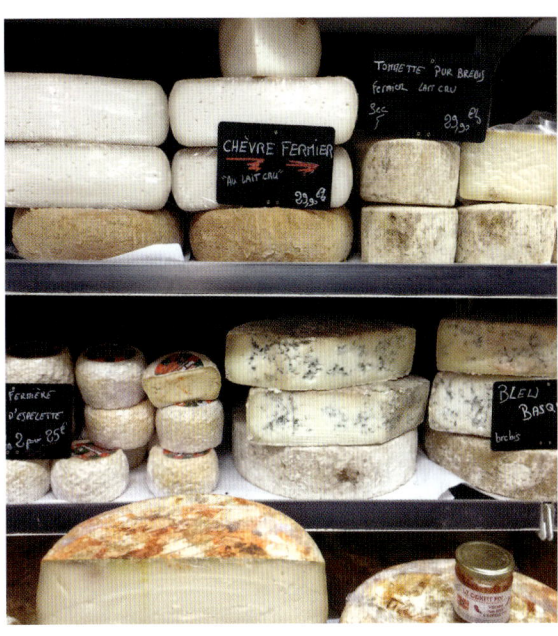

While not the best option for everyone, whole fat, organic, raw (unpasteurized) cheese and dairy products are nutrient dense and flavorful and, of course, consumed in great quantity by the French. Just because Paleolithic man may not have necessarily harvested or consumed dairy doesn't mean we should preclude it from our diet today, unless we have an individual intolerance. Some people are much more sensitive to the casein proteins or even the estrogenic effects of dairy and must use caution. French cheese connoisseurs and producers recognize that a cheese made from unpasteurized or raw milk (*au lait cru*) has more depth of flavor due to its aromatically diverse population of bacteria. With pasteurization, the good and the bad bacteria are annihilated, similar to the effect antibiotics have on the diversity of our gut microflora. For those who cannot handle cow cheeses, they may be able to eat sheep and goat cheeses without issue, and there are so many wonderful kinds to choose from in France, the best being *au lait cru*.

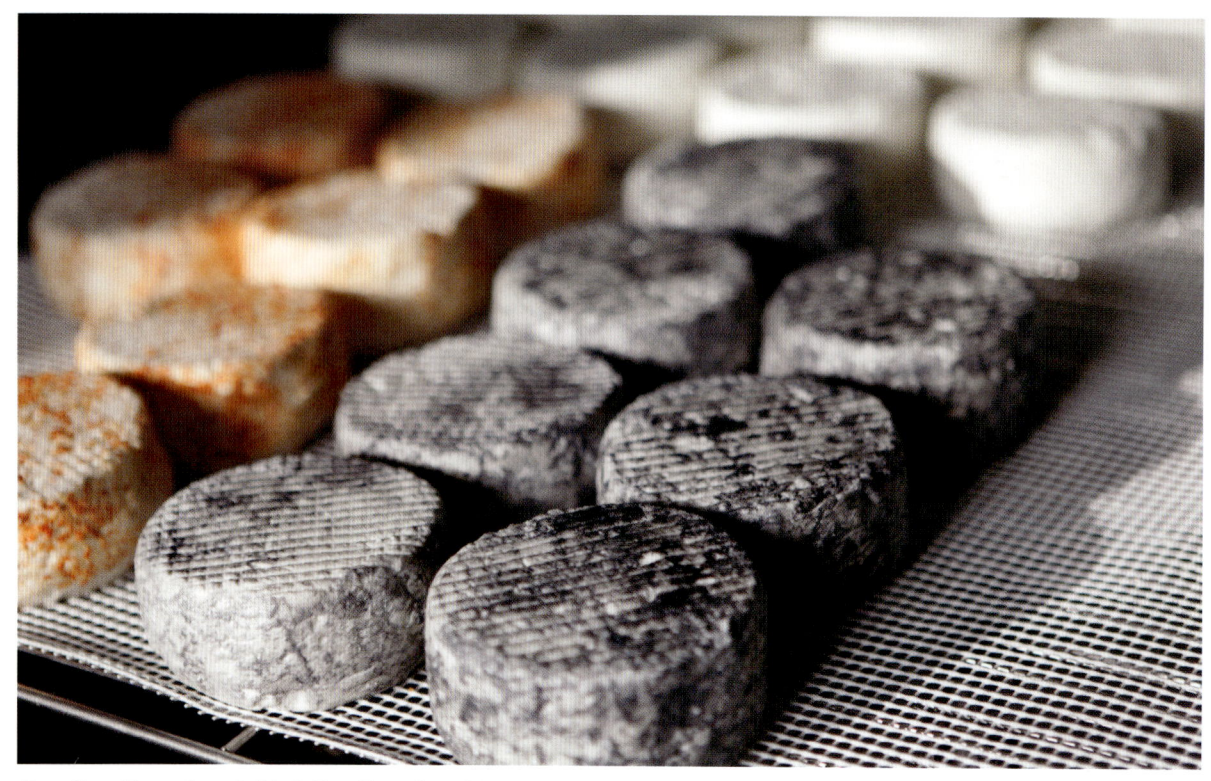

Raw Goat Cheeses from the Teulé Goat Farm Outside Bordeaux

Because they come from circadian rhythmic organisms (the cow, goat, and sheep, who follow seasonal mating, birthing, and lactating cycles), cheeses have seasons, too, when they are either at their best flavor or simply not produced. Some cheeses, however, like *Comté* (or *Gruyère-Comté*), a hard, yellow cow's milk cheese matured (*affiné*) in wheels 21 to 30 inches (53 cm to 76 cm) in diameter, do not necessarily have a particular "best season" and can be enjoyed year-round. The seasons have an effect on the forage eaten by the milk-producing cows, goats, and sheep. The concept of *terroir* (a combination of the effects of local climate, vegetation, geography, and yes indeed, soil microflora on a particular "product") is very much in play with dairy and cheese as it is with other foods and wine.

According to the French artisan master of cheese (*maître artisan de fromage*) Dominique Bouchait who grew up on a cheese making farm in southwestern France, "The many regions of France vary in climate and vegetation, supporting natural treasures and richness of pasture that follow the season."[93]

His observation is that springtime announces abundance and renewal with tender grasses and rich perfumed milks and is the season of highest productivity for traditional cheese makers. The summer abundance of flowers and herbs alike contribute to the milk aromas, while the climate can affect both the quantity and dilution of milk, depending on the amount of heat or rain in a given area. Fall generally brings an end to lactation, the vegetation is drier and less abundant. With a natural drop in milk production, supplemental forage is often required to meet certain demand. Some cheese making comes to a halt for the season, which allows what has been already made to mature, and is restarted in the spring. This is why seasonal cheeses appear in the cheese counter only at certain times of year, such as *Vacherin*, a soft cheese sold between September and May and which is enjoyed sometimes on New Year's Eve. Milk produced in the winter is aromatically rich thanks in part to the carotene-rich, dried forage given to the animals in the stable when fresh grasses are gone.

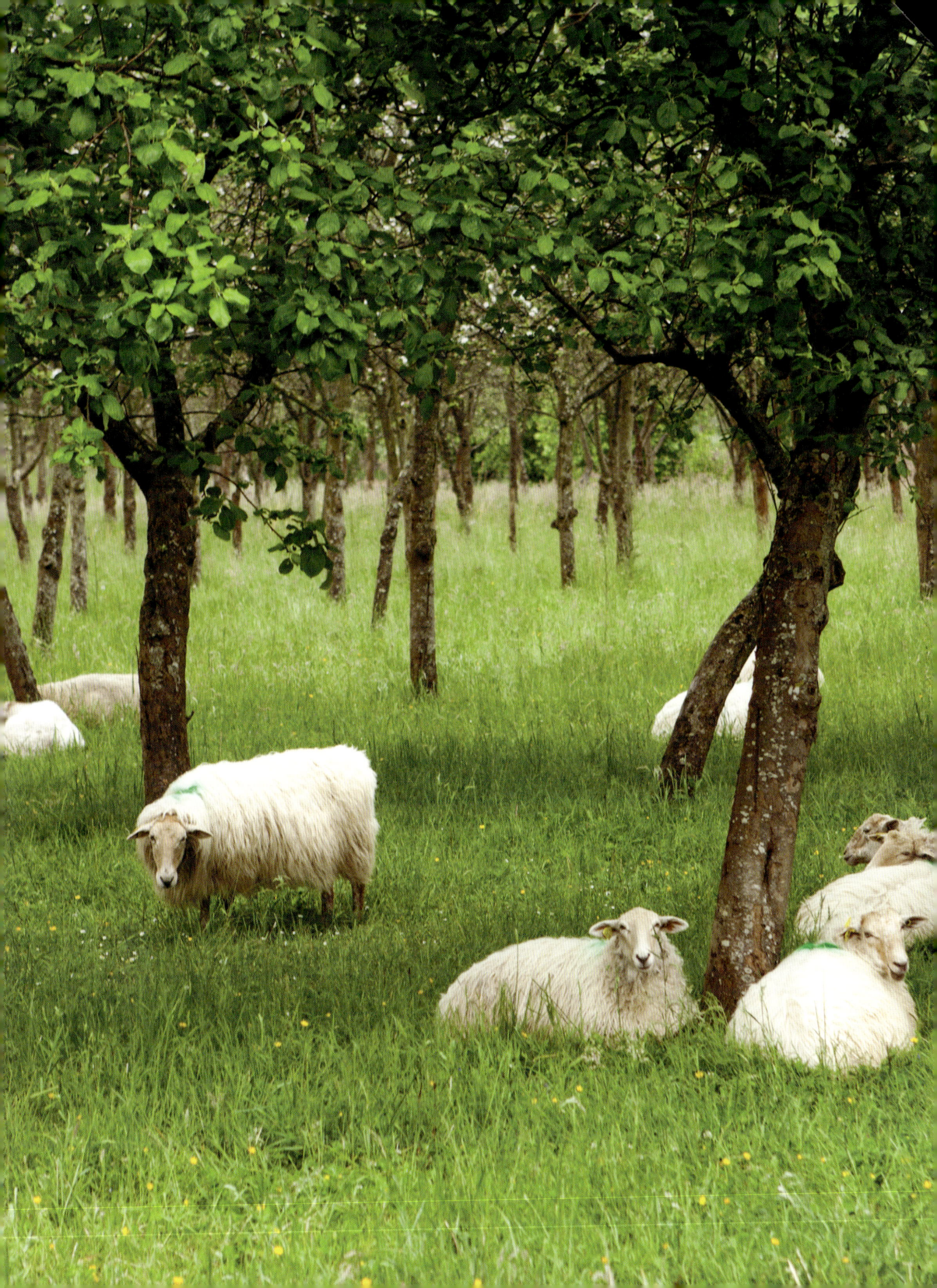

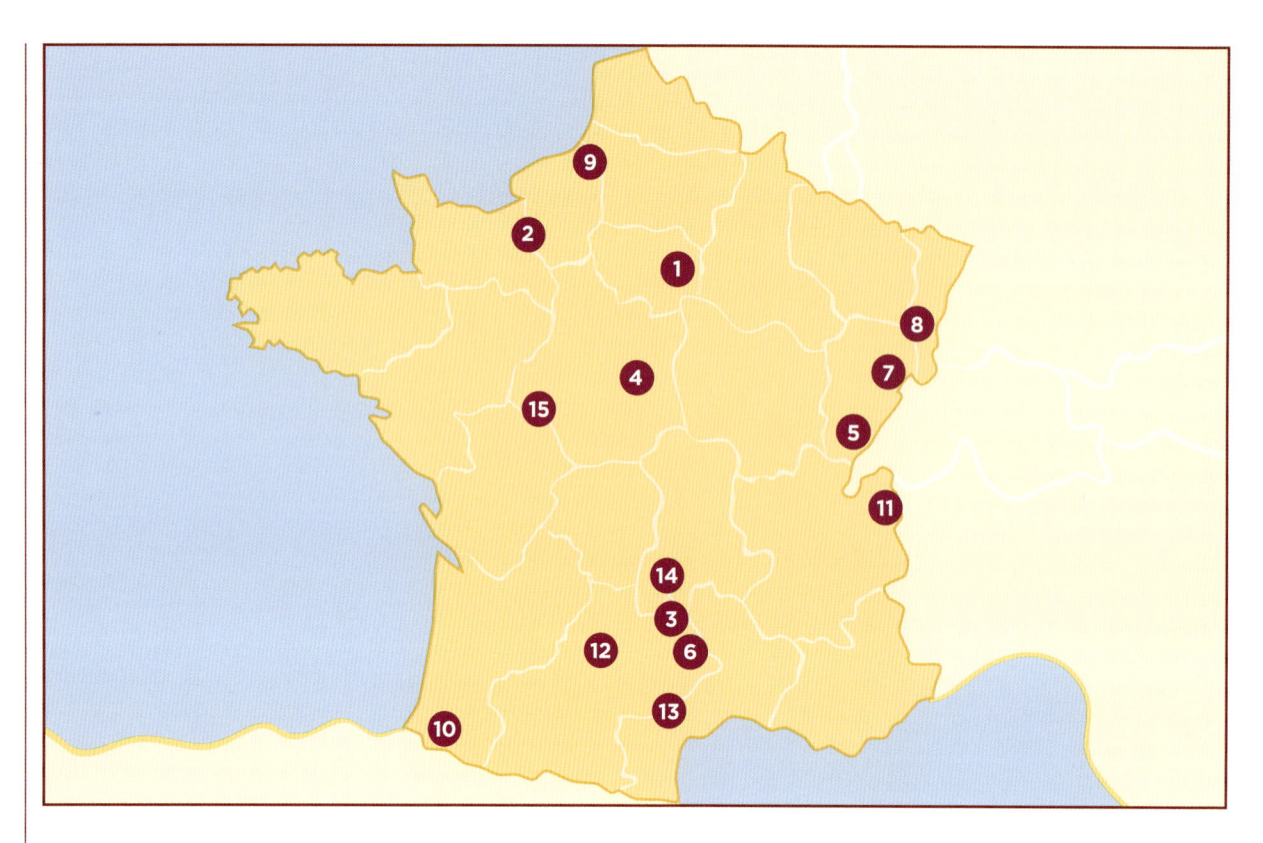

Every Cheese Has a Season

In his 2016 book *Fromages*, Dominique Bouchait, artisan master of cheese and best cheese craftsman of France (*Meilleur Ouvrier de France*) in 2011, states that cheeses have seasons when they are best to eat, a function of the cycles of grass and forage availability, maturation, climate and *terroir*. Here is a selection of the 45 French cheese AOPs (*Appellations d'Origine Protégées*) and their seasons. (Their numbers correspond to the Cheese Map of France above.)

1) Le Brie de Meaux – Summer, Autumn, Winter. Cow (*vache*), from North Central France. Creamy bouquet with aromas of mushroom. Pair with a fruity and structured red wine such as a Burgundy from Côte de Beaune or a dry white from the Loire Valley.[94]

2) Le Camembert de Normandie – Summer, Autumn, Winter. Cow, from Normandy, Northwestern France. Soft texture with flavors of fresh cream and slight mushroom aroma. Pair with cider or a dry white from the Loire Valley.

3) Le Cantal – Year-round. Cow, from the Massif Central, South Central France. A hard cheese that is aged (*affiné*), with buttery and vegetal aromas. Good for grating. An "everyday" kind of cheese for its approachability and inexpensive cost. Pair according to age. The older the Cantal, the bolder the wine.

4) Le Chavignol or **Crottin de Chavignol** – Spring, Summer, Autumn. Goat (*chèvre*), from Central France, Loire Valley. Can be eaten fresh (softer goat aromas) to aged (stronger goat aromas and flavors). Pair a young Chavignol with a Loire Valley dry white, such as a Sancerre and an aged Chavignol with a dry, not tannic Loire Valley red, such as a Sancerre Rouge.

5) Le Comté – Year-round. Cow, from the Jura in East Central France. Hard cheese aged in a 99-pound (45 kg) wheel. Fruity, floral, nutty, and buttery aromas. Pair regionally with a wine from the Jura.

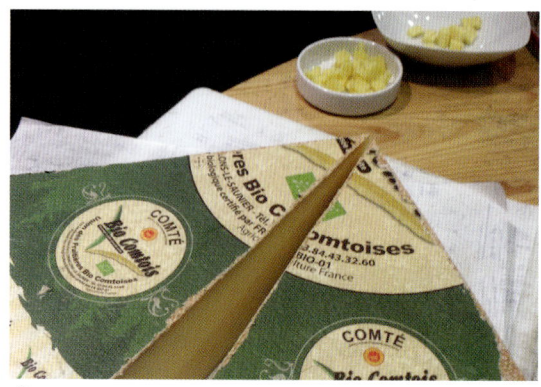

Comté

6) Le Laguiole – Year-round. Cow, from the easternmost edges of the French Southwest, known since the Middle Ages for its close link to its terroir. Hard cheese, aged in a round, hard-crusted wheel with a stamp or brand on it. Aromas of dried hazelnuts. Eaten young or aged. Bouchait recommends this "goldilocks" cheese (not too salty, not too acidic, not too bitter) be paired regionally with red wines from the Southwest. He suggests a "light" approachable Bergerac, Gaillac, or Limoux for a young Lagiole cheese, and a more structured Marcillac for an aged cheese, or else a red tannic Cahors. A "marvelous," non-regional pairing would be with an Alsatian Gewürztraminer.[95]

7) Le Mont d'Or (or Vacherin du Haut-Doubs) – Late summer, Autumn, Winter, Early Spring. Cow, from the Jura in East Central France. Spreadable and sold in a balsa wood container. Creamy, unctuous texture and buttery aromas. Pair with a wine from the Jura region.

8) Le Munster (or Munster-Géromé) – Summer, Autumn, Winter. Cow, from the North-Eastern Vosges mountain range. Medium-hard cheese, sold young or aged. Pair with an Alsatian wine.

9) Le Neufchâtel – Mid-Spring, Summer, Autumn. Cow, from Normandy in the North of France. Represented most often in heart-shaped form (created during the Hundred Years' War as a gift from French girls to English soldiers), its texture is similar to brie and camembert. Mild, milky flavor. Pair with light or medium-bodied wines from the Loire Valley, according to the cheese's age.

10) L'Ossau-Iraty – Spring, Summer, Autumn. Sheep (*brebis*), from the Basque country in the deep French Southwest. Aromas of lanolin, served with dark cherry marmalade. Pair according to age with regional wines, a sweet Jurançon or white Irouléguy for younger Ossau-Iraty and an Irouléguy red for aged Ossau-Iraty.

11) Le Reblochon de Savoie – Summer, Autumn, Early Winter. Cow, from the mountainous Savoie region of Eastern France. Medium-hard cheese with strong grassy and nutty aromas. Good for melting. Pair with Savoie white wines.

12) Le Rocamadour – Spring, Summer, Autumn. Goat, from the French Southwest region around the town of Rocamadour, a town hewn into the rocky hillside. Small but flavorful and creamy, with slightly buttery and nutty aromas. Pair with a sweet or dry white or light-bodied red from the Southwest or Côtes du Rhône.

13) Le Roquefort – Year-round. Goat, from the French Southwest in the Langedoc-Roussillon region. Strong "blue" cheese, that melts in your mouth, with fresh, strong mushroom and buttery aromas. Pair with a red from Langedoc-Rousillon, Côtes du Rhône or a sweet wine from Bordeaux or Jurançon.

14) Le Saint-Nectaire – Mid-Spring, Summer, Autumn, Mid-Winter. Cow, from the Massif Central, Central France. Hard cheese with earthy aromas. Pair with either medium or full-bodied and fruity regional red or white wines from Burgundy, Côtes du Rhone or the Southwest.

15) Le Sainte-Maure-de-Touraine – Spring, Summer, Autumn. Unpasteurized goat, from the Loire Valley. Delicate aromas of vegetation, hay, hazelnut, and cream. Fresh or aged, long and cylindrical, and traditionally rolled in ash. Pair with a dry white or a light-bodied red wine from the Loire Valley.

In France, cheese is served as part of an apéritif or after dinner, either before dessert or as dessert. Sometimes it is even served with more wine or another wine, depending on how lavish the dinner. When it comes to pairing wine with cheese, like with French food, when in doubt, pairing regional cheeses with regional wines is your best bet. Somehow, a white Jura wine goes best with Comté cheese from that eastern, mountainous region of France, accentuating the fruity aromas and flavors of the cheese.

Cheese in France is named after its origin, where it was made and what animal it came from. A selection of cheeses will arrive on a platter, usually containing a goat or sheep cheese in addition to the cow milk cheeses, along with a variety of hard or soft, fresh, or aged cheeses. Cut off and serve pieces of cheese in a way that leaves behind the original shape of the cheese.

GOAT CHEESE FARM IN BOULIAC

In the spring of 2016, we discovered a wonderful goat dairy farm outside of Bordeaux upon the recommendation of Chef Célia at Le Saint James, a Michelin one-star restaurant, which serves the cheeses from Mr. and Mrs. Teulé's goat farm. (Photo A shows the Teulés with their newest member of the farm, baby Max.) What started out as a quick run to see the goats being milked and to buy some cheese turned into repeated interesting, fun-filled visits. On our first visit, we were lucky enough to arrive when a group of cute baby goats was being bottle fed separately, as they were the runts and had not grown as quickly as the rest. We had a wonderful tour of the modest facility by the hardworking family members of mother, father, son, and daughter-in-law. Their raw goat cheese starts out as *faiselle*, looking like watery cottage cheese, which is drained in cups with holes over a couple of days and then left *au nature* or rolled in herbs, ash, or spices. (Photo B) *Faisselle* is a style of goat or sheep cheese that is cured with rennet, an enzyme in the stomachs of ruminant mammals such as the goat or sheep, and is left to age. (Photo C) Faisselle can be eaten fresh on its own, "sweet" (*sucré*) with honey or jam or other sweeteners, or salty (*salé*) with salt and pepper, shallots, garlic, or chives, much like cream cheese in the U.S.

CHEESE AND VITAMIN K2

The bacteria that makes brie cheese has a high amount of K2, as do goose liver pâté and fermented foods, particularly natto, that helps protect people from heart disease, according to Canadian Dr. Kate Rhéaume-Bleue. On Dr. Mercola's YouTube channel on January 13, 2013, Dr. Rhéaume-Bleue comments on the French Paradox: "We used to consider [it] the French Paradox, the supposed contradiction between their high intake of saturated fat and creamy rich food and low risk of heart disease. Well, it turns out that goose liver pâté, brie cheese, butter, and egg yolks are some of the highest foods in vitamin K2 when they are produced properly. So there really was no French Paradox, the French were simply happily stuffing themselves with this nutrient that would clear out their arteries." Researchers Stephan Guyenet[96] and Chris Masterjohn[97] and clinician Beverly Meyer[98] (who discusses K2's presence in Australian Walkabout Emu oil) all have helpful websites with abundant information on vitamin K2 as well.

> One cheese I found had such an impressive sounding title: "Camembert de Normandie AOC (Appellation d'Origine Contrôlée) Fromagerie de la Vie, St. Loup de Fribois (Gold Medal Winner Paris 2013 by the Ministry of Agriculture)." You know you're in France when the name of the cheese takes up three lines of text!

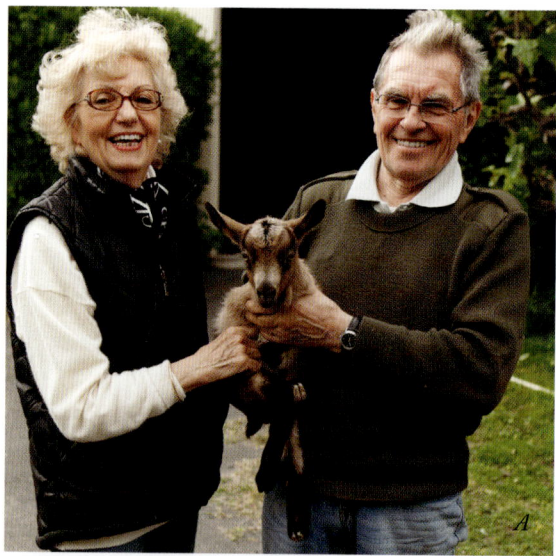

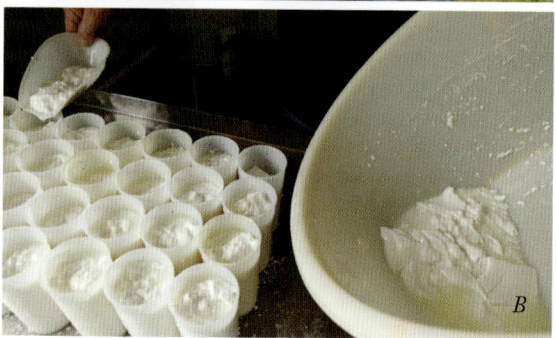

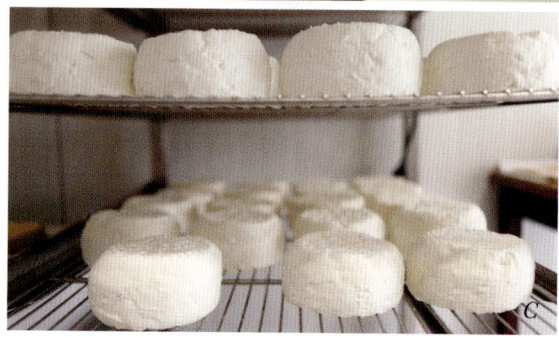

THE BORDEAUX KITCHEN

How My Plum Tree Taught Me to Make Marmalade: An Allegory for Living by the Seasons

Plum trees are native to the French Southwest. The *Pruneaux d'Agen*, prunes from around the city of Agen in Southwestern France, are famous for their bountiful flavor and their luscious texture. All manner of desserts and confection are made with these prunes. As a result of this ubiquitous fruit, plums and prunes play a key role in cooking, baking, and stuffing in traditional French recipes. (See page 308 for a recipe on **Prune-Stuffed Pork Loin with Bacon**.)

Watching how the decades old, thick-trunked plum tree (*le prunier*) in our backyard changed year-round with the seasons exemplified to me what season we were in: the fall leaves changing their color in the autumn, the thinning out of the leaves as we moved into winter, the bare branches in winter, the hopeful, barely visible buds of the late winter, the bright white flowers as an early signal that spring was coming, the almost neon green leaves bursting out from around the tree, the green beginnings of small plums, and the dark purple beauty of the ripe plums as they hung on the tree or fell off once sufficiently ripened. After about two weeks of harvesting many buckets of plums as they fell softly into the grass from the tree, the tree enjoyed many weeks of a majestic green splendor in the garden through the summer, until the cycle began again. The magic of experiencing the changes of a garden is that one sees how certain blossoms, like the plum, bloom early after winter, then giving way to the next flower and the next, keeping bees truly busy, until the fruit comes, keeping the harvester, like me, truly busy.

And when the plums were ripe, there was no waiting. There was no convincing the tree, "Tree, I have an exam to study for, you'll have to hang on to your plums." The plums just dropped from that tree, and I could not bear to let them all go. The worms and birds got some, but I did, too.

Dehydrated Fruit: I dehydrated some in the oven at 122°F (50°C) for 24 hours after laying them out in the sun. (You can easily do this with apple slices, without laying them out in the sun.) But the plums were so small, it was impossible to destone them before drying them, as they would end up as mush.

Homemade Plum Preserves: While the world went about its business, with people racing to and fro, I was at home with my purple hands immersed in plum mush, unable to tear myself away from the work for four solid days. I destoned the rest of my harvest, for several days in a row, making several batches of plum jam, *confiture de prunes*, without sugar. I boiled and re-boiled each batch four times, allowing to cool between batches. I filled sterilized jars, placing them again in the oven at 212°F (100°C) for a few minutes to create a vacuum seal. (I could have also just turned the jars upside down while they were still hot, I later realized.)

I used the preserves in sauces and served it warmed with **Orange Duck Breast** (page 351). I gave some jars away to neighbors and friends, refrigerated others, and froze a few, for safety purposes, just in case my canning techniques were incorrect. As it turned out, most jars that remained at room temperature made it without molding up. Everybody loved the jam, a real *confiture*, fruit preserved in its own juices and sugars. All this joy (and work) from just one tree. I can't imagine the amount of work even a small orchard would produce. Having a year to rest up for the next harvest as well as to enjoy the preserves while looking forward to the next bounty is the beauty of the seasonal cycle. One thing is for sure: the seasons change. Nature won't wait.

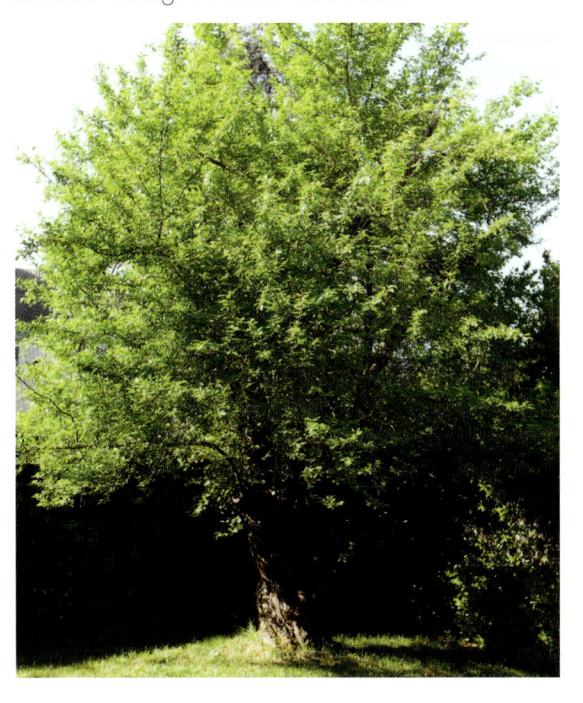

THE SECRET TO FRENCH COOKING #3: THE CAST-IRON POT (AND OTHER KITCHEN ESSENTIALS)

The French ancestral approach to cooking is rooted in the use of fresh, local ingredients as the foundation of all recipes. It is an approach that genuinely supports our health with the most nutrient-dense varieties of food. This approach also informs the choices in quality and type of equipment and utensils one uses to prepare and store one's food. The following are recommendations regarding tools that I use in my French cooking and ancestrally-minded, modern-day kitchen.

HEAVYWEIGHT CHAMPION: THE CAST-IRON POT (A.K.A. DUTCH OVEN)

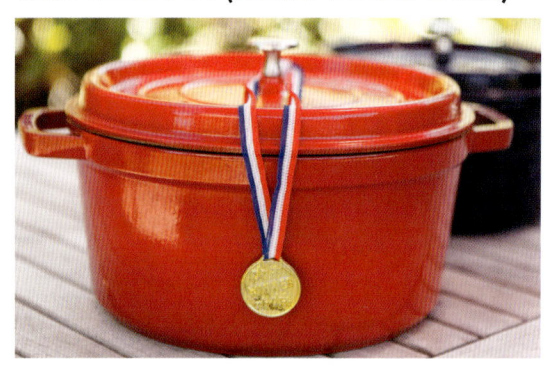

Much of French cooking is founded on the process of slow cooking. In fact, most dishes, and the ones with the most flavor, are those in which the meat has been slow-cooked in the family cast-iron pot (*la cocotte en fonte*) and includes a long-cooked stock or broth (*un fond*) or a healthy dose of animal fat. The bonus of such long-cooking meals, of course, is the collagen extracted from the meat, bones, and cartilage, useful for our own collagen production, in addition to nutrients like gut-healing glycine and other amino acids and minerals. Using a cast-iron pot (two famous French brands are *Staub* from Alsace and *Le Creuset*, for example) in slow cooking is one of the secrets for success in French cuisine. The cast-iron pot cooks evenly, retaining both flavor and heat, and it is heavy and thick, a serious utensil for seriously nutritious cooking! Handle these with great care so as not to drop them on your feet or on other utensils, as even the smaller cast-iron pots are heavy and could do damage. Every good restaurant around the world follows the basic French culinary principle of always brewing an iron stock pot full of broth (though many restaurants use stainless steel vats for greater volume), whether it's a combination of bones and flavors, or a specific type of broth, such as **Veal Stock** (page 415) to use as the foundation for sauces, gravy, or extra flavoring for dishes. This kind of flavoring takes time, hence the importance and beauty of slow cooking the French way.

SAUCY SECRETS

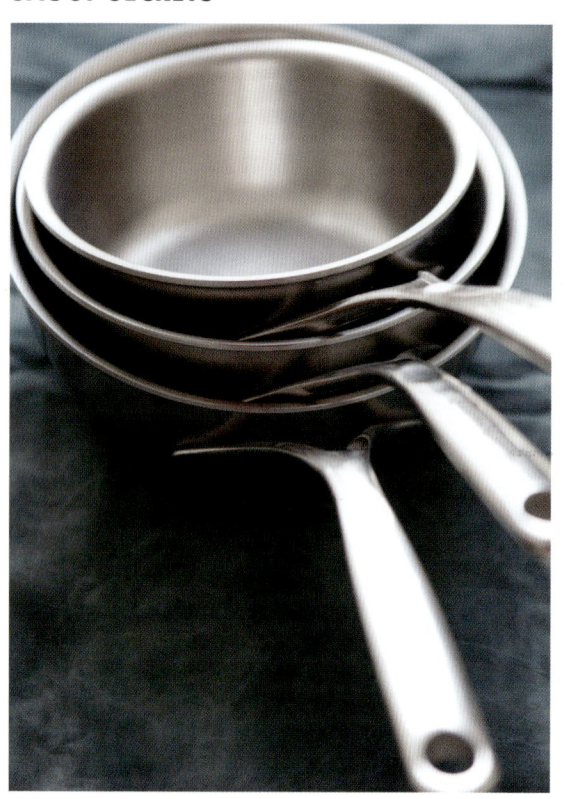

Demeyere Saucepans

Yet another secret to French cooking is the vast array of sauces that seem from the outside to be so complicated. Often these are made with fat-rich ingredients like cream and eggs, but also, as you will see, with stocks and broths for their deep flavors. I have tried to break these sauces down as much as possible in the Stocks and Sauces chapter, but one of the main tools for successful sauces are thick-bottomed saucepans or saucepots. I use

Demeyere's seven-ply stainless steel saucepans which eliminate the need for a double boiler and greatly increase my rate of success in a sauce that will not be burned or boiled too quickly in a thin pan or pot. Perhaps knowing that melting chocolate for **Chocolate Mousse** (page 490) is a breeze with one of these thick saucepans will convince you that it is time to have one of these in your kitchen. I have three sizes: seven-inch (18 cm), eight-inch (20 cm), and nine-inch (23 cm) in diameter, and I often wish I had one or two more!

SORRY, TUPPERWARE, THE PARTY'S OVER!
Before plastic was invented, people used paper, tin cans, iron, glass, and wood. The transfer of toxic chemicals from plastic to food was not an issue because it did not exist. Instead, people used utensils such as wooden spoons, spatulas, and cutting boards, non-plastic mortar and pestle, metal knives, glassware, ceramics, porcelain, and pottery for cooking and storing food, as well as cast-iron pots. I advocate using these same materials to match this kind of traditional cooking.

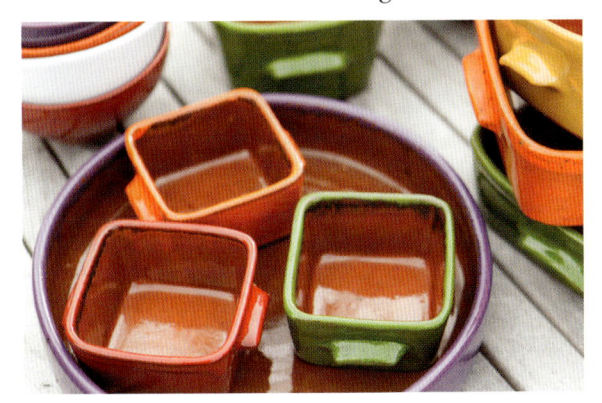

Terafeu Dishes

My favorite oven-safe cooking dishes are those made in the Basque region of Southwestern France by *Terafeu*. They are hand-thrown using red terra cotta clay and come in beautiful, earthy colors. Revol is a French company that makes ceramic cooking dishes (and ramekins for **Crème Brûlée**—page 505). I have a set of French *Duralex* tempered-glass nested mixing bowls that I have used for almost two decades. My daughters play with the smallest bowls, which are tiny, for their mini-stuffed animals. In 1939, the Duralex company invented tempered glass, which is less likely to break and more heat resistant than "normal" glass. I use Pyrex glass dishes for storing, roasting, and baking. They generally come with lids (made of plastic, but I make sure the plastic lid is not in contact with the food) and in many sizes, and they are affordable, reusable, oven-safe, and hard to break, if a bit heavy for travel. I have managed to break a few large nesting Pyrex bowls. (Tip: do not store glass or breakable bowls on top of the refrigerator!) I have used the same *Zyliss* (Swiss-made) salad spinner for 15 years—it is a gem!

DITCH THE PLASTIC
Nowadays we have stainless steel pans, silicone spatulas, food processors, blenders, mini-choppers, and cooking thermometers, which I use as needed. But we also have easy access to the poorer quality and cheaper but ubiquitous choices of Teflon-coated pans, plastic cutting boards, plastic containers and utensils, and microwave ovens. I do not advocate using any of these, except in dire cases. Teflon-coated and non-stick surfaces are toxic to us when heated.[99] Rather than risk exposure to the toxic chemicals, such as BPAs, in these and other plastic materials, would it not be wise to choose from the options our ancestors had at their disposal, prior to the development of petrochemicals and plastics? The extremes of heat and cold cause chemicals to become active, therefore heating or freezing items made of plastic causes their chemicals to leach into our food through direct contact and condensation. While using a food processor to grind up meat at room temperature for a pâté is efficient and relatively benign, the reheating of leftovers in a plastic container or freezing foods in plastic is not recommended. Links have been made between BPA and thyroid autoimmunity.[100] BPAs are also risky for those with brain multiple sclerosis.[101] Plus, as we all know, even "recycled" plastic takes years and years to degrade. Minimize it everywhere in your life.

FOILED AGAIN: BANNING ALUMINUM

I use as little aluminum foil as possible, as aluminum only accumulates in our bodies, is toxic to us, and has been linked to Alzheimer's and other diseases, sensitivities, and conditions.[102] I don't let it touch my food. An exception might be when roasting a head of garlic, which is in its skin anyway, but parchment paper can be used as well. Aluminum in any product is harmful to us, such as anti-perspirants, vaccines (where it's used as a preservative), and baking powder. Find aluminum-free versions of antiperspirants and baking powder. Vaccines, well that's a whole other ball of wax and not within the scope of this book.

CHIP-CHOP-CHIP!

One blade I use to chop rosemary in particular is my *mezzaluna* single-bladed cutter that is rounded and has two ends that fold out. The Italians use these to make pesto, and larger ones to slice pizza. I find my small one gets the herb-cutting job done in minimal time and is a fun motion to make with both hands bobbing up and down like on a see-saw. This is much more efficacious than the small food grinder I use which is better suited for larger quantities of garlic cloves, for example.

Rosemary grows plentifully in the South of France, and its aroma is savory and soothing. For emergency purposes, I have kept chopped rosemary in a glass container in my freezer and a glass jar of chopped garlic in my fridge (preserved with bit of olive oil, as noted previously in this chapter) in case I am in a rush and need these ingredients immediately. As I have gotten faster with my *mezzaluna* knife, I just harvest the rosemary from our bush in the garden, something I recommend everyone to have, even if it's just in a little pot in your kitchen. No need to wash it if it's from your garden or organic, as washing will dilute the aromatic oils on the surface of the herb. Just remove the rosemary needles in one stroke, pulling down against the upward growing leaves and chop it up in 30 seconds, fresh for the recipe!

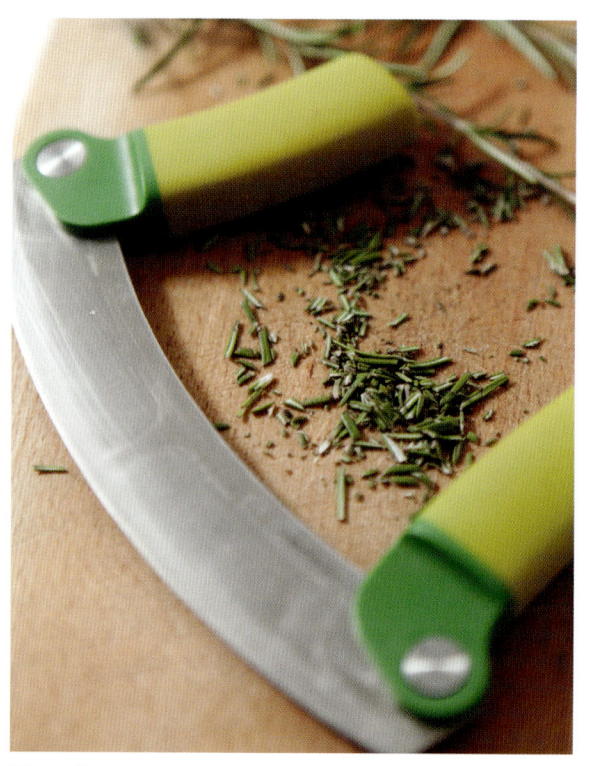

Mezzaluna Knife

THE APRON AND THE KITCHEN TOWEL – *LE TABLIER ET LE TORCHON*

It sounds like the title to one of Jean de La Fontaine's[103] famed fables, but the protective apron and the weathered kitchen towel are both handy tools in the kitchen. The apron (*le tablier*) keeps you from getting your clothes splattered, especially when cooking and butchering. Somehow regular aprons are not particularly "sexy" unless it's a nice maroon apron slung over one shoulder of your handsome butcher with his black *chemise* underneath. The French cotton or linen kitchen towel is essential and only improves with age and use. Some of my *Jacquard Français* towels are fraying at the edges after over 15 years of use, but they are soft and absorbent, much more economical and infinitely less wasteful than paper towels. (I have used French cotton and linen towels as props throughout this book for their lovely and inspiring colors and designs.) Let us also not forget the most essential oven mitts. You will need ones you can trust with the heat and your ability to grip hot items.

STOCKING YOUR PANTRY

Now that you know what to use and what not to use, go through your pantry and find a new home for iodized table salt, industrial seed oils, packaged "foods" that have a list of unwanted ingredients in them, and any industrially refined flours and sugars, as well as canned or boxed drinks. Replace these with fresh, local, in-season organic foods, where possible. Find Celtic or Himalayan salts in various forms (fine, coarse, and *fleur de sel*). Any canned or packaged items should ideally contain only one ingredient, such as "nori" or "tomatoes" or "honey." Some packaged goods invariably require sea salt, oil, or vinegar as a preserving agent, or even a bit of non-GMO cane sugar, such as in marmalades, "sardines in olive oil," or preserved lemons. Use your best judgment and be ready to change as you learn more. Certain olive oils are better in taste and quality than others. Source ones that assure you they are actually 100% olive oil. Spices are often irradiated, so learn to look out for non-irradiated, organic ones. As you get to know new ingredients and how often you use them, you will be able to let go of the old ones, along with old habits, and let go of the poorer quality, more refined products that are often expensive and potentially harmful. Investing in your pantry is investing in your health.

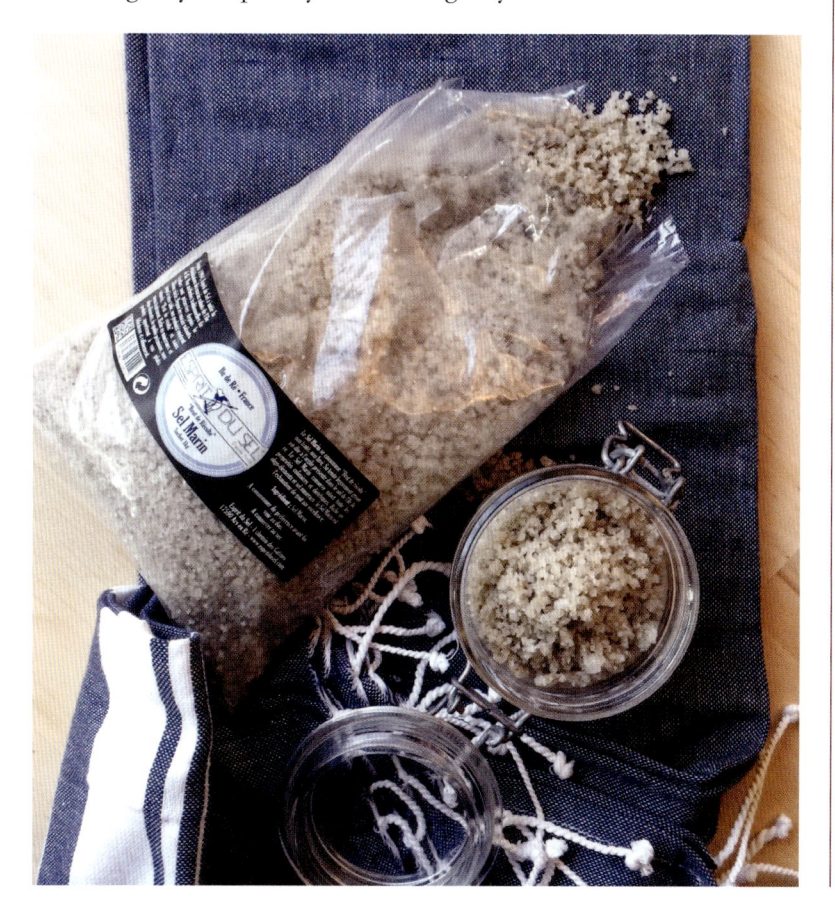

The French Great-Grandmother's Kitchen Routine

Here is what a French great-grandmother (*arrière-grande-mère*, or just "Mamie") would have done after preparing a meal in her cast-iron pot using a wooden spoon to stir. Mamie would have stored the sauce and vegetables in glass or clay jars. She would have wrapped the meat up in cloth or paper, or else have stored the meal in the pot itself, to be reheated at the next mealtime or the next day. With enough natural fat in the pot, such as butter, duck or goose fat, lard or tallow, the meat would remain preserved in a cool spot, if not kept on low on the stove overnight. In fact, many meals, like the **Boiled Beef Stew "Pot-Au-Feu"** (page 123), a long-cooked stew, would remain in the pot on the stove for days, or even the entire week, feeding the family a soothing, nutritious meal without a lot of hassle and with ever-increasing flavor. Any garden herb, vegetable or leftover meat from another meal could easily go into the pot, adding to and modifying the flavor from one meal to the next. This freed up the cook to do other things.

THE BORDEAUX KITCHEN FRENCH ANCESTRAL DIET CHART

ORGANIC FOODS	INCLUDED	ALTERNATIVE(S)
Poultry, Meat, Offal	Yes	
Fish, Seafood	Yes	
Vegetables	Yes	
Roots, Spices	Yes	
Dairy Products	Yes, raw, (unpasteurized) organic, full-fat, and grass fed	
Oils	Yes: olive, coconut oil, avocado oil, macadamia nut oil No: industrial seed oils (canola, corn, soy)	Limited: grapeseed oil
Fruits	Limited	
Nuts and Seeds	Limited	
Lentils, Peas, Beans	Limited	
Other Legumes	No	
Starchy Vegetables	Not to be consumed in excess	
Seaweed	Yes	
Grains, Flours, Rice, Corn, Soy, Glutens, Oats, Buckwheat, Quinoa	No	In limited quantities: chestnut flour, almond flour, coconut flour, arrowroot, rice and rice flour (very limited)
White Sugar	No	In limited quantities: honey, raw sugar cane, coconut sugar, pure stévia, maple syrup
Salt	Yes: sea salt, Himalayan, or underground (mountain) salts No: NaCl/table salt	
Wine	Yes, occasionally and in sensible quantities	
Animal Fats: Lard, Tallow, Duck and Goose Fat	Yes, organic and grass fed	

HEALTH BEGINS IN THE KITCHEN

The kitchen is more than the living place for our kitchen appliances. It is really the heartbeat of the home. In many cultures, the kitchen is where life unfolds, discussions are held, and life's stories are shared. The kitchen is where the family's health is sustained. If you think of your equipment, utensils, and pantry from this perspective, the choice of what to use to prepare and cook meals becomes clear. And the beauty of cooking from scratch is that you can improvise on the spot, depending on the season, your tastes, and what's right there in your pantry.

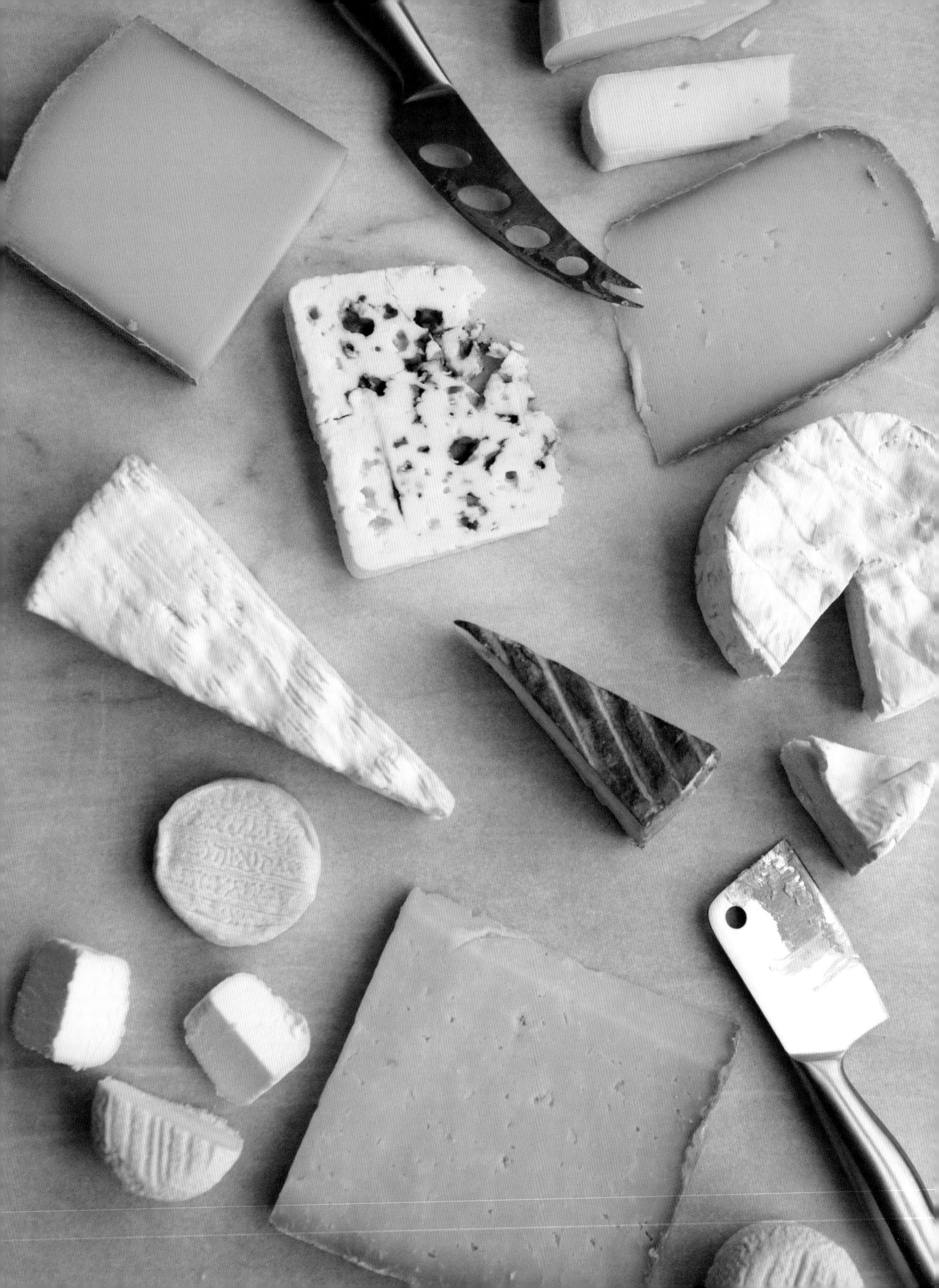

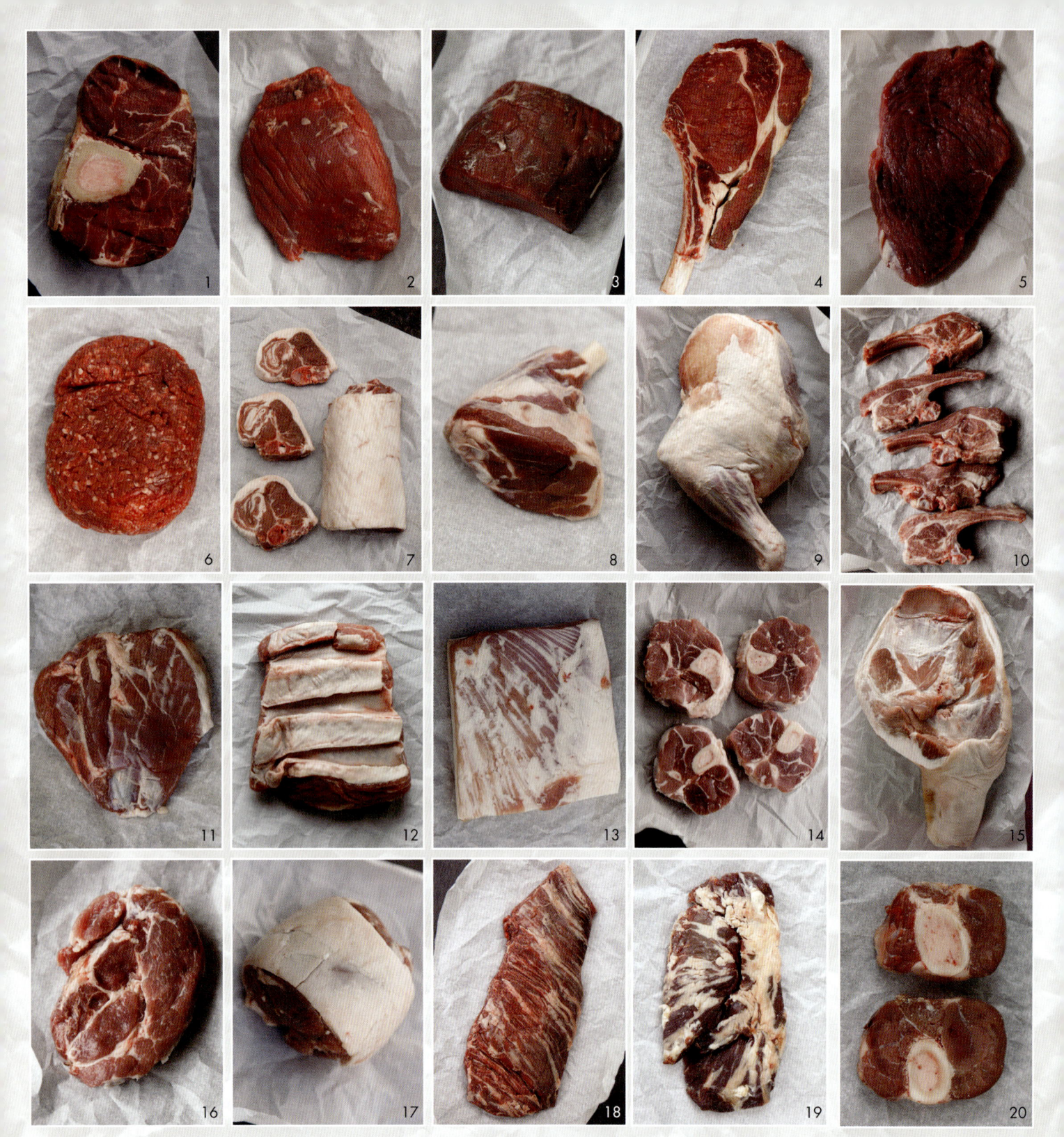

From top left to right: 1. Beef Shank *(Jarret de Boeuf)* 2. Beef Shoulder *(Paleron)* 3. Beef Sirloin *(Rumsteck)* 4. Bone-in Prime Rib *(Côte de Boeuf)* 5. Flank Steak *(Bavette)* 6. Ground Beef *(Steak Haché)* 7. Lamb Loin Roast & Chops *(Côtes Filet)* 8. Lamb Shank *(Souris d'Agneau)* 9. Lamb Shoulder *(Épaule d'Agneau)* 10. Lamb Shoulder Chops *(Côtes Découvertes)* 11. Lamb Topside Roast *(Noix d'Agneau)* 12. Plate (Beef Short ribs) *(Plats-de-Côtes)* 13. Pork Belly *(Carbonnade de Porc)* 14. Pork Knuckle *(Jarret de Porc)* 15. Pork Lower Shoulder and Shank *(Épaule et Jambonneau)* 16. Pork Shoulder *(Échine de Porc)* 17. Rolled Lamb Saddle *(Selle d'Agneau Roulée)* 18. Skirt Steak *(Hampe de Boeuf)* 19. Spider Steak *(Araignée de Boeuf)* 20. Veal Shank *(Jarret de Veau)*

CHAPTER 5
BUTCHERY BASICS:
KNOW YOUR CUTS AND HONE YOUR KNIVES

"The cave paintings of prehistoric grottos lead us to believe that the profession of the butcher is one of the oldest in the world." [1]
—Jean-Francois Mallet

BUTCHERY: PUTTING THE PIECES TOGETHER

To cook delicious, satisfying, and healthy meat dishes, you need to know the basics about where your meat comes from. This means knowing how the animal was raised and what part of the animal you are preparing. Knowing about butchery will help you make better decisions about what cuts of meat to look for and how you can save money by buying lesser known pieces. To start, it's worth getting to know your butcher. Putting my money where my mouth is, I asked my local organic butcher in Bordeaux if he would take me on as an apprentice for a few months so that I could learn where each cut of meat came from on the animal and why some pieces require more cooking time or preparation than others. That way I would understand, as will you, why certain cuts become steaks and why other cuts of meat go best into long-cooking recipes, roasts, and so on. In return, I worked for free, served customers, and cooked **Sarlat Sautéed Potatoes** (page 468) with steak at lunchtime for the other butchers.

INTRODUCING BUTCHERY – *LA BOUCHERIE*

In butchery (*la boucherie*) and the other related arts such as sausage-making, curing and drying meat (*la charcuterie*), or working with fowl (*volailler*), the necessary skills are transferred from artisan to apprentice. As with general cooking, it is both rewarding and economical to learn some of these techniques. At the same time, it is a great help and relief when one has an excellent butcher or other culinary artisan in the neighborhood. In France, the number of butchers are in decline, and continued customer support is needed for these skills to flourish. They take pride in their work, and I learned that they are often quite happy to share their knowledge with those who ask questions and show interest. As with any artisanal profession (*métier d'artisanat*), learning takes time and practice. Even so, my several-month-long apprenticeship gave me a new way of looking at meat and the animals who provide it. I am grateful to now share the basics of butchery that I was able to learn during those inspiring few months.

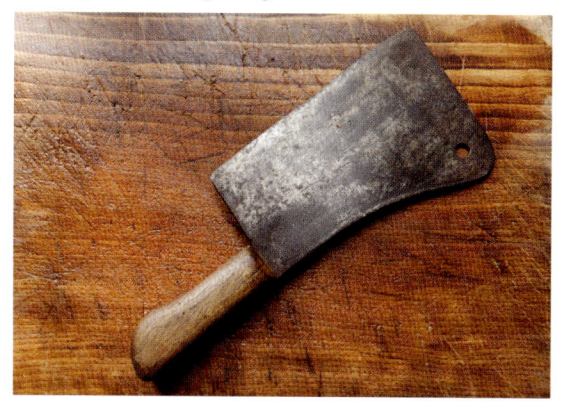

A BUTCHER'S UNDERSTANDING OF TASTE: FLAVORS AND CUTS

If anyone knows about taste, it's an experienced butcher (*le boucher*). Taste is based on the age of the animal when slaughtered and the amount of maturation time (*la maturation*) given to each piece of meat. Even the season during which the animal is raised, which often determines the type of feed, forage, or grasses (*l'alimentation*) the animal eats, affects the quality of its fat and thus the taste. Butchers understand intimately how the fat in meat gives it its flavor. They understand how fattening (*l'engraissement*) animals, especially cows during the last month before slaughter, affects the taste and marbling (*le persillage*) of the fat in the muscle meats. Butchers know how to age meat, grade it, and carve it according to its marbling. In fact, certain breeds of cow are selected for their ability to produce fat by consuming a given type of feed or grass. In addition, butchers, like trained chefs, are influenced by consumer demand, regional preferences, economics, current dietary beliefs, and the widespread industrial food system, even in France.

Unfortunately, most beef in France is grain-finished, and most butchers understand meat primarily from this grain-finished perspective. There are a few farmers in France who raise "grass-finished" or "100% grass-fed" cows. This is a result of market demand and economic dynamics, which hopefully will change as people come to realize the benefits of consuming "grass-finished" versus "grain-finished" beef. (More on grass-fed beef later in this chapter—page 88.)

A French butcher will recommend a cut of meat based on its flavor, the amount of fat, and the tenderness of the cut, as well as its availability in his and farmers' inventories. There are certain cuts of meat that always sell depending on the clientele, therefore butchers must be creative about suggesting other cuts of meat that are less popular but delicious when prepared in certain ways. An experienced butcher also understands the freshness and hygiene conditions required for certain cuts of meat to be served raw or seared on the outside and raw on the inside (*bleu*).

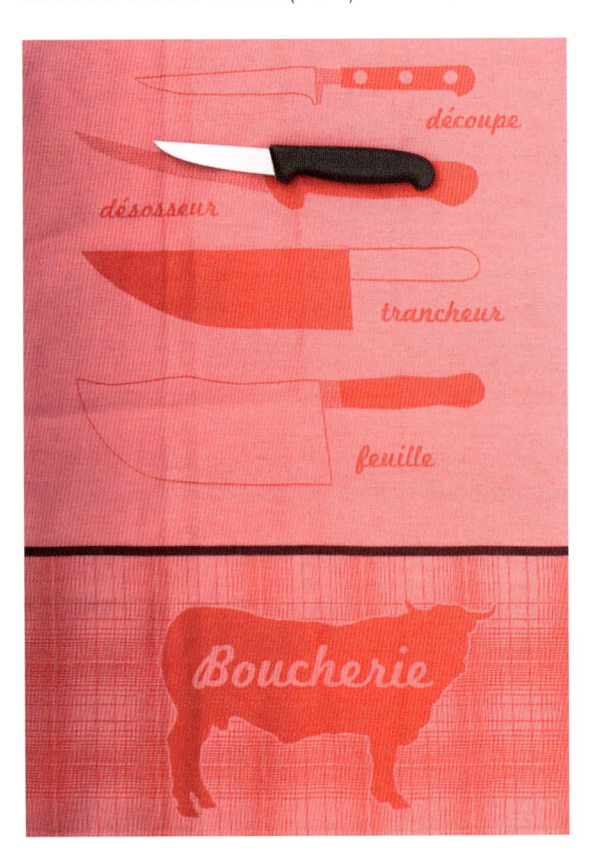

SEASONAL BUTCHER ECONOMICS

An enterprising butcher is a repository of recipes and will be able to suggest the proper cooking style for any cut of meat you purchase. His suggestions not only demonstrate his understanding of flavors, it also helps him sell excess cuts of meat he may have in stock at any given time. A butcher receives meat deliveries in entire halves or

THE BORDEAUX KITCHEN

quarters, and aims to sell all the meat, not just the most popular cuts. (I say "him" because the reality is that most butchers in France are male, though I hope there are exceptions as I know there are in the U.S. and the U.K.) Like farmers and gardeners, butchers have to adapt with the seasons. They must find ways to match the customer demand for meat with the supply from farms. In the winter, their customers tend to make more soups, stews, and "slow-cooked recipes" (*recettes de longue cuisson*), while in warmer months customers prefer sausages or meats for grilling or for easy stir-fries (*sauté de boeuf, sauté de porc*, etc). Certain butchers in Paris specialize only in certain cuts of meat, as their upscale clientele has narrowed its tastes over the years. This has driven up their prices. Nevertheless, a butcher must guide his clients in terms of his own needs and inventory balanced with his clients' wishes and preferences in order to stay in business and not waste resources. Understanding the seasonal and economic issues a butcher faces can help inform your own choices and reduce your costs. Buying more of what is in stock at a lower price and freezing it for later use is one way of reducing costs per pound or kilogram of meat.

In general, the front part of the cow, calf, lamb, or pig is generally tougher and requires longer cooking. The front half of a grazing animal is where it tends to place its center of gravity as it bends its head and neck down to forage or eat. Forward cuts tend to be less expensive but more collagenous and fatty, and therefore tastier. The back end of these four-legged creatures is where you find the loins and specialty steaks. These cuts are often more expensive but require shorter cooking times. The more you understand what you are consuming, the more ways you can find to save money. Throughout the recipe sections, this book provides you with diagrams of cuts from each animal in English and French to understand where each cut of meat comes from. (Find the Beef Cuts Diagram on page 106, the Lamb Cuts Diagram on page 188, the Pork Cuts Diagram on page 284, and the Veal Cuts Diagram on page 418.)

BYOB – BE YOUR OWN BUTCHER

If cooking for oneself is self-sufficiency, then butchering for oneself is self-empowerment. Asking your butcher about cuts of meat and recipes that go with them is a great way to start planning your dinner menu. There are many videos online as well as good books and classes on butchery. If you understand that certain cuts, such as those from the leg or other tough muscle meats are less expensive, then you can buy them in bulk, freeze, and then cook them when you know you will have time to make a stew or a long roast. Organ meats such as sweetbreads, on the other hand, are more delicate and in France can be more expensive because they are limited in quantity per beast. In the U.S., certain purveyors like US Wellness Meats sell organ meats at reasonable prices. Your local butcher or farmer might be very happy to sell you organ meats at reasonable prices, as these pieces may otherwise be difficult to sell in a society that has shied away from organ meats in recent decades. Previously, dishes of liver and onions, for example, were on menus across America and prepared at home (not to mention dishes of sweetbreads, calf's head, and calf's brains).[2] Buy organ meats when you can consume them right away, or bake them into a *terrine* or *pâté*, which can be stored for longer in the refrigerator or freezer. (If you are going to freeze liver, for example, first slice it into single-serve portions, wrap each in butcher or parchment paper, and store in a sealable container or a plastic bag, for thawing as needed.) Learning how to debone or separate certain cuts of meat is very helpful when you buy a half a pig or lamb or a quarter of a cow as part of a cow share or direct from a farmer. I have bought half pigs and half and whole lambs in this manner and saved money. But you have to be willing to devote time to the deboning and butchering, and then even curing. This does take a commitment of time… and some physical endurance!

THE SURGICAL PRECISION OF THE BUTCHER

The phrase in English "butchering something" connotes that one has messed something up, such as a speech, a translation, or even the cutting of a piece of meat or a beautiful cake. However, butchers are actually (thankfully) very precise, whether sawing, chopping, or slicing meat. How else could he get people to buy his meats if they were not beautifully cut and displayed in his showcase (*vitrine*)?

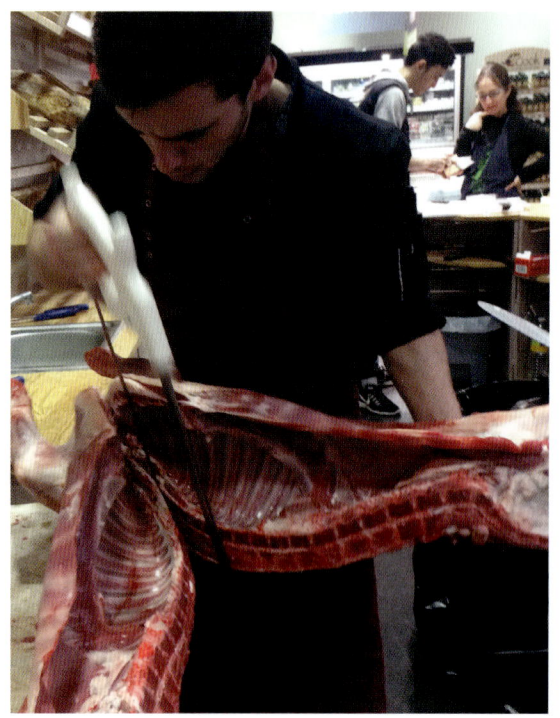

Florent Breaks Down a Lamb

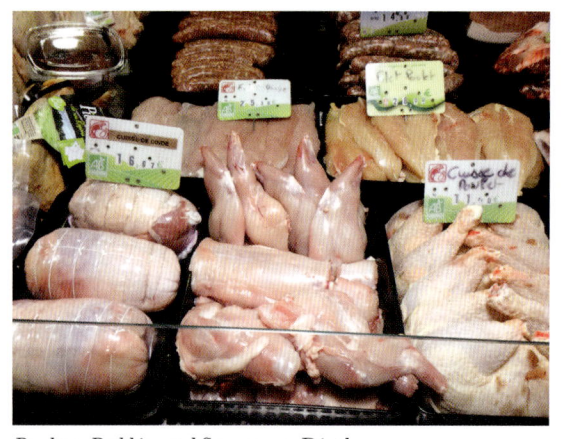

Poultry, Rabbit, and Sausage on Display

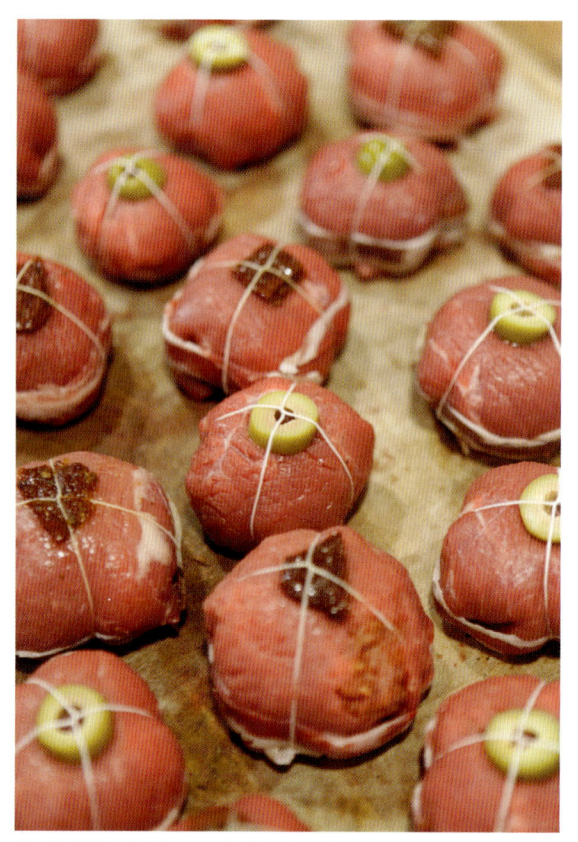

Stuffed Veal Cutlets at the Butcher Shop

One thing I learned while watching the team of butchers at work in Bordeaux was the way they moved through the meat almost effortlessly at times with their ever-honed knives. Once a piece had been sawed and then deboned using a short deboning knife, they would "follow the fascia" in order to cut out each muscle with delicate precision using the same knife or a slightly longer one. Obviously, they knew where they were going on each carcass, along each muscle. Experience really pays for a butcher, as the "breaking down" (*casser*) of the carcass becomes over time a natural, automatic art form with each carcass and cut of meat. The longest length knives are used to cut neat slices of meat (such as tied-up roasts or slippery veal liver), slicing once forward and once backward in one meaningful and connected stroke, akin to the movement of a cello player on a long note. To finish a piece of meat, the butcher will expertly shave off excess fat, depending on the cut, but also to make a piece more presentable and less fatty (*moins gras*), as is the conventional norm. You can request that your butcher shave off less fat, or none at all. If you are cutting down your own meat, you can leave as much fat on it as you like, remembering to keep in mind the suggested length of cooking time for particular cuts. The fattier the meat surrounding a roast, the juicier the roast will be. Some pieces are so lean that French butchers will sell them wrapped in slices of lard, to keep the meat from burning or drying out on the outside. More on this "barding and tying" (*barder et ficeller*) technique in the photo tutorials on "How to Tie a Roast (without Stuffing or Barding)" (page 82) and "How to Stuff, Wrap, and Tie a Roast" (page 83).

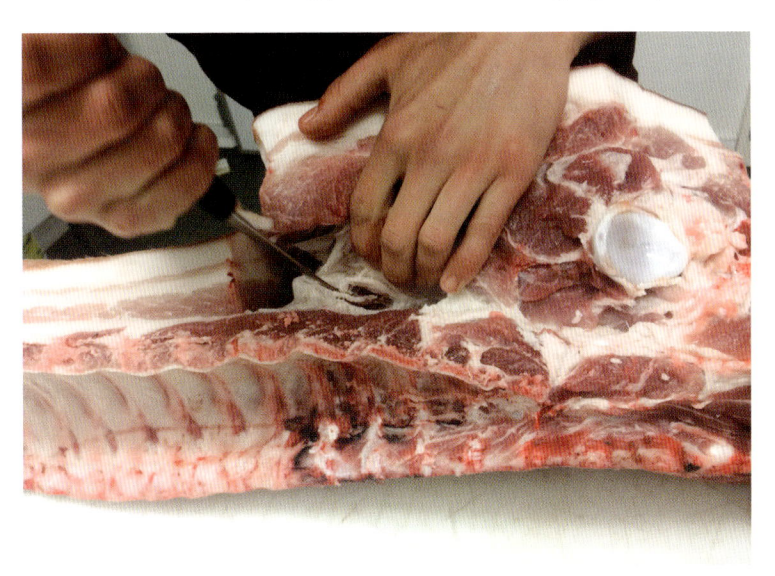

Following the Fascia

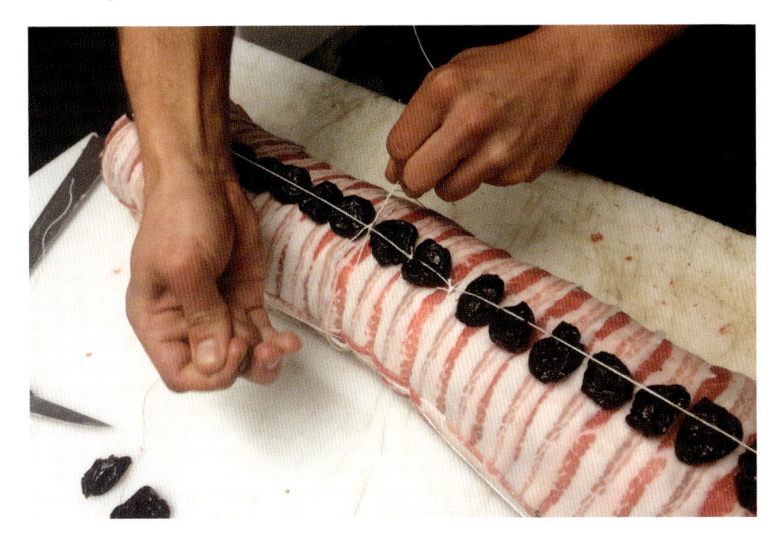

Florent Ties a Prune-Stuffed Pork Roast

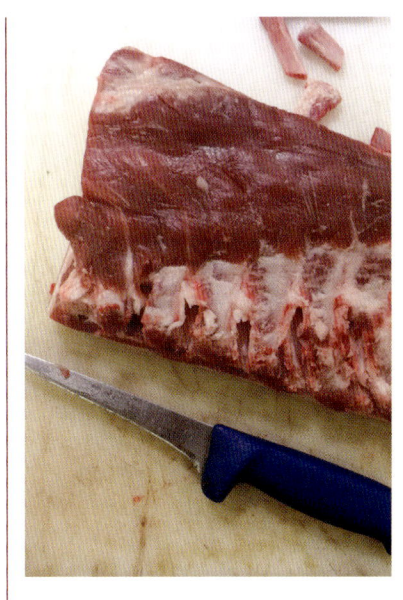

Don't Cry Wolf

The Basque (*Euskadi*) butcher, Florent Carriquiry, who kindly allowed me to learn from him over the course of a few months, admonished me as I practiced how to properly debone a pork belly (*poitrine de porc*): "It must not look like the wolf (*le loup*) had been there," he exclaimed, as I wrangled with several pork bellies, trying to learn where to crack off the bone so as not to puncture a hole in the meat and thus open the door to external microbes.

CHAPTER 5

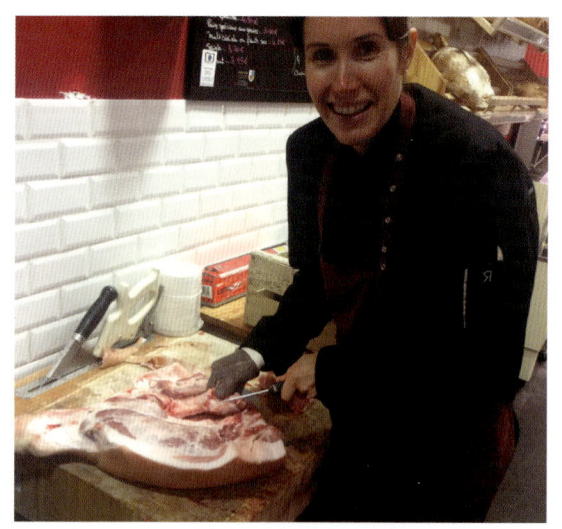

Tania Deboning a Pork Leg Photo Credit: Florent Carriquiry

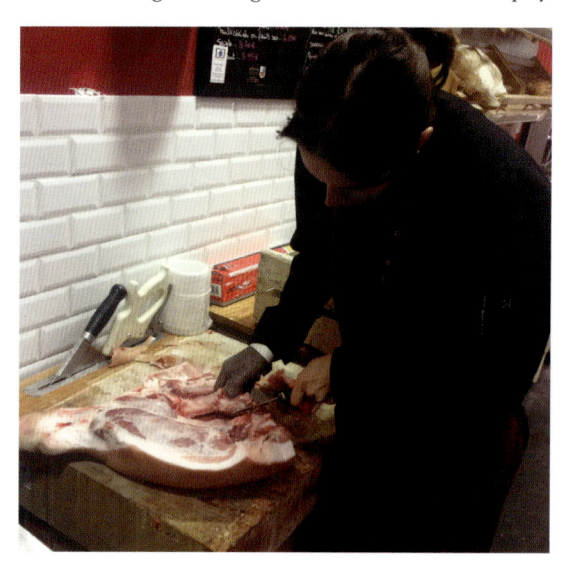

In the time it took me to debone a single turkey leg, Florent the butcher deboned six legs while serving several customers in between drumsticks! Here I was, the foreigner (*étrangère*) with the funny French accent, playing butcher's apprentice and receiving curious looks from customers who took pity on me by repeating things in loud voices if I did not catch their rapid-fire request the first time around. Florent had me introduce myself to the customers and explain who I was and why I was there. By the end of my "apprenticeship," I got to know many of the regular customers and took on the jovial manner of the butcher in asking how they were doing and taking pride in serving customers whom I had come to know a bit. The customers were often grandmothers purchasing chicken, offal, or rabbit for themselves or cooking veal steaks or sausages for their grandchildren. Sometimes they were young mothers or fathers in need of easy-to-cook steaks, sausages, ground beef, or sautés.

THE ART OF SYMMETRY

During my brief apprenticeship at the butcher shop, I learned that butchers cut animals in a symmetrical, formulaic way that keeps the cuts consistent. The cow, pig, and lamb are cut into quarters. At the butcher shop, we usually received the beef and veal in quarter pieces or smaller, as even a quarter is unwieldy and enormous. (Lifting, carrying, and sawing meats in cold temperatures is a workout all on its own!) Pig carcasses arrived by the half (*une longe de porc*) and were sliced down the middle from neck to hind leg, minus the head, tail, and feet. (These last pieces were not being ordered frequently enough and are not part of the slaughtering norm, even in the organically certified French slaughterhouse from which the store ordered its meats.) Lambs arrived whole but eviscerated, except for the kidneys. These are hidden inside the lamb, each within a ball of hard visceral fat called suet (*suif*), which when rendered is useful as tallow. In France, lamb is considered mutton from 12 months of age at a weight of about 66 pounds (30 kg). Before that, there are certain gradations of lamb: small milk-fed lamb (*agneau de lait*) – five to six weeks in age and weighing 13 to 18 pounds (6 to 9 kg); large milk-fed lamb (*agneau*) – three to four months of age, weighing about 31 to 40 pounds (14 kg to 18 kg); and weaned and pastured lamb (*agneau sevré, agneau de pâturage*) – four and a half months to 12 months of age, weighing 44 to 66 pounds (20 kg to 30 kg). A special designation (*agneau de pré-salé*) is given to weaned lambs who have spent at least three months pastured in the salt meadow estuaries of Brittany and Normandy, the most famous of which is that of Le Mont-Saint-Michel and whose "season" is September and October.

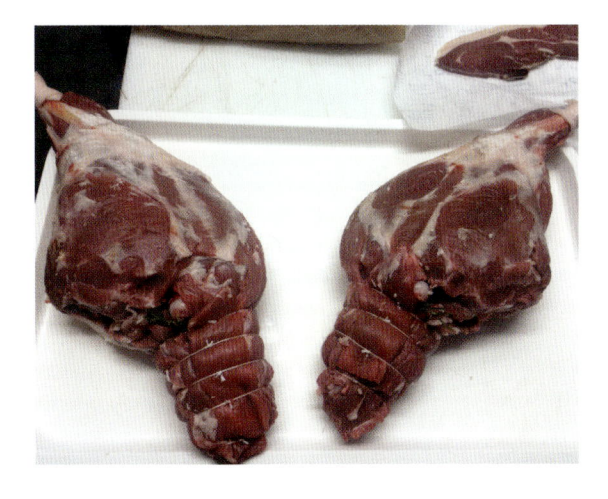

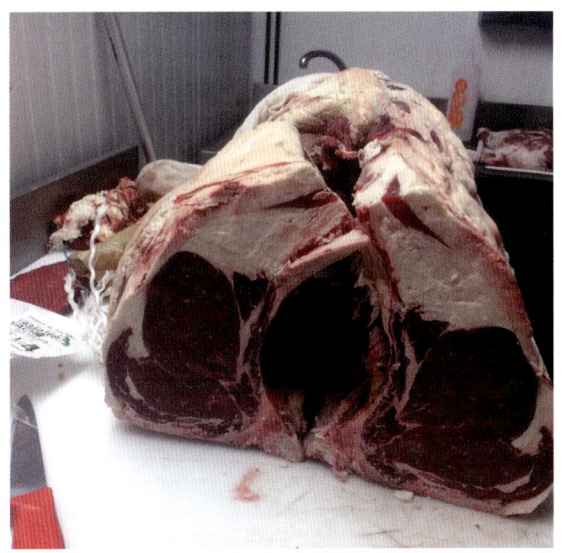

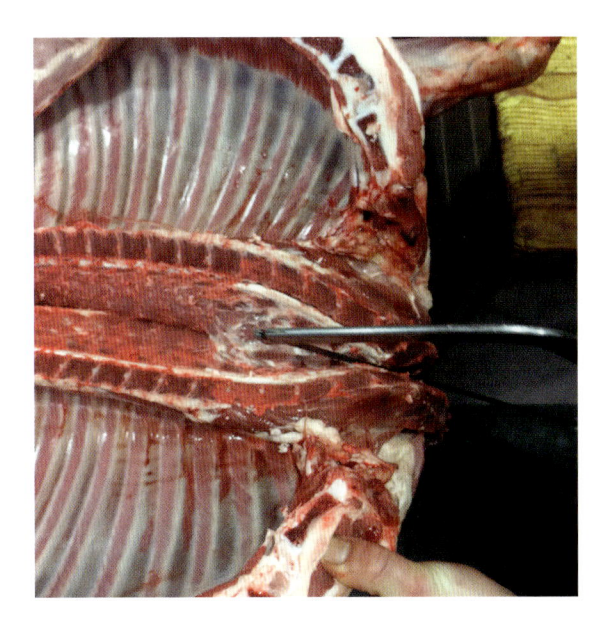

To break down the lamb carcass (*casser l'agneau*), we used a D-shaped "American" hand saw (*scie à l'américaine*) to saw down the middle of the lamb spine. It takes a strong shoulder and is truly an art form to cut properly. Remaining precisely centered while sawing along this fine length of spine makes for proper-looking lamb cutlets later on in the butchering process. An expertly cut lamb chop commands a handsome price. If it looks like "the wolf has been there," the butcher will have to eat the cost (and the chop) himself. The D-shaped saw was also used to divide the ribs of a half pig carcass in two as well, as shown in the photo below.

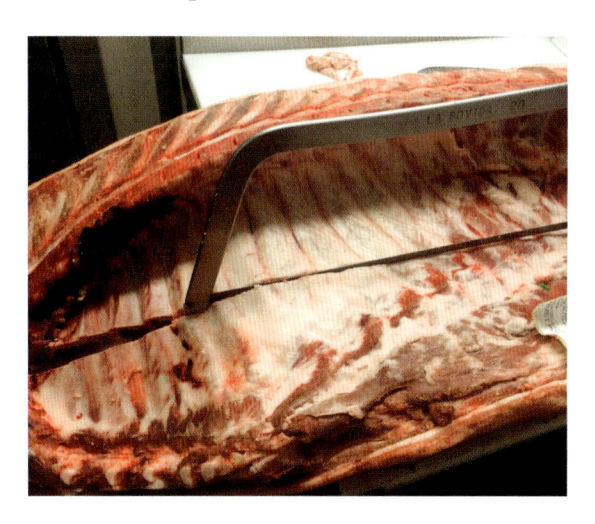

Depending on the cut, the meat is stored for several days in a walk-in freezer or cold chamber (*la chambre froide*) at 32°F (0°C) either on the carcass or as individual cuts sometimes vacuum-packed in plastic (*sous vide*) for freshness preservation. I do not particularly like the use of *sous vide* because of the potential for the xeno-estrogens in the plastics to leech into the meat, but the reality of the bottom line in a modern butcher shop (and even for the modern farmer) calls upon the use of such modern technology. A butcher essentially "finishes" the meat by allowing beef and veal to age on meat hooks in the freezer (*la chambre froid*) and storing items vacuum-packed on shelves.

CHAPTER 5

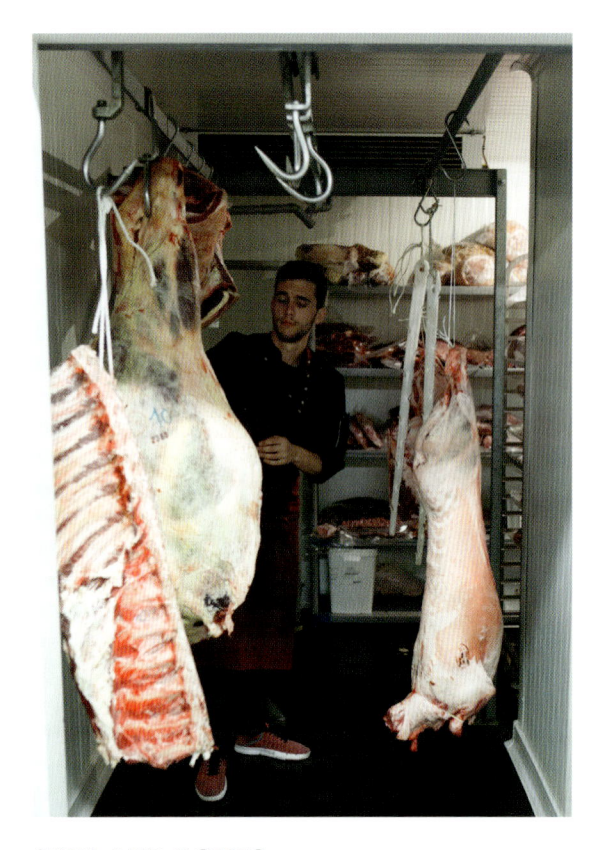

SKIN AND BONES

Even at an organic butcher shop, skin, bones, fat, and scraps were discarded in the interest of time, money, or for lack of demand. It was not economical or feasible to hang on to bones for soup, skin for pork rinds, or fat for rendering. Hating to see quality meat go to waste, I would save some of these scraps in the chilled back room (*le labo*) to take home, as the butchers suggested. This was how I became acquainted with rendering lard and tallow, how to make **Crispy Pork Rinds** (page 240), a favorite of my younger daughter's, and what to do with cracklings. It also allowed me to make rich bone broths for my family on a weekly basis.

PARISIAN-STYLE CUTS – *LA DÉCOUPE PARISIENNE*

La découpe Parisienne is a standardized style of cutting down meat for the customer into neat, eye-pleasing, but more expensive morsels. This technique became the norm in Paris several centuries ago due to busy, demanding city dwellers who had small ovens and kitchens and could not manage larger pieces of meat. It also set the standard for cutting each carcass in the same manner, symmetrically, to achieve repeatable, clean, and saleable results. This practice, however, can result in many wasted scraps. Therefore, even if they have neat pre-cuts of meat on display, many butchers will take the time to cut a fresh slice of steak in front of the customer in order to keep the meat fresh until the last minute.

ECONOMICAL SAUSAGE MAKING

Visually, every piece of meat sold at the butcher counter must look appetizing and, even in France nowadays, "not too fatty" in order to appeal to the modern customer. Any piece of meat that does not look adequately trimmed of fat goes into the sausage-making pile. Only twice during my butcher apprenticeship did I make sausage in the 4° Celsius (39°F) "cold room" (*laboratoire*, or *labo*). It can feel like a punishment to be sent to the *labo*, but luckily the butchers usually took pity on me and allowed me to chip away at my pork shoulder or pork belly behind the counter where it was warmer! (Mixing cold ground sausage meat with your bare hands is not necessarily what I would call fun. My fingertips periodically needed to be thawed while working with the sausage meat.)

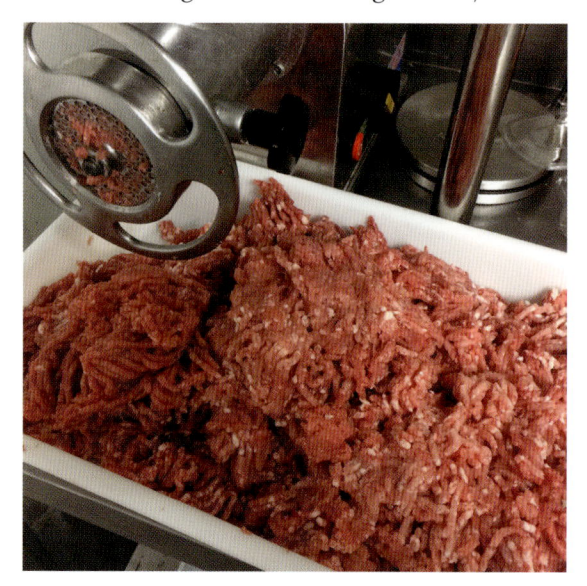

Ground Sausage Meat

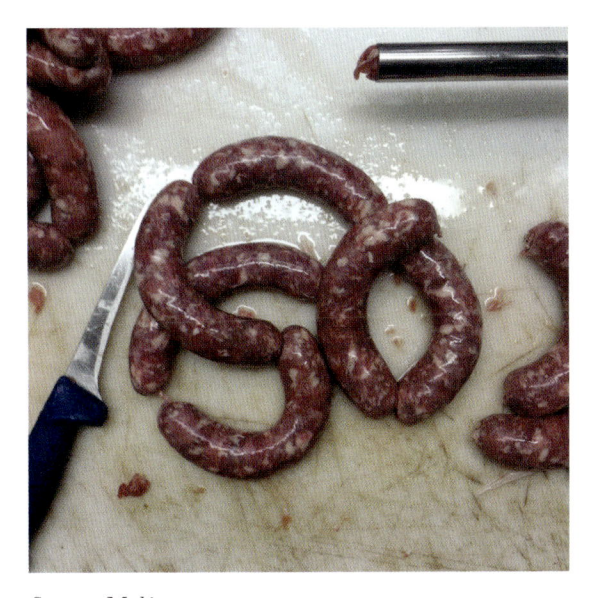

Sausage Making

A butcher will typically make large amounts of sausage at a time, because cleaning the meat-grinding and sausage-making machines afterwards in itself is also no picnic. Freshly made sausages are popular and sell out fast because they are such an easy food for customers to cook up at home. A batch of pork sausage might look something like this: 11 pounds (5 kilograms) of ground pork, 2 ounces (60 grams) of fine salt, 4-½ teaspoons (18 grams) ground black pepper, and 4-½ teaspoons (18 grams) of powdered garlic. Stuffing the encasings with a hand-cranked sausage-making machine and tying each sausage off by hand is its own art form, but it is one of the first things apprentices must learn to do.

HONING AND SHARPENING YOUR KNIFE

Knives are essential to good cooking as well as good butchery. In order to be precise, you need a sharp knife. Things really started coming together for me when I learned how to hone a knife using the honing steel (*le fusil à affûter*) at the butcher shop. I learned to use the *fusil* to sharpen my knives prior to each use, as the butchers do.[3] Theirs was a flat rod, probably a diamond steel (covered in diamond dust), but the most common kind is a round rod made of stainless steel.[4] At home, I was able to use the honing steel that came with my wedding gift knife set. Our knives had gotten so dull that I had to have them professionally sharpened at a knife shop in town where they use a rotating sharpening stone. In France there used to be at least one butcher shop and one knife shop in every village. This is no longer necessarily the case, especially for knife shops. If you are friendly with your local butcher, he might sharpen your knives for you. A newly sharpened knife makes for much more joy in cutting and chopping and actually reduces the risk of injury from pressing too hard or from slippage (as long as you keep your thumb and fingers out of the way). You can keep your knife honed with the honing steel in between annual or semi-annual trips to the professional knife shop (or sharpen it yourself on a water stone, or whetstone—literally a moistened, flat stone).[5] Every once in a while, the butchers would pull out their knife-sharpening wheel and really "sharpen" their knives, as shown here.

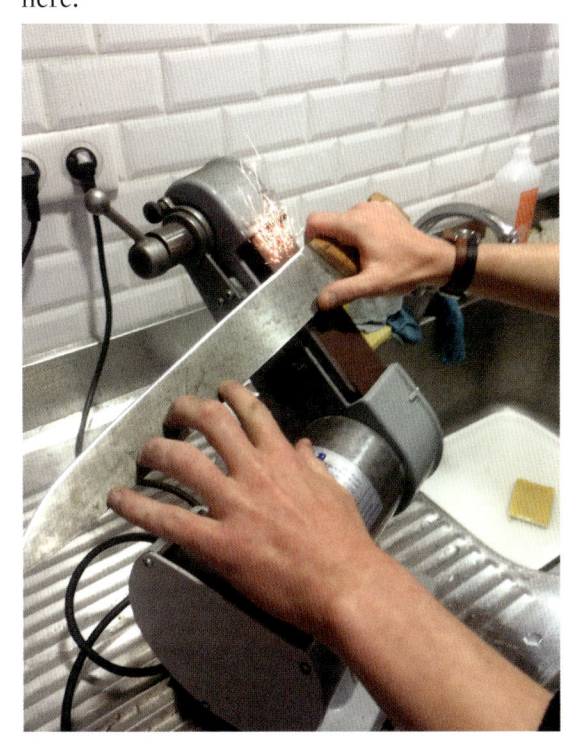

CHAPTER 5

How to Hone a Knife

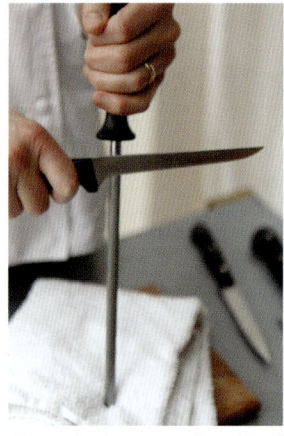

Grasp the honing steel and knife firmly in each hand. Press the edge of the blade at the base at a 30- to 45-degree angle against the top of the honing steel.

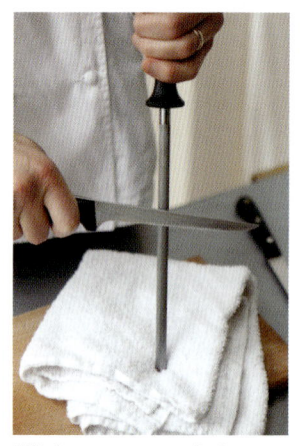

While pressing into the honing steel, move the blade down the length of the steel toward the tip of the blade.

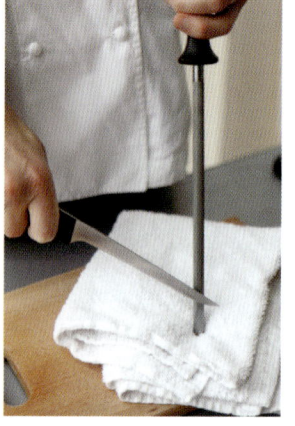

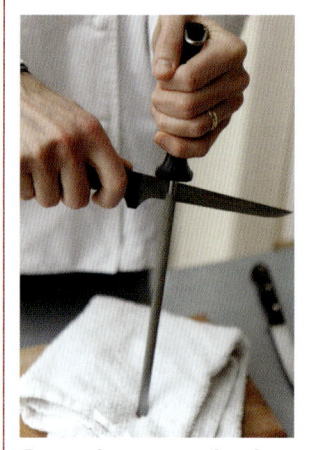

Repeat these steps on the other side of the blade.

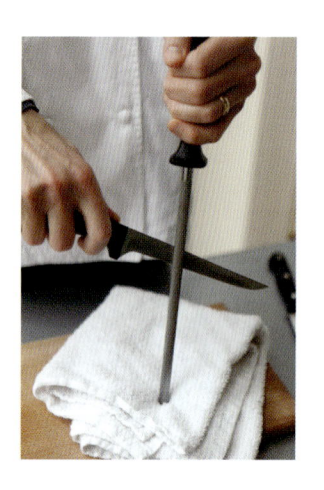

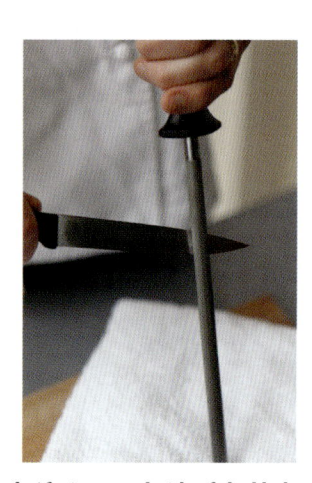

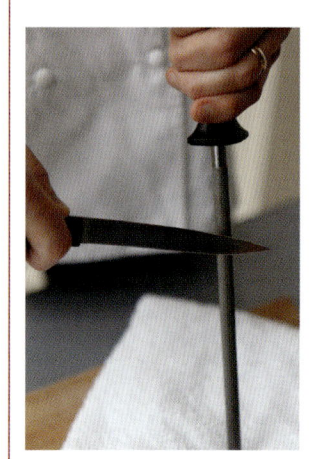

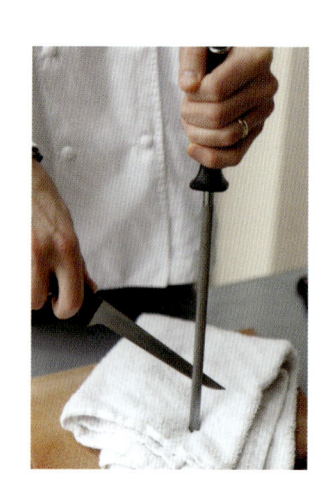

Additionally, if desired, you can hone just the knife tip on each side of the blade.

THE BORDEAUX KITCHEN

It is recommended to have the right knife for each purpose: A small-bladed paring knife (*petit couteau* or *couteau à éplucher*) for handling garlic, peeling apples, or removing fascia or layers of film on meats like sweetbreads; a flexible blade (*couteau à lame flexible* or *un désosseur*) for filleting a fish or deboning meat; an inflexible, four-inch (10 cm) deboning knife; a long blade to slice thin, large pieces of meat (*un trancheur*); a cleaver (*une feuille*) to chop through bones to make things like lamb and pork chops (this needs to be very heavy and carefully handled, or else left to the butcher to use); and of course the all-purpose chef's knife or kitchen knife to chop, slice, and dice (*un découpeur* or *un couteau de cuisine*). Knives of stainless steel or carbon steel are generally what the butchers use, which they hone frequently by hand. Every so often, butchers sharpen all their knives on a rotating electrical stone wheel at the butcher shop, bright orange sparks shooting out from the blade. Ceramic knives, on the other hand, require a fine diamond sharpener.

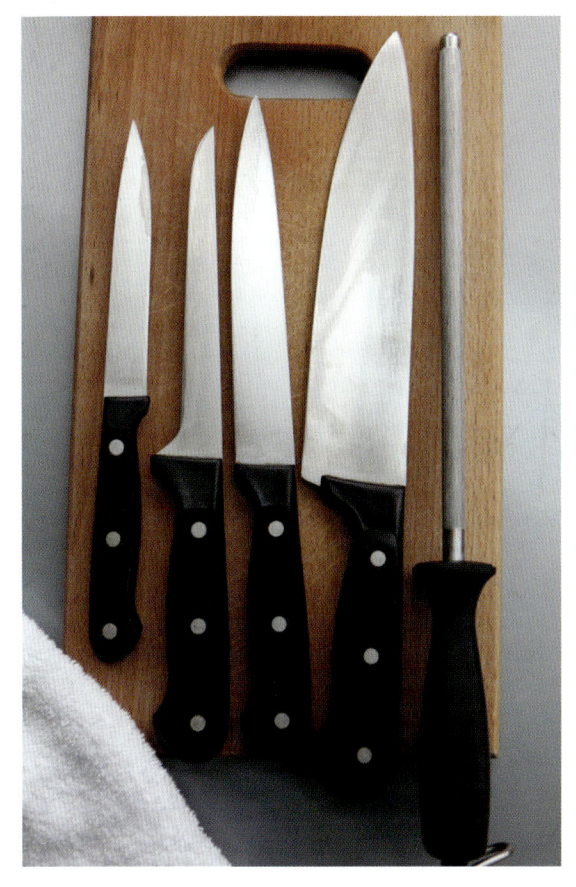

As an apprentice, I was required to wear a steel mesh glove on the hand that was not doing the cutting. The best way to do this was to don a surgical glove and then cover it with a mesh glove followed by another surgical glove. This practice keeps meat and fat out of the mesh glove and away from direct skin contact. At home, I use a protective glove as well since I have no time for random cuts on my hands to stop me from cooking! As for taking care of your knives, wash and dry the "good knives" by hand. Keep them out of the dishwasher, or they will become dull too fast. When scraping vegetables or meat off of your cutting board, be sure to use the back of the knife blade instead of the blade side or you will dull your knife's edge in double time. Research carbon versus stainless steel knives, to see what works best for your needs and budget. As with all your equipment, get the best quality you can afford.

USING BUTCHER'S STRING – *FICELLER*

Learning to use butcher's string or thread is an art in its own right and makes for a lovely presentation of meat. It serves the dual purpose of adding value to the meat and holding the meat together, as it will expand or change shape when heated. It also keeps the meat from burning or drying out on the outside. Butchers generally use a paring or other small knife to cut the string as they go. Many butchers will add their flourish of bacon strips, decorative olives, dried tomatoes, prunes, or herbs to remind themselves of what a meat may have been stuffed with, as well as to make an eye-pleasing package for the customer. The bacon strips also serve to keep the meat from drying out, a technique called "barding" (*barder*). Keeping these in place requires butcher's thread (*la ficelle*) in such preparations as **Stuffed Veal Cutlets** (page 427) or **Pork Roast Stuffed with Prunes and Tied** (page 308). If the cut of meat is lean, such as in a beef loin roast, then a border of pork or beef fat (*la barde*) is added around the edges to keep the meat from burning or becoming too dry. Another option is to stuff

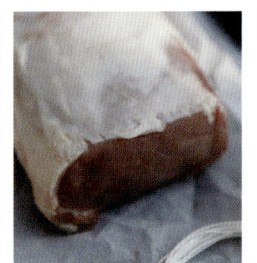

How to Tie a Roast (without Stuffing or Barding)

This series shows you simply how to tie a roast to help it to cook more evenly. The piece of meat pictured here happens to be a boneless pork loin roast (see **Pork Roast with** *Herbes de Provence* on page 305), but this technique may be applied to beef, lamb, or other pork roasts, as well as when you are preparing **Stuffed Rabbit Saddle** (page 368) and **Stuffed Veal (or Chicken) Cutlets** (page 427).

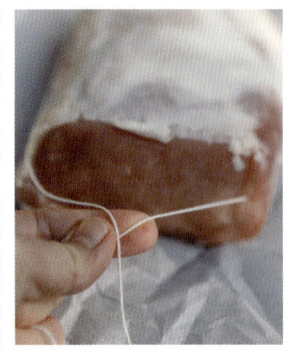

Wrap a string around the sides of the roast from the back end to the front end (nearest you), and criss-cross the string.

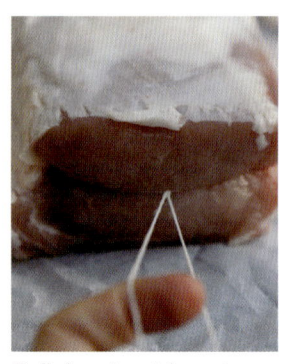

Pull the string tight against the front of the roast.

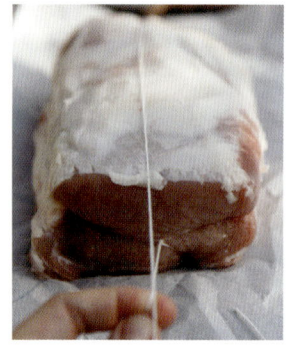

Wrap the string underneath the roast toward the back and bring it over the top of the roast toward you again, much like you would tie a ribbon around the sides of a package.

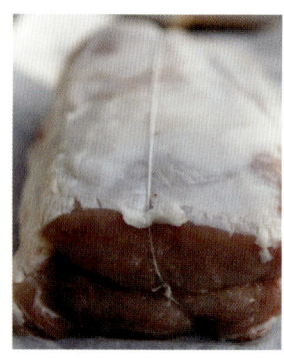

Tie a knot at the front, and cut the string close to the knot.

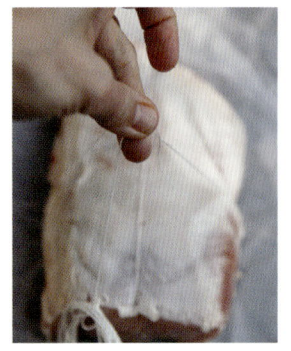

Place the butcher's string underneath the center of the meat and bring both ends of the string to the top.

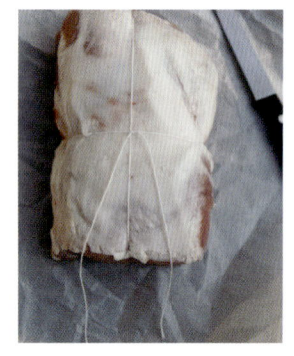

Tighten the string around the meat, make a knot at the top of the meat, and cut the string ends close to the knot.

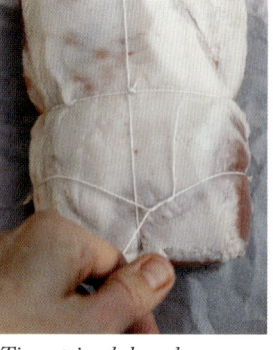

Tie a string below the center string towards the midpoint between the edge of the meat and the center string. Tighten the string around the meat, make a knot, and cut the string close to the meat.

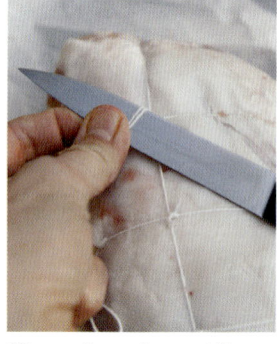

Tie another string equidistant from the center and the top edge of the meat, for a symmetrical look. Tighten the string, tie a knot, and cut the string close to the meat.

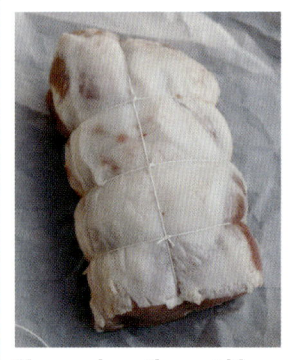

You may leave the roast like this or continue tying strings at the midpoint between the edges of the meat and the other strings, again, for symmetry.

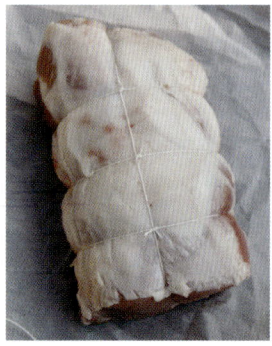

This roast is sufficiently tied and ready for seasoning and roasting.

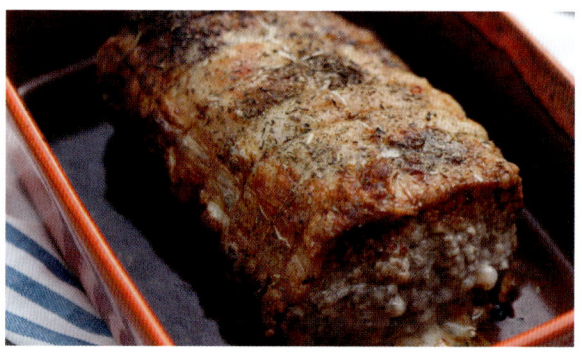

The finished roast, using the Pork Roast with Herbes de Provence recipe (page 305).

THE BORDEAUX KITCHEN

How to Stuff, Wrap, and Tie a Roast

This series shows a pork loin being stuffed with prunes and then topped with bacon slices, but the same principle can be used for other types of stuffing with other roasts of beef, lamb, pork, veal, and poultry, with or without bacon on top.

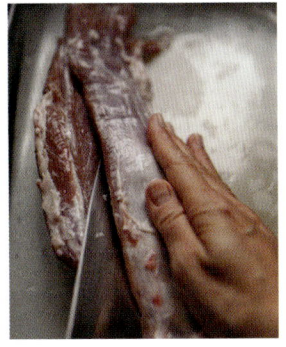

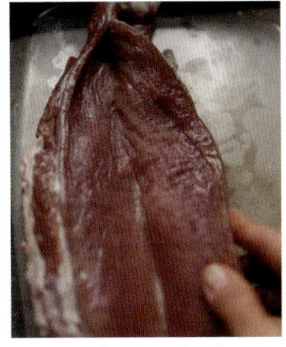

Slice into the meat lengthwise, cutting it sandwich-style, almost to the edge, but leaving the two pieces attached.

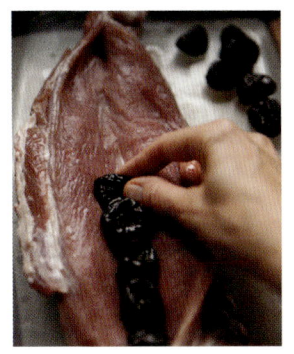

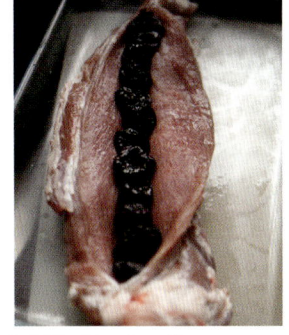

Line the inner edge of the open "sandwich" with a line of prunes. Sprinkle a pinch of salt along the line of prunes (optional).

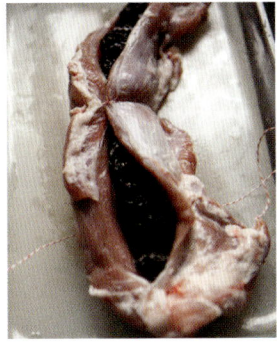

Close up the "sandwich" of prune-stuffed meat. (This roast needs string to hold it together, to make a surface for the bacon on top. Other larger roasts may close more easily, in which case you may place bacon strips on top before tying to save tying the roast twice.) Place a piece of butcher's string underneath the center of the meat and bring both ends to the top. Tighten the string around the meat, make a knot at the top of the meat, and cut the string ends close to the knot.

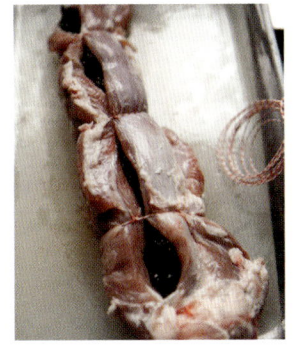

Use the string to tie knots near both ends of the piece of meat to hold the two halves and prunes in place.

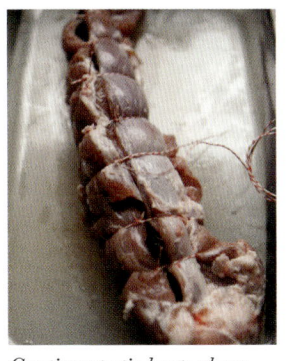

Continue to tie knots along the entire length of the piece of meat, tying off at every inch or two (every 2.5 cm to 5 cm), centering them between the first three knots you tied, until you are satisfied with how the meat looks.

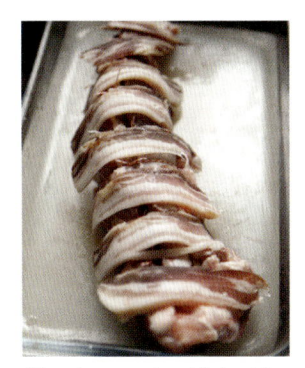

Place bacon strips side by side, crosswise, along the top of the meat.

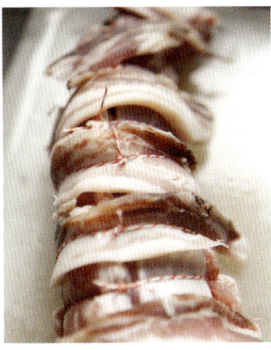

Use the butcher's string again to secure the bacon to the meat. The roast is ready for the oven.

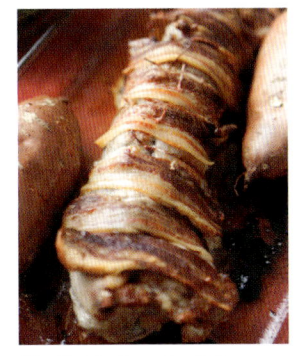

The finished roast whole.

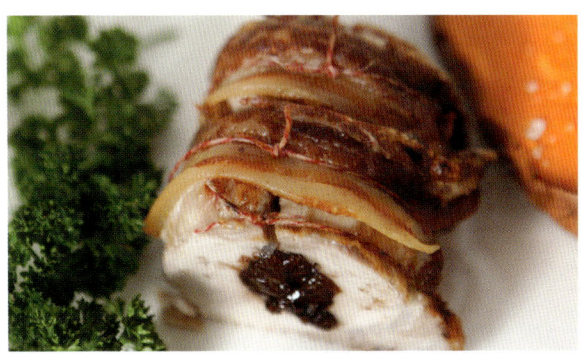

The finished roast sliced.

CHAPTER 5

the pork or beef fat inside a roast or else thread it with pieces of fat, called "larding" (*larder*) to add to the taste. Grass-fed beef is less marbled and fatty and benefits from some extra fat around the edges for cooking and flavor. You can also choose to not trim as much fat off of your cuts of meat as is "traditionally" done, or else ask your butcher if he will keep as much fat as possible on the meat. See preceding pages for two photo tutorials about using butcher's string for tying roasts.

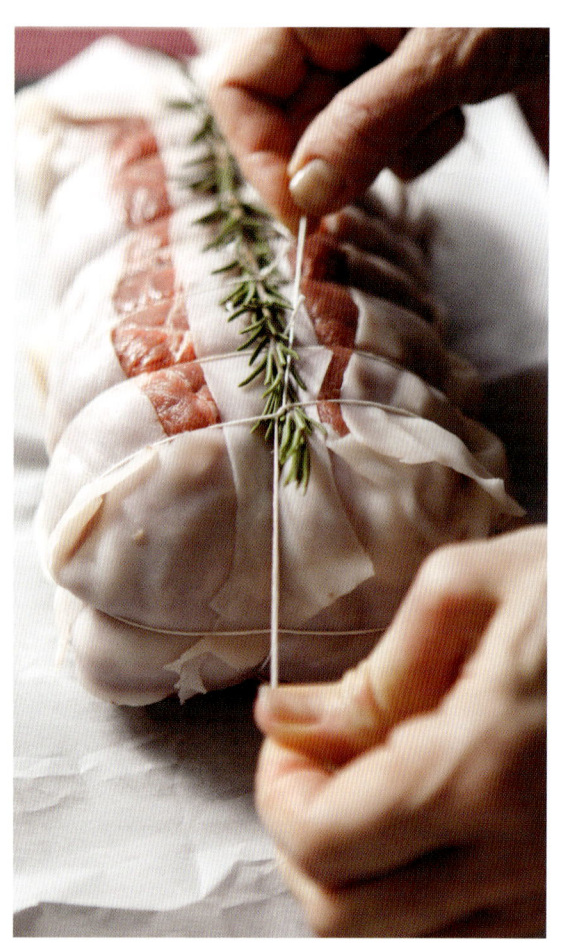

BUTCHER'S PAPER, NOT PLASTIC

While apprenticing at the butcher shop, I also sold meat to the clientele. I learned to package each order of meat in butcher paper and place it in a brown paper bag with the store's logo. Some clients preferred their meat vacuum-packed in plastic (*sous vide*), which would allow the meat to last several more days without exposure to air. For the butcher, vacuum sealing has become the norm for preserving meat, as it reduces waste. Many chefs even cook meats in vacuum-sealed plastic, a practice that I find worrisome given the dangers of the chemicals in the plastics leeching into the heated food. The irony is that this method is used in fine dining restaurants, and you might not know it unless it is specified on the menu or you have inspected the kitchen yourself! But for the chefs using this method, it is a matter of flavor, and for butchers, a matter of extending the freshness of food, thereby wasting less. Fortunately, though, some butcher shops still wrap meat in special butcher's paper rather than plastic, as was the case for generations before plastics became ubiquitous.

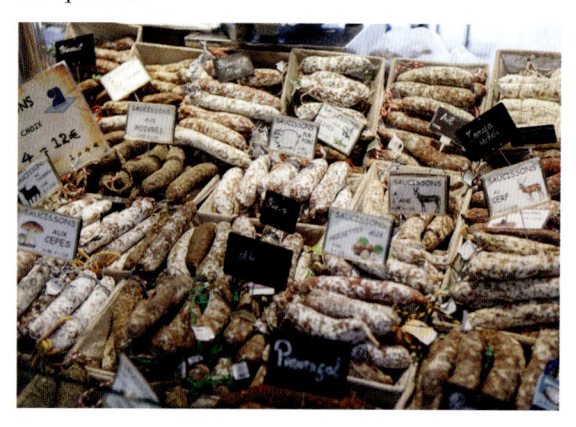

CHARCUTERIE

The art of what we call "delicatessen meat" or "cured meats" (*charcuterie*), is another economical way of preparing meat, as the cured meats can be saved for sale and consumption in the future. In France, charcuterie is its own specialty performed by the *charcutier*, sometimes also a butcher, whose knowledge is passed down from one generation to the next. French butcher shops (*boucheries*) and delicatessens or gourmet food shops (*épiceries fines*) offer charcuterie for sale, as do larger grocery stores. Many restaurants and wine bars around France sell charcuterie platters (*planches de charcuterie*), an assortment of cured and preserved meats. These platters are a fun way to get to know different kinds of charcuterie by region and curing style, just ask the waiter for an explanation. The same goes for cheese platters (*planches de fromages*).

Knowing the person who made the sausage, however, makes all the difference in the taste and experience. Making it oneself provides the ultimate satisfaction, though it does require the knowledge and tools, and not everyone is interested in taking the time. When I apprenticed with Florent, a skilled butcher, qualified chef, *and* charcutier, I learned about meats from this triple perspective of butcher-charcutier-chef. I saw how certain cuts and bits of meats not presentable (*noble*) enough to sell were transformed into sausage, sautés (prepared with spices and vegetables, but sold uncooked for customers to cook at home), and pâtés. Not only did these strategies make use of any and all of the pork, lamb, veal, chicken, duck, turkey, or beef being sold at the butcher counter, it created variety for the customer and higher value-added products to sell. That's genuine butcher economics!

In general, curing meats from scratch requires cold temperatures, salt, vinegar, spices, garlic, and a variety of tools, or the use of smoke, one of the oldest forms of preserving meat known to humans. Nowadays, people can buy smokers or other tools to help them cure meats. It is mostly a question of time, patience, and sourcing the right ingredients. There is a whole world of knowledge to gain from books and videos or asking someone who knows about curing and smoking meats. (See the Resources and Further Reading appendix for a list of relevant books.)

Charcuterie is traditionally stored in a cool basement or dedicated meat pantry. A native of Bayonne, Florent says that the *jambon de Bayonne*, the beloved dried ham of the surrounding Bayonne and Basque region (the Spanish side has its own similar product, known as *jamón Ibérico*), is so important to the Basque (*Euskadi*) culture that they wouldn't think of doing anything else with the hind legs of the pig other than dry-cure them whole. There is no cutting up of these fine legs into various roasts, as is done further north and east in France and in much of Europe. Instead, the jambon de Bayonne is prepared in the time-honored way in which the whole leg is cured with salt from the ancient saltpans of the the neighboring region of Béarn (*Salies-de-Béarn*) and the skin is rubbed with the Basque ground red pepper powder, *piment d'Espelette,* before drying. The town of Espelette celebrates an annual festival for its prized pepper, and indeed, the entire Basque region is adorned with strung-up bunches of this skinny, dark red vegetable. (Beware to those who are sensitive, as this is also a nightshade vegetable.)

SALT-CURING BACON

Florent taught me the following recipe for salt-cured pork (also called salt pork or dry-cured, or *la poitrine sèche* or *la ventrèche séchée* in French) that is hung to dry to use as bacon or for bacon pieces (*lardons)*:

Debone 2 pork bellies (without poking into the flesh beyond the edge of the bone). Rub them in a mixture of 4.5 pounds (2 kg) large grain sea salt (*gros sel de mer*), a handful of juniper berries (*baies de genevrier*), one bay leaf (*feuille de laurier*), several cloves of minced garlic or several teaspoons of powdered garlic, a few teaspoons of powdered sweet red chili (*piment d'Espelette*), and one cup to one-and-a-half cups of white vinegar. Allow the pork bellies to bask in this mixture for three days in the lab (refrigerator) at 39°F to 43°F (4°C to 6°C). Desalinate by plunging into cold water and soaking for 15 minutes for every day the pork bellies spent in the mixture, or roughly 45 minutes. Hang on a meat hook in the lab at 39°F to 43°F (4°C to 6°C) for five days. Transfer to the cold chamber at 32°F (0°C) for five days. Hang to dry in ambient temperature for 3 to 4 weeks.

As Joel Salatin explains in his book *Folks, This Ain't Normal*, when curing pork, the fresh pork must remain cold but not freeze so that the curing agents can move through the meat via its juices. Therefore, we kept slabs of bacon that were curing in the lab between 39°F to 43°F (4° to 6°C) until they were ready to be hung up to dry for another few weeks. The cooler and drier the climate, the faster the pork will dry.

Salt-Curing Pork Belly

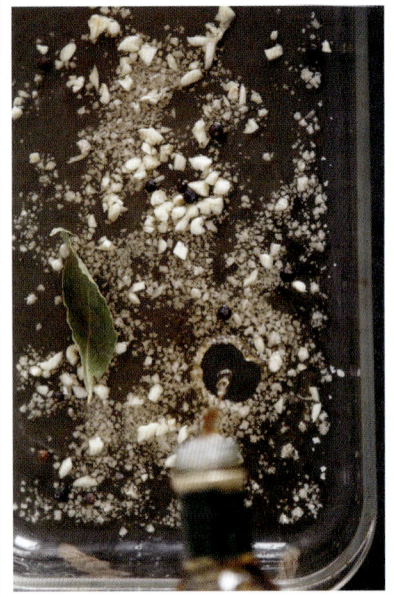

Mix aromatics, minced garlic, salt, and vinegar in a large dish.

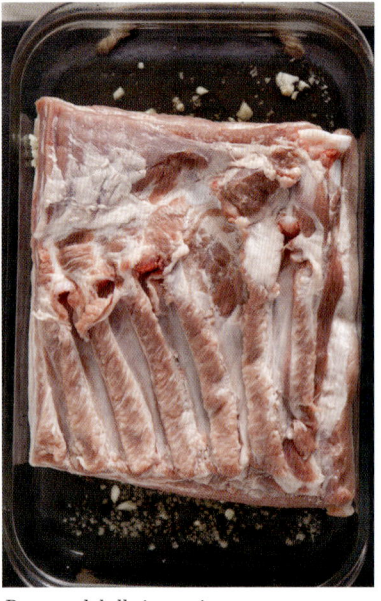

Press pork belly into mixture.

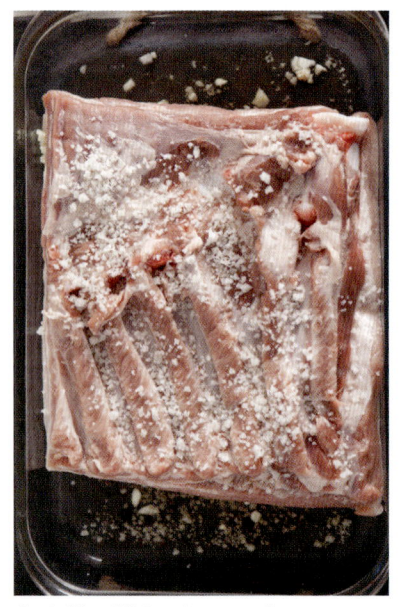

Sprinkle additional coarse salt on top.

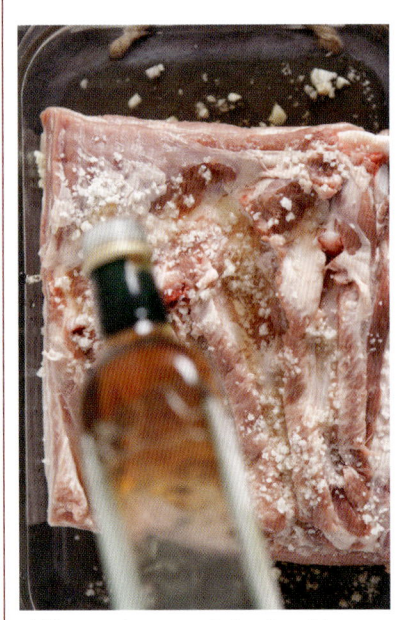

Add more vinegar, and place in refrigerator.

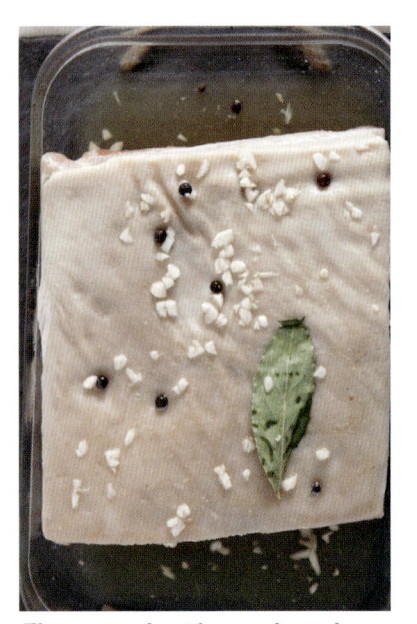

Flip over to other side every day so that each side is remoistened every 24 hours.

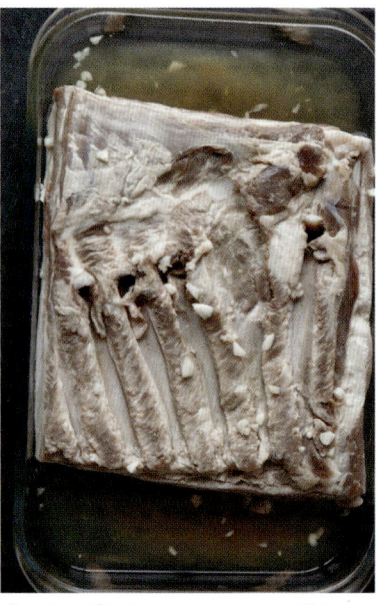

Continue flipping over once every 24 hours. After a couple of days, the pink colors of the meat will become dulled and grey as the vinegar and salt seep through the meat.

The way I did it at home was to change the proportions and lengths of time due to various circumstances: I used less salt (because I had less in my pantry) but used just as much vinegar. I stored my one pork belly in a large Pyrex glass casserole dish with a cover in the refrigerator for 4 days, before soaking it in cold water for one and a half hours. Next, I kept it in the refrigerator at 39° F (4°C) for one and a half weeks (because I was waiting for my meat hook to arrive by mail). During the refrigeration time, I patted dry the top, bottom, and sides of the pork belly using a paper towel to keep it dry and turned the pork belly over about once a day, allowing each side to have a chance to air dry. The refrigerator smelled like vinegar as a result of the pork belly chilling out in there. My solution was to cover the pork belly in its glass dish with a paper bag to muffle some of the vinegar smell but not cut off the air supply. Then I hung it to dry in the cellar for several weeks. You know it's ready when the pork belly is hardened up and the colors have darkened. When it is dry like this, it is also very hard to cut or slice, therefore always wear a protective glove, at least for the hand that is not doing the cutting. This is where a mechanical meat slicer like they have at the butcher shop would be handy! But you can still manage to cut slices or make bacon cubes (*lardons*). Save the skin or rind (*la couenne*) to flavor soups such as **Bone Broth** (page 394) and stews such as **Beef Stew with Carrots** (page 116).

At one point, I saw that white mold was growing on the outside of the pork belly because the ambient temperature was a bit too warm (low 70°s, high 60°s F). Florent instructed me to wipe off the pork belly with a cloth soaked in vinegar and to allow the pork belly to continue its drying process. When finally hardened, it was very difficult to slice into bacon slices, but it tasted great. And I had the great satisfaction that I had made this "bacon" myself without any industrial chemicals.

In another attempt, I used a mixture of white wine vinegar and regular white vinegar, leaving the pork belly basking for 12 days in the salt, spice, and vinegar mixture. Thereafter, I left it in the refrigerator for 12 days and then hung it on the meat hook to dry in the cellar in much cooler air, as the season had changed from warm, early fall to cool, late fall temperatures. Again, the "bacon" was a success, if a bit salty. A shorter time in the salt and vinegar mixture and a longer time for desalination might have gotten get me closer to the original recipe and resulting salt-cured and dried pork belly (*la ventrèche séchée*).

On another occasion, upon receiving half a pig (which I paid to have deboned so I could write instead of spending the day carving out bones and butchering meat), I immediately cut the pork belly in half, "marinating" both pieces for only 5 days this time and desalinating each for one hour. I kept them stacked in separate glass casserole dishes, patting them dry and flipping them over once every day or so for 11 days. It took them about 3 weeks to dry. The result was less salty, perhaps because they had marinated for a shorter time. The fact is, the saltiness seems to be a bit unpredictable, at least for a novice like me. But at least I know there are no weird salts or preservatives in my ingredients. Just the pork belly in all its glory!

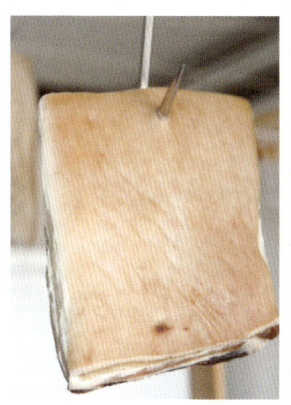

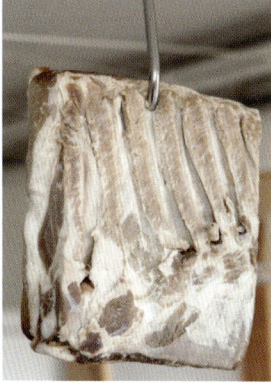

IN THE PASTURE

"The quality of the pastures, and thus the food of the bovines, is of primordial importance to obtain savory meat," says Jean-François Mallet in his French meat cookbook *Viandes*.[6] Joel Salatin would take this one step further and remind us that it is the richness of the *soil*

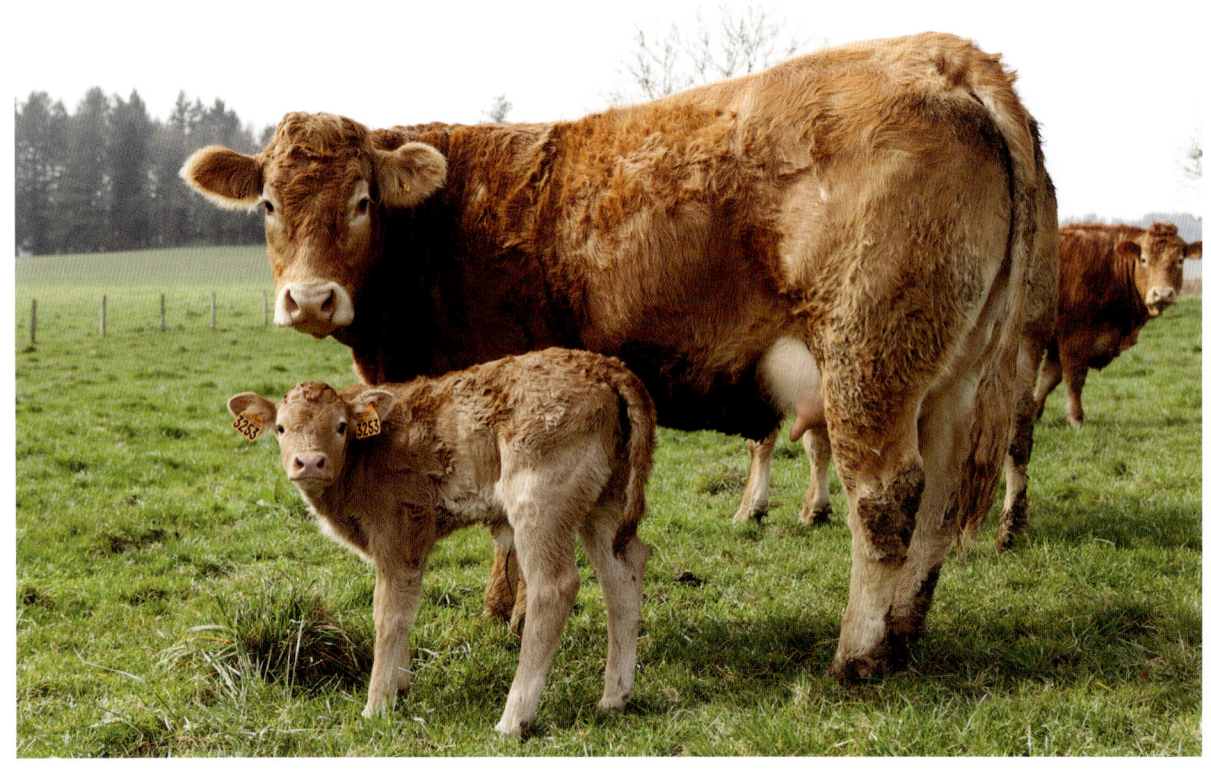

Organic Grass-Fed Limousine Cow and 3-Day Old Calf, Southwestern France

in the pasture that makes all the difference.[7] This biological ecosystem, starting with the soil and ending with the health of our bodies and communities, provides the foundation of an ancestral lifestyle. Animals in the pasture were meant to be there, and our proper management of these animals and lands are critical to the survival of this healthy soil-to-human ecosystem. French farmers, butchers, and cooks understand the link between pastured animals, quality, and taste and pride themselves on supporting this process to the best of their ability.

GRASS-FED VERSUS GRASS-FINISHED

Unfortunately, even France is not immune to the temptations and commercial "necessities" of using pesticides, antibiotics, and the widespread use of grains for the fattening up of animals before slaughter. Though much of France's "organically raised" livestock is grass-fed on pesticide-free grasses, it is still difficult to find grass-finished, as mentioned previously. Even French organic livestock farmers generally supplement with a mix of organic grains, particularly during that last month before slaughter. Visually, grass-fed beef fat is yellower than grain-fed beef thanks to the beta-carotene from the grass.[8] Compared to grain-fed beef, grass-fed beef is much higher in conjugated linoleic acid (CLA), a polyunsaturated omega-6 fatty acid that acts much like an omega-3 acid by lowering inflammation in the body and helping us to burn fat and regulate levels of our hunger hormone ghrelin and thus lower our risk of cancer.[9,10,11] Grass-fed beef is less marbled than grain-fed. Grass-fed beef tends to be leaner and tougher because the cow is not artificially "fattened" by grains. Grass-fed cows are allowed to graze on what they evolved eating, namely grasses. Grains fatten up herbivores, much like they fatten up humans. Also, most grains today are hybridized, and in the U.S., many grains are cross-contaminated with GMOs (genetically modified organisms), if not GMOs themselves. This is all the more reason to seek out grass-fed meats.

Note that grass-fed steaks tend to cook more quickly, and you should adjust the searing and cooking times accordingly. With a bit of experience and experimentation, you will find the right cooking times for your grass-fed beef.

When it comes to lamb in France, most fall under the category of 100% grass-fed and are slaughtered having reached a specific age or weight. Grass-fed lambs are taken to slaughter not long after they have been weaned and have transitioned to eating grass (technically, when they have reached adolescence). Certain types of lamb are milk-fed only (*agneau de lait*) and sold as such. A French butcher will stock lamb year-round but particularly around Easter for Easter lamb and springtime lamb dishes. (See **Springtime Lamb Stew** on page 213 and **Milk-Fed Lamb Roast** on page 205.) In France, the kind of meat required for a dish is a question of taste, tradition, and season, and the local butcher is attuned to this rhythm and tradition more so than the grocery chains are.

MEAT PROCESSING IN FRANCE

The general meat processing cycle begins with an animal that is raised for slaughter by the farmer and then sent to a certified slaughterhouse (*abattoire*). Organic abattoires have their own certifications, as do the farmers who supply them. A complicating factor is that by law, due to bacterial risk, poultry must be slaughtered separately from other species of animals. This adds to the loss of product in some instances, as well as the expense of dealing with more than one slaughterhouse if a farmer raises more than one species of animal. Indeed, at the butcher shop, I was instructed to thoroughly wash my hands after handling chicken before handling other meats again. The meat is distributed from abattoires to chain stores, some of which carry both conventional and organically raised meats. Organic food stores have their own supply chain and often receive meat from organically certified slaughterhouses, particularly if they have an in-house butcher, which not all have. Independent butchers have suppliers, or they go to markets in or outside their towns to purchase their meat.

A SENSE OF COMMUNITY AND ECONOMY

My friend Chef Fréd explained to me that right up until the 1980s, French villagers slaughtered their own pigs, making their own products and preserves to last through the winter and eat year-round. My own German relatives did this, up until around the year 2000. My German aunt and uncle slaughtered a village pig annually and created their own sausages to eat year round. This was a most economical and quality-assured way to feed one's family, as they knew the farmer who raised the pigs as well as his farm. It also brought the family together, with my uncle's brothers joining to help, each with his own skill set to contribute to the sausage, meat, and preserves production in the cellar of my aunt and uncle's home. In France, this is no longer allowed in villages. Pigs must be taken to special slaughterhouses, which of course costs the individual much more. This admirable annual ritual of making homemade, nutrient-dense, storable sausages and pâtés exemplifies the economical way of eating nose-to-tail while bringing members of the family together for a common purpose.

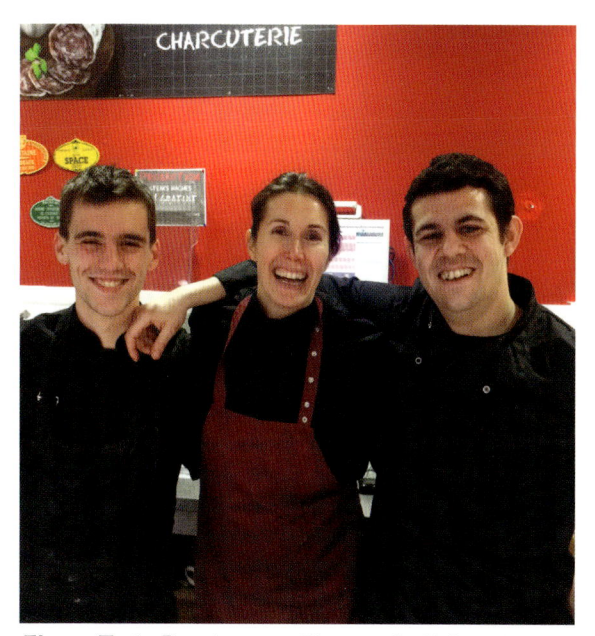

Florent, Tania, Romain Photo credit: Jérôme Mazurier

CHAPTER 5

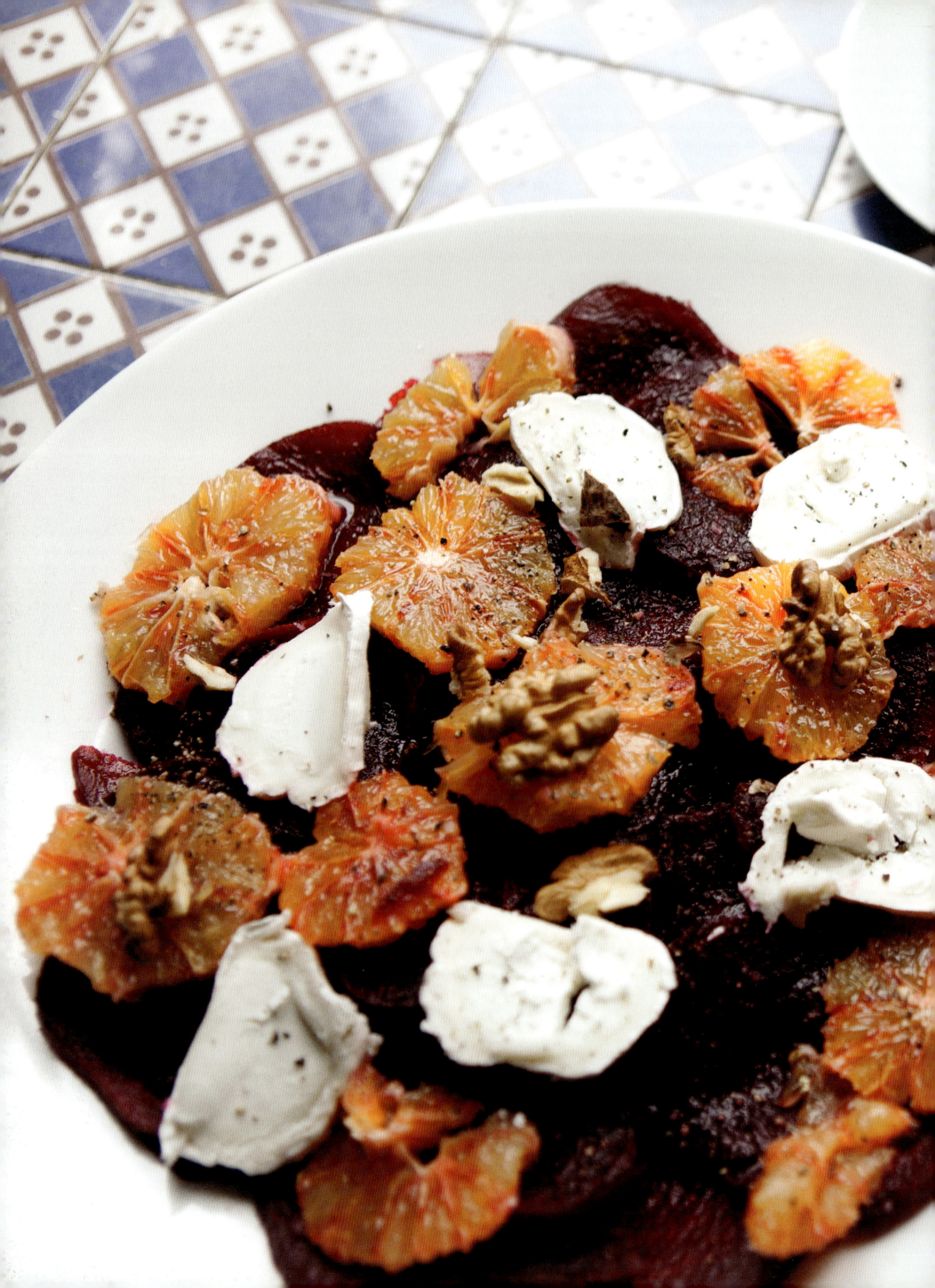

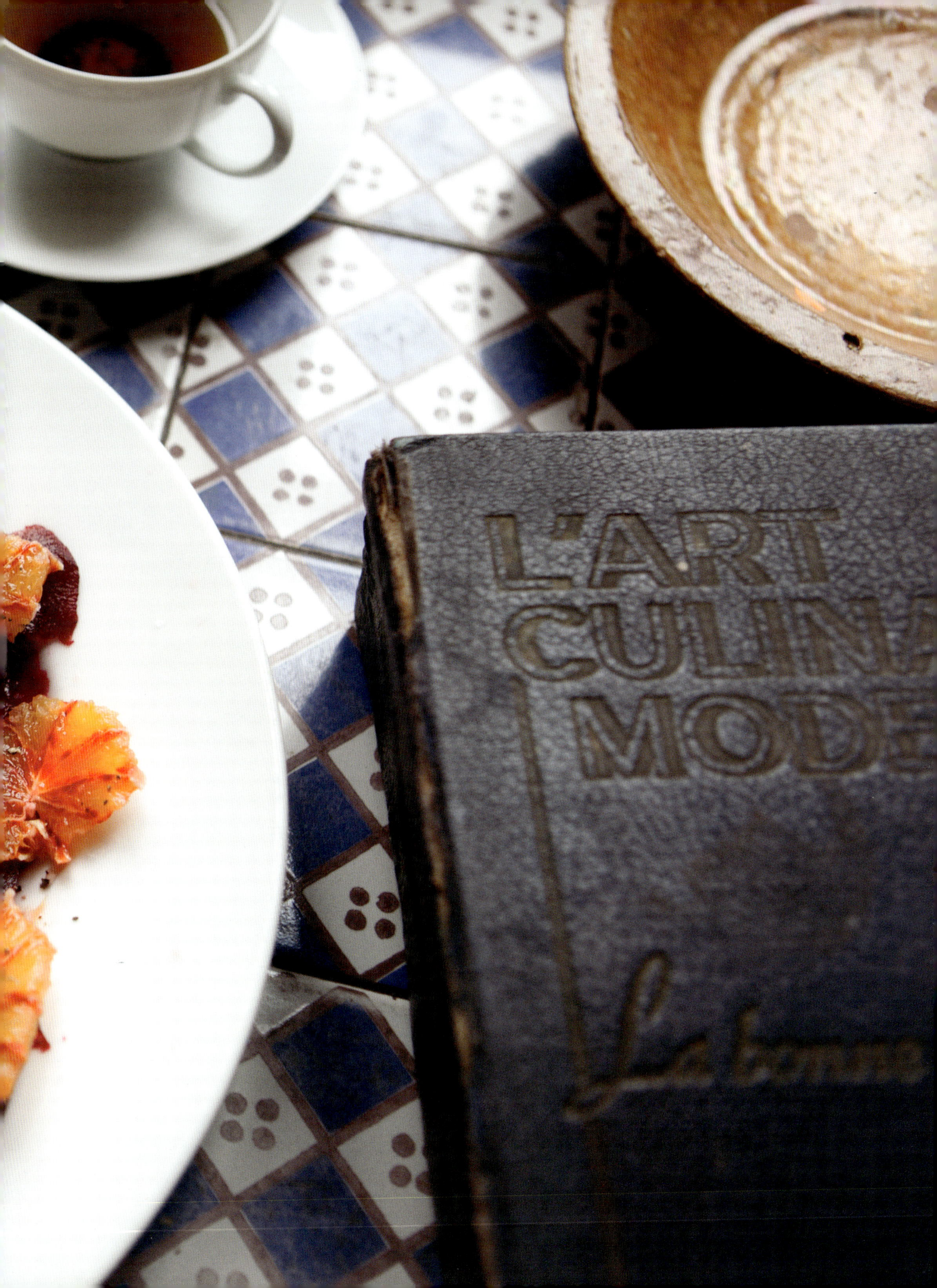
L'ART
CULINA
MODE
La bonne

RECIPES

Beef – *Le Boeuf* 107

Fish and Seafood – *Les Poissons et les Fruits de Mer* 159

Lamb – *L'Agneau* 189

Offal and Fats – *Les Abats et les Graisses* 217

Pork – *Le Porc* 285

Poultry, Eggs, and Rabbit – *La Volaille, les Oeufs, et le Lapin* 333

Stocks and Sauces – *Les Fonds, Bouillons, et Sauces* 381

Veal – *Le Veau* 419

Vegetables – *Les Légumes* 437

Desserts – *Les Desserts* 483

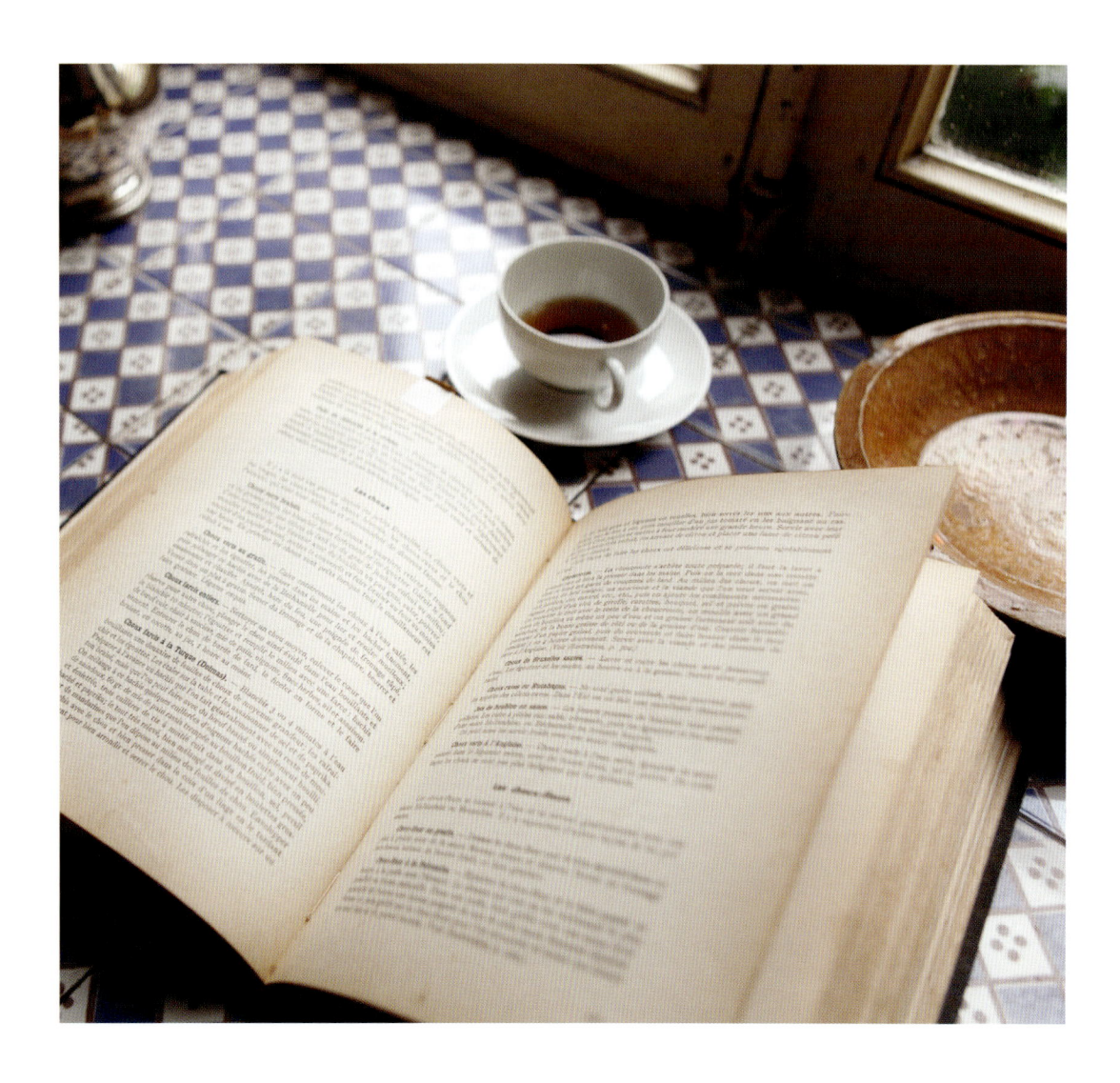

CHAPTER 6
RECIPES, STORIES, COOKING TIPS, AND WINE PAIRINGS

A FEW NOTES ON THE RECIPES

Here we arrive at the traditional French recipes of *The Bordeaux Kitchen*. At their core, the recipes, their ingredients, and how they are cooked follow the Tenets of the Bordeaux Kitchen as discussed in Chapter 2 (page 8). As I have explained, I have modified many of these recipes to align with a health-promoting primal-paleo approach while remaining true to the ancestral secrets of French cooking that I shared in Chapter 4: "farm fats," fresh ingredients, and cast-iron pots, along with wooden spoons and spatulas for stirring and sautéing, bone broths and stocks for sauces and soup bases, natural salts and spices that allow the ingredients to shine, and pairing the meal with an appropriate French wine. But before I set you loose in the kitchen, here are a few notes to help you make the most of each recipe with the right ingredients and equipment, background knowledge, and mindset.

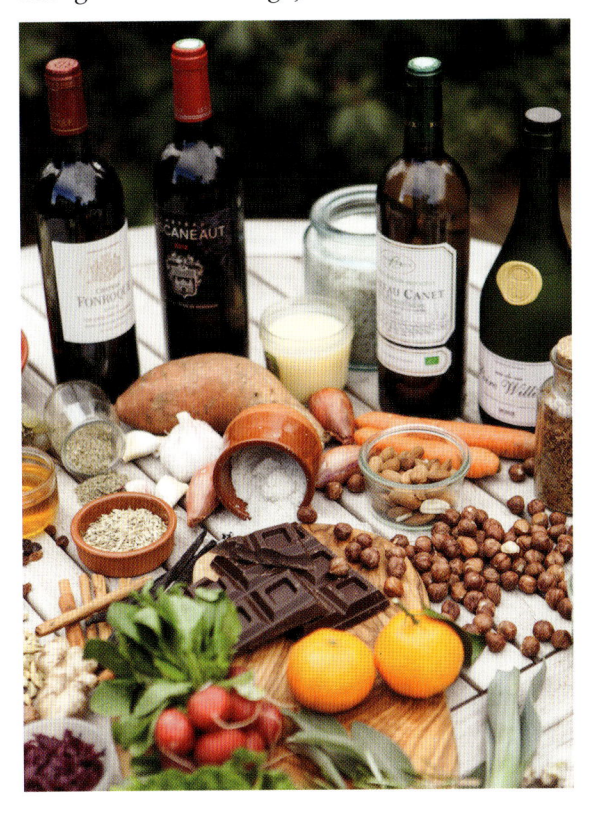

MAXIMIZE NUTRITION, CELEBRATE FLAVOR!

The recipes in *The Bordeaux Kitchen* represent the essence of French traditional cooking that maximizes nutrition while celebrating flavor. I have chosen specific ancestral French recipes that can be prepared in the primal-paleo spirit and with a "slow food" perspective which merits our renewed attention.

ENGLISH – *FRANÇAIS*

Throughout *The Bordeaux Kitchen*, I have in many cases provided French terms alongside the English ones for those who wish to learn some *authentic* French cooking and butchering terminology. You will also find a bilingual Cooking Glossary on page 597.

RECIPE ORGANIZATION

To bring the recipes to life, I have included anecdotes about the person from whom I learned the recipe, its history or regional origin, or some background information where possible. I have included some background about the cuts of meat, which are detailed in the corresponding animal diagrams. I have drawn from a number of disparate sources to create these unique reference diagrams of meat cuts in both English and French, something I could not find anywhere else. Personally, I find it very useful to be able to visualize where each cut comes from and therefore how it might best be prepared. As mentioned in the Butchery chapter, a rule of thumb primarily for beef and veal is that the front section (shoulder, neck, legs) are the tougher pieces of meat, requiring longer cooking times. (The pieces of meat from the front of the animal are tougher largely because these muscles are used more by the animal, as its center of gravity is forward as it bends down to feed on grass.) The mid-section and rear of the animals are the less tough and more expensive steak pieces which require less cooking time (unless it is the shank or tail, whose "meat on the bone" require longer cooking times).

THE CONCEPT OF PROPORTION

If you were to refer to traditional French cookbooks, you would find recipes in paragraph form, without many quantities specified other than "a little" or "several." A certain level of cooking knowledge was assumed, and cooks worked in proportions. In *The Bordeaux Kitchen*, as in all modern cookbooks, quantities are specified and amounts are measured out, though you will find an occasional ingredient such as a "handful" (of parsley), "several" of something, and most often a "pinch" (of salt, pepper or spice), which are remnants of a way of cooking that demand thinking in proportions. If an extra serving is needed for a dish for example, you will know how much of which ingredients to add. Over time, you will begin to "feel" or "sense" the right proportions required and customize the cooking and recipes to your needs.

MODERATION – *LA MODÉRATION* VS. THE PRIMAL-PALEO APPROACH

When I initially began collecting and learning recipes, it was difficult for me to convince cooks to modify their recipes according to my needs. Certain "traditions," even if only one lifetime deep, become embedded and are hard to change. It is difficult to get around the common French notion of *la moderation*, "a little of everything." (Farmer and sustainability advocate Diana Rodgers reminds us to think about who is benefitting from "everything in moderation."[1] To this I would add to think about upon *whose* moderation are you basing your limitations and excesses?) It is difficult to not sound extreme, for example, when I recommend avoiding all grains, especially to someone like my friend Chef Frédéric who says, "I am French, I must have my bread!" But even a little of something like gluten can mean a lot of problems for some individuals. At first I was worried about this, especially when we used ingredients such as dairy or alcohol that I knew might give *me* an immediate reaction. So, I examined every recipe and each ingredient to consider how I could adapt it to my dietary needs and a primal-paleo perspective. Overall, things turned out just fine, and they will for you, too! You'll figure out what works best for you, and you'll adapt ingredients as necessary based on the recipe or even the season of the year. There is also the other French adage, "Be moderate in your moderation."

SEASONS – *LES SAISONS*

For each recipe I note the most appropriate season for preparing the recipe, based on the availability and freshness of ingredients. Many grilled and some stewed meats can be eaten year-round. It is the availability of vegetables and certain fish that fluctuate most with the seasons. Even certain meats and cheeses, due to animal growth and birthing rhythms, have seasons when they are more readily available and at their most flavorful for consumption.

PREPARATION TIME – *TEMPS DE PRÉPARATION*

Don't set your clock by the "Preparation Time," as it is more of a rough guide. Preparation time is going to be different for each person and each set of ingredients. Some people read, organize, or chop faster than others, depending on their personal experience with reading recipes, their ability to function in the kitchen, and even the sharpness of their knives. (I now make a point of honing my knives before almost every use, especially since it really only takes a few extra seconds of time. Cutting and chopping are so much more pleasant as a result.) The "Preparation Time" estimates are often just my "best guess," because I am inevitably cooking (or doing) other things simultaneously, as you will likely be doing. Unless you are microwaving a TV dinner (unlikely, if you are reading this book!), you will be making several things at once in the kitchen in a juggling act that can be challenging, but ultimately satisfying. For me what seems to take a lot of time is collecting the necessary ingredients. So, I try to line those up on the counter and prep them ahead of time—the French call this *mis en place*—to ease the time crunch later.

If you take the time to slow down, "Preparation Time" can also be a time for reflecting on and anticipating the meal, preparing your body for good digestion, and transitioning into a parasympathetic state, where the body is in the "rest-and-digest" mode (as opposed to the sympathetic "fight-or-flight" mode) and ready to receive and absorb nutrients. Therefore, the longer you take, and the slower and more deliberate you are, the more time you will have to transition into "chill out" mode, not to mention the more pride you will have in the nutrient-dense meal, packed with love, that you will have prepared for yourself and your family. If you are in a bit of a hurry making dinner, however, preparing ingredients may not be so relaxing. But, you can at least be thinking about those who will enjoy the meal and who may be adventurous, or squeamish, about trying a particular dish. While my husband will eat just about anything with great pleasure, my children are a tougher crowd to please. Therefore, when the kids like it, I know it tastes good and that my repetitive food introduction strategies have worked! (For more on this, see Chapter 8 for a discussion of family food organization and meal planning.)

Factor in ample time to prepare your recipes whenever possible. Guests invariably go for seconds when you have put a little extra time, care, and lots of fresh ingredients into the preparation of your meals. I now understand the great sense of satisfaction with which my grandmothers, aunts, and parents prepared special meals for me. Feed someone a good meal, and they will likely always remember it.

COOKING TIME – *LA CUISSON*
Temperatures for ovens and stoves and pots and pans (made of different metals, layers, and thicknesses) will vary, and therefore cooking times and results will vary. You can calibrate your oven temperature using an oven thermometer to ensure accuracy, as they are not always properly calibrated. This will give you a sense of how high or low you should set your oven. I have "learned" my oven's temperatures (and temperament) by noting how long something takes to cook at a certain temperature. By getting to know your equipment you will know what the temperature gauge means for your cooking time in the oven and on the stove. Experiment and increase or decrease the heat accordingly. Every time we move, it takes a month or two, sometimes longer, to understand the idiosyncrasies of our "new" kitchen appliances. We have moved 11 times in 20 years, so I know that it takes a while to adapt! I often employ a dial meat thermometer for checking internal temperatures when cooking roasts.[2] I have supplied charts for "Degrees of Doneness" and cooking temperatures in the respective recipe sections for beef (page 119), lamb (page 193), and pork (page 307), and also in the Cooking Glossary (page 597). Sometimes I use a digital thermometer with a probe that goes into the oven to stick into terrines or pâtés (or into a pot when making sauces to make sure a certain temperature is not breached). The digital attachment remains outside the oven to give you the internal temperature. Unlike baking, cooking home meals in many cases can be less precise and more like an experiment. Rather than feel intimidated, I see it as an opportunity to use what I have in the kitchen and to try out new things, allowing room for "mistakes." What's the worst that can happen? Most of the

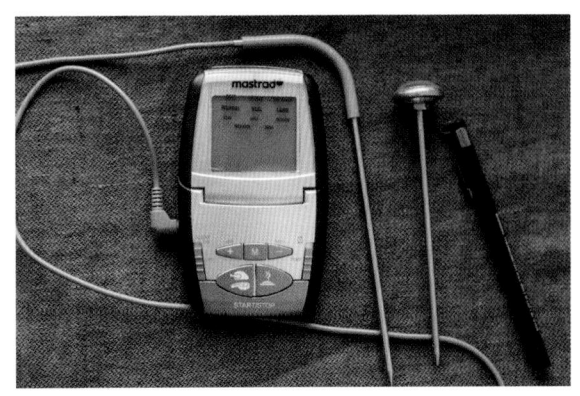

time, if you are not checking your social media accounts while searing a steak, you will not burn your food.

Those with time constraints might tend to shy away from "complicated and time-consuming" recipes under the false belief that there is not enough time and that the challenge is too great. But if we understand that the reward of a good meal goes beyond its consumption, we can see that it is worth taking the time to gather all the interesting and fresh ingredients and incorporate them into a meal, like a work of art, and to share this with family and friends. Cooking becomes an anticipatory, confidence-boosting process, with the potential to create memorable meals to relish again and again. What cook isn't proud after mastering a new technique or method? This is positive reinforcement at work, and a great example for children and for potentially doubtful family members. I encourage you to take the time and try something new. It's the only way to learn and expand, with mysteries solved and discoveries made along the way! Fall back on your stand-bys on days when time is truly short.

A FEW NOTES ABOUT SERVINGS
The number of servings and serving sizes can vary if you or those you are serving eat smaller or larger portions than the "average" calculated for each recipe. Since everyone has varying portion preferences depending on the meal, the time of day, or whether it is being served as an appetizer or a main dish, etc., "serving size" is a bit ambiguous. But after you have made a recipe once or twice, you will get to know how many servings it will actually make for *your* family and *your* situation.

In general, I have accounted for about a minimum of 5 to 7 ounces (150 grams to 200 grams) for an adult serving (much less for the desserts and starchy carbohydrates). Thus, a 2.2-pound (1 kilogram) piece of meat will feed five to six people or a family of four with leftovers for one or both parents' lunches the next day. If you are used to smaller portions, then this amount of meat will last you longer. In fact, those following a low-carb and nutritionally ketogenic diet (fat burning, mitochondrially boosting) for the prevention and reversal of modern-day chronic metabolic (cancer, diabetes) and neurodegenerative diseases (Alzheimer's, MS, rheumatoid arthritis), will cycle their protein serving sizes to as low as 1 gram per kilogram of calculated bodyweight (0.035 ounces per 2.2 pounds of lean body mass).[3] For most adults, this works out to about 30 to 60 grams (one to two ounces) of protein per day (thus, a smaller serving size or sizes), while they also restrict carbohydrates to under about 50 grams (1.8 ounces) or less per day.[4] (A low-carb approach may count protein in a range from 1.2 g to 1.8 g per kilogram (0.042 to 0.063 ounces per 2.2 pounds) of "ideal" lean body mass (or 25% to 30% of calories from protein), a somewhat larger serving size or sizes of protein per day, along with a slightly higher amount of carbohydrates (60 to 70 or more grams, or 2.1 to 2.5 ounces) per day (not counting the fiber content of the carbohydrates, and depending on the individual's needs).[5] Following such a regimen therefore, the number of servings of meat or fish, for example, noted in each recipe in this book could be doubled or tripled. Everything depends on your dietary needs. And as I have noted previously, once you have made a recipe once or twice, you will see how long it lasts you, based on your family's needs. When you have leftovers, these may be frozen in family-size or individual-size portions. Freezing leftovers is also helpful if you are histamine-intolerant, as the growth of histamine-producing bacteria on meats halts in the freezer, but continues in the refrigerator. You can also feel free to halve or double any recipe, depending on how many leftovers you want or need.

Keep in mind that each meat or fish dish, prepared with delicious fats, will likely be served with raw, cooked, roasted, steamed, or sautéed vegetables, also accompanied by delicious fats. In fact, as you increase the amount of quality animal fats and olive and coconut oil in your meals, you will probably find that you need less protein and fewer starches, and have fewer cravings, because *you will feel satiated sooner and longer.* Thus, your serving size(s) might very well decrease as your body becomes adapted to ingesting and burning higher proportions of fat, a condition called "keto-" or "fat-adapted."

INGREDIENTS AND MEASURING

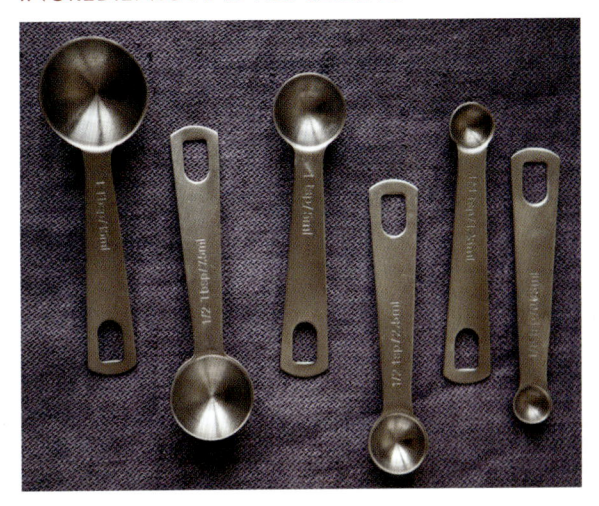

The amounts and quantities of ingredients may vary as well, depending on a person's taste and sensitivities, the seasonality, or the availability in the pantry. I have tried to write the recipes listing the ingredients in the order of their use in the dish. While I do not specifically indicate that ingredients should be organic, please know that I am referring to organic products. For fats, meats and dairy, I suggest "organic and grass-fed" sources, according to your ability to find them and your desire to use them.

The recipes and ingredients are measured in U.S. measurements for quantity and volume, but I have also provided the metric conversions. The French use teaspoons (*cuillère à café*) and tablespoons (*cuillère à soupe*) in their recipes, therefore I have not converted these. Something I have found very useful, thanks to recommendations by my chef friends Frédéric Schueller and Dewey Markham, Jr., who are more precise than I am in their cooking, is a kitchen scale. I now have a digital scale that converts metrics into the U.S. standard measurements for weight and volume. When I am cooking recipes I know by heart, I go by what looks and feels like the right amount of one ingredient or another. If you are not already there in your cooking, you will get there, too!

Before attempting a recipe, scan the list of ingredients; they are generally listed in the order they are needed. Gather and prepare each item (such as garlic minced, carrots chopped, etc.) and line them up in bowls or on cutting boards on your counter if this helps you visually. Then it is a matter of following the directions, step by step. I will admit that I myself do not always carefully read through every step or ingredient list and then find I am stuck without something or running out of time. Things get easier when you become accustomed to making a particular recipe and learn the ingredients by heart, or even have some garlic or herbs chopped ahead of time. In general, I recommend having cubed bacon pieces (*lardons*) and chicken stock (or some sort of bone broth or stock) on hand at all times, as these figure in so many recipes. It is also easy just to have a cup of bone broth or sauté up some lardons with a chopped green vegetable as an easy meal or side dish.

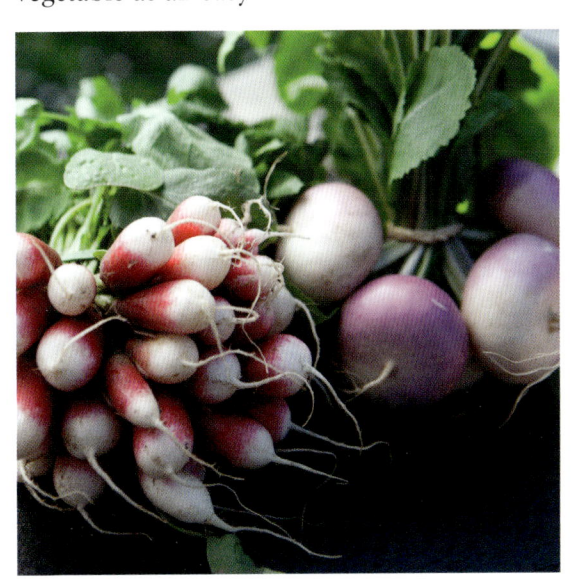

Radishes and Turnips

If ingredients will be sautéed or boiled together, I sometimes recommend cutting ingredients (such as carrots, onions, potatoes, turnips, parsnips) in a uniform size so that they cook through at a similar rate. Other times I may recommend adding certain ingredients, such as mushrooms, potatoes, or sweet potatoes, toward the end of the cooking time so they do not fall apart during the long-cooking duration of the rest of the dish.

IT STARTS WITH FAT

I begin many recipes instructing you to "melt the tallow" or "melt the butter," and by this I mean to allow these to melt and bubble a bit so you know they are hot and ready to receive the meat or vegetable. Whenever I list "olive oil," I mean organic, extra-virgin olive oil. With regard to butter, I use raw, organic sweet cream butter, adding salt to the dish separately. If you choose to use salted butter, you may need to add less salt in a particular dish. Clarified butter and ghee are very similar and are sometimes used or suggested in recipes as alternatives, but feel free to substitute them for butter or other fats, as their smoke point is higher than butter and they are both generally more tolerable to people who react to butter, thanks to the lower casein protein content.

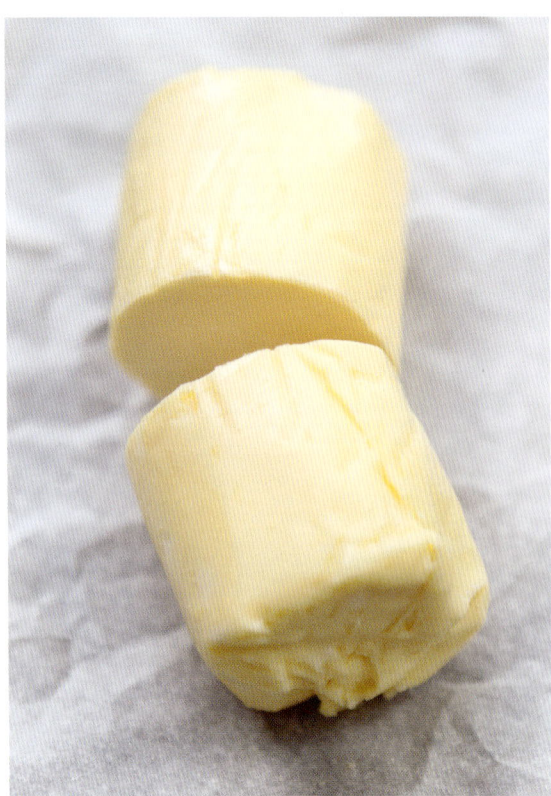

French Butter

FARM FATS: WHY DOES ONE RECIPE CALL FOR ONE TYPE OF FAT AND NOT ANOTHER?

When I recommend a certain amount or kind of fat to melt in the pan, feel free to add *more* fat or another fat that you have in stock, such as replacing butter with ghee, tallow with lard, or lard with butter. For example, adding olive oil to fish, meat, or vegetables or allowing bacon fat to melt over any of these foods directly after cooking can add to the flavor and to the healthy fat content of the meal.

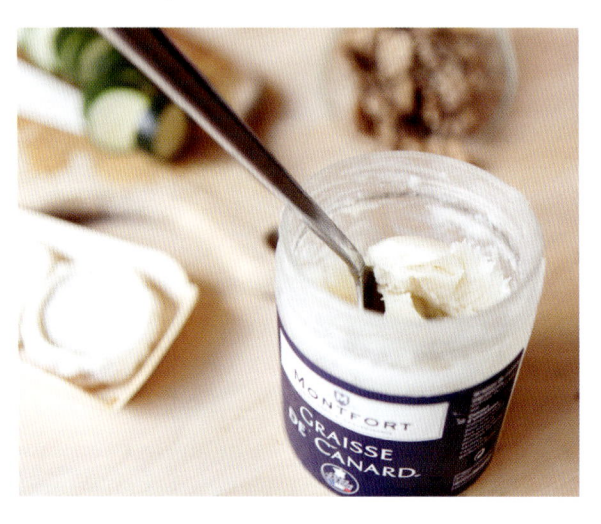

While each recipe calls for a certain kind of fat, depending on the regional origin (remember from Chapter 1 Waverley Root's four fat regions of France, and tallow, the Fifth Fat?), ingredients, and cooking methods, you can always experiment, especially when food sensitivities and allergies or dietary restrictions must be taken into account. Butter is the optimal flavoring and cooking fat in many French dishes, but certainly not the only possibility. Clarified butter, ghee or entirely non-dairy options like coconut oil, avocado oil, or a virtually tasteless rendered lard, are all good choices, depending on the recipe or inclination of the cook. There is evidence in the early French cookbooks and documents which review them of multiple types of fat being used for one dish, either to augment flavor, or in response to economic viability or overall availability.[6]

Many recipes call for olive oil, which is inevitably heated. I keep my oven temperatures usually to a maximum of 365°F (185°C) when oven cooking with olive oil to prevent the olive oil from burning, while retaining the flavor and allowing for a reasonable (not too long) cooking duration. For certain fish recipes, where the fish are sautéed in olive oil (mackerel or sardines, for example), it is a matter of taste originating from the Atlantic, Basque, or Mediterranean coastal areas. Use your own judgment in the case of heating olive oil. Oils such as macadamia nut oil or avocado oil, with higher smoke points, could serve as replacements. Where sautéing with olive oil is concerned, you decide when you prefer to use olive oil or other fats based on your own needs and tastes. Historically, olive oil and butter have been mixed with other fats to enhance flavor (and increase the smoke point, as discussed on page 39) if available and economically viable.

A good French butcher who keeps "like with like" will offer in his shop window beef roasts wrapped in raw, thinly-sliced leaves of tallow and pork roasts wrapped in thinly-sliced strips of lard. However, I have been surprised to find that even the meat-centered, butcher-endorsed French cookbooks of today list vegetable oil, olive oil, or butter for cooking in the recipes, but almost never tallow and very rarely lard as the cooking fat. Pieces of bacon end (*bout de lard* or *bout de ventrèche séchée*) are used in some recipes for flavor enhancement, and as it turns out, this is another secret and undeniable tenet of French cooking. Rendered lard, however, is not usually called for in actual sautéing, searing, or frying food. It is very rare to find a French recipe these days using beef tallow. Using tallow, lard, and animal fats, however, was necessary from the end of the Middle Ages up to when margarine was invented in France in 1869. People *had* to use animal fats, as that is what they had at their disposal. Cooks also used fats such as butter for pastries or olive oil in cooking certain dishes according to familial, regional, and societal tastes and availability (which often depended on social class during certain periods of French history and the fashions of the times).[7] I like to imagine a local Southwest French butcher recommending our French great-grandmother a **Springtime Lamb Stew** (page 213) using *suif*, lamb tallow as the cooking fat, but also perhaps along with some duck fat, butter, or olive oil for added flavor.

Whatever "farm fat" we use, keeping in mind the concept of nutrient density and diversity will help guide us in our ancestrally-minded cooking. Using what is available and fresh and cooking with minimal waste are both key elements in considering what to cook, an economical and environmental way of approaching our food.

SALT AND PEPPER

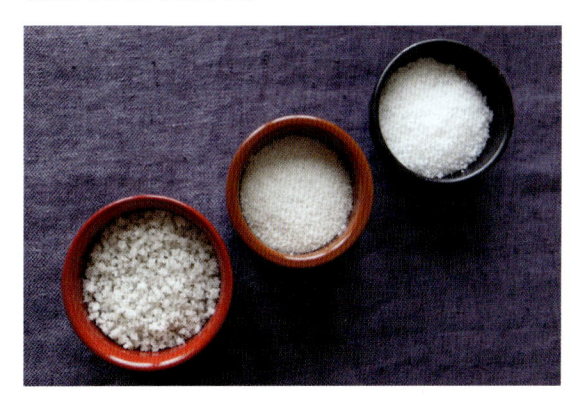

Sea Salts Left to Right: Coarse, Fine, and Fleur de Sel

I learned from French chef Frédéric Schueller that a "pinch" is using your thumb and first two fingers to grab salt, pepper, or a ground spice; this turns out to be slightly less than ⅛ teaspoon. The best way to get a pinch is to have your salt, pepper, or spice in a small bowl, ready with space enough for you to be able to dip in your fingers and pinch what you need. When a recipe calls for "salt," I mean "Celtic sea salt" (sea salt from France, *bien sûr!*), and I will indicate whether it should be fine (*sel de mer fine*) or coarse (*gros sel de mer*). If not, use what salt grain size you have on hand. Fine or coarse pink Himalayan salt or American-mined pink Redmond "Real Salt" sea salt from Utah may be substituted if you prefer this type of "ancient sea" salt or do not have Celtic sea salt. Both pink and Celtic salt are mineral-dense. *Fleur de sel*, the

CHAPTER 6   99

top layer of Celtic sea salt that dries on the surface of seawater in a salt bed and is hand harvested and highly valued, is made of fine, crunchy salt crystals, does not taste as "salty," and is crunchy and beautiful. It makes for a wonderful garnish. You may wish to garnish every dish, even sweet ones, with *fleur de sel* (I do!) Flaky and kosher salt variants exist as well. You will find your favorite among the many types and over time understand how they enhance the flavor of your dishes.

When I say "pepper," I am talking about "freshly ground black pepper," unless otherwise indicated, which you can either grind out of a pepper mill or grind by hand using a mortar and pestle. Grind pepper as you need it, because the peppercorn oils are delicate and go rancid easily. The flavors of freshly ground pepper are much enhanced when compared with pepper that has been sitting, already ground, in a jar for weeks or months on end. If I mean for you to use whole peppercorns, I specify these in the ingredients list.

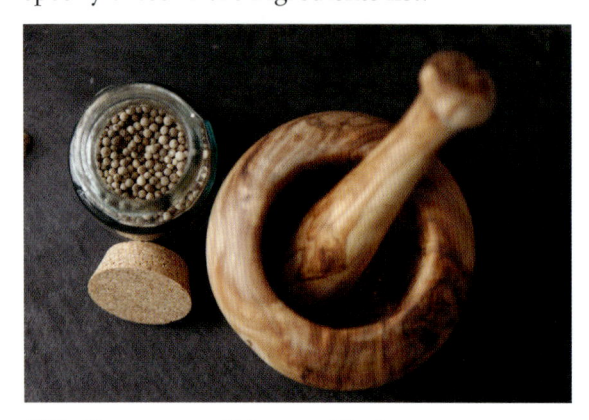

White Peppercorns and Mortar and Pestle

Black peppercorns are harvested unripe and sun-dried, turning them black and giving them that slightly smoky aroma and peppery flavor. White peppercorns have been allowed to ripen, then are fermented and the skins are removed. The aromas and flavors of white peppercorns are more subtle, but also more complex and vegetal. White pepper is often used in recipes to "hide" the pepper in white-colored foods, such as potatoes. If you have a favorite pepper mix of multi-colored peppercorns, please feel free to use it, experimenting with the amount needed for the intensity you wish to achieve. There is some evidence that pink peppercorns are less allergenic than black or white,[8] but they are also in the cashew (tree nut) family. I go easy on the pepper for dishes I cook for my children, as their palates are more sensitive to spices.

When a recipe calls for "salt and pepper to taste," I mean for you to add as much or as little as your palate desires. I find that even coarse sea salt can be generously applied to fresh food, as it elevates the flavor without the need for sauces or common American condiments like relish, mayo, and ketchup.

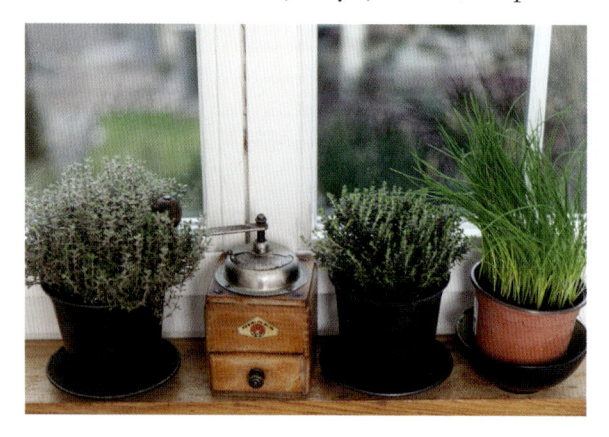

HERBS: FRESH VS. DRIED

For simplicity and flexibility, I have often listed "fresh or dried" for my two favorite and most frequently employed herbs, rosemary and thyme, without making any distinction in quantity to be used in the recipe. Some say to use ⅓ or ½ dried to one part fresh because the aromatic oils are more concentrated in dried herbs, and they are denser with flavor than a fresh herb. I find fresh herbs more potent in aroma and flavor and less prickly in the mouth, especially fresh rosemary. My preference is usually to use fresh herbs, but I tend to use about the same amount of a dried herb such as thyme as that of a fresh herb. When it comes to a larger leafy herb like sage, I usually use only fresh sage. You might actually want to add more dried sage in cases where fresh sage is called for. Sage when dried is quite shriveled without its water content. Try to find fresh sage (or grow it) if possible; the flavor it adds to a dish like **Chicken**

Hearts (page 230) really makes the dish. If you have an herb garden, which I highly recommend even if it is a small windowsill pot, you will not have to rely on expensive store-bought herbs and can always have fresh herbs on hand. Remember that the freshness of ingredients is one of the secrets to French cooking!

> **Chef's Tips** – *Astuce du Chef*
> Here and there I will give culinary or related tips straight from the chefs with regard to the recipes I have learned from the chefs themselves.

"SERVE WITH" SUGGESTIONS
Though you may always choose your own favorite accompanying vegetables, for most meat and fish dishes, I have noted common, in-season side dishes served with each dish, but preferably cooked or dipped in rich amounts of "farm fats!"

VARIATIONS
I offer variations on the recipe, ingredients to include or swap, and optional (*facultatif*) ingredients or procedures. Keeping the options varied, you can base your cooking on what you have available or what you might like to try. This opens the door to more experimentation (*experimentation*), improvisation (*improvisation*), and creativity (*créativité*)!

WINE PAIRING TIPS
Eating food and sipping wine is a sensory-dense experience, slowing you down to enjoy the meal. As my friend, and cooking and wine professional Dewey Markham, Jr., says, when it comes to food and wine pairing, "the most important thing is to *avoid the horrible*. After that, it's all experimentation and finding what you like." Choosing a wine to go with a food (or a food to go with a wine) can seem daunting, but, as Dewey says, "Whether you are in a restaurant in front of a wine list or in a wine shop, chances are you'll hit on something *okay*. Anyway, is this a beauty contest or are you hungry and want to order a drink?" So do not worry too much about the plethora of choices. When you are in good company, pretty much any good quality wine will do.

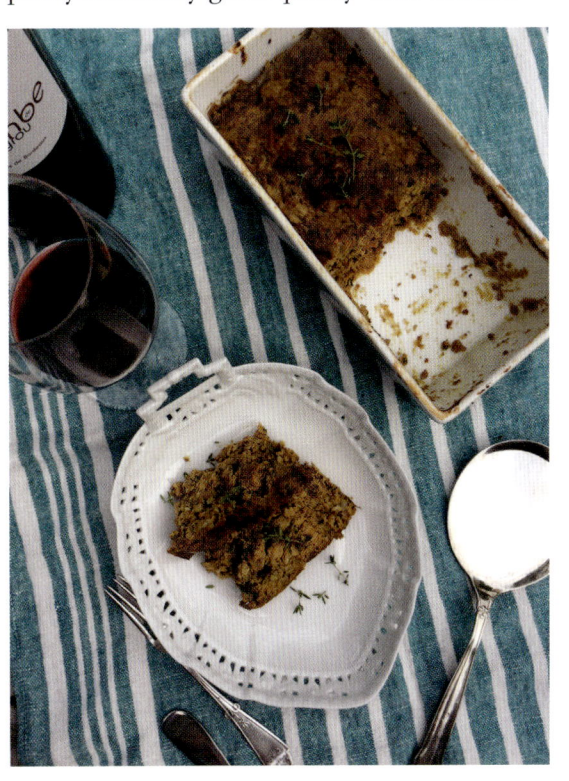

With regard to pairing wine with the recipes in this book, I have drawn upon my experience from my year-long professional wine tasting "DUAD" course in Bordeaux, where we tasted, rated, and discussed local and regional French wines, as well as some international wines. I have also asked my esteemed Bordeaux wine professional friends and my fellow wine course classmates for their pairing recommendations. For certain wine pairing tips, I have researched recommendations by international sommeliers and French and English language wine and cooking websites and other resources. I have also referred on occasion to Julia Child's *Mastering the Art of French Cooking*. And in some cases, I will have tasted certain meals with certain wines with friends and family and can recommend those. All wine recommendations are for French wine. After all, *c'est la France*! Use these recommendations as a guide when ordering wine online or purchasing wine from a wine shop, whether the recommendations name a specific wine, a grape variety, or a region. Again, the suggestions are for French wines, but you may find something similar by asking the wine purveyor what they might recommend based on these suggestions and your preferences. That way, you will be more likely to find the French wine you are looking for or an international or American equivalent.

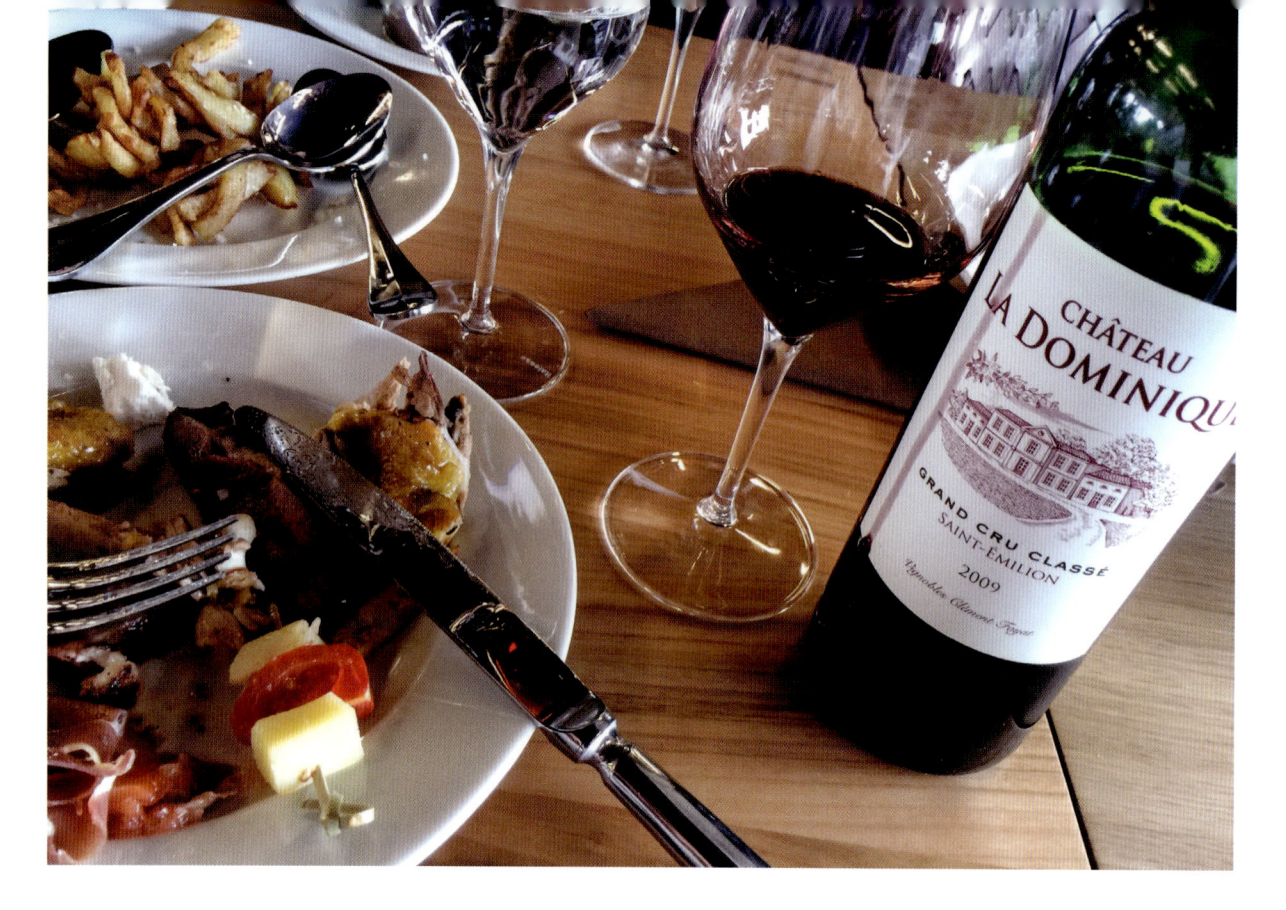

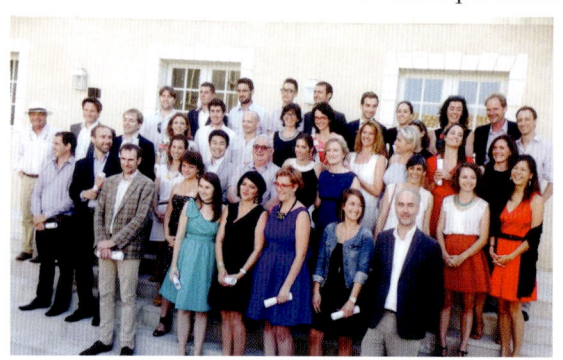

2015 DUAD Graduates and Professors

When organizing a menu for family or friends, Dewey recommends putting all the ingredients together in your mind and imagining them with the wine or wines you are thinking about serving (or ordering, if you are in a restaurant). If you have a budget large enough, you can even try a wine or two before deciding which one to buy more of for your guests. Once you have made your match, allow yourself to focus on the sensory and emotional experience of the wine, especially when it's combined with food and good company.

FOOD AND WINE PAIRING: A SOMMELIER'S APPROACH

Annabelle Nicolle-Beaufils, one of my very astute and resourceful University of Bordeaux DUAD[9] wine course classmates, a professional sommelier (*sommelière*), cellar master (*caviste*), wine competition tasting judge (*jurée degustation – concours de vin*), and former restaurateur, helped me with many of the food and wine pairings for this book. The many food and wine pairing recommendations for specific recipes Annabelle has provided are often based upon whether the meat (or fish) has been roasted, stuffed, covered in a sauce, braised for several hours, or grilled for several minutes, as all these cooking techniques affect both the meal and one's perception of the accompanying wine. Annabelle spent three years recommending wines at her restaurant in Bordeaux to go with the delectable creations her husband, Chef Jean-Luc, made daily for lunches and dinners. I have much confidence in and gratitude for her thoughtful suggestions.

According to Annabelle, the first question when pairing a wine with food is to first ask yourself (or the customer, in Annabelle's case), *what wine do you like*? If the answer is a type of grape or wine or region, then she makes suggestions on that basis. Otherwise, if there is no particular preference and a recommendation is requested, she will offer the most typical wine pairing with the particular dish in her experience as the sommelier at her restaurant. Or, she will suggest a wine that goes well with some aspect of the dish, for example, one with a spicy, fruity, creamy, or acidic sauce. (To learn more about French wines, refer to Chapter 7: Know Your French Wines, How to Taste Them, and How to Pair Them with Food.) The only problem with a delicious wine pairing is that you will want to take a sip with each bite, which can add up to more wine than you might initially have wanted to drink!

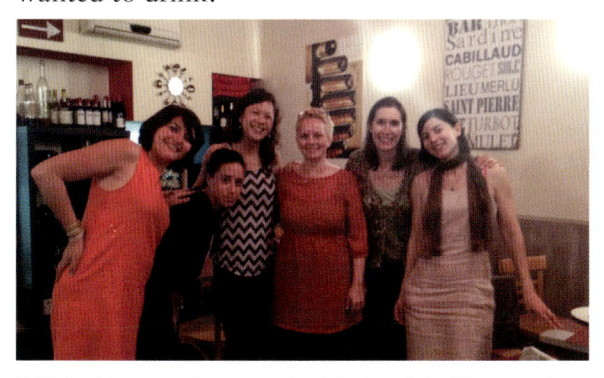

DUAD Classmates Laeticia, Elsa, Vy, Annabelle, Tania, and Anne at Annabelle's Restaurant in Bordeaux

KITCHEN UTENSILS AND EQUIPMENT – *MATÉRIEL DE CUISINE*

When I say "pan," I mean either a cast-iron pot (*une cocotte en fonte* or *une marmite*), a cast-iron pan (*une poêle en fer*), or a stainless-steel pot (*une casserole*) or pan (*une poêle en inox*). If you do not have a cast-iron pot with a lid, please go buy one now. I recommend a *Staub* or *Le Creuset*, as they will last you for life and can be passed on to the next generation, just as they have been in French families for generations. (Chef Frédéric uses his grandmother's cast-iron pots.) The pot may be enameled on the outside and the inside, though I prefer no enameling on the inside where the food cooks. I have two such (large) circular pots, 11 inches (28 cm) and 10 inches (26 cm) in diameter, and one (medium) oval pot, 10.6 inches (27 cm) in diameter, and sometimes I need to use a fourth! No family should be without one.

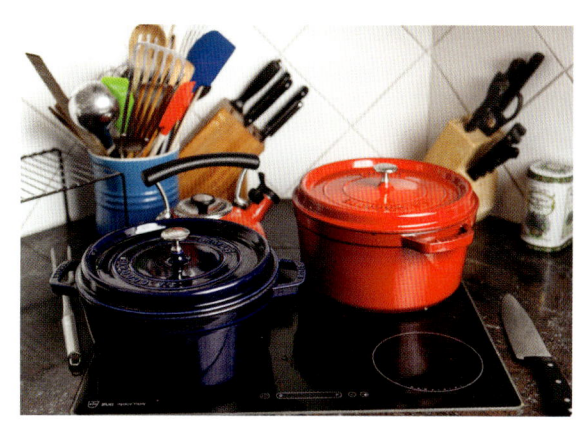

I do not recommend ever using cheap "polytetrafluoroethylene" or other coated pans, as the food is more easily burned in a cheap, thin pan, and the toxic plastics flake and wear off, going into the food. Who knows how much toxic transfer there is from these heated plastics while we are using them to cook? Unfortunately, I used these kinds of pots and pans for years before I understood their toxic hazards. The same goes for plastic spatulas. I use silicone spatulas for scraping fat out of jars and cooled pans, but not for stirring in a hot pan. For stirring hot food in hot pans and pots, I use wooden, flat-edged spatulas or spoons, or else stainless-steel slotted spoons and ladles. I use wooden cutting boards which will not dull one's knife like glass or ceramic boards. I only use a large plastic cutting board while I am butchering raw meat, as I do not have a wooden cutting board large enough for this task. The plastic cutting board generally goes into the dishwasher for disinfection on these occasions, though butchers will still use wooden butcher's blocks and scrape these clean with a sharp-edged scraper on a daily basis. For sauce making and sautéing, I use multi-layer saucepans because they are thick enough to make sauce in them without burning it, including melting chocolate, forgoing the need for a double boiler. I use the seven-layer *Demeyere* (from Belgium) saucepans for sauces, and their frying pans for searing and much of my "faster" cooking. Otherwise, I have a couple of good old American "Lodge" cast-iron skillets 8-inches (20 cm) and 11-inches (28 cm) in diameter, along with several smaller round and oval *Staub* cast-iron skillets. Feel free to try some recipes using a slow cooker or an Instant Pot, though the timing and results will likely vary.

A FEW OTHER NOTES ON COOKING

Following are a few of my recommended techniques. See also the Cooking Glossary for cooking terms (in English and French) as well as "doneness" (*la cuisson*) of meats and other terms to help guide you.

WHY PREHEAT THE OVEN?

Preheating the oven gets the oven to the right cooking temperature *before* you put the food in. So turn that oven on as you walk into the kitchen (some ovens take longer than others to heat up to the desired temperature).

WHY USE GLASS?

For the oven, I recommend using oven-safe glass, clay (terra cotta) dishes, and ceramic or cast-iron pots and pans as much as possible to reduce the toxic load from treated metallic pans such as "cookie sheets," as these usually have some coating which essentially is a plastic. Plastics and other coatings leach their toxins into food, especially when heated or frozen.

Allow food to cool off before putting it in the refrigerator or freezer. One technique suggested by Dewey, who is a trained chef, is to place, for example, a freshly made pot of hot soup in a sink filled with cold water and ice (essentially giving the pot an ice bath) before putting it in the refrigerator. If this is not possible, then he recommends placing a wooden spoon beneath the pot to allow air to circulate for swifter cooling of the soup and pot. I pour my hot soups in glass containers and place those on flat, raised racks, which also allow air to circulate underneath the containers to cool the soups more quickly.

I recommend freezing meats, vegetables, broth, and sauces in glass containers, and not filling them all the way, as the liquids will expand as they freeze. Wrap up any meat in butcher's or parchment paper when possible before wrapping them in plastic, if glass is not an option. When I am freezing bones and vegetable ends for future bone broth or stock making, I place them in paper bags from the organic store and, if I am really organized, sometimes I label the contents. Then when I go to make the broth, I can easily spot the bags in the freezer and know what is in them.

THAWING FROZEN FOODS

When thawing food, allow sauces or vegetable dishes to thaw on the counter. Meat thaws slowly but safely in the refrigerator overnight. If the piece of meat is more than one-and-a-half pounds (680 g), then it may need 24 hours to thaw completely. For a quick thaw of smaller amounts of meat, including ground meat or sausages, a half-hour in a bowl or tray of room temperature or cold water works as well. Make single-serve or family size portions ahead of time and freeze them in glass containers for easy thawing when you need a meal quickly. When I'm really pressed for time, I have found that even frozen portions of these "ready meals" in thick glass containers need only a few minutes on the counter before heating in the oven. This is not ideal because the outside of the food will heat more quickly and dry out, but it's better than nothing.

EXPERIMENT!

Remember that there is room for experimentation, especially after you have done a recipe once or twice. Some of the dessert recipes where eggs or cream are involved might need adhering to a bit more strictly. However, there is always room for more or less sweetener, again depending on one's tastes and needs. In many of the recipes, I have offered variations and options, where I have thought of them, but you may find your own ideas, adding flourishes of your own. This is part of the fun of being the cook!

Just get the basics down and then go from there. Got meat or fish, some vegetables, salt, and fat? It's all good food, just apply heat, and you will make it work! My family and I have come a long way from packaged cereal (though my children still have some granola or oatmeal occasionally), soy chicken nuggets, and pasta. It was not so long ago that we had juice and bread with jam for breakfast and my children would only eat the whites of eggs. Now they spread liverwurst on either store-bought organic spelt crackers or grain-free **Seedy Crackers** (page 501) at breakfast (and sometimes for dessert), and that's a step in the nutrient-dense direction, even though the store-bought crackers are not grain-free. (Their diet is not always my diet.) It has been about a three-year process to come to a place where our meals are as nutrient dense as they are today, and there is still more to be incorporated. Although my husband and I would love to take credit for our girls' good behavior and attentiveness in school, I think it is more thanks to their breakfasts of bacon, eggs, liverwurst, and raw vegetables every morning that they start the day off right and carry through with adequate motivation and concentration, after having also had a hearty warm dinner the night before, no screen time at night, and a good night's sleep.

GOOD FLAVOR TAKES TIME
Remember that "quick and easy" is not necessarily better. As we have discovered, French cooking is founded on the process of slow cooking. And most dishes, and the ones with the most flavor, are those that have either been slow-cooked in the family cast-iron pot or that incorporate a long-cooked stock or broth. Chefs and cooks around the world who follow the basic French culinary principle of always having a stockpot full of broth brewing to use as the foundation for sauces, gravy, or as extra flavoring for their dishes understand that good flavor takes time.

ONE RECIPE AT A TIME
While there is no need to feel like you must make an award-winning meal every time you cook, the key is to feel capable of adapting as you go. I, and the people I have cooked with, almost invariably swapped ingredients, left things out, modified amounts, and added ingredients, depending on the parameters within which we were working. Try not to allow the feeling of intimidation to get the better of you. How does anyone, even Julia Child back in the day, learn to cook? *One recipe at a time.*

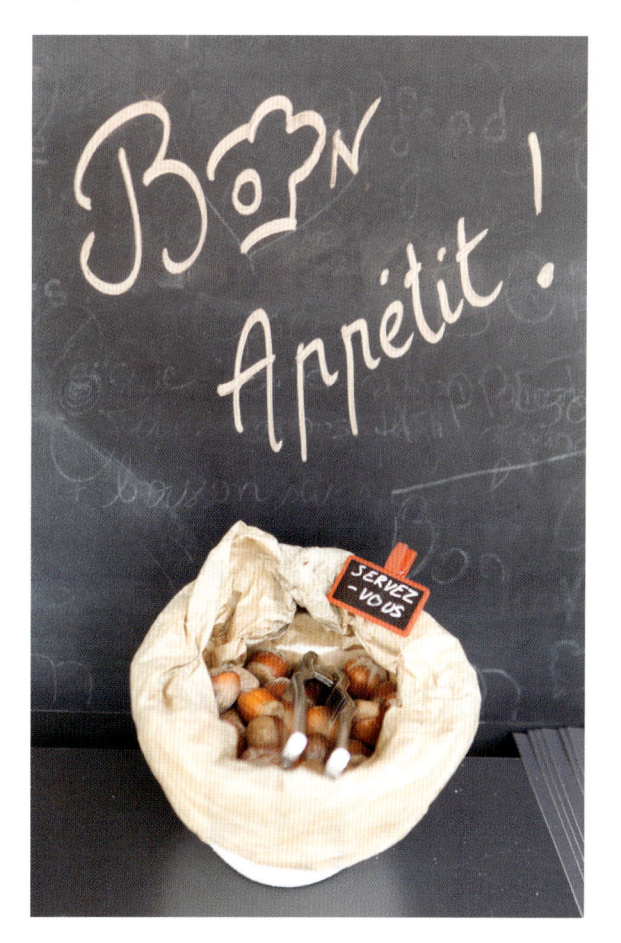

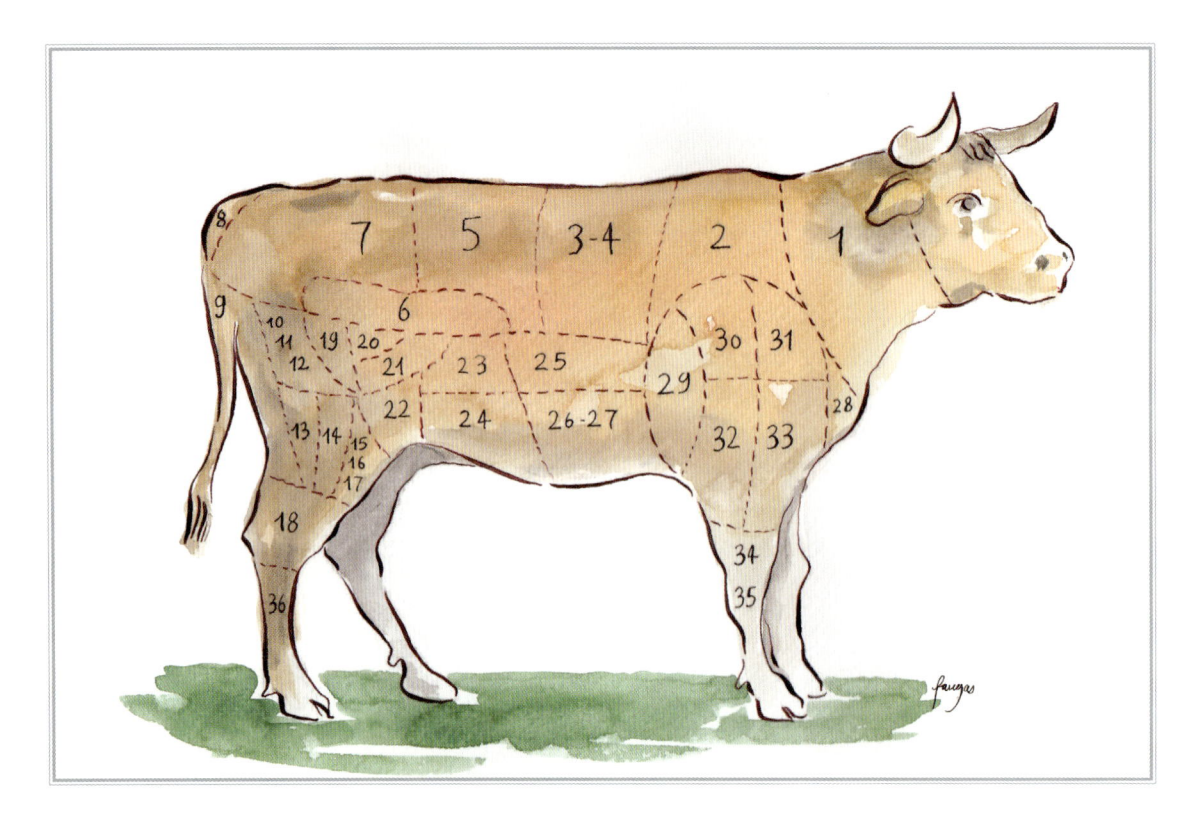

BEEF – *LE BOEUF*
DIAGRAM KEY

1. Neck – *Collier* (Use: Ground, Roast, Stew)
2. Fore Chuck or Upper Chuck – *Basses Côtes* or *Entrecôtes Découvertes* or *Train de Côtes* (Use: Chuck Roast, Steak)
3. (Bone-In) Prime Rib Steak – *Côte de Boeuf* (Use: Roast, Steak)
4. (Boneless) Rib Eye Steak – *Entrecôte* (Use: Roast, Steak)
5. Top Loin, Top Sirloin or Strip Loin – *Faux-Filet* (Use: Roast, Sauté in Pieces, Steak)
6. Beef Tenderloin – *Filet de Boeuf* (Use: Roast, Sauté in Pieces, Steak)
7. *Coulotte* (Top Sirloin Cap) or Sirloin (Top Sirloin Butt) – *Rumsteck* (Use: Roast, Sauté in Pieces, Steak)
8. Oxtail – *Queue* (Use: Stew)
9. Round – *Rond de Gîte* (Use: Carpaccio, Ground, Roast, Steak, Tartare)
10. Inside Topside – *Tende de Tranche* (Use: Roast, Steak)
11. Sirloin or Topside – *Poire* (Use: Roast, Steak)
12. Sirloin or Topside – *Merlan* (Use: Roast, Sauté, Steak)
13. Eye of Round, Round or Thick Flank – *Gîte a la Noix* (Use: Ground, Roast, Steak, Stew, Tartare)
14. Spider Steak – *Araignée* (Use: Steak)
15. (Inside) Round – *Plat de Tranche* (Use: Steak)
16. (Inside) Thick Flank – *Rond de Tranche* or *Tranche Grasse* (Use: Steak)
17. (Inside) Round – *Mouvant* (Use: Sauté in Pieces, Steak)
18. Hind Shank – *Gîte* or *Jarret Arrière* (Use: Stew, Marrow)
19. Tri-Tip (Bottom Sirloin Butt) – *Aiguiette Baronne* (Use: Roast, Steak)
20. Hanger Steak – *Onglet* (Use: Steak)
21. Skirt Steak – *Hampe* (Use: Steak)
22. Flank Steak – *Bavette d'Aloyau* (Use: Steak)
23. Flank Steak (Bottom Sirloin Butt) – *Bavette de Flanchet* (Use: Steak)
24. Flank Steak and Suet – *Flanchet et Suif* (Use: Ground, Steak, Stew, Tallow)
25. Plate (Short Ribs or Thick Ribs) – *Plats-de-Côtes* (Use: Grill, Stew)
26. Breast, Brisket or Plate – *Tendron* (Use: Ground, Steak, Stew)
27. Breast, Brisket or Plate – *Milieu de Poitrine* (Use: Ground, Stew)
28. Brisket – *Gros Bout de Poitrine* (Use: Ground, Stew)
29. Brisket Beefsteak or Chuck Steak – *Macreuse à Bifteck* (Use: Steak)
30. Brisket, Chuck or Thick Ribs (Shoulder) – *Paleron* (Use: Steak, Stew)
31. Brisket Beefsteak or Chuck Steak – *Jumeau à Bifteck* (Use: Steak)
32. Brisket or Chuck – *Macreuse à Pot-Au-Feu* (Use: Stew)
33. Brisket or Chuck – *Jumeau à Pot-Au-Feu* (Use: Stew)
34. Fore Shank or Shin – *Gîte* or *Jarret Avant* (Use: Stew, Marrow)
35. Fore Knuckle or Shank or Shin – *Crosse* or *Gîte* or *Jarret Avant* (Use: Stew)
36. Hind Knuckle or Shank – *Crosse* or *Gîte* or *Jarret Arrière* (Use: Stew)

BEEF
Le Boeuf

Beef Burgundy – *Boeuf Bourguignon* 109

Beef Roast – *Rôti de Boeuf* 113

Beef Stew with Carrots – *Boeuf Carottes* 116

Beef Tagine Stew – *Tajine de Boeuf* 121

Boiled Beef Stew "Pot-Au-Feu" – *Pot-au-Feu* 123

Bone-In Prime Rib – *Côte de Boeuf* 125

Braised Oxtail – *Queue de Boeuf* 127

Flambéed Sirloin Steak with Cream Sauce – *Pavés de Rumsteck Flambés, Sauce à la Crème* 129

Flambéed Sirloin Steak with Sautéed Vegetables – *Pavé de Rumsteck Flambé avec Garniture de Légumes à la Poêle* 131

Flank Steak with Shallots – *Bavette à l'Échalote* 133

Grilled Rosemary Beef Skirt Steak – *Hampe de Boeuf au Romarin* 135

Ground Beef Parmentier – *Hachis Parmentier* 137

Peppered Roast Beef – *Rosbif au Poivre* 141

Roquefort Sirloin Steak – *Pavé de Rumsteck au Roquefort* 143

Sage Butter Sirloin Steak – *Pavé de Rumsteck au Beurre à la Sauge* 145

Slow-Cooked Beef Shank – *Jarret (Gîte) de Boeuf* 146

Spider Steak with Orange – *Araignée de Boeuf à l'Orange* 148

Wine-Braised Beef Stew with Orange – *Daube de Boeuf à l'Orange* 151

Wine Trader's Rib Eye Steak – *Entrecôte Marchand de Vin* 155

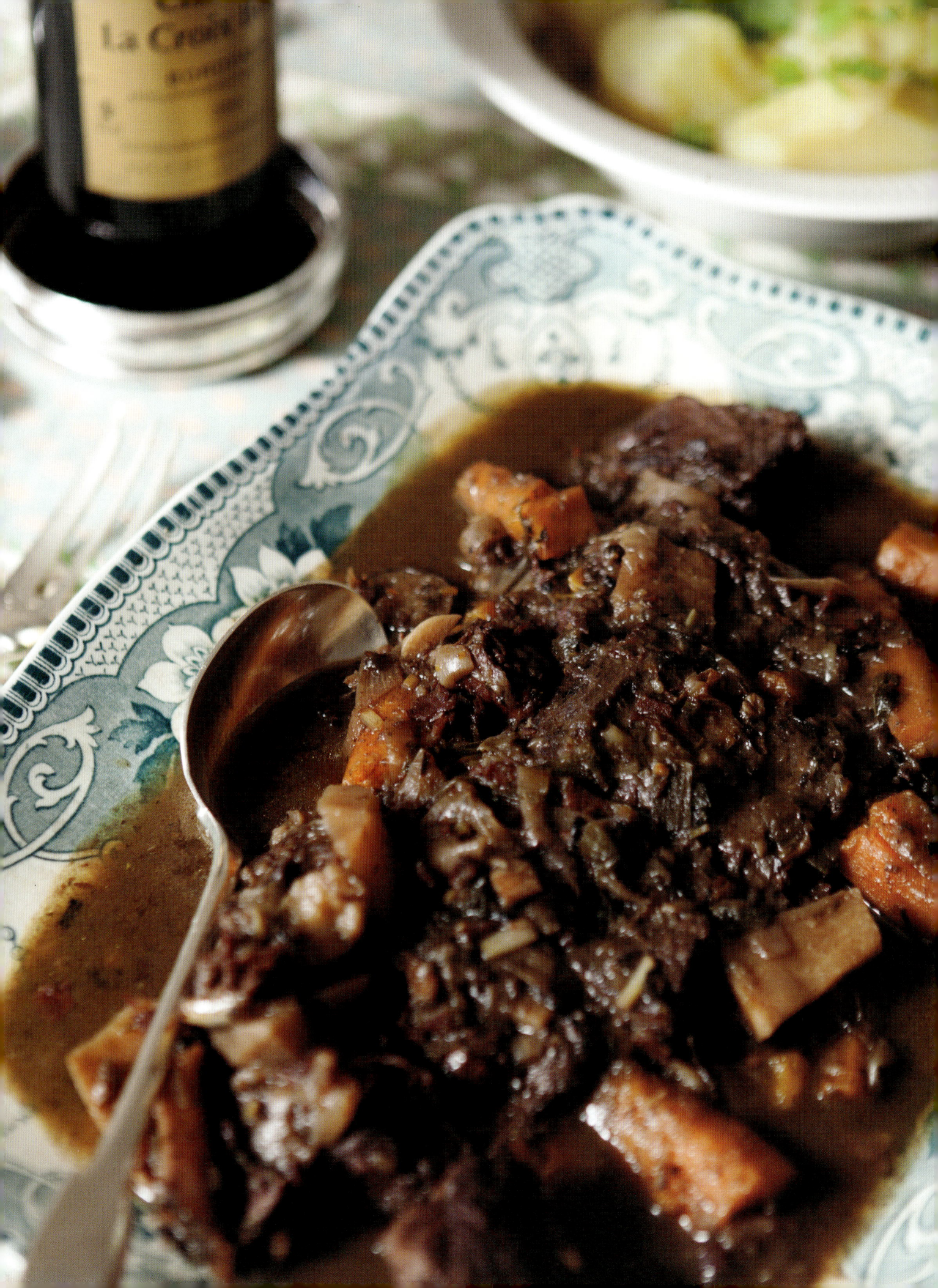

BEEF BURGUNDY
Boeuf Bourguignon

Season Autumn and Winter   **Preparation Time** 30 minutes
Cooking Time 2 hours minimum, preferably 3 to 4 hours   **Serves** 6

We begin the beef chapter with perhaps the best-known French recipe, which also is seen to be more complicated than it needs to be. Following this simplified version step by step should alleviate this worry. A long list of ingredients need not mean that a recipe is complicated or difficult. Bourguignon is the adjective for Bourgogne, Burgundy, whose wine (particularly from the northern Burgundy regions of Côte de Beaune and Côte de Nuits, both of which make up the famous Côte d'Or, or "Golden Slope" of Burgundy), made from the Pinot Noir grape, figures in the original recipe, along with beef from the Charolaise cow, also from the Burgundy region. Of course, over the centuries, cooks have taken liberties, as they do, to experiment with adaptations of the original. Here, my lovely friend Joelle Luson, a mother, grandmother and cook, used a Bordeaux wine, as we were cooking in Bordeaux. Originally from Nice, Joelle and her English husband, Peter, lived for many years in Belgium and England, but Joelle never forgot her roots, always preparing French traditional dishes for her family and friends.

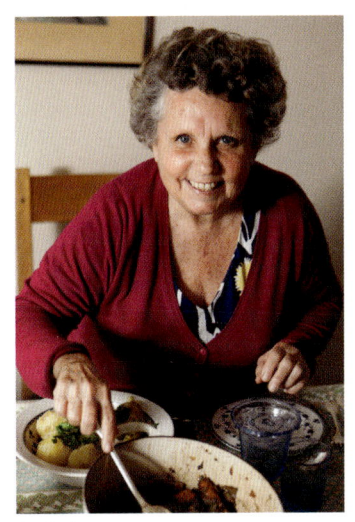

Joelle Luson

This truly classic French country dish uses tougher cuts of meat, from the breast (*flanchet*, *tendron* or *poitrine*) or neck, "blade," or shoulder area of the cow (*paleron* or *macreuse*), and is at its best when cooked for at least two hours or more in a cast-iron pot. The longer a meat cooks on low, the more tender it becomes. (In fact, this dish can cook on low through the night and will be even more flavorful the next day.) Note the following butcher's meaty secret: Remove the meat from the refrigerator and allow it to come to room temperature before heating it, so as to cook it evenly as well as to not give the meat a thermal shock, causing the muscle fibers to contract and harden.[1] To augment the flavor in many French dishes, including this classic recipe, cured pork belly cut into small pieces or ½-inch (1 cm) cubes (*lardons*) is often added. Canadian bacon or "regular" bacon strips cut into smaller pieces may be substituted. If you are avoiding mushrooms, add another onion to this recipe. Butter is traditionally used in this recipe, but ghee, olive oil or tallow (*suif*) certainly could be used instead, each bringing its own flavors to the end result. We also replaced the usual white flour with local, organic chestnut flour. According to Joelle, adding a square or two of dark chocolate reduces the acidity of the dish. It also intrigues the chocolate lovers among us! ➤

BEEF – LE BOEUF

4 tablespoons butter

9 ounces (250 g) carrots, chopped into circular pieces (*rondelles*)

7 ounces (200 g) bacon cubes (*lardons*)

9 ounces (250 g), about 6 to 8 small mushrooms, wiped off and sliced

2 onions, chopped

3.3 pounds (1.5 kg) chuck roast, cut into 1-inch (2.5 cm) cubes

4 tablespoons chestnut flour, for flouring the meat cubes

Bouquet garni (see the side bar on the next page)

1 celery stalk

Optional: 2 squares of dark chocolate

2 garlic cloves, crushed

1 tablespoon fresh or dried parsley, chopped

8 peppercorns

Pinch of sea salt

5 to 6 shallots, chopped, or 12 pearl onions

2 cups (½ L) beef or veal stock

1 or 2 turnips, cut into eighths

2 cups (½ L) red wine, usually a Pinot Noir from Burgundy

Melt two tablespoons of the butter in a pan over medium-high heat, and then brown the carrots, *lardons*, mushrooms, and onions.

Melt the other two tablespoons of butter in a cast-iron pot over medium-high to high heat. Roll each cube of meat in the chestnut flour and add to the pot, browning on each side. (The flour creates an unctuous texture around the meat, but it may be avoided if desired. But do not forget to brown the cubes, regardless!)

Transfer the vegetables and *lardons* from the pan into the cast-iron pot with the meat. Add the *bouquet garni*, celery, chocolate, garlic, parsley, peppercorns, sea salt, shallots, stock and turnips. Pour in the wine last. Stir and cover the pot. Cook for a minimum of two hours on low. (Three to four hours is even better, or else overnight, on very low heat.)

Remove the *bouquet garni* before serving in a beautiful dish. Serve with boiled potatoes garnished with minced parsley, or serve with other prepared vegetables.

WINE PAIRING TIP My wine course buddy and experienced restaurateur and sommelière Annabelle Nicolle-Beaufils, who recommended wines to her clientele in her family-owned restaurant for more than three years, suggests powerful and structured wines to go with this flavorful dish, such as Merlot and Cabernet Franc blends, heavy with ripe red berries, from St. Emilion or Pomerol in the Bordeaux region, a spicy Bandol from Provence, a tannic Cahors from the Southwest with notes of cherry and cedar, or a spicy, full-bodied red from the Rhône Valley. You can also finish off the wine you used to cook with, whether a Burgundy or a Bordeaux, or do like the pros do, and buy two bottles of the same wine, cooking with one, drinking the other!

Garnished Bouquet
Bouquet Garni

A bouquet garni is a small bundle of aromatic herbs, usually comprised of bay leaf, leek, parsley, rosemary, thyme, and/or savory, tied together with string or in a cheesecloth.

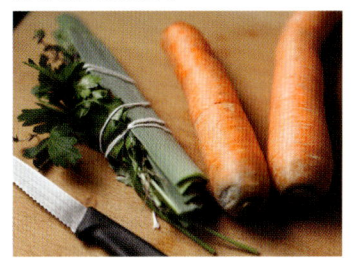

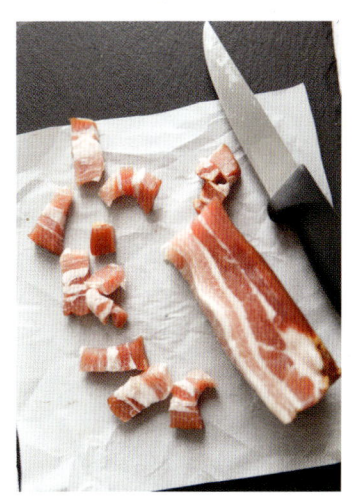

Lardons

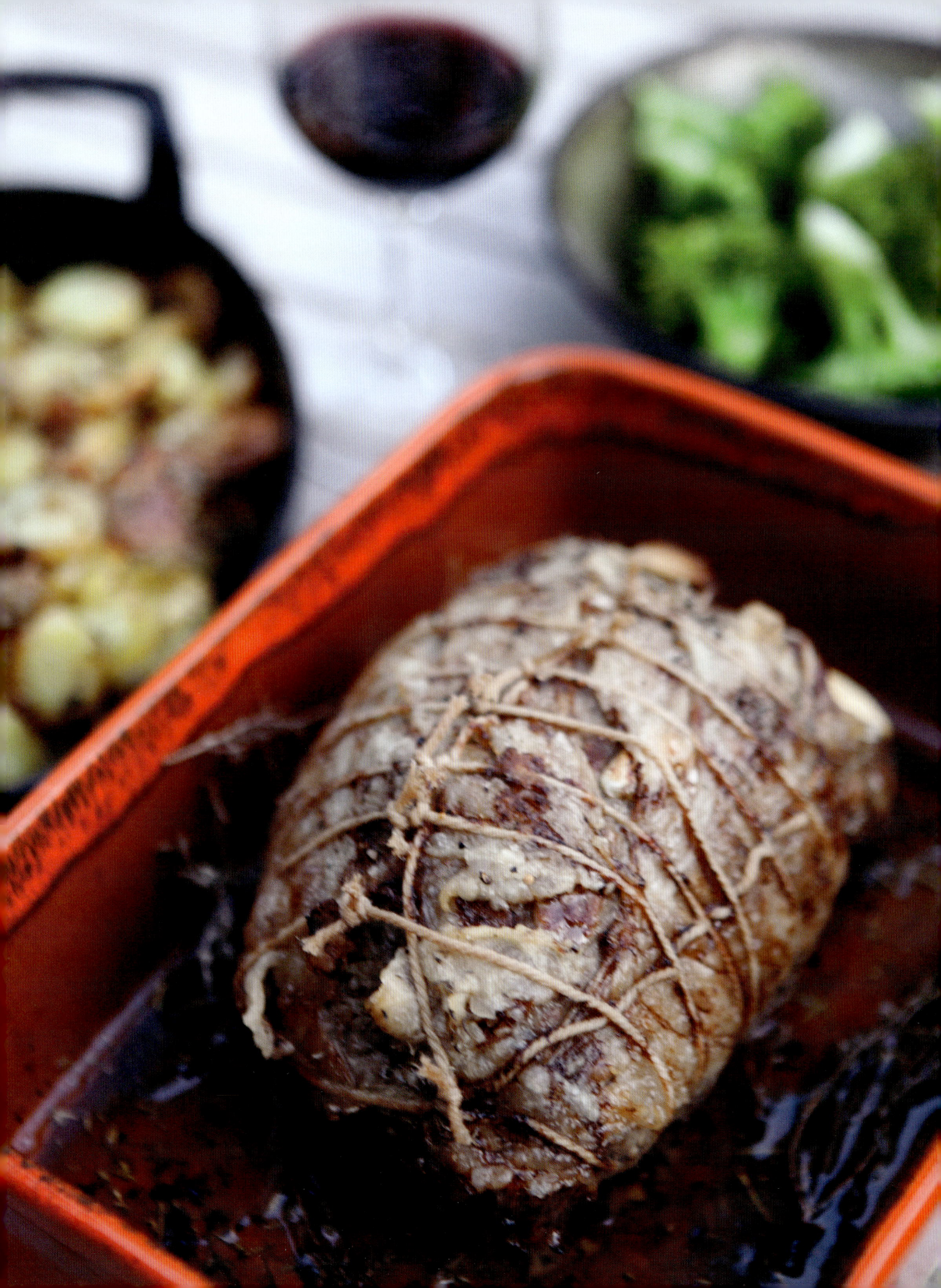

BEEF ROAST
Rôti de Boeuf

Season Year-round   **Preparation Time** 10 to 15 minutes to bard and tie up the roast
Cooking Time 8 minutes to brown, 30 to 35 minutes in the oven   **Serves** 6

This preparation of beef loin (*longe*, *filet* or *faux filet*), using thinly-sliced pork "fatback" lard, bacon fat, or beef fat with which to wrap or "bard" (*barder*) the meat, is also commonly used for other French meat roasts of lamb, pork, and veal. In the case of a veal roast, usually cuts from the rump (*quasi*) or the round (*noix*) are used. The technique using fat and string (*la barde et la ficelle*) makes for an eye-pleasing package in the butcher's window or on your dinner table, it maintains the shape of the roast during cooking, and it provides a bit of fat around otherwise lean pieces of meat that might burn or dry out on the edges without the added layer of fat. (See pages 82 and 83 for photo tutorials on using "butcher's" or "cooking" string to tie a roast.)

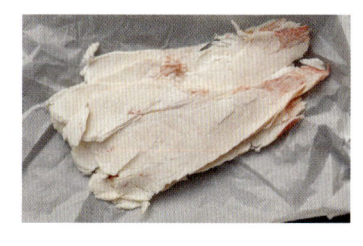

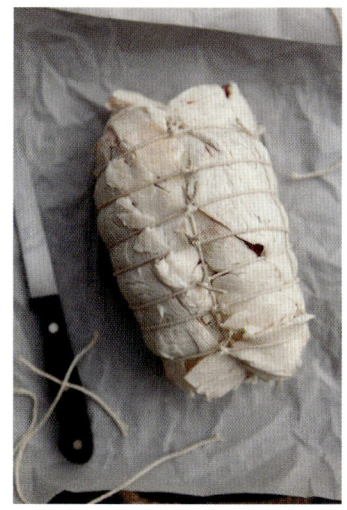

A butcher will sometimes use slices of beef fat (shown here) in which to wrap a roast beef, as opposed to slices of pork back fat, to keep "like with like." Usually, however, because thinly-sliced pork fat is more plentiful, easier to work with, and less crumbly, butchers will wrap their roasts in the pliable pork fat (as shown in the **Peppered Roast Beef** recipe on page 141), or else they will use thin slices of cured or fresh pork belly, essentially bacon. Usually, a butcher will wrap only the circumference of the roast, leaving the top and bottom of the meat visible. I have wrapped roasts in this way, but I have also wrapped top and bottom, covering the entire piece of meat of a beef shoulder roast (as shown here and in the finished recipe photo) wrapped entirely in thinly sliced beef fat. Either way, the roasts have come out delicious and juicy.

Pinch of salt, plus more to taste

Pinch of pepper, plus more to taste

2.2 pounds (1 kg) roast beef

Several thin slices of beef fat, lard or bacon for barding (*barder*)

Butcher's string

1 tablespoon tallow (*suif*) or lard (*saindoux*)

Preheat the oven to 395°F (200°C). Remove the meat from the refrigerator 20 to 30 minutes before cooking to allow it to come to room temperature. This is for the purpose of uniform cooking throughout the roast and not toughening the meat. Season the meat with the salt and pepper, and wrap or bard the sides (top and bottom, also, if desired) with the slices of pork lard. Tie the meat with string, using knots to secure the string. ➤

Chef's Tip
Astuce du Chef

A reminder that a pinch (*une pincée*) is using three fingers. For fine salt (*fleur de sel*), pepper, and spices this turns out to be slightly less than ⅛ teaspoon. For the coarser grains of sea salt, it might be slightly more.

Butcher's Tip
Astuce du Boucher

Cook roasts for about 15 minutes per 1.1 pounds (500 g), thicker roasts for about 20 minutes per 1.1 pounds (500 g)

Melt the tallow over medium-high to high heat in a cast-iron pot or pan, and brown the top, bottom, and sides of the roast on high heat for about two minutes each side, using stainless-steel tongs or a large meat fork and a wooden spatula to help you turn the roast. Place the pot in the oven, uncovered, for about 35 minutes.

Check the inner temperature of the roast using a meat thermometer to see whether the center of the roast has reached the temperature for the desired degree of doneness (refer to the chart on page 119). Leave the roast in 5 to 15 minutes longer for a less rare "doneness" (*cuisson*). Remove from the oven when the desired doneness has been reached. Larger roasts will take longer.

Allow the roast to rest for 5 minutes before carving to allow the temperature to level off and to keep the juices from escaping too quickly. The roast may be served hot with the sauce from the pot, sliced and sprinkled with coarse sea salt and freshly ground pepper. Or it may be served with a **Béarnaise Sauce** (page 391), or as cold "roast beef" in thin slices with **Homemade Mayonnaise** (page 406). Serve with sides of **Oven-Baked French Fries** (page 459), **Fennel with Red Onion** (page 445), **Oven-Baked Sweet Potatoes** (page 460), or a small helping of **Kabocha Squash Soup and Chestnut Soup** (page 454).

VARIATIONS You can roast the beef as is without barding or browning, though both of these techniques add to the flavor and make the difference between this recipe and regular roast beef (which is also delicious, of course). For a large roast of 3.5 to 4 pounds (1.6 kg to 1.8 kg), place in preheated oven at 395°F (200°C) for 15 minutes then turn down to 355°F (180°C) for another 30 to 45 minutes to reach an internal temperature of 140°F (60°C, medium), or another 45 minutes to one hour to achieve an internal temperature of 150°F (66°C, medium well) or another one hour to one hour and 15 minutes for 160°F (71°C, well done). Another option for a very tender roast is the "low and slow" cooking method of roasting the 3.5 to 4-pound (1.6 kg to 1.8 kg) piece of beef for four to four and a half hours in the oven at 240°F (115°C) for "well done," as you would roast a **Slow-Cooked Leg of Lamb** (page 209).

WINE PAIRING TIP With simple dishes you can pair complex wines. For example, the complexity of Pomerol wines with their tobacco and peppery notes, are an aromatic match with this dish. You can also try a red Grenache Noir wine, with its notes of black cherry, white pepper, tobacco, and dried fig from the regions of Côtes du Rhône or Languedoc-Roussillon, but watch out for its high alcohol content. I have tried this dish with a fruity, medium-bodied Bergerac, made using Cabernet Franc, ➤

Cabernet Sauvignon, and Côt (Malbec), similar to certain Bordeaux blends. Restaurateur and sommelière Annabelle recommends red wines with good tannic structure but not quite full-bodied, such as a fruity Anjou from the Loire Valley or a Grenache-based Gigondas or Vacqueyras, with notes of berries and spice, from the Rhône Valley. See also the wine suggestions under the **Peppered Roast Beef** recipe on page 141. If you are making this roast using veal, Annabelle recommends pairing it either with a fresh and sweet white Premières-Côtes-de-Bordeaux, with notes of acacia, peach or vanilla, or a powerful red wine, such as a Saint-Aubin, with notes of dark berries and cherries from the Côte de Beaune in Burgundy, or a lightly herbal and full-bodied Corbières from Languedoc-Roussillon (a velvety pairing I have tried and can recommend as well, especially with caramelized strips of lard enveloping the roast, namely an organic Château Pech-Latt Grande—and this wine makes dark chocolate taste like cherry liqueur!).

BEEF STEW WITH CARROTS
Boeuf Carottes

Season Year-round   **Preparation Time** 5 to 10 minutes
Cook Time 2 hours minimum, preferably 3 to 4 hours   **Serves** 8

Made with chuck roast (*paleron* or *macreuse*) from the neck, "blade," or shoulder area of the cow, a tough but flavorful cut, this is an easy, slow-cooking, French-family-everyday kind of dish. Put beef and chopped carrots in a cast-iron pot or a slow cooker, and it's dinner a few hours later! My friend, Stephen Davis, a transplanted Englishman in France since 1989, showed me this classic dish. He owned a bookstore in Montpellier for many years, where he amassed lots of great knowledge about life in general and a collection of books, including many cookbooks. He is a sensible, economically-minded father of five, who also happens to be a great cook of French cuisine, a great dad, and a great friend.

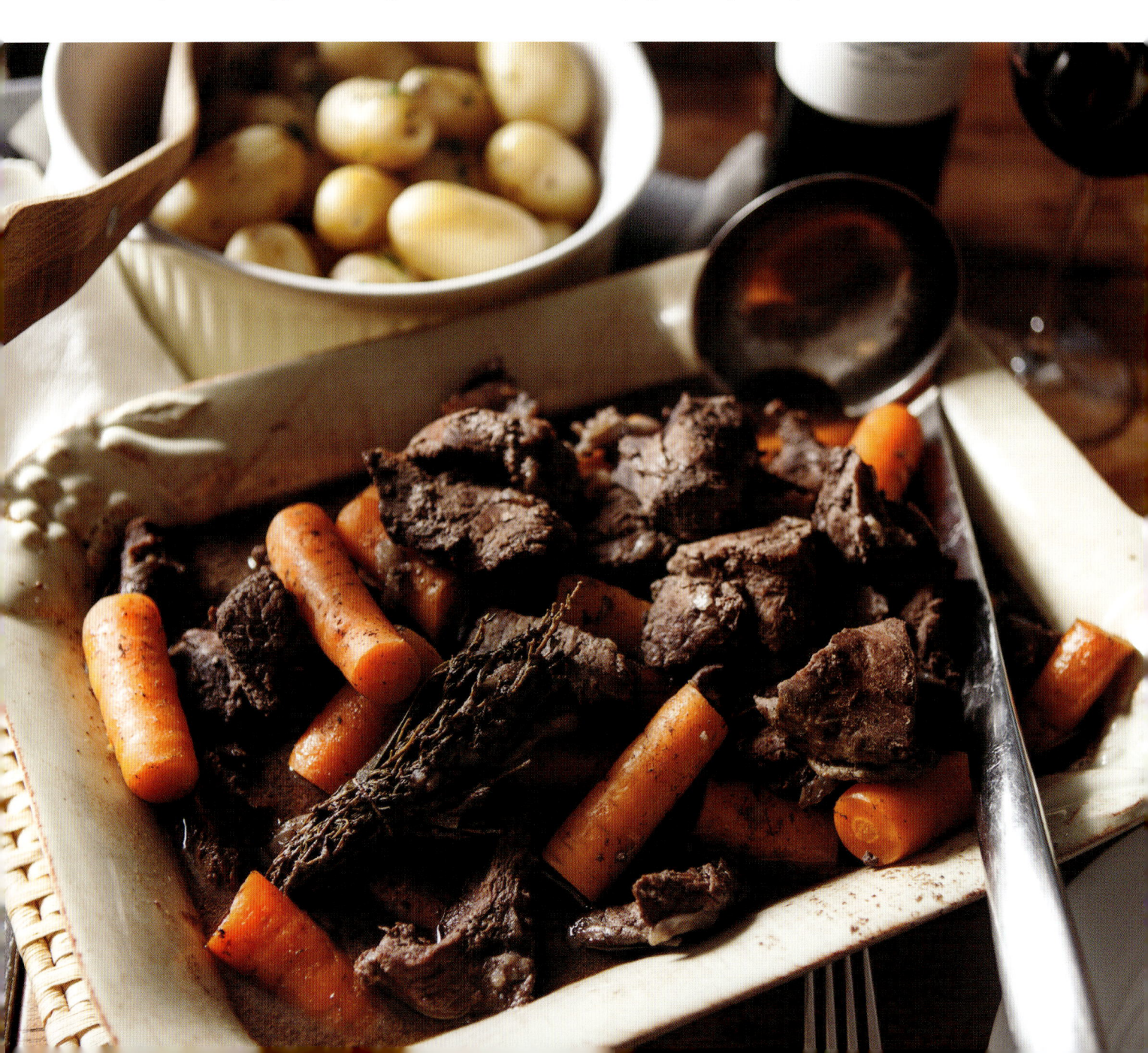

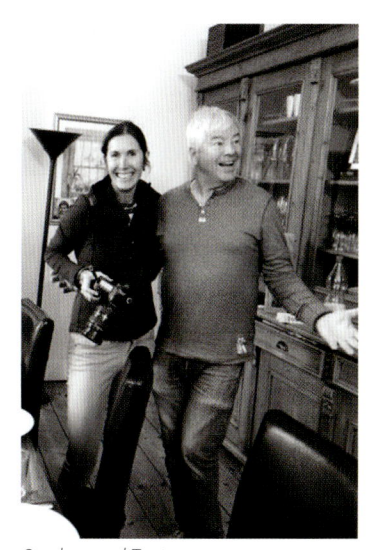

Stephen and Tania Photo Credit: Pascale Davis

3.5 pounds (1.5 kg) chuck roast

2.2 pounds (1 kg) carrots, chopped

1 onion, sliced (yellow or red, red is less potent)

1 piece of bacon rind (*bout de poitrine séchée* or *bout de ventrèche séchée*), or else a few strips of bacon, for taste

½ bottle red wine

2 cups (½ L) beef or veal stock

Bouquet garni

Pinch of sea salt

Pinch of pepper

Place all the ingredients in the cast-iron pot and cook on low for at least 2 hours, or for about 6 hours in the slow cooker, as Stephen did.

Serve with a side of boiled potatoes or other vegetables. Enjoy the other half of the bottle of red wine with the meal. For dessert we had an array of cheeses: Papillon Roquefort (in the red wrapper), Cheddar, Stilton, Tomme de Brebis (sheep), Comté, Grana Padano and fresh Chèvre (goat). The red Pessac-Léognan we had with the meal also went well with these cheeses. ➤

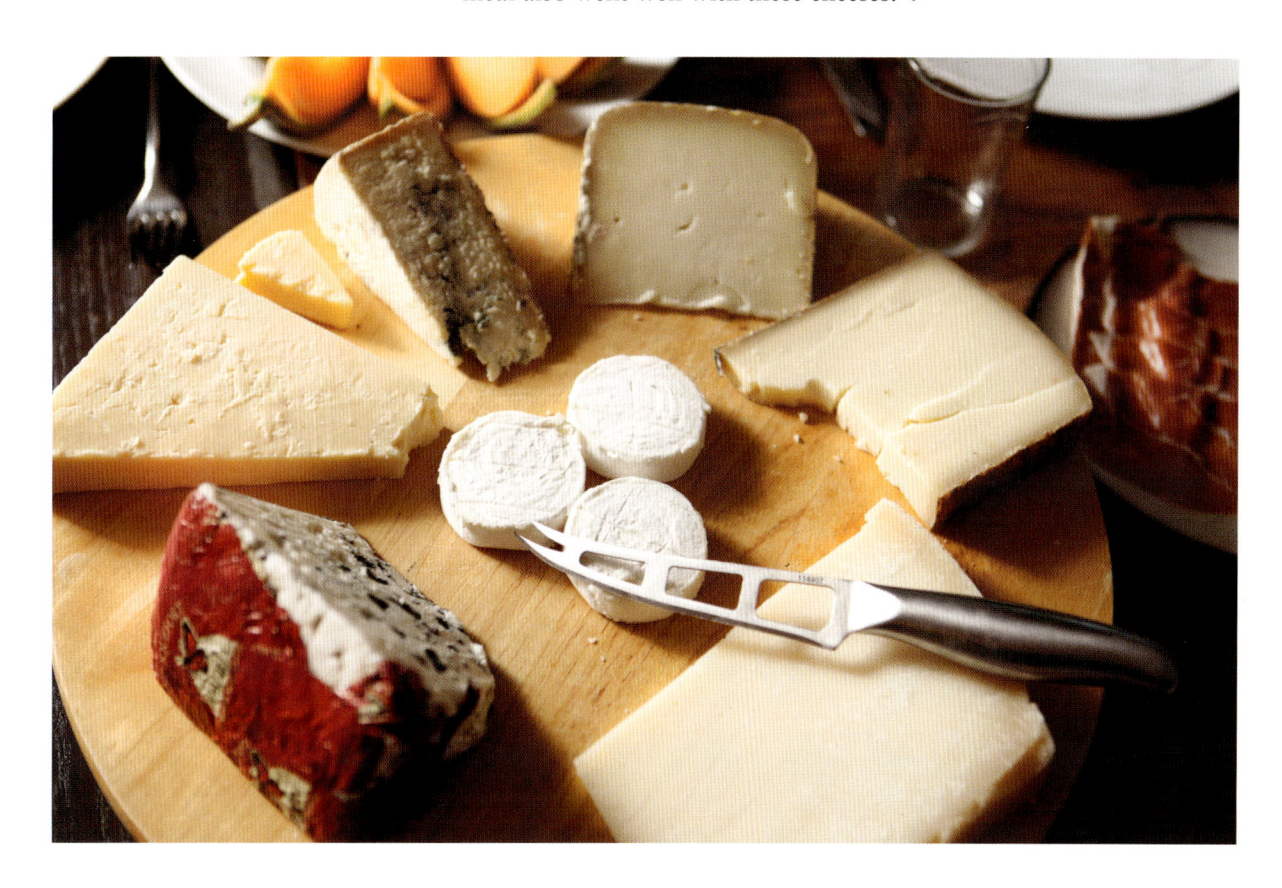

Nothing is Wasted

In traditional French cooking, everything is used. We hear the refrain that nothing is wasted. Even bacon ends (the dried end of the pork belly, not quite neat and straight enough for bacon strips) and bacon rind (the dried skin part, too hard to chew) are used in stews and stocks for flavor, even when they cannot be easily eaten. When you have a nice piece of cured pork belly (see photo A), cut away the rind, or skin (see photo B), and use the skin for a stew such as **Beef Stew with Carrots** or freeze for later use in a **Bone Broth** (page 394). The remaining bacon may be sliced or diced into cubes or rectangles (*lardons*), as shown in photo C, to fry up as needed in a multitude of recipes. Everything has its use.

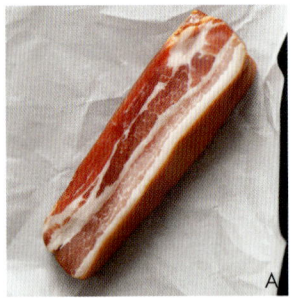

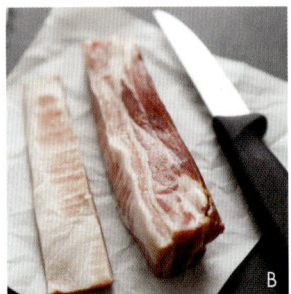

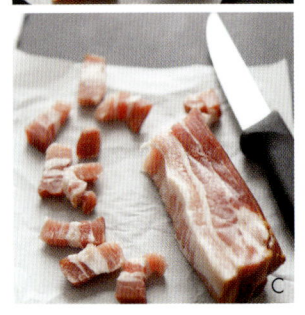

VARIATIONS This recipe is so basic, it can be added to or subtracted from easily. Like potatoes? Throw them in during the last half hour of cooking. Kids don't like the subtle taste of wine in their stew? Replace the wine with extra broth. Can't live without tomatoes or garlic? Add them to the mix and see what you get!

WINE PAIRING TIP With this meal, we drank a 2011 Château Le Pape from the region just South of Bordeaux, Pessac Léognan (part of the Graves region of gravely soil); we used a different Bordeaux red for the cooking. The reds from this region are versatile and flavorful, but not overpowering. Because of the strength in flavor of the meal, you can also go for more tannic wines, like those of Bordeaux's left bank from the Médoc, which are blends with a majority of the hearty Cabernet Sauvignon grape. You can also try wines from Bordeaux's right bank, St. Emilion, Castillon, and Pomerol, where Merlot comprises the majority percentage of the blends. If you add tomatoes to the stew, try a rustic Cahors, a region East of Bordeaux, made from the Malbec grape, or a Malbec blend from Bordeaux itself.

TABLEAU DES TEMPÉRATURES
de cuisson à cœur après saisie (°C)

VIANDES & POISSONS

	BLEU	SAIGNANT	A POINT	BIEN CUIT
Bœuf	45-50	50-55	60	>60
Porc	-	-	65	80
Agneau	55	60	68	75
Veau	-	-	68	75
Canard	48-50	55	>62	
Lapin	-	-	68	
Bar / Daurade	-	51	54	

TERRINES

	CUIT	MI-CUIT
Foie gras	62	48
Campagne	80	-
Volaille	72	-
Poisson	70	-

Meat Temperatures at Atelier des Chefs, Bordeaux

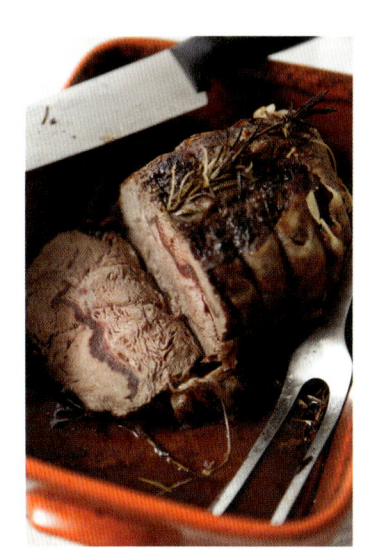

Grass-fed Beef Roast, Well Done

Butcher's Tip
Astuce du Boucher

Cook roasts for about 15 minutes per 1.1 pounds (500 g), thicker roasts for about 20 minutes per 1.1 pounds (500 g)

Degrees of Doneness for Beef
Températures de Cuisson à Coeur or Stades de Cuisson pour le Boeuf

First of all, note the following butcher's meaty secret: Remove the meat from the refrigerator and allow it to come to room temperature before heating it. This is so it will cook evenly throughout as well as to not give the meat a thermal shock, which causes the muscle fibers to contract and harden.[2] This goes for all meats, but most of all for roasts, which are larger pieces of meats requiring a bit of time to come to room temperature throughout. To assess the "degree of doneness" (*stade de cuisson*), use a meat thermometer, placed into the center of the roast to determine the inner temperature of the meat. The duration of cooking will depend on the size of the roast, so checking every 10 to 15 minutes after the initial recommended cooking time will help you gauge when to remove your roast from the oven. Roasts may actually be removed from the oven once they have reached 5°F to 10°F (3° to 6°C) lower than the desired temperature, as the inner temperature (*temperature à coeur*) will continue to rise for several minutes outside of the oven. It helps to experiment with your oven, your thermometer, and different sizes of roasts to see how long they take to reach your desired degree of "doneness." Approximate temperatures are as follows:[3]

Bloody or Extra Rare – *Bleu* (briefly seared on the outside, raw on the inside): 113°F to 122°F (45°C to 50°C)

Rare – *Saignant* (cool red center): 122°F to 131°F (50°C to 55°C)

Medium Rare (warm red center): 135°F (57°C)

Medium – *À point* (warm pink center): 140°F to 144°F (60°C to 63°C)

Medium Well (slightly pink center): 144°F to 150°F (63°C to 66°C)

Well Done – *Bien Cuit* (little or no pink, cooked through): 151°F to 160°F (66°C to 71°C)

Note: Americans' "well done" is often considered already "overcooked" (*trop cuit*).

BEEF – LE BOEUF

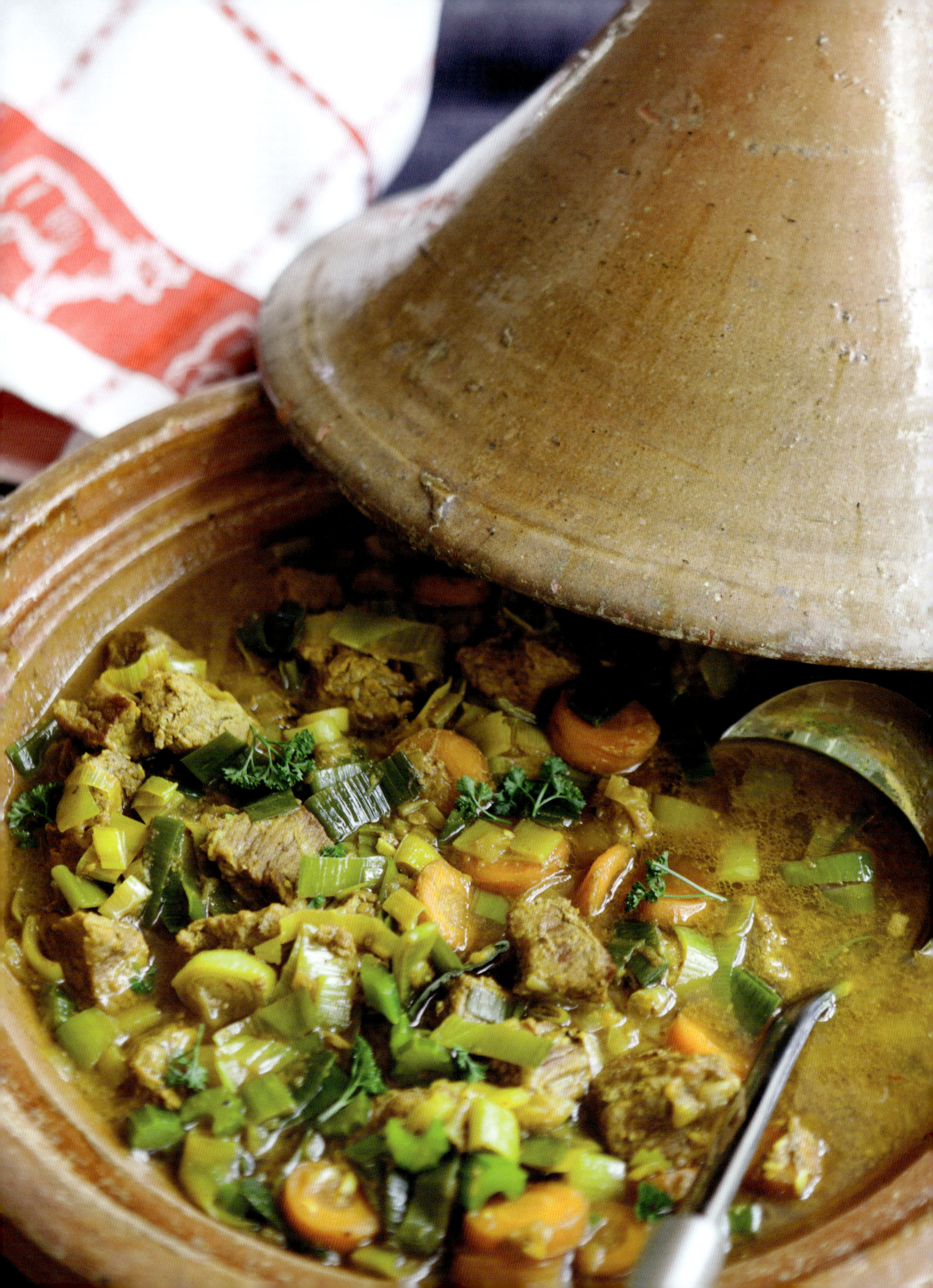

BEEF TAGINE STEW
Tajine de Boeuf

Season Year-round **Preparation Time** 15 minutes
Cooking Time 1 hour (up to two hours) **Serves** 6

The tajine originates from North Africa and there are many variations. With its anti-inflammatory ingredients of turmeric and ginger, this recipe is gut-friendly. This dish can be made in a cast-iron pot or in the traditional tagine clay dish, shown here, and as seen in the recipe for **Veal Stew Tagine** (page 431).

- 2 tablespoons beef tallow
- 2.2 pounds (1kg) chuck roast, cut into 1.5-inch (2 to 3 cm) cubes
- Sea salt to taste
- Pepper to taste
- 1 onion, chopped
- 2 garlic cloves, crushed
- 2 cups water
- 2 tablespoons olive oil
- 1 leek chopped into rounds (*rondelles*)
- 2 carrots, chopped into rounds
- 1 bay leaf
- 1 celery stalk, chopped
- 1 tablespoon fresh or dried turmeric (*curcuma*)
- 2 teaspoons fresh or dried ginger
- Parsley, for garnish

Melt the tallow in a cast-iron pot over medium high to high heat. Salt and pepper the beef cubes. Brown the cubes in batches, then brown the onion and garlic in the pot. Transfer to a terra cotta dish, if you have one, being sure to use a metal grill made to protect the tajine dish underneath the dish to keep it from cracking. Otherwise leave the beef in the pot. Add the remaining ingredients, and bring to a boil. Cover and simmer for 2 hours.

VARIATIONS Add three cloves (or ¼ teaspoon ground clove) and 1 to 2 star anise. This is not a flavor my children love (yet), but if the dish is for grown-ups, these spices round out the aromatics of the dish. If more vegetables are desired, add in-season vegetables, zucchini, and tomatoes, if available, or tomato paste.

WINE PAIRING TIP I recommend trying a fruity, medium to full-bodied Merlot-based Castillon – Côtes de Bordeaux from the Bordeaux region, a Languedoc-Roussillon blend containing the fruity grape variety of Cinsault, or else a fresh mint tea with honey, following the meal. To match up with the strength of this recipe's flavors, restaurateur Annabelle recommends powerful, well-structured red wines from the Southwest such as a meaty, cherry-spiced Cahors or a tannic Madiran, made from the Tannat grape. To match the spiciness of the recipe, Annabelle also recommends a hearty Bandol from Provence, made from the red Mourvèdre grape that has spice and character, or a rich and complex Crozes-Hermitage from the Rhône Valley.

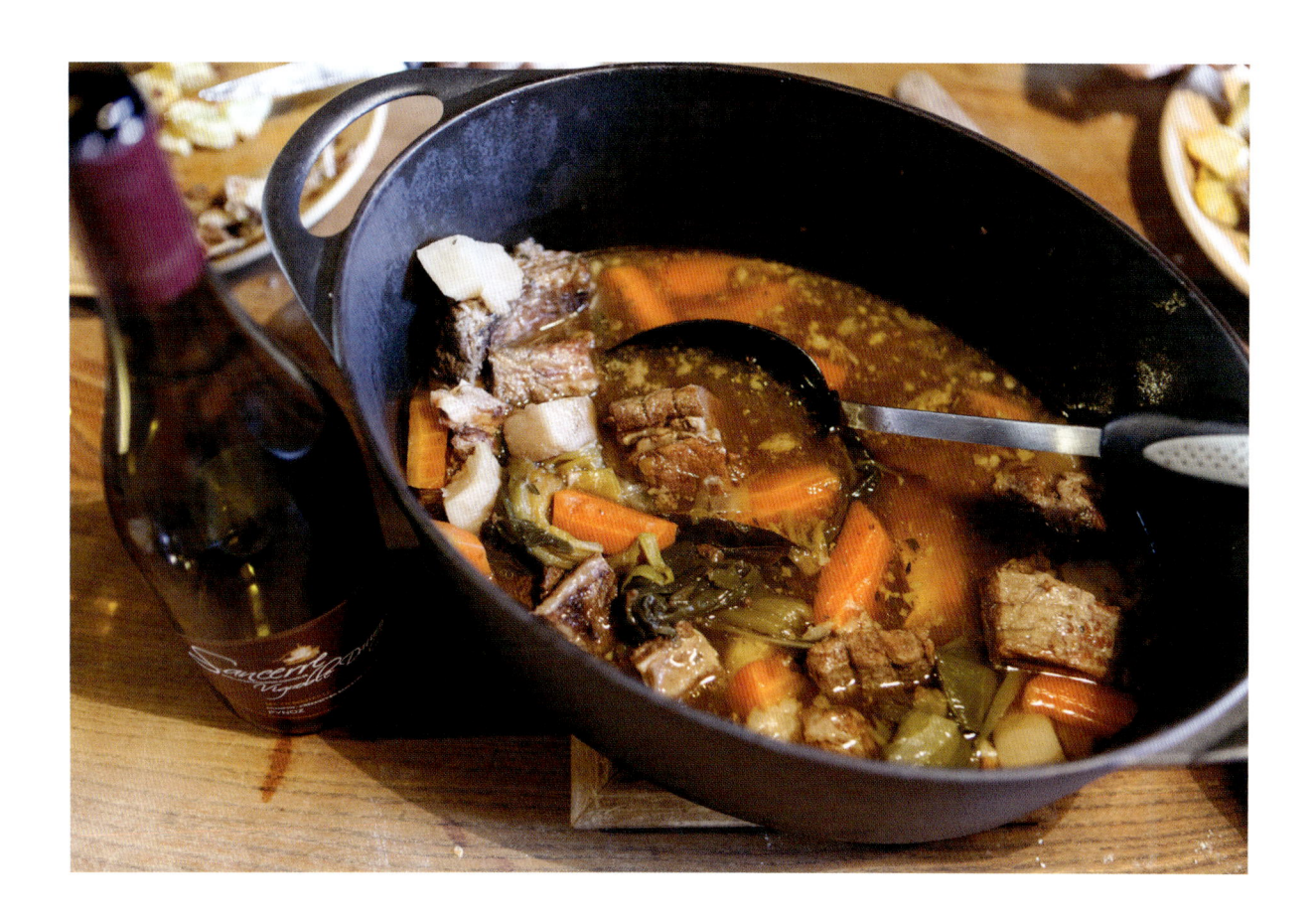

BOILED BEEF STEW "POT-AU-FEU"
Pot-au-Feu

Season Year-round, ingredients vary with the seasons   **Preparation Time** 10 minutes
Cooking Time From 3 hours to all week long!   **Serves** The Whole Family (about 6)

This quintessential French meal, made for centuries, was cooked in a round pot and always on the low fire or embers, bubbling through the night and through the week. Meats and vegetables were tossed into the pot as the week went on. Organic Limousin veal livestock farmers Joel and Josiane Sardenne in Peyrissac, part of the Corrèze region of Southwestern France, often have a *Pot-au-Feu* brewing on their stove throughout the week. They generously served my knowledgeable co-pilot (and fellow DUAD classmate) Vy Nguyen and me this delicious meal on a visit to their farm in 2016. We met with the Sardennes because I wanted to photograph their organic grass-fed cows and calves. This is the Sardennes' recipe as we had it that day, though many variations of this meal exist. Feel free to improvise according to your favorite ingredients! Use flavorful meats that require long, slow-cooking, such as short ribs (*plats de côtes*), chuck (*paleron* or *macreuse*), or other slow-roast pieces from the front of the animal, including "bottom round" (*gîte à la noix* or *noix de gîte*). This recipe calls for a *bouquet garni*, which includes a bay leaf, thyme, the green leaf sheath of a leek, and parsley if you have it.

2.2 pounds (1 kg) slow-roast meat

Bouquet garni

1 celery bunch or several stalks

Several carrots, chopped

2 to 3 root vegetables, chopped (turnips shown in recipe photo)

Water or stock, enough to cover the ingredients in the pot

Salt to taste

Place all the ingredients into a large pot and cover with water or stock of any meat or vegetable. Bring to a simmer and leave covered, reducing heat to low for the duration of the cooking time. Add meat as you have it during the week, as the Sardennes do for a perpetually ready meal. With *Pot-au-Feu*, the broth and vegetables are sometimes served separately from the meat, but the pot is usually brought right to the table and serves as the table centerpiece.

VARIATIONS Depending on the ingredients in the pot, the flavor profile of the dish will of course vary. If the ingredients are a combination of beef, pork, chicken, sausage, and vegetables, then, according to Julia Child, this is called a *Potée Normande*, and she recommends cooking 5 hours before serving.[4] If it is only chicken in the pot, then the dish is aptly named *Poule au Pot*.

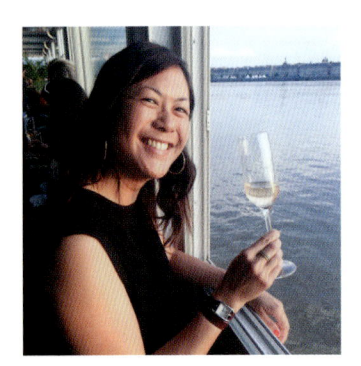

WINE PAIRING TIP We shared a cherry-and-orange-flavored Sancerre Rouge Pinot Noir from the Loire Valley with this meal after taking a tour of the farm. The French website www.platsnetvins.com, a handy resource for wine pairings, recommends a Cahors, or an elegant and spicy Côte-Rôtie, a fruity but balanced Crozes-Hermitage, or a pepper-and-spice Saint-Joseph from the Rhône Valley. Julia Child recommends a red Bordeaux, a Beaujolais, or a chilled rosé.[5] For this very traditional dish, sommelière Annabelle recommends rounded and supple wines, such as a Saint Emilion, Lalande de Pomerol, or Pomerol, or else a crisp Saumur-Champigny from the Loire Valley, made mostly with the herbaceous and spicy Cabernet Franc grape, sometimes smelling of pencil shavings (*retaille de crayon*).

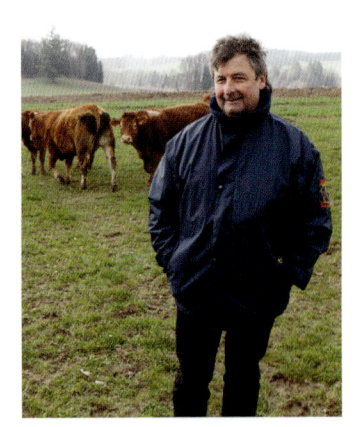

Organic Veal Farmer Joel Sardenne with his Grass-fed Cows

My Co-Pilot Vy, Off Duty

BONE-IN PRIME RIB
Côte de Boeuf

Season Year-round **Preparation Time** 1 minute
Cooking Time 12 to 20 minutes **Serves** 2

This is a large, fatty steak, potentially requiring a few extra minutes in the oven, preheated to 400°F (200°C), to cook through, unless you prefer a rarer steak. You can also just grill this steak without the herbs and serve the steak with **Béarnaise Sauce** (page 391). (Additional fat is usually not used on a barbeque grill.) Prime rib, from the mid-section of the cow, is also known as rib eye in English. In French, the boneless steaks between the ribs are called *entrecôtes* and are thinner. (See the recipe for **Wine Trader's Rib Eye Steak** on page 155.)

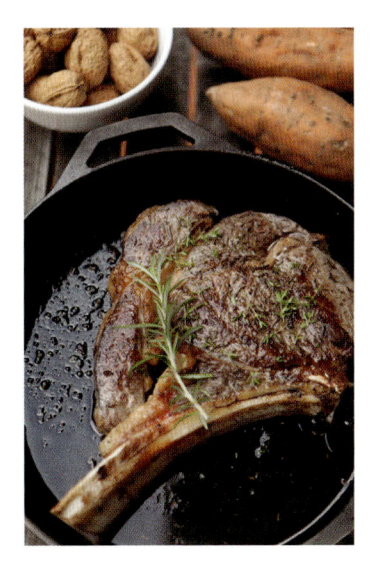

2 tablespoons tallow (*suif*) or butter

Fine salt and ground pepper for seasoning

1 teaspoon fresh or dried rosemary

1 teaspoon fresh or dried thyme

1 bone-in prime rib steak

Melt the tallow over high heat in a flat pan or grill pan if you like the grill lines. Season the steak with the salt, pepper, rosemary, and thyme. Sear the steaks for several minutes on each side, while basting them with the herbs and liquid tallow sauce in the pan. Tip the pan and use a spoon to retrieve the sauce for basting.

Place the steak into the oven for several minutes to achieve the desired "doneness" (per the Degrees of Doneness for Beef guide page 125).

VARIATIONS This type of steak begs to be grilled. For a guide on grilling, check out *Paleo Grilling* by Tony Federico and James Phelan. The Bordelais grill steaks in the winter on cut-and-dried vine shoots (*sarments de vigne*), particularly from the Cabernet Sauvignon grapevine, whose smoke enhances the flavors in the meat.

WINE PAIRING TIP This steak also begs to be paired with a Cabernet Sauvignon-dominated and full-bodied Médoc from North of Bordeaux. Sommelière Annabelle suggests full-bodied wines with rounded tannins, such as a Syrah-based Hermitage from the Northern Rhône Valley or a lesser-known, fruitier but also full-bodied Pécharmant from Bergerac in the French Southwest. For another French Southwestern regional pairing, Annabelle also recommends a tannic Madiran, Gascony's signature red wine.

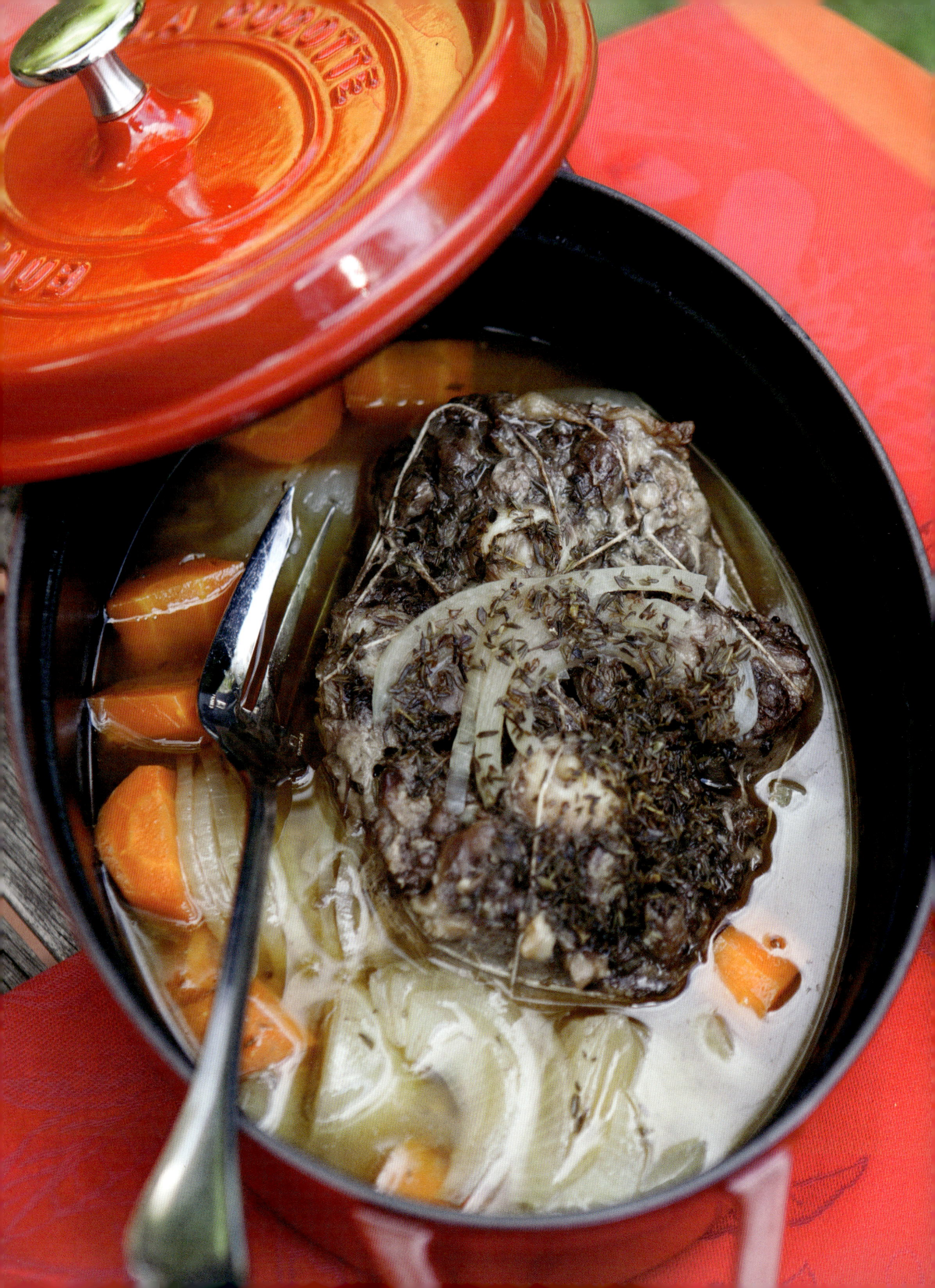

BRAISED OXTAIL
Queue de Boeuf

Season Autumn through early Spring   **Preparation Time** 30 minutes
Cooking Time 3 hours   **Serves** 4

In France, oxtail (the tail of the cow) is usually sold chopped (severed between the joints) and already neatly tied up in a circle with butcher's thread (*la ficelle*), which makes it easy to handle when browning. Sold along with other meat cuts, oxtail nonetheless technically falls into the offal (*abats*) category in France. Oxtail is very hard to eat off the bone if it has not cooked long enough; it truly necessitates slow cooking for three hours minimum. I have tried cooking it only two hours and was sorely disappointed! The flavor amplifies the longer the oxtail cooks and has even more flavor the next day, as with most slow-cooking recipes. Braising a meat essentially means browning it in a pot and then slow-cooking it.

WINE PAIRING TIP Try a medium to full-bodied red Côtes du Rhône Villages from the Rhône Valley, made with the Syrah grape. Or try a Syrah from the Languedoc region, which can also be added to the sauce. Sommelière Annabelle recommends structured red wines to go with this dish such as: a Grenache-majority, robust Gigondas, with notes of red and black fruit or a red-fruited Châteauneuf-du-Pape, both from the Rhône Valley, or else a rich, structured and herbaceous Corbières from Languedoc, with notes of red fruit, ripe black fruit, licorice, pepper, and thyme.

6 tablespoons beef tallow

Salt and pepper for seasoning

2.2 pounds (1 kg) oxtail

1 medium onion, halved and thinly sliced into semi-circles

3 cloves

1 medium onion, quartered, and pierced with the cloves

1 carrot, cut in 1-inch (2.5 cm) cylinders (*rondelles*)

1 small fresh rosemary twig

1 teaspoon fresh or dried thyme

1 bay leaf

Melt three tablespoons beef tallow in a cast-iron pan over medium-high heat. Salt and pepper the oxtail. Brown the bound pack of oxtail (or each individual piece if they are not bound together) on each side. Remove the meat and set aside for the moment. Add the sliced onion to the pan to soften it in the fat for a few minutes.

Reduce the heat to low, adding the meat back to the pot, as well as the remaining ingredients. Cover and allow to simmer for three hours.

VARIATIONS For extra flavor, add a piece of pork rind or browned bacon pieces (*lardons*) along with the remaining ingredients to simmer for three hours. You might also try adding a cup of white or red wine during the simmering phase. You can also add 1.5 cups of soaked and sprouted lentils for the last 40 minutes of cooking.

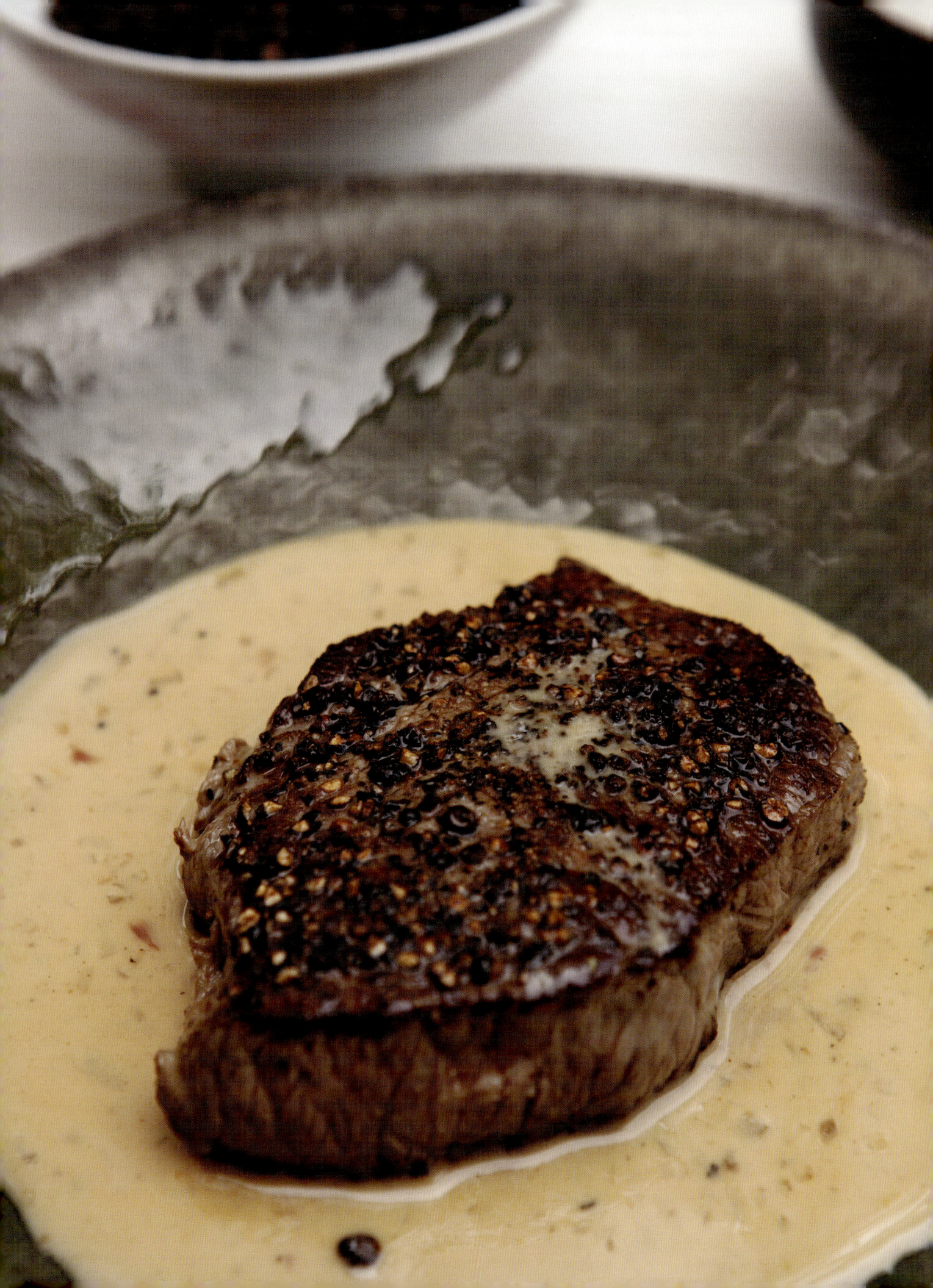

FLAMBÉED SIRLOIN STEAK WITH CREAM SAUCE
Pavés de Rumsteck Flambés, Sauce à la Crème

Season Year-round   **Preparation Time** 5 minutes
Cooking Time 20 minutes, depending on how rare or well done you like your steaks   **Serves** 3

The sirloin steak (or "rump" steak) comes from the back end of the cow between the short loin and the round (back haunch). Other steaks can, of course, also be used in this recipe. The sirloin steak (*rumsteck* or *bifteck de surlonge*) is commonly served in France, often with **Oven-Baked French Fries** (page 459.) I needed practice with flambéing (setting food with alcohol on fire very briefly), so I asked my friend Chef Jean-Luc to demonstrate his way of preparing flambéed steaks. He also showed me how to "smash" (*écraser*) fresh pepper without a pepper mill or mortar and pestle: between the bottoms of two pots. This recipe uses **Veal Stock** (page 415), but other stocks or broths may be used. The creamy sauce in this recipe is divine, but the cream can be skipped if necessary. In that case, reduce the sauce a few minutes longer. The steaks made for a nice lunch for Chef Jean-Luc, his wife Annabelle (also my DUAD wine course classmate and wine pairing advisor extraordinaire), and me. Both Annabelle and Jean-Luc are from the Calvados "department" of Normandy, known for its apple brandy and the Normandy beach landings of World War II. Annabelle was born in Bayeux, city of the famous 11th Century 68-meter (almost 75 yards) long Tapestry of Bayeux.

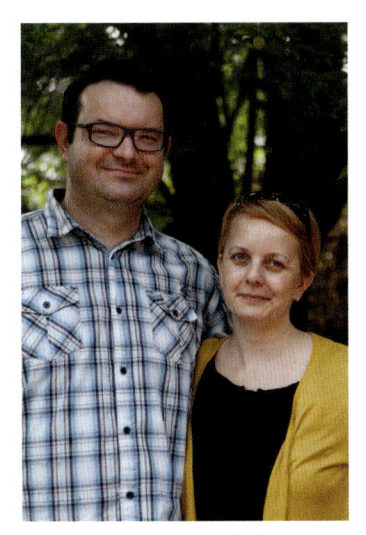

Chef Jean-Luc and Annabelle

1 tablespoon lard (*saindoux*) or tallow (*suif*)

2 tablespoons peppercorns, smashed (*graines de poivres écrasées*)

Pinch of fine salt

2 to 3 steaks

1 tablespoon Cognac or whiskey

1 shallot (*échalote*), diced

2 tablespoons white wine (*vin blanc*)

4 tablespoons veal stock (*fond de veau*) or other meat stock

2 tablespoons sour cream (*crème fraîche*) or heavy cream (*crème liquide*)

Melt the lard or tallow in a pan over high heat. Mix the salt and pepper together and rub the mixture onto both sides of each steak. Sear (*saisir*) the steaks for one to two minutes on each side until the edges are browned.

With the steaks still in the pan, pour the Cognac into the pan, turn off the stove and the ventilation fan above, if it is on. Keeping your face and body away from the pan (not hunched over it), bring a match or a kitchen flame-torch to the edge of the pan to ignite the alcohol. Immediately remove your hand as the flame catches. Shake the pan back and forth until the flames die out (the sign that the alcohol has burned off). Move the steaks temporarily to a plate.

Turn the heat back on to medium high and add the shallots to the pan, stirring for a minute and making sure they do not burn. Stir in the wine and scrape the flavorful, caramelized solids at the bottom of the pan to deglaze (*déglacer*) the pan. Pour in the veal stock, gently whisk in the cream, and allow to reduce (*réduire*) for several minutes. Add the steaks back into the pan to finish cooking (*finir la cuisson*) for several minutes.

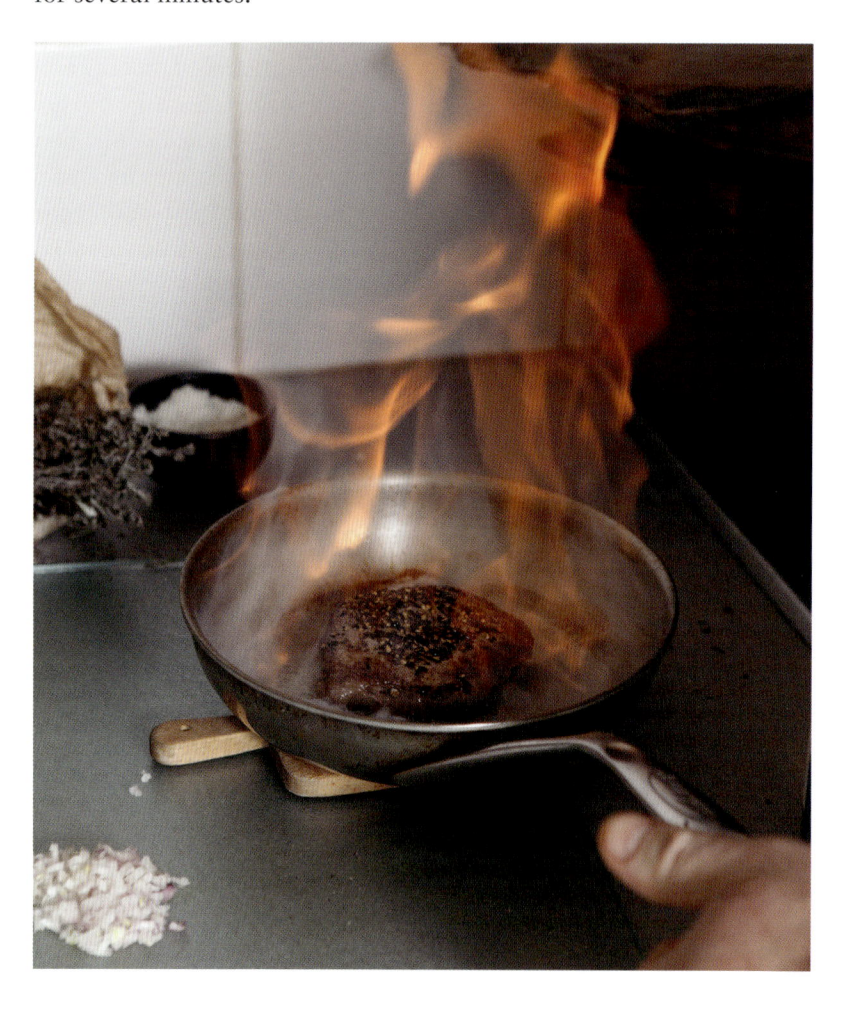

WINE PAIRING TIP To match this dish's powerful flavors, try medium or full-bodied reds with Grenache, Malbec, or Syrah, such as a Malbec-heavy Cahors wine from the Southwest, a Syrah from the Rhône Valley, or else a Grenache-majority wine, such as Pic-Saint-Loup from Languedoc-Roussillon. Annabelle recommends well-structured Cabernet Sauvignon-majority wines from Bordeaux's Haut-Médoc, or else from Languedoc-Roussillon, where Grenache, Mourvèdre, and Syrah grapes, infusing spice and character, are used in wines such as Faugères, Minervois, and Saint-Chinian.

FLAMBÉED SIRLOIN STEAK WITH SAUTÉED VEGETABLES
Pavé de Rumsteck Flambé avec Garniture de Légumes à la Poêle

Season Year-round   **Preparation Time** 10 minutes
Cooking Time 10 to 15 minutes   **Serves** 1 to 2

Since steaks are such an easy meal, here is another sirloin steak recipe, but one slightly more daring than the **Sage Butter Sirloin Steak** (page 145), as it is flambéed with cognac like the previous recipe **Flambéed Sirloin Steak with Cream Sauce** (page 129). My friend Chef Frédéric showed me the flambé trick, which requires some practice. I admit it is a bit scary to do yourself at first, but after a few tries, it actually works. The key is to do it swiftly (staying out of the way of the flames) while the food, alcohol, and pan are still hot enough to make igniting the alcohol easier. Chef Frédéric says the reason for flambéing the meat is to burn off the alcohol, which would otherwise become bitter (*amer*) in the cooking process, leaving only the aroma (*le parfum*) of the alcohol, in this case the cognac. This recipe can be multiplied easily, depending on the number of people to feed.

Fine salt and pepper for seasoning

One 6- to 8-ounce (170 g to 230 g) sirloin steak

2 tablespoons olive oil

1 tablespoon beef tallow

1 capful of cognac

Handful of mixed in-season vegetables, sliced

Pinch of fine salt

Season the steak with salt and pepper and one tablespoon of olive oil. Melt the tallow in the pan over high heat. Sear the steak for one to two minutes on each side until the edges are browned.

Add the capful of cognac and allow it to distribute in the pan. To flambé the steak, remove the pan from heat and ventilation, hold it at an arm's length, and hold a lighted match or kitchen blowtorch (*chalumeau*) to the edge of the pan, immediately pulling back your hand as the alcohol lights. Shake the pan back and forth a little to help the alcohol burn off. It will burn out on its own after several seconds.

Remove the steak from the pan and place it in an oven-safe dish in a preheated oven at 320°F (160°C) for five minutes to finish the cooking process. (See the **Degrees of Doneness for Beef** chart on page 125.)

Add the other tablespoon of olive oil to the pan, the vegetables, and the pinch of salt. Sauté the vegetables in the steak juices and oil for several minutes until cooked through. Add them on top of the steak after it has come out of the oven, and garnish with thin strips of raw vegetables.

> WINE PAIRING TIP To match the steak's strong flavors, try a Syrah from the Côte-Rôtie, known to produce elegant, complex, and powerful wines in the Northern Rhône Valley, or a full-bodied Côtes-du-Rhône-Villages from the Southern Rhône Valley. A "left bank" Cabernet Sauvignon blend from the Médoc region of Bordeaux, such as Saint-Estèphe, Saint-Julien, Pauillac, or Margaux, is also an excellent pairing choice. For a less tannic, but flavorful pairing, try a red Graves – Pessac-Léognan such as Château Haut Bailly or Château Olivier.

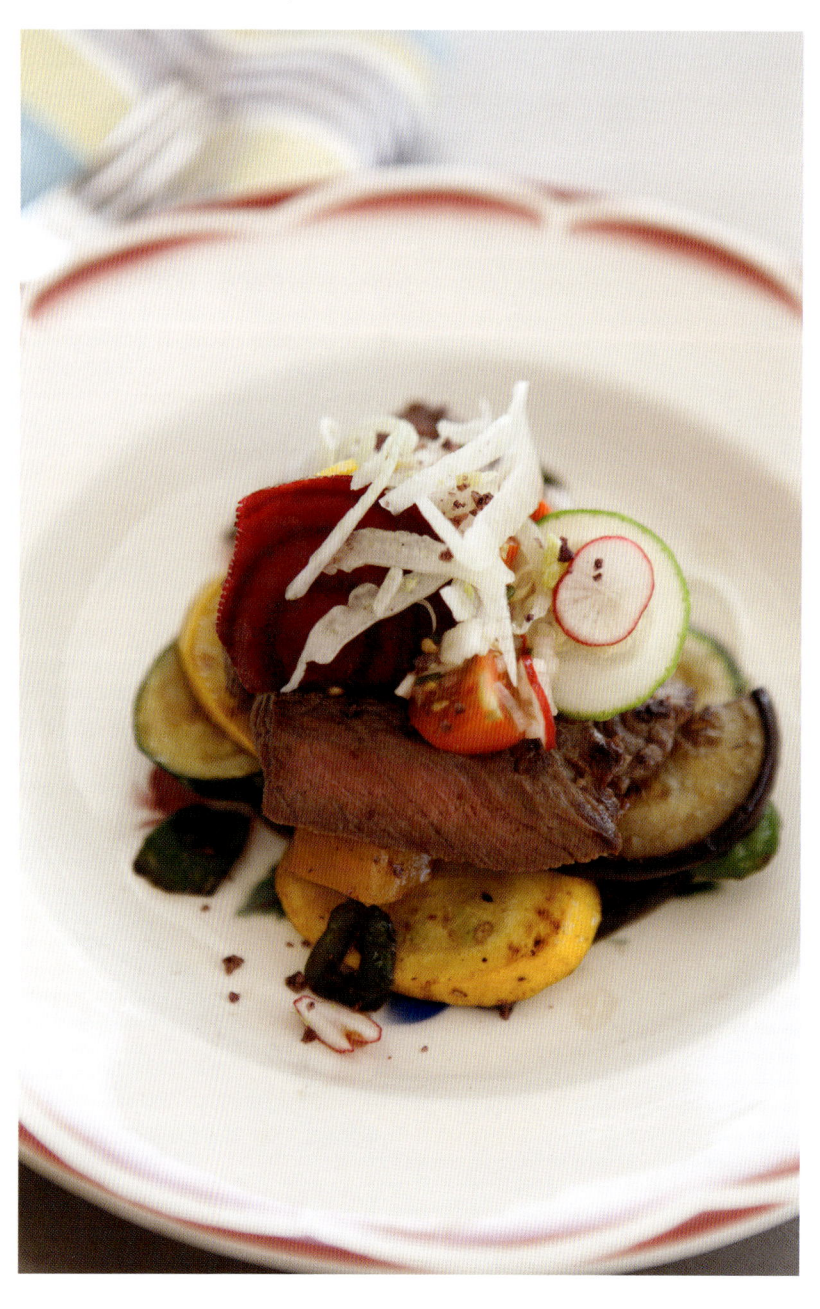

Flambéed Sirloin Steak with Sautéed Vegetables ›

FLANK STEAK WITH SHALLOTS
Bavette à l'Echalotte

Season Year-round   **Preparation Time** 5 minutes
Cooking Time 10 to 15 minutes   **Serves** 1 to 2

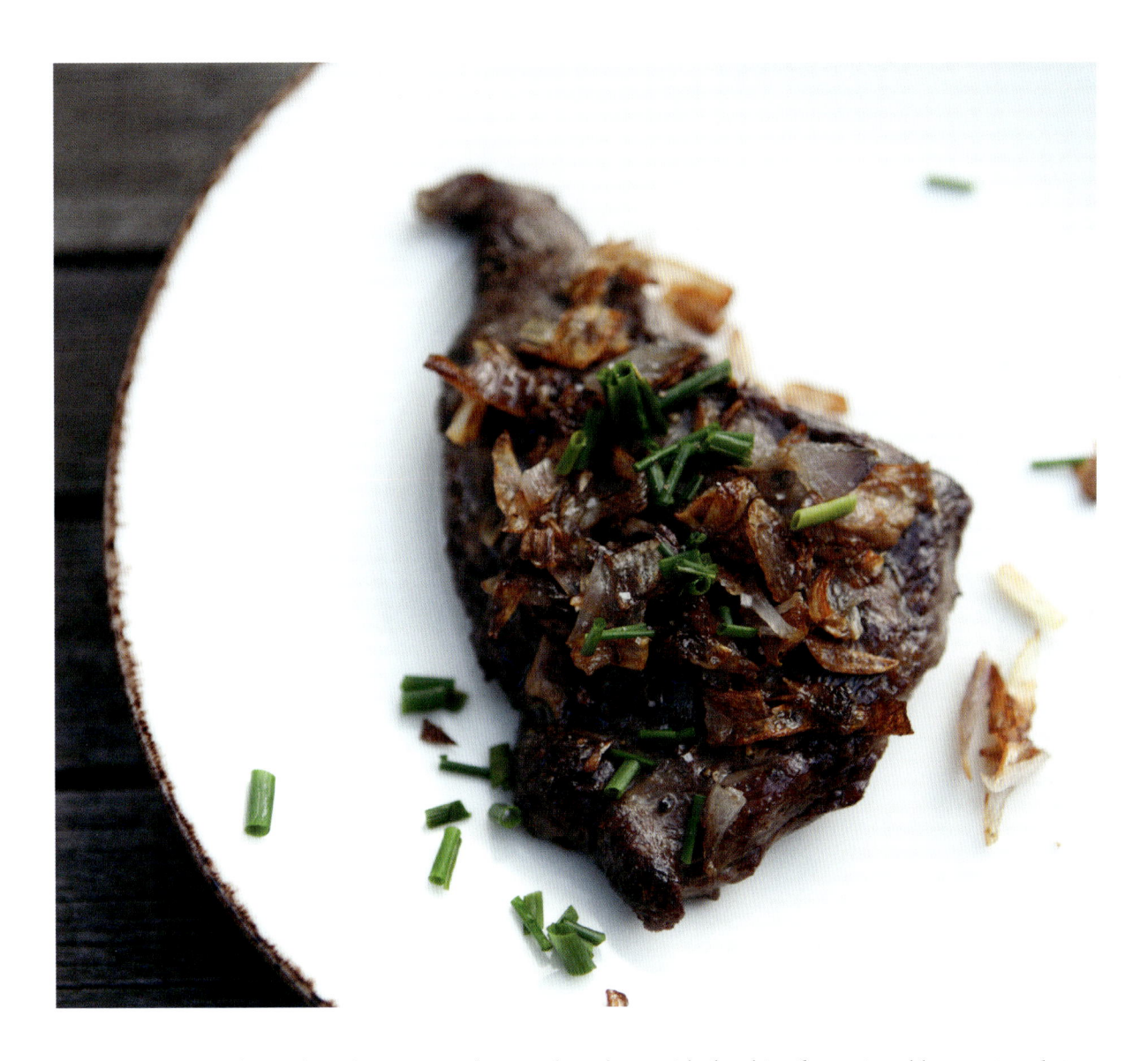

The flank steak (often referred to as "London Broil"), along with the skirt (*hampe*) and hanger (*onglet*) steaks, seems to be a standard butcher's cut that the butcher might keep for himself to easily grill up for his lunch or dinner. A whole flank steak weighs between one and two pounds (450 g to 910 g). During my apprenticeship at the butcher shop, for lunch we would throw a few slabs of these steaks (or else the end pieces of meat or leftover sausages) in a pan and sauté some **Sarlat Sautéed Potatoes** (page 468) or **Baked French Fries** (page 459) on the side. (There was a mandatory shop closing for lunch for one and a half hours, so we often had time to cook a real meal.) This recipe with shallots is an easy one for any steak, as shallots go well with pretty much any red meat.

1 tablespoon tallow or duck fat, plus 1 teaspoon

Pinch of salt

1 shallot, minced

1 tablespoon butter

Fine salt and pepper for seasoning

6 to 7 ounces (185 g) flank steak

Melt the tallow in a flat cast-iron plancha or stainless-steel pan on medium high to high heat. Add a pinch of salt along with the minced shallot, and allow the pieces to brown.

Transfer the shallot to a plate or bowl, and add the teaspoon of tallow plus the butter to the pan. Salt and pepper the steak, and sear it on each side for three minutes. Reduce heat and continue to cook for five minutes, turning once. Serve with grilled, roasted or sautéed vegetables.

> **WINE PAIRING TIP** If one could easily afford a red Château Haut Brion, from the Northern Graves region of Pessac-Léognan in Bordeaux, I would recommend it. Alas it is one of the very few and most expensive "first growths" of the Bordeaux wine region, one that even Thomas Jefferson famously adored in 1787. But there are many good red Graves wines from Pessac-Léognan to discover. Otherwise, try a heavier Cabernet Sauvignon from the Médoc region North of Bordeaux, including Haut-Médoc, Listrac-Médoc and Moulis-en-Médoc, among others, or a robust Côte-Rôtie from the Northern Rhône Valley. This steak can handle it!

GRILLED ROSEMARY BEEF SKIRT STEAK
Hampe de Boeuf au Romarin

Season Year-round, but especially for summer grilling!   **Preparation Time** 5 minutes   **Cooking Time** 10 minutes   **Serves** 3 to 4

Skirt steak (hampe de boeuf) is technically placed in the "offal" (*Abats*) category in France. This recipe can be used for any steak, really, including the skirt (*hampe*) or "inside skirt" (which has more fat), but also flank (*flanchet*), rib or "prime rib" (*côte*, *entrecôte*, or *faux-filet*), sirloin (*rumsteck* or *bifteck de surlonge*), and beef tenderloin (*tournedos*), which in France is often topped with a slab of foie gras and called tournedos Rossini. To me, the basic combination of garlic, fresh rosemary, and salt, together with a mixture of animal fat and olive oil makes for an impact of flavors that delivers every time.

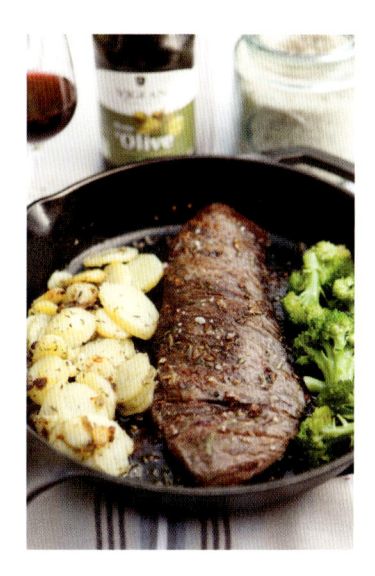

Pinch of sea salt (fine or coarse, depending on your preference)

Pinch of pepper

1 tablespoon fresh or dried rosemary, minced

1 clove garlic, minced

1 tablespoon olive oil, plus a bit more to drizzle after grilling

14 to 16 ounces (400 g to 450 g) skirt steak

1 tablespoon tallow, lard, or butter

Salt and pepper for seasoning

Rub the salt, pepper, rosemary (fresh rosemary is most flavorful, if you have it), garlic, and olive oil onto the meat. (This can be done the night before or from several hours to right before cooking. The longer it marinates, the longer the aromas and flavors are able to infuse into the meat.)

Melt the fat over high heat in a cast-iron grill pan or flat pan (*plancha*). Sear the steak on each side for two to three minutes, then turn the heat down to medium-high and turn the steak again once or twice, if needed, depending on thickness of the piece and how raw or cooked you like your meat.

Transfer the steak from the pan to a plate, drizzle with olive oil, and sprinkle a bit more salt and pepper on the meat. (I like to garnish almost everything, including steaks, with some crunchy *fleur de sel*.)

Serve with salad, other grilled vegetables, sautéed potatoes, **Oven-Baked French Fries** (page 459), sweet potato fries, or an **Oven-Baked Sweet Potato** (page 460).

WINE PAIRING TIP If you are doing "steak frites," that is, steak with white or sweet potato fries, try a Beaujolais, which is by definition young and fruity, an herbaceous Loire Valley Chinon or Saumur, or else go with a hearty, tannic Cabernet Sauvignon blend from Bordeaux or a robust, tannic, and expressive Madiran from "Gascon" country in the French Southwest.

BEEF – LE BOEUF

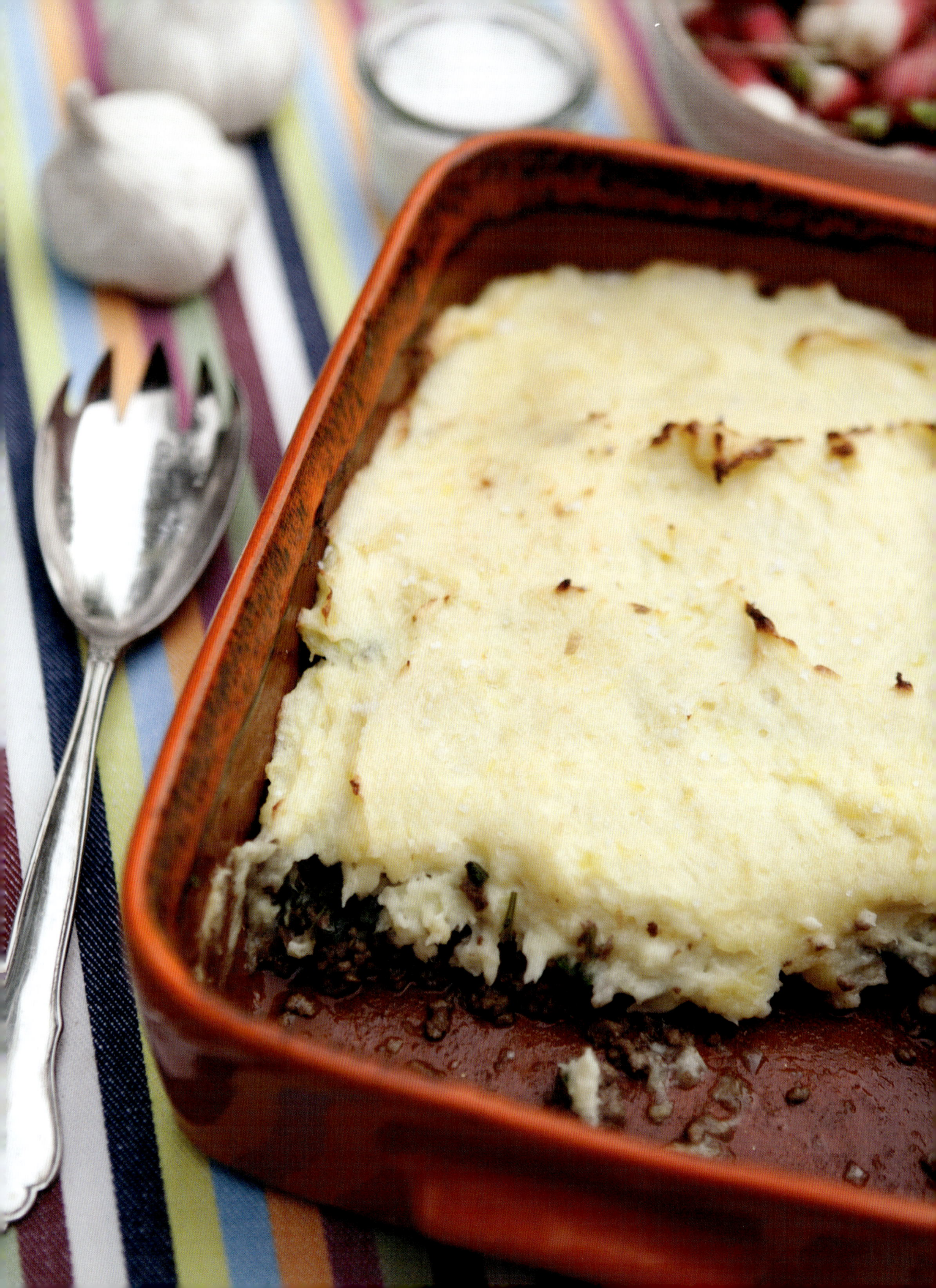

GROUND BEEF PARMENTIER
Hachis Parmentier

Season Autumn and Winter   **Preparation Time** 30 minutes
Cooking Time 50 minutes   **Serves** 6

Antoine-Augustin Parmentier was a French nutritional chemist and pharmacist who was instrumental in rousing public interest in the potato as food for humans in the late 1700s, during a time of famine from poor harvests, when it had been considered only for animal feed and thought to cause disease. He planted a garden of potatoes guarded by watchmen who left at night, cleverly allowing for people's curiosity to get the better of them and snatch potatoes to try them out. His strategy worked, as potatoes began showing up in dishes in Parisian homes and nobility, eventually influencing the French in the countryside. For better or for worse, he was able to convince academia and society to accept the potato as food in his royally-condoned "Treatise on the Culture and Use of the Potato, Sweet Potato and Jerusalem Artichoke"[6] on the eve of the French Revolution. Whether or not you like his contributions to "modern progress," Parmentier's name is frequently invoked with several potato dishes in France, including this one. This dish is basically a British "cottage pie" or "shepherd's pie" using ground beef (*steak haché*) and can either be cooked in individual ramekins (*mini-cocottes*) or in one larger casserole dish. This particular version is inspired by one of my favorite French cookbooks by Parisian butcher Hugo Desnoyer who uses more parsnips than potatoes. The more "traditional" Parmentier recipes generally call for only potatoes (which is what my children prefer and is described in "Variations" on this recipe below and shown in the accompanying photo), as the parsnips flavor the potatoes enough for them to notice. Potatoes are a nightshade and have a high glycemic effect on blood glucose levels, therefore I like replacing them partially with parsnips as in this recipe, but you may not win over your children by using parsnips. Try it out both ways and see who likes what. I also use white pepper in this recipe to "hide" it visually in the white parsnip-potato purée, while still providing the complex and vegetal aromas and flavors that white pepper can give to a dish. Desnoyer uses lamb meat, and less of it, in his recipe. (See page 197 for **Ground Lamb Parmentier**.) See also Variations below for other possibilities for adaptation besides type of meat and the ratio of parsnips to potatoes. For this recipe I have used my favorite hand-thrown terra cotta Basque "Terafeu" casserole dish. The colors of these dishes are earthy, lively, and appealing. (Their only drawback is that they are fragile. Soak them in cold water for two hours before using the first time and every two months that they go unused.)

FOR THE PARSNIPS AND POTATOES:

1.5 pounds (600 g to 700 g) parsnips (*panais*), chopped into 1-inch (2.5 cm) cubes

⅔ pounds (300 g) potatoes, peeled and chopped into 1-inch (2.5 cm) cubes

⅓ cup (80 g) butter

Optional: 2 tablespoons sour cream (*crème fraîche*) or 4 tablespoons whole milk (*lait entier*),

Fine salt to taste

White pepper to taste

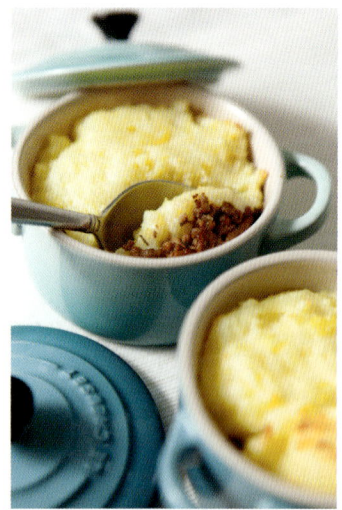

You can fill the mini-cocottes and store them in the refrigerator overnight without baking them until the next day when needed. The mini-cocottes are easy to reheat. Directly out of the fridge, I reheat them at 400°F (200°C) for 20 minutes. Quick, easy lunch or dinner! The advantage of mini-cocottes is that kids love to eat out of them like little cats out of their kibble bowls. The colors are bright and fun, and the portions are scalable to your child's appetite. You can also make the layer of parsnips and potatoes as thick or thin as you like, depending on how much carbohydrate you desire, and even add slabs of butter on top for extra fat.

FOR THE MEAT:

2 tablespoons tallow or duck fat

1 small onion, minced

3 shallots, minced (optional, for flavor; my children prefer fewer)

Pinch of fine salt

Pinch of pepper

2.2 pounds (1 kg) ground beef

4 garlic cloves, minced

Optional: Small handful parsley

Optional: 1 tablespoon olive oil

Place the parsnips and potatoes (chopped to similar size, 1- to 2-inch pieces) in boiling, salted water. Boil until they are easy to prick with a fork, about 20 minutes. Drain. If you have a hand-operated stainless-steel food mill (*moulin à legumes*), you can run the parsnips and potatoes through the mill to purée them (in this case, the potatoes don't even need to be peeled). Otherwise, use a hand mixer and a bowl, adding the butter and optional sour cream or milk and the salt and pepper to taste as you mix.

Preheat the oven to 365°F (185°C). Melt the tallow or duck fat in a pan over medium heat. Sauté the onions (and optional shallots) with the salt and pepper for several minutes before adding the ground meat, garlic (and optional parsley), and stirring with a wooden spoon for several more minutes, until the meat is just cooked. (If you are using tallow and parsley, you might consider drizzling about a tablespoon of olive oil over the meat at the end after turning off the stove. It makes for a nice flavor combination!)

Distribute the meat in a large casserole dish or fill several mini-casserole dishes halfway with the meat mixture. Spread an even layer of the parsnip-potato mixture over the meat layer.

Place in the oven uncovered, and allow to bake for 30 minutes for a large casserole dish or 20 minutes for ramekins/mini-cocottes.

You can also make this recipe in advance and store in the refrigerator overnight. When reheating the next day, allow the dishes to come to room temperature for 10 to 15 minutes before cooking, or else bake them at 400°F (200°C) for about 30 minutes for a large dish or 20 minutes for small dishes.

VARIATIONS There are so many ways to make this dish, depending on your taste preferences and what's in your pantry.

- Solely potatoes may be used in lieu of the parsnips. This would be more aligned with the "original" style of this dish named after Parmentier. If you are only using potatoes and you do not have a food mill, you can boil the potatoes skin on and then peel them when they are done, but allow them to cool them off first by putting them in a bowl of cold water. Peeling is easier because the skin comes off easily, but boiling them whole takes longer, especially if you have larger potatoes (up to 45 minutes!).

- Two tablespoons of olive oil or butter can be used in place of or in addition to the tallow or duck fat when sautéing the onions and meat to augment the fat content of the dish.

- Two or three minced shallots may be added to the pan to brown in addition to or in lieu of the onion.

- Six tablespoons of tomato paste may be added to the meat as it's being sautéed in the pan for a more Bolognese spaghetti-and-meatballs flavor.

- An egg yolk may be added to the cooked meat before it goes into the oven, along with some grated hard cheese of your choice.

- A teaspoon of *herbes de Provence* may also be mixed into the pan after the meat has been cooked before transferring the meat to the baking dish, especially if you are using tomato paste.

- Sneak in a tablespoon of liver powder!

- Ground lamb or even duck meat may replace the ground beef, or else you may replace about half a pound (250 g to 300 g) of the ground beef with ground pork. See **Ground Lamb Parmentier** (page 197) for Lamb and Duck Parmentier variations with potatoes.

WINE PAIRING TIP I recommend a fruity but full-bodied St. Emilion or Castillon – Côtes de Bordeaux, or else a medium-bodied Pinot Noir from Burgundy. Restaurateur Annabelle also recommends red wines that are fruity, fresh, and warm (expressive and filled with character), such as an Alsatian Pinot Noir, a Beaujolais, or a Burgundy Pinot Noir such as an Irancy (located just West of Chablis), a Cabernet Franc-powered spicy and berry-fruited Saumur-Champigny from the Central Loire, an aromatic and rustic Quincy or Reuilly Pinot Noir from the Eastern Loire Valley, or a soft red Lirac from the Southern Rhône Valley.

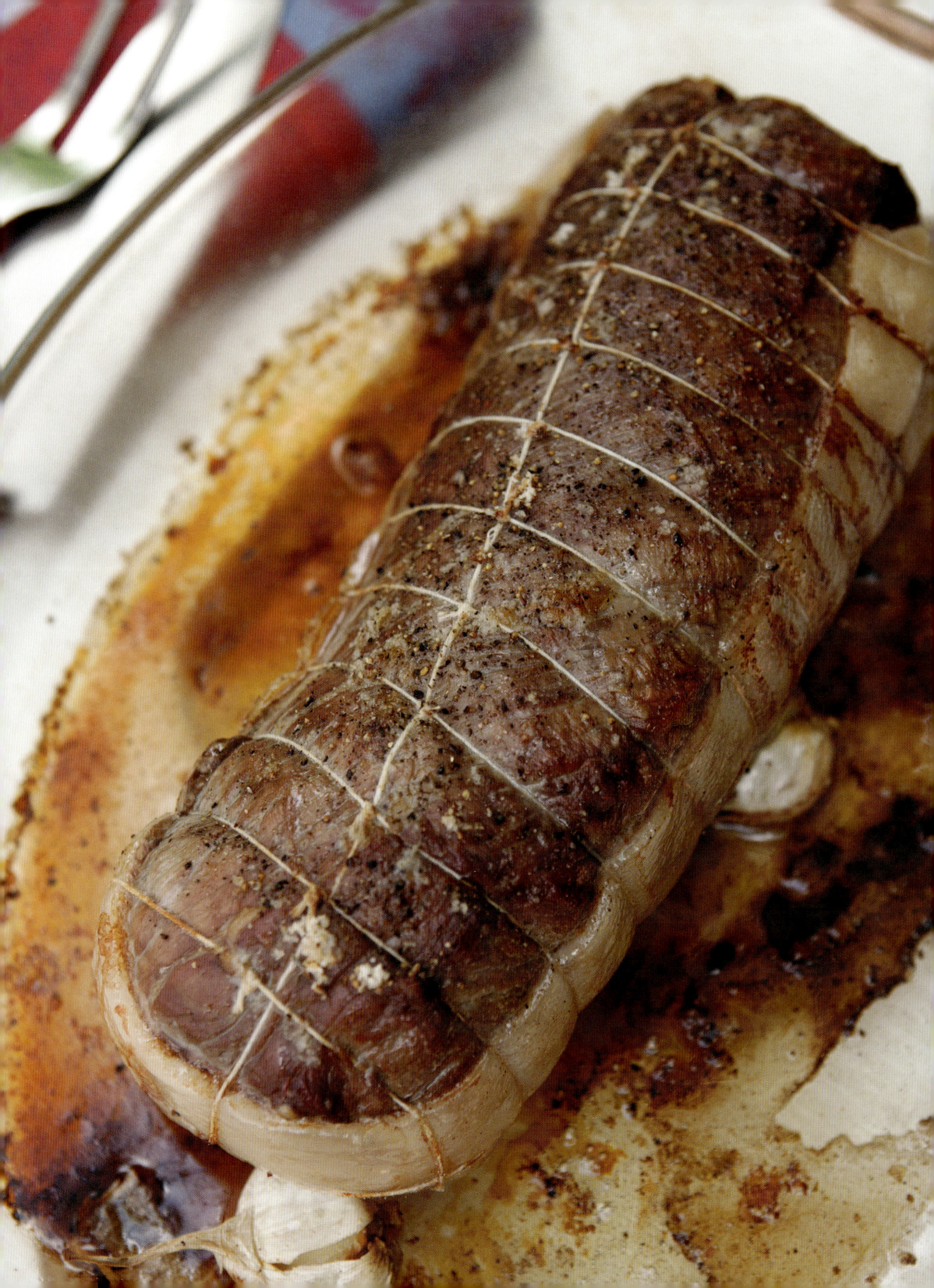

PEPPERED ROAST BEEF
Rosbif au Poivre

Season Year-round   **Preparation Time** 15 minutes, plus 15 minutes (optional) for wrapping and tying the roast   **Cooking Time** 25 minutes   **Serves** 5 to 6

This dish is simple, fast, and delicious, if you like eating beef rare. If not, you just cook it longer. (See the **Degrees of Doneness** for Beef chart on page 119). This dish can be served hot or cold. It calls for a tender cut of beef, such as the loin (*longe*, *filet*, or *faux filet*). It makes for an easy meal when you are in the middle of a project and need a quick fix. If this peppered version is too much for more tender palates (i.e., children), then try the other **Beef Roast** recipe (page 113). Roast beef can be wrapped or "barded" (*bardé*), wrapped in slices of fatback lard or bacon, and tied (*ficellé*), like in the Beef Roast recipe, or cooked without these extra steps. The wrapping and tying hold the roast in place make it more visually appealing (for guests, for example) and increase the fat content, and therefore the juiciness, of the dish.

- 2.2 pounds (1 kg) beef loin
- Optional: 1 tablespoon olive oil
- Pinch of fine salt
- Up to 3 tablespoons of ground black, white, or combination of peppercorns
- 1 tablespoon lard (or tallow or olive oil)
- Sprig of rosemary *(branche de romarin)*
- 3 garlic cloves, peeled and crushed
- ¼ cup water (60 ml)
- Additional salt and pepper to taste

Preheat the oven to 465°F (240°C). Pat the meat dry. Rub the olive oil around the surface of the meat (optional). Sprinkle the salt on the meat. Roll the meat in the ground pepper, or else sprinkle the pepper on the meat if you only are using a little bit of pepper. Wrap and tie the roast, if desired.

Smear one tablespoon of lard or tallow in the bottom of a casserole dish. Place the rosemary and garlic cloves in the pan and lay the meat on top of them.

Pour the ¼ cup water into bottom of the dish and place in the oven. After 10 minutes, turn the oven temperature down to 410°F (210°C) and allow to roast for 15 more minutes. (If you find this is still too rare, continue cooking for five to ten minutes until you find the desired "doneness" of the roast. Again, refer to the **Degrees of Doneness for Beef** chart on page 119.

Serve hot with **Potato Gratin "Dauphinois"** (page 463), baked potatoes, sweet potato fries, or cold with warmed **Béarnaise Sauce** (page 391), **Homemade Mayonnaise** (page 406), **Old-Fashioned Mustard** (page 410), or Primal Kitchen Mayo.

WINE PAIRING TIP Try a complex leather, plum, and tobacco Pomerol from Bordeaux, the aromatic berry, spice, and pepper of a Syrah from the Rhône Valley, or a peppery and dark-fruited Grenache from Languedoc-Roussillon. For roasts that are less cooked and more rare, Sommelière Annabelle recommends red wines that are tannic but not full-bodied, such as a Bordeaux Côtes de Bourg or a Bordeaux Supérieur, or a Pinot Noir from Burgundy's Côte de Beaune such as a Santenay, with notes of licorice, rose petals, and red berries. See also the wine suggestions under the **Beef Roast** recipe on page 113.

ROQUEFORT SIRLOIN STEAK
Pavé de Rumsteck au Roquefort

Season Year-round   **Preparation Time** 3 minutes   **Cooking Time** 6 to 10 minutes, depending on how rare you like your steak (Use the Degrees of Doneness for Beef chart on page 119.)   **Serves** 4

Pavé means thickly cut, about 1- to 1.5-inches thick (2 cm to 3 cm). A meat lover's favorite, the *pavé de rumsteck* is a "topside" or "rump" steak that comes from the hind quarter or rump of the cow. Roquefort cheese, usually eaten at room temperature, is made from sheep's milk that is inoculated with the local soil's mold spores, *Penicillium roqueforti*, seasoned with sea salt and aged in caves[7] in Languedoc-Roussillon, bordering Southwestern France.[7]

VARIATIONS To add crunch and flavor, sprinkle on a few grilled or toasted chopped nuts. Paula Wolfert suggests a mixture of pine nuts, walnuts, and blanched (peeled) almonds in a similar dish, inspired by Gascon chef André Daguin, in her wonderfully authentic cookbook from 1983 (revised in 2005), *The Cooking of Southwest France*.[8]

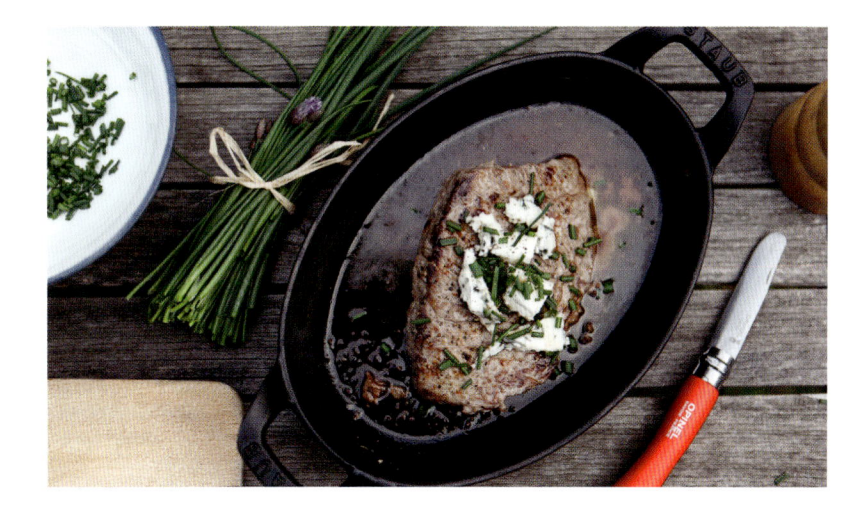

WINE PAIRING TIP In the presence of a strongly flavorful Roquefort, you can pair this dish with a sweet desert wine from the Southwest (Barsac, Loupiac, Monbazillac, or Sauternes), or else try a more traditional regional pairing with a Languedoc-Roussillon red, as Roquefort cheese is made in this region.

1 tablespoon beef tallow (*suif*)

1 tablespoon butter

Salt and pepper for seasoning the steaks

1.5 pounds (700 g) steak (makes 4 steaks)

1 tablespoon Roquefort cheese, crumbled

1 teaspoon chives, minced

Optional: 1 tablespoon parsley, minced, for garnish

Melt the tallow and the butter over high heat in a flat cast-iron pan or plancha pan. Salt and pepper the steaks. Sear the steaks for several minutes on each side, using a spoon to baste (*arroser*) them with the juices.

Remove from heat and sprinkle with the crumbled Roquefort and chives. Garnish with optional parsley. Serve with white or sweet potato fries and sautéed or roasted vegetables.

BEEF – LE BOEUF

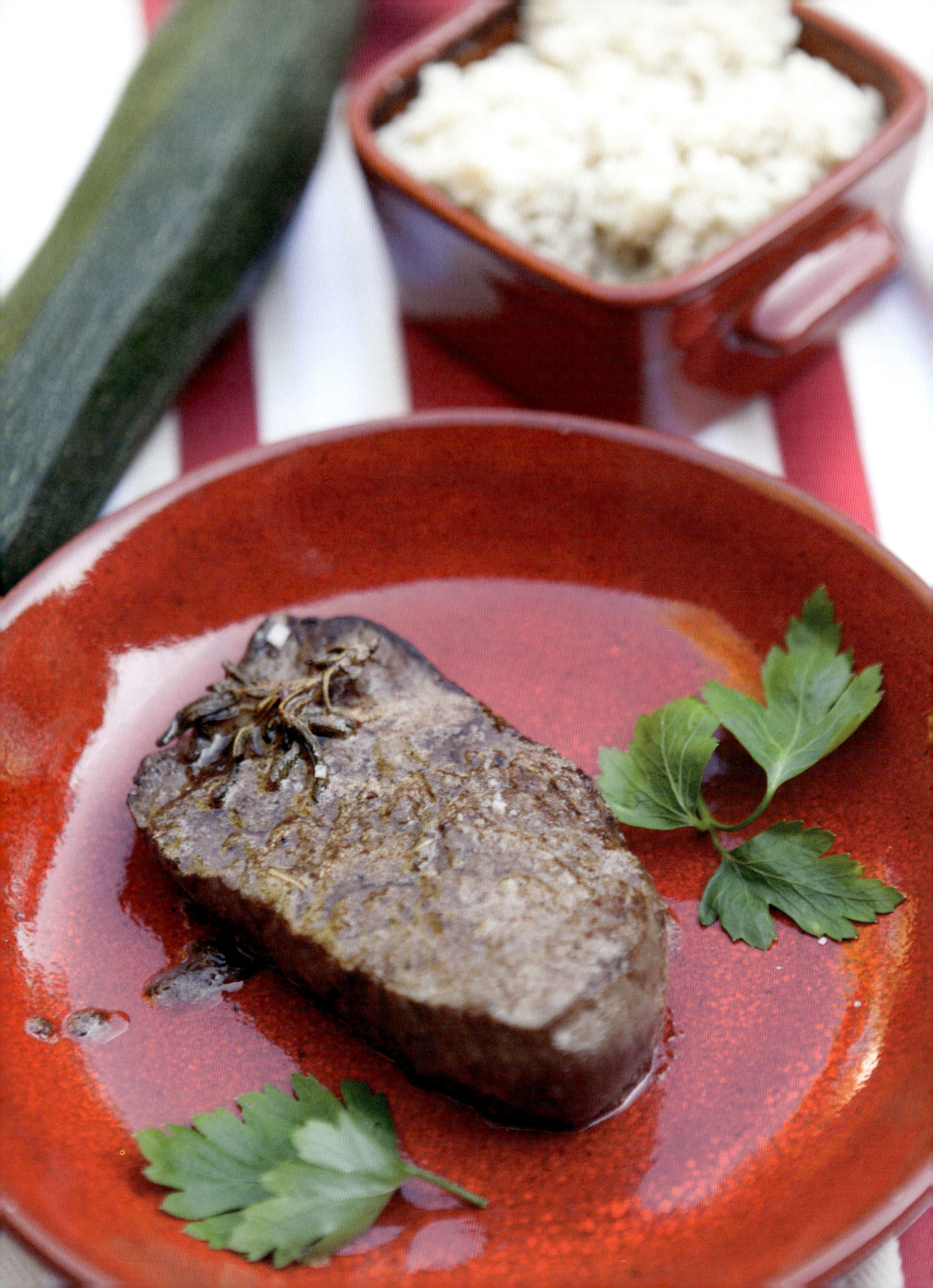

SAGE BUTTER SIRLOIN STEAK
Pavé de Rumsteck au Beurre à la Sauge

Season Year-round **Preparation Time** 2 minutes
Cooking Time 6 to 10 minutes, depending on how rare you like your steak **Serves** 4

French chefs tend to put herbs in butter to augment the flavor of a dish. If you would like to make an herbed butter to place on the side of a dish and to use for spreading, blend chopped butter at room temperature and chopped herbs in a food processor or blender, adding fine salt if desired. Scrape the "herbed" butter into a nice little ramekin or roll it with parchment paper, cool in the fridge, and cut into eye-pleasing round disks. In this dish, the butter and sage are mixed together in the pan. You can dream up any combination of butter and spices and it will probably taste great on this steak, or any steak cut I have mentioned in previous recipes. The *pavé de rumsteck* comes from the "rump," or the "topside." Remember that a *pavé* is a thickly cut steak and will be rarer in the middle than a regular steak, thus might need additional time to cook in the oven. (Refer to the **Degrees of Doneness for Beef** chart on page 119.)

1 tablespoon butter or ghee

Fine salt and pepper for seasoning the steaks

1.5 pounds (700 g) steak (makes 4 steaks)

1 tablespoon dried sage, chopped

Melt the butter over high heat in a flat or plancha pan. Salt and pepper the steaks. Add the sage to the pan. Sear the steaks for several minutes on each side while basting the steaks with the sage and butter. Serve rare in the middle, or place in the oven preheated to 375°F (190°C) for 5 to 12 minutes.

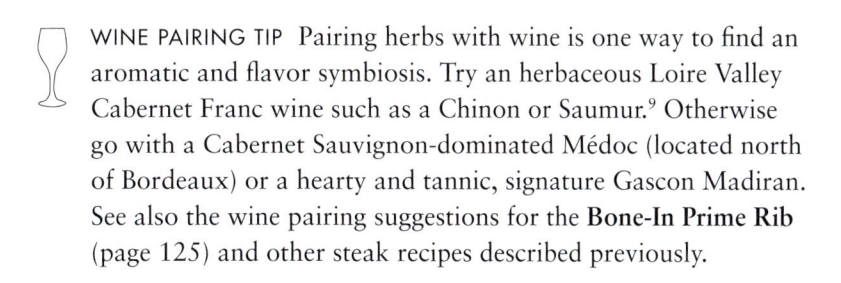

WINE PAIRING TIP Pairing herbs with wine is one way to find an aromatic and flavor symbiosis. Try an herbaceous Loire Valley Cabernet Franc wine such as a Chinon or Saumur.[9] Otherwise go with a Cabernet Sauvignon-dominated Médoc (located north of Bordeaux) or a hearty and tannic, signature Gascon Madiran. See also the wine pairing suggestions for the **Bone-In Prime Rib** (page 125) and other steak recipes described previously.

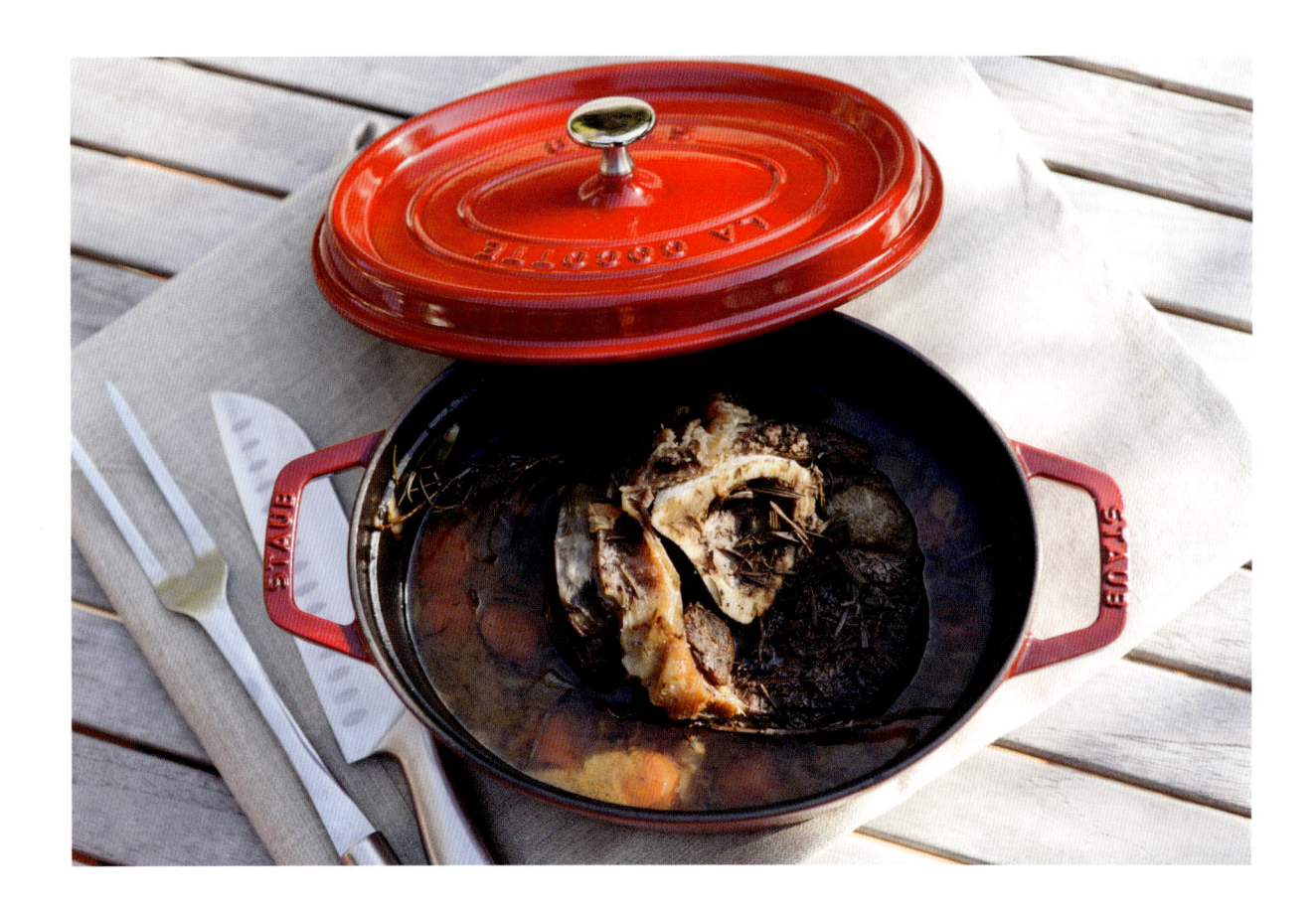

SLOW-COOKED BEEF SHANK
Jarret (Gîte) de Boeuf

Season Year-round, but usually Autumn, Winter, or early Spring   **Preparation Time** 20 minutes   **Cooking Time** 3 hours minimum   **Serves** 5

The beef "shank" (*le jarret* or *la gîte*) is the leg, technically extending from the ankle to the knee of the cow, and is a tough bite to eat, requiring a long cooking time. According to Basque butcher Florent Carriquiry, *gîte* is the nationally recognized term for shank, while *jarret* is the regional or colloquial term. Braising (*braiser*) is the method by which a meat is browned on high heat and then cooked slowly in broth, fat, water, wine, or its own juices. The extra bonus from this particular piece of meat is the collagenous tissues it contains and the marrow in the bone. A thick cut of shank, as well as the whitish marrow it contains, will both be rendered tender and soft (*moeulleux*) from the long cooking. Slow cooking softens and extracts the collagen for us to easily consume in the meat and broth. This dish is another good example of nose-to-tail eating. If you have more shank meat on hand, feel free to double the recipe.

2 tablespoons tallow

2 to 3 slices (60 g) bacon, cut in pieces (*lardons*)

2.2 pounds (1 kg) beef shank

3 pinches of salt

3 cloves of garlic (*gousses d'ail*), unpeeled (*en chemise*) but smashed

2 shallots, minced

1 cup (240 ml) bone broth

1 cup (240 ml) water

1 bay leaf

2 sprigs of rosemary

1 teaspoon thyme

2 carrots, chopped

Optional: 1 tablespoon apple cider vinegar

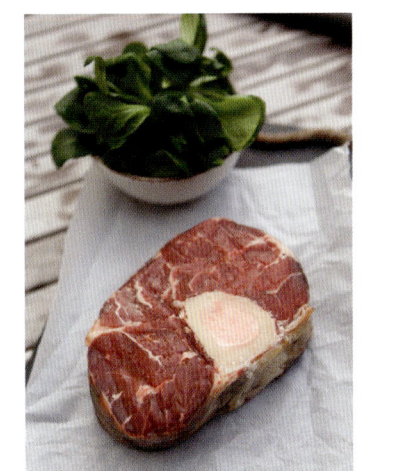

Melt the tallow in a pan over medium-high heat. Brown the *lardons* for up to 10 minutes, stirring now and then to brown them evenly. Transfer the *lardons* to a bowl, turn the heat to high, and brown the meat for two to three minutes on each side. Turn the heat down to medium-low and add the remaining ingredients. Cover and cook for 3 hours.

Serve with roasted or sautéed in-season vegetables, boiled or roasted potatoes, roasted root vegetables, or baked sweet potatoes.

WINE PAIRING TIP To match the more subdued flavors of this slow-cooked dish, try an aromatic and delicate Volnay Pinot Noir, with notes of cherry, flowers, spice, and stewed prunes, from Burgundy's Côte de Beaune, or a well-structured, berry fruits Givry from Burgundy's Côte Chalonnaise. Otherwise go with a bolder, more tannic red from Bordeaux's "right bank" of Saint Emilion, Pomerol or Lalande de Pomerol. To underscore the rosemary and thyme in this dish, my DUAD wine course classmate and sommelier friend Natalia Youreva recommends going with a spicy, elegant Syrah from the Northern Rhône Valley (try a fruity and well-balanced Crozes-Hermitage), or else a more rustic Syrah from the Southern Rhône Valley such as from Châteauneuf-du-Pape. In particular, Natalia recommends organic and sustainably-minded Château de la Gardine's red wines with melty tanins and stewed fruits. See also the wine pairing suggestions for **Braised Oxtail** (page 127).

Raw Beef Shank

SPIDER STEAK WITH ORANGE
Araignée de Boeuf à l'Orange

Season Late Autumn and Winter **Preparation Time** 10 minutes
Cooking Time 15 minutes **Serves** 1 (with a bit left over)

The spider steak (*araignée*) is a flavorful, rare piece of beef often set aside by the butcher for his own consumption (*pièce du boucher*) rather than sold to customers. Other such pieces, often reserved for the real meat *connoisseur*, are the *merlan* and the *poire*, both from the sirloin (*surlonge*) or "topside." The reason the spider steak is often kept by the butcher is because the piece is replete with nerve tissue, forming a kind of spider's web through the muscle that gives the piece its name (as seen in the raw spider steak photo below). The many fibers are difficult to remove without a lot of care and time to make the steak presentable. This extra effort makes it too expensive to be worth the trouble to sell. Spider steaks comes from the hip joint of the cow. There is one on each side, weighing about 1.3 pounds (600 g) each. Having befriended and apprenticed with my local organic butchers, I asked them for a part of this piece to give it a try. We did not bother to remove all the nerve tissue (which contains collagen), and it was delicious! Perhaps that is the real reason butchers save it for themselves.

FOR THE ORANGE SAUCE

Zest of half an orange

Juice of one orange

Pinch of sea salt

1 tablespoon duck fat

Pinch of sea salt

3 shallots, finely chopped

FOR THE STEAK

Fine salt and pepper for seasoning the steak

11 ounces (315 g) spider steak

2 tablespoons butter

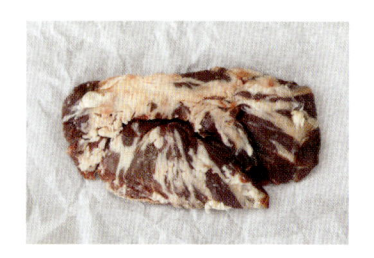

Raw Spider Steak

Place the ingredients for the orange sauce into a small saucepan, and allow to reduce for several minutes on medium-low heat. Meanwhile, melt the duck fat in a pan over medium heat, add the salt, and brown the shallots for several minutes. Scrape the shallots out of the pan and mix into the orange sauce in the small saucepan. Keep the sauce warm on low until the steak is ready.

Salt and pepper the steak. Allow the butter to melt in the same pan used for the shallots on high heat. As the butter begins to turn slightly caramel colored (*noisette*), add the steak. Sear each side for two to three minutes, drizzling (*arroser*) the butter sauce over the steak. Turn the heat down to medium-high, and flip the steak over a few times to cook through for a few more minutes, if desired, while you continue to drizzle the butter sauce over the steak. Remove the steak from the pan and top with half of the orange shallot sauce, putting the other half in a small ramekin or dish for dipping.

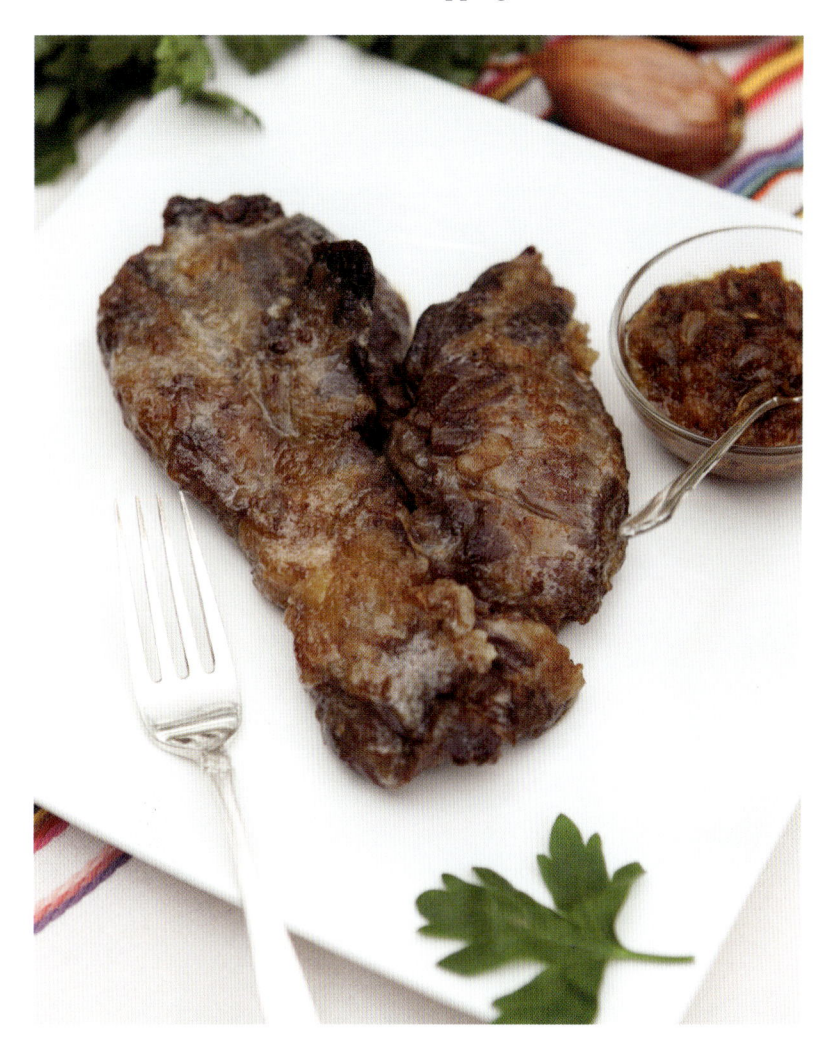

WINE PAIRING TIP To play up the fruit in this dish, try a young, also fruity Beaujolais or a flavorful but less tannic Graves – Pessac Léognan from Bordeaux. Otherwise, restaurateur Annabelle recommends wines that are well-structured, oaked (spicy, smoky, or vanilla-flavored), tannic and powerful, in contrast to the subdued flavors in this dish. She suggests the dark berry-flavored wines from Saint Emilion or the leather and tobacco wines of Pomerol, both from Bordeaux, or else a spiced Syrah from the Côtes du Rhône, or a Côtes du Roussillon with notes of dark fruits and spice, or an aromatic Saint-Chinian from Languedoc, with notes of cacao, raspberry, red currant, and spice.

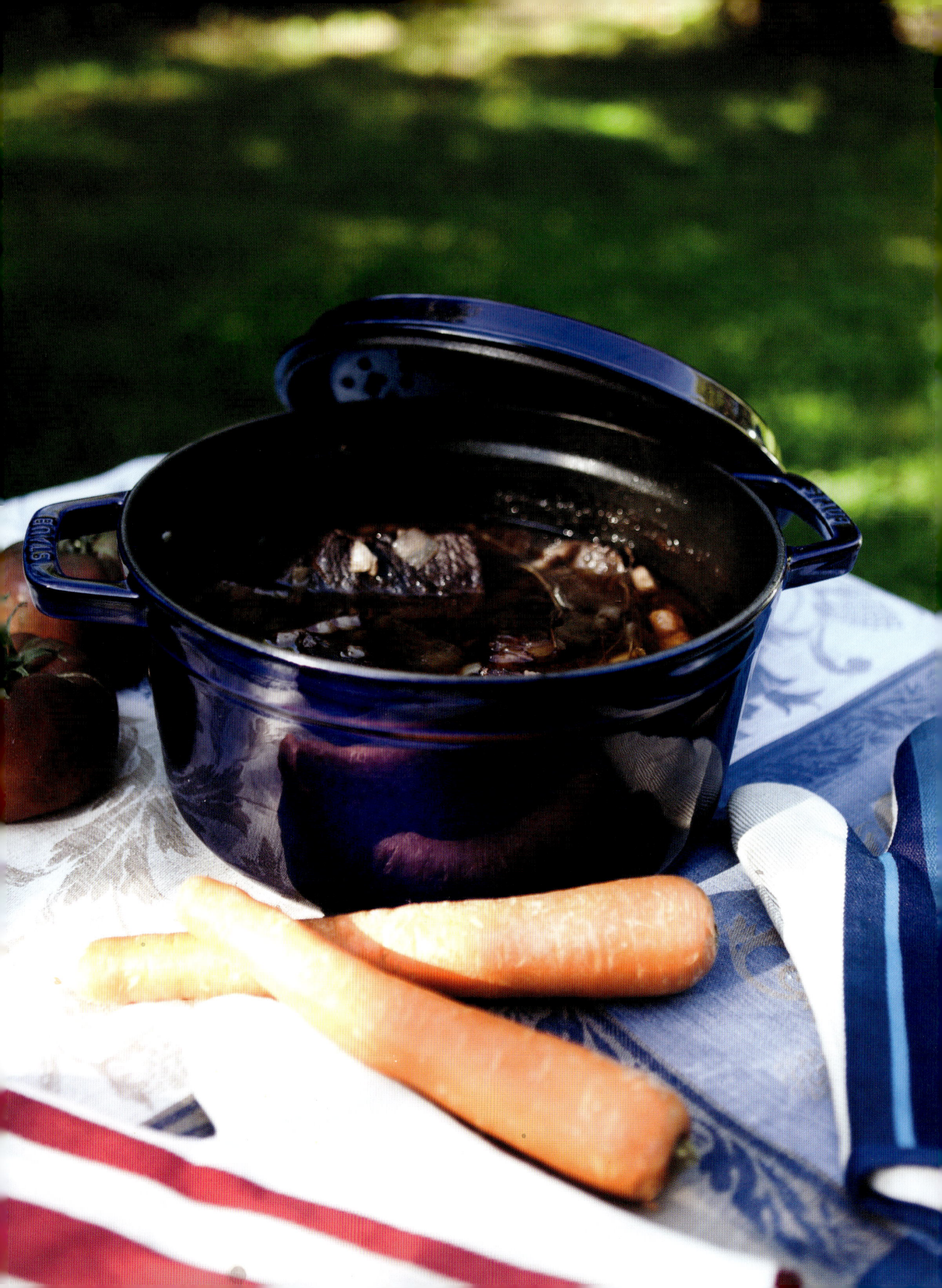

WINE-BRAISED BEEF STEW WITH ORANGE
Daube de Boeuf à l'Orange

Season Late Autumn through Winter   **Preparation Time** 25 minutes, plus overnight marinating
Cooking Time 3 hours minimum   **Serves** 8

This is another slow-cooking recipe, and depending on the region, the ingredients, particularly the wine used, will vary. Braising (*braiser*) is essentially to slow-cook a meat, usually after it has been browned. This is a variation on the classic with added orange zest, inspired by Parisian butcher Hugo Desnoyer, who magnificently presents dozens of recipes in his lovely book, *Morceaux Choisis* ("Chosen Pieces"), which was proudly displayed at the butcher counter where I apprenticed for the customers to view and gain inspiration. Tough meats, such as chuck (*paleron*) or even beef cheeks (*joues de boeuf*) can replace the round or rump steak (*noix de gîte*). Note again the following butcher's secret: Remove the meat from the refrigerator and allow it to come to room temperature before heating it so as to cook it evenly and also not give the meat thermal shock, causing the muscle fibers to contract and harden.[10] The magic of this dish is in the marinating overnight in the vegetables, spices, and wine.

- 1 large onion or 2 small onions, red or yellow, thinly sliced
- 4 cloves of garlic, minced
- 1 carrot, cut in rounds (*rondelles*)
- 1 branch of celery, diced
- ½ pound (200 g to 250 g) smoked bacon (*poitrine fumée*), diced, or pre-cut bacon pieces (*lardons*)
- 1 sprig of thyme, fresh or dried
- 2 bay leaves
- 2 cloves
- 1 tablespoon olive oil
- Bottle of red wine
- Pinch of sea salt
- Pinch of ground pepper
- 1.5 to 2 pounds (750 g to 900 g) round or rump steak, cubed
- 2.2 pounds (1 kg) plate meat, bone-in
- Zest of half an orange
- 4 tablespoons tallow (beef or lamb)
- Optional: Cinnamon stick

BEEF – LE BOEUF

Place all ingredients except the tallow and cinnamon stick into a large cast-iron pot with a cover or into an oven-safe terra cotta dish. Douse everything with the wine. Allow to marinate, preferably overnight.

Remove from the refrigerator half an hour before cooking. Melt the tallow in a large pan over high heat. Remove the meat cubes and plate meat from the marinade and brown them on all sides in the pan in batches along with the *lardons*. Transfer them back to the cast-iron pot, add one cup of water to the pot, and bring to a boil. Add the cinnamon stick, cover the pot, and allow to simmer for a minimum of three hours. This is one of those dishes that has even more flavor the next day!

VARIATIONS If you have any marrow bones, you can add them at the beginning of cooking. You can add a handful of black olives, zest of one lemon, and a few peeled and diced tomatoes, or a tablespoon of tomato sauce, to the pot before cooking. This makes it a Provençale beef stew (*daube de boeuf à la provençale*), with ingredients originating from Provence.

WINE PAIRING TIP Try a Côtes du Rhône, Vacqueyras, or Châteauneuf-du-Pape, from the southern Rhône region. If you add tomatoes, go for a wine made with Malbec grapes, such as Côtes de Bourg and Côtes de Bordeaux Blaye, where Malbec is found in greatest percentage in a Bordeaux blend (*assemblage*). Or, for a more Provençale pairing, try a Bandol that can have notes of dark fruits, leather spice, and vanilla. See also Annabelle's wine recommendations for the **Spider Steak with Orange** on page 149.

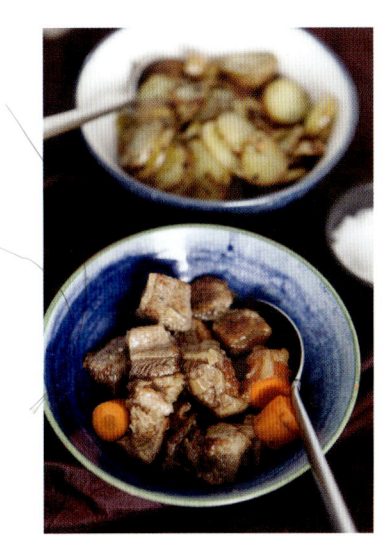

Simplest Beef Stew

Simple Braised Beef Stew with Orange
Daube de Boeuf à l'Orange Simple

This is another, simpler version of the braised beef stew, using 2.2 pounds (1 kg) of stew meat (chunks of chuck beef), if you are lacking in or do not want to add red wine and/or the bacon pieces and do not have time to marinate. Season the meat chunks with two or three pinches each of salt and pepper. Brown several pieces of beef at a time on all sides over medium-high to high heat (about three minutes per batch) in five tablespoons of beef tallow (or duck fat), giving each batch an additional pinch of salt as you put them in the pot. Once all the pieces are browned on the outside, return them to the pan, reduce the heat to medium-low, and add some chopped onion (about 2.2 ounces or 60 g), one chopped carrot (about 3.5 ounces or 100 g), one diced celery stalk, four cloves of minced garlic, a bay leaf, one more pinch of salt, one teaspoon thyme, pepper to taste, and the zest of one orange. If you have it, add some dry bacon rind. Cover everything with one part water to one part veal stock or bone broth, and simmer on low for a minimum of three hours. Garnish with coarse sea salt. I have paired this stew with a fruit-forward Bergerac from the French Southwest—fruit on fruit, delicious! I have also paired this stew with an organic red, smoky, mocha, leather and cinnamon-spiced 2005 (nicely aged) Château Lagarette Cuvée Renaissance from the Premières Côtes de Bordeaux (whose appellation changed to Cadillac – Côtes de Bordeaux in 2009). See also the wine pairing suggestions for the **Wine-Braised Beef Stew with Orange** on the previous page. Need even simpler beef stew? Are oranges out of season? Just brown the beef and add chopped onions and carrots, salt, pepper, and a cup of water. Cover and simmer for two to three hours. Simple! See the finished product for "Simplest Beef Stew" shown above. Serves 6 to 7.

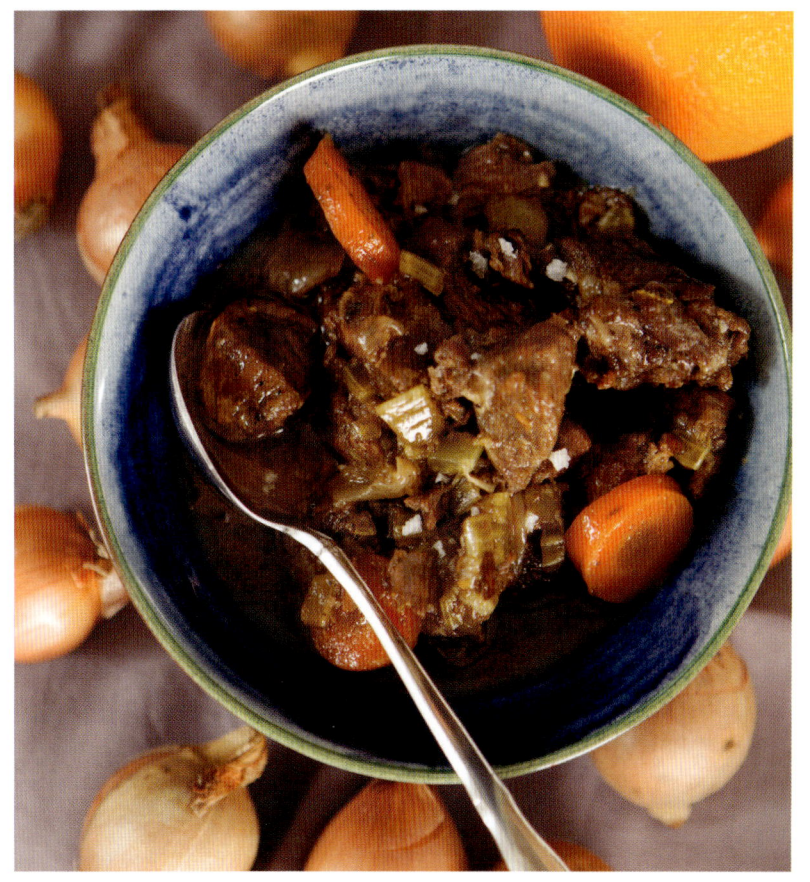

Simple Beef Stew with Orange

BEEF – LE BOEUF

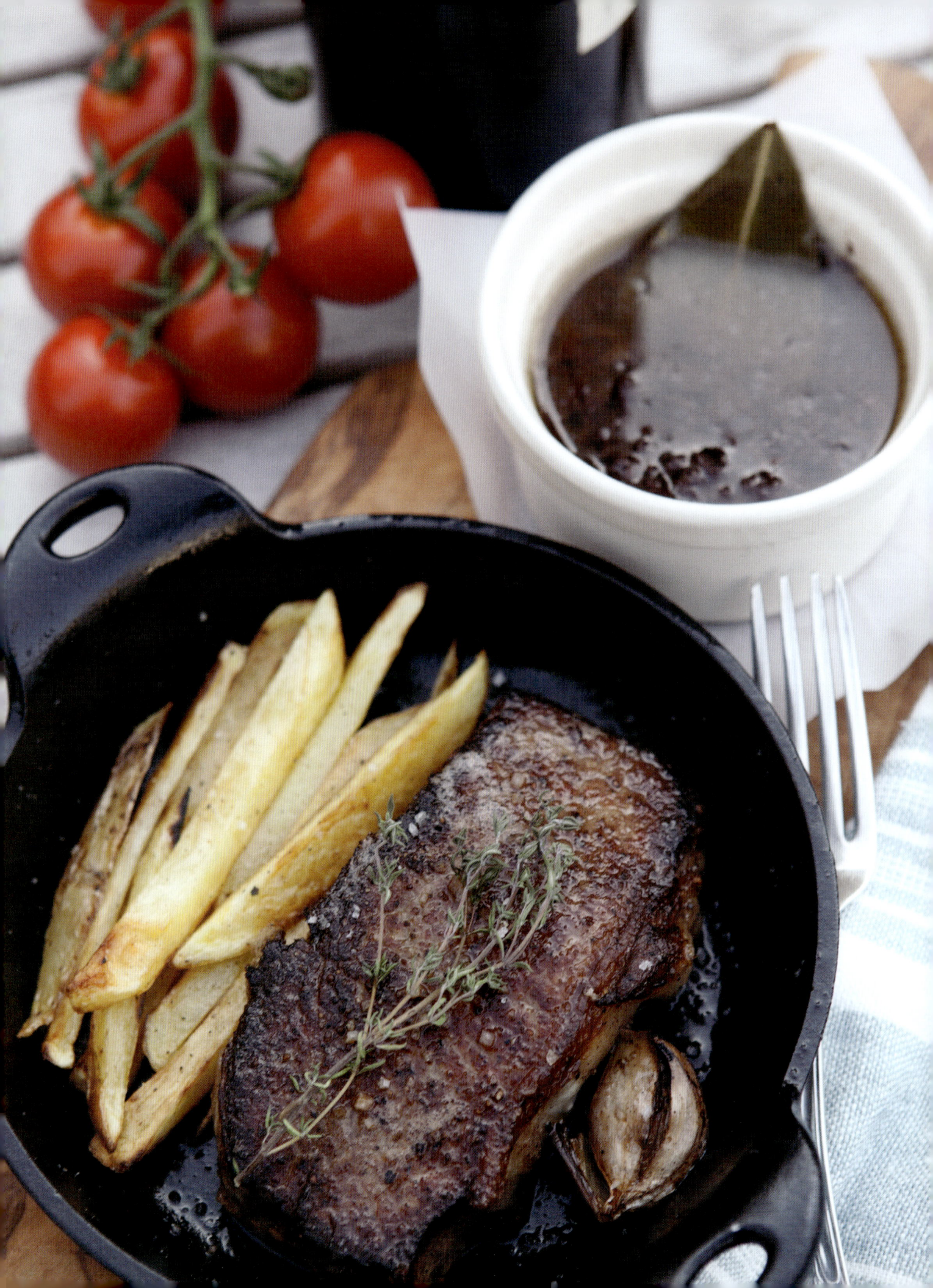

WINE TRADER'S RIB EYE STEAK
Entrecôte Marchand de Vin

Season Year-round   **Preparation Time** 35 minutes
Cooking Time 45 minutes for the sauce, 7 to 15 minutes for the meat   **Serves** 4

Inspired by one of my favorite French cookbooks, *Viandes*, by Jean-Francois Mallet, this recipe is the perfect example of a regional food matched with a regional wine (i.e., Bordeaux and Bordeaux!), as Bordeaux wine is used in the preparation of this dish. The wine sauce is essentially a "Bordeaux wine sauce" (*sauce bordelaise*) minus the beef bone marrow. If you have bone marrow on hand, you can add about three tablespoons (poach it in gently boiling water for about 5 minutes first) to the sauce as it stews and reduces down; you will have an official *sauce bordelaise*. Otherwise, the sauce is called as it is here, "wine trader's sauce" (*sauce marchand de vin*), using a wine from Bordeaux, which is historically famous for its wine traders (known as négotiants in Bordeaux). If you were in Southwestern France, you would order a Bazas or Limousin beef steak, not necessarily just rib eye. Other cuts of steak will do. If a steak has a side rim of fat, score (*taillader*) the fat side to keep the steak from curling, or ask the butcher to do this. Make the wine sauce with any Bordeaux red, and then drink the rest of the bottle with the meal, making a perfect match. For a Bordeaux wine connoisseur this means almost too broad a choice of reds, as they vary so much in their blends (*assemblages*), styles, and terroirs across the Bordeaux region. On the other hand, this choice opens up the door to experimentation, even beyond the traditional, tannic red grape varieties of Bordeaux, democratizing the dish, and opening the door of opportunity to try other regional pairings.

Since the wine is heated, some of its original magic gets cooked off. However, the rule of thumb is to always use a good wine, one you actually like, not "just a cooking wine." As my wine connoisseur friend Dewey Markham, Jr. reminds us, "specially packaged 'cooking wines' have added salt to make them a condiment and thus avoid taxes and other assorted duties that alcoholic beverages are subject to. This is why you don't want to drink the stuff." Just like everything else in life where you get what you pay for, the taste of the finished dish will reflect the quality of the wine. A lot of ingredients go into making this sauce, but the richness and buttery smoothness of the sauce is well worth the effort, particularly for guests. As with so many beloved French recipes, butter is called for here for its flavor. Ghee is a good substitute. If you cannot tolerate even ghee, then replace the butter or ghee with tallow. This recipe would then call for a total of about 15 tablespoons of tallow. If you do not have enough tallow for the recipe, use lard. The subtle flavors of each of these fats will change the taste of the sauce, which is part of the fun of experimenting! ➤

FOR THE WINE SAUCE (MAKES ABOUT 1 CUP OF SAUCE)

1 tablespoon beef tallow

9 to 10 tablespoons butter

5 shallots, minced

1 sprig of fresh or dried thyme

2 bay leaves

Optional: 1 teaspoon organic brown sugar, honey, or maple syrup

⅔ to 1 cup (150 to 240 ml) red wine

½ cup (120 ml) beef or veal stock

Salt and pepper to taste

FOR THE STEAKS

4 tablespoons butter (1 tablespoon for each steak)

1 tablespoon tallow

1 garlic clove, unpeeled (*en chemise*) and crushed

Fine salt and pepper for seasoning

4 rib-eye steaks, about 7 ounces (200 g) each

Sea salt to taste

Freshly ground pepper to taste

A few small sprigs of fresh or dried thyme for garnish

Deglazing *(déglacer)* is the process of un-sticking or scraping the stuck "sugars" from the bottom of the pan. It is one of the secrets to delicious sauces in French cooking!

To prepare the sauce, melt the tallow and 3 to 4 tablespoons of the butter in a saucepan over medium-high heat. Brown the shallots, adding the sprig of thyme, bay leaves, and optional sweetener. Reduce the heat and allow to stew (*compoter*) and caramelize for 8 to 10 minutes, stirring occasionally. (If you have beef bone marrow, you would add it now.) The trick here is to allow the sugars and juices from the shallots to stick a bit to the bottom of the pan, but not to burn. This caramelization is called the Maillard reaction. Deglaze the pan with the wine using a wooden spatula while pouring in and mixing the wine with the syrupy mixture.

Allow the sauce to reduce by about a quarter over medium-low heat (this takes about 6 to 10 minutes). Add the beef stock, and allow the sauce to reduce again by about half (this can take about 20 minutes). Try the sauce, adding salt and pepper to taste. Be generous with these seasonings. Add the rest of the butter, stirring it in with a whisk. If you find the sauce is a bit bitter, add a bit more sweetener. Rather than let the sauce boil again at this point, keep the sauce warm until the steaks are ready by putting the pan into another pan with hot water (*bain-marie*), or keep the saucepan over a very low heat if the pan is thick enough. (Chefs often use five-ply or seven-ply saucepans, meaning seven layers of metals, such as Demeyere, which are thick enough to make sauces without burning them.)

For the steaks, melt the butter and tallow in a pan over medium-high heat. Add the crushed garlic clove. Season both sides of the steaks with salt and pepper. Sear the steaks for two to three minutes on each side while spooning (*arroser*) the butter and tallow sauce from the pan over each steak. The steaks will be rare on the inside. To further cook the steak if necessary, place it in a dish into a preheated oven at 375°F (190°C) for 8 to 10 minutes for medium, 10 to 12 minutes for well done. (See the **Degrees of Doneness for Beef** chart on page 119.)

Sprinkle the steaks with additional salt and pepper to taste and garnish with the thyme. Serve the steaks with the wine trader's sauce on the side for dipping. Combine the steak with your favorite sautéed vegetables. Traditionally, this dish is eaten with sautéed potatoes or fries or grilled vegetables. Because the sauce is made with plenty of fat, it will preserve for a week in an oven-safe glass or ceramic container in the refrigerator, easily reheatable in the oven for subsequent meals.

VARIATIONS To make this a traditional Sauce Bordelaise, gently fold two to three tablespoons of poached, diced beef bone marrow (the fatty filling inside the leg bones) into the sauce after you have whisked in the last of the butter. (Poaching the marrow requires removing it from the bone, preferably in one piece or in spoon-sized pieces, and placing it in gently boiling water for three to five minutes.) Have your butcher slice the bones lengthwise for you, or else chop them carefully yourself with a cleaver, being careful to remove any bone splinters from the marrow. Sometimes leg bones will be sold in two-inch pieces cut cross-wise, the marrow should be easy to remove with a spoon.

WINE PAIRING TIP The rich sauce in this recipe calls for a hearty red Bordeaux wine with structure and character, and there are so very many from which to choose. I initially used Château Haut-Bailly's "second wine," La Parde, from 2010, an excellent year in Bordeaux and one of Haut-Bailly's best vintages, to make the sauce and pair the dish. Their blend is Cabernet Sauvignon, Merlot, and Cabernet Franc in decreasing order. Try also the Merlot-majority wines of Castillon or other Côtes de Bordeaux, Côtes de Blaye, Côtes de Bourg, Graves de Vayres, or St. Emilion, or else the Cabernet Sauvignon-dominated wines of the Médoc. A slightly less tannic red Graves – Pessac Léognan from Bordeaux, like Haut-Bailly, blends careful amounts of both of these grapes, often along with the Cabernet Franc grape, for a lovely Bordeaux pairing with this dish as well.

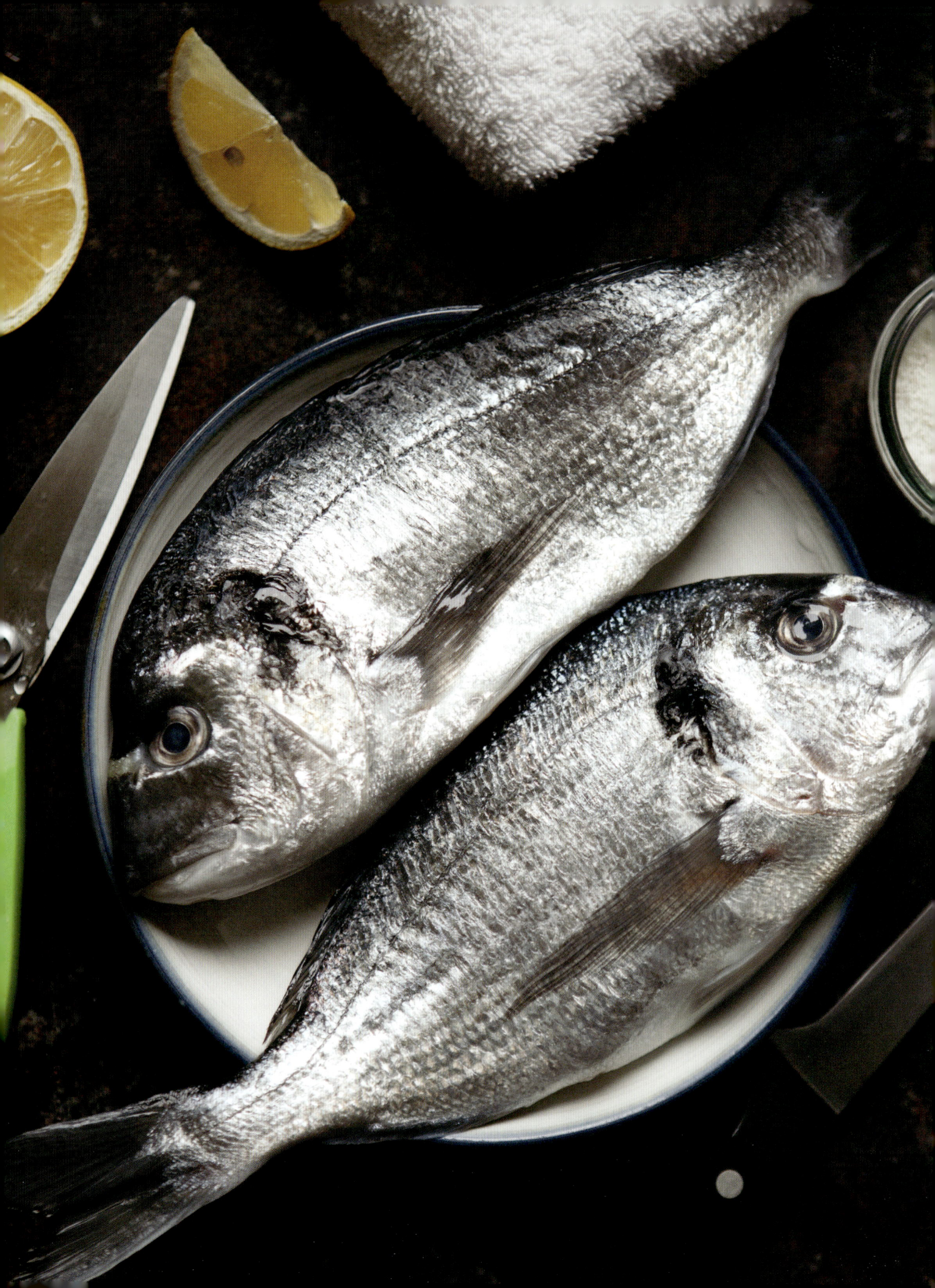

FISH AND SEAFOOD
Les Poissons et les Fruits de Mer

Basque Grilled Squid – *Chipirons à la Plancha* 160

Bordeaux Oysters with Pork and Shallot Meatballs – *Huitres à la Bordelaise, Crépinette de Porc à l'Échalote* 163

Butter-Fried Scallops – *Coquilles Saint Jacques au Beurre* 167

Catch of the Day – *Marmite de Poisson* 170

Grilled Sardines with Garlic and Parsley – *Sardines Grillées à l'Ail et au Persil* 173

Mackerel with Garlic and Shallots – *Maquereau à l'Ail et à l'Échalote* 175

Marinated Cuttlefish – *Blanc de Seiche Mariné* 178

Salmon Tartare – *Tartare de Saumon* 180

Sea Bream Fillets with Grilled Pine Nuts – *Filets de Daurade aux Pignons de Pin Grillés* 184

Spreadable Fish Paste – *Rillettes de Poisson* 186

BASQUE GRILLED SQUID
Chipirons à la Plancha

Season Late Autumn through early Spring   **Preparation Time** 35 minutes
Cooking Time 30 minutes   **Serves** 2

Squid (*encornet*) is a kind of cuttlefish (*seiche*). Chipirons (called *chipirones* in Spanish) are a small type of squid in the cuttlefish family that are caught along the Basque coast (*la Côte Basque*) and are grilled in a similar manner, with olive oil and garlic. But in the Basque recipes they add parsley, red or green bell peppers, and sometimes vinegar, onion, *piment d'Espelette* (a sweet, sometimes slightly spicy powdered chili pepper and hallmark of Basque cooking), and white wine to deglaze the pan. You can make this dish using fresh or frozen squid, but for actual chipirons, you will have to make the pilgrimage to the Basque coastal region. Basque chipirons are best in the winter but are available in late Autumn and early Spring as well. This is a great dish to make as an appetizer and serve with Champagne. Chipirons are usually cooked on a flat iron grill or iron skillet (*plancha*).

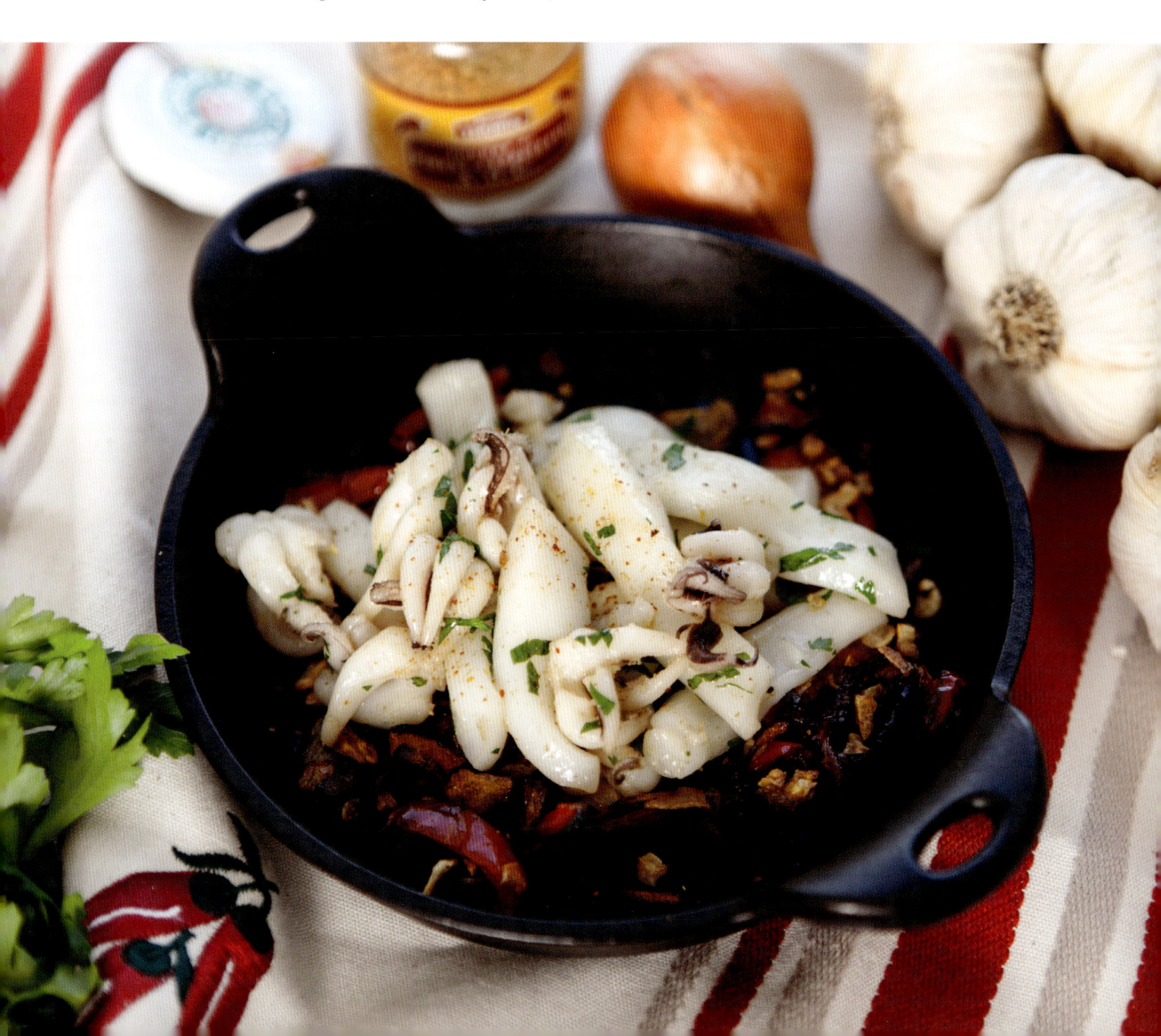

4 tablespoons olive oil

1 small onion minced (about 1.3 ounces or 35 g)

½ red or green bell pepper (about 2 ounces or 55 g), thinly sliced into 1-inch (2.5 cm) pieces

3 garlic cloves, plus one more, minced

1.1 pounds (500 g) squid, cleaned, outer film removed, sliced into bite-sized rings and pieces

Pinch of fine sea salt

3 sprigs parsley, stems removed, minced

1 tablespoon white wine vinegar (or 2 to 3 tablespoons white wine)

Optional: *piment d'Espelette*

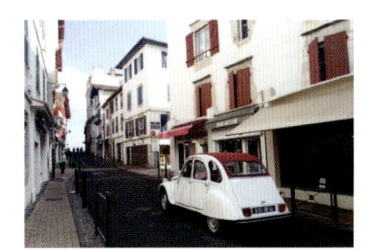

St. Jean de Luz, Basque Coast

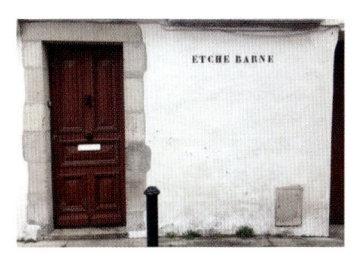

Barne House, a residence in St. Jean de Luz

Heat two tablespoons of olive oil in a pan over medium heat, and add the onions and peppers. Allow them to soften, stirring occasionally, about 15 minutes. Remove from the pan and set aside in a bowl.

Add the garlic and one tablespoon olive oil to the pan, and allow the garlic to brown for four to five minutes.

Transfer the garlic to the bowl with the peppers. Increase the heat under the pan to high, and add the squid, salt, and the last clove of minced garlic. As the water from the squid begins to steam off, add one more tablespoon of olive oil and cook for five to seven more minutes. Remove from heat, stir in parsley. Serve over the pepper-onion-garlic mix. If you wish to deglaze the pan (by stirring in a liquid to remove the browned juices stuck to the pan), you would do this now with either one tablespoon of white wine vinegar or two to three tablespoons of white wine, scrape the pan, and spoon this over the squid. (Not shown in recipe photo.) Top with *piment d'Espelette*, if desired.

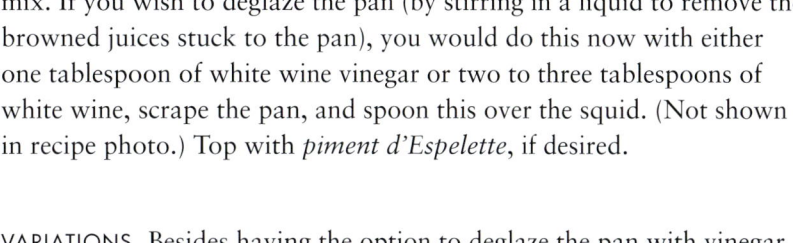

VARIATIONS Besides having the option to deglaze the pan with vinegar or white wine, you can also add bits of chorizo to increase the savory umami profile of this dish.

WINE PAIRING TIP For a regional pairing, try a white, full-bodied, and fruity Irouléguy from the Basque country or a predominantly Merlot, dry Côtes de Bergerac from the Southwest. Otherwise, try a dry white Graves or Entre-Deux-Mers from the Bordeaux region; a Champagne, Bordeaux Crémant, or other sparkling wine could work as well, if you like "bubbly."

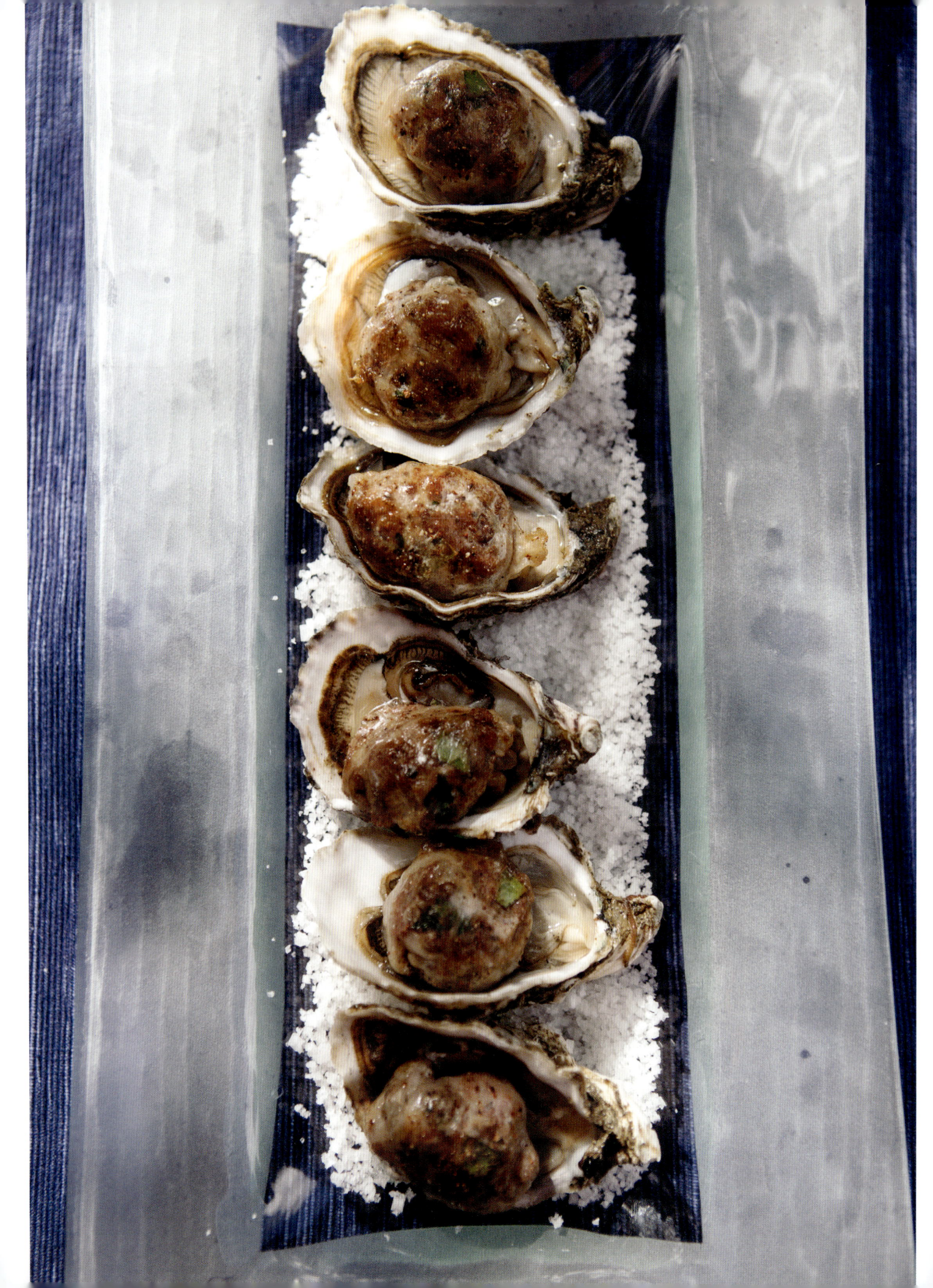

BORDEAUX OYSTERS WITH PORK AND SHALLOT MEATBALLS
Huîtres à la Bordelaise, Crépinette de Porc à l'Échalote

Season Autumn through early Spring   **Preparation Time** Several minutes to open the oysters, 45 minutes for the meatballs   **Cooking Time** 15 to 20 minutes   **Serves** 6

My French chef friend Chef Frédéric, from whom I initially took several cooking classes, came to my kitchen in Bordeaux one day to teach me this amazing, nutrient-dense combination of shellfish and pork, surf and turf. This recipe incorporates the ancestral notion of eating the whole animal to derive the most nutrient density and economical potential from the animal. Why would you waste any of it? So many parts of the whole with which to create delicious meals! No waste! Economical! When you eat oysters, you are eating the whole animal. As for the meatballs in this recipe, as you can see from the ingredients list, so many parts of the pig, even the liver, are included. Pork has a long history of being a rich man's and a poor man's food in societies over the centuries. *Lesser Beasts: A Snout-to-Tail History of the Humble Pig* by Mark Essig is a great book about just that. Pork is available year-round, so you can make the meatballs any time. And the lard and fat in a dish like this really satiate as cooler fall weather arrives.

French oysters come from the northern coasts of Brittany and Normandy, the Loire estuary, La Rochelle and the Island of Ile de Ré (where some of the best hand-harvested French sea salt comes from), the Bay of Arcachon, and the French Mediterranean coasts, including Corsica. The Bay of Arcachon, *Bassin d'Arcachon*, produces 8,000 to 10,000 metric tons of oysters annually. During the months of June, July, and August, the oysters are not eaten and thereby given the chance to reproduce. The people of Bordeaux, *les Bordelais*, eat oysters from Arcachon, a seaside town an hour from Bordeaux, known for its oyster growing, between October and March. They have oysters by the seaside, oysters at the market, oysters for New Year's. Some families eat oysters once a week, often on Sundays, when the oyster vendors are out on neighborhood street corners selling various sizes (*calibres*). The bang for your buck (or Euro) with oysters is powerful: Vitamin B12, Selenium, Zinc, Magnesium, Molybdenum, Iodine, Niacin, DHA, Phosphatocholine, and omega-3 fatty acids are some of the essential nutrients we gain from oysters. Check out the post on Mark's Daily Apple for more on the most nutrient-dense foods, like oysters; maybe that will help convince you to try them.[1] This is also a prime example of eating "nose-to-tail," even though the oyster doesn't really have a nose. You are eating the *whole* creature. Now *that's* a *whole food*. To your health! *À votre santé!*

I admit oysters are a bit slithery in the mouth. It took a harvest lunch at Château Biac in Langoiran, a town to the south of Bordeaux, where I was shooting the picking of grapes, for me to try oysters. The twenty others around the table were delighted to see the large platters of oysters going around the table. I had worked up an appetite, and not wanting to disappoint my generous and patient hosts, the Asseilys, I put two oysters on my plate. I was told that one can eat them either by squeezing lemon on them or else with a **Shallot and Vinegar Dip for Oysters** (page 413). I tried one of each. They were a bit cold and slimy, but tasty. Paired with their unique barrel of house dry white wine, I was on my way to appreciating how the French eat oysters in the Southwest. From then on, I dared again and again, knowing these were so nutrient dense, starting with only one or two. Now I can eat a dozen oysters on my own, along with a sip or two of crisp white wine, and feel happy about the nutrients I am getting.

Despite the fact that this recipe looks complicated with lots of steps, it's basically oysters and meatballs! You can eat either of these separately, but also together (who knew?) to pack a one-two nutrient-dense punch for your health because it combines zinc and selenium-rich oysters with the nutrient-dense pork meatballs, containing pork fat, meat from the fatty neck (*gorge de porc*), and liver (*foie*). And let's not forget the all-powerful but under-exploited vitamin-rich herb, parsley. Plus, you can double the recipe, make bunches of meatballs in advance, and freeze them for future snacks and meals when you have less time to prepare a meal. So, make this recipe on a day you have set aside several hours for prepping meals ahead for the week. One key to success during the busy times of the week is having prepared, homemade food! The oysters must be consumed immediately, of course, particularly once opened. This is a fun way to invite some friends over and share a meal, making sure one of them knows how to open an oyster (a skill I have yet to master). This dish can be served as an appetizer (*entrée*) or a main course (*plat*). The unrendered fatback lard (*lard*) called for in this recipe is the subcutaneous fat between skin and muscle on the back of the pig. Leaf lard (*saindoux*) is the highest-grade lard rendered from pork belly and fatback lard. This recipe calls for another unusual ingredient: pork caul (*crépine*), also known as "lace fat." Pork caul is a web-like membrane that holds the viscera of pigs, also cows and sheep, in place. Because it is thin and malleable, it is helpful in holding things together like the ground meat of a meatball, as in this recipe. Caul is a specialty item to be ordered from the butcher and may be frozen in small quantities in airtight containers for up to a year. You can make the meatballs without the caul, as I do in the **Pork Meatballs** recipe (page 301). As with many Southwest recipes, you can replace any fat with the venerable duck or goose fats.

Oyster Size

Oyster size (*calibre*), ranges from smallest, "number 5," weighing only 1 to 1.5 ounces (30-45 g) to the largest size, "number 0," weighing more than 5 ounces (150 g). In exceptional cases there are sizes "00" and "000." The larger the size, the more expensive the oyster, usually.

FOR THE OYSTERS

36 oysters (6 per person)

Large sea salt crystals

Open the oysters carefully with the appropriate dull, thick blade of an oyster knife, or else have the fishmonger at least crack them open for you, so it will be easier to open them at home. The oysters will need to be double-bagged however, as they will leak sea water.

Place the oysters on each plate over some large sea salt crystals, it looks pleasing, and holds the half shell in place!

FOR THE MEATBALLS

1.7 cups or 14 ounces (400 g) pork caul

3 shallots, minced

1.5 cups or 12.5 ounces (350 g) pork liver

1.3 cups or 10.5 ounces (300 g) fatback pork lard, unrendered

1.3 cups or 10.5 ounces (300 g) pork neck

Handful of flat parsley, stemmed

3 pinches of fine sea salt

3 pinches of ground pepper

Pinch of ground nutmeg (freshly ground or already powdered)

4 tablespoons unsalted butter, or duck or goose fat or lard

2/5 cups or 3.5 ounces (100 g) rendered leaf lard (*saindoux*)

Optional: Bay leaf (*feuille de laurier*), torn into small pieces

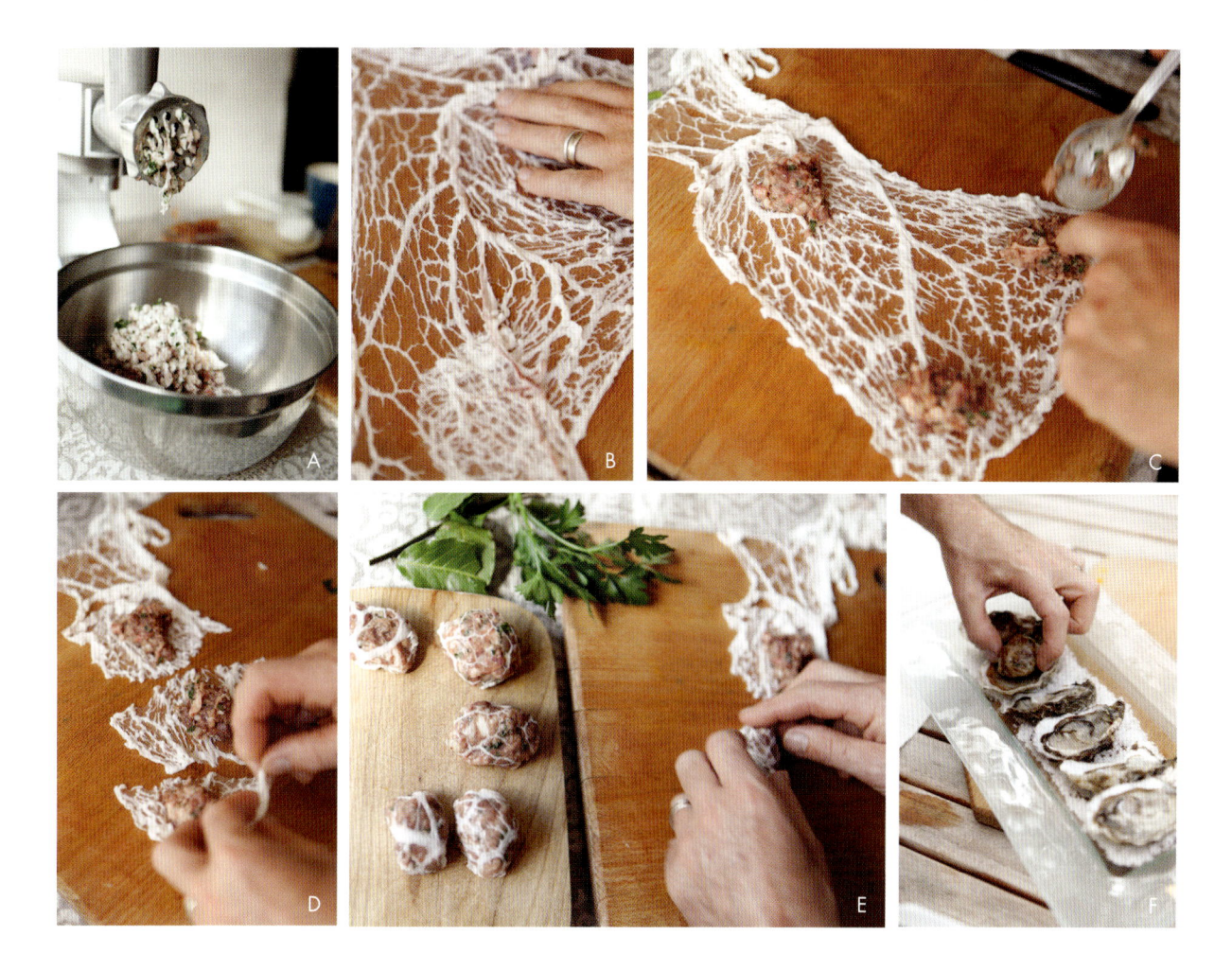

Rinse the pork caul in cold water and set aside.

Place the shallots into a large mixing bowl. Grind the liver, fatback, pork neck, and parsley leaves in a meat grinder (Chef Frédéric had brought his own) or food processor to a medium consistency (not too fine, see photo A) and add to the mixing bowl. Add the salt, pepper, and nutmeg, and mix everything well with your hands.

Spread the pork caul out on a large cutting board. (See photo B.) Form meatballs of about one teaspoon to one tablespoon in size and place them on the pork caul, leaving enough pork caul around each meatball to envelope it. (See photo C.) The pork caul will be your "envelope," or covering, around the meatball. As an optional step, place a small torn piece of bay leaf at each spot on the pork caul where you will place a meatball. The laurel leaf adds to the flavor and aroma of the finished product. Cut the pork caul around each meatball. (See photo D.) Envelope each meatball in the pork caul. (See photo E.)

Melt the fat in a large frying pan over medium-high heat. Place the meatballs in the pan and sauté them for several minutes on each side until they are cooked through. (You can also place them, covered, in the oven to finish cooking for several minutes at 365°F or 185°C.)

Place the finished meatballs, one on each oyster. (See photo F.) Serve immediately. The warm flavor of the pork meat contrasts nicely with the fresh, cold, salty, iodized flavors of the oyster. ➤

FISH AND SEAFOOD – *LES POISSONS ET LES FRUITS DE MER*

VARIATIONS If you have read this recipe all the way to here, thank you for your attention! I know the pork part of this recipe looks very complicated, but you could actually just form some ground pork and onions into little balls. See also my recipe on **Pork Meatballs** (page 301). Again, as with most recipes, you can improvise! I actually don't like following intricate recipes. Maybe it's an inability to focus on the page or to take the time to read and prepare all the ingredients. Sometimes the fun part is in just mixing whatever ingredients you have and fitting a recipe to that.

WINE PAIRING TIP For a regional Bordeaux pairing, try a crisp white Bordeaux Graves (always a delightful blend of Muscadelle, Sauvignon Blanc and Sémillon), or a dry white from the Entre-Deux-Mers or Côtes de Bordeaux, or else a Bordeaux sweet wine (*liquoreux*). Wines from the *Entre-Deux-Mers* ("between two waters"—the Garonne and the Dordogne rivers) region of Bordeaux are most commonly paired in Bordeaux with oysters from Arcachon. Oysters also go well with a crisp, citrusy, and mineraly Sancerre Sauvignon Blanc from the Central Loire Valley, or a Chablis from Burgundy, with notes of gunflint, lemon, and white peach. For Château Biac's dry white wine, *Felix*, you will have to go to the château itself, which you would not regret in the least, as it has the most magnificent view of the Garonne River from the vineyard, and the Asseilys are warm, wonderful, and welcoming. They even have a lovely guest house with rooms next to the vines. In addition to its reds and whites, Château Biac even makes "Secret de Biac," a sweet wine in the Côtes de Bordeaux Cadillac Appellation. So many reasons to try a Bordeaux oyster!

Opening an Oyster—Safely

There are videos online that will show you how to open an oyster properly.[2,3] In both of these videos, they say to hang onto the water in the oyster and to detach the oyster from its shell upon opening. They emphasize using a towel to protect your hands, as my friend Chef Craig demonstrates in the photo on the left. You can also use a protective or even chainmail glove, like I used at the butcher shop. Chef Frédéric did not use a towel to protect his hand, as shown in the other photo here, but don't try this at home! He says there is no need to hang onto that first water that sprays or drips out of the shell upon opening. Also, the French leave the detaching of the oyster from its half shell to the consumer of the oyster by supplying them with a nice oyster fork! This ensures freshness upon consumption if you are eating the oyster raw.

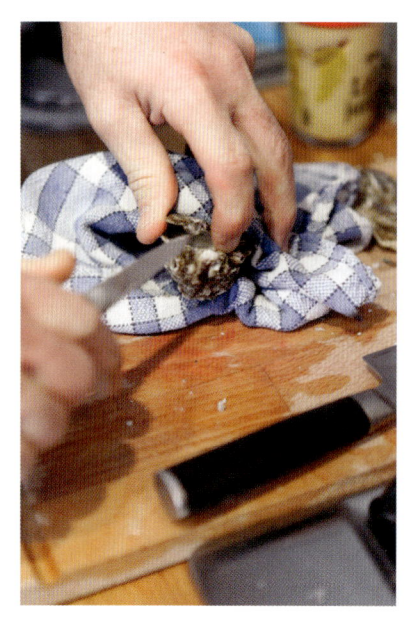

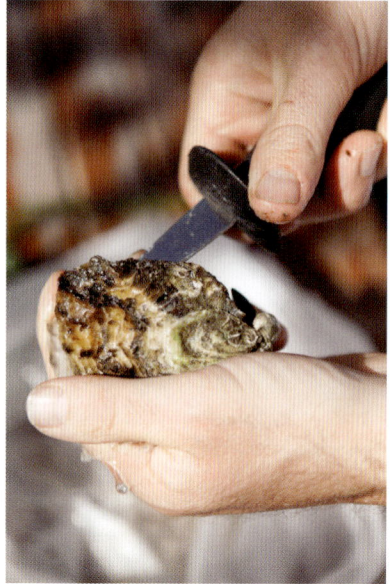

THE BORDEAUX KITCHEN

BUTTER-FRIED SCALLOPS
Coquilles Saint Jacques au Beurre

Season Autumn through early Spring (best in December)   **Preparation Time** 1 minute
Cooking Time 6 minutes   **Serves** 2 for a meal, 4 for an appetizer

Like other shellfish, scallops are a good source of iodine, magnesium, potassium, and vitamin B12. This dish is so simple to make and can be served as an appetizer (*une entrée*) or a main course (*un plat*). Scallops can be eaten from September until April, but the height of the season is December. My friend Océanne Auffret told me about this recipe, which, in its simplicity, accentuates the delicate flavors of the scallops. Being a Bretonne (woman from Brittany), she recommends using salted butter—butter with added Celtic sea salt, a regional product famously used in many Breton dishes. I used unsalted butter but added salt to the recipe. Either way, the salt and butter combination helps bring out the richness of the scallops. Scallops are usually sold in the US as just the white part of the scallop, a muscle. Sometimes, scallops are sold with the orange organ (a gonad) attached, which can be eaten as well and cooked up attached and in the same browning manner with the white muscle. Try to find scallops that are "MSC-approved" (Marine Stewardship Council) to be assured that you are consuming sustainably harvested scallops. Scallops do not reproduce until about the age of four years and need protection from pre-mature harvesting so they have time to grow.

1 tablespoon butter per 6 scallops

2 pinches of fine sea salt

12 sea scallops

Several parsley leaves, whole and minced, for garnish

Melt the butter in a stainless-steel or cast-iron pan over medium-high heat until it is bubbling. Sprinkle a pinch of salt on the butter then brown the scallops for three minutes on each side, turning again if additional browning is desired. Sprinkle the scallops with another pinch of salt.

Serve immediately. Garnish with parsley on top or on the side, or serve with lamb's lettuce (*la mâche*). You can also drizzle the remaining butter from the pan over the scallops. ➤

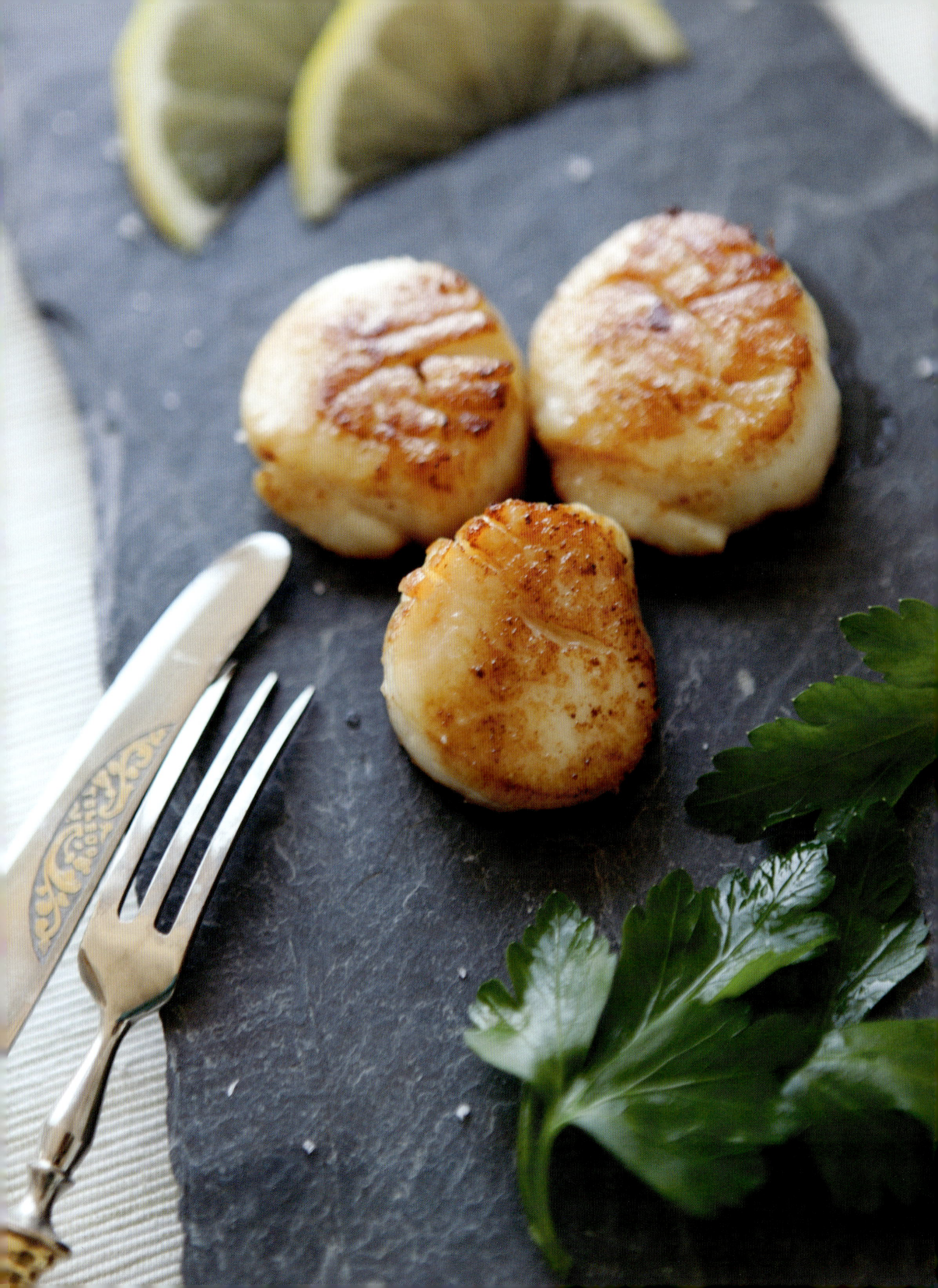

VARIATIONS Though this dish does not require anything else, some optional frills include:

- Drizzling few drops of lemon juice over the scallops.
- Adding a ⅕ cup (65 ml) of white wine to the pan before adding the scallops.
- Mincing two cloves of garlic and sautéing those with the scallops.
- Crushing two unpeeled garlic cloves and allowing them to heat with the butter to infuse the butter with garlic flavor.
- Sprinkling minced parsley over the butter in the pan before browning the scallops.
- Garnishing each scallop with one or two small, thin strips of cooked bacon or raw dry-cured ham (*Jambon de Bayonne* or French *prosciutto*).

WINE PAIRING TIP There are many options to try: a white Graves from the Bordeaux region, a flinty Chablis with high acidity from the northernmost and coolest wine region of Burgundy, or a buttery, mineral and citrus Meursault from the Côte de Beaune region of Burgundy. Others to try: a Chardonnay such as Pouilly-Loché from the Mâconnais region of southern Burgundy; a dry Sauvignon Blanc from the Loire Valley such as Pouilly Fumé or Pouilly Louché; a Loire Valley Chenin Blanc blend from Saumur, with notes of white flowers; or a dry white from the Entre-Deux-Mers ("between two waters," or between the two rivers Garonne and Dordogne) region of Bordeaux. As this is a good appetizer, try serving it with a good Champagne, Bordeaux crémant or other dry sparkling wine.

CATCH OF THE DAY
Marmite de Poisson

Season Year-round   **Preparation Time** 15 minutes
Cooking Time 20 minutes   **Serves** 6

A marmite is an earthenware dish or cauldron used for cooking, and a cast-iron pot is perfect for cooking this meal. It is usually a mix of four types of fish from the "catch of the day." It is the "surf" equivalent to the "turf" recipe *Pot-au-Feu* (page 123) using whatever meat is available that day. Because of the different ingredients being cooked or boiled, you may end up using all your burners for this recipe. My good friend Stephen Davis showed me this dish, which his children, having grown up with it, do like to eat, as they get to pick their favorite types of fish and shellfish out of the pot. Stephen is English but spent almost two decades in the French southern town of Montpellier, just kilometers from the Mediterranean Sea. As this dish is usually served with boiled potatoes, I have included them in the recipe, but other serving suggestions are mentioned below.

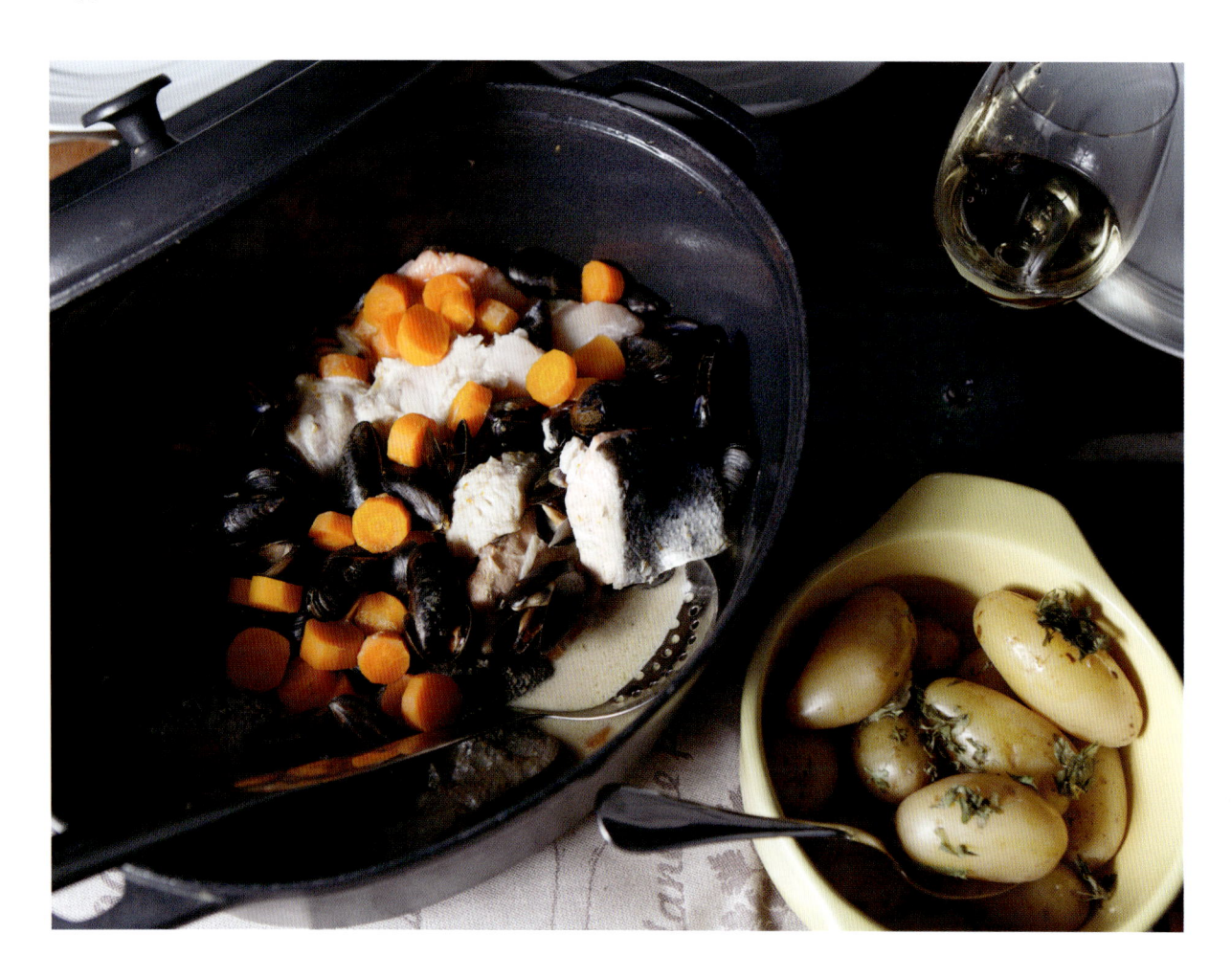

2.2 pounds (1 kg) potatoes, peeled

1.1 pounds (500 g) carrots, chopped into 1-inch (2.5 cm) pieces

2 tablespoons olive oil

1 red (or yellow) onion, minced

2 cups (½ L) **Fish Stock** (page 403)

1 cup (125 ml) white wine

⅘ cup (240 ml) heavy cream

Ground pepper to taste

Handful of parsley, minced

1.1 pounds (500 g) cockles

1.1 pounds (500 g) mussels

1.1 pounds (500 g) salmon fillet, cut into large chunks

1.1 pounds (500 g) mackerel fillet, cut into large chunks

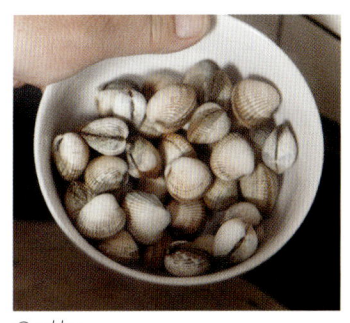

Cockles

Boil 2.2 pounds (1 kg) potatoes in a pot of salted water for 20 to 30 minutes. Poke the largest among them to see if it is soft enough to eat. Meanwhile boil the carrots in a separate pot for about 20 minutes. Also check the cockles and mussels and discard any that are already open to avoid bacterial contamination.

Heat the oil in a pan over medium heat, and brown the minced onion for about 10 minutes.

Combine the fish stock, wine, cream, pepper, and parsley into the marmite or cast-iron pot and heat to a boil. Add the cockles before other shellfish and fish, as they take the longest to cook, and bring the pot to a boil again. The cockles are cooked when they have opened. Add the fish, shellfish, and carrots and bring back to a boil before adding the mussels to the pot. Allow to simmer for a few minutes until the mussels open.

Serve with the boiled potatoes, or else with roasted or sautéed or raw vegetables (*crudités*).

> WINE PAIRING TIP We paired this meal with a fruity and light Bergerac Blanc Sec (dry) 2015, an excellent year for the Southwest wines in general, including all the Bordeaux wines. Any dry white Bordeaux blend of Sauvignon Blanc, Sémillon, and Muscadelle, especially from Graves or Entre-Deux-Mers will match up nicely with the varying blends of flavors you can come up with combining various types of shellfish and fish. Or else try a famed, aromatic white Châteauneuf-du-Pape from the southern Rhône Valley.

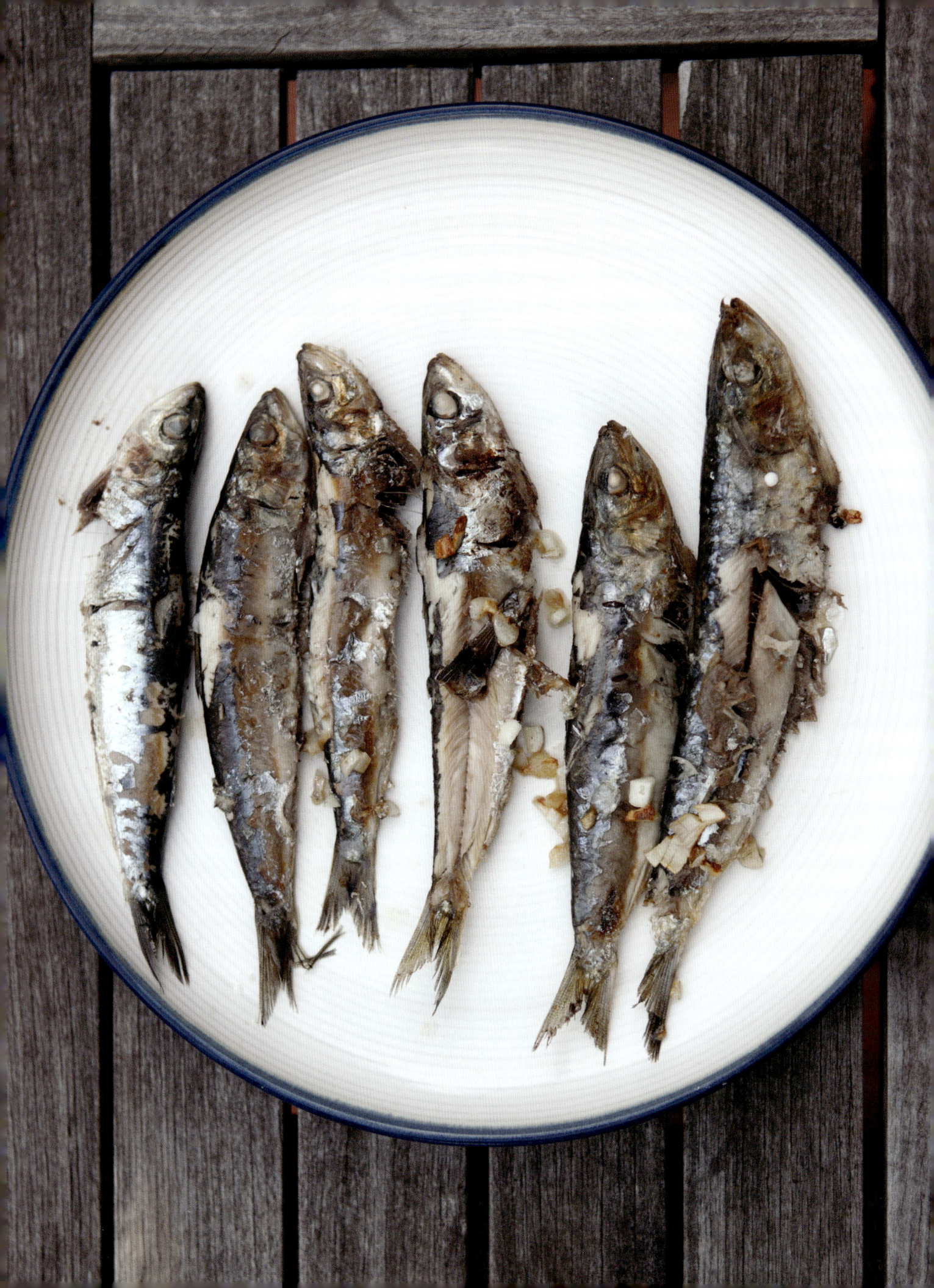

GRILLED SARDINES WITH GARLIC AND PARSLEY
Sardines Grillées à l'Ail et au Persil

Season May through October (for fresh sardines in France)   **Preparation Time** 5 to 10 minutes
Cooking Time 7 to 10 minutes   **Serves** 2

Fresh sardines are an unsung hero in the fish world. They are very low on the food chain and thus do not live long enough to bio-accumulate many toxins as larger fish might. They provide us with lots of omega-3 oil, and they are indeed delicious when freshly grilled. Fresh sardines are incredibly economical: I once paid 1.27 Euros, the equivalent of $1.50 at the time, for 10 sardines. They are a fitting example of eating nose-to-tail, as they are grilled whole in the French Southwest. This recipe is very simple, and you could just use olive oil, salt and garlic if you had nothing else. One French (lady) fishmonger told me *not* to wash the sardines before cooking them, *nor* to eviscerate them, so as to retain all of their fishy-ness. I usually do wash and eviscerate them, but you can decide not to if you so desire. Eating fish whole respects the whole animal.

- 10 to 12 medium sardines (about 1 pound or 500 g), eviscerated
- 2 tablespoons olive oil, plus more to drizzle on after grilling
- 2 to 3 garlic cloves, minced
- 1 teaspoon fresh parsley, minced, plus extra for garnish
- Pinch of fine sea salt, plus extra to taste
- Optional: Slice of lemon

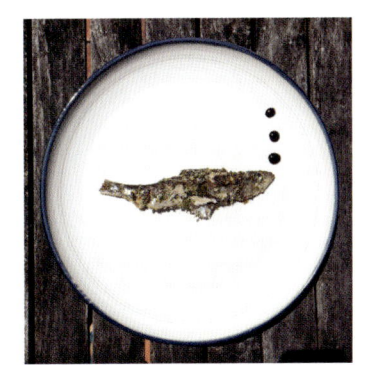

Heat one tablespoon of olive oil in a pan over medium-high heat. Combine the ingredients except for the lemon, and rub gently all over the sardines. Lay each sardine in the pan, giving each enough room to fry for about 4 minutes per side. Garnish with the lemon, parsley, salt, and olive oil.

VARIATIONS   Try mixing and matching ingredients such as those above with coconut oil, shallots, ground flax, *piment d'Espelette*, garlic, fenugreek, thyme, minced rosemary, or ground almonds. You can also sprinkle or stuff ingredients into eviscerated sardines and bake them in the oven at 375°F (190°C) for 10 minutes.

WINE PAIRING TIP   According to *What to Drink with What You Eat*, an award-winning book by Andrew Dornenburg and Karen Page, grilled sardines go particularly well with a Muscadet, from the Nantes region of the Loire, a Pinot Gris from Alsace, or a Sancerre from the Central Loire Valley. I would suggest either a rosé or a white Sancerre, or a white Vermentino from the French Mediterranean island of Corsica (*la Corse*).

FISH AND SEAFOOD – LES POISSONS ET LES FRUITS DE MER

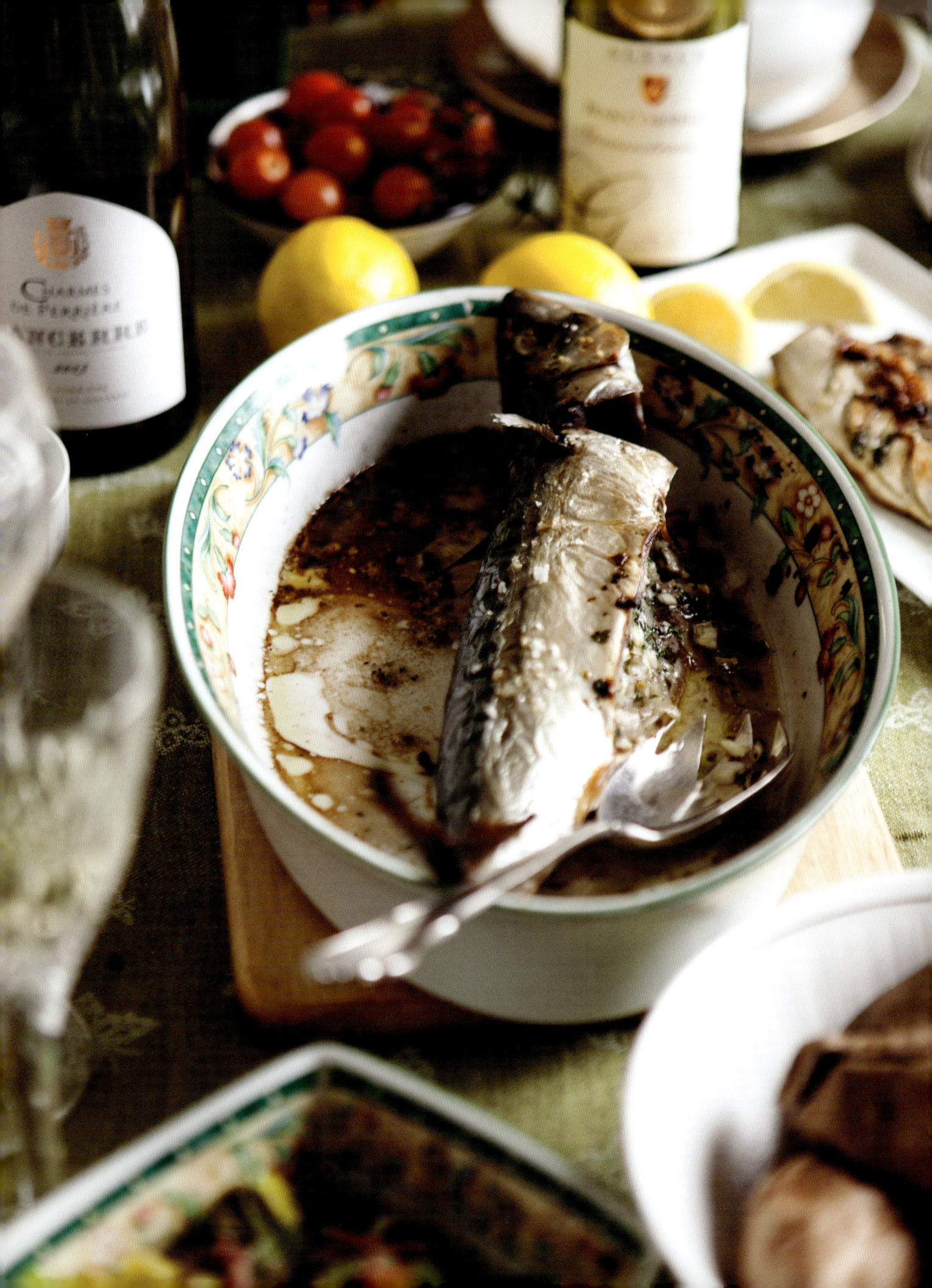

MACKEREL WITH GARLIC AND SHALLOTS
Maquereau à l'Ail et à l'Échalote

Season Spring is the best season for wild-caught mackerel
Preparation Time 25 minutes if you are fish-mongering, otherwise 10 minutes
Cooking Time Baked: 20 minutes, Grilled: 7 to 10 minutes   **Serves** 2 to 4, depending on the size of the mackerel

Mackerel do not generally receive the high status or respect they should, even in France. They are oily, flavorful cold-water fish that are abundant in nutrients and inexpensive. My husband calls this "Mackerel Economics." At 4 to 7 Euros a kilogram (about $4 to $7 for about 2 pounds), you just can't go wrong! Below are two basic recipes, plus variations on ingredients, for baked whole mackerel and for grilled mackerel fillets. A single mackerel fillet also makes for a good starter (*entrée*), as fish is usually served first in a multi-course meal, its flavors being more delicate than meat and the fillet size small enough to whet the appetite but not ruin it, all while giving your guests and you some hearty nutrients. See the photo tutorial on **How to Fillet a Whole Fish** on page 182, or else have the fishmonger gut and fillet the fish for you. (Or just gut the fish if you are eating it whole.) I encourage you to try gutting and filleting a fish yourself with a honed filleting knife. After a few tries, you will get the hang of it. For both the whole and the filleted fish, this recipe calls for a "garnished bouquet" (*bouquet garni*), a traditional French combination of herbs, either freshly minced or dried and ground, containing any of the following ingredients: basil, bay leaf, celery, parsley, rosemary, savory, and thyme.

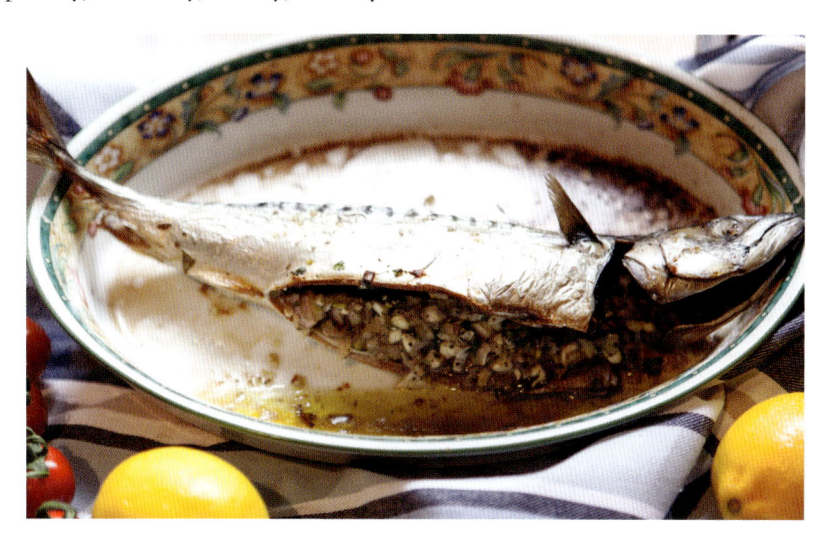

FOR BAKED WHOLE MACKEREL

4 whole mackerel, de-scaled, de-finned, and gutted (see photo tutorial on page 182) or else have the fishmonger do this, but leave the fish whole)

4 teaspoons garlic, minced

4 teaspoons shallots, minced

1 teaspoon *bouquet garni*

2 pinches of coarse sea salt or *fleur de sel*

2 tablespoons olive oil, plus extra for garnish

Quarter of a lemon, for garnish

FISH AND SEAFOOD – *LES POISSONS ET LES FRUITS DE MER*

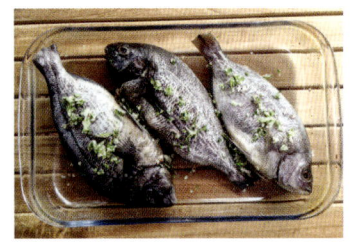

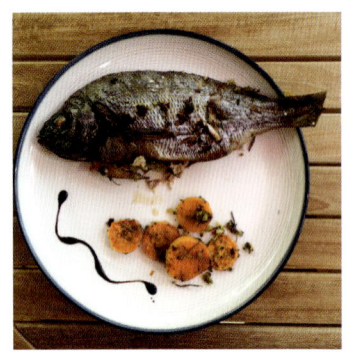

Preheat the oven to 395°F (200°C). In a small bowl, combine the garlic, shallots, *bouquet garni*, salt and olive oil, and stuff each mackerel in the gutted abdominal cavity.

Place the fish in an oven-safe dish and bake for 20 minutes. Garnish with squeezed lemon, extra olive oil, and/or *fleur de sel*, as desired.

VARIATIONS Use this recipe for sea bream—swap the herbs for simple chopped parsley and add extra stuffing as a topping to accompanying sweet potato slices, as shown here. Stuff the mackerel with the additional spice of fenugreek, tahini, and sesame seeds. Or try a combination of orange zest, parsley, and ground almonds. Freeze the fish bones (tails and heads) for making **Fish Stock** (page 403.) You can also try the fallback spice mixture of *herbes de Provence*, which has some of the same herbal ingredients as the *bouquet garni*.

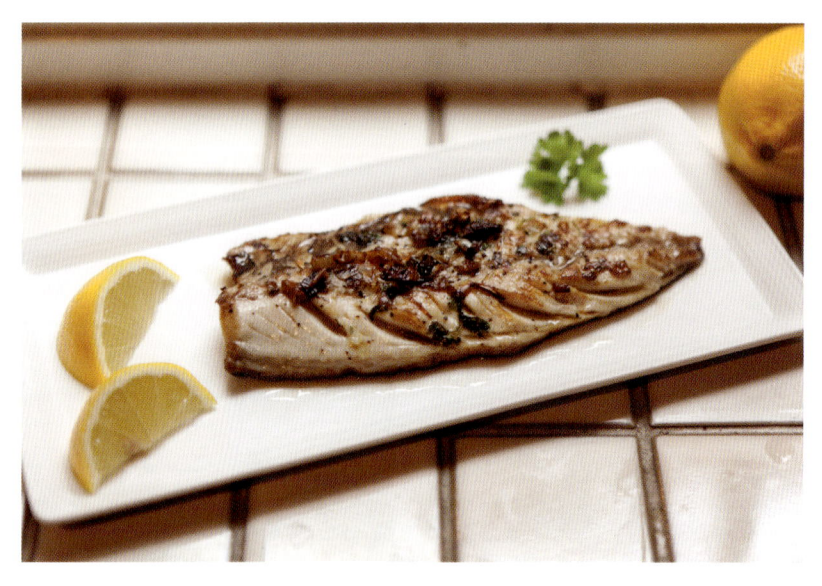

FOR GRILLED MACKEREL FILLETS

8 mackerel fillets, prepared by fishmonger or else by you (see photo tutorial on **How to Fillet a Whole Fish** on page 182)

2 tablespoons olive oil for the fish, plus 2 tablespoons for the pan

4 teaspoons garlic, minced

4 teaspoons shallots, minced

1 teaspoon *bouquet garni* (use an unbundled, dried, ground spice mixture that contains four out of the following ingredients: basil, bay leaf, celery, parsley, rosemary, savory, and thyme)

2 pinches of *fleur de sel* (or small grains of coarse sea salt)

Quarter of a lemon

Heat two tablespoons of olive oil in a pan over medium-high heat. Lay all the fillets skin side down on a plate. Drizzle them with two tablespoons of olive oil and distribute the ingredients, except for the lemon, over the fillets. Place the fillets skin-side down in the pan and cook for about five minutes, then carefully flip them over and cook the other side for another minute or two. (Some chefs will only cook the fillets on one side, which means you may need to keep the fillets in the pan longer, but the garlic may remain quite raw. This can be avoided by adding the garlic to the pan *next* to the fillets and then adding it later as a topping once cooked.)

Garnish with squeezed lemon, extra olive oil, and/or *fleur de sel*, as desired.

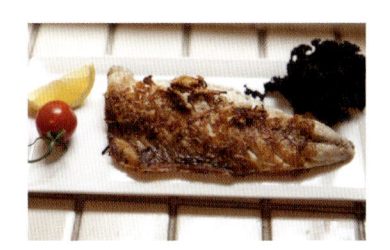

VARIATIONS Try using a combination of coconut oil, coconut flakes, olive oil, sea salt, and grated fresh ginger for your fillets (as shown here). This combination can also be stuffed into whole mackerel. If you are trying another kind of whole fish, such as sea bass or sea bream, try a combination of minced shallots (or onion), garlic, parsley, rosemary, thyme, olive oil, and salt for the stuffing. Don't forget to drizzle the fish with extra olive oil before (and, if desired, after baking), as well as sprinkling a bit of *fleur de sel* on top. If I have extra stuffing, I sprinkle it on top as well before baking.

WINE PAIRING TIP Try a dry white Muscadet from the Pays Nantais region of the Loire Valley, a Provençale rosé, a chardonnay from Burgundy, Languedoc-Roussillon or the Southwest, a medium-bodied, floral Sauvignon Blanc from the Loire, such as a Sancerre, or a full-bodied, herbal white Cassis from coastal Provence. I have also had a robust, Merlot-heavy Saint Emilion, with its slightly salty and metallic character matching those of the fish.

FISH AND SEAFOOD – *LES POISSONS ET LES FRUITS DE MER*

MARINATED CUTTLEFISH
Blanc de Seiche Mariné

Season Mid-Autumn through mid or late Winter, sometimes in Summer **Preparation Time** 20 to 30 minutes, depending on whether you are cleaning the cuttlefish yourself or have had the fishmonger do it. Prepare and marinate overnight or just before cooking. **Cooking Time** 10 to 12 minutes **Serves** 4 to 5

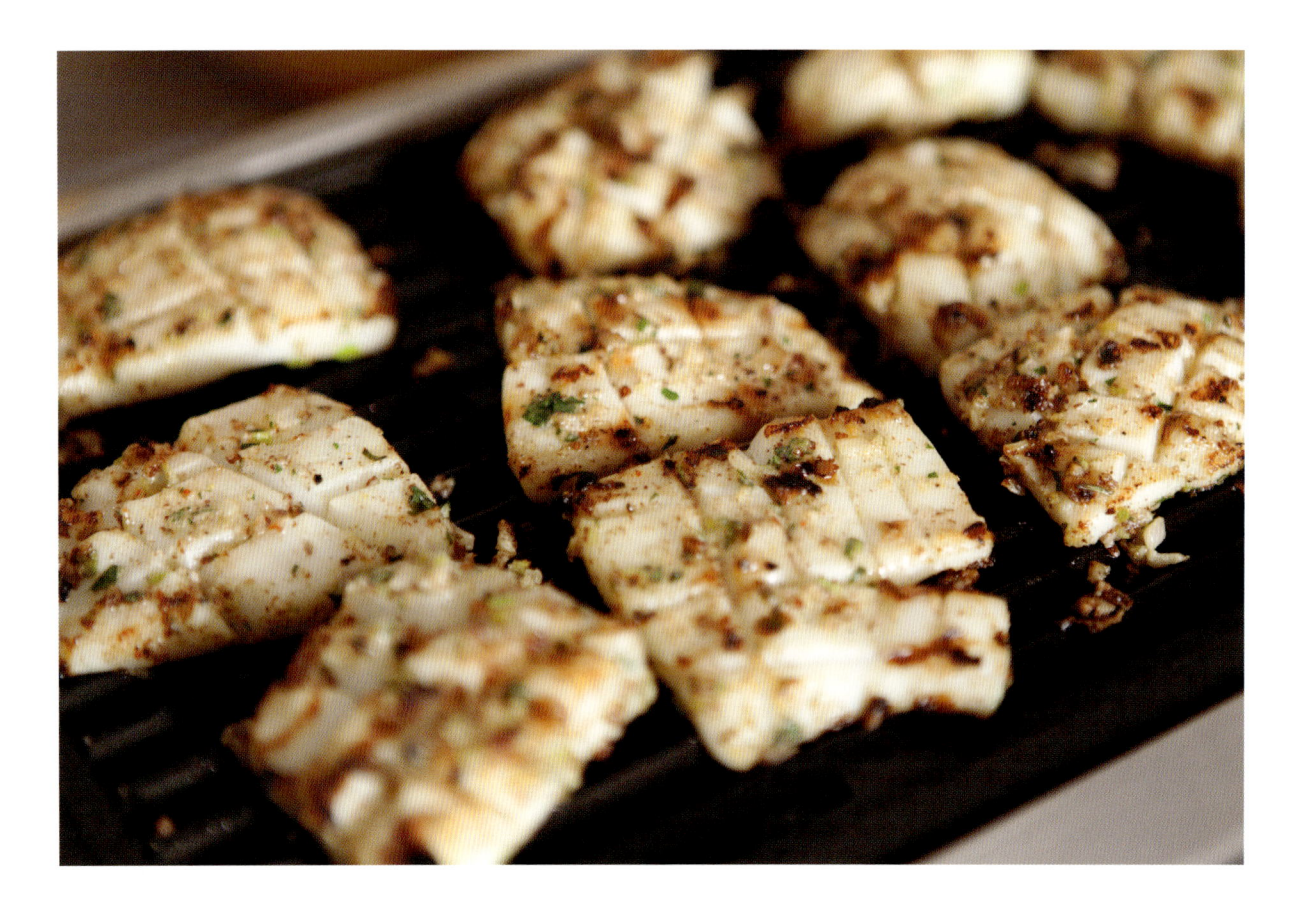

My good friend Craig Dennis, a transplanted Francophile from Jackson, Mississippi, is a trained chef *and* masseur. What better skills to have in life? He and his lovely French wife, Frédérique, have raised two teenagers near the Southwestern coastal town of La Rochelle, where Craig has become a local who knows the "fish guy" (*le poissonnier*) as well as the neighboring island Ile de Ré sea salt cultivators, including Thomas Citeaux and his wife Marie-Marie, among other locals, who harvest sea salt by hand every summer. Craig swears by this sea salt, as do all the locals. I have become a devoted convert myself, now that I have seen how painstakingly the salt is harvested. Craig cooks, gives massages, maintains his house, paints, and surfs on the weekends and travels to Paris during the week to give lucky Parisians and clients from around the world massages. We have known Craig since 2002 when we lived in Paris, and whether it's a massage or a meal, time with Craig is always too short. Bilingual and bi-cultural, Craig's repertoire of delicious culinary creations is endless, as is his modesty and generosity.

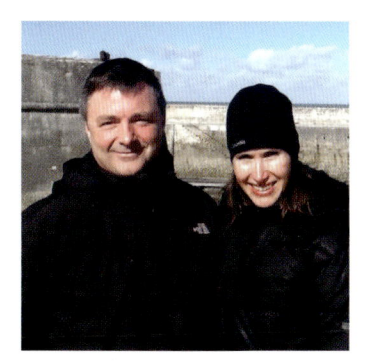

Craig and Tania

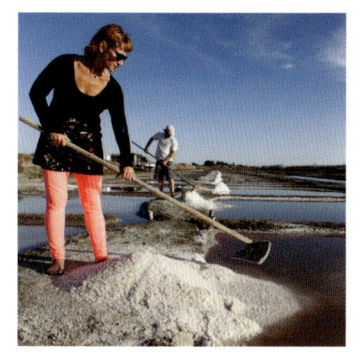

Marie-Marie Citeaux

Chef's Tip
Astuce du Chef

Scoring medium or large pieces of cuttlefish keeps them from curling but also serves to capture the ingredients. The cuttlefish or squid picks up all the flavors, which is why marinating overnight or for several hours will enhance the complexity of the dish.

This recipe is a mixture (*mélange*) of ingredients that reflects Craig's cooking experience in the U.S. and France: spices often used in the American South combined with seafood and ingredients from the French Southwest. Cuttlefish are in the *Cephalopoda* class along with octopus and squid, either of which you could use instead in this recipe. These are all mollusks, without the outer shell. The season for cuttlefish is October through January, sometimes through March, in the North Atlantic and English Channel for certain species, and again in summer for other species. Cilantro is in season June through August, but if you have an indoor herb garden, you can have it any time of year. This dish can be served as an appetizer (*entrée*) or as the main course (*plat*).

2.2 pounds (1 kg, about 3 adult cuttlefish) cuttlefish or squid, cleaned (beak and pen or backbone removed, outer skin pulled off), cut into 3- to 4-inch squares, and scored

¼ cup (60 ml) olive oil, plus extra for the pan

3 shallots, minced

7 ounces (200 g) pecans (or pine nuts), finely chopped

6 tablespoons fresh cilantro, minced

1 tablespoon Dijon or **Old-Fashioned Mustard** (page 410)

2 teaspoons *fleur de sel*

½ teaspoon ground black pepper

Optional: Pinch of cayenne pepper

Pinch of ground pink peppercorns (*baies roses*)

1 teaspoon lemon zest (or lime zest mixed with cumin)

1 sprig green onion, finely chopped

Mix all the ingredients together and marinate the cuttlefish in this mixture, if possible, overnight or for several hours. Heat a barbeque grill, grill pan, or a flat iron pan (*plancha*), adding olive oil to the pan if desired, and sear for several minutes on each side until cooked through. The cuttlefish will become whiter as it cooks. Try not to overcook, as this renders the cuttlefish very chewy.

> WINE PAIRING TIP Try pairing this dish with a dry white from Bordeaux's Entre-Deux-Mers or Graves regions, a Chardonnay from the Mâconnais region of Burgundy, a dry white or rosé from Corsica, a Muscadet from the Loire Valley, or a rosé from Languedoc-Roussillon. To satisfy the sweet tooth, you might also try a sweet wine from the French Southwest, such as a Béarnaise Jurançon.

FISH AND SEAFOOD – *LES POISSONS ET LES FRUITS DE MER*

SALMON TARTARE
Tartare de Saumon

Season July through October   **Preparation Time** 20 minutes   **Serves** 4

Because the salmon is served raw, this is one of the more daring recipes that I learned at Atelier des Chefs, Bordeaux's cooking school for regular people who want to learn to cook specific dishes. In the summer, this dish appears on menus around France, as it is served cool and, of course, raw. The season for wild-caught Alaskan salmon is July through October. Finding wild-caught salmon in France, however, is truly challenging and seemed only to be available around New Year's, even though the season is only through October. If you are not familiar with the fishing seasons, it can be confusing. But when you do find fresh wild-caught salmon, this cooling dish is a delight to eat, especially in the summer. The trick with the salmon is to slice it or buy it already cut into thin steaks. Hold one of the thin edges firmly while using a sharp knife to scrape beneath the pink flesh along the skin to remove the flesh from the silvery skin. Then dice the fish flesh. You can freeze the skin for your next batch of **Fish Stock** (page 403.) This recipe calls for **Preserved Lemons** (page 53), which adds a citrusy, salty tang. But there are many variations on salmon tartare; preserved lemon is not a requirement.

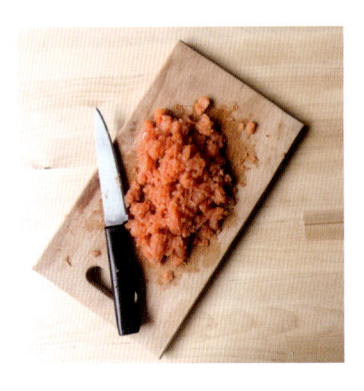

1.3 pounds (600 g) fresh salmon, diced into small cubes

2 shallots, minced

½ preserved lemon rind (lemon pulp removed), minced

8 sprigs of chive, minced, plus extra for garnish

4 teaspoons **Old-Fashioned Mustard** (page 410)

2 tablespoons olive oil, plus extra for garnish

2 pinches of fine sea salt, plus extra to taste

2 tablespoons sour cream (*crème fraîche*) or mascarpone

1 teaspoon liquid whole cream

Optional: 4 pinches of *piment d'Espelette*

Gently mix all of the ingredients together before adding the salmon cubes. Top with extra minced chives, olive oil, and salt, as desired. Serve with arugula leaves.

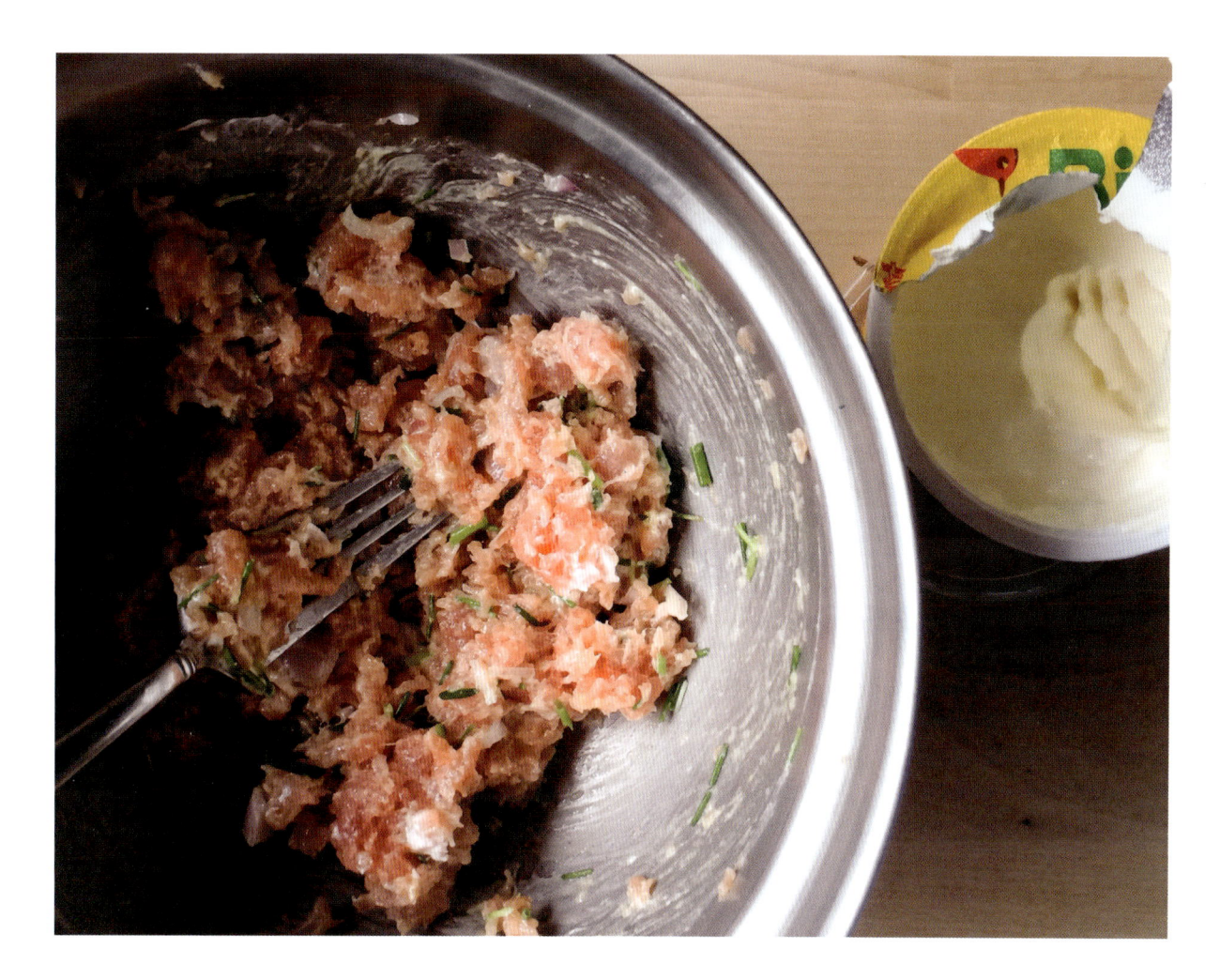

VARIATIONS You can use one teaspoon freshly grated horseradish in addition to or instead of the mustard. You can also add the juice of one orange along with one teaspoon orange zest. For a dairy-free version, try using two tablespoons of a dairy-free **Homemade Mayonnaise** (page 406), or else Primal Kitchen's organic mayonnaise in place of the mascarpone and liquid cream, or leave out the mayonnaise or dairy entirely and augment the olive oil to reach the desired "creaminess." You can also mix in a bit of high-quality smoked salmon with the raw salmon. This dish can also be made using raw wild-caught sea bass or sea bream.

WINE PAIRING TIP According to the pairing website, www.platsnetvins.com, the French will pair this dish with an array of wines from around the country: an Alsatian Pinot Blanc-Klevner or Riesling; a Chardonnay from Burgundy from the Côte de Beaune or the Côte Chalonnaise; a Champagne, a dry (*sec*) white Jurançon; a white Cassis from Provence; a Picpoul de Pinet from the Mediterranean edge of Languedoc-Roussillon; or a crisp Sauvignon Blanc from the Loire Valley such as the well-loved, flinty Pouilly-Fumé, with aromas of flowers and grapefruit.

FISH AND SEAFOOD – *LES POISSONS ET LES FRUITS DE MER*

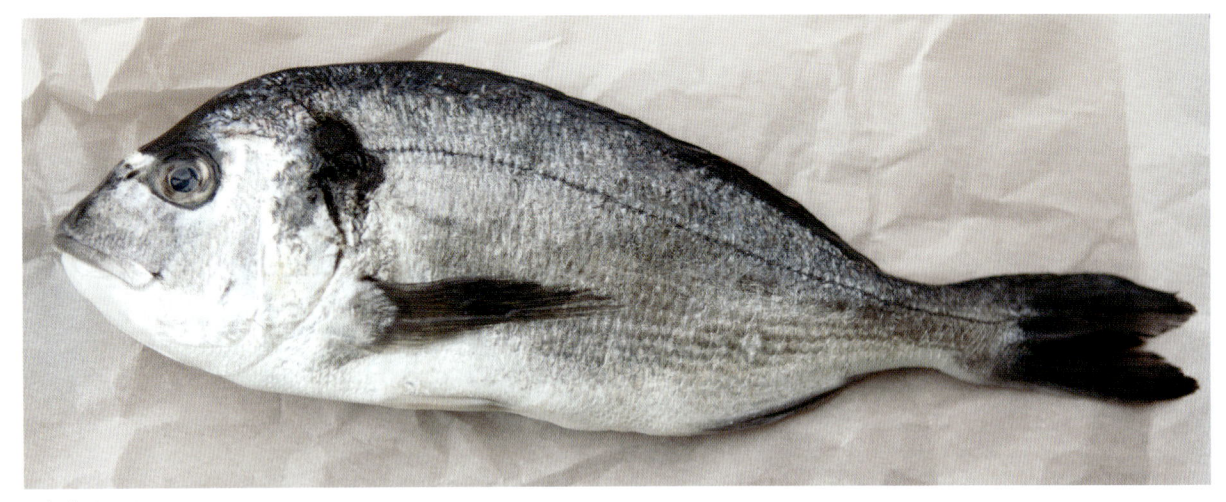

Whole Sea Bream

How to Fillet a Whole Fish

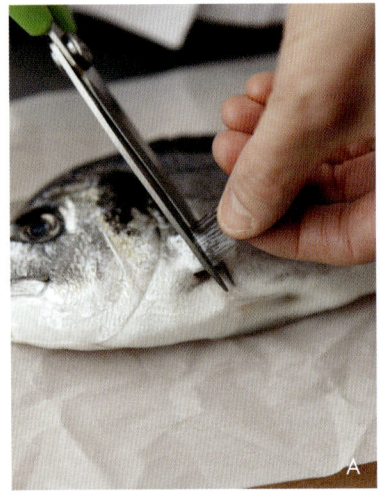

Cut off all the fins. (photos A through E)

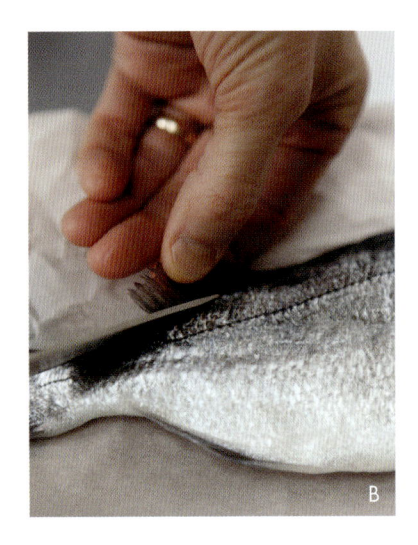

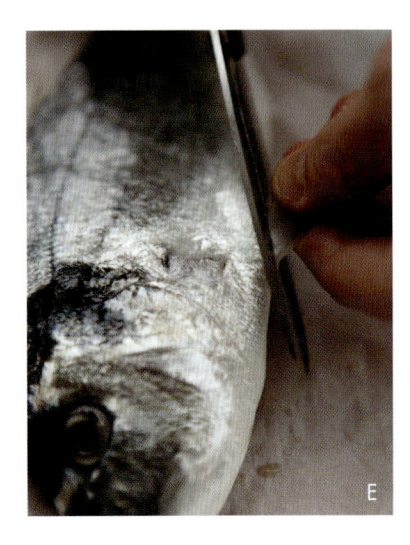

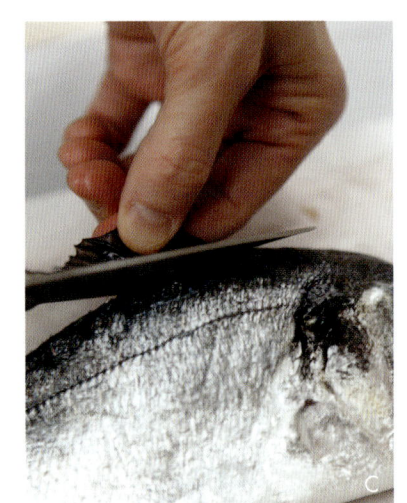

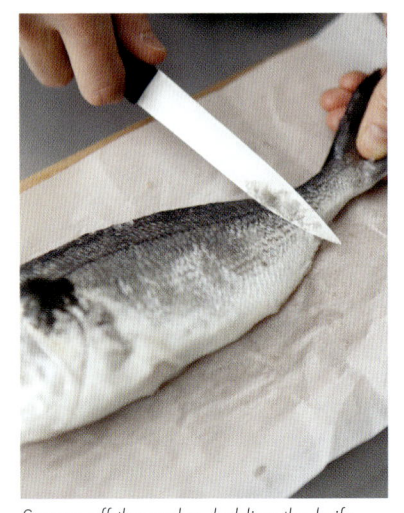

Scrape off the scales, holding the knife blade almost parallel to the fish.

182   THE BORDEAUX KITCHEN

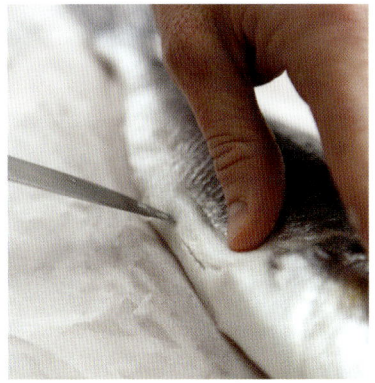

Cut along the belly of the fish. Then remove the guts using your index finger or a small spoon to scoop out them out while holding the fish over a sink (not shown here).

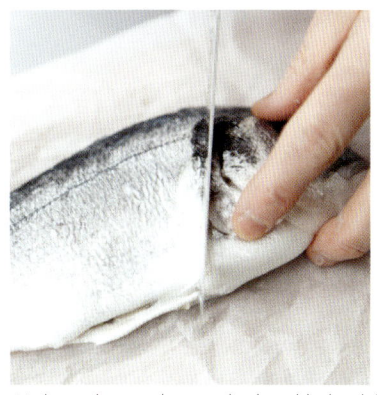

Make a diagonal cut at the head behind the gills to the spine.

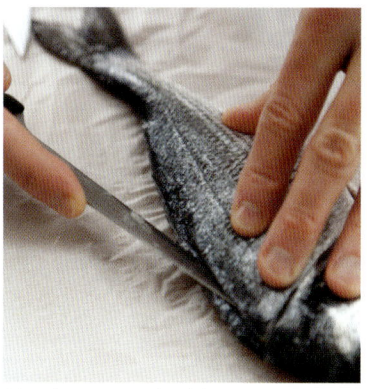

Cut along one side of the spine.

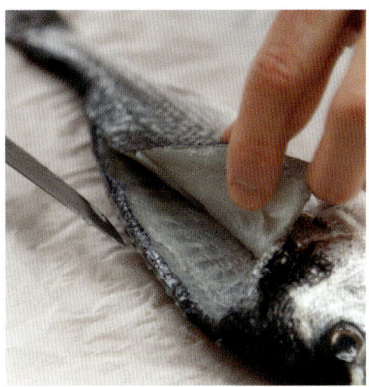

Pull the fillet away from the fish as you cut from the dorsal side to the belly.

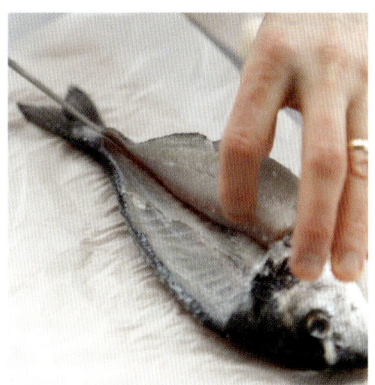

One side is filleted.

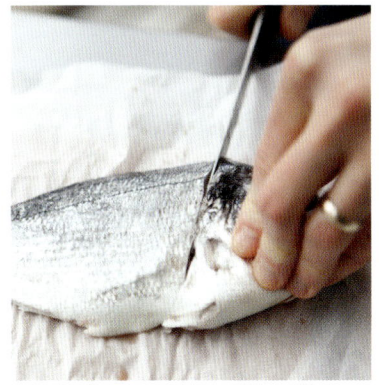

Flip the fish over and repeat the same steps on the other side.

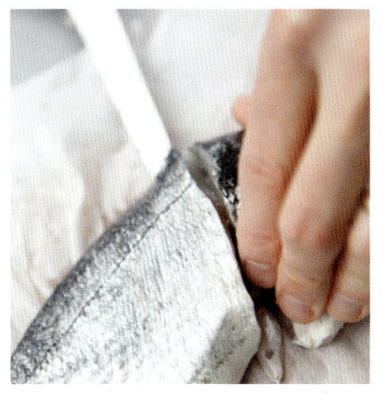

The second side is trickier. Hold the fish head firmly and move the knife blade along the top edge of the spine from the head toward the tail, pulling the fillet as you go.

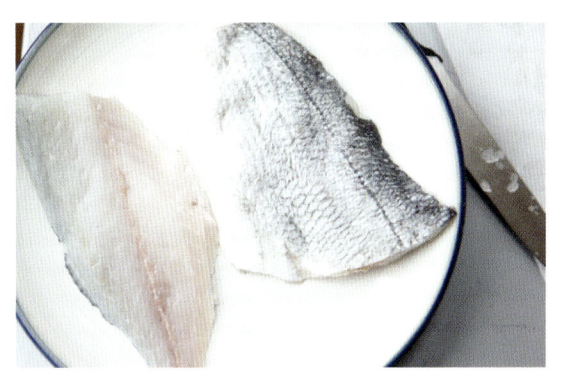

Two fillets are ready for cooking.
Use the fish carcass for **Fish Stock** (page 403.)

FISH AND SEAFOOD – LES POISSONS ET LES FRUITS DE MER

183

SEA BREAM FILLETS WITH GRILLED PINE NUTS
Filets de Daurade aux Pignons de Pin Grillés

Season Year-round except mating season in March   **Preparation Time** 20 minutes (if filleting the fish yourself)   **Cooking Time** 5 minutes   **Serves** 2

Sea bream (*daurade* or *dorade*) is a mild tasting white fish, as is sea bass (*bar*), which can be easily substituted in this recipe. The coastal French eat a lot of ocean fish, while the inland French eat river fish, such as trout (*truite*), which could also be substituted in this recipe. The pine nuts, a beloved Southwest condiment, add a nice crunch and extra flavor but can be omitted if desired. (See page 50 for **Grilled Pine Nuts** recipe.) For help on **How to Fillet a Whole Fish**, see the photo tutorial on page 182, in which a sea bream fish is used as the model, along with my husband's hands.)

Pinch of fine sea salt

Pinch of ground pepper

2 whole fish, filleted (see photo tutorial) or 4 fillets

2 teaspoons olive oil, plus more for garnish

2 garlic cloves, minced

Several leaves of parsley, minced

1 tablespoon water or fish stock

1 tablespoon white wine vinegar

1 tablespoon grilled pine nuts

Pinch of *fleur de sel*, for garnish

Optional: Quarter of a lemon, for garnish

Salt and pepper the fillets, and drizzle olive oil on both sides. Distribute the garlic and parsley over the fillets, saving a bit for garnish.

Heat the olive oil in a pan on medium-high heat, and add the fillets skin side down, searing them for about two to three minutes on each side.

Remove the fillets from the pan when done, and deglaze the pan with water or fish stock and white wine vinegar. Spoon the sauce onto the fillets. Garnish with parsley, grilled pine nuts, and fleur de sel. Squeeze some lemon juice over the fish if desired.

VARIATIONS For flavor variations, try adding powdered fenugreek or drizzling tahini on the fillets. You can also try deglazing the pan with one tablespoon white wine instead of white wine vinegar. Some of the ingredients from this recipe (*fenugreek*, grilled pine nuts, lemon, minced garlic, olive oil, and parsley) may be drizzled and sprinkled onto haddock (*églefin*) or cod (*cabillaud* or *morue*), but these thicker fillets are better baked in the oven at 365°F (185°C) for about 20 minutes. You might try baking them with chopped hazelnuts and rosemary. *Herbes de Provence* can also be lightly sprinkled on any of these white fish, baked or pan-fried, if you are in need of an easy change of flavor. Serve with steamed French-cut green beans slathered in olive oil or butter, or with roasted or sautéed vegetables.

WINE PAIRING TIP Trying pairing your white fish with a Burgundy Côte de Beaune Chardonnay or a crisp Chablis with notes of gunflint, lemon, and white peach, or else try a dry white from the Loire Valley. My wine class buddy and former restaurant owner and cellar master Annabelle Nicolle-Beaufils suggests pairing with these white fish white wines that are full-flavored, spicy and fruity, such as a Lirac from the Southern Rhône Valley or an aromatic Saint-Joseph from the Northern Rhône Valley. Annabelle also recommends coastal red wines traditionally paired with fish, such as those from Provence and Corsica.

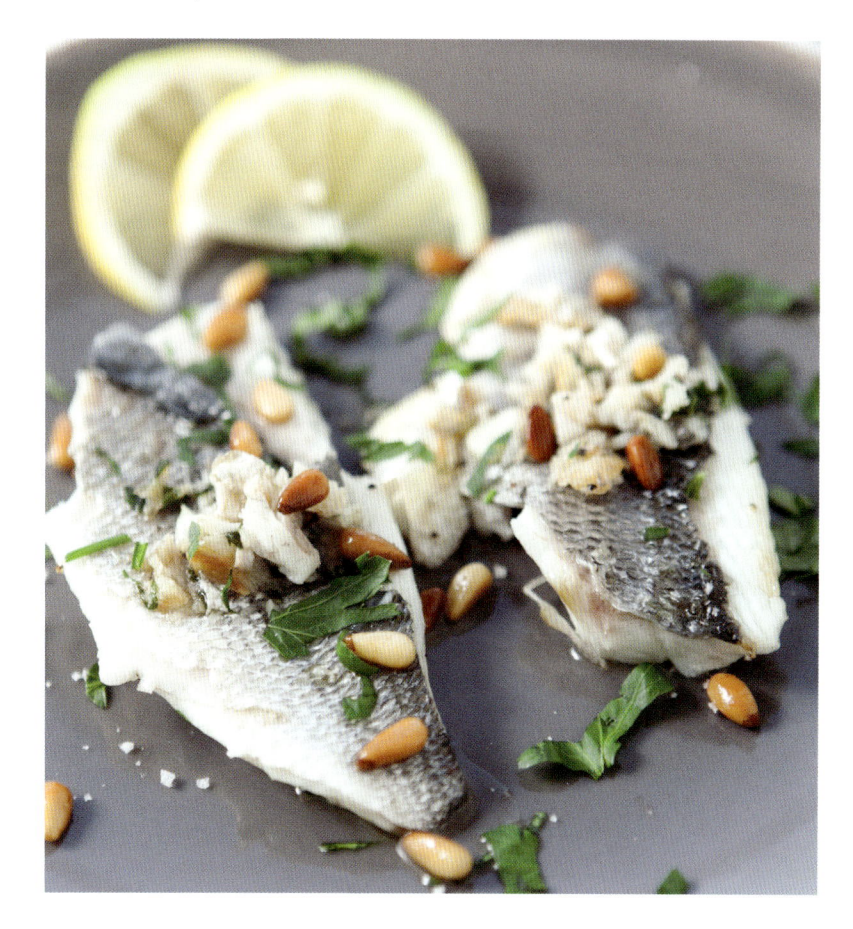

SPREADABLE FISH PASTE
Rillettes de Poisson

Season Year-round, depending on the catch of the day   **Preparation Time** 10 minutes
Cooking Time 20 minutes   **Serves** 6, as an appetizer

Similar to a pâté, *rillettes* is a spreadable paste of chopped fish or meat (usually pork or duck), salted, and cooked in fat. In this case, my friend, master home cook, Stephen Davis, had fresh mackerel on hand. Stephen says he learned it from an elderly fellow, now in his late 90s, in Montpellier, while living there for 20 years. This dish is often made using mackerel, sardines, salmon, or else the "catch of the day," and it makes a tasty appetizer or salad topper. The great thing about mackerel (and sardines) is that they are oily, cold water fish, teeming with omega-3 fatty acids and they are generally not farmed nor very expensive. If the fish comes with its roe, that can be added to the *rillettes* preparation as well. What makes this dish is the *rémoulade*. Basically tartar sauce, *rémoulade* is a combination of mustard, mayonnaise, and eggs flavored with garlic and herbs or spices. (See Stephen's **Tangy Seafood and Salad Dressing (Tartar Sauce) – Sauce Rémoulade** recipe on page 414.) As with most recipes, there is room for experimentation here to add or subtract favorite ingredients. Stephen makes his own mustard and mayonnaise, both of which go into his homemade *rémoulade*. (See page 410 for his **Old-Fashioned Mustard** recipe and page 406 for his **Homemade Mayonnaise** recipe.)

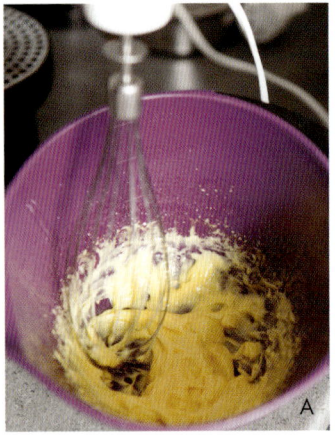

2 medium-sized whole mackerel (fresh or thawed overnight in the refrigerator), gutted, dorsal and tail fin removed

⅓ cup (80 ml) tartar sauce (*sauce rémoulade*)

½ teaspoon *herbes de Provence*

Optional: Pinch of sea salt

Preheat the oven to 395°F (200°C). Place the fish onto a piece of parchment paper (try not to rely on foil for cooking in general because of the dangers of heated aluminum foil[4]) large enough to fold over the fish like a puffy envelope, called a *papillote*. This locks in the flavor and juices during baking.

Bake the fish for 20 minutes or until cooked through.

While the fish is baking, you can make the mayonnaise (see photo A) that goes into the *rémoulade*, if you do not have any on hand. (The best store-bought mayonnaise I have tasted is of course Primal Kitchen Mayo, made with avocado oil and organic egg yolks.) Whisk in the *herbes de Provence* and the salt to the *rémoulade*.

Remove the fish from the oven and carefully unwrap the parchment paper. Pour the juices into the *rémoulade* and mix. Then add the flesh of the fish, including some skin and the thinnest bones, as these have calcium and other nutrients. Use a fork to break apart the pieces of fish into a textured paste (see photo B). You can eat it warm and by the spoonful if you've worked up your appetite! Usually, *rillettes* are served cold. Serve on celery sticks, on warmed sweet potato or beet chips, or on grain-free **Seedy Crackers** (page 501).

VARIATIONS In a pinch, you can also use canned fish, such as canned mackerel or sardines. You can also replace the *rémoulade* with sour cream (*crème fraîche*) or cream cheese, or else add just a bit of either of these in addition to the *rémoulade*.

WINE PAIRING TIP To go with the savory fish, garlic, and herbs in this recipe, try a full-bodied, crisp Chenin Blanc such as a Vouvray with notes of apricot and honey, or a crisp and aromatic Sauvignon Blanc-based Sancerre, both from the Loire Valley. Other suggestions include: a dry Chardonnay from Burgundy; a dry white Bergerac from the Southwest; a Côtes du Jura with notes of almond and flowers; a light-to-medium-bodied Pinot Noir from Burgundy; or a crisp rosé from Provence. Sommelière Annabelle suggests white wines that are fresh and fruity, such as a crisp and light-bodied Muscadet with floral and mineral notes, or a crisp and refreshing Sancerre with citrus and grassy notes, both from the Loire Valley, or else a fresh and lively Chablis Premier Cru from Burgundy.

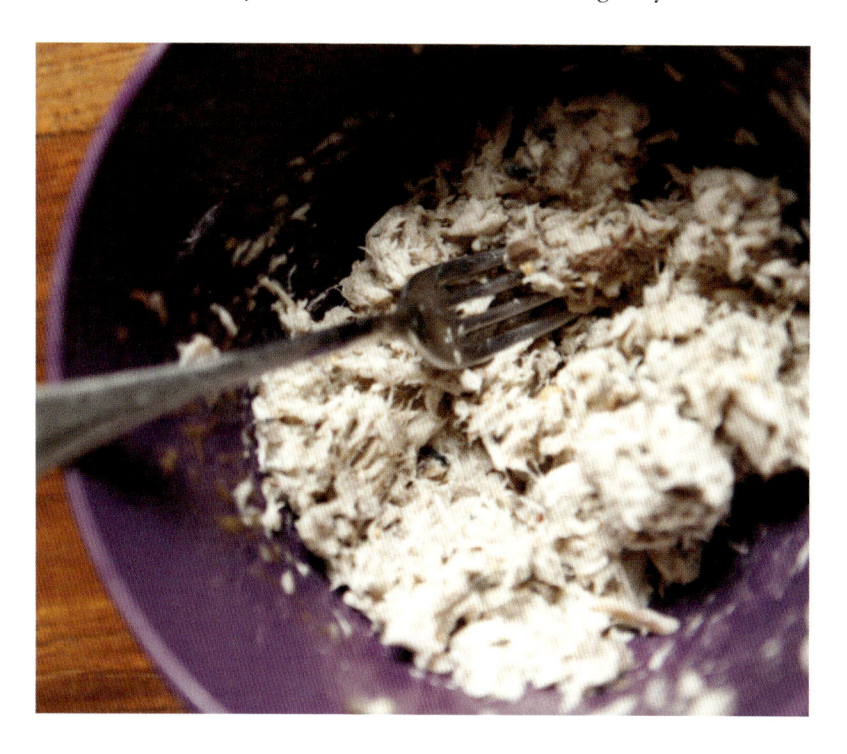

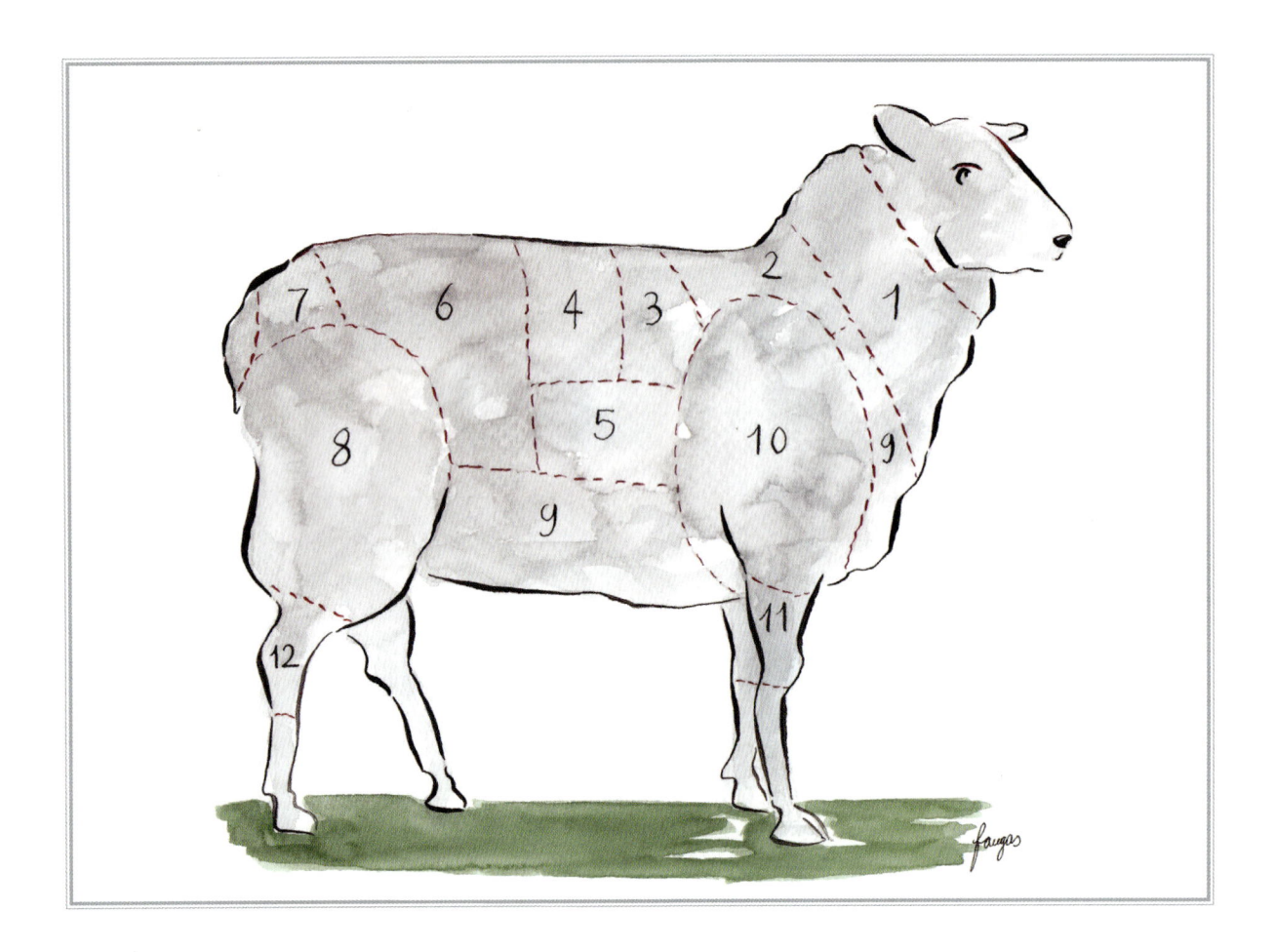

LAMB – *L'AGNEAU*
DIAGRAM KEY

1. Neck - *Collier* (Use: Ground, Roast, Sauté, Stew)
2. Shoulder – *Côtes Découvertes* (Use: Chops, Rack Roast)
3. Loin – *Côtes Secondes* (Use: Chops, Rack Roast)
4. Loin – *Côtes Premières* (Use: Chops, Rack Roast)
5. Loin – *Haut de Côtes* (Use: Chops, Rack Roast)
6. Tenderloin and Loin – *Filet et Côtes Filet* (Use: Chops, Rack Roast, Sauté)
7. Saddle or Sirloin – *Selle* (Use: Roast, Steak)
8. Leg – *Gigot* (Use: Roast)
9. Belly – *Poitrine* (Use: Rolled and Grilled, Ground, Roast, Stew)
10. Shoulder – *Épaule* (Use: Roast, Stew)
11. Fore Shank – *Souris Avant* (Use: Roast, Stew)
12. Hind Shank – *Souris Arrière* (Use: Roast, Stew)

LAMB
L'Agneau

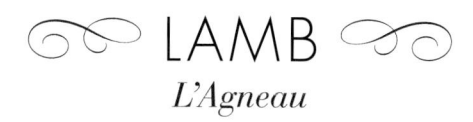

Garlic and Rosemary Lamb – *Agneau à l'Ail et au Romarin* 191

      T-Bone Lamb Chops or Loin Chops – *Côtelettes de Filet or Côtes Filet* 194

      Shoulder Chops – *Côtes Decouvertes* 194

      Rack of Lamb – *Carré d'Agneau Découvertes* 194

      "Frenched" Rack of Lamb or Bone-In Loin Roast – *Carré d'Agneau Côtes de Filet (or Carré de Cotes Premières)* 194

      Rolled Lamb Saddle – *Selle d'Agneau (or Quasi d'Agneau) Roulée* 195

      Rolled Rack of Lamb or Deboned Loin Roast – *Carré d'Agneau Côtes de Filet Roulé* 195

      Topside Roast – *Noix d'Agneau* 195

      Bone-In Lamb Shoulder Roast – *Épaule d'Agneau Entier Rôti* 195

      Deboned Lamb Shoulder Roast – *Épaule d'Agneau Entier Rôti Désossée* 196

Ground Lamb Parmentier – *Parmentier Hachis à l'Agneau* 197

Herbed Rack of Lamb – *Carré d'Agneau aux Herbes* 199

Lamb Meatballs – *Kefta d'Agneau* 202

Milk-Fed Lamb Roast – *Rôti d'Agneau de Lait* 205

Nut-Encrusted Lamb Shank – *Souris d'Agneau en Croûte de Noix* 207

Pyrénées Seven-Hour Slow-Cooked Leg of Lamb – *Gigot D'Agneau des Pyrénées Cuisson Sept Heures* 209

Simple Lamb Stew – *Agneau Mijoté* 211

Springtime Lamb Stew – *Navarin Printanier* 213

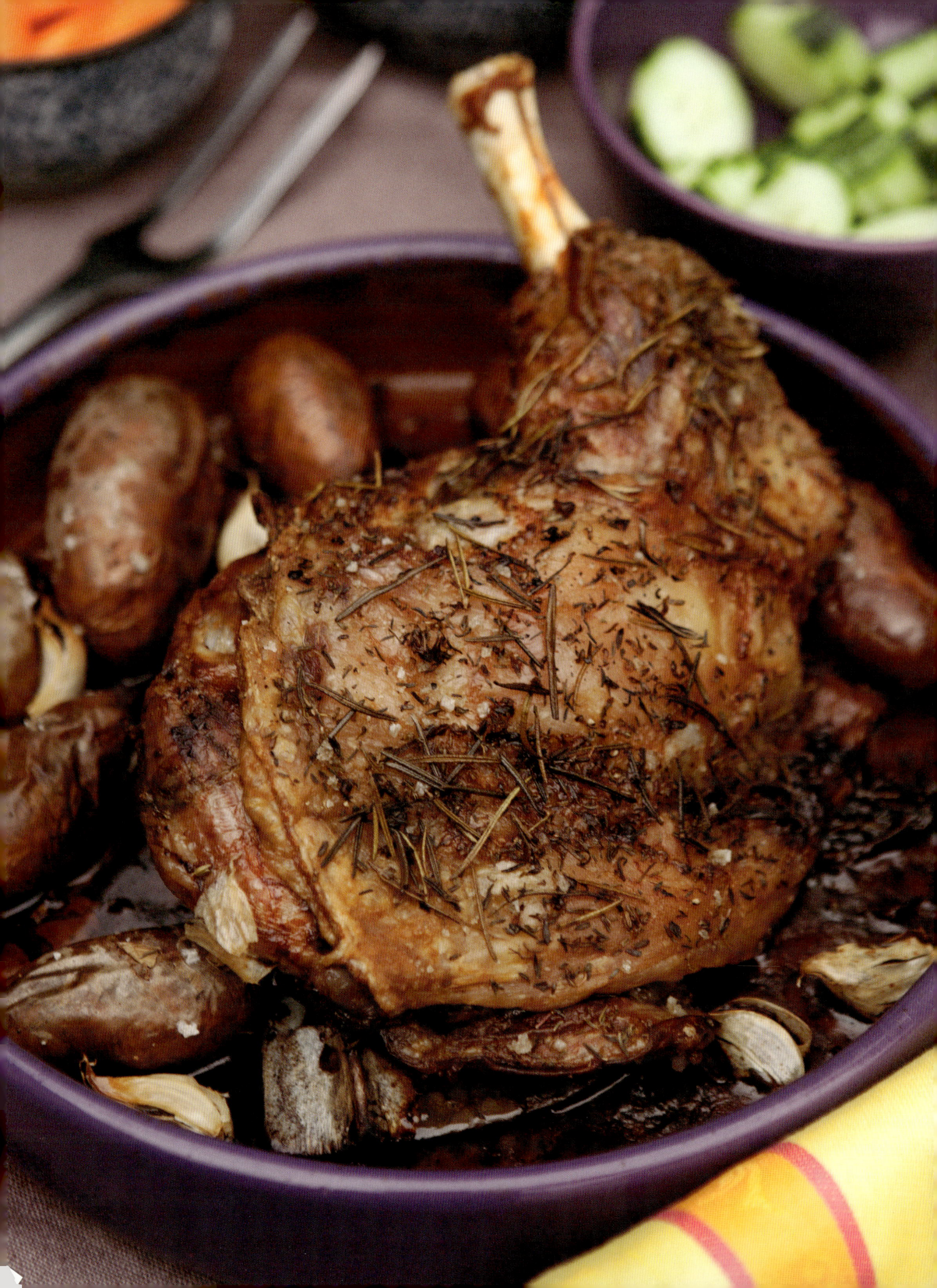

GARLIC AND ROSEMARY LAMB
Agneau à l'Ail et au Romarin

Season Year-round **Preparation Time** 10 to 15 minutes
Cooking Time See each cut for advised cooking time **Serves** (see serving size notes below for each cut)

Garlic and rosemary are a magic flavor combination when it comes to lamb. You can roast or grill any piece of lamb with this mixture, and it will be delicious. Following are some of the cuts of lamb, roasted in the oven or grilled in a pan, with cooking instructions.

The five ingredients are the same throughout these first lamb recipes: minced garlic, chopped rosemary, coarse sea salt, ground pepper, and optional olive oil drizzled over all sides of the meat. If by chance you do not have rosemary, thyme (especially fresh thyme) is a good substitute. It has a different flavor profile, but it is still aromatic and well-suited to lamb dishes.

The five ingredients are the same throughout these first lamb recipes: minced garlic, chopped rosemary, coarse sea salt, ground pepper, and optional olive oil drizzled over all sides of the meat. If by chance you do not have rosemary, thyme (especially fresh thyme) is a good substitute. It has a different flavor profile, but it is still aromatic and well-suited to lamb dishes.

You can eyeball the amounts and adjust whether more or less is needed, depending on the size of the piece of meat. If the meat is frozen, remember to allow it to thaw overnight. Once thawed, you can then marinate the meat in the ingredients mixture overnight or for several hours prior to cooking. Remember to remove meat to be roasted from the refrigerator 20 to 30 minutes prior to cooking to allow the meat to come to room temperature so that it will cook through evenly. Steaks are thinner and require only 5 to 10 minutes to come to room temperature.

With garlic and rosemary lamb, whether grilled or roasted, I recommend serving roasted root vegetables or potatoes or sautéed in-season vegetables. **Sarlat Sautéed Potatoes** (page 468) are always a good choice!

Several garlic cloves, minced

Several teaspoons fresh or dried rosemary, minced

Several pinches of coarse sea salt

A pinch or two of ground pepper

Several tablespoons olive oil

GENERAL DIRECTIONS FOR PAN GRILLING

Warm the olive oil in the pan over medium-high heat. If you would rather not use olive oil, replace it with one tablespoon of beef or lamb tallow, duck fat, or lard, which you would melt in the pan over medium-high heat. Brown the steaks on each side for 3 to 5 minutes. If more cooking is desired, place in a preheated oven (at 365°F or 185°C) for 5 to 10 minutes.

GENERAL DIRECTIONS FOR ROASTS

Preheat the oven to the suggested temperature given for each style of roast, and remove the meat from the refrigerator. While you wait for the meat to come to room temperature, you can prepare the ingredients if you have not already marinated the meat in them. To assess the "degree of doneness" (*stade de cuisson*), use a meat thermometer placed into the center of the roast to determine the inner temperature of the meat. The duration of cooking will depend on the size of the roast (and whether you have multiple items in the oven at once), therefore checking every 10 to 15 minutes after the initial recommended cooking time will help you gauge when to remove your roast from the oven. Roasts may actually be removed from the oven once they have reached 5°F to 10°F (3° to 6°C) lower than the desired temperature, as the inner temperature (*temperature à coeur*) will continue to rise for several minutes outside of the oven. It helps to experiment with your oven, thermometer, and different sizes of roasts to see how long they take to reach your desired degree of "doneness." (See approximate temperatures for **Degrees of Doneness for Lamb** on the next page.) For roasts, a butcher's rule of thumb is to cook roasts for about 15 minutes per 1.1 pounds (500 g), thicker roasts for about 20 minutes per 1.1 pounds (500 g).

Butcher's Tip

Astuce du Boucher

Cook roasts for about 15 minutes per 1.1 pounds (500 g), thicker roasts for about 20 minutes per 1.1 pounds (500 g)

Meat Temperatures at Atelier des Chefs, Bordeaux

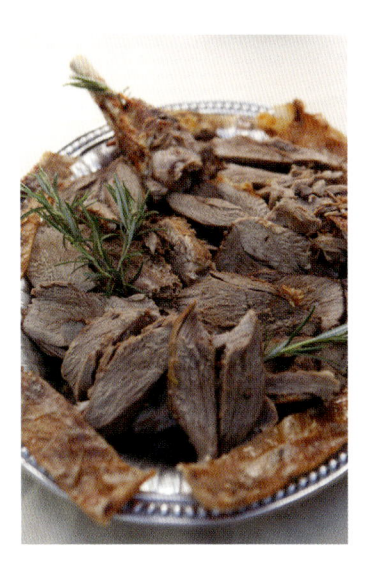

Degrees of Doneness for Lamb
***Températures de Cuisson à Coeur* or *Stades de Cuisson pour l'Agneau*[1]**

Bloody or Extra Rare – *Bleu*: 131°F to 135°F (55°C to 57°C)

Rare – *Saignant*: 140°F (60°C)

Medium Rare: 140°F to 149°F (60°C to 65°C)

Medium – *À point*: 149°F to 158°F (65°C to 70°C)

Medium Well: 158°F (70°C)

Well Done – *Bien Cuit*: 158°F to 167°F (70°C to 75°C)

Note: When trying for "well done" it is easy to overcook meat (*trop cuit*). One sure way to avoid doing so is to check frequently using a thermometer (as described in **General Directions for Roasts** on the previous page.

LAMB – *L'AGNEAU*

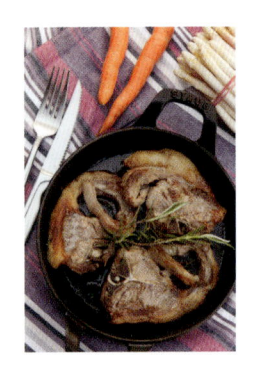

T-BONE LAMB CHOPS OR LOIN CHOPS
CÔTELETTES DE FILET OR CÔTES FILET

Serves 2 chops per person

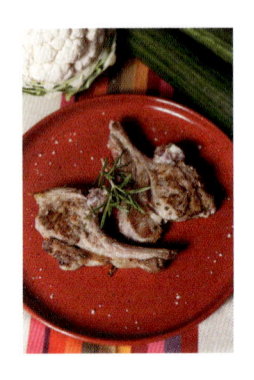

SHOULDER CHOPS
CÔTES DECOUVERTES

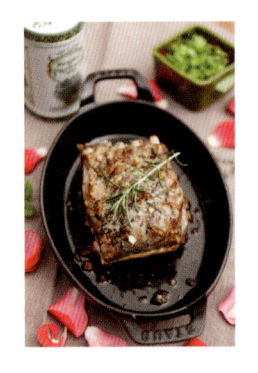

Serves 2 chops per person

RACK OF LAMB
CARRÉ D'AGNEAU DÉCOUVERTES

Serves 2 to 3

Roast at 365°F (185°C) for 40 minutes.

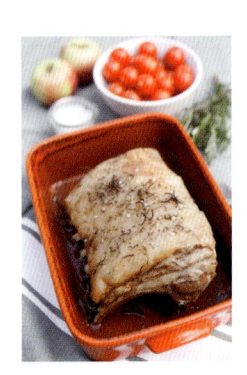

"FRENCHED" RACK OF LAMB OR BONE-IN LOIN ROAST
CARRÉ D'AGNEAU CÔTES DE FILET (OR CARRÉ DE COTES PREMIÈRES)

Serves 4

Roast at 365°F (185°C) for 40 minutes. See also **Herbed Rack of Lamb** (page 199).

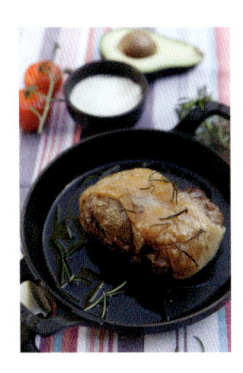

ROLLED LAMB SADDLE
SELLE D'AGNEAU (OR QUASI D'AGNEAU) ROULÉE

Serves 3 to 4

Roast at 395°F (200°C) for 20 to 25 minutes.

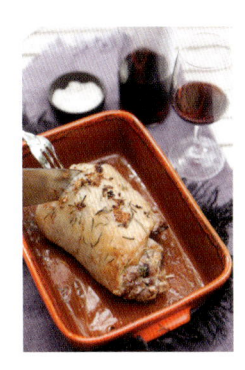

ROLLED RACK OF LAMB OR DEBONED LOIN ROAST
CARRÉ D'AGNEAU CÔTES DE FILET ROULÉ

Serves 4

Roast at 395°F (200°), 20 to 25 minutes or at 375°F (190°C) for 30 minutes.

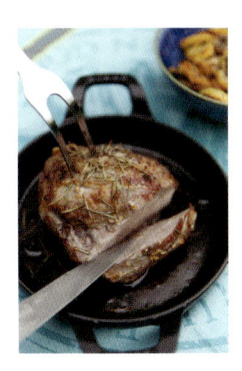

TOPSIDE ROAST
NOIX D'AGNEAU

Serves 4 to 5

Roast at 395°F (200°C) for 20 to 25 minutes, or roast at 395°F (200°C) for 10 minutes, then reduce heat to 365°F (185°C) and roast for another 35 to 40 minutes. The latter cooking time creates a browner crust on the outside of the meat.

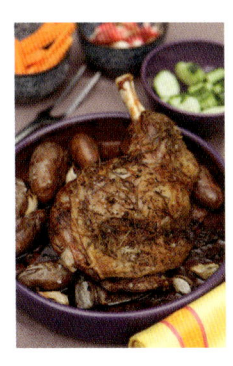

BONE-IN LAMB SHOULDER ROAST
ÉPAULE D'AGNEAU ENTIER RÔTI

Serves 4 to 5

For about 2 pounds (900 g), cook for 10 minutes at 395°F (200°C), then for 35 to 40 more minutes at 365°F (185°C).

LAMB – *L'AGNEAU*

DEBONED LAMB SHOULDER ROAST
ÉPAULE D'AGNEAU ENTIER RÔTI DÉSOSSÉE
Serves 4 to 5

The deboned shoulder roast is traditionally prepared in two ways: "melon" (shown, unroasted, to the left, bottom) or "rolled" (shown, unroasted, to the left, top). For either style roast of about 1.8 to 2 pounds (850 g to 900 g), cook for 10 minutes at 395°F (200°C), then for 40 more minutes at 340°F (170°C). Then turn off the oven, but leave the roast in for 10 additional minutes. Butcher Florent Carriquiry recommends basting (*arroser*) the roast in its juices several times during cooking to keep the roast moist.

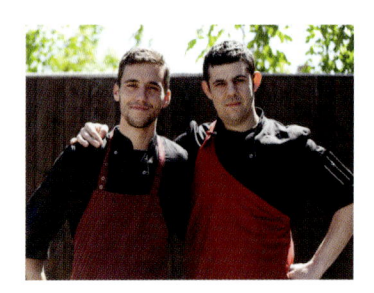

Butchers Florent and Romain

WINE PAIRING TIP I have had **Garlic and Rosemary Lamb** with elegant red wines from around Bordeaux, but also more rustic and fruity wines, such as from the Côtes du Rhône, the "hillsides" of the Rhône Valley. My Bordeaux University wine course classmate Annabelle Nicolle-Beaufils, who ran a restaurant with her chef husband for several years and is a professional sommelière and cellar master, recommends a wide range of red wines to go with these lamb dishes.

For **grilled lamb**, Annabelle proposes red wines that are aromatic, fruity, rounded, and ranging from lighter to more powerful: a fruity Beaujolais Nouveau; an aromatic and supple Bordeaux Clairet, halfway between a red wine and a rosé; a warm and full-bodied Tavel rosé, with notes of almonds and stone fruits, or a spiced Côtes du Rhône Villages, both from the Rhône Valley; a Saint-Chinian with notes of cacao and roasted coffee beans, or a Faugères with notes of coffee, red fruits, smoke, and vanilla, both from Languedoc-Roussillon; a fruity and tannic Gascon Madiran from the Southwest; or a full-bodied, well-structured Mercurey Pinot Noir, with notes of cocoa, red fruits, and tobacco undergrowth (*sous-bois*), from Burgundy's Côte Chalonnaise.

For **lamb roasts**, Annabelle suggests full-bodied, well-structured, savory, and tannic red wines from Bordeaux's Haut Médoc and Margaux (Pauillac wines also make a superior pairing with lamb), or else slightly less tannic red wines from other regions around France: a Côtes-du-Roussillon from Langeudoc-Roussillon, with notes of spice and stewed fruits, made primarily from the Grenache, Mourvèdre, and Syrah grapes; a rustic, leather-scented, and slightly herby Fitou from Languedoc made with similar grapes in addition to the Carignan grape; a Ventoux, with notes of red fruits, licorice, and spice and flavors of game and leather, or a Crozes-Hermitage, with rounded tannins and notes of licorice and red and dark fruits, both from the Rhône Valley.

GROUND LAMB PARMENTIER
Parmentier Hachis à l'Agneau

Season Late Spring through late Winter   **Preparation Time** 40 minutes
Cooking Time 30 minutes   **Serves** 4

In the notes for the **Ground Beef Parmentier** recipe (page 137), you can read about how Antoine-Augustin Parmentier used reverse psychology in the late 1700s to incite interest by the French in the potato—a traditionally suspect food source. The white potato, a member of the nightshade family, is not now considered the healthiest of vegetables, as it is capable of spiking insulin levels or flaring auto-immune responses. Nevertheless, the white potato seems to be tolerated (and adored) by many, and if eaten in small portions along with healthy doses of fat, this dish can be an easy choice for weeknight cooking. The **Ground Beef Parmentier** recipe uses a combination of parsnips and potatoes, but here I give you the "potatoes-only" version. March and April are the two months out of the year when potatoes are not in season in France. At the butcher shop in Bordeaux where I apprenticed, we usually sourced our meat for ground lamb from scraps of various parts of the lamb, including cuts from the breast and flank (*poitrine*), also called the "belly section." These "scraps" contain more fat and collagenous tissue than meat, but ground lamb can also come from the front shoulder (*épaule*) or back leg (*gigot* and *selle*) or neck (*collier*).

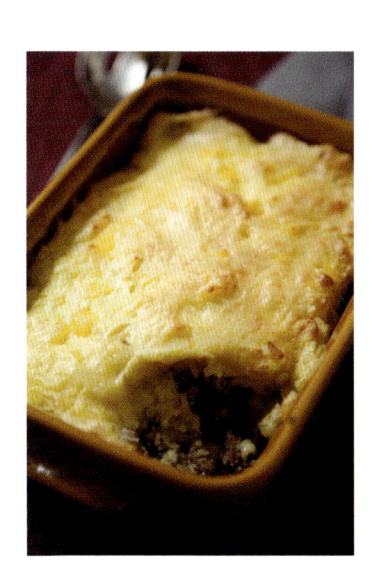

FOR THE MEAT

1 tablespoon lamb or beef tallow

1.3 pounds (600 g) ground lamb meat

1 tablespoon fresh or dried rosemary, minced

1 teaspoon fresh or dried thyme, minced

2 shallots, minced

3 pinches of fine salt

Pinch of pepper

Optional: 1 tablespoon parsley, chopped

FOR THE POTATOES

1.1 pound (500 g) white potatoes

1/3 cup (80 ml) milk

1 tablespoon butter

Pinch of fine sea salt

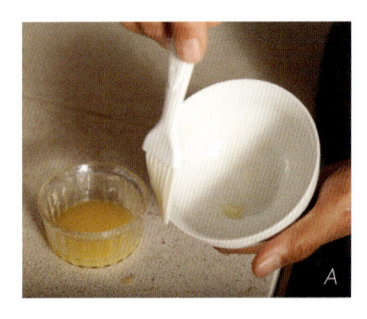

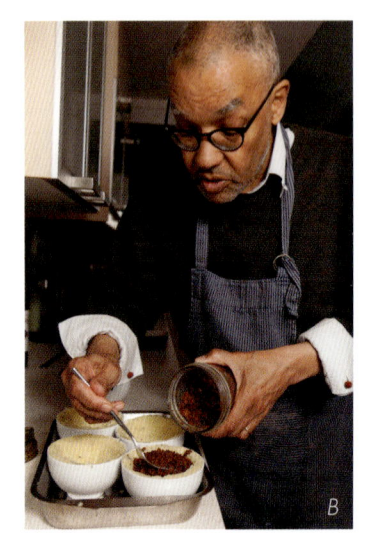

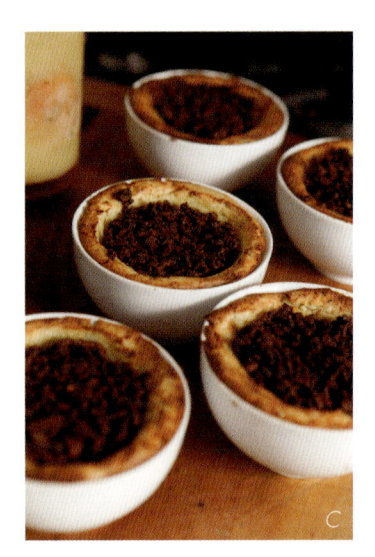

Preheat the oven to 365°F (185°C). Melt the tallow in a large pan over medium to medium-high heat, and combine all the ingredients in the pan. Sauté, stirring occasionally, for 10 to 12 minutes. Distribute evenly in a casserole dish.

Boil potatoes in salted water for 20 minutes, drain, and allow to cool. Peel and mash using a mixer while adding in the milk and butter. Scrape out the potatoes and spread them over the ground lamb mixture in the casserole dish. Place in the oven for 30 minutes.

VARIATIONS   As with **Ground Beef Parmentier** (page 137), you can also make this dish with a mixture of puréed turnip and potato in a ratio of about ⅓ or ¼ turnip to potato. The photos here depict bowls for **Duck Parmentier** with mashed potatoes using duck meat (*grattons*), as demonstrated to me by my good friend and experienced cook Dewey Markham, Jr. (shown left). The bowls may be turned upside down to form an individual dome of **Duck Parmentier** for each hungry guest if the bowls are adequately buttered (see photo A), preferably with two layers of butter, before filling the bowls with a layer of mashed potatoes and duck meat (see photo B). Cook the bowls in a bain-marie (tray filled with hot water) at 395°F (200°C) for 25 to 30 minutes and allow them to cool off a bit before serving (see photo C).

WINE PAIRING TIP   Sommelière Annabelle recommends flavorful wines such as a complex Pomerol from Bordeaux, with notes of dark fruits and leather, or else a much simpler, lighter-bodied wine made from the Gamay grape that offers freshness and notes of red fruit, from Touraine in the Loire Valley, or from Beaujolais, such as a Juliénas with additional floral and spicy aromas. (See also the wine pairing suggestions for **Ground Beef Parmentier** on page 139).

HERBED RACK OF LAMB
Carré d'Agneau aux Herbes

Season Spring   **Preparation Time** 15 minutes
Cooking Time 30 minutes   **Serves** 6

My former wine class buddy, Malika Faytout, kindly invited me to her family estate, Château Lescaneaut, in the appellation of Castillon east of the city of Bordeaux, on several occasions to cook together. The rack of lamb (*carré d'agneau*) is a springtime delicacy and looks very regal indeed. A French butcher prepares the rack by pushing down the tissues from the rack bones toward the bulk of the meat, or removing the tissue entirely, to reveal the thin rib bones of the rack. In English, this is known as a "French rack," shown on the next page. For the sake of easier cutting between bones, it is advisable to request the butcher to cut into each joint of the rack while maintaining the rack intact so that there is less work to do separating the cutlets once the rack has been cooked. You can get about 12 cutlets, two per person, out of an entire rack of lamb.

In this recipe we used Moutard de Meaux Pommery, which is a traditional French brand without preservatives, only vinegar. It is made from whole mustard seeds and comes in a stone jar with a wax seal. It is a good choice if you are not making your own mustard (see page 410 for **Old-Fashioned Mustard** recipe). With so many ingredients to mince in this recipe, it is handy to use a small electric chopper (*mini robot*). That way you can mix the herbs, shallots and garlic in one go or in batches, depending on the size of the chopper.

2 cloves of garlic, smashed but unpeeled (*en chemise*)

1 rack of lamb

3 tablespoons olive oil

Salt and pepper to taste

3 tablespoons mustard

Handful each of a variety of herbs, such as parsley, tarragon, and thyme, minced

4 shallots, minced

Preheat the oven to 465°F (240°C). Place the garlic cloves in a casserole dish. Lay the rack in the dish with the bones facing down, and slather (*badigeonner*) the meat with olive oil. Add salt and pepper, and slather on the mustard.

Mix the herbs and shallots in a bowl, and then press them onto the meat of the rack. ➤

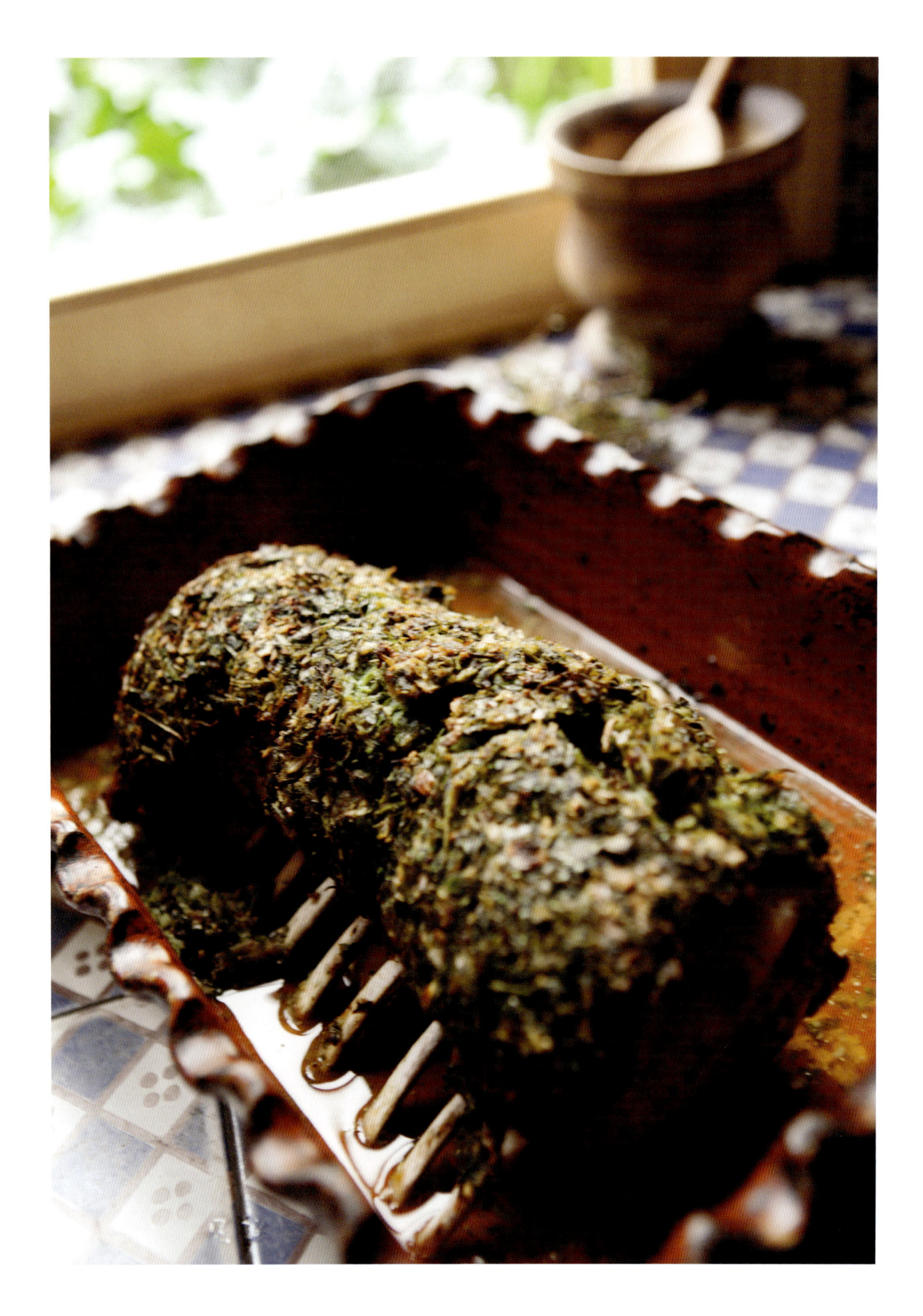

Place the roast in the oven for 15 minutes to solidify the herbed crust around the meat. Reduce the heat to 355°F (180°C) for another 15 minutes. Use a meat thermometer to check the roast (*vérifier la cuisson*), or make an incision in the middle of the roast to see for yourself what it looks like, and continue cooking if it is still too raw. (See **Degrees of Doneness for Lamb** chart on page 193.)

This dish was served with the **Field Potatoes** (page 449). You can also serve it with roasted vegetables and salad.

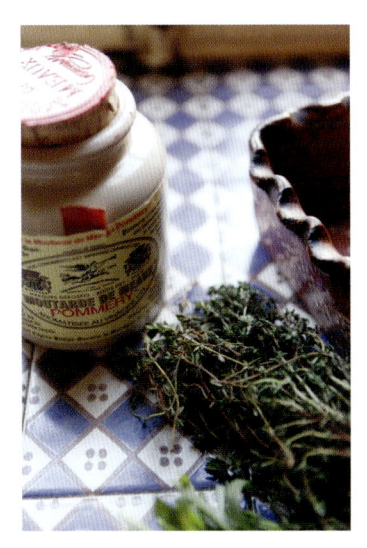

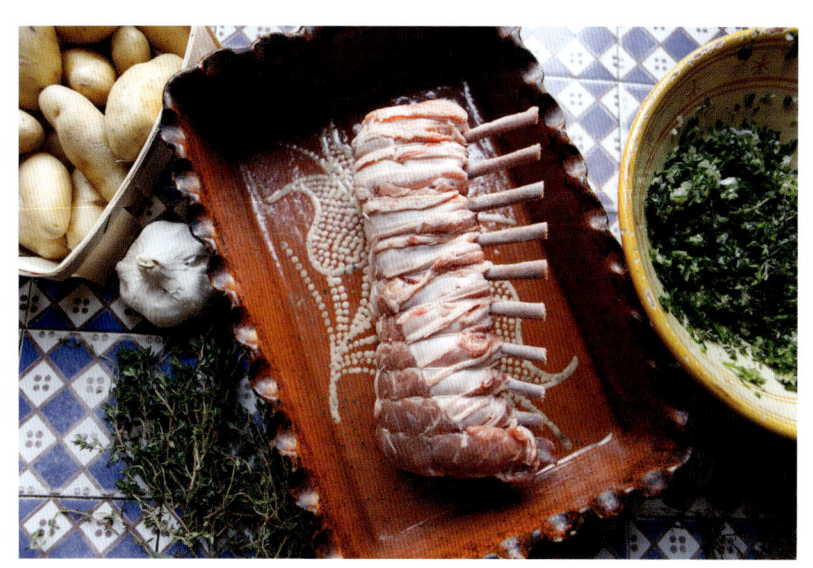

Moutard de Meaux Pommery

Frenched Rack

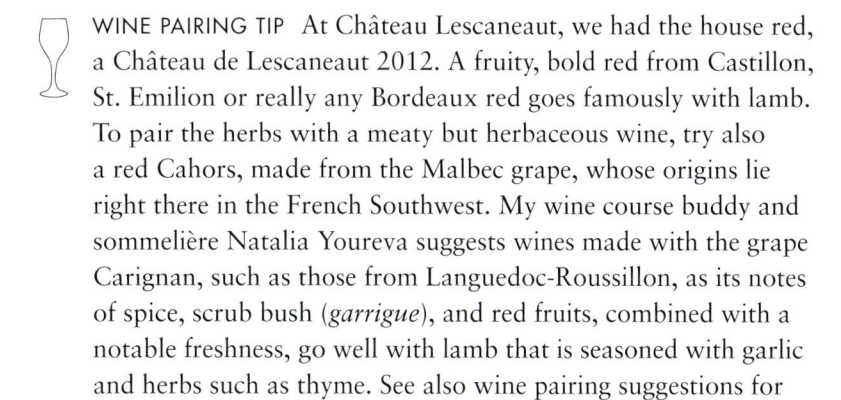

WINE PAIRING TIP At Château Lescaneaut, we had the house red, a Château de Lescaneaut 2012. A fruity, bold red from Castillon, St. Emilion or really any Bordeaux red goes famously with lamb. To pair the herbs with a meaty but herbaceous wine, try also a red Cahors, made from the Malbec grape, whose origins lie right there in the French Southwest. My wine course buddy and sommelière Natalia Youreva suggests wines made with the grape Carignan, such as those from Languedoc-Roussillon, as its notes of spice, scrub bush (*garrigue*), and red fruits, combined with a notable freshness, go well with lamb that is seasoned with garlic and herbs such as thyme. See also wine pairing suggestions for **Garlic and Rosemary Lamb Roasts** (page 196).

LAMB MEATBALLS
Kefta d'Agneau

Season Summer   **Preparation Time** 10 minutes
Cooking Time 35 to 40 minutes   **Serves** 5 to 6

My butcher friend and apprenticeship guide Florent Carriquiry showed me this recipe that he learned from his *patron*, a master French butcher, during his own apprenticeship. One of my first projects at the butcher shop in Bordeaux was to make kefta meatballs of about 1.8 ounces (50 g) each for the shop window (shown uncooked on the next page). Not so much a French dish as it is Balkan, Central Asian, Mediterranean, Middle Eastern, or South Asian, *kefta* (or *kofta* or *kofteh*) are meatballs of ground meat, in this case, lamb, mixed with spices. For the meatballs, we collected scraps from the breast and belly (*poitrine*), the neck (*collier*), hind leg (*gigot*), and small pieces from the loin and tenderloin (*onglet* and *hampe*) to keep the larger, more "noble" pieces intact. But all deboned parts of the lamb are useable in this recipe. This can be served as an appetizer (just add toothpicks after cooking) or as a main course. Fresh mint and cilantro are in season in the summer, but you can add them dried during other seasons or leave them out. A handful of fresh or dried parsley may be added in addition to or in lieu of cilantro. I have mentioned as optional several ingredients with which I have made kefta: powdered collagen (for extra collagen), two eggs (for holding the meatballs together), and one tablespoon of olive oil (for taste and additional fat).

5 cloves garlic minced

3 pounds (1.4 kg) ground lamb

5 pinches of fine sea salt

Pinch of ground pepper

Handful of cilantro, stemmed and minced

1 teaspoon fresh mint, minced

1 teaspoon ground nutmeg

Optional: 3 tablespoons powdered collagen

Optional: 2 eggs

Optional: 1 tablespoon olive oil

4 tablespoons lamb or beef tallow or duck fat

Fleur de sel, for garnish

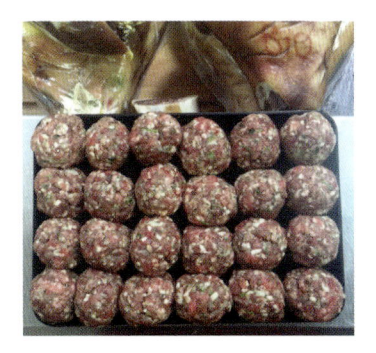

Combine all the ingredients except the tallow into a large bowl, and mix well with both hands. Form small handful-sized balls of about 1.8 ounces (50 g) each, and flatten (*aplatir*) each ball.

Melt the tallow in a large cast-iron pan over medium-high heat. Cook the meatballs in batches for five to seven minutes on each side, making sure they are cooked through.

Makes 25 to 28 meatballs. Garnish with *fleur de sel*. Serve with **Barbeque Sauce** (page 389), **Homemade Mayonnaise** (page 406), or **Old-Fashioned Mustard** (page 410), olive oil, and/or the liquid fat from the pan.

> WINE PAIRING TIP Sommelière Annabelle suggests a range of red wines, from an aromatic Bordeaux Clairet to a complex, fresh, and lively Merlot-dominated Bordeaux Supérieur, with notes of red and black fruits, leather, vanilla, and violet. She also recommends warming and fruity red wines, such as a Southwestern Côtes-du-Marmandais (where the dominating grapes are Cabernet Franc, Cabernet Sauvignon, and Merlot), or an aromatic Côtes du Rhône with rounded tannins, or an herbaceous Côtes de Provence, with notes of licorice, rosemary, and thyme.

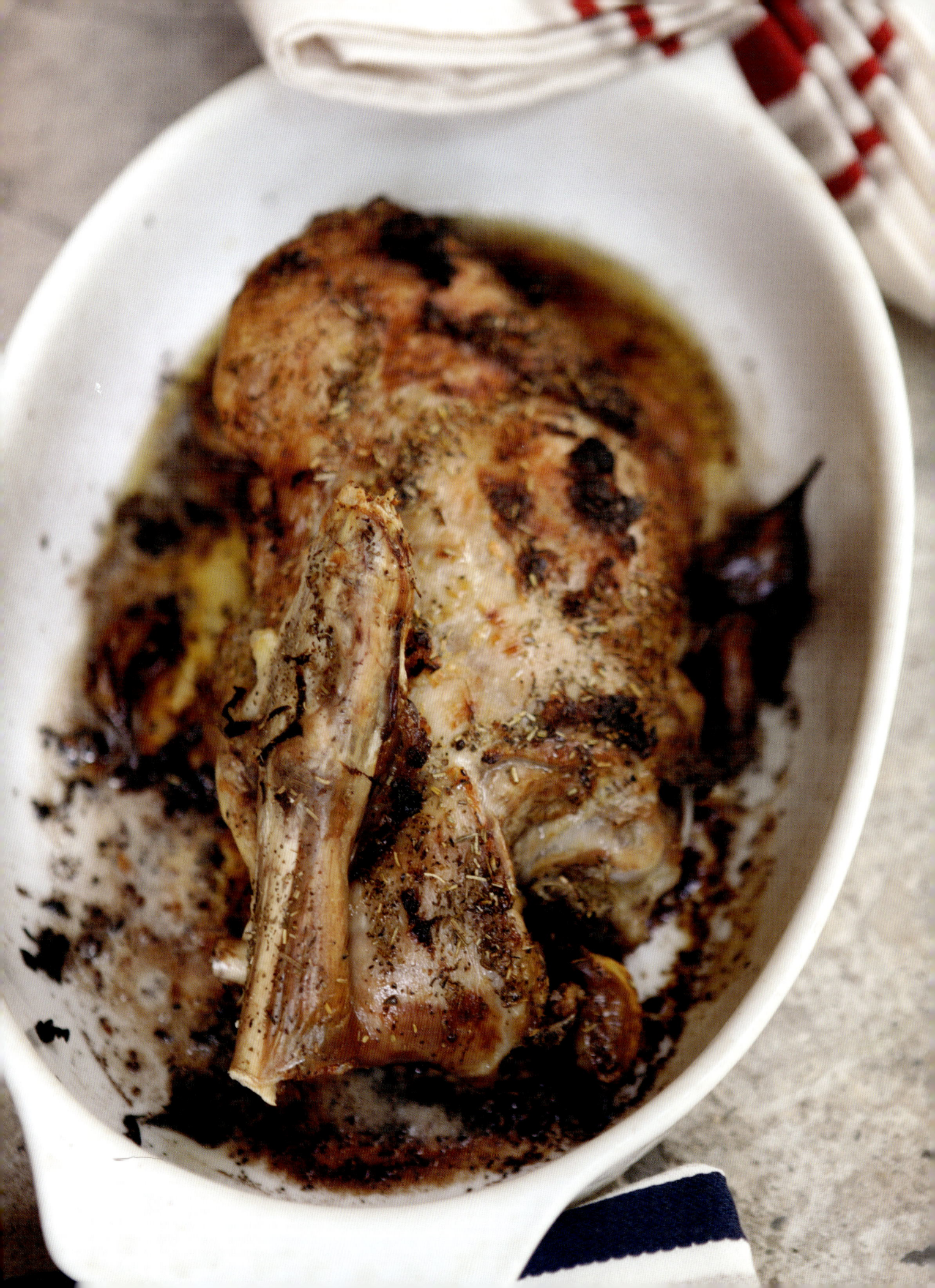

MILK-FED LAMB ROAST
Rôti d'Agneau de Lait

Season Spring   **Preparation Time** 5 minutes
Cooking Time 30 to 35 minutes   **Serves** 5 to 6

This recipe was shown to me by my Basque friend, Lilou Leonard. It is delicious in its simplicity. Milk-fed lamb is smaller than "regular" lamb in France, as it has not yet transitioned to eating grass, though its mother is grassfed. My preference is lamb that is older with bolder flavors, but this is an example of a specialty served around Easter, the spring birthing season of lambs.

1 leg of milk-fed spring lamb

2 tablespoons olive oil

1 tablespoon *herbes de Provence*

2 pinches of coarse sea salt

7 teaspoons unsalted butter

Preheat the oven to 430°F (220°C). Remove the leg of lamb from the refrigerator, and allow it to come to room temperature for about 20 minutes. Rub the olive oil onto the leg of lamb and lay it in an oven-safe casserole dish. Sprinkle on the *herbes de Provence* and the salt. Distribute the butter in teaspoon-sized knobs on the meat.

Cook for 30 to 35 minutes. Using a meat thermometer, check the center of the leg for the desired degree of doneness. (Refer to **Degrees of Doneness for Lamb** on page 193.) Serve with spring potatoes or roasted vegetables.

> **WINE PAIRING TIP** A red Bordeaux from Pauillac or Margaux is a standard, no-fail recommendation for this roasted lamb, but reds from across the Rhône Valley would make for a very flavorful pairing as well. Sommelière Annabelle recommends elegant, fruity wines with a moderate tannic structure, such as a Burgundy Pinot Noir from Vosne-Romanée from the Côte de Nuits, with notes of cherry and dark fruits, or a fresh and floral Anjou from the Western Loire Valley, with notes of red fruits. She also recommends a complex Bordeaux Saint-Julien (known for its capacity to age well, thanks to its solid tannic structure from the Cabernet Sauvignon grape), with notes of caramel, cocoa, dark berries, prunes, tobacco, vanilla, and violet. This wine is a meal unto itself!

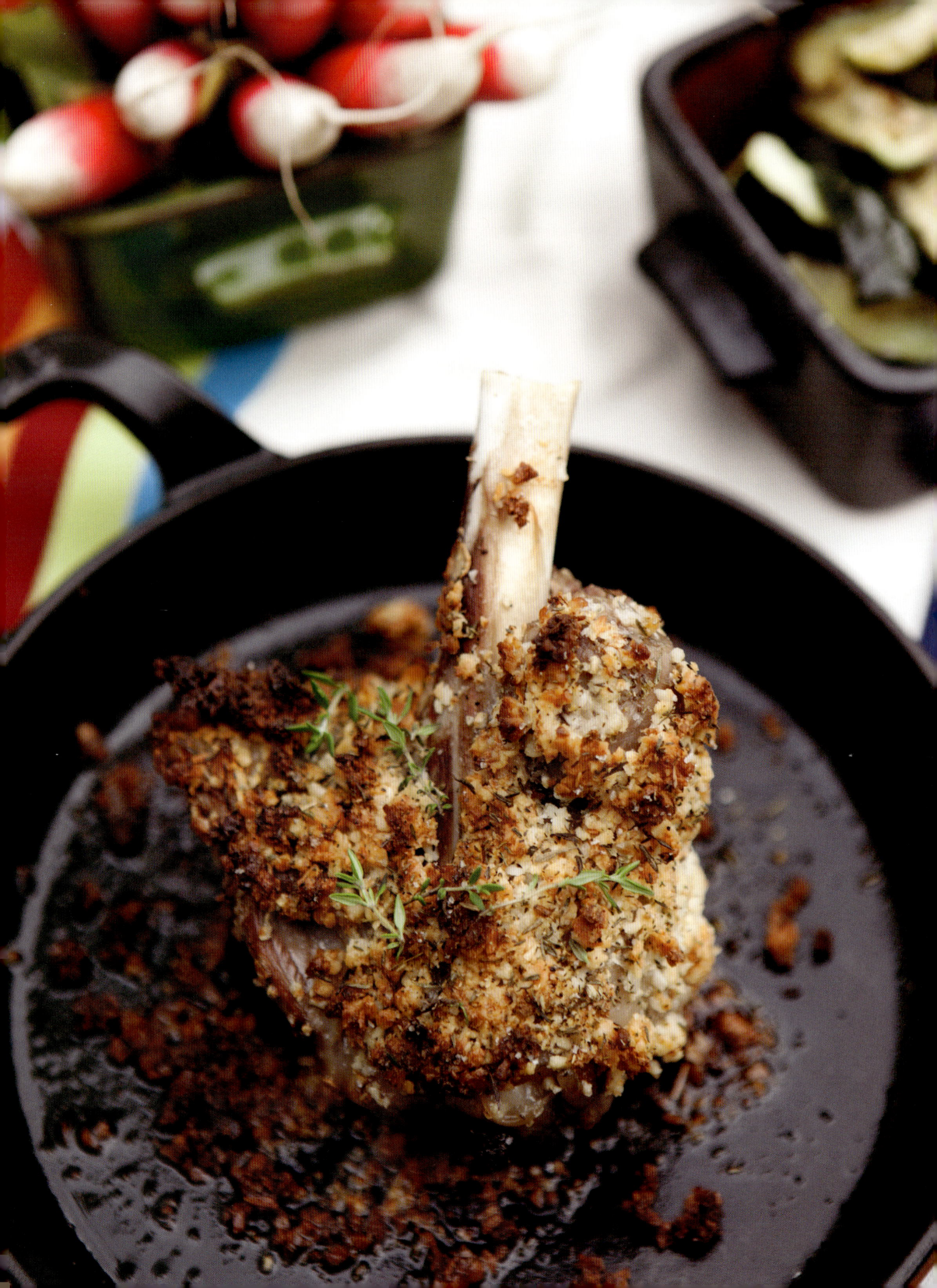

NUT-ENCRUSTED LAMB SHANK
Souris d'Agneau en Croûte de Noix

Season Year-round   **Preparation Time** 10 minutes   **Cooking Time** 40 minutes   **Serves** 1 to 2

Shown here using macadamia nuts (much loved in the primal/paleo community for their high monounsaturated fat and mineral content and low phytate content[2]), this recipe provides flavor and crunch while using a popular French lamb cut, the shank. Depending on how high it is cut, a lamb shank (leg piece with bone) can weigh between 7 and 14 ounces (200 g to 400 g). I do not soak, sprout, or dehydrate macadamia nuts, though you may decide to do so. You can make this recipe, however, with soaked and dehydrated pine nuts or walnuts (both native to the French Southwest), almonds (widely cultivated in neighboring Spain), hazelnuts (originating in Turkey, brought to France by the Romans, and now widely cultivated in the French Southwest and on the French island of Corsica), cashews, or pistachios. Go nuts!

1 tablespoon macadamia nut oil or olive oil

1 lamb shank

Handful (9 to 12) macadamia nuts, chopped

3 garlic cloves, minced

1 teaspoon fresh or dried thyme

Pinch of fine sea salt

Preheat the oven to 365°F (185°C). Rub the shank with the macadamia nut oil.

In a small bowl, mix the garlic and chopped nuts. Spread the mixture uniformly around the shank. Place the shank in an oven-safe dish, and sprinkle the herbs and salt over the meat. Cook in the oven for 40 minutes.

> **WINE PAIRING TIP** As with all wine pairings for lamb, the lamb's strong flavors need to be supported by the accompanying wine. For this recipe, my trusty Bordeaux wine course classmates have a few recommendations for red wines. Sommelière Natalia Youreva advises the most popular pairing with lamb, a Pauillac wine from the Médoc region of Bordeaux—you can't ever lose pairing a Pauillac with lamb, as the region is known for both its wine and its lamb. Natalia also proposes a spiced and generously flavored Fitou from Languedoc. Organic wine buff Vy Nguyen suggests a red organic wine from the Bordeaux Supérieur appellation and located just a few miles from Saint Emilion. In particular, she recommends Château Vieux Mougnac, a wine with character to match the nut, garlic, and lamb flavors in the dish. Winemaker Malika Faytout advises a powerful wine with flavors of stewed fruits, usually an older wine. From the Bordeaux region, you will find these hailing from appellations such as Pessac-Léognan, Pomerol, Saint Emilion, and Saint Julien. Or else try an aged Pinot Noir from Burgundy.

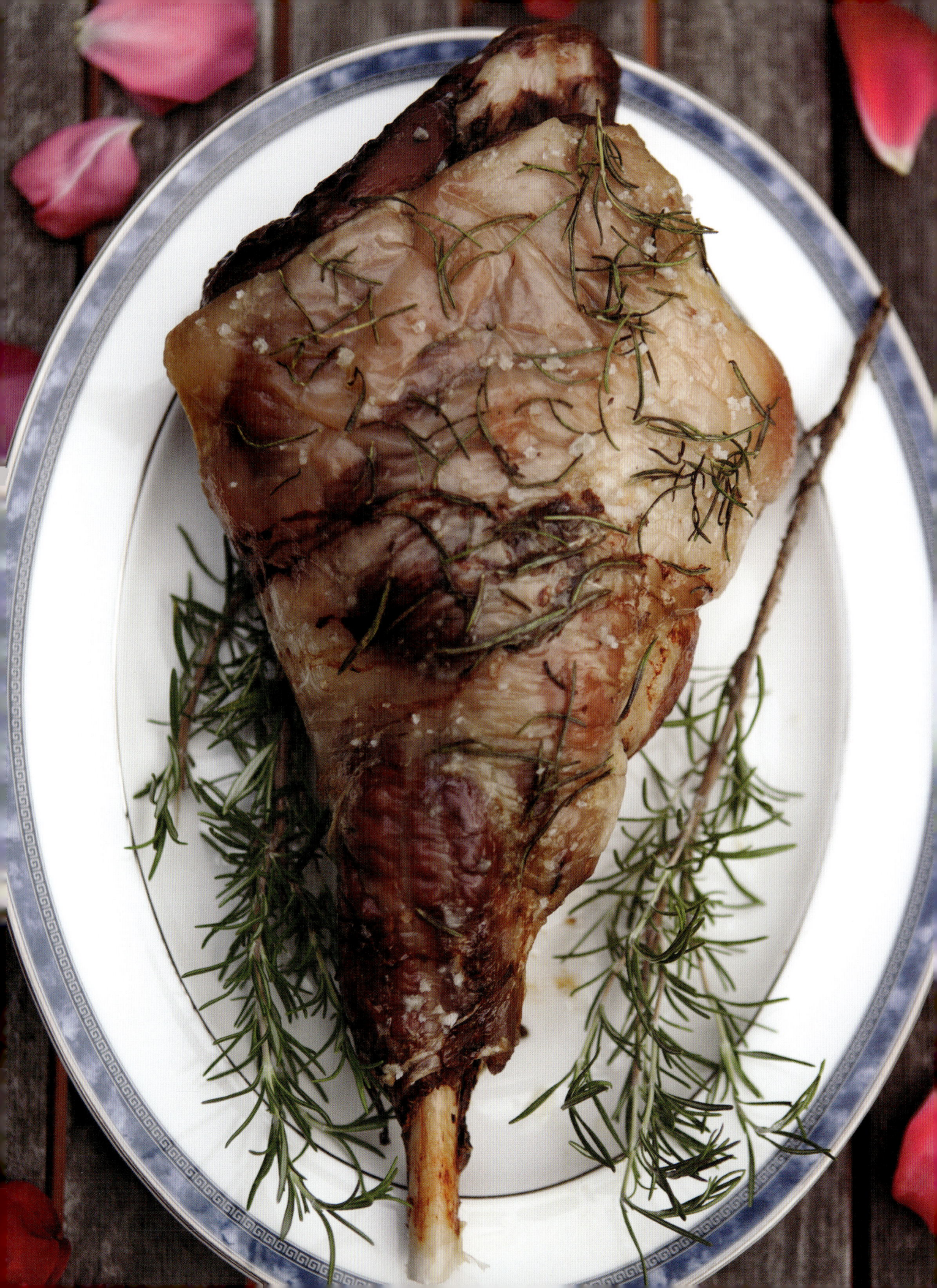

PYRÉNÉES SEVEN-HOUR SLOW-COOKED LEG OF LAMB
Gigot D'Agneau des Pyrénées Cuisson Sept Heures

Season Year-round   **Preparation Time** 20 minutes
Cooking Time 7 hours   **Serves** 6 to 7

My husband and I had this dish for the first time with my good friend Béatrice Pontallier and her family at their home in Bordeaux. The four of them glowed with happiness when the father brought out the finished leg of lamb in a lovely dish and set it on the table. They enthusiastically explained to us how the lamb had been in the oven all day, with the aromas wafting through the house, and they were glad to be able to finally eat it! They explained how they prepared it, and since then, I have been making this dish, with several modifications, whenever I can get my hands on a *gigot*. In the photo shown here, olive oil was used, but employing duck or goose fat, and lots of it, is truer to the original recipe, with the dish originating from the Pyrénées in Southwestern France, after all! Also, Béatrice had covered the leg of lamb in sliced onions, which fell into the gravy, adding to the flavor of the dish. The cooking time may be shortened, but the original idea of the seven-hour leg of lamb adds tenderness and flavor to the dish while supporting the idea and charm of slow food and fellowship around good food and wine at the end of the day.

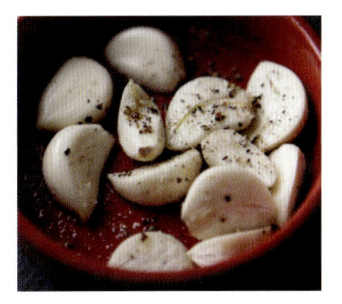

1 leg of lamb, bone-in

Optional: 1 to 3 sprigs of fresh rosemary

7 garlic cloves (optionally rolled in salt and pepper)

1.5 cups (360 ml) water

3 tablespoons olive oil (or duck or goose fat)

Chef's Tip
Astuce du Chef

Rolling the garlic cloves in salt and pepper is a trick I learned from butcher Florent Carriquiry. I have added the trick of drizzling a bit of olive oil on the garlic to make the salt and pepper stick, as shown here.

Preheat the oven to 210°F (100°C). Using a sharp knife, make several slits on top of and beneath the leg of lamb, and place a garlic clove in each slit. Lay the leg of lamb in a large casserole dish on top of the rosemary sprigs. Add the water to the dish and drizzle the oil over the lamb. The water combined with the garlic and rosemary will steam flavor into the lamb and makes for a nice gravy. Cook at 205°F to 210°F (95°C to 100°C) for seven hours. Shorter cooking time alternatives are 230°F (110°C) for six hours, 250°F (120°C) for five hours, 275°F (135°C) for three-and-a-half to four hours. Times will vary depending on the size of the leg of lamb and the oven used. Use a meat thermometer to help you determine the internal temperature of the meat if you are unsure. (See **Degrees of Doneness for Lamb** on page 193.) The idea here is to experiment, not letting the amount of time or temperature keep you from enjoying a leg of lamb. It's a very easy dish to prepare, and once it's in the oven, you are free to go about doing other things! ➤

LAMB – L'AGNEAU

Serve with **Sarlat Sautéed Potatoes** (page 468), salad, and/or other cooked vegetables, as shown here on the plate. You will find that everyone will like this dish, from children to grandfathers. Leg of lamb is traditionally served sliced on a platter. This dish is shown on page 193 as sliced by butcher Florent Carriquiry from a whole lamb I bought and we "broke down" (*casser*, a butchering term for cutting up a carcass) to feed some of my *Bordelais* friends.

WINE PAIRING TIP We enjoyed a very elegant wine from Bordeaux's legendary Margaux appellation with Béatrice's family, but another Cabernet-Sauvignon-weighted Bordeaux red from the Médoc's many appellations will go marvelously as well. For this dish, restaurateur Annabelle recommends powerful red wines with rounded tannins such as an elegant Syrah-based red from the Rhône Valley's Côte Rôtie, or a Grenache-Mourvèdre-Syrah blend from Languedoc-Roussillon, such as a rustic but rich Corbières, a Faugères with notes of coffee and vanilla, a medium-bodied Fitou, or a supple Minervois, with spicy notes of cinnamon and vanilla. I have paired this dish with an organic Bergerac from the Southwest, which is similar in composition to a powerful Bordeaux blend of Merlot, Cabernet Sauvignon, and Cabernet Franc, but is less tannic and overpowering, allowing it to cradle the subtle flavors of the tender leg of lamb.

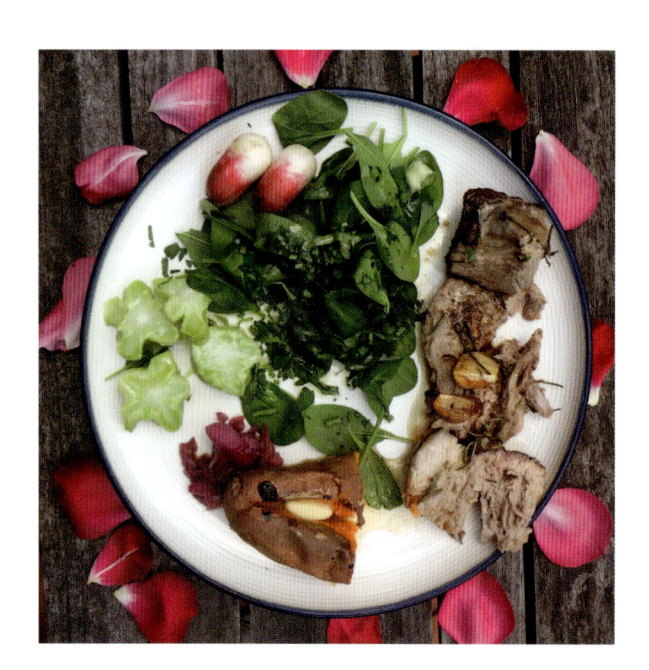

SIMPLE LAMB STEW
Agneau Mijoté

Season Year-round   **Preparation Time** 35 minutes
Cooking Time 2 to 3 hours   **Serves** 5

This easy, flavorful stew can be made with lamb pieces on the bone as well, just use more lamb, as the weight of the bones displaces some of the weight of the edible meat. Like the **Springtime Lamb Stew** (see page 213), usually the neck and shoulder cuts are used, but any cuts of lamb will do. What makes it so flavorful is a combination of the browning of the meat, the fresh herbs (otherwise use dried), the garlic, and the slow cooking of the meat. This dish is easy to throw together if you have planned ahead a bit on your timing: prepare it in the morning for a weekend lunch or after lunch for the evening meal. If you add chopped vegetables (such as carrots, leeks, onions, peppers, potatoes, sweet potatoes, or tomatoes) during the last hour or so of cooking, it is called a lamb *ragoût*. If you add curcumin, ginger, and vegetables, it is essentially a lamb *tajine*.

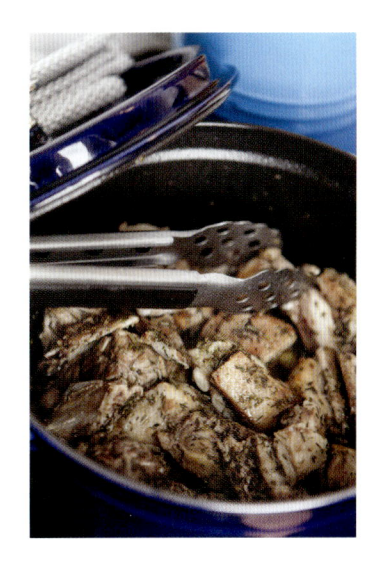

1.8 pounds (800 g) lamb meat, cut into 1- to 2-inch (2.5 cm to 5 cm) cubes

3 tablespoons lard or duck fat

Several pinches of fine sea salt

½ cup (120 ml) water

4 garlic cloves, minced

1 tablespoon fresh or dried rosemary, minced

1 teaspoon fresh or dried thyme, minced

Melt the fat in a cast-iron pot over medium-high to high heat. Brown the pieces in batches for two to three minutes on each side, sprinkling a pinch of fine salt over each batch.

Add ½ cup water, bring briefly to a boil, then reduce the heat to medium-low or low. Stir in the garlic, rosemary, and thyme. Cover the pot, and allow to simmer for 3 hours.

> **WINE PAIRING TIP** To match the bold flavors of this stew, try a red wine from the Côtes du Rhône, such as an aromatic Duché d'Uzès, with notes of licorice, pepper, and spice, or a classic and complex Châteauneuf-du-Pape. For stewed lamb, restaurateur Annabelle suggests strong wines that are meaty and spiced, such as a Saint-Chinian, made with the Grenache and Syrah grapes and a bit of Carignan, with notes of cacao and roasted coffee beans, or a Faugères with notes of coffee, red fruits, smoke, and vanilla, or a supple Minervois, with notes of cinnamon, vanilla, and violet, all from Languedoc-Roussillon, or else a fruity and tannic Fronton from France's Southwest, with notes of violet.

LAMB – L'AGNEAU

THE BORDEAUX KITCHEN

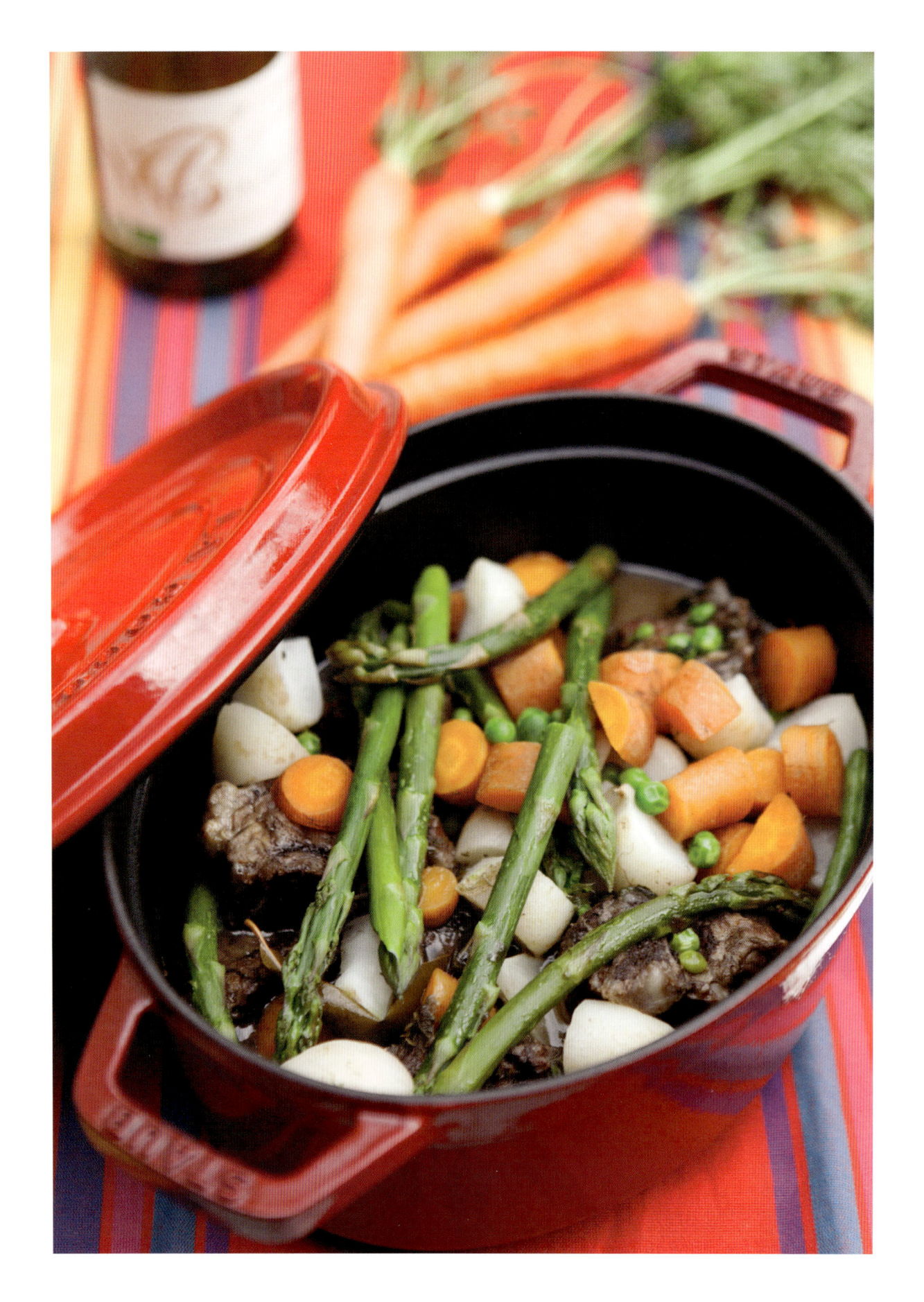

SPRINGTIME LAMB STEW
Navarin Printanier

Season Spring **Preparation Time** 35 to 40 minutes
Cooking Time 1 hour 15 minutes to 2 hours **Serves** 4

This dish is an undeniable French springtime classic. Much like the **Boiled Beef "Pot-Au-Feu"** (page 123) and the **Chocolate Mousse** (page 490), every cook has his or her own slightly personalized version of this stew. I was inspired by recipes from my two favorite French cookbooks, *Morceaux Choisis* by Hugo Desnoyer and *Viandes* by Jean-François Mallet, but also by recipes from my friends, Basque butcher Florent Carriquiry, and Nice native Joelle Luson. There are many ways to make this dish: browning or not browning the vegetables; using flour (in this case chestnut flour, *farine de châtaigne*) in which to roll the meat before browning it; not using flour before browning the meat; or using certain herbs and spices and not others. It depends on what you have available to you at the market or in your pantry and your tastes and preferences. Below is the recipe as I have made it, and under Variations you will find Florent's and Joelle's minor adaptations. What makes this a springtime stew, besides the lamb, are the spring vegetables: springtime asparagus, carrots, green peas, and turnips. The meat used in this dish generally comes from the neck (*collier*), in-bone, as the bones are cut and smaller, or from the deboned shoulder (*épaule*), as the shoulder bones are sizeable.

Fine salt and pepper, for seasoning the meat

1.8 to 2.2 pounds (800 g to 1 kg) lamb neck or shoulder, cut into 1- to 2-inch inch (2.5 to 5 cm) cubes

1 tablespoon chestnut flour

4 tablespoons lamb or beef tallow

1 leek, white part chopped into ½-inch (1¼ cm) rounds

1 onion, chopped

3 pinches of fine sea salt

½ cup (120 ml) white wine

5 garlic cloves garlic, crushed but unpeeled (*en chemise*)

½ cup (120 ml) water

1 teaspoon fresh or dried thyme

1 teaspoon fresh or dried rosemary

Handful of fresh parsley, chopped

2 medium-sized carrots, chopped into ½-inch (1¼ cm) rounds

3 small turnips (*navets*), quartered

1 ounce (30 g) green peas (*petit pois*)

3 ounces (85 g) green asparagus (about nine stalks), bottom halves snapped off

Sprinkle salt and pepper on all the pieces of meat. Place the flour in a dish and roll each piece of meat in the flour. Melt two tablespoons of the tallow in a large cast-iron pot over medium-high to high heat, and brown the meat cubes for two to three minutes on each side.

Set the meat aside in a bowl, and melt two more tablespoons of tallow. Brown the white leek rounds and onion for several minutes, until they become translucent, adding a pinch of salt. Save the green sheaths of the leek for another recipe or freeze them, chopped into four-inch (10 cm) pieces for future garnished bouquets (*bouquets garnis*).

Deglaze the pot using ½ cup (120 ml) white wine (I used a rich Côtes du Rhône Blanc for the recipe as shown in the photo) and a wooden spatula to scrape off the browned pieces stuck to the bottom of the pot.

Reduce the heat to medium-low, transfer the meat back to the pot, and add the garlic, ½ cup (120 ml) water, another pinch of salt, and the thyme, rosemary, and parsley. Cover and cook for a minimum of one hour and 15 minutes, and up to two hours.

Meanwhile, boil a pot of water with a pinch of salt, and boil the carrots for five minutes. Then add the turnips, and continue boiling for five minutes. Add the peas and asparagus to the boiling vegetables for five more minutes to blanche them. Drain out the water, and add the vegetables to the pot containing the meat for the last 10 minutes of cooking.

VARIATIONS Joelle includes a teaspoon of butter, four shallots, several springtime potatoes (*rattes*), and sometimes three tablespoons of tomato concentrate in her recipe, while Florent adds juniper berries (*baies de genévrier*), a bay leaf (*feuille de laurier*), and several whole cloves (*clous de girofle*).

WINE PAIRING TIP For the Springtime Lamb Stew, restaurateur Annabelle recommends red wines that are rounded, supple, and expressive, like the flavors of the stewed meat itself. From Bordeaux she suggests an Haut-Médoc, with notes of ripe red fruits, a Médoc with notes of chocolate and fruits, a smoky Pauillac, with notes of leather and vanilla, or a delicate Saint-Julien, all wines with excellent aging potential, thus never a poor choice. From the Rhône Valley she suggests the Côtes du Rhône Villages, with aromas of dark fruits and spice. From Burgundy she suggests Pinot Noir reds from the Côte de Beaune, either a tannic Beaune, with notes of blackberry and black currant, red fruits, and leather, or a rich Corton, with notes of dark berries, cherry, leather, undergrowth (*sous-bois*), and violet. And from Beaujolais she recommends a fleshy and fresh Crus-du-Beaujolais with notes of red fruits, flowers, and herbs.

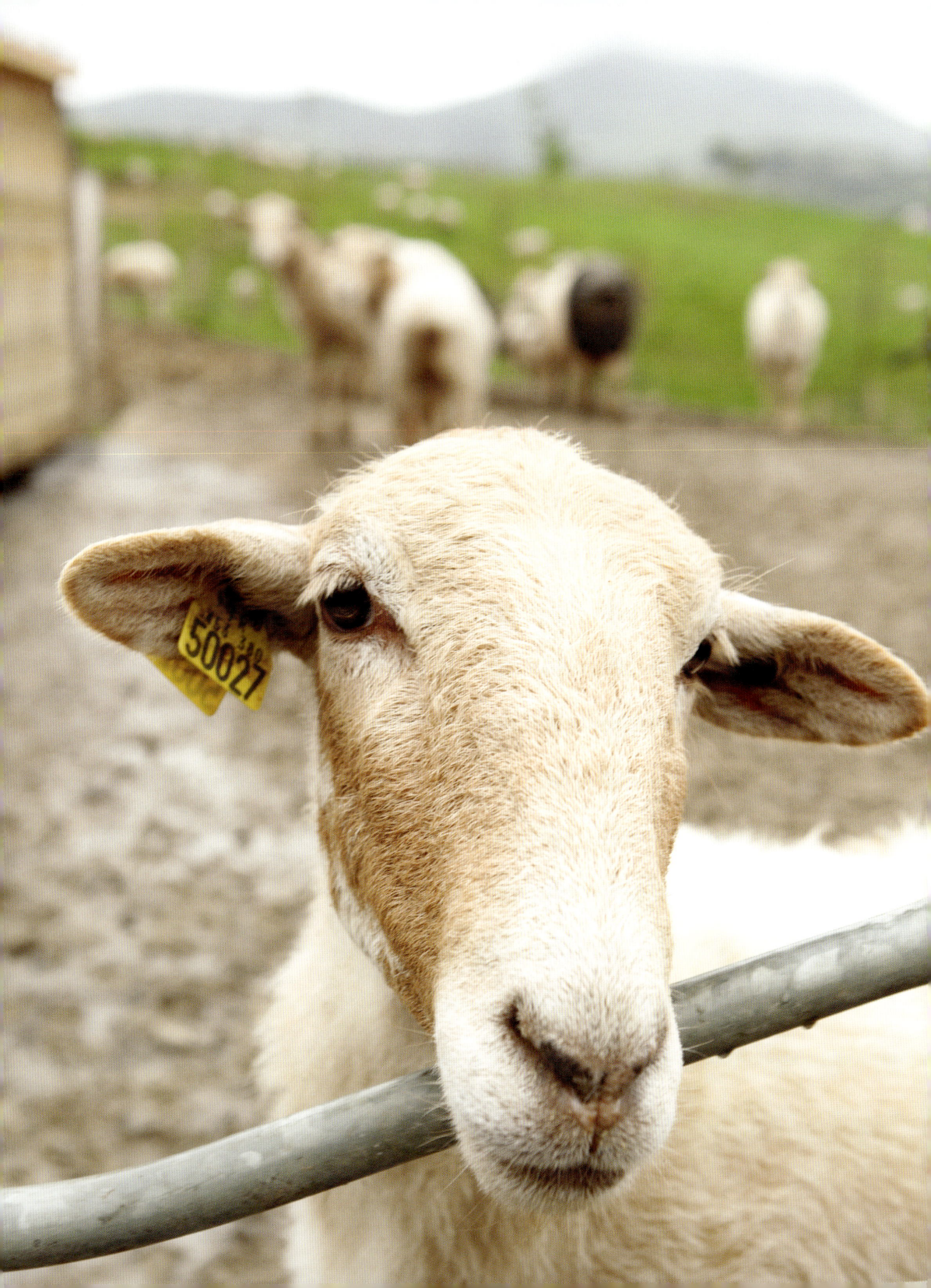

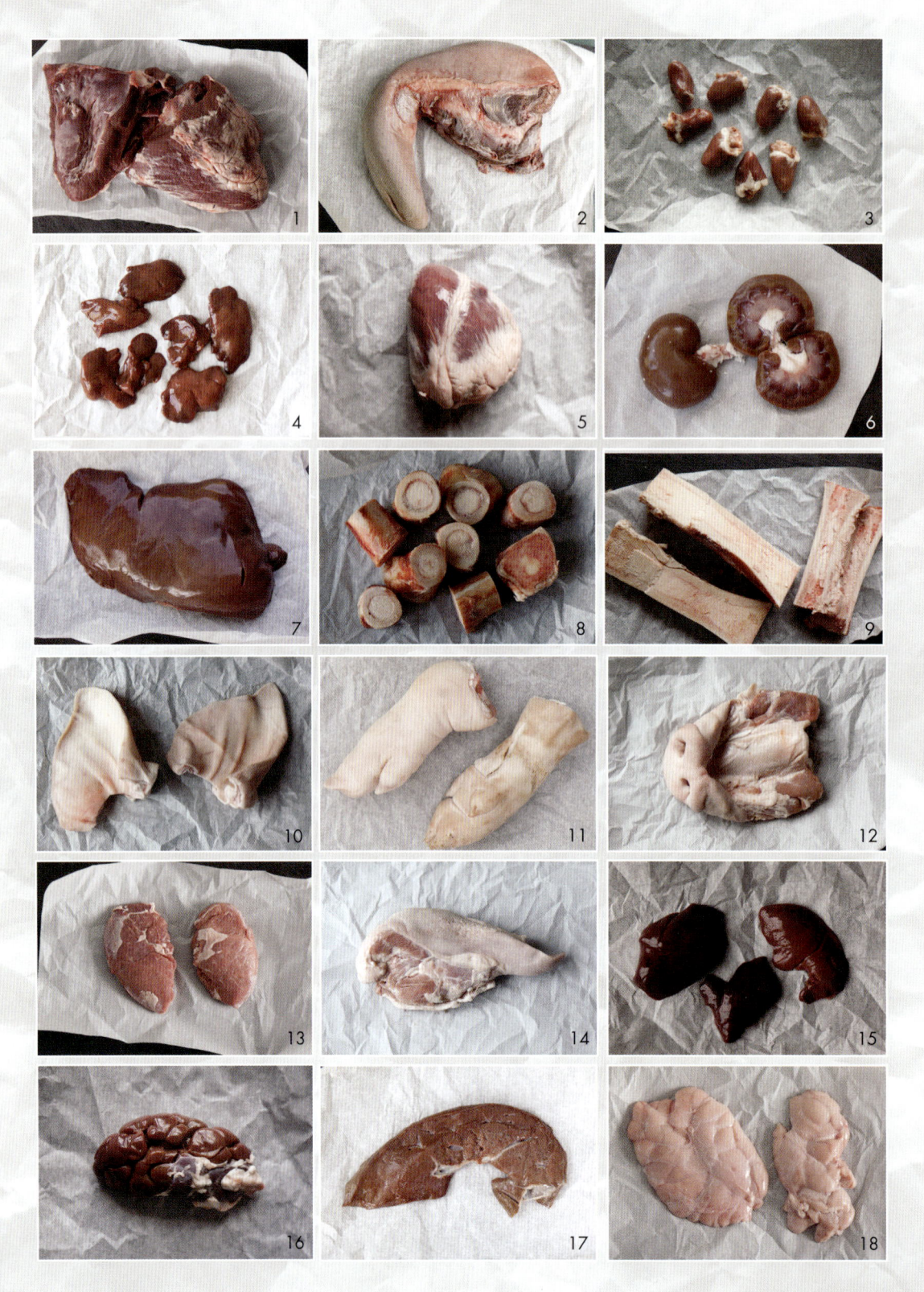

From top left to right: 1. Beef Heart *(Coeur de Boeuf)*, 2. Beef Tongue *(Langue de Boeuf)*, 3. Chicken Hearts *(Coeurs de Volaille)*, 4. Chicken Livers *(Foies de Volaille)*, 5. Lamb Heart *(Coeur d'Agneau)*, 6. Lamb Kidneys *(Rognons d'Agneau)*, 7. Lamb Liver *(Foie d'Agneau)*, 8. Marrow Bones (Cut Crosswise) *(Os à Moelle)*, 9. Marrow Bones (Cut Lengthwise) *(Os à Moelle)*, 10. Pig's Ears *(Oreilles de Cochon)*, 11. Pig's Feet *(Pieds de Cochon)*, 12. Pig's Snout *(Hure de Cochon)*, 13. Pork Cheeks *(Joues de Porc)*, 14. Pork Tongue *(Langue de Porc)*, 15. Turkey Livers *(Foies de Dinde)*, 16. Veal Kidney *(Rognon de Veau)*, 17. Veal Liver Slice *(Tranche de Foie de Veau)*, 18. Veal Sweetbreads *(Ris de Veau)*

OFFAL AND FATS
Les Abats et les Graisses

Alsatian Pig's Snout and Ears – *Hure et Oreilles de Cochon à la Façon Alsacienne* 220

Beef Heart Jerky – *Coeur de Boeuf Seché* 223

Beef Tongue – *Langue de Boeuf* 224

Breaded Veal Sweetbreads "Meunière" – *Ris de Veau Meunière* 227

Chicken Hearts with Garlic and Parsley – *Coeurs de Volaille en Persillade* 230

Chicken Liver Cake with Crab Sauce – *Gâteau de Foies de Volailles Sauce aux Crabes* 233

Chicken Livers with Bacon – *Foies de Volaille aux Lardons* 236

Chicken Liver Dip – *Sauce aux Foies de Volaille* 238

Crispy Pork Rinds – *Grattons de Porc Croustillants* 240

Duck Liver Pâté – *Pâté de Foie de Canard* 242

Foie Gras with Figs and Armagnac – *Terrine de Foie Gras aux Figues et à l'Armagnac* 244

Lamb Heart with Sage – *Coeur d'Agneau à la Sauge* 248

Lamb Kidneys with Butter and Garlic – *Rognons d'Agneau au Beurre et à l'Ail* 250

Lamb Kidneys with Old-Fashioned Mustard – *Rognons d'Agneau à la Moutarde à l'Ancienne* 252

Lamb Liver with Onion Chutney – *Foie d'Agneau, Chutney d'Onions* 254

Lamb Liver with Orange – *Foie d'Agneau à l'Orange* 257

Pig's Feet Sliders – *Galettes de Pieds de Cochon* 259

Poached and Sautéed Lamb Brains – *Cervelles d'Agneau Pochées et Sautées* 262

Rendering Farm Fats: Duck Fat, Lard, and Tallow – *Fondre la Graisse des Animaux de la Ferme* 265

    Rendering Duck (or Goose) Fat – *Fondre la Graisse de Canard (ou de l'Oie)* 266

    Rendering Lard (Pork Fat) – *Fondre le Saindoux* 267

    Rendering Tallow (Beef Fat) – *Fondre le Suif* 268

Roasted Marrow Bones – *Os à Moelle* 269

Slow-Cooked Beef Cheeks – *Joues de Boeuf* 271

Slow-Cooked Pork Cheeks with Apricots – *Joues de Porc aux Abricots* 272

Turkey Liver Pâté with Figs – *Pâté de Foie de Dinde aux Figues* 274

Veal Kidneys in Old-Fashioned Mustard Sauce – *Rognons de Veau à la Moutarde à l'Ancienne* 277

Veal Kidneys with Pickled Pears – *Rognons de Veau, Pickles de Poires* 280

Veal Liver – *Foie de Veau* 282

Offal (*abats* or *produits tripiers*) has a special, lofty place in French cuisine, as evidenced by the common practice of eating organ meats as well as their frequency around the country on menus in restaurants, in the home, and in cookbooks, historically and today. These organ meats are very delicate but packed with nutrients. In fact, organ meats are the most nutrient-dense foods we can eat, and everyone can benefit from their nutrients.[1] The word "offal," or that which has "fallen off," is similar to the German "*Abfall*," literally "off-fall," but meaning trash or rubbish in German. ("Offal" in modern German is *Innereinen*, literally "inner ones.") Nevertheless, these are rarer pieces, often requiring special attention, and therefore can sometimes be more expensive to purchase from the butcher or to order at a restaurant. Organs from smaller animals (such as chicken hearts and livers) are usually less expensive.

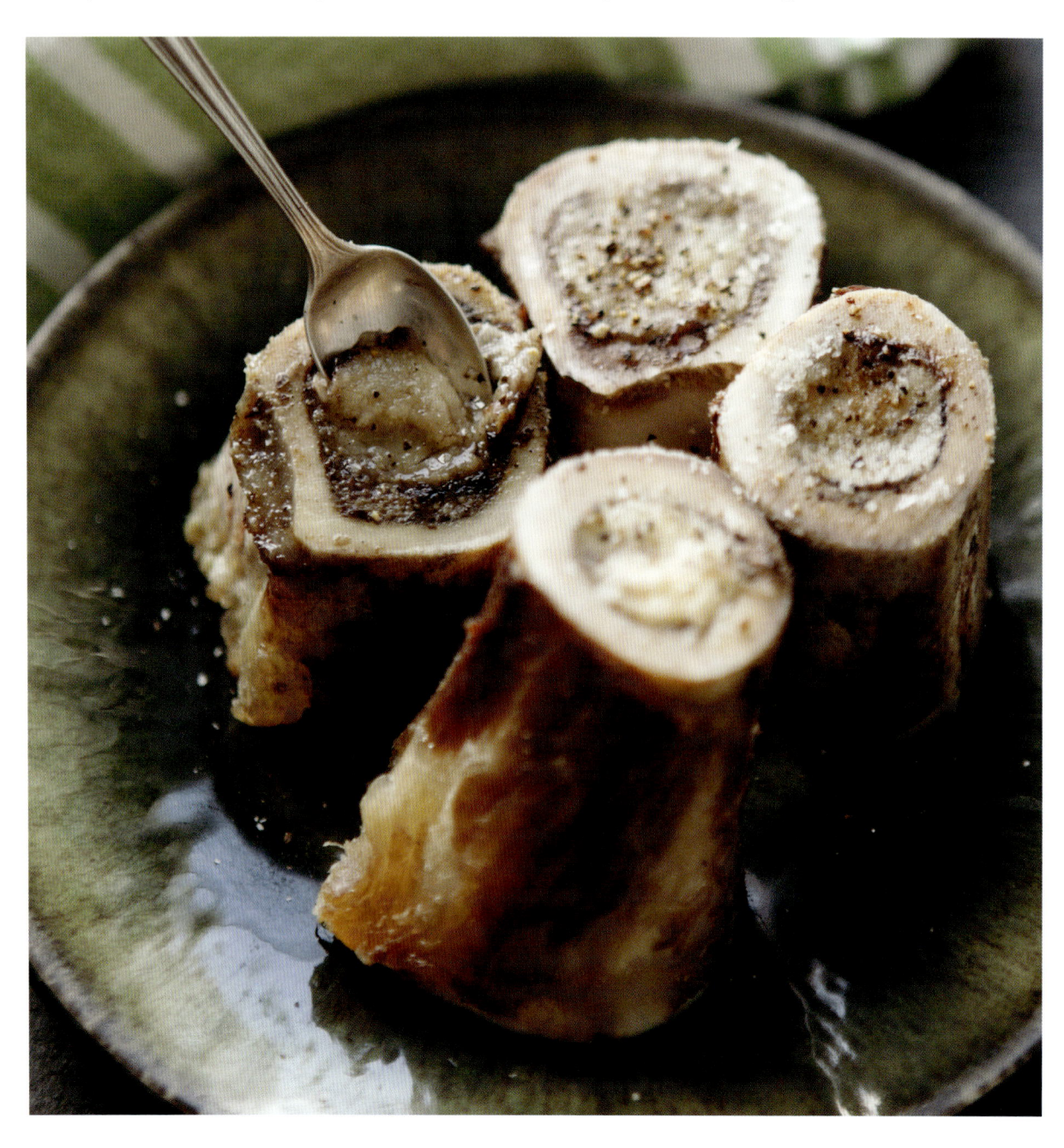

Both *The Big Fat Surprise*, by Nina Teicholz, and *Primal Fat Burner*, by Nora Gedgaudes, refer to numerous studies and research regarding indigenous and hunter-gatherer societies who went for the fat first or only killed animals that were fat enough to eat. The *fat and viscera* (organ meats) were the first to be consumed, while the muscle meat, typically too tough and tasteless to eat, was only consumed as a last resort or left to the dogs. Nora Gedgaudes carries the argument even further, claiming that our consumption of animal fats over the past several hundred thousand years was *central to our health* and what *made us human* in the first place.[2]

Considered the "fifth quarter" (*le cinquième quartier*) in butchery, meaning neither flesh (*chair*) nor muscle (*muscle*), organ meats (*les abats*) are used frequently in French cooking. Entire shops (*triperies*) used to be devoted to organ meats, and they were sold by a tripe vendor (*tripier*). Sometimes you can find organ meats in the supermarkets wrapped in plastic and Styrofoam, looking somehow less appetizing than fresh from the butcher's counter. Today there are far fewer shops in France devoted to just organ meats; rather, these are more commonly sold in butcher shops or supermarkets. The French word for offal (*abat*) is related to the word for slaughterhouse (*abattoir*).

The "red" organ meats (*les abats rouges*), meaning they are red when raw, include brain (*cervelle*); bull, lamb, or ram testicles (*animelles* or *testicules*); cheek (*joue*); heart (*coeur*); kidney (*rognon*); liver (*foie*); lungs (*poumons* or *mou*), used less today than in Escoffier's time in the early 1900s; snout (*museau* or *hure*); spleen (*rate*); and tongue (*langue*). The "white" organ meats (*les abats blancs*) include calf's head (*tête de veau*); ears (*oreilles*); feet (*pieds*), intestinal membrane (*fraise*); spinal marrow (*amourette* or *moelle épinière*); thymus gland or "sweetbreads" (*ris*); tripe (*tripes*) or rumen from the cow, including stomach, "paunch" or "rumen" (*panse* or *pansette*, *rumen*, and *gras double*, the thickest part of the stomach), honeycomb tripe or "reticulum" (*reticulum* or *bonnet*), omasum or "bible tripe" (*feuillet*); and udder (*mamelles*).[3] Abdominal and flank fat (*gras*), blood (*sang*), caul fat (*crépine*), marrow bones (*os à moelle*), thick skirt steak (*onglet de boeuf*), thin skirt steak (*hampe de boeuf*), oxtail (*queue de boeuf*), and skin (*peau*) are also considered by French butchers to be in the organ meats category.[4]

Some odd bits, such as beef or pork cheeks, while not cheap, are still less expensive than more sought-after steak meats. Other items like chicken livers, pigs' feet, and beef tongue tend to be less expensive. Brain, heart, kidney, and thymus gland, among other bits, are much more nutrient dense than muscle meats, and liver is the ultimate nutrient-dense food.[5,6] The energy-intensive brain and heart contain among the highest concentrations of mitochondria (energy-producing organelles) per cell compared to other cells in the body, and eating these organ meats helps fuel our own mitochondrial energy production. Organ meats, like eggs, are also rich in choline, needed for methylation (gene expression) and are rich in minerals and vitamins A, the B vitamins, including B12 (folate), D, E, K2 and other essential nutrients which the mitochondria require. Mitochondria, consisting of fatty membranes, require fat to function optimally. High-quality animal fats are both nutrient-dense, energy rich, and provide the right kind of fat for optimal mitochondrial function.[7] Rendering your own animal fats will allow you to better control the quality and quantity of these fats in your cooking. I like to have multiple jars each of duck fat, lard, and tallow in my freezer to take out as I need them.

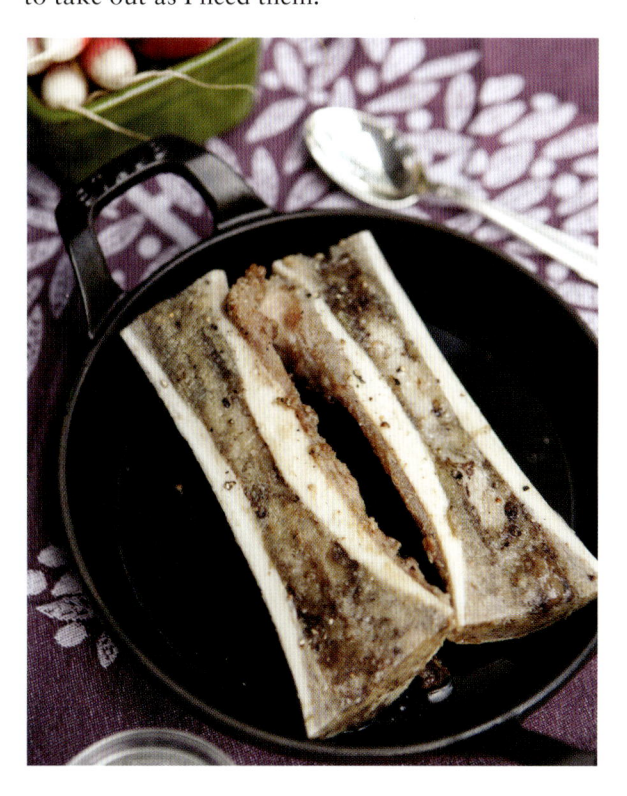

OFFAL AND FATS – *LES ABATS ET LES GRAISSES*

ALSATIAN PIG'S SNOUT AND EARS
Hure et Oreilles de Cochon à la Façon Alsacienne

Season Year-round   **Preparation Time** 15 minutes
Cooking Time 4 hours   **Serves** 12

Respecting the whole animal, we are eating snout to tail here, starting with the snout and ears (use pig tails in **Bone Broth**, page 394). This recipe is from an Alsatian master butcher, imparted to me by a French-German-Swiss butcher in Bern, Switzerland, who apprenticed with the master in Alsace, France decades ago. This recipe may include other parts of the pig's head. In this recipe, I have used the snout and ears (as pictured) but the ears are quite chewy, definitely an acquired taste and texture. The cartilage base of the ears are best cut away and cooked in a bone broth for all their collagen, and the rest of the ears sliced into strips for this recipe or else baked like pork rinds. Ryan Farr, author of *Whole Beast Butchery*, recommends cutting the ears into very fine strips and adding them atop salads for their crunch. The broth with cabbage and potatoes in this recipe is delicious and absolutely packed with collagen. The snouts are meatier and augment the flavor and are akin to pigs' feet, soft and collagenous when cooked. After cooking this recipe, allow it to sit overnight in the refrigerator. This makes the snout and ears softer to eat, yet they are still quite chewy. To make the resulting liquid more diluted (it sets to a hard gel like aspic or *glace*), just add water when reheating the dish. See **Soupy Vocabulary Explained** (page 396) for the differences in stock consistencies, from thinnest (*bouillon*) to thickest and most collagenous (*glace*). See page 417 for **White Poultry Stock** or page 394 for **Bone Broth**, to help you make the stock. Any bone broth or vegetable stock may be substituted if you do not have chicken stock. (A vegetable stock usually has no bones, only vegetables.)

1 head of cabbage (about 1.5 pounds or 680 g), chopped

1 pound (450 g) potatoes, chopped into ½-inch (0.6 cm) slices

2 pig snouts, chopped into bite-size pieces

2 to 4 pig ears, sliced into bite-size pieces

2 pinches of coarse salt

2 cups (475 ml) *demi-glace* chicken stock

1 cup (240 ml) water

Preheat the oven to 230°F (110°C). Place the cabbage in the bottom of a cast-iron pot. Place the chopped potatoes in next.

Place the snouts and ears on top, and sprinkle on the salt. Cover the meat and vegetables with the broth. Cover the pot and place in the oven for four hours. Place in refrigerator overnight and reheat before serving to soften the meat.

WINE PAIRING TIP Pair this dish with an Alsatian white wine, such as a crisp and fleshy Muscat, a fruity and floral Pinot Blanc, a Riesling, with notes of fennel, lemon, peach, and silex (flint or gunpowder), or a Sylvaner with notes of citrus and white flowers. I have paired this dish with a citrus and floral Côtes de Provence rosé, which is refreshing and adds sweetness to the dish.

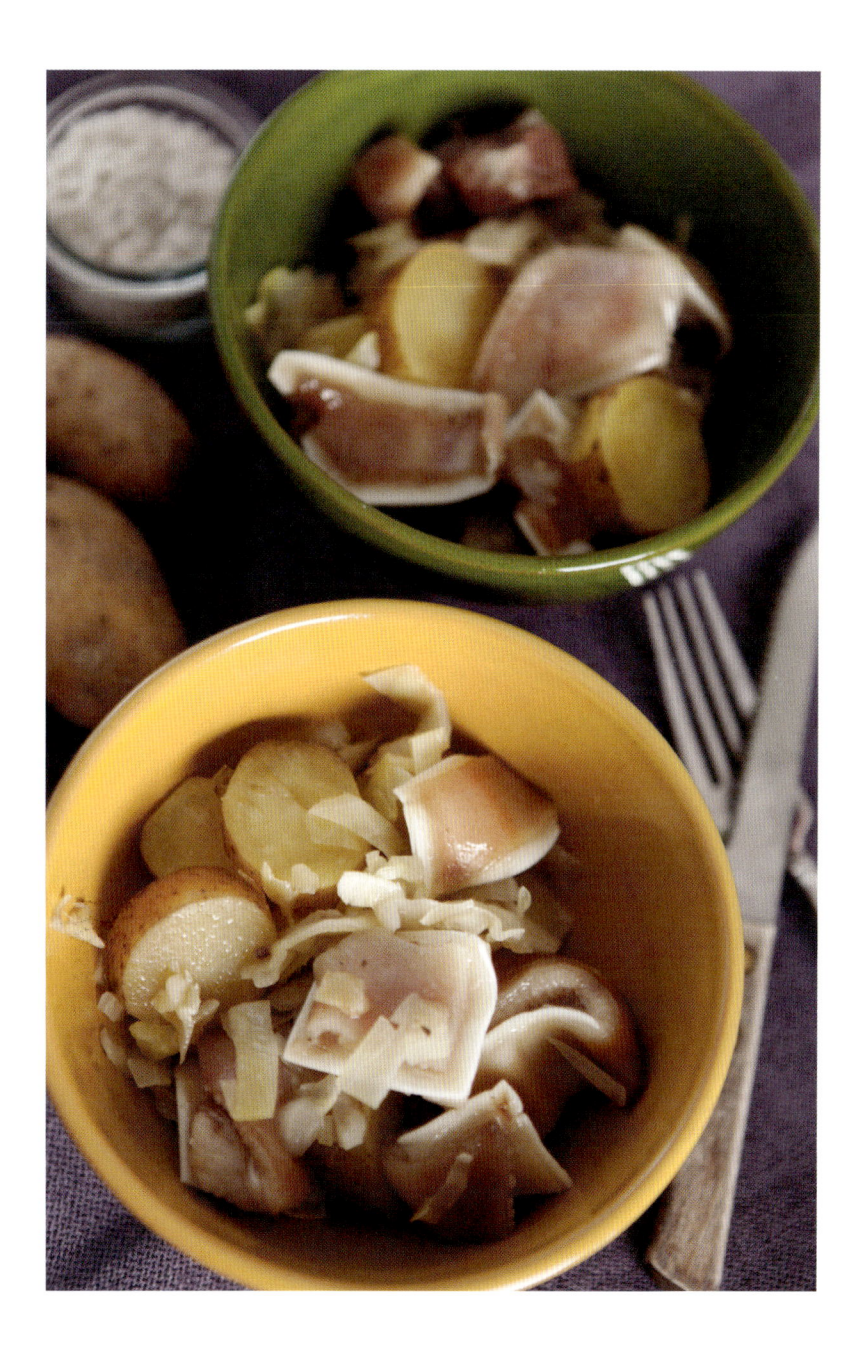

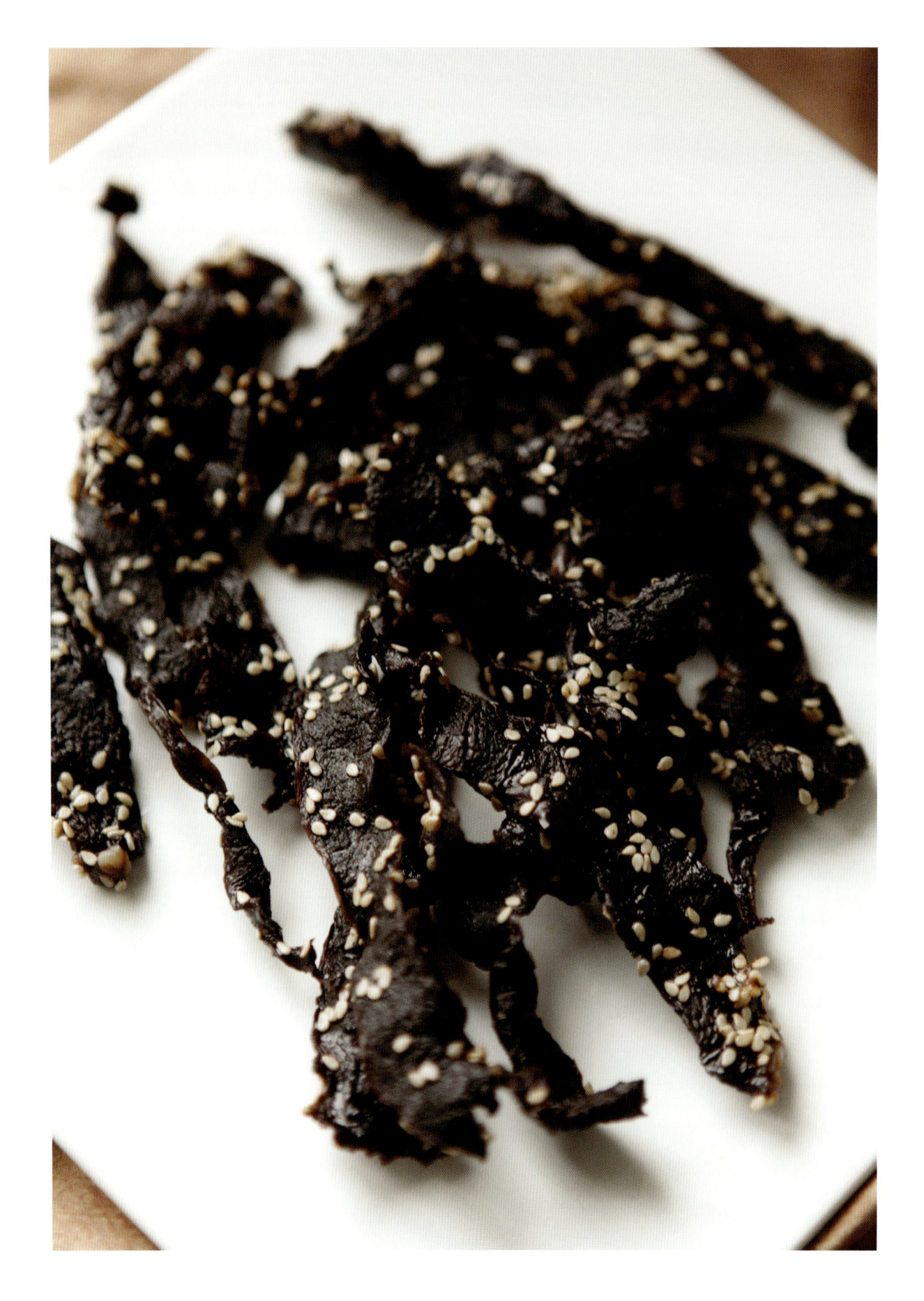

BEEF HEART JERKY
Coeur de Boeuf Seché

Season Year-round   **Preparation Time** 10 minutes, plus marination
Drying Time 3 to 4 hours   **Makes** about two dozen jerky strips

Beef Heart Jerky is a nutritious snack if you are on the go, as it is economical and so easy to make. Dehydrating the meat takes a few hours, but the preparation is quite short. A whole beef heart can weigh almost three pounds (1.3 kg), so for one batch of jerky, you really only need ¼ of a beef heart, or about 11 ounces (310 g), sliced thinly. One trick is to cut the raw heart into four pieces and partially freeze the piece that will be sliced into jerky. This allows for easier slicing into strips (along or against the grain). If the heart is already frozen, then allow it to partially thaw until you can make thin slices. You can marinate the meat in your favorite oil and spices (such as turmeric, ginger, coriander, cinnamon, or clove) overnight or for as little as an hour before placing into the oven. Some oils to try are olive oil, toasted sesame oil, and macadamia nut oil. The longer the marination, the greater the flavor. For their flavor and texture, I like to use sesame seeds that I have soaked, sprouted, and dehydrated (instructions for this process for nuts and seeds is on page 48).

¼ beef heart, cut into thin strips about ⅛-inch (0.3 cm) thick

2 tablespoons toasted sesame oil

4 pinches of fine salt

Pinch of pepper

Optional: other spices

1 tablespoon sesame seeds

Marinate the meat from one hour to overnight in the oil, spices, and seeds.

Lay the strips to dry on a rack in the oven for three to four hours at 195°F (90°C). Store in the refrigerator for up to 10 days, or tightly sealed up to at least two months in the freezer.

> **WINE PAIRING TIP** This is more of a "snack" food to tide you over, and as I have said before, the French do not traditionally snack. Nevertheless, you could try a medium-bodied red from the Southern Rhône Valley or from Languedoc-Roussillon, or else a flavorful, dry, full-bodied Chenin Blanc from the Loire Valley.

BEEF TONGUE
Langue de Boeuf

Season Year-round, most commonly Autumn and Winter   **Cooking Time** 4 hours 30 minutes
Preparation Time 30 minutes for submerging in vinegar and water, plus 5 minutes   **Serves** 6 to 7

Beef tongue (*langue de boeuf*) is a relatively inexpensive meat that is wonderfully tender and flavorful when slow-cooked. This uncomplicated recipe was again inspired by one of my favorite French cookbooks, *Morceaux Choisis*, by Parisian butcher Hugo Desnoyer. Having no idea how to cook beef tongue otherwise, I referred to his recipe, which gave me a basic foundation, as did instructions from the organic butcher shop in Bordeaux where I sourced my first beef tongue. As usual, I made timing and ingredient tweaks and left out the mayonnaise and egg sauce (*sauce gribiche*), which is often used for calf's head dishes. Beef tongue weighs between two and three pounds (900 g to 1.4 kg) and requires submerging in vinegar and water for half an hour. This, along with the long cooking time should be factored into your timing. Pork tongue (*langue de porc*) may be prepared similarly. This recipe calls for piercing an onion with cloves (*clous de girofle*). This is done to gain the flavor of the cloves while not losing them in the stew, as they are a potent spice when bitten into directly.

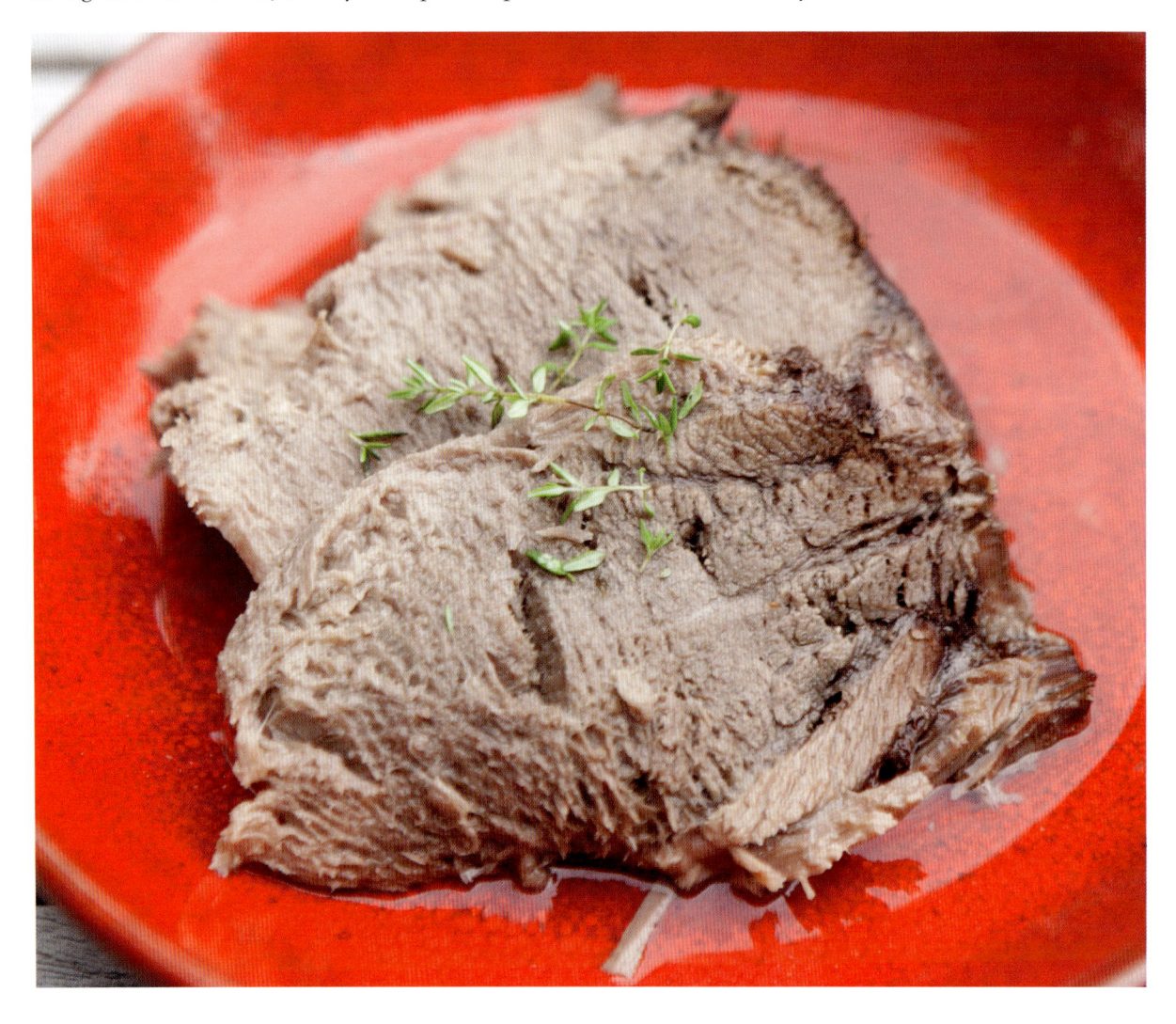

1 beef tongue

½ cup (about 120 ml) white vinegar

1 onion (red or yellow), peeled, halved, and pierced with 4 cloves

1 cinnamon stick

1 teaspoon nutmeg

3 bay leaves

6 black peppercorns

Several sprigs of thyme

1 tablespoon coarse sea salt

Fleur de sel, for garnish

Place the beef tongue in a large bowl, add half of the vinegar, and cover with cold water. Allow the tongue to remain submerged for half an hour. Rinse the tongue under cold water.

Combine the tongue and remaining ingredients, including the remaining vinegar, in a large crock pot (*cocotte*), and cover with water. Cover and bring to a boil briefly over high heat, then reduce the heat to medium-low or low and allow to simmer for four and a half hours. The long cooking time ensures really tender meat.

After cooking, remove the tongue from the pot and peel the whitened skin from the tongue. Cut in slices and return to the pot. Serve hot in bowls with a bit of the broth over the meat and garnished with *fleur de sel*.

> WINE PAIRING TIP To underscore the subtle but rich and spiced flavors of the slow-cooked beef tongue, restaurateur Annabelle recommends red wines that are powerful, well-structured, and spiced. Among these from the Southwest are a rounded and warming Côtes de Bourg, or a Cabernet Sauvignon-dominated and full-bodied Médoc, or a fruity, mocha and spiced Graves, all three of these from the Bordeaux region, or else a Basque Irouléguy, with a floral fruity nose combined with notes of undergrowth (*sous-bois*). I have paired beef tongue with an aromatic Rhône Valley red wine from the UNESCO-protected Ventoux AOP (appellation of protected origin). With notes of red berries, leather, licorice, and spice, this medium-bodied, silky wine frames the dish with its tannic structure, giving the meal a balance to the mild but subtly spiced flavors. (Incidentally, Ventoux reds pair nicely with fresh goat cheese, which may be served after this dish for the cheese course or for dessert.)

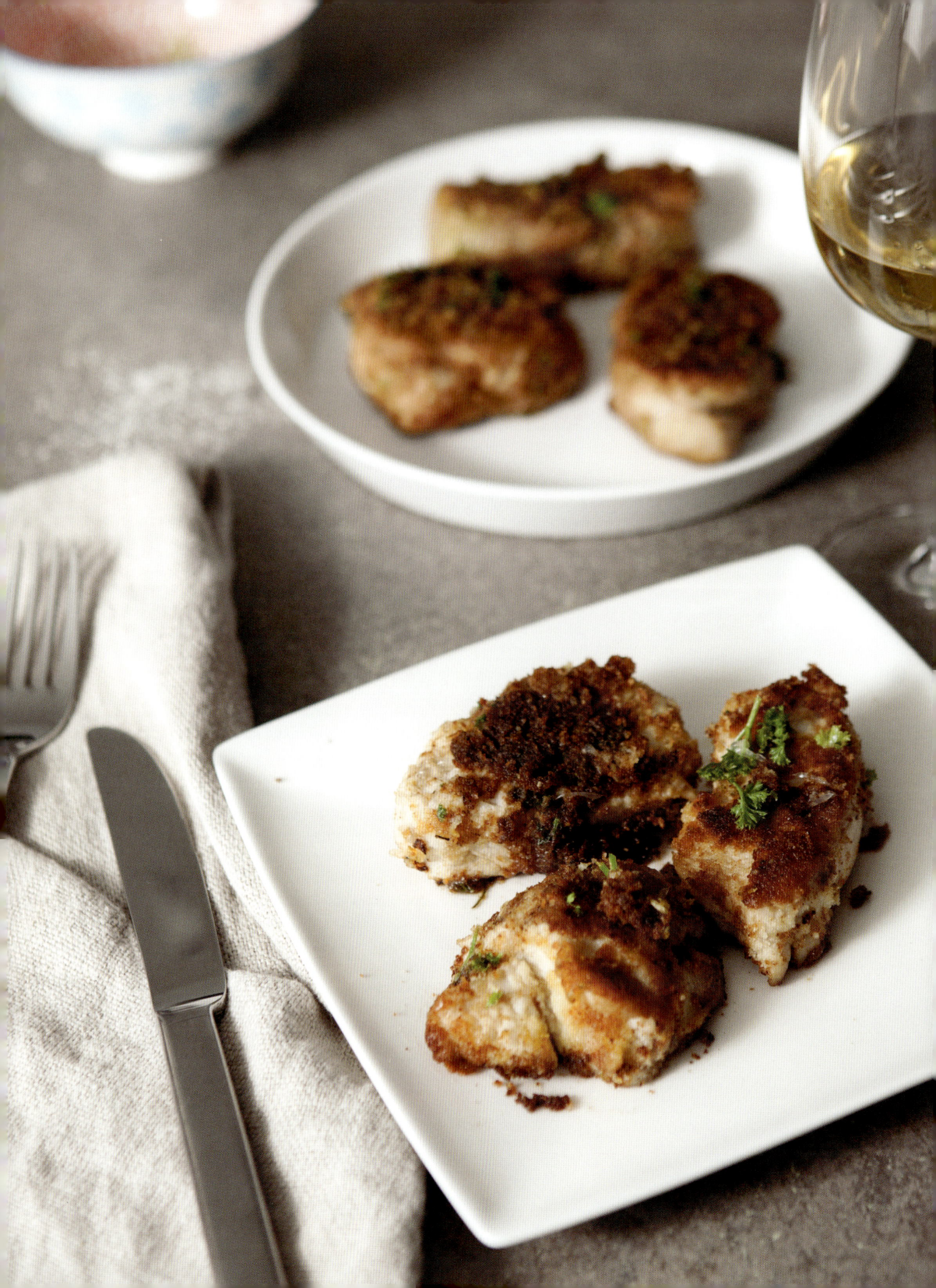

BREADED VEAL SWEETBREADS "MEUNIÈRE"
Ris de Veau Meunière

Season Year-round   **Preparation Time** 35 minutes (plus up to one hour if you wish to soak the sweetbreads in water first)   **Cooking Time** 10 to 15 minutes   **Serves** 4

Sweetbreads are the thymus gland of the animal, part of the lymphatic immune system. They have a light texture, like very tender meat, and are not chewy unless they are cooked too long. In France, they are a delicacy, as they have a very subtle flavor. They are rare relative to the muscle meats, and are very nutrient dense. They are also expensive, as there is only one pair of thymus glands per animal. This recipe can be used for veal or lamb sweetbreads (lamb sweetbreads are smaller and require less time to poach and to cook), and may be served either as an appetizer (*une entrée*) or a main course (*un plat*).

According to *Le Répertoire de la Cuisine*, by Louis Saulnier, first published in 1914 as a handbook on French culinary terms, recipes, and preparations, *meunière* means a fillet of meat that is breaded and browned on both sides in butter and topped with lemon juice and parsley. This is a variation on that theme. I first made this recipe with my neighbor Rébecca Pinsolle who is originally from Dijon and grew up eating offal at her grandmother's house. We tried both chestnut and coconut flour, and, in a taste test, the chestnut flour won out, only because the coconut flour masked the delicate flavor of the sweetbreads themselves. Both variants were delicious, however, and are shown in the recipe photo opposite, with the coconut flour variant in the foreground, chestnut in the background. We are both moms with small children and despite being under time pressure we were able to finish this recipe in an hour, including photographing each step! Then we had time to enjoy the meal for a few minutes over a small glass of wine.

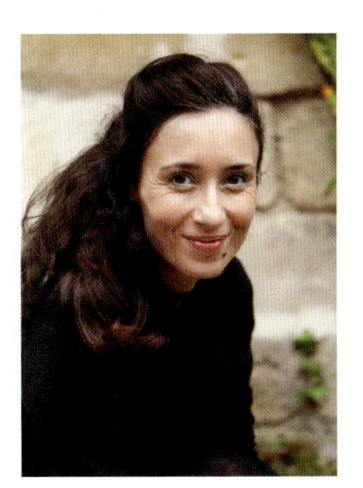

Rébecca Pinsolle

2 lobes veal sweetbreads (or about 12 to 14 ounces or 350 g to 400 g)

2 pinches of fine sea salt

2 ounces (about 8 tablespoons or 50 g) chestnut flour or coconut flour

2 tablespoons butter or ghee

Optional: 1 tablespoon olive oil

Juice of ½ lime

Zest of ½ lime

2 tablespoons parsley, minced

Rinse the sweetbreads in cold water. (If there is blood residue, place the sweetbreads into a bowl of cold water for 20 minutes to one hour, changing the water once every ten minutes. This process removes any visible "impurities." (We rinsed but did not do the soaking.)

Bring a pot of water containing two pinches of salt to a gentle boil. (Reminder, a "pinch" is using two fingers plus your thumb to pick up the salt.) Using a slotted spoon, place the sweetbreads in the pot, and allow them to poach (*pocher*) or "blanche" (*blanchir*) for 15 to 20 minutes. (Lamb sweetbreads need only 8 to 10 minutes.) ➤

228 THE BORDEAUX KITCHEN

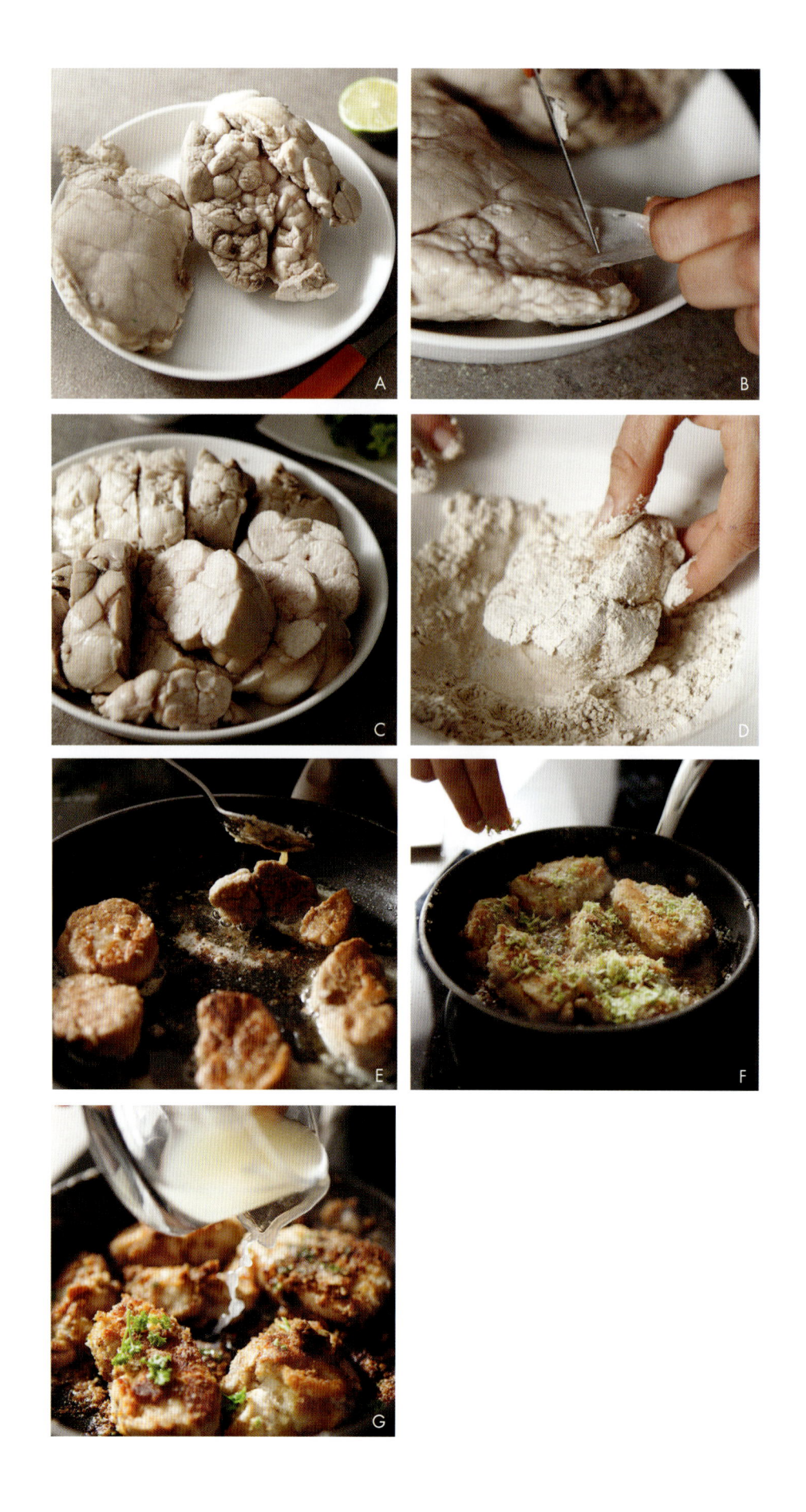

Gently remove the poached sweetbreads from the pot, and allow them to cool a bit on a plate, or place them in a bowl of cold water for half a minute to "shock" them without cooling off the interior. (See photo A.) Gently remove the thin outer skin of the sweetbreads with the help of a small paring knife. (See photo B.) This may take a few minutes.

Slice the sweetbread lobes into about five thick slices each, like cutting a loaf of bread. (See photo C.) (Skip this step if using lamb sweetbreads, since they are small enough already.)

Roll each piece in the flour. (See photo D.) The flour helps hold the sweetbreads together and gives them a slightly crispy exterior texture when cooked in the pan, in contrast to the interior, unctuous texture.

Melt the butter in a pan on medium-high heat, allowing it to brown slightly. This is called "hazelnut butter" (*beurre noisette*), giving the butter a lightly nutty flavor.

Add the pieces of sweetbreads, allowing them to brown for a few minutes in the butter before turning them over, sprinkling salt on each side. Using a spoon, drizzle each piece every few minutes with the butter sauce. (See photo E.) Add the olive oil if the pan seems dry, or else a bit more butter.

Sprinkle lime zest onto both sides as you turn the sweetbreads again in the pan. (See photo F.) After 10 to 15 minutes of cooking in the pan (for lamb sweetbreads only 8 to 10 minutes cooking time), add the parsley and lime juice, allowing another minute cooking time before turning off the heat. (See photo G.) Remove the sweetbread pieces from the pan and serve them hot with a small side of baked sweet potato and a green salad.

VARIATIONS I have used a combination of duck fat and chestnut flour and not added lime, and that tastes good, too. Using a bit of lime or lemon juice (or zest), however, does give the sweetbreads a bit of extra pizzazz, helping to elevate their subtle flavor. I will usually drizzle on extra ghee or olive oil as the sweetbreads become a bit dry in the pan during cooking. See more variations in the following wine pairing tip.

WINE PAIRING TIP Try accompanying the sweetbreads with a dry white wine, such as a Sauvignon Blanc. Rébecca and I shared a Sauvignon Gris from the Francs Côtes de Bordeaux appellation. Sweetbreads made with coconut flour are fabulous with a Pinot Gris from Alsace. I have had sweetbreads with walnut flour and macadamia nut oil and fresh lemon, which goes well with a Jura Chardonnay. I have also paired sweetbreads cooked in almond flour, lemon, butter, and olive oil with a white Côtes du Jura, offering its own notes of apple, biscuit, lemon, lime, oak, and vanilla.

CHICKEN HEARTS WITH GARLIC AND PARSLEY
Coeurs de Volaille en Persillade

Season Year-round   **Preparation Time** 15 to 20 minutes
Cooking Time 15 to 20 minutes   **Serves** 2 to 3

Where do all those hearts go from the multitudes of chickens Americans eat? In France, chicken hearts are easy to obtain, and this recipe is so very easy to prepare. I made this dish with my lovely friend and neighbor, Rébecca Pinsolle on a Wednesday morning, when her kids were home from school. French school children usually have Wednesdays free from school or else they only have half days, to allow for extracurricular activities outside of school. This requires mothers to either work "part-time" to be home with children, or else be very organized in terms of babysitters, drop-offs, and pick-ups if they have a job outside the home. Rébecca knew this dish from childhood, having eaten it at her grandmother's house in Dijon on numerous occasions. Rébecca's children joined us to taste the chicken hearts and liked them, as they had eaten this dish before and it was therefore not off-putting to them. The hearts have a milder flavor than liver and are a very nutrient-dense organ meat. Eating heart is a great way to feed your own mitochondria, as the heart, along with the brain and the eyes, contain the highest amount of mitochondria in animals and in humans. Cooked *en persillade* (a combination of parsley, garlic, and usually butter or olive oil, and sometimes vinegar), they are buttery, garlicky morsels! Pretty much anything cooked *en persillade* is easy to make and delicious. Add to that the shallots, and this dish is just bursting with flavor. In this very basic recipe, we used *piment d'Espelette*, a sweet chili powder from the French Basque region, but this is an optional ingredient, not central to the dish, unless you are Basque! I have had this dish without the parsley and it is still good. Olive oil, butter, or ghee confer to the dish a lot of flavor, but duck fat works well, too.

1 pound (450 g) whole chicken hearts

2 tablespoons olive oil, butter or ghee

Pinch of sea salt

2 garlic cloves, minced

2 shallots, minced

Handful of parsley, minced

Optional: *piment d'Espelette*, for garnish

Wash the hearts in cold water to remove the blood. Cut off the large outer vein from the end of the hearts (as shown on the next page, top), and cut each heart in half. Do not remove the fat on the hearts, as this adds to the flavor. Rébecca says it is the charm of the dish (*le charme du plat*).

Heat the oil or fat in a pan over medium-high heat, and sauté the heart halves for about three minutes, stirring them frequently. Stir in the salt, garlic, and shallots, stirring frequently for about three more minutes. Turn down the heat to medium. Stir occasionally for about 10 more minutes, until the hearts, shallots, and garlic look cooked through. Add the parsley, stir, and remove from heat. Garnish with *piment d'Espelette*, if desired.

VARIATIONS I have tried using ghee as the fat in this dish, as well as a mix of olive oil and lard; both are tasty. I have also replaced the parsley (first because I did not have any parsley on hand and then because I liked the sage flavor better) with two tablespoons of minced fresh sage leaves (about six leaves), which I threw in a few minutes after the garlic and shallots. It turns out, I like the sage flavor even better than the parsley! Give each a try and see what you prefer.

WINE PAIRING TIP Rébecca and I had a Japanese-inspired sweet wine from Alsace. If a sweet wine is not to your liking, try a red wine with low tannins, such as a Pinot Noir from Burgundy, or else a dry white from Alsace, such as a crisp, medium-bodied Pinot Blanc, a lower-acid Pinot Gris or Muscat, or a full-bodied, aromatic Gewürztraminer. Sommelière Annabelle recommends strong, aged (*évolués*), dry reds, such as a tannic Bordeaux Médoc or a Plan de Dieu, "God's Plain," from the Rhône Valley, whose vines grow in a sparse, dry scrubland, carrying notes of bay leaf and thyme, or a spiced Côtes du Rhône Villages, with notes of dark fruit.

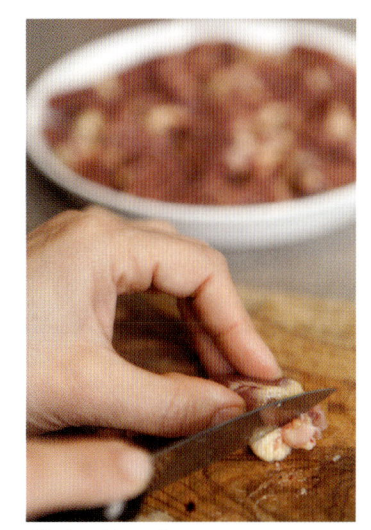

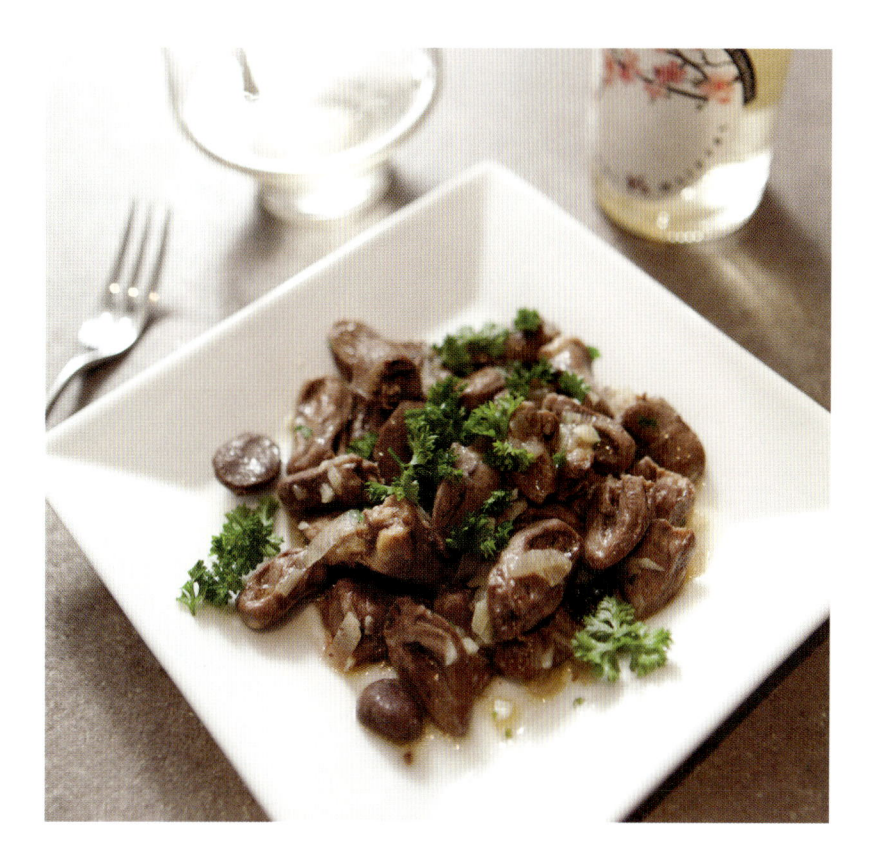

Chicken Heart Artery

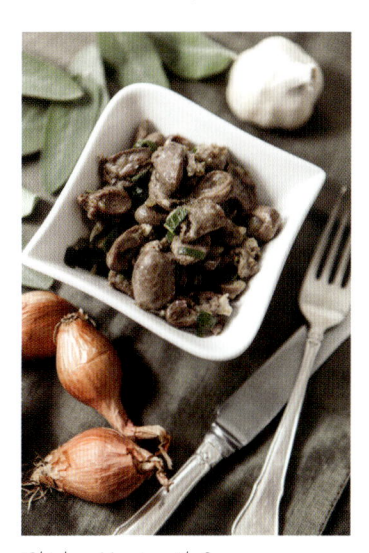

Chicken Hearts with Sage

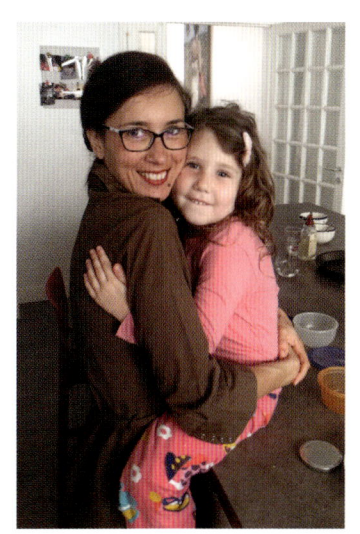

Rébecca with Her Daughter

OFFAL AND FATS – *LES ABATS ET LES GRAISSES*

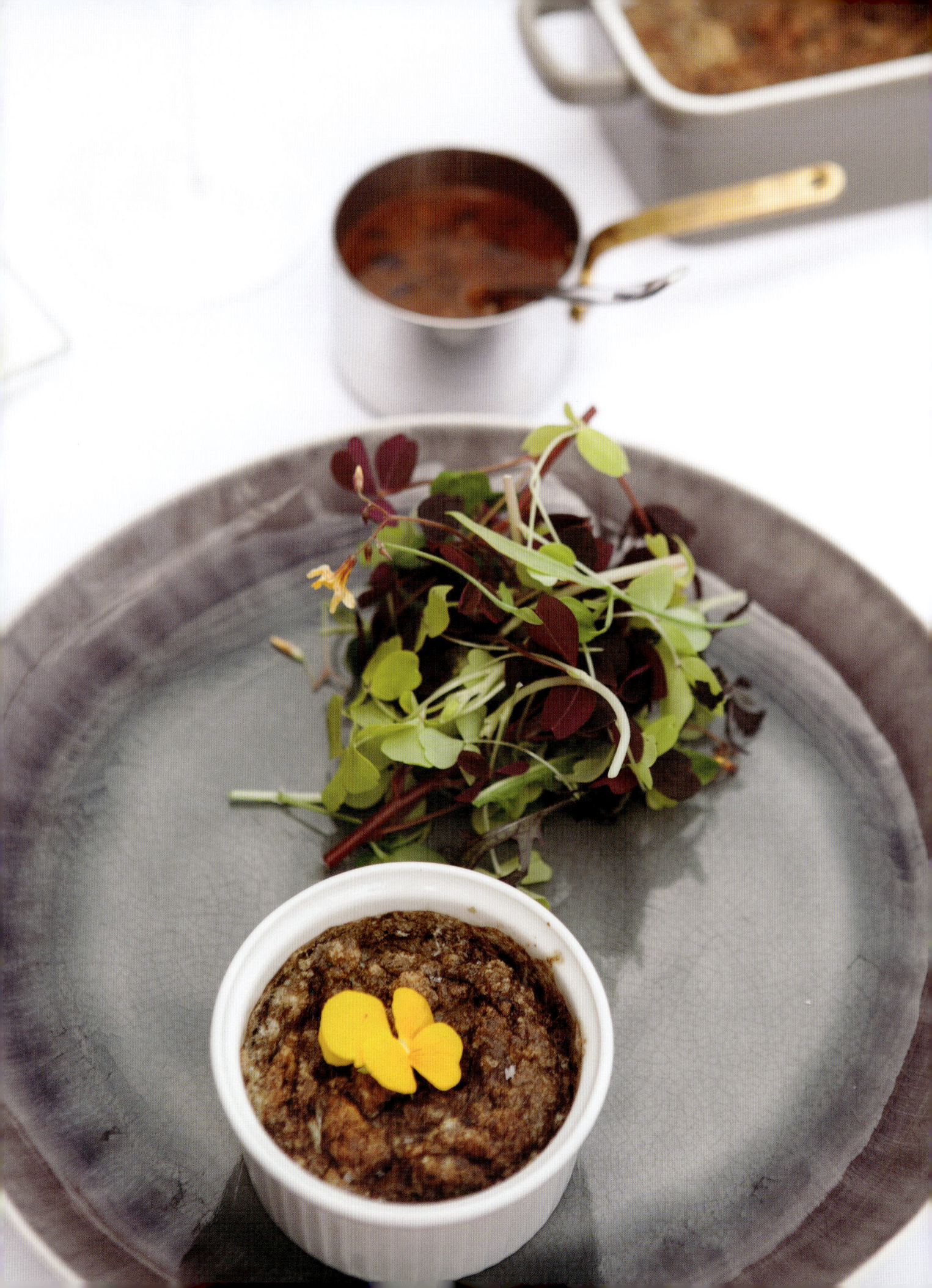

CHICKEN LIVER CAKE WITH CRAB SAUCE
Gâteau de Foies de Volailles Sauce aux Crabes

Season Year-round   **Preparation Time** 30 minutes
Cooking Time 15 to 35 minutes   **Serves** 4

There is no shortage in France of ways to make liver pâtés. This recipe comes from a grandmother called "VonVon," originally from the Piémont Alps of Italy, who moved to Lyon, France around the time of World War II. She is the maternal grandmother of Chef Célia Girard, who is from Gap, in the French Alps. Chef Célia is the instructor at the cooking school *Côté Cours* that is part of the Relais & Châteaux St. James Hotel and Restaurant in Bouliac just outside Bordeaux. One-star Michelin Chef Nicolas Magie runs the restaurant's kitchen, while Chef Célia runs the hands-on cooking courses. Thanks to my thoughtful classmate Anne Perez, two cooking classes were gifted to me by a group of my generous, thoughtful, and dedicated Bordeaux University DUAD wine course classmates whom I so admire and who knew I was eager to learn more French cooking techniques.

This is not a dairy-free pâté, there are other recipes for pâté in this chapter without dairy, but feel free to try dairy-free variations of this recipe, if you are so inclined. In this recipe, we replaced the usual wheat flour with chestnut flour, but even the chestnut flour may be replaced by one egg. If made in small ramekins, this dish can serve as an appetizer, but in a larger mold, it may be sliced and served on a plate, one slice as an appetizer, or several slices as a meal. The accompanying **Crab Sauce** can be found on page 400.

Chef Célia

9 ounces (about 250g) whole chicken livers

1 garlic clove, crushed

Handful of parsley, stems removed

3 eggs, separated (yolks and whites separated)

1 tablespoon chestnut flour (or 1 whole egg)

2 tablespoons butter

2/5 cup (100 ml) heavy cream

4/5 cup (200 ml) milk (use only half if replacing flour with whole egg)

1 tablespoon cognac or Armagnac

Pinch of nutmeg

Pinch of fine sea salt mixed with *piment d'Espelette*

Pinch of fine sea salt

Preheat the oven to 320°F (160°C). Mix the livers, garlic, and parsley in a food processor for about 30 seconds until combined together and creamy. Scrape into a large mixing bowl. ➤

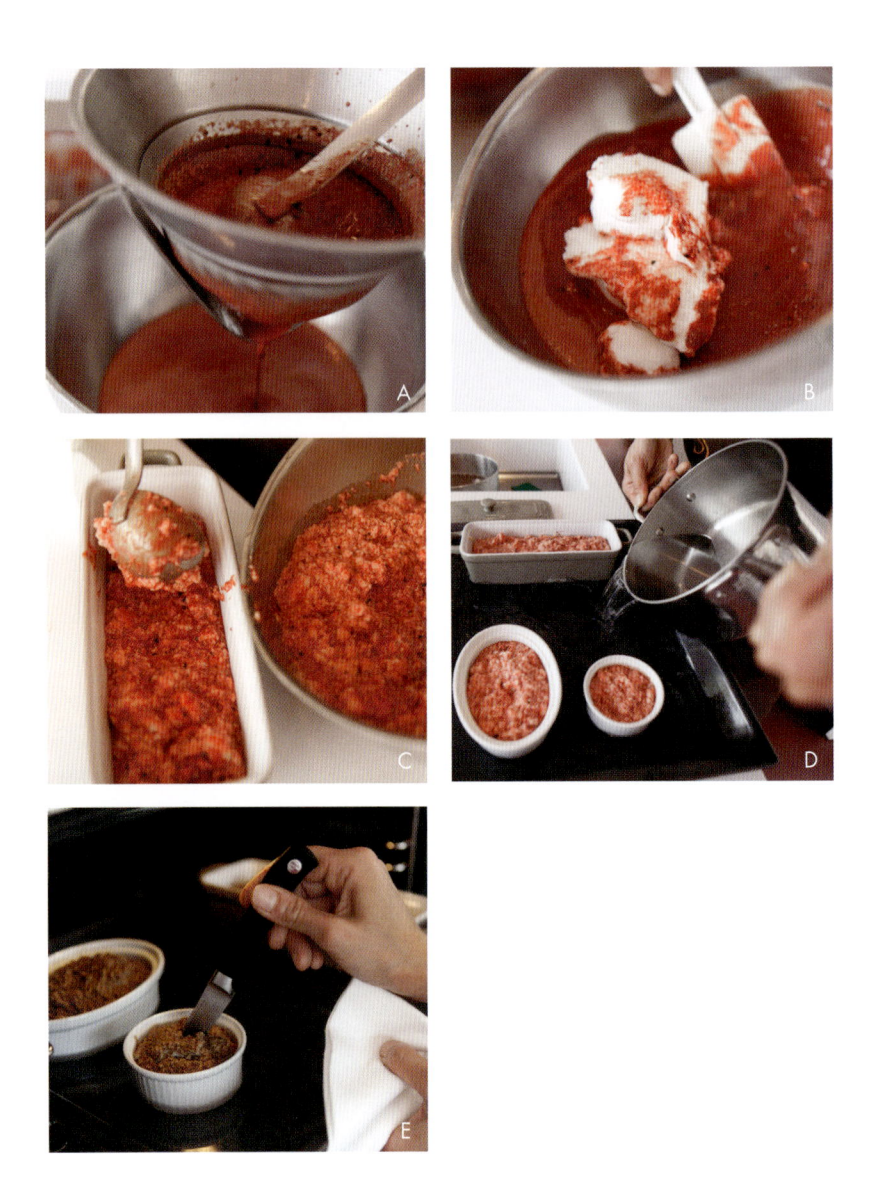

In a separate bowl, mix the 3 egg yolks (and extra egg if not using flour), flour (if using), butter, cream, milk, cognac, nutmeg, and salt and *piment* mixture with a hand mixer. Pass through a sieve, rubbing the inside of the sieve with a soup ladle to achieve a smooth consistency of the mixture (photo A). The sieve step is optional.

Pour the egg whites into another separate bowl, and use a hand mixer to "whip the egg white to a snow" (*faire monter en neige*), adding a pinch of salt. To check if the egg whites are whipped enough, turn the bowl upside down. If they stay put, they're ready! Using a spatula, gently incorporate the egg whites into the liver mixture in the large mixing bowl (photo B).

Butter several small ramekins or one larger pâté mold (*terrine*) before pouring the egg and liver mixture into the baking dish(es), filling each to about ¾ full (photo C).

THE BORDEAUX KITCHEN

Heat a pot of water to boiling. Place the ramekins or mold uncovered in a tray with high sides, and fill the tray with the hot water to about half way (photo D).

The ramekins will heat in this hot water bath (*bain-marie*). Place the tray in the oven and cook for 15 to 35 minutes. (The length of time will depend on the size of the ramekins or mold.) Using a knife (if it pulls out clean, the liver cake is ready), check frequently, as smaller ramekins will cook faster than larger ones (photo E). Our two-ounce ramekin (about 50 g) only took 20 minutes, while the two-cup (½ liter) and three-cup (¾ liter) dishes took each about 30 and 35 minutes, respectively.

Serve with Célia and VonVon's accompanying **Crab Sauce** (page 400) or **Onion Marmalade** (page 411) and a green salad. Eat within five to seven days.

WINE PAIRING TIP With this recipe, I sampled a crisp and fragrant white Bordeaux from Entre-Deux-Mers in Célia's *Côté Cours* teaching kitchen at the St. James Restaurant and Hotel. Sommelière Annabelle recommends a range of dry white wines to match the delicate flavors of the "cake" and accompanying sauce, including: a dry Cru Classé (a wine that has achieved a classified or high status) from Bordeaux's Pessac-Léognan; a full-bodied Condrieu, the northernmost white wine Rhône appellation; a fresh and aromatic Côtes du Rhône made from a variety of white grapes; or a Northern Rhône white made from the Marsanne and Roussanne grapes, such as a floral and nutty Crozes-Hermitage or Saint-Péray, and Hermitage, with notes of apricot and hazelnut, or a Saint-Joseph, with notes of flowers and apricot. Dry Burgundy Chardonnays recommended by Annabelle include a Mâconnais from Southern Burgundy that goes well with salty foods and is often served with appetizers, a rich Mersault from Burgundy's Côte de Beaune, or a Mercurey, with notes of almond, spice, and white flowers, from Central Burgundy's Côte Chalonnaise.

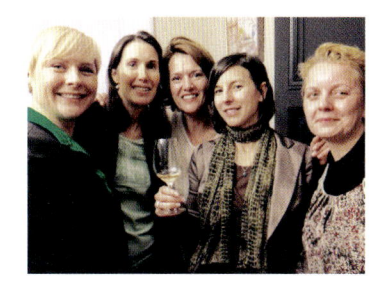

DUAD Support Team: Natalia, Tania, Malika, Anne, Annabelle

OFFAL AND FATS – *LES ABATS ET LES GRAISSES*

CHICKEN LIVERS WITH BACON
Foies de Volaille aux Lardons

Season Year-round **Preparation Time** 5 minutes
Cooking Time 15 to 20 minutes **Serves** 4 to 5

Chicken livers are another unsung hero in cooking, but the French eat them frequently sautéed, as in this recipe, baked into patés and terrines (see recipe for **Duck Liver Paté** on page 242), or ground into a sauce (see recipe for **Chicken Liver Dip** on page 238). Chicken livers are also very economical. They pack a nutrient-dense punch and are, at least in France, relatively inexpensive. (Three Euros—about 3 U.S. Dollars—for nine livers, for example, makes an easy dinner for two! For a kilogram I usually paid just shy of 9 Euros or about 9 U.S. Dollars.) Like our own livers, chicken livers have a larger lobe and a smaller lobe. Sometimes these separate during cooking, which does not matter for the recipe. I have made chicken livers weekly now for quite some time, and they can be made in many ways: plain, with or without bacon, with or without garlic, with or without parsley. What you need most is fat and salt. Something akin to this recipe was first shown to me after my first year in Bordeaux by my good friend Béatrice Pontallier who grew up in the village of Saint Emilion with her school next door and surrounded by vineyards. Once she showed me how to cook up chicken livers, I was off on a mission to cook them more frequently and to learn more about how to cook organ meats in general. I have her to thank for getting me started!

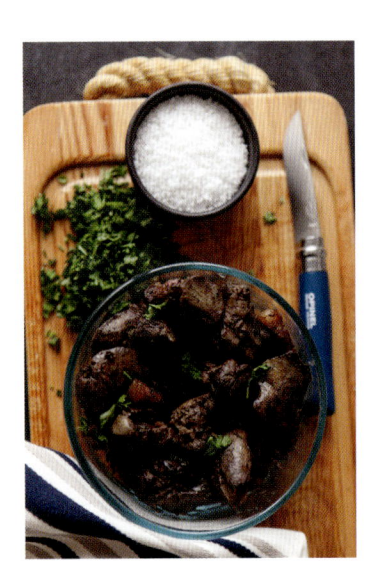

35 ounces (about 4.5 cups or 1 kg) chicken livers

2 tablespoons bacon fat, lard or duck fat

10 to 12 ounces (285 g to 340 g) bacon pieces *(lardons)*

1 tablespoon garlic, minced

4 pinches of fine sea salt, plus extra for garnish

Optional: Pinch of pepper

Optional: Parsley, for garnish

Melt the fat in a large pan over medium-high heat. Stir in all the ingredients, allowing the livers to stick a bit to the pan, caramelizing for a bit of added flavor. Reduce the heat to medium after a few minutes, and keep the pan uncovered. A loose mesh splatter screen may be used, but an odor-absorbing screen will also retain the water and steam the livers rather than sauté them.

Cook for about 15 more minutes until the livers no longer look red on the outside. Test one to see if it is cooked through by cutting through the middle of it. Make sure the livers are adequately salted, as it really makes the recipe. Serve with eggs and bacon for breakfast, topped on a green salad for lunch, or with baked sweet potato for dinner (my favorite way).

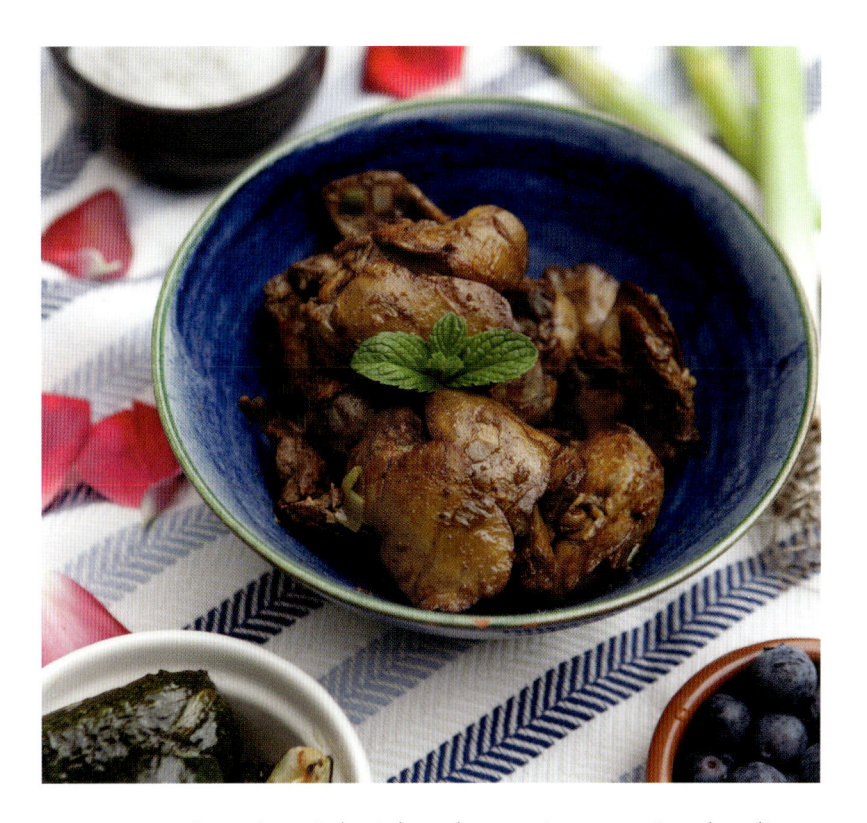

VARIATIONS Sometimes I don't have bacon pieces or minced garlic to add to the chicken livers. Plain liver with fat and salt works fine, but you can also top them with cinnamon. Or try sautéing the livers with chopped spring onions, as shown here, instead of or in addition to garlic. You can also deglaze the pan with ¼ cup (60 ml) water (or white wine) to make a bit of sauce.

WINE PAIRING TIP I have paired chicken livers with a crisp, oaked Chardonnay from the Côtes du Jura, with notes of apple, biscuit, citrus and, vanilla. I have also paired chicken livers with a young (2015), fleshy, biodynamic Domaine Cazes Marie–Gabrielle from Côtes du Roussillon, which essentially magically turned the livers into chocolate-covered fruits in the mouth (*en bouche*)! Restaurateur Annabelle has a concurrent recommendation for chicken livers: warming and full-bodied red wines or wines that are "fleshy" (like biting into a ripe fruit). For French Southwest pairings, she suggests a Bordeaux Clairet, with notes of red fruits and grenadine, or a Buzet, also with notes of red fruits, made with the same grapes as typical Bordeaux blends: Cabernet Franc, Cabernet Sauvignon, and Merlot. Further afield, Annabelle also proposes a Côtes du Roussillon, often with notes of stewed fruits or marmalade, a fruity Côtes du Rhône or a structured and elegant Lirac from the Southern Rhône Valley, made from a blend of Cinsault, Grenache, Mourvèdre, and Syrah grapes. I have also had chicken livers with a fruity and vivacious Brouilly from Beaujolais, which sweetened the flavor of the livers.

CHICKEN LIVER DIP
Sauce aux Foies de Volaille

Season Year-round   **Preparation Time** 5 minutes
Cooking Time 10 to 15 minutes   **Serves** 4

This recipe was originally taught to me by my good friend Malika, who was the first person I met in line on the first day of my Bordeaux University wine course. We sat next to each other in the first row throughout the academic year, and she ended up being the top student in our class. Luckily, some of her smarts rubbed off on me, and I was able to pass the course, too. Malika was taking the wine course to be able to play a more central role in her family's organic vineyard, Château Lescaneaut, in Castillon, a Bordeaux region next to St. Emilion, which produces fruity, bold Merlot-based wines, a delicious accompaniment to the liver dip!

This recipe is versatile in that you can eat it warmed, room temperature, or chilled, with a variety of raw vegetables, such as endive leaves as we did, or on top of lettuce, and with a thicker or thinner consistency. It is a great way to eat nutrient-dense chicken livers. This recipe can be halved or doubled as your ingredients allow. It can be served as a party dip, an appetizer, or as a meal. When we made this recipe together, it was spring, so we used local spring onions (*oignon aillé*), but garlic may also be used. Shown in the photo below is the sauce on the left and a bowl of extra whole chicken livers on the right, served along with the sauce at lunch.

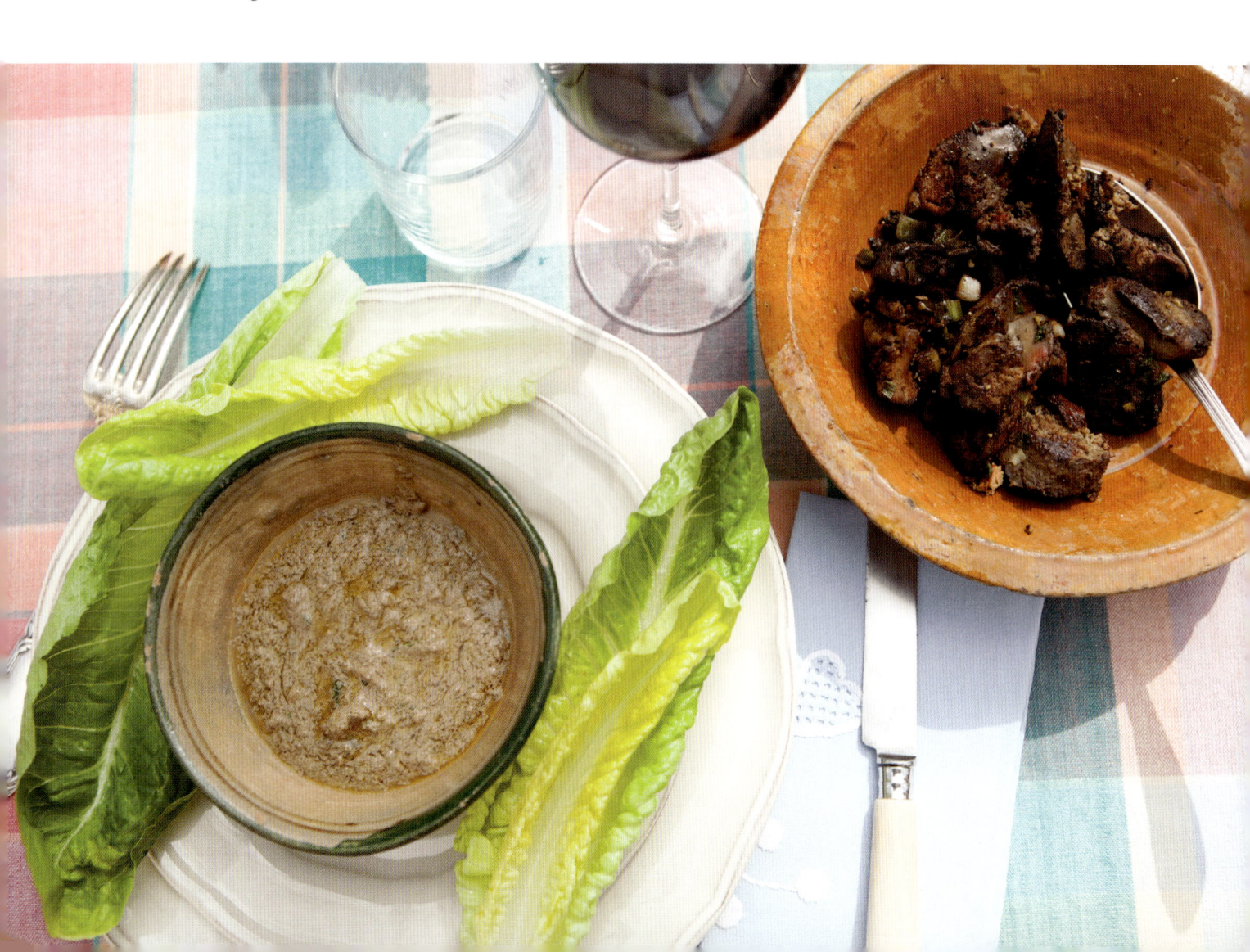

2 tablespoons bacon fat (or duck fat)

15 whole chicken livers (12.5 ounces or 350 g)

1 tablespoon spring onion or garlic, minced

3 pinches of sea salt

¼ cup (60 ml) water

3 tablespoons red wine vinegar

½ cup (about 120 ml) extra virgin olive oil

2 teaspoons mustard

Fine salt and ground pepper to taste

VARIATIONS If you leave out the vinegar and water, you will get a much thicker dip, as shown here.

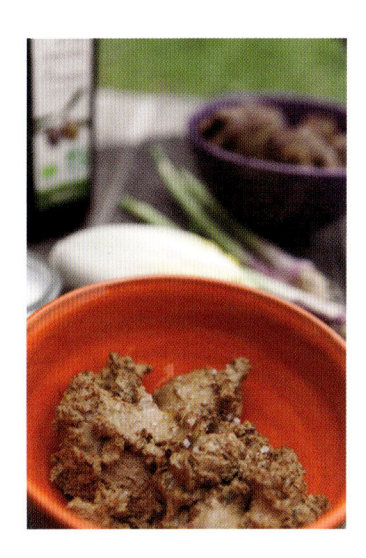

Melt the fat in a large pan over medium-high to high heat. Add the chicken livers, garlic (or spring onion), and salt. Allow the livers to stick a bit to the pan, letting them caramelize a bit.

Reduce the heat to medium, then stir every few minutes until the livers are cooked through (12 to 15 minutes).

Remove the livers, allowing them to cool in a bowl for several minutes. Deglaze the pan with ¼ cup (60 ml) water (removing the caramelized material stuck to the pan), and add this liquid to the bowl of livers.

Mix the livers in a food processor, in batches if needed, adding the mustard, vinegar, and olive oil, until you reach the desired consistency. (This step should take less than a minute). To increase the liquid consistency of the sauce, add a bit more water and/or olive oil. Adjust the taste by adding salt and pepper as needed.

Serve while still warm, chilled, or at room temperature with romaine or endive leaves, with carrot or celery sticks, homemade beet chips, or on **Seedy Crackers** (page 501)! I prefer eating the dip warmed.

WINE PAIRING TIP Malika's family and I had their house wine, a flavorful 2012 Château Lescaneaut from Bordeaux's Castillon appellation. For another regional Southwest pairing, sommelière Annabelle suggests a dry white Pacherenc du Vic-Bilh Sec (though this area, located between Bordeaux and the Pyrénées foothills of Pau, is more known for its sweet wines, which are also worth a try). Otherwise she proposes either an effervescent white Muscat from Languedoc-Roussillon or a Champagne. See also the wine pairing suggestions for Duck Liver Paté (page 243) and Chicken Livers with Bacon (page 237).

CRISPY PORK RINDS
Grattons de Porc Croustillants

Season Year-round   **Preparation Time** 10 minutes
Cooking Time 25 to 30 minutes   **Serves** 4

When you have pork skin, you can make crispy pork rinds. The thickness of the rind depends on how much fat you or the butcher have left attached to the skin. Butchers and slaughterhouses (*abattoirs*) have machines that slice this subcutaneous fat (usually from the back, called fatback), into strips of lard which can be used for wrapping or "barding" (*barder*) lard around meat roasts. Rinds, literally "scraps" or "scrapes" (*grattons*), derived from the verb "to scrape" or "to scratch" (*gratter*), are the fatty skin of the pig and the adipose tissue of the duck, goose, and chicken cooked or baked in their own fat. Other French names for *grattons* include: *fritons, gratons, gratterons, greubons, griaudes, grillaudes, grillons,* or *rillons*. Many cultural cuisines have their own versions, including Belgium, Canada, Mexico, the Netherlands, the Philippines, Spain, Switzerland, Thailand, the United States (pork rinds), and Vietnam.

Whenever I have a piece of pork (the shoulder, leg, back, or belly) that still has the skin attached, and if I am not curing pork belly, I remove the skin from the fat and meat and slice the skin to make pork rinds, a crispy, crunchy homemade fatty chip. If the skin has been frozen, it will tend to be chewier and may need longer in the oven to achieve crispiness. The liquid fat left in the dish is perfect lard, this may be poured into a jar and saved in the refrigerator for later use.

2 handfuls of pork skin

Pinch of fine sea salt

Preheat the oven to 340°F (about 170°C). Cut the pork skin into ½-inch (1.25 cm) by 2- to 3-inch (5 to 8 cm) strips (photo A). Place the rinds side by side in an oven-safe dish (photo B). Sprinkle a pinch of salt over the rinds. Allow them to bake for 25 minutes, stirring once or twice. Check to see if they have browned enough (a light brownish-orange color or darker orange color if baked longer) for your liking (photo C). If not, continue to bake. Sometimes it helps to pour off the liquid lard during the cooking process to allow the rinds to become crispy. Watch so they do not turn too dark brown.

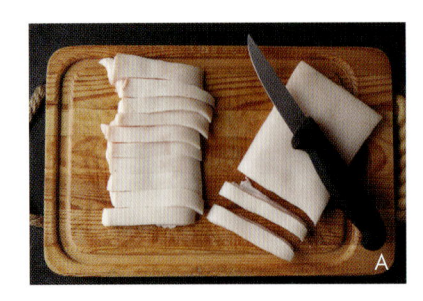

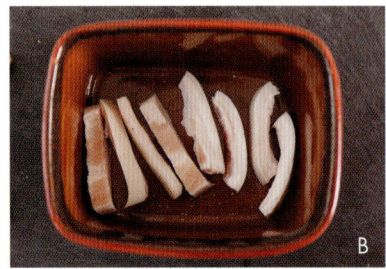

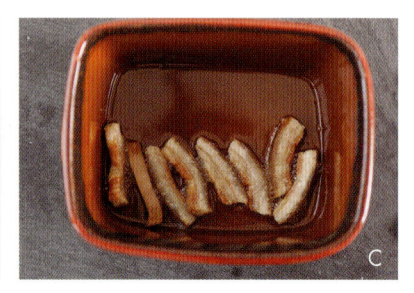

Pour off the liquid lard into a glass jar and save for cooking. Serve the rinds while they are hot, as they become chewier as they cool off. Pork rinds may be stored in the refrigerator and reheated, though reheating makes them progressively chewier. I have experimented with other cooking times: 40 to 45 minutes at 300°F (about 150°C) and 35 to 40 minutes at 325°F (160°C). The timing depends more on how crowded the rinds are in the dish than the temperature, but do check the rinds to make sure they do not become too dark.

WINE PAIRING TIP I do not recommend pairing this with wine, as the delicate, salty flavor of the pork rinds are lost to the alcohol in the wine.

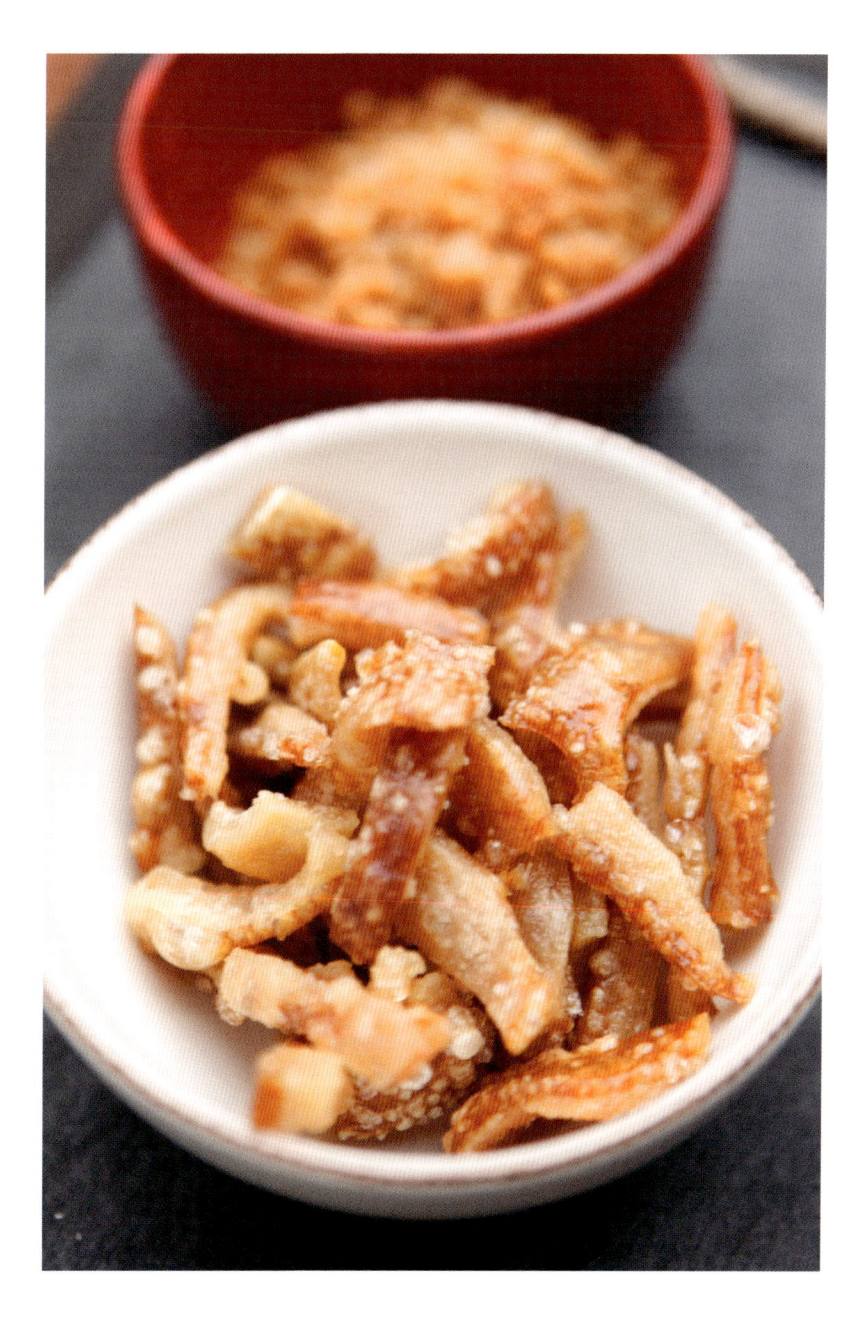

DUCK LIVER PÂTÉ
Pâté de Foie de Canard

Season Year-round **Preparation Time** 25 minutes
Cooking Time 30 to 45 minutes **Serves** 6

When you get a hold of duck livers, make a pâté! These livers are not "fatty" as the livers are in *foie gras* (see the next recipe for **Foie Gras with Figs and Armagnac**) and are much smaller. Livers are the most nutrient dense of all foods and are most palatable in the form of a pâté. In this recipe I have combined the duck livers with chicken livers to vary the nutrients and flavors and to fill a sizeable mold, such as the one shown on the next page alongside a bottle of pear brandy from the French Southwest. This pâté has a lightly moussy consistency. It is reminiscent of the taste of *foie gras* even though these duck livers are from ducks that have not been stuffed to harvest *foie gras*.

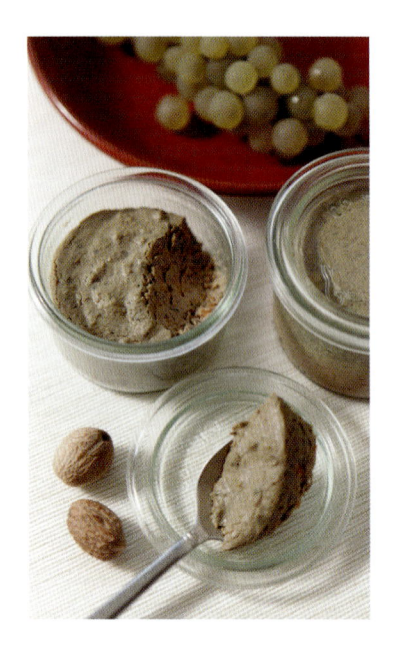

2 tablespoons duck fat, plus 1 teaspoon

1 carrot, finely chopped

1 garlic clove minced

3 shallots, minced

9 ounces (250 g) chicken livers

23 ounces (660 g) duck livers

1 teaspoon thyme, fresh or dried

½ teaspoon nutmeg

4 pinches of fine sea salt

¼ cup (60 ml) pear brandy (*eau de vie de poire*)

2 eggs

1 tablespoon parsley, minced

Preheat the oven to 320°F (160°C). Place a pan inside filled halfway with water and large enough to fit your pâté mold(s). Melt two tablespoons of duck fat in a pan on the stove over medium-high heat and brown the carrot, garlic, and shallots for a minute before adding the livers. Stir once or twice, and allow the ingredients to caramelize in the pan for five minutes.

Add the thyme, nutmeg, and three pinches of the salt, and reduce the heat to medium. Cook the livers for another five to seven minutes until they are lightly rosy on the inside. (Test one by cutting it in half to see how pink it is inside.) Scrape the livers into a large bowl to allow them to cool off. While the pan is still hot, deglaze the pan with the pear *eau de vie*, and add this to the bowl of livers.

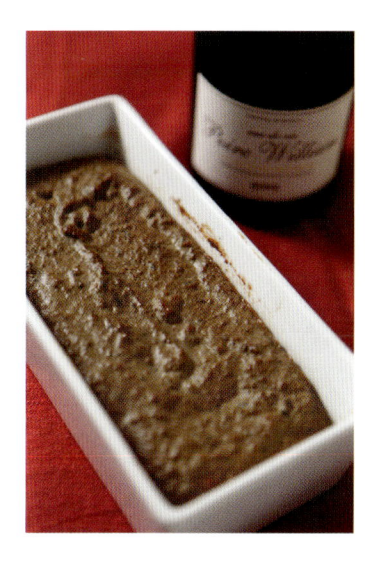

Whisk the eggs and parsley together in a separate bowl, then add them to the livers. Run the entire mixture through a food processor to obtain a smooth consistency.

Line the mold(s) with one teaspoon of duck fat. Fill each mold (*terrine*) or ramekin ¾ full, and carefully place into the water-filled pan in the oven. As each mold reaches 175°F (80°C), remove it from the oven and allow to cool. (Use a meat thermometer to determine the internal temperature of each *terrine* of pâté.) Depending on the size of the mold(s), cooking time can take from 30 to 45 minutes. Serve on **Seedy Crackers** (page 501), sweet potato or beet chips, or serve with raw vegetables such as carrot or celery sticks. Eat within five to seven days.

> WINE PAIRING TIP *Foie gras*, made from fatty duck livers, is usually served with a sweet wine in Bordeaux, such as a Barsac or a Sauternes. This pâté, made from non-fatty duck livers (as well as chicken livers) could also be served with a Bordeaux Sauternes or Southwest sweet wine, such as a Jurançon from the Pyrénées. Otherwise, sommelière Annabelle offers a number of options from around France, powerful but unoaked whites such as a fresh and complex Lubéron, a mix of several white grape varieties with notes of citrus and white peach, from the South-Eastern Rhône Valley. Burgundy wines in this category that she suggests include a Chablis with notes of gunflint, lemon, and white peach; a Mâcon with notes of citrus, verbena, and white flowers; a Mercurey Chardonnay from the Côte Chalonnaise with notes of white flowers and almonds; a crisp, complex, and much-loved Mersault from the Côte de Beaune; a crisp, aromatic and mineraly Pouilly-Fuissé, with notes of white peach, from the Maconnais region; or a citrus and floral Fixin from the Côte de Nuits. For red wines, Annabelle proposes light-bodied to medium-bodied reds, such as a Chinon from the Touraine region of the Loire Valley; a Samumur-Champigny, with notes of red fruits, made predominantly from the Cabernet Franc grape in the Anjou region of the Loire Valley; an aromatic and fruity Marsannay from Burgundy's Cote d'Or; a well-structured, floral, and fruity Santenay from Burgundy's Côte de Beaune; a fresh, floral, and fruity Volnay also from Burgundy's Côte de Beaune; or a Vougeot Pinot Noir, with notes of red fruit and violet, from Burgundy's Côte de Nuits.

FOIE GRAS WITH FIGS AND ARMAGNAC
Terrine de Foie Gras aux Figues et à l'Armagnac

Season Late Autumn through Winter   **Preparation Time** 45 minutes (including 30 minutes of marination)   **Cooking Time** 20 minutes   **Serves** 6

Like it or not, foie gras is part of French culture as much as many other delicacies and "weird" things the French eat. While I don't care for the way ducks are fed in order to enlarge their livers for our consumption, I will tell you that if you cannot find a fresh, smooth-textured liverwurst, foie gras is the next best thing (though in a class of its own), as a "gateway drug" to eating liver, especially when topped with a bit of crunchy *fleur de sel*. I grew up on German liverwurst (*Leberwurst*), so the transition to foie gras in France was natural for me. I only have foie gras rarely, as it is pricey, and it is "fatty" liver, not a regular, healthy liver, therefore it is more of a food for a special occasion. Most foie gras in France is consumed over the holidays as a festive appetizer passed around at social gatherings. My children actually like foie gras spread on an oat or spelt cracker, a non-primal/paleo tradeoff I am willing to live with if they get used to the taste of liver, or else on **Seedy Crackers** (see page 501). You can spoon it onto a cracker, a vegetable chip or even raw vegetables, though the French tend to eat it on slices of bread or spiced bread, *pain d'épices* (made with spices such as cinnamon, cloves, ginger, and nutmeg), especially around the holidays. My children are less fond of the extra figs and alcohol, though, and this recipe can easily be made without those (*au nature*). For adults, however, the Armagnac (or Sauternes, a Bordeaux dessert wine) adds extra flavor and sophistication, while the figs add sweetness and a mildly crunchy texture from their tiny seeds, to contrast with the rich creaminess of the foie gras. Foie gras is available at www.dartagnan.com, whose CEO, Ariane Daguin, is the daughter of the famous Gascon two-Michelin-starred chef André Daguin and carries the torch of Southwestern French culinary tradition in the U.S.

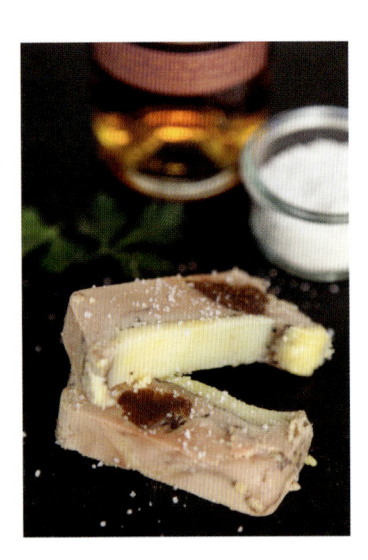

According to my friend Chef Frédéric, from whom I initially learned several ways of preparing foie gras while he was a chef at *Atelier des Chefs* in Bordeaux, the ducks are naturally fattest in February, so that is the best season for making and eating this delicacy. You may not want to leave a party, or your own *terrine*, until you have eaten every last morsel of foie gras, it's that good. You will impress your friends and family because it will taste great and because they will have no idea how easy it was to make! If you purchase whole foie gras (the whole liver), you might also want to try searing a few slices (*escalopes de foie gras poêlées*) seasoned with a bit of *fleur de sel* for one minute on each side over high heat (no extra oil needed in the pan), and deglaze the pan with a teaspoon or two of balsamic vinegar (pour this over the foie gras). Serve over a bed of arugula, as shown on page 247, in spring or fall. Foie gras sliced and seared this way is a delicacy much loved by the French. May be served with a dollop of **Onion Marmalade** (page 411) or a piece of grilled stone fruit (such as apricot or peach), or served atop a rolled piece of beef, famously known as *Tournedos Rossini*. (See wine pairings below for the seared foie gras option.)

1 pound (450 g) raw "fatty" duck liver (foie gras)

3 to 4 dried figs

Fine salt

Ground pepper

Pinch of cinnamon

⅓ cup (75 ml) Armagnac

Fleur de sel, for garnish

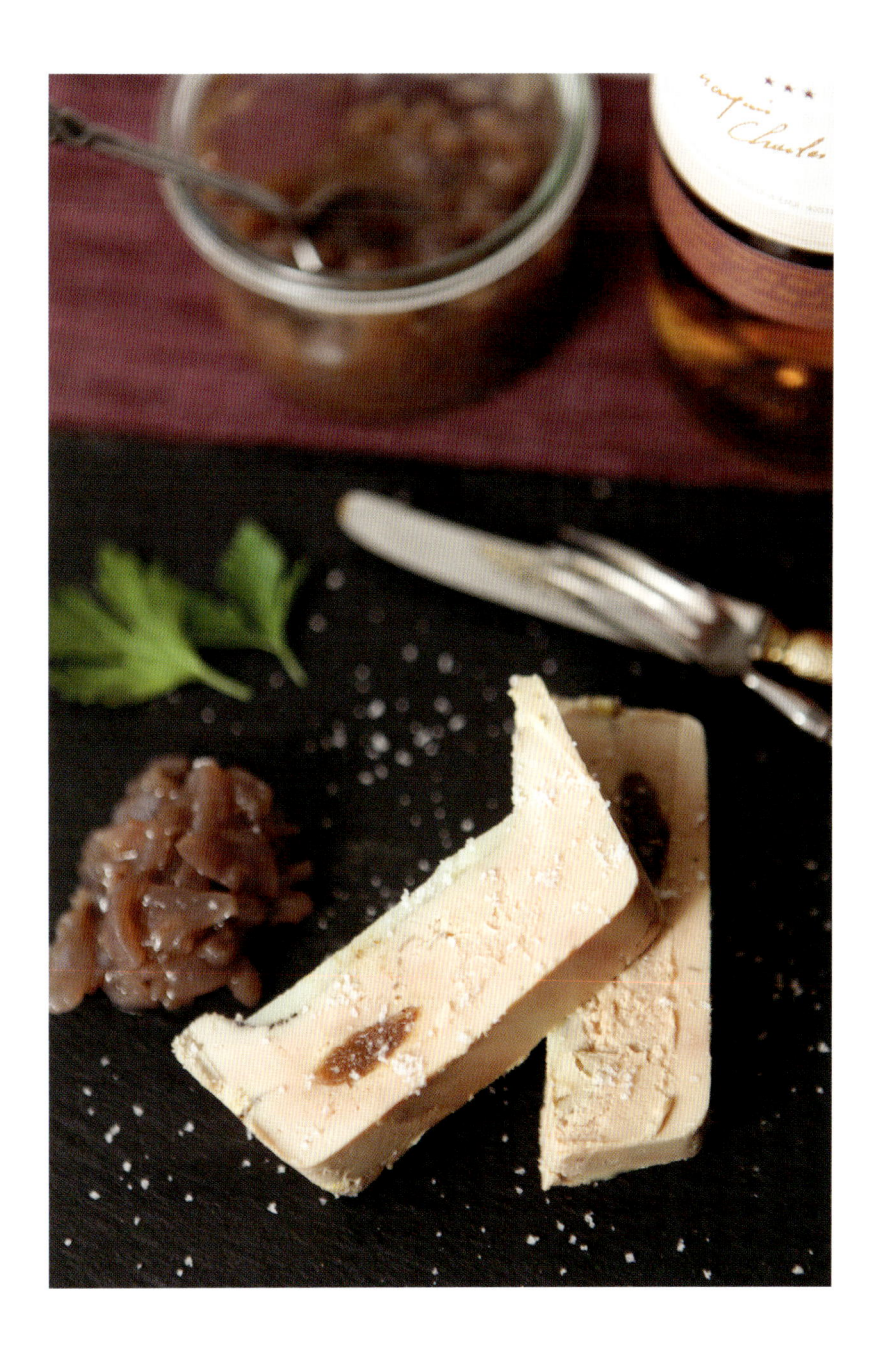

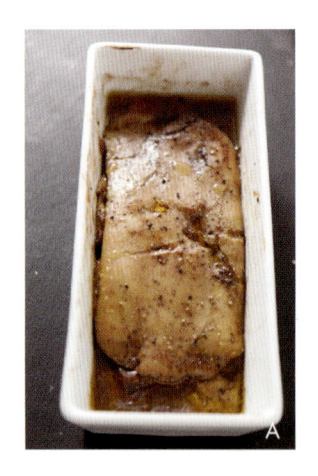

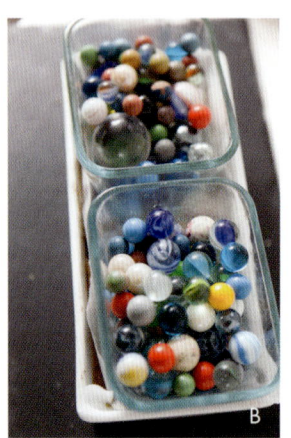

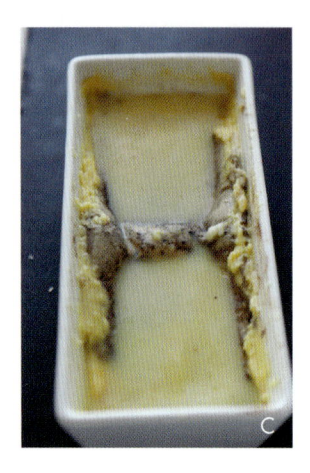

Remove the liver from the refrigerator and place in a bowl of cold water for an hour. The other option is to soak the liver in a mixture of one-part milk to one-part water for an hour to render the liver very supple and cleanse the veins. But if you are avoiding milk, then just use water, which will soften and cleanse the liver and bring it to room temperature. (If the liver has not been deveined, you can devein it yourself by following the veins into and along each lobe and gently pulling the veins upward out of the liver using your fingertips. If the liver ends up in several pieces, it's okay, it's all going into a ceramic mold or *terrine*, anyway.) In France, you can buy liver that is deveined (more expensive) or not yet deveined (less expensive).

If the figs are hard, place them in boiling water for 7 minutes to soften and rehydrate them. Slice each fig in half.

Preheat the oven to 320°F (160°C). Place a large baking dish with sides that are at least two inches (5 cm) high in the oven, and fill it ¾ with water. (Filling with hot water speeds up the process.) This will be the bath (*bain-marie*) into which you will place your liver-filled mold or terrine.

Slice the liver in half lengthwise. Salt and pepper the liver on all sides. Sprinkle on the cinnamon as well or just on top, as desired. Place one half of the liver in a mold (*terrine*), spreading it along the bottom so it creates a layer covering the mold. Line the fig pieces along the middle of the liver. Place the other half of the liver on top and squash it down a bit, spreading it along the dish. Pour the Armagnac over the liver and allow it to marinate for 30 minutes. You can also marinate the liver overnight, making the alcohol flavors more potent.

Pour off the marinade liquid (and save it in the refrigerator for a stew of game meats or beef). Sprinkle a bit of extra pepper and fine salt on top of the liver in its mold, then place the mold into the larger baking dish with heated water in the oven.

Allow to cook in the oven for about 20 minutes. After 20 minutes, check the temperature of the middle of the foie gras using an oven-safe digital thermometer whose indicator screen remains outside the oven. This is a handy device I recommend so that you are sure of the meat's inner temperature. "Half-baked" (*mi-cuit*), the most flavorful and exquisite cooking of foie gras, is 118°F to 122°F (48°C to 50°C), but do not worry if your thermometer goes into the higher 120s°F (low to mid-50s°C). "Fully cooked" (*cuit*) is 144°F (62°C) for foie gras. Remove the terrine from the oven upon reaching the desired temperature. Allow the dish to cool for an hour. (See photo A.) Carefully remove the larger baking dish filled with water, and carefully pour out the water. Inevitably, you will be interrupted by one of your children while you are doing this.

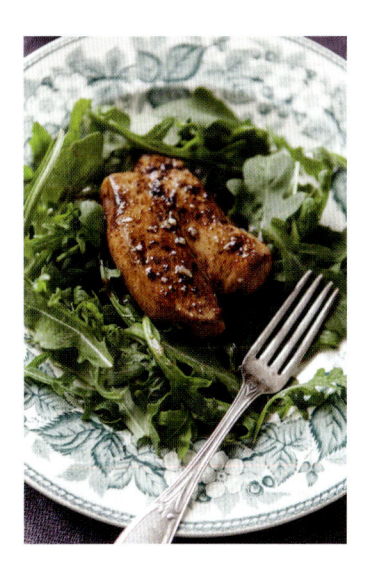

After the terrine has cooled, place a piece of parchment paper over the top and add a flat weight, preferably something that covers the entire surface of the foie gras, to weigh it down so that the fat rises. (I used two rectangular Pyrex dishes filled with marbles, not having a board or slate narrow enough to fit into the terrine. (See photo B.) Allow this weight to remain on the foie gras for several hours in the refrigerator until the fat has hardened and the foie gras has cooled completely before removing them. (See photo C.) To best conserve the foie gras, scrape off the fat where it is thickest, melt it in a pan, and pour it evenly over the entire foie gras to protect it from oxidation. If you need additional fat to be able to entirely cover the top of the foie gras, melt a couple tablespoons of duck fat (always have a jar handy!)

Wait two to four days for your homemade foie gras to "cure" before cutting into it, but eat it within 12 days. Once you have broken the fat layer, finish it within 48 hours. This will not prove difficult. Serve at just below room temperature with *fleur de sel* on top for the added texture and enhanced flavor. This is a must! Serve also with **Onion Marmalade** (page 411) as shown in the recipe photo on page 245.

> WINE PAIRING TIP The Bordelais generally serve foie gras with a dessert wine from Barsac or Sauternes. Further south they might serve a Jurançon from Béarn. Foie gras, a specialty of the French Southwest, is in a class of its own when it comes to pairing. Here is what two *Bordelais* say about pairing foie gras with wine: Veronique Sanders of Château Haut-Bailly in the Graves–Pessac-Léognan appellation says, "I enjoy foie gras with a fine and fruity red like our second wine La Parde Haut-Bailly. It brings freshness and spices." Aline Baly of Château Coutet in Barsac says, "The traditional liver pâté and Sauternes association is enhanced by the presence of fig. It is a bit of a contrast pairing, since an older Château Coutet (say 1997) will have more mineral and dried fruit characteristics. But what's great about a sweeter fruit like the fig in this pairing is that it will bring out the younger notes of the wine, such as fresh pitted fruits and nectars."
>
> Should you sauté a few slices of foie gras rather than bake them into a terrine, a very common practice in France, pair the foie gras slices with aromatic dry white or semi-sweet (*demi-sec*) wines, such as a Cotes-de-Bordeaux-Saint-Macaire sweet (*moelleux*) from Bordeaux, or else from the Loire Valley: a famed white Bonnezeaux, with notes of apricot, beeswax, and dried fruit; a Coteaux de L'Aubance, with notes of pear and apricot; a floral and citrus Coteaux du Layon; a floral and fruity Jasnières; or a Montlouis (sweet or *demi-sec*), with notes of tropical fruits, all of which are made from the Chenin Blanc grape affected by the *botrytis cinerea* fungus to create and concentrate their sweet aromas and flavors.

LAMB HEART WITH SAGE
Coeur d'Agneau à la Sauge

Season Year-round   **Preparation Time** 30 minutes
Cooking Time 30 minutes   **Serves** 4 to 5

Heart happens to have among the highest concentrations of mitochondria and nutrients and is therefore an excellent source of nutrients for humans to eat. Lamb heart is a less-strongly flavored meat than is lamb meat itself. The French often cube lamb heart and skewer it for grilling. Sage goes well with lamb meat as well as lamb heart. Fresh or dried sage leaves may be used. Here is yet another reason to have your own herb garden if possible. Being able to harvest herbs year-round is very rewarding and supports your creative spontaneity to use them in a dish. The arteries should be removed (usually already done by the butcher), but leave the fat on the outside of the hearts. This recipe calls for grainy, traditional "Dijon" mustard, an ingredient that comes up frequently in French recipes and that contributes to very flavorful sauces. There is a recipe for **Old-Fashioned Mustard** on page 410 that you can use. This dish may be served as an appetizer (*entrée*) or as a main dish (*plat*).

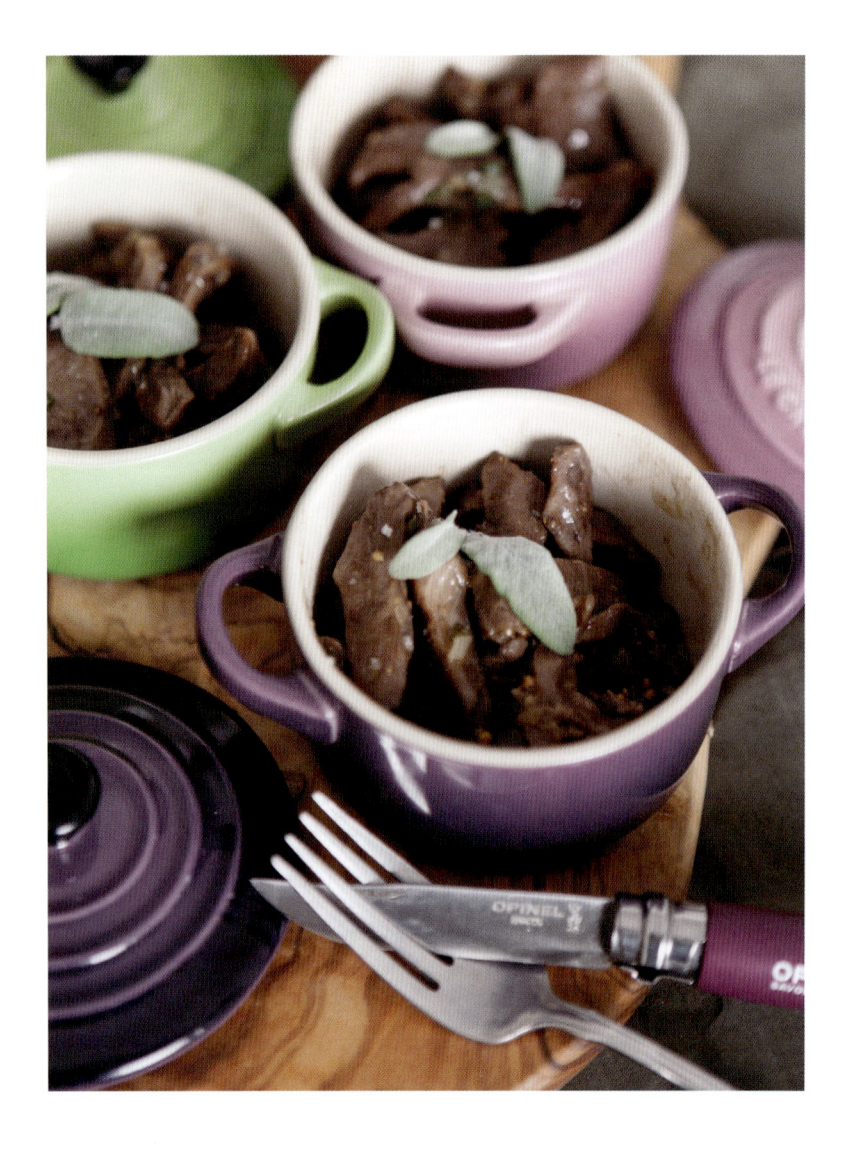

4 tablespoons duck fat

3 pinches of fine salt

2 to 3 shallots (about 2 ounces or 55 g), minced

½ cup (120 ml) lamb or other stock

2 tablespoons fresh sage leaves, coarsely chopped, plus extra for garnish

2 teaspoons grainy, **Old-Fashioned Mustard** (page 410) or traditional "Dijon" mustard

2 lamb hearts, halved and cut lengthwise in ¼-inch (0.6 cm) strips (*lanières*)

½ teaspoon white pepper, coarsely ground (*mignonette*)

Fleur de sel, for garnish

Melt one tablespoon of duck fat in a pan over medium-high heat. Add a pinch of salt, and brown the shallots for three to four minutes until they are translucent. Deglaze the pan with ½ cup (120 ml) stock, and allow the liquid to reduce for three minutes. Reduce heat to the lowest setting, and stir in the sage leaves and mustard.

Season the strips of lamb heart with two pinches of fine salt and the pepper in a bowl. In another pan, melt three tablespoons of duck fat over medium-high heat, and sauté (*rissoler*) the lamb heart strips, in batches if necessary, for about five minutes per batch until the pieces are browned but not thoroughly cooked through. Set aside the cooked strips in a bowl, and go on to brown the next batch. Return all strips to the pan, and stir in the shallot, sage, and mustard sauce from the first pan. Reduce the heat to medium or medium-low, and allow to simmer for 12 to 14 minutes until cooked through. Garnish with *fleur de sel*. Serve with baked sweet potato, **Sarlat Sautéed Potatoes** (page 468), or sautéed vegetables.

VARIATIONS Deglaze with ½ cup (120 ml) dry white wine instead of the stock. Replace the sage with parsley.

WINE PAIRING TIP Try a peppery and bold, medium-bodied Saint Joseph from the Northern Rhône to boost the flavors of shallot and sage with the sautéed heart, or else try a generously-flavored Côtes-du-Rhône Villages made with 50% Grenache grape, lending notes of spice and dark fruits to the combination, or else a lightly-tannic Saumur-Champigny with notes of berry and spice. See also wine pairing suggestions for **Veal Kidneys in Old-Fashioned Mustard Sauce** (page 279) and **Lamb Kidneys with Old-Fashioned Mustard** (page 410).

LAMB KIDNEYS WITH BUTTER AND GARLIC
Rognons d'Agneau au Beurre et à l'Ail

Season Late Spring through Winter   **Preparation Time** 10 minutes
Cooking Time 10 minutes   **Serves** 1 main course or 2 starters

The winning combination of butter, garlic, and salt is an easy formula to apply to many organ meats. For a similar flavor, ghee works as well, but so do lard and tallow (and suet, the fat surrounding the kidneys). Butter and ghee give that buttery, nutty flavor that goes so well with garlic. Lamb kidneys have the scent of lamb but are less pungent than lamb liver. As we know, organ meats are the most nutrient-dense parts of the animal. When lamb kidneys arrive at a butcher shop in France, they are usually sold quickly, as they are valued and rare. In order to have enough, I always order mine in advance from my butcher. Sautéing organ meats such as liver, kidney, and heart in butter, garlic, and parsley is a very common combination in France called *en persillade*. A dash of balsamic or red wine vinegar is often also added. This dish makes a good starter because of the small size of the kidney, with either a half or a whole kidney per person.

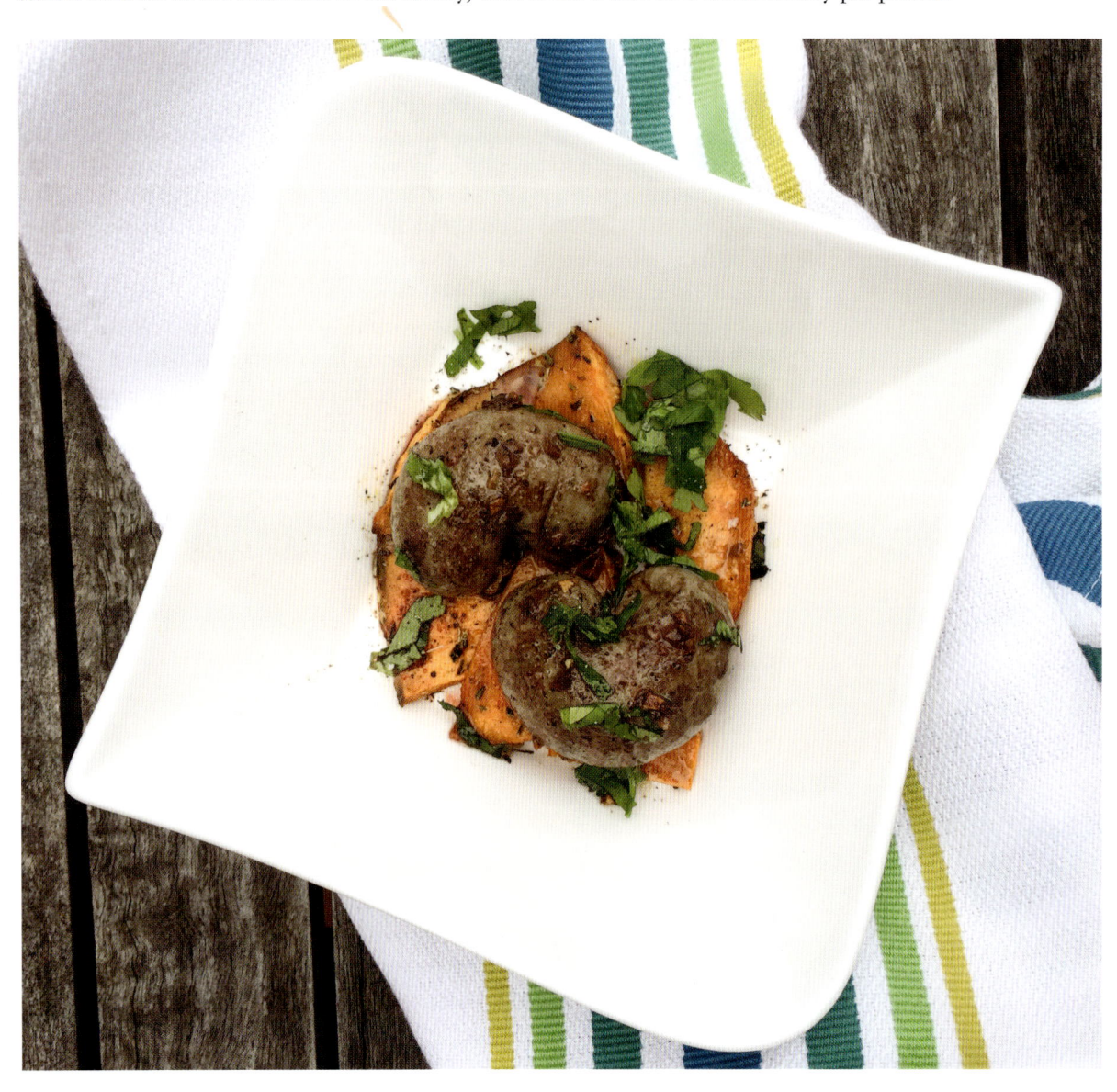

2 lamb kidneys

1 tablespoon butter (or ghee)

1 teaspoon garlic, minced

Fine sea salt, for seasoning

Freshly ground pepper, for garnish

A few stems of fresh parsley, leaves removed and chopped, for garnish

Course sea salt or *fleur de sel,* for garnish

Rinse the kidneys in cold water, peel the outer visceral skin with the help of a sharp paring knife, and slice each kidney in half lengthwise. Remove the inner white tubular tissue with the paring knife.

Melt the butter in a pan over medium-high heat and add the garlic. Salt both sides of each kidney half and place the kidneys in the skillet. Sauté for several minutes on each side, allowing for a light caramelization on each side. Reduce the heat by a notch to allow the kidneys to cook through without burning for two or three more minutes.

Remove the kidneys from the pan, and dress them with sauce from the pan, fresh parsley and freshly ground black pepper. Adding a bit of coarser salt grains on top accentuates the salty flavors and gives a tiny amount of crunch. *Fleur de sel* (the cream of the crop when it comes to sea salt bed harvesting) is particularly special because of its mild saltiness, lovely purity, cubical shape, and crunch.

Serve hot, with baked sweet potato, as shown in the recipe photo, or with **Onion Marmalade** (page 411).

> WINE PAIRING TIP So as to not overpower the flavors of the lamb kidneys, I would recommend serving lamb kidney with a low- to medium-bodied (medium tannic) red wine, such as a Bordeaux Pessac-Léognan or a medium-bodied Pinot Noir from Burgundy. Restaurateur Annabelle recommends red wines that are fleshy (like biting into a ripe fruit) and structured, offering fruity aromas: a fruit-driven, Merlot-dominant Saint Emilion; a crisp and lightly-spiced Cabernet Franc-dominated Saumur-Champigny from the Loire Valley; or a rich and spicy Côtes du Rhône or an elegant, flowery, and robust Crozes-Hermitage from the Rhône Valley.

LAMB KIDNEYS WITH OLD-FASHIONED MUSTARD
Rognons d'Agneau à la Moutarde à l'Ancienne

Season Year-round   **Preparation Time** 20 minutes
Cooking Time 20 minutes   **Serves** 1 to 2

I first made this dish with my friend and former neighbor, working mom, and cook, Rébecca Pinsolle, originally from Dijon, where she grew up. Rébecca often ate at her grandmother's house, where her grandmother prepared all sorts of dishes that are even a bit foreign to modern-day French people, such as lamb brains, chicken hearts, and lamb kidneys. We attempted recipes of all of these organ meats together, all featured in this chapter. Since Rébecca is from Dijon, we based our recipe on a mustard sauce. We were inspired by a recipe on the French cooking website www.cuisineactuelle.fr to flavor this recipe additionally using a red Pineau des Charentes, or Pineau Charentais, a *vin de liqueur* from the Charentes and Charentes-Maritimes (Cognac) regions in Southwestern France, north of Bordeaux. Pineau is made by combining Cognac *eau de vie* (a distilled fruit brandy made from the fermentation of macerated fruit) and fresh grape must (freshly pressed juice containing the seeds, skins, and stems) of the current vintage.[8] Pineau des Charentes is a French apéritif that comes in white, rosé, or red and is sweet like a port or sherry. Pineau alcohol has fruity aromas akin to cognac, making it amenable for cooking. I don't tolerate mushrooms very well, so we did not include them, but for flavor, they make a nice addition to this recipe. If you are adding mushrooms, drizzle the lemon juice over them after slicing them to keep them from turning brown (oxidizing). This recipe can be easily doubled, tripled, or quadrupled, and the kidneys may be served as a meal or as an appetizer.

2 lamb kidneys

Sea salt & pepper to taste

2 tablespoons butter (or ghee)

Optional: ¼ cup (1.8 ounces or 50 g) mushrooms, sliced

¼ lemon, juiced

⅕ cup (50 ml) Pineau des Charentes

¼ cup (60 ml) whole cream

1 tablespoon **Old-Fashioned Mustard** (page 410)

Cut each kidney in half lengthwise, and remove the fat and the white tubing inside each half kidney. Salt and pepper the kidneys. Melt one tablespoon of the butter or ghee in a pan or cast-iron pot over medium-high heat, and sauté the kidneys for two to three minutes on each side. Transfer the kidneys from the pan to a covered bowl or plate and keep them warm.

If you are using mushrooms, add them to the pan along with the remaining butter. Otherwise, just add the remaining butter to the pan, and save the lemon juice for later in the sauce-making process.

Add the Pineau to the pan, and allow it to come to a gentle boil. Add the cream, and decrease the heat to medium. Allow the cream to reduce by about one third while stirring. This only takes a few minutes. Stir in the mustard. Add the kidneys back to the pan, and stir in the lemon juice now if you are not using mushrooms and therefore have not yet incorporated the lemon juice. Heat the pan again on medium-high, allowing the sauce to boil briefly before removing it from the heat.

Place the kidneys on small plates and spoon some extra mustard sauce over them. Garnish with lemon verbena, chopped parsley, mint or sage, if desired. Serve immediately.

VARIATIONS Try sautéing shallots and/or garlic and sage for several minutes in the butter before adding the kidneys. Feel free to try this dish using duck fat, lard, or tallow.

WINE RECOMMENDATION Serve with more Pineau, it pairs deliciously. See also wine pairing suggestions for **Lamb Kidneys with Butter and Garlic** (page 251).

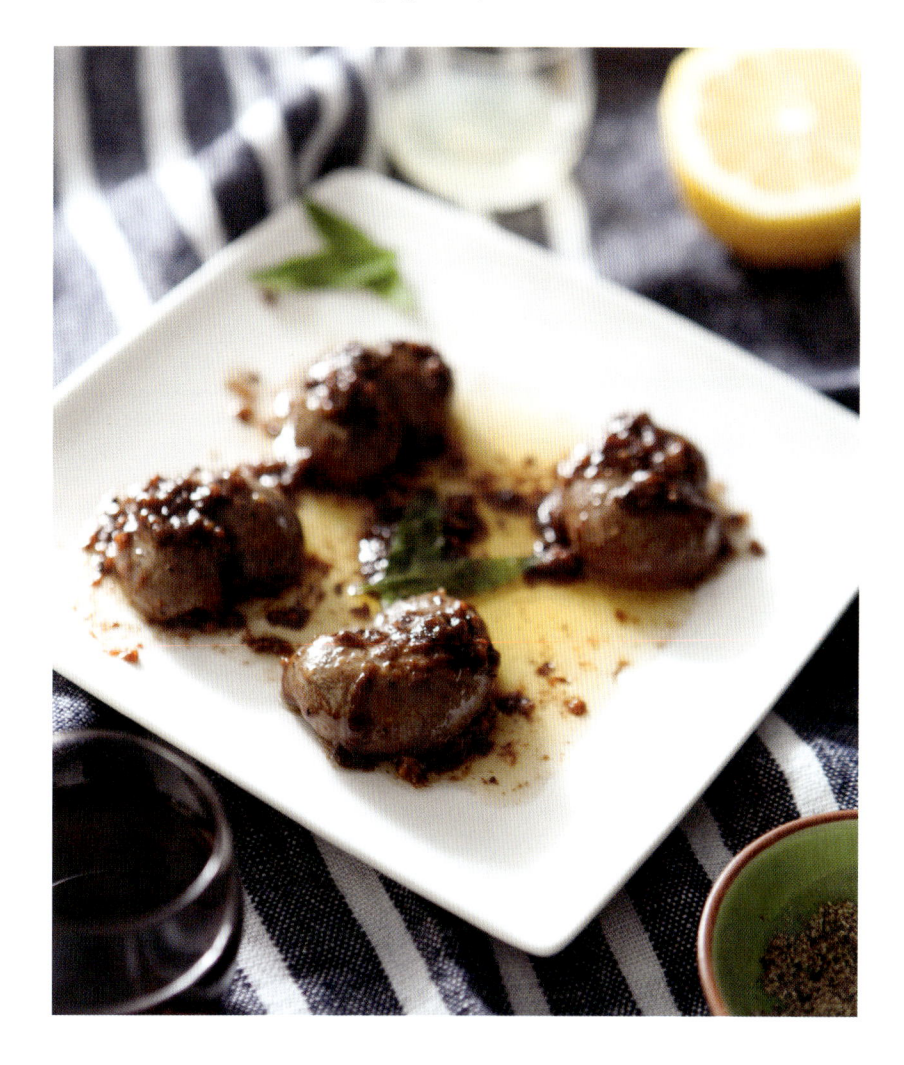

LAMB LIVER WITH ONION CHUTNEY
Foie d'Agneau, Chutney d'Onions

Season Spring through Autumn   **Preparation Time** 15 minutes
Cooking Time 15 minutes   **Serves** 4

Besides the usual *persillade* of parsley, garlic, and butter in which one can prepare lamb liver, lamb kidneys, lamb brains, and veal liver, there are fancier ways of dressing up an already strong-flavored organ meat such as lamb liver. Adding a touch of sweetness to anything makes it go down more easily. That is just our nature as humans, to enjoy sweetness. Inspired by a recipe found at *Atelier des Chefs* online, I made this special dish with my organ meats cooking buddy and neighbor, Rébecca Pinsolle. Our taste testers, her two children of four and six years at the time, liked the liver, but *really* liked the chutney. Chutney is a spiced and sweet condiment originating in India. In this case, it sweetens the deal to help the liver go down. To spice the chutney, we used a grouping of "five spices" (*cinq épices*): cinnamon, clove, fennel, black pepper, and star anise, but you can also include cardamom or ginger. We used olive oil in this recipe, but other fats will do as well. The chutney calls for grilled almonds, which add crunch and toasted aromas and flavors to the dish. Grill (*griller* or *torréfier*) the almonds gently in a pan over medium heat by stirring often for several minutes until they begin to change color. Rather than use plain sea salt, we used a mixture of fine sea salt and *piment d'Espelette*, sweet chili powder from France's Basque country with which Rébecca likes to cook, as it adds a flavor nuance along with color. We used a raspberry-infused vinegar for the added fruity flavor, but apple cider vinegar will provide ample flavor as well.

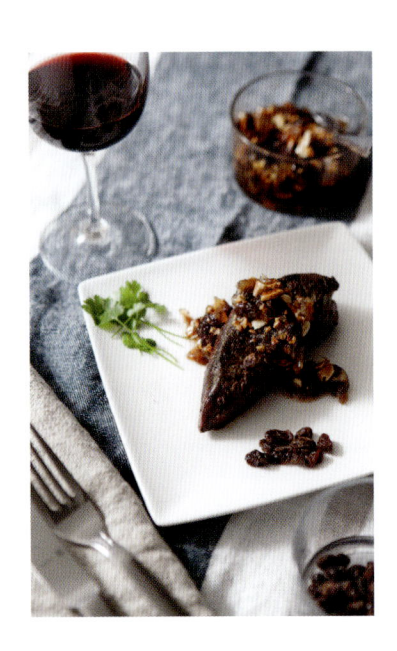

FOR THE LIVER

1 lamb liver

1 teaspoon fine sea salt

4 teaspoons olive oil, butter, ghee, tallow, or coconut oil

Ground pepper, for seasoning

FOR THE CHUTNEY

2 small onions, minced

2 tablespoons honey

½ teaspoon "Five Spices" (*cinq épices*)

Pinch of sea salt, or sea salt and *piment d'Espelette* mixture

3 tablespoons raspberry-infused vinegar or apple cider vinegar

2 tablespoons peeled almonds, chopped

2 tablespoons golden raisins

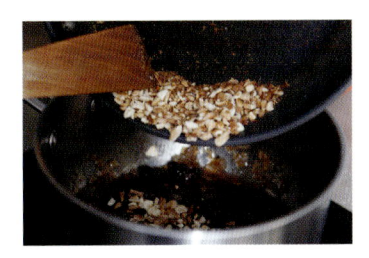

Grilled Almonds

Cut the lamb liver into six to eight slices and cover each piece with salt on both sides.

Heat the oil in the pan over medium-high heat, and brown each side of the liver slices for two to three minutes per side. (Finish off in an oven-safe dish in a preheated oven at 365°F or 185°C for five to eight minutes, if needed.) Transfer the liver pieces from the pan to a plate, and sprinkle each piece with ground pepper. Cover and keep warm.

Cook the onions, honey, *cinq épices,* and salt on low in a covered saucepan for five minutes. Add the raspberry vinegar, and stir until the mixture becomes a bit syrupy. Remove from heat and stir in the almonds and raisins, as shown here.

Serve the liver with a dollop of the chutney on top or on the side, and top everything with a sprig of fresh cilantro or parsley.

VARIATIONS I have sautéed lamb liver in macadamia nut oil and duck fat as well. For the chutney, try adding chopped fresh or dried apricots, or just use apricot marmalade instead as a sweet topping, as it sweetens the strong flavors of the lamb liver like the chutney does. Otherwise, try a combination of shallots and fresh cilantro instead of the chutney.

WINE PAIRING TIP To contrast the chutney's sweetness, while supporting the robust flavors of this dish, sommelière Annabelle recommends pairing it with dry, powerful red wines such as a fleshy Canon-Fronsac from the Bordeaux region, lesser known than other Bordeaux appellations, and therefore more economical; a Pic-Saint-Loup with notes of leather, ripe fruits, and spice from Languedoc; or a medium-bodied Beaumes-de-Venise from the Rhône Valley with aromas of berries, licorice, leather, resin, and spice and made from the Grenache and Syrah grapes.

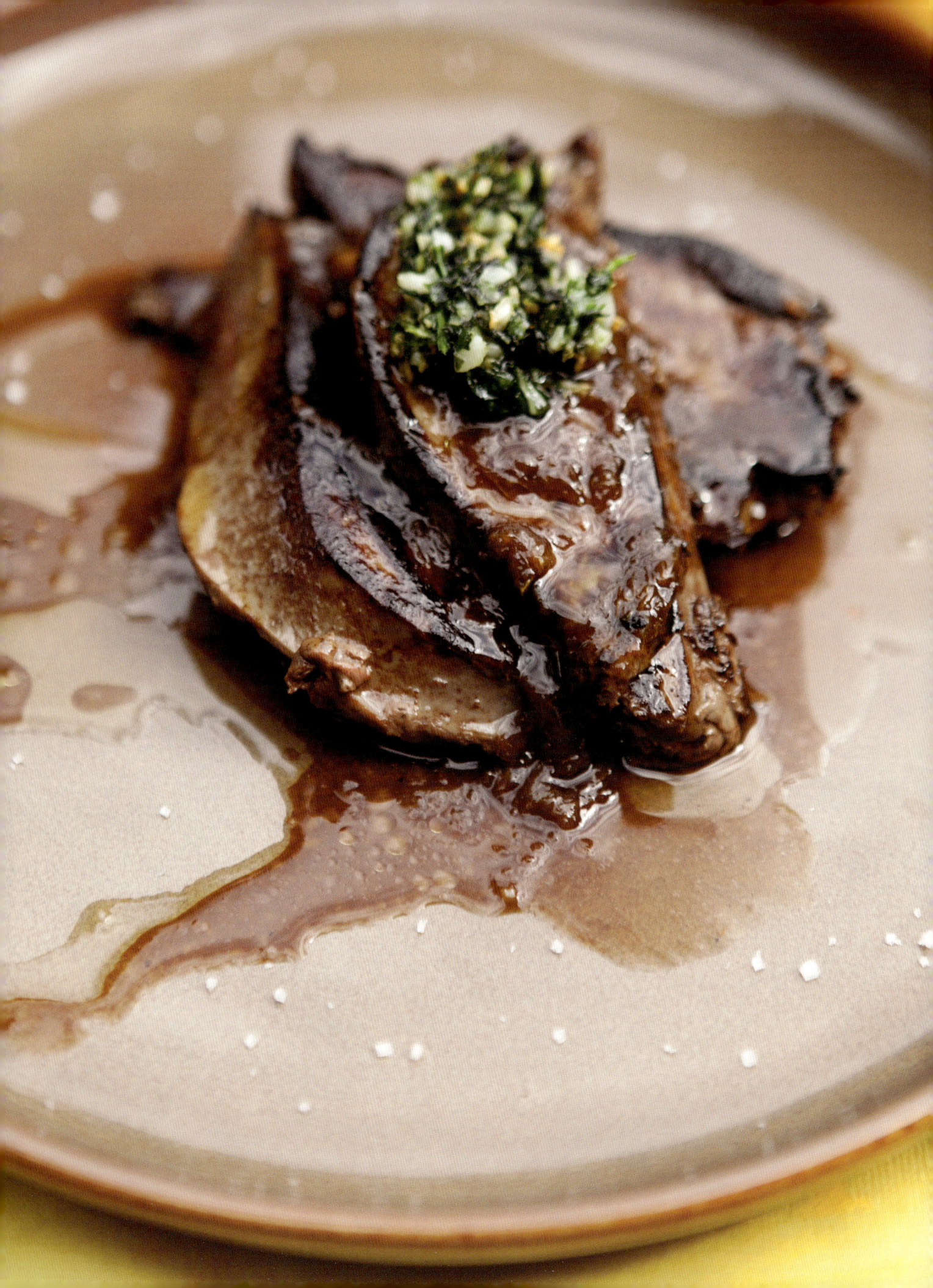

LAMB LIVER WITH ORANGE
Foie d'Agneau à l'Orange

Season Late Autumn through early Spring   **Preparation Time** 15 minutes
Cooking Time 15 minutes   **Serves** 4

The flavor and sweetness of the freshly-squeezed oranges cut the strong flavors of the lamb liver in this dish, which I concocted in order to be more enthusiastic about eating lamb liver. Even my husband enjoyed it.

2 oranges, juiced (keep pulp)

2 tablespoons balsamic vinegar

Pinch of fine salt

1 tablespoon, plus 1 teaspoon duck fat (or ghee)

1 lamb liver

Salt and pepper, for seasoning

3 garlic cloves, minced

2 tablespoons chopped parsley

Fleur de sel, for garnish

Olive oil, for garnish

Juice the oranges to make about ½ to ¾ cups (120 to 175 ml) orange juice, including the pulp (minus the seeds). Combine the juice, vinegar, and salt in a saucepan, and reduce the liquid over low heat until it is syrupy (7 to 10 minutes).

Meanwhile, melt a tablespoon of duck fat in a pan over medium-high heat. Slice the liver into four pieces, season with salt and pepper, and sauté on each side for 3 to 5 minutes. Finish off in an oven-safe dish in a preheated oven at 365°F or 185°C for five to eight minutes, if needed.

In a small pan, melt one teaspoon of duck fat over medium-high heat and sauté the garlic and parsley for about five minutes.

Top the liver with the orange juice syrup, the garlic, and parsley, and garnish with *fleur de sel* and olive oil, if desired.

> **WINE PAIRING TIP** As with the **Orange Duck Breast** (page 353), try a Southwest regional pairing that matches the robust flavors of the dish, such as a darkly-colored Cahors, with notes of cinnamon, dark fruits, and licorice; or a tannic Madiran, with notes of raspberry and made from the Tannat grape in a part of the French Southwest that has been cultivated for its wine since Roman times. See also the wine pairings for the previous recipe, **Lamb Liver with Onion Chutney** (page 255).

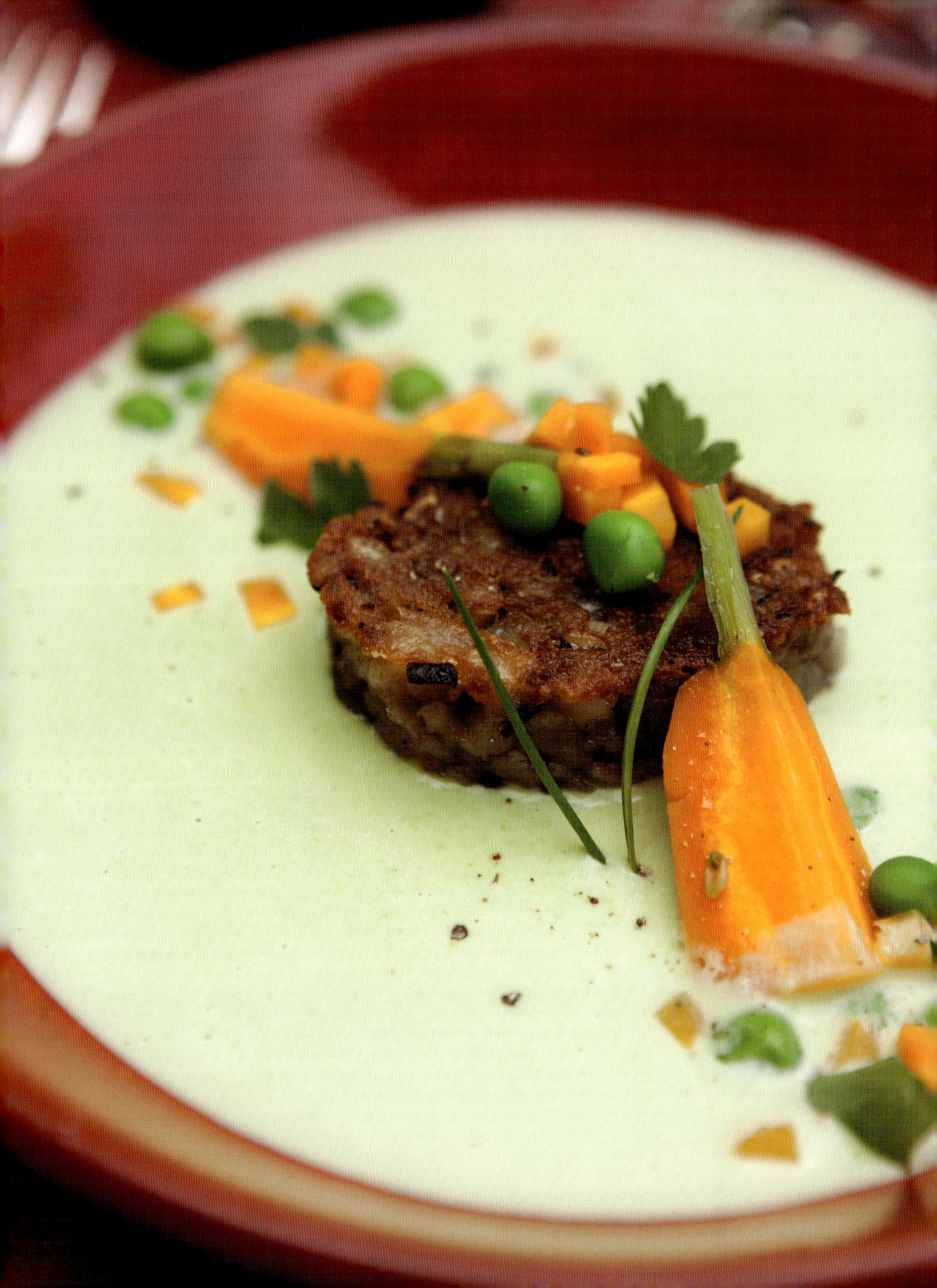

PIG'S FEET SLIDERS
Galettes de Pieds de Cochon

Season Year-round   **Preparation Time** 10 minutes for the stock, 30 minutes for the feet   **Serves** 4
Cooking Time 3 hours for the pig's feet stock, 15 minutes to sauté the chopped pig's feet,
30 minutes to overnight to chill, 4 to 6 minutes to sauté the sliders

This recipe is an original and delicious way to get a large dose of gelatin and make use of the pig's feet (*pieds de cochon*). This is my favorite dish by Chef Jean-Luc Beaufils, who visited my kitchen in Bordeaux to show me how it's done. His dynamic and talented wife, Annabelle, a sommelière and cellar master with her own wine tasting and tour company, *Voyages Autour du Vin*, helped me with a great many of the wine pairings throughout this book. Chef Jean-Luc now runs a restaurant with two friends in Saint-Christoly-Médoc, North of Bordeaux called *La Maison du Douanier*, where he is the "Chef de Cuisine." Jean-Luc has had his recipes featured in a number of French cookbooks. He introduced me to the phrase, "A meal without wine is called breakfast." But even in France, you might find wine, or at least Champagne, at breakfast (*le petit déjeuner*) or brunch (*le brunch*). This dish can be served as an appetizer for four or a full meal for two, especially if served over a vegetable purée. As it was springtime when we made this recipe, Jean-Luc also showed me how to make a fresh **Cream of Green Peas** (page 443), into a bowl of which he placed one slider for each of us for lunch after we spent the morning cooking.

Because the sliders (*galettes*) are so very flavorful and delicious, you will inevitably want more. My recommendation is to double the recipe to four pig's feet, once you have gotten the hang of the recipe. Do note that the pig's feet must simmer in a broth for three hours. This may be done a day or several hours in advance and the resulting pig's foot or "trotter" stock may be used in recipes calling for stock. The meat must also be rolled and chilled, which will take 30 minutes in the freezer or several hours (or overnight) in the refrigerator, and then sliced (see raw slider slices below) therefore it is helpful to plan ahead when making this recipe. In a true "snout-to-tail" effort, I have also made this recipe using two pork snouts (which are slightly meatier but also very collagenous) prepared along with the four pig's feet, resulting in a larger batch of delicious sliders. Just add a little bit more of each of the other ingredients, and this makes an excellent and economical way to make use of pork snouts as well. ➤

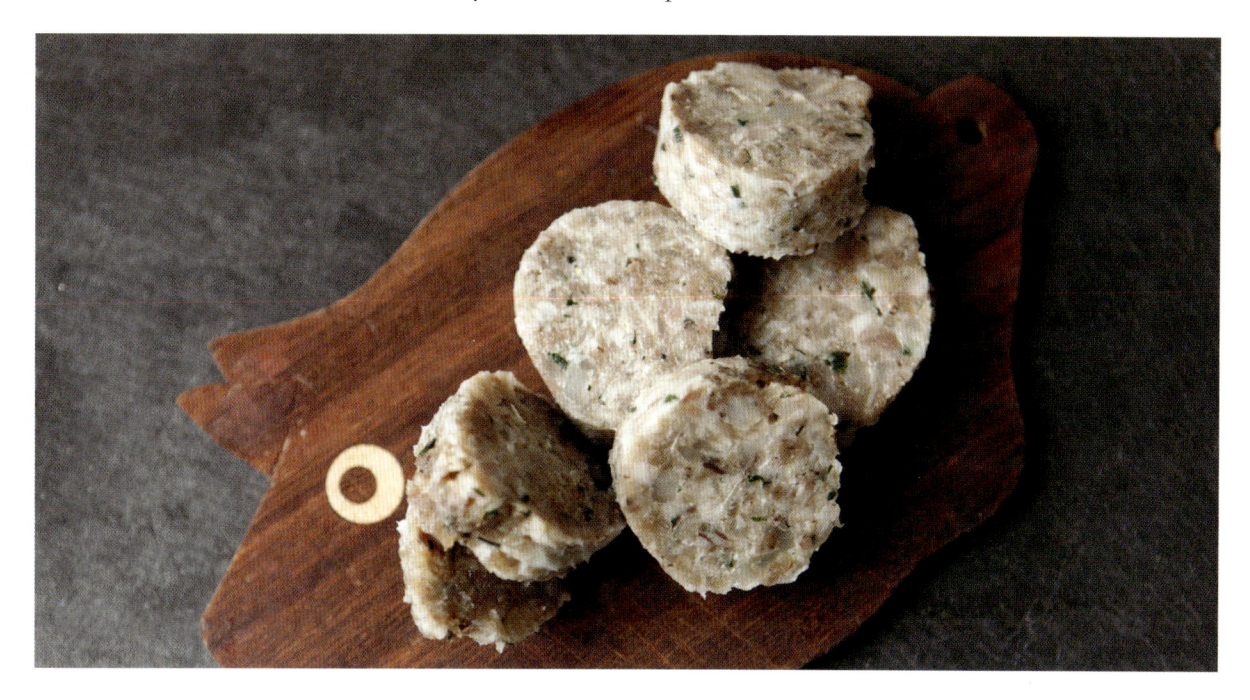

OFFAL AND FATS – *LES ABATS ET LES GRAISSES*

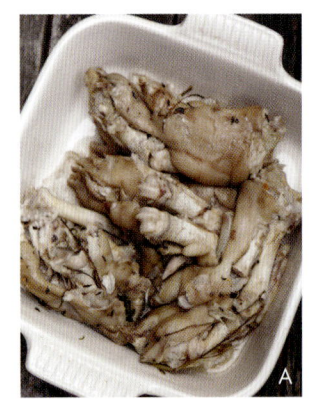

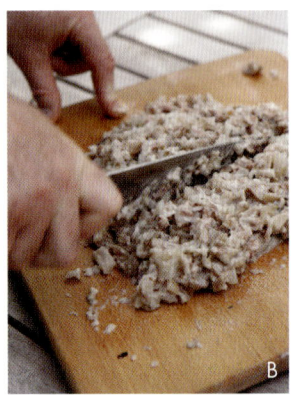

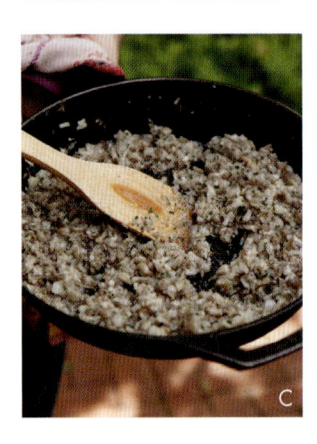

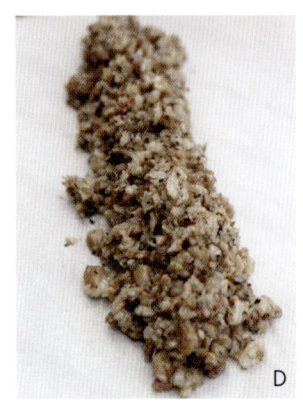

FOR THE PIG'S FEET STOCK

4 pig's feet

2 shallots, peeled and halved

3 to 4 parsley sprigs

2 bay leaves

2 sprigs of thyme

Onion, halved and poked (*implanté*) with 2 cloves

Carrot, broken in half

Garlic clove, peeled

1 tablespoon coarse sea salt

FOR THE SLIDERS

5 tablespoons lard (*saindoux*)

1 teaspoon fine salt, plus more for seasoning

1 teaspoon ground pepper

10 scapes of chive (*ciboulette*)

If the butcher has not already done the job, use a kitchen torch to burn the hairs off the pig's feet. Use a knife to scrape off the hairs, if necessary. Combine all the ingredients for the stock in a pot, cover with water, and bring to a boil. Reduce the heat to low, cover the pot, and simmer for 3 hours.

Remove the feet from the pot, leaving the "soup" in the pot. (See photo A.) Debone (*désosser*) the feet of all the large and tiny bones. This takes about 7 to 10 minutes. Place the bones back in the pot, and continue cooking on low heat for the rest of the day for a gelatinous broth you can have for sauces or as soup.

Chop (*concasser*) the skin and gelatinous meat by hand with a large chef's knife; this way you will feel it if you run into any small bones you missed. They will tend to stick to the knife. Remove them carefully as you go along, chopping for about six to eight minutes. (See photo B.)

Melt three tablespoons of the lard in a pan on medium-high heat, and add the chopped meat along with the salt and pepper. The pepper heightens (*relever*) the mild flavors of the dish. Allow the meat to cook for about 10 minutes, stirring and scraping the caramelized meat on the bottom of the pan. Reduce the heat to medium, add the chives, and stir for an additional few minutes. (See photo C.)

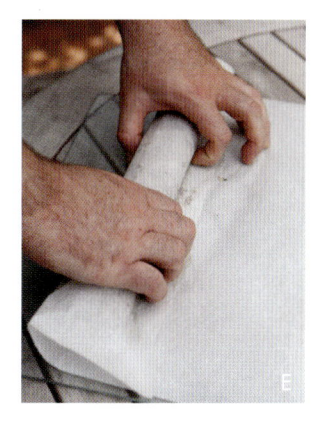

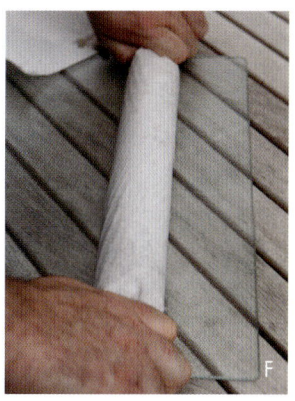

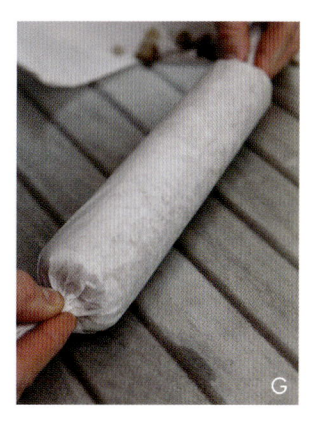

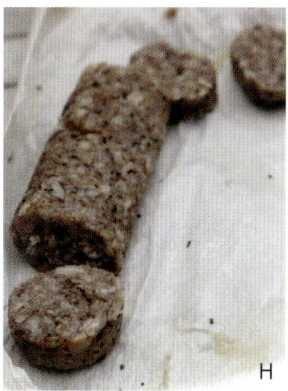

Remove from heat and allow to cool to room temperature before spreading the mixture about 10 inches (25 cm) from the edge of a piece of parchment paper, forming a rectangular pile. (See photo D.) Roll the mixture into cylindrical form inside the parchment paper, tucking the shorter side in after enveloping the chopped meat. (See photo E.) Roll all the way to the end of the parchment paper to form a cylindrical log, and twist off the ends of the paper. (See photos F & G.) Place the log on a plate in case of leakage, and chill in the refrigerator for half a day (or overnight), or else for 30 minutes in the freezer before unrolling the paper and cutting thick slices. (See photo H.)

Season both sides of each slider with salt. To cook the sliders, melt the remaining two tablespoons of lard in a pan over high heat and place the sliders in the pan. Allow them to fry for two to three minutes on each side to achieve a caramelized crust. Be sure to use a wire mesh cover over the pan to keep from getting splattered.

Serve the sliders over a vegetable purée or a green salad.

WINE PAIRING TIP When Chef Jean-Luc cooked the sliders, he, Annabelle, and I shared a fresh and fruity Touraine from the part of the Loire Valley dotted with many of the famous Loire châteaux. As this dish is one of Chef Jean-Luc's specialties, Annabelle has had much experience recommending wines to go with pig's feet cooked in this manner. She suggests supple reds such as an Alsatian Pinot Noir; a subtly smoky and spiced Côtes de Bergerac from the Southwest; an aromatic Crus du Beaujolais, an appellation comprised of ten different communes or vineyard areas producing the highest quality wine in Beaujolais; or else dry reds that are powerful but not oaked such as a fruity and medium-bodied Languedoc (formerly called Coteaux du Languedoc), or a smooth Côtes du Ventoux from the Southern Rhône Valley in the UNESCO-protected "biosphere" of the Mount Ventoux area.

OFFAL AND FATS – *LES ABATS ET LES GRAISSES*

POACHED AND SAUTÉED LAMB BRAINS
Cervelles d'Agneau Pochées et Sautées

Season Spring through Autumn   **Preparation Time** 20 minutes to soak the brains in water
Cooking Time 20 minutes   **Serves** 2

I know this may literally be tough to swallow at first, but as I have said before, organ meats are the most nutrient-dense foods we can eat. Add butter, which is rich in K2 and saturated fat, and sea salt, which has a delicious blend of many of the trace minerals we need, and you've got yourself a power-packed meal. I can say that it was a little hard for me to swallow the first bite or two, as the scent of cooked lamb brain was subtle but new to me, the texture a bit mushy, and the idea a bit off-putting thanks to my "brain-washed" disgust of mushy organs. To my offal-cooking buddy and former Bordeaux neighbor Rébecca Pinsolle, the scent of cooked lamb brains takes her back to her childhood days visiting her grandmother in Dijon. It's all about what you grow up experiencing. Rébecca's grandmother used to prepare lamb brains for her as a nutritious treat, and Rébecca says she never thought of this as an odd thing to eat. She was just content to eat it when visiting her grandmother. I find that the French who grew up on offal and other foods Americans might find "strange" had the good fortune of just that: growing up with these foods so that they never thought of them as strange and as a result never missed out on the nutrients, not to mention the convivial feeling of eating a warm dish prepared by their grandmother. This is the same effect that smooth pork liverwurst has on me: it transports me to my childhood when I would smear that liverwurst on dark German bread for my breakfast. I am truly grateful for that small indoctrination into "strange" foods, as I think it has helped me enjoy other foods like chicken liver pâté or just plain old liver.

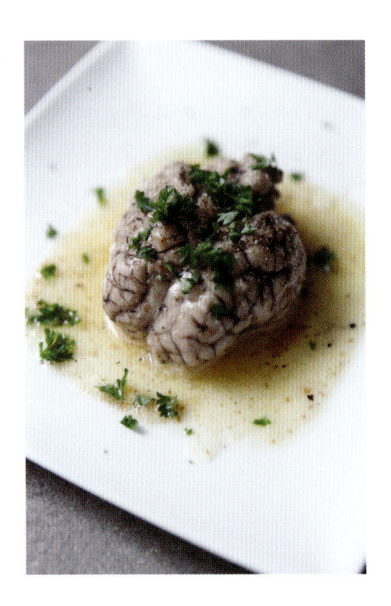

I will admit that it can be difficult to eat more than just a forkful or two of lamb brains on one's first attempt. But as I have said, I am motivated by the quest to heal my gut, strengthen my body, and accept those foods which keep me on that path, and lamb brains are just one example of the rich diversity of French traditional cuisine to be discovered.

Brains are extremely fragile and may fall apart a bit as you handle them during each step. But this is only a problem when you are trying to photograph the finished product or serve it to a very discerning customer. This recipe shows you how to poach and then sauté lamb brains, though as mentioned, they risk falling apart a bit from the cooking. Another way to do this recipe so that the brains do not fall apart is to poach them and then drizzle them with heated butter on a plate. After a taste test, however, Rébecca and I both agreed that the light caramelization effect of sautéing the brains in the butter in the frying pan added texture and flavor to a dish that is otherwise mushy in texture, especially if one is not used to it. Like many organ meats, soaking them in water ahead of time helps remove residual blood.

2 lamb brains

6 tablespoons apple cider vinegar

Pinch of salt

4 tablespoons butter or ghee

4 tablespoons parsley, minced

Sea salt and pepper, for seasoning

Soak the brains in a bowl of cold water and two tablespoons of the vinegar for 15 to 20 minutes to remove impurities (residual blood).

Bring a pot of water with a pinch of salt to a boil over high heat. Reduce the heat to medium-low or low, and simmer the brains for 10 minutes without bringing the water back to a boil. Remove the poached brains from the water, allowing them to drip excess water onto a plate (shown below, left).

Melt the butter in a pan over medium-high heat, and gently place the brains into the pan to sauté them lightly on the bottom and top for a few minutes on each side. Stir in the rest of the vinegar, mixing it with the butter. Use a spoon to drizzle (*arroser*) the melted butter and vinegar over the brains while they are sautéing. Remove the brains from the pan and place gently on a plate.

Sprinkle with sea salt and pepper to taste, and garnish with parsley. (The crunchy crystals of *fleur de sel* also make a nice garnish.) Serve immediately. ➤

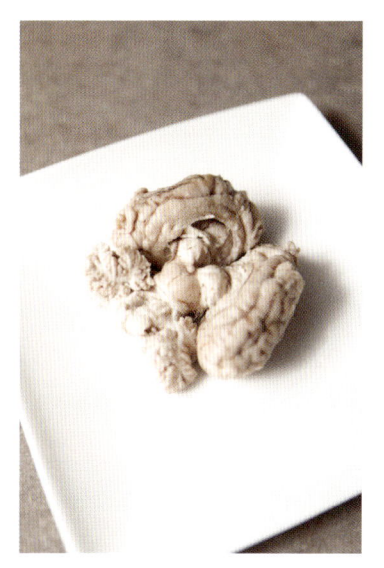

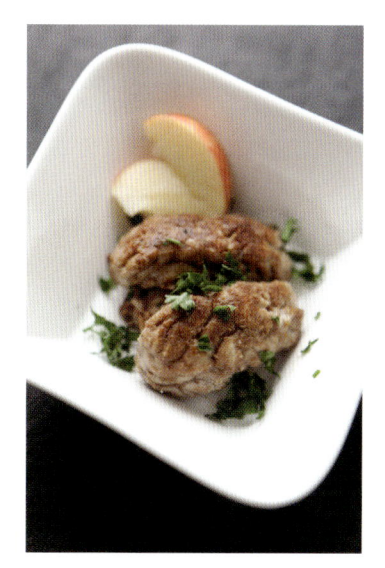

Poached Lamb Brain

Lamb Brain with Chestnut Flour

VARIATIONS I have made "breaded" (*meunière*) lamb brains on several occasions, similar to breaded sweetbreads, rolling the brains in a tablespoon of chestnut or coconut flour after poaching them for 10 minutes. Using two tablespoons olive oil (adding more to the pan as the brains soak up the oil—brains need fat, remember?), I sauté the brains with a pinch of salt in a pan over medium-high heat for up to 10 minutes on each side to cook through. The coconut confers more of a "nuggets" flavor, but I prefer the subtler flavors of chestnut flour with lamb brains (shown on the previous page). Prepared this way, the lamb brains go well with an Alsatian Pinot Gris.

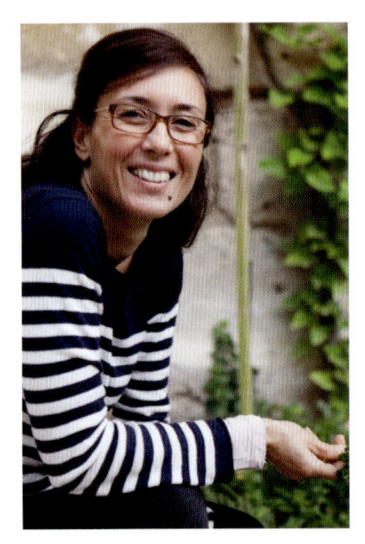

WINE PAIRING TIP Go for a medium red, either a Bordeaux Graves or Côtes de Castillon, for example, something balanced between Merlot and Cabernet Sauvignon, so as not to overpower the dish. Or try a crisp white—I love the Bordeaux Graves dry wines myself. Or else try something that is less floral and more buttery, such as an almond and citrus Saint-Véran from Burgundy to bring out the buttery flavors of the dish. Sommelière Annabelle recommends dry, light whites, such as a mineral and floral Loire Valley Saumur Blanc, made from a minimum of 80% of the Chenin Blanc grape; a honey and lemon medium-bodied Cheverny, also from the Loire Valley; or a citrus and verbena Mâcon or a lightly fruity and floral Aligoté, both from Burgundy. Alternately, Annabelle suggests flavorful and fruity reds, such as a well-structured Beaujolais-Villages or a velvety and lightly spiced Saumur-Champigny from the Loire Valley.

Rébecca Pinsolle

RENDERING FARM FATS: DUCK FAT, LARD, AND TALLOW
Fondre la Graisse des Animaux de la Ferme: La Graisse de Canard, du Porc, et du Boeuf

I like to keep different types of cooking fats in glass jars in my refrigerator so that I am not limited in flavor or cooking combinations. I try to make sure I always have one stick or container each of butter, duck fat, lard, olive oil, and tallow. I get nervous when I am missing one! Each has its particular flavor and use. Rendering duck (or goose) fat, lard, and tallow are quite easy, and takes only about an hour to an hour-and-a-half of your time. Below are instructions for each.

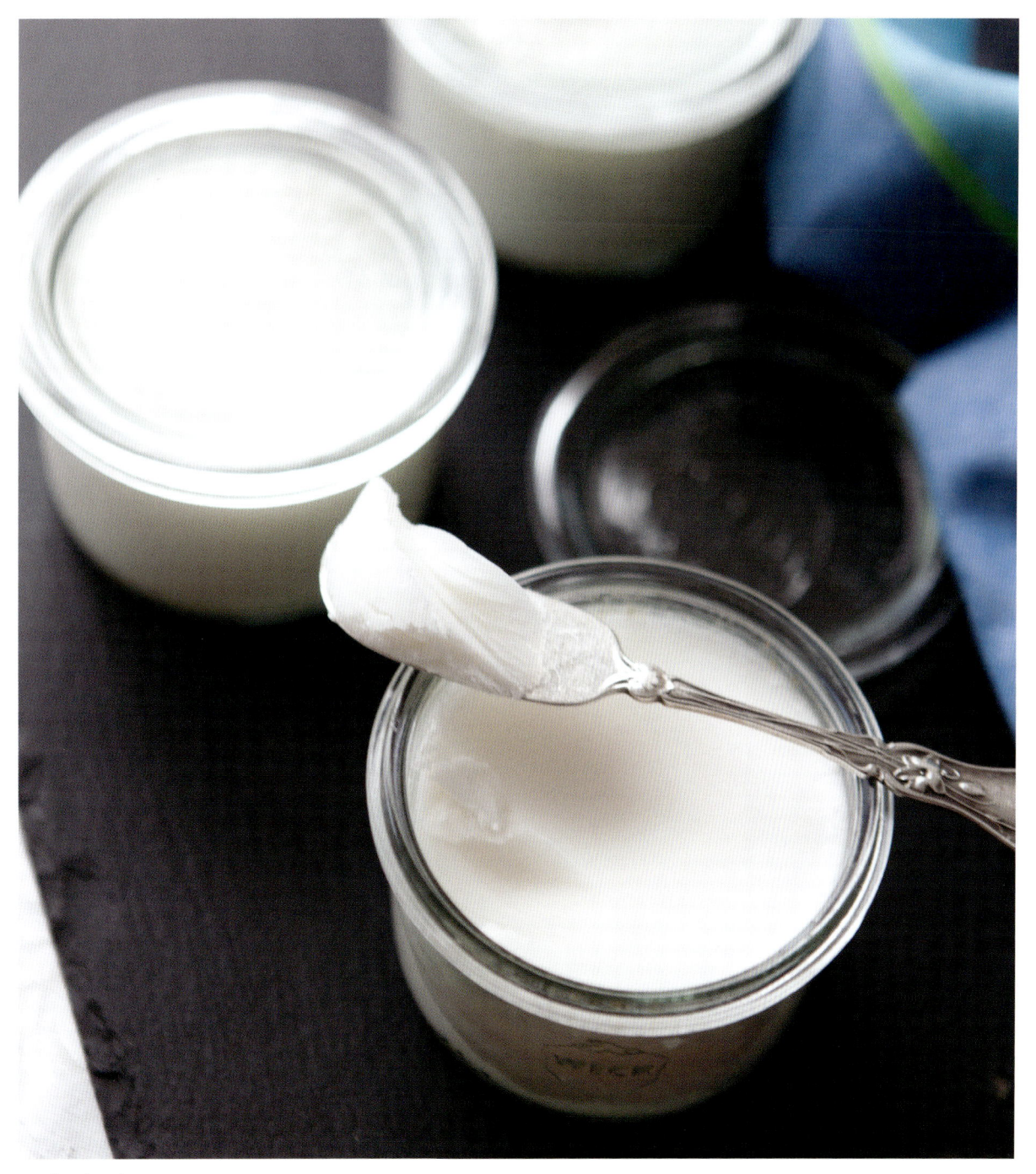

Rendered Lard

RENDERING DUCK (OR GOOSE) FAT
Fondre la Graisse de Canard (ou de l'Oie)

Cooking Time 1 hour to 1 hour, 15 minutes
Makes 6.5 cups (1560 ml) rendered duck fat and 3.5 ounces (100 grams) of cracklings

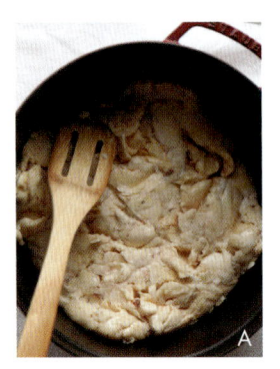

3.3 pounds (1.5 kg) duck fat

½ cup (120 ml) water

Salt and pepper, for seasoning

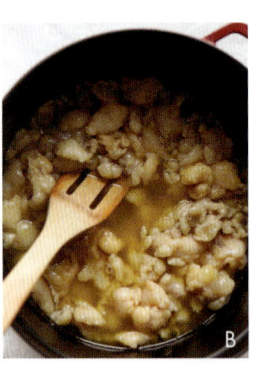

Pour the water into a large crock pot and place the duck fat in the pot, partially covered to allow the water to evaporate (photo A). Cook over medium heat. When you hear the water boil and the duck fat begins to sizzle, reduce the heat to medium-low or low to avoid burning the fat. You will see liquid fat begin to form around the solid fat (photo B). Stir every few minutes to keep the fat from sticking to the bottom of the pot. After about half an hour (photo C), you can begin to ladle out the liquid fat into glass jars (photo D). When you have ladled out most of the liquid, by about the 45-minute mark, you will have the remaining protein "cracklings" (*grattons*) left in the pot (photo E). Increase the heat to medium again, and allow the cracklings to brown slowly, stirring every few minutes (photo F). Continue to ladle or spoon out the liquid fat as it accumulates in the bottom of the pan. Don't worry about little brown specks in the fat, as they will sink to the bottom. These are just duck proteins, edible, like the *grattons*. Makes 6.5 cups (1560 ml) rendered duck fat. At about the one-hour mark, you will have about 3.5 ounces (100 g) of cracklings (photo G). Continue to brown them for a few minutes, if desired. Season them with salt and pepper, and eat them mixed with sautéed vegetables on salads or on their own, like pork rind chips. Store them in the refrigerator for up to a week or freeze them. (See **Duck Rinds** recipe in the side bar on page 359 for their further use.) When you are more comfortable with this process, you can skip using water as long as you cook on low heat.

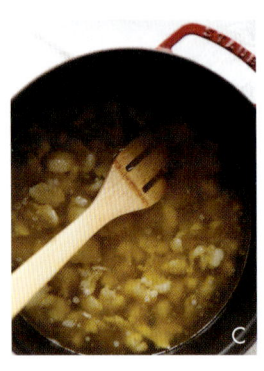

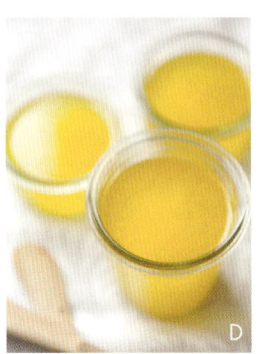

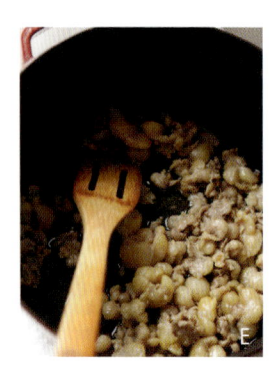

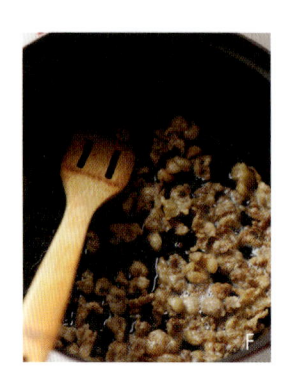

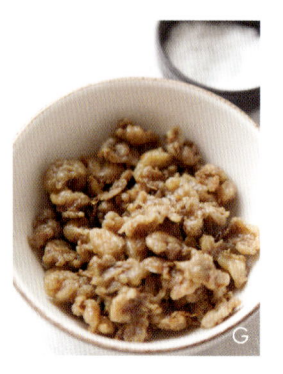

RENDERING LARD (PORK FAT)
Fondre le Saindoux

Rendering pork fat into lard is just as easy as rendering duck fat. You will need to grind up the pork fat (either from the viscera, called "leaf lard," or from the back, called "fat back" or "back fat") in a meat grinder, or else run it through a food processor for a minute or two until it reaches the consistency of a paste, if this has not already been done for you by the butcher. (Often, you can request ahead of time that the butcher grind the pork fat for you.) Otherwise you can chop it up with a knife (photo A). Machine-ground pork fat makes the rendering process in the pot a bit more efficient and even. Place the pork fat in a large, uncovered, or partially covered cast-iron pot over medium-low to low heat (photo B). Using a wooden ladle, break apart the clumps of fat as they melt to liquid (photo C). Stir the lard and scrape the bottom of the pot now and then to keep the cracklings from sticking to the bottom of the pot. Ladle out the liquid lard as it becomes rendered or strain the lard using a fine mesh sieve to separate it from the cracklings. Use a ladle to press on the cracklings in the sieve to push out the liquid fat, as there is less liquid and you have more cracklings than fat (photo D). Increase the heat by a notch to brown the cracklings, and keep scraping the bottom of the pot, as they will stick to it (photo E). You may also place the pot in the oven at 300°F (150°C) so the heat is not coming only from the bottom of the pan but from all around. I like to be able to stir and keep an eye on my lard as it is rendering, so I keep it on the stove. Another option is combining the pork fat with a half cup of water in the pot to avoid burning the fat as it begins to melt. With the pot uncovered or only partially covered, the water will evaporate. I have found, however, that if the heat is low enough, water is not necessary. The entire process can take up to two hours, depending on how much fat you are rendering, but usually, it takes me about an hour for 3.3 pounds (1.5 kg) of lard. The protein cracklings (photo F), or greaves, (*cretons*) remaining in the bottom of the pot can be browned further (like duck cracklings) and sprinkled over salads like bacon bits, or mixed in with sautéed vegetables or potatoes.

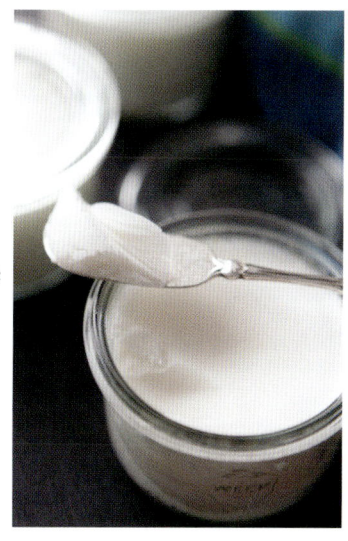

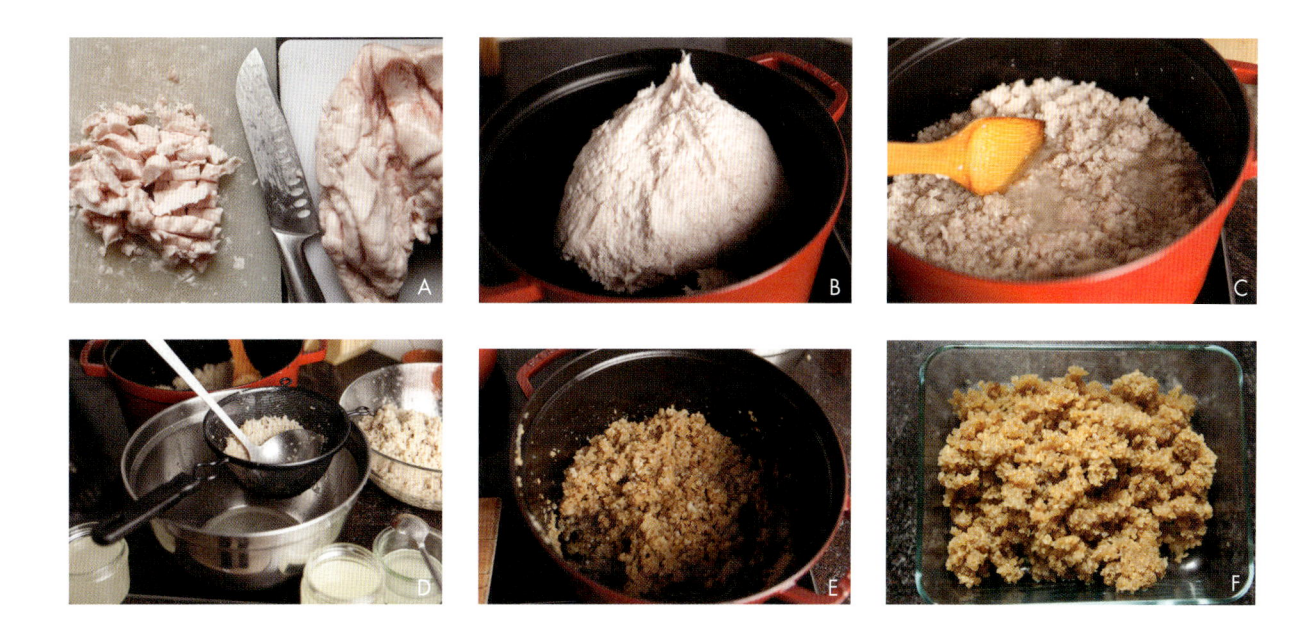

OFFAL AND FATS – *LES ABATS ET LES GRAISSES*

RENDERING TALLOW (BEEF FAT)
Fondre le Suif

Makes four and a half 14-ounce (400 g) jars of rendered tallow from 4.5 pounds (2kg) of beef fat

Beef fat (as well as lamb fat) is called "suet" (*suif*) before it is rendered into tallow (blanc de boeuf). Chop it up into small pieces (photos A & B), if it has not been ground using a food processor or meat grinder. I render beef tallow without water, setting the heat to medium-low, uncovered, so it melts very slowly, without burning. Using a wooden ladle, break apart the clumps of fat as they melt to liquid and the cracklings turn brown (photo C). Scrape the bottom of the pan now and then to keep the cracklings from sticking. You will see liquid fat begin to form around the solid fat (photo D). Strain the fat using a fine mesh sieve to separate it from the cracklings. Beef cracklings, or greaves (*cretons*), are delicious in broths or sautéed with leeks or chard. Rendered tallow may be used in cooking but also to make one's own skincare balms when mixed with other oils.

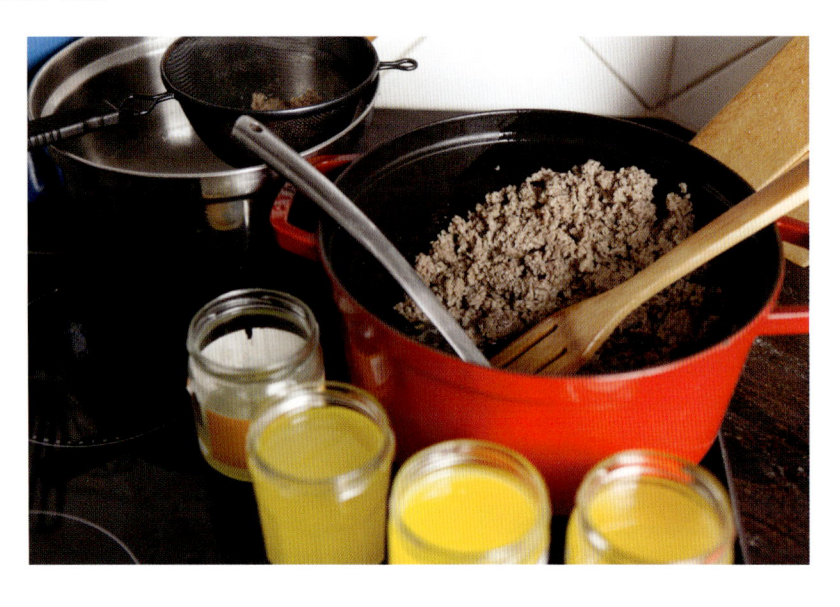

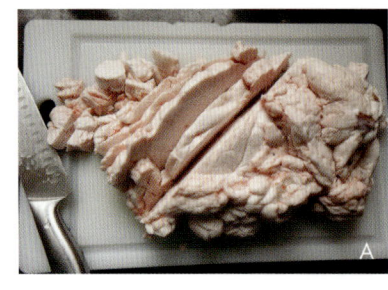

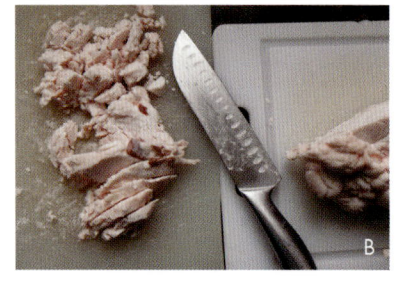

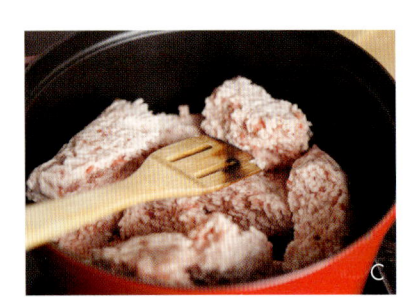

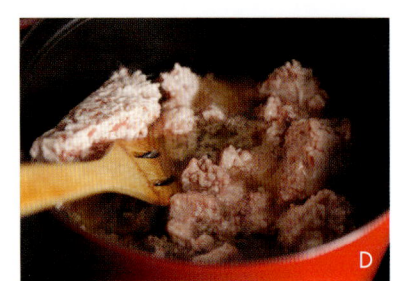

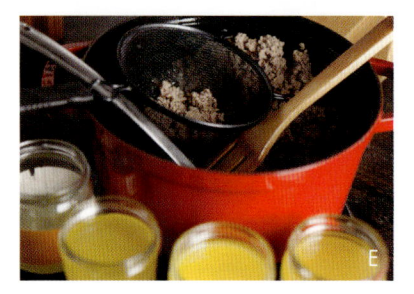

268

THE BORDEAUX KITCHEN

ROASTED MARROW BONES
Os à Moelle

Season Year-round   **Preparation Time** 1 minute
Cooking Time 15 minutes   **Serves** 1

Bone marrow is a delicacy which can be eaten right out of the marrow bones (leg bones of the cow) or can be scooped out and poached. This recipe is for eating roasted marrow right out of the leg bones cut lengthwise, as shown in the top photo below, or else crosswise, as shown in the bottom photo below, in which case a thin spoon is needed. This is a nutritious and easy recipe that can be served as an excellent appetizer.

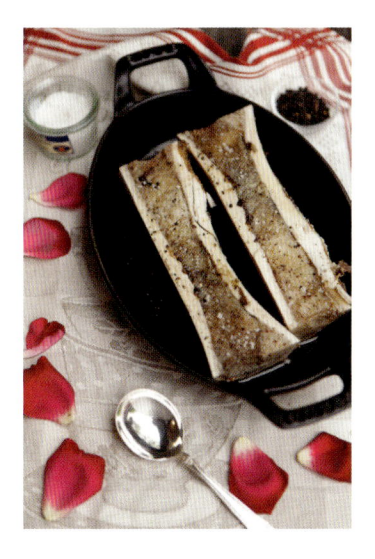

Two 6- to 8-inch (15 to 20 cm) beef leg bone sections, sawed in half

Salt and pepper, for seasoning

Fleur de sel, for garnish

Preheat the oven to 395°F (200°C). Lay the bones flat, marrow side up in an oven-safe dish. Sprinkle with salt and pepper. Cook in the oven for 15 minutes. Garnish with *fleur de sel*.

VARIATIONS Basque butcher Florent Carriquiry recommends adding minced garlic before placing in the oven. Traditionally, in some areas of France, this dish is topped with a pat of butter!

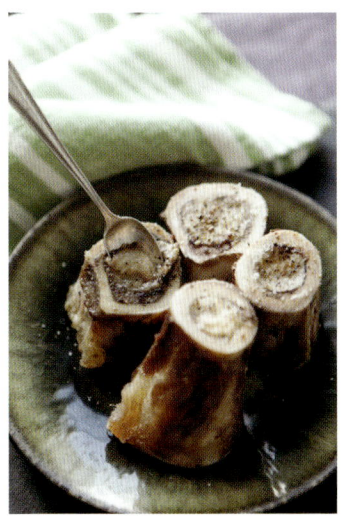

WINE PAIRING TIP A red Bordeaux will pair deliciously with marrow, such as with the organic, mocha, leather, and cinnamon-flavored 2005 (nicely aged) Château Lagarette Cuvée Renaissance from the Premières Côtes de Bordeaux (now called Cadillac–Côtes de Bordeaux). The subtle flavors of the marrow combined with the wine make for a long, rich aftertaste. Sommelière Annabelle recommends powerful whites, whose rich flavors will support the equally rich flavors of the marrow, such as a complex, aged Pessac-Léognan from Bordeaux, a gourmet and elegant Côtes du Rhône Villages, an aromatic and mineral Pernand-Vergelesses from Burgundy's Côte de Beaune, or a rich Faugères from Languedoc-Roussillon, with notes of apricot.

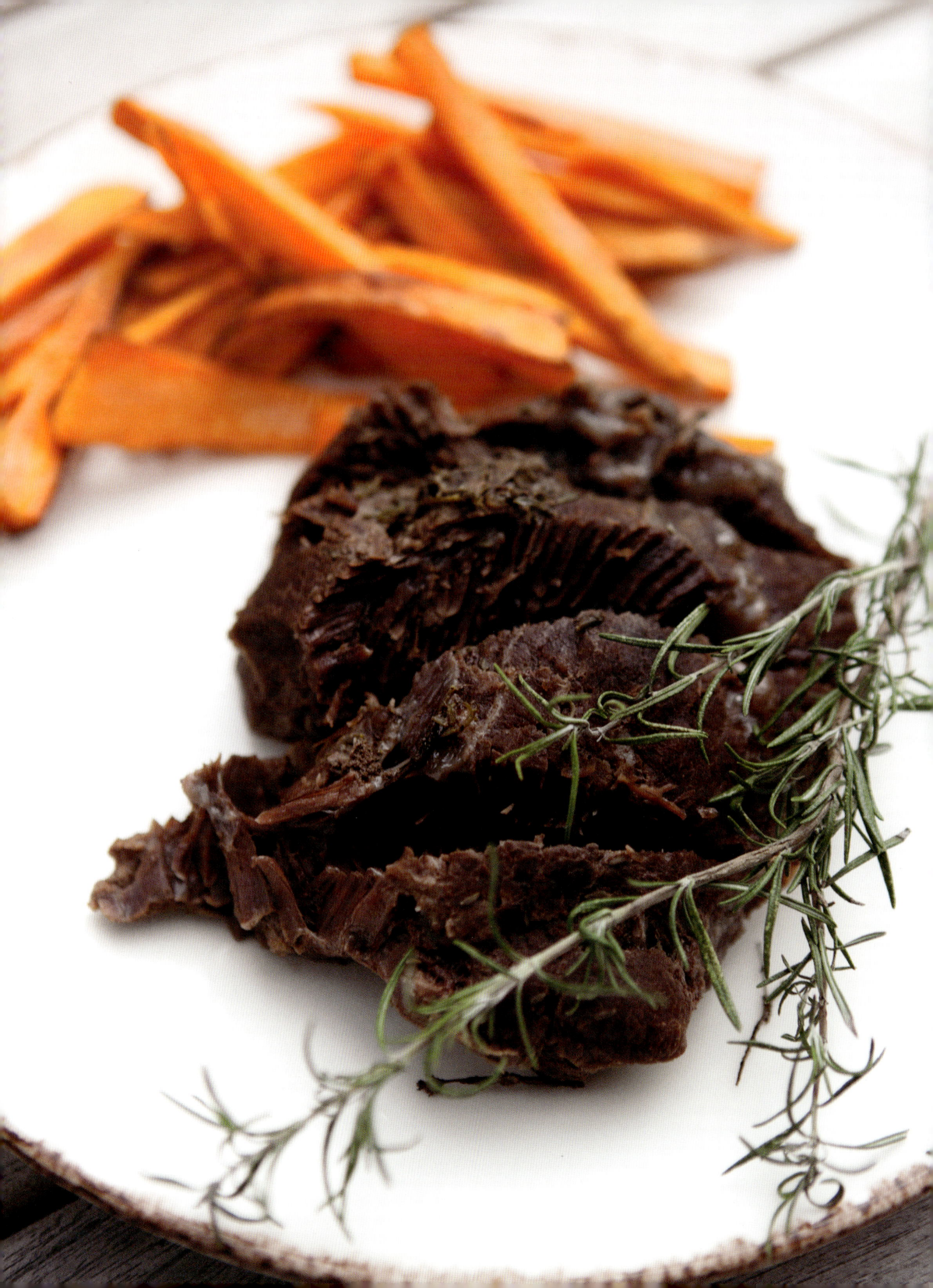

SLOW-COOKED BEEF CHEEKS
Joues de Boeuf

Season Year-round   **Preparation Time** 30 minutes
Cooking Time 3 hours   **Serves** 4 to 5

Beef cheeks require time to cook to tenderness but cost less than most other cuts of meat. Beef cheeks are flavorful and full of healthful collagen. I learned about this recipe from a French butcher's cookbook and then asked my local butcher about it. I always like to mix and modify, based on the ingredients I have on hand and the style of cooking I would like to try, and this recipe was the result. This is one of my favorite recipes for both taste and value. It is also great reheated for lunch the next day.

WINE PAIRING TIP So as not to overpower the tender flavor of the beef cheeks, serve with a light red, such as a Burgundy Pinot Noir, or a berry and cherry Sancerre Rouge or a light- to medium-bodied, fresh Touraine, both from the Loire Valley. Sommelière Annabelle recommends supple and light reds such as a crisp, aromatic Cabernet Franc-dominated Bourgueil from the Loire Valley, with notes of cherry, red berries, undergrowth, and licorice; or a light, fruity, and approachable Beaujolais Primeur (also known as Beaujolais Nouveau), released annually on the third Thursday in November and meant for immediate drinking; or else a full-bodied Bordeaux, such as one from the Médoc appellation.

2.2 lbs. (1 kg) beef cheeks

¼ cup (60 ml) white vinegar

1 leek, chopped into 1-inch (2.5 cm) rounds

2 carrots, chopped into 1-inch (2.5 cm) rounds

1 onion, peeled and halved

2 cloves, one stuck into each onion half

2 tablespoons thyme, fresh or dried (or a bit of each)

1 or 2 bay leaves

Handful of parsley stems (save the leaves for a salad), to flavor the broth

2 pinches of sea salt

Place the cheeks in a large bowl and cover with cold water, adding ¼ cup (60 ml) white vinegar for 30 minutes to remove blood and impurities.

Rinse the cheeks and place in a cast-iron pot. Add the leek, carrots, onion with clove, thyme, bay leaf, parsley, and salt to the pot, and cover the ingredients with water. The key here is to submerge the beef such that it is just covered with water. Cover and bring to a boil.

Reduce the heat and simmer covered at a low gurgle for three hours. (An additional hour or two of cooking will make the meat even more tender, but three hours are sufficient.) Uncover for the last 30 minutes if you wish to reduce the liquid.

Slice the meat, pour some of the sauce over the meat if desired, and add a dash of salt and pepper to taste.

Serve with white potatoes, sweet potato fries, green salad, or sautéed vegetables.

OFFAL AND FATS – *LES ABATS ET LES GRAISSES*

SLOW-COOKED PORK CHEEKS WITH APRICOTS
Joues de Porc aux Abricots

Season Year-round   **Preparation Time** 5 minutes
Cooking Time 1.5 hours   **Serves** 4

This is another great recipe adapted from one of my all-time favorite French cookbooks by Parisian butcher Hugo Desnoyer. Pork cheeks cooked slowly are tender but chewy. They are much smaller than beef cheeks, and serve about two per person. One trick to keep in mind is to rinse and pat the cheeks dry so that the caramelization in the pot happens without producing steam from excess water on the meat.

8 pork cheeks, rinsed and patted dry

3 tablespoons lard

2 tablespoons duck fat (or butter or ghee)

3 pinches of fine salt

2 to 3 sprigs of thyme (or 1 teaspoon fresh or dried)

Pinch of pepper, for seasoning

8 dried apricots, cut into quarters

Optional: Toasted pine nuts

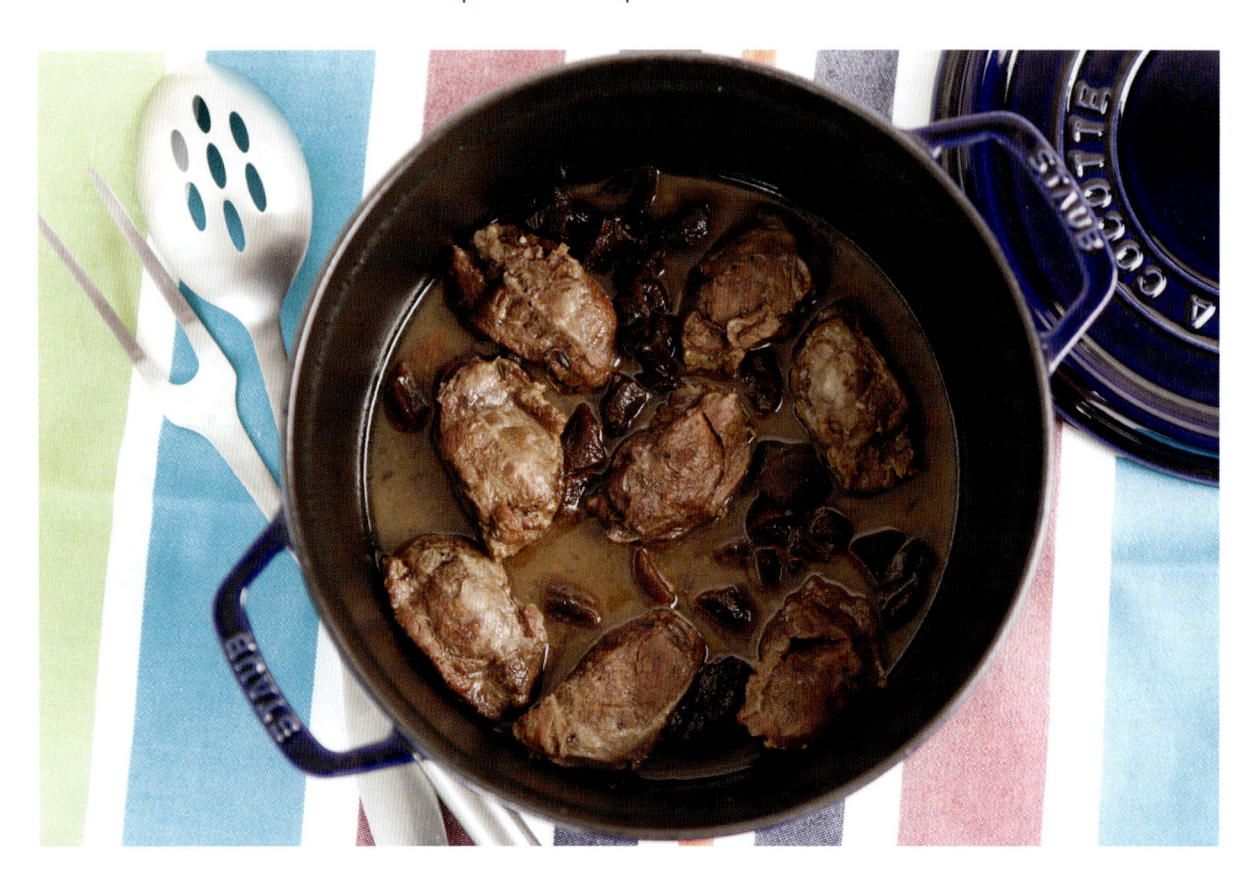

Melt two tablespoons of the lard and one tablespoon of the duck fat in a cast-iron pot over high heat. Divide the meat into two batches. Place the first batch in the pan, season with a pinch of salt, and sear the cheeks for one minute on each side. Transfer the first batch to a plate to make room in the pot for the second batch. Add another pinch of salt with the second batch of cheeks, and sear for one minute on each side.

Add the first batch of cheeks back to the pot, and reduce the heat to medium-low or low and add one tablespoon more each of the lard and duck fat (or butter or ghee), thyme, pepper, and one more pinch of salt. Allow to bubble slowly for an hour and a half, turning the cheeks occasionally. During the last 15 minutes, add the chopped apricots. For extra flair, add toasted pine nuts.

Serve hot on a plate with a bit of sauce and apricots, along with roasted or sautéed vegetables.

> WINE PAIRING TIP To contrast the stewed apricot flavors of this dish, try pairing it with a red Bandol from Provence, made with 50% Mourvèdre, giving the wine spice and personality. For a French Southwest pairing, try a hearty red wine from the Southwest: a rich Béarn, made from the tannic grape, Tannat; a Bergerac with rounded tannins and notes of blackcurrant and cherry; a Côtes de Bergerac, with notes of ripe red fruits, coffee, and cocoa; a Cahors, made largely from the Malbec grape, with notes of cinnamon, dark fruits, hazelnut, and licorice, or a Côtes de Bourg or a Fronsac, both of which have notes of red and black fruits, vanilla and chocolate; or a Sainte-Foy-Bordeaux, with notes of ripe red and black fruits, cedar, and graphite. See also the wine pairing suggestions for **Braised Veal Shanks** (page 426), a slow-cooking recipe that also incorporates apricots into the cooking.

TURKEY LIVER PÂTÉ WITH FIGS
Pâté de Foie de Dinde aux Figues

Season Year-round   **Preparation Time** 20 minutes
Cooking Time 10 minutes in the pan, 7 to 15 minutes in the oven   **Serves** 4 to 5

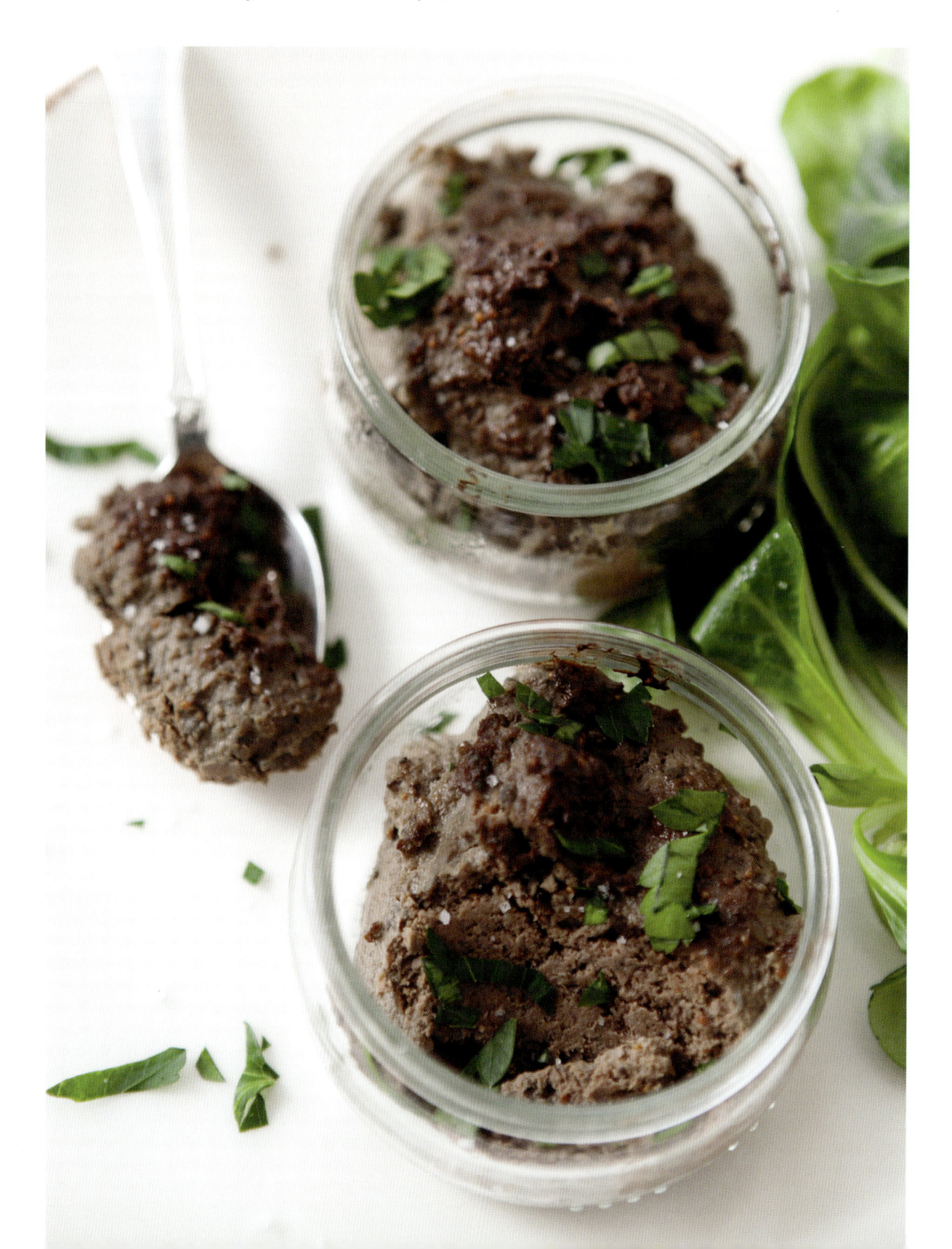

Figs, fresh or dried, are a much-loved fruit in France, used in tarts, terrines, appetizers, main courses, and desserts. Here I have incorporated dried figs into an easy turkey liver pâté, but chicken, duck, or goose livers may also be used. The sage leaves go well with the turkey flavors. If you do not have fresh sage, use the equivalent in dried sage leaves. Like all pâtés, this one may be served as an appetizer (*entrée*) or a main course (*plat*).

2 tablespoons goose fat (or duck fat)

18 ounces (about 500 g) turkey livers

2 garlic cloves, minced

10 fresh sage leaves, chopped

1 teaspoon thyme, fresh or dried

2 pinches of fine salt

Pinch of ground pepper

4 figs, finely chopped

2 eggs

Fleur de sel, for garnish

VARIATIONS For added fat and flavor, add three slices of finely chopped bacon (*lardons*) to the pan when you add the livers.

Melt the fat in a pan over medium-high heat. Combine the livers, garlic, sage, thyme, salt and pepper, and cook for about 10 minutes until the livers are no longer raw inside. (Cut into one of the lobes to check to see if it still raw.) Set aside in a bowl for 10 minutes to cool.

Preheat the oven to 365°F (185°C). Stir the figs into the liver mixture. Combine the liver mixture with two 2 eggs in a food processor, and mix until blended into a thick, sauce-like consistency. Pour into ramekins, and place in the oven, uncovered, for 8 to 15 minutes, depending on the size of the ramekins, or for about 20 minutes for one larger mold (*terrine*). For the eggs to fully cook, the internal temperature of each ramekin or mold must reach 158°F (70°C). Check the temperature with a digital or meat thermometer if you are unsure of the cooking time.

Remove from the oven, and allow to cool. Sprinkle with *fleur de sel*, and serve hot or lukewarm (*tiède*) in individual ramekins or in slices, accompanied by a green salad and/or baked sweet potato, if desired.

WINE PAIRING TIP With a liver pâté such as this, you cannot go wrong with a few sips of a richly flavored but fresh Barsac or Sauternes from Bordeaux. Otherwise, try a darkly-colored Cahors from the French Southwest, with notes of black currant, hazelnut, licorice, and violet. See also the wine suggestions for the **Chicken Liver Cake** (page 235) and **Duck Liver Pâté** (page 243) and **Foie Gras** (page 247).

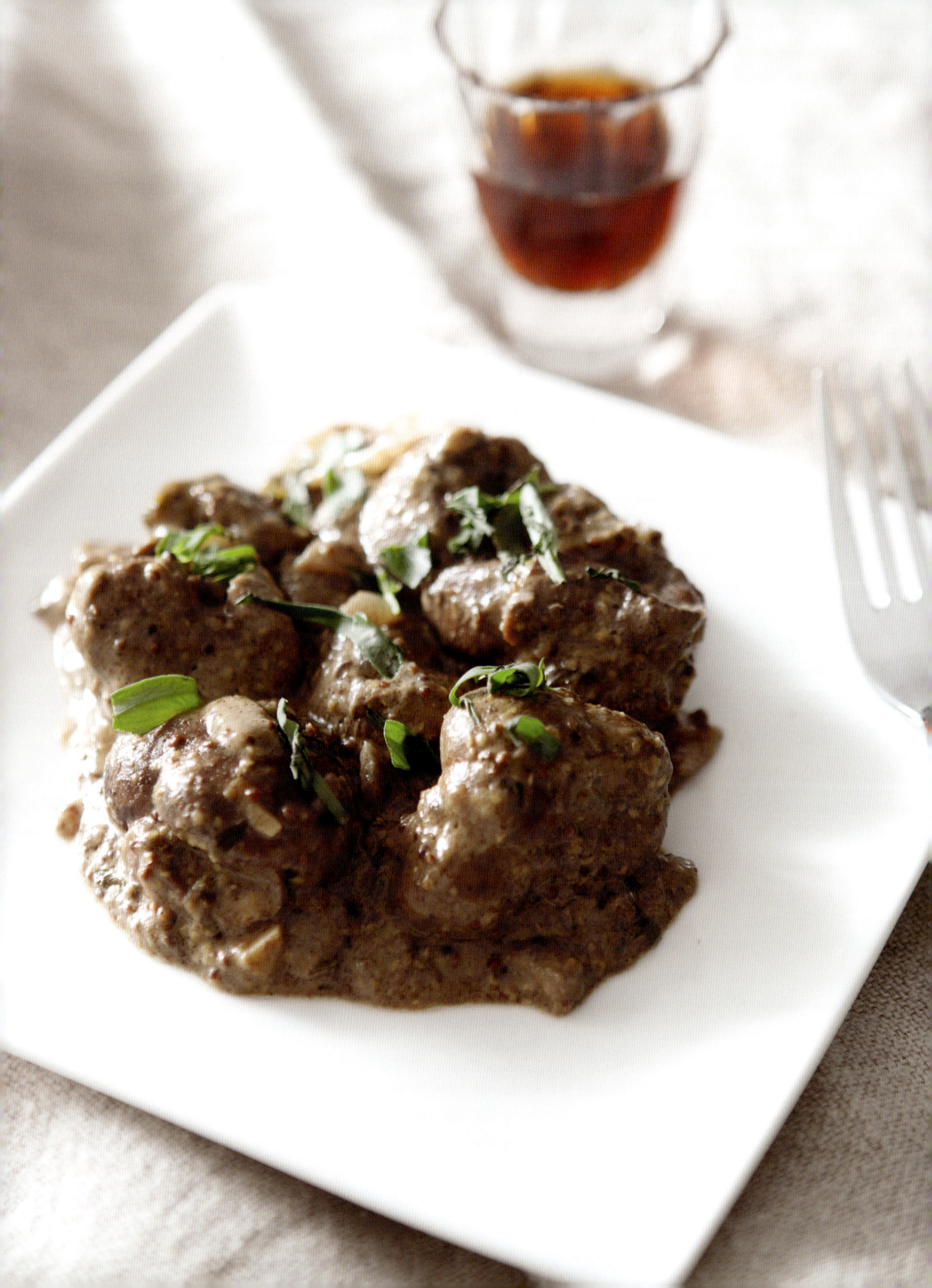

VEAL KIDNEYS IN OLD-FASHIONED MUSTARD SAUCE
Rognons de Veau à la Moutarde à l'Ancienne

Season Year-round **Preparation Time** 20 minutes
Cooking Time 35 to 40 minutes **Serves** 4

Once again, my "offal" cooking buddy Rébecca Pinsolle and I adapted this recipe, with a little help from the great French cooking website Marmiton (www.marmiton.org). This recipe calls for two "exotic" ingredients: powdered vanilla and Madeira (*Madère*), a fortified wine flavored by the rich volcanic soils upon which it grows on the islands off of the coast of Portugal. In France, Madeira was reputed and valued for its rich flavor as early as the 1600s. Replacements for Madeira would be a Porto or other fortified red wine, such as a Rivesaltes from Languedoc-Roussillon.

Like lamb kidneys, veal kidneys are tucked inside visceral fat which is usually cut and peeled away by the butcher (photos A, B, and C). Sometimes the butcher will also peel away the thin outer membrane on the kidney if you request it (photos D and E). Like sweetbreads, veal kidneys are generally soaked in water (or buttermilk) ahead of time. To prepare veal (or beef) kidneys for cooking, submerge them in water for an hour to remove residual blood. They may also be soaked in buttermilk for between one and four hours to tenderize them and reduce the strong kidney odor. Use a sharp knife to cut out the largest portion of white nerve tissue left on the inside of each kidney without cutting the kidney into pieces. You may choose to remove the thin outer membrane around the kidney lobe, but it can be left intact so that the kidney does not fall apart during the cooking process. The bits of white fat on the kidney may be used as cooking fat for the kidney.

This recipe utilizes **Old-Fashioned Mustard** (page 410). The herb tarragon (*estragon*) is also called for in this recipe, which we used fresh but for which you could substitute about one tablespoon of dried tarragon. In France, tarragon is in season April through October, but it is an herb that can be used dried during the rest of the year. ➤

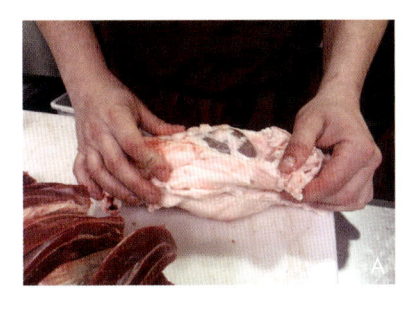

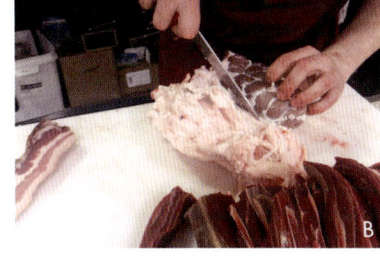

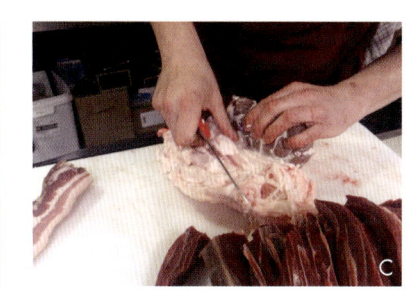

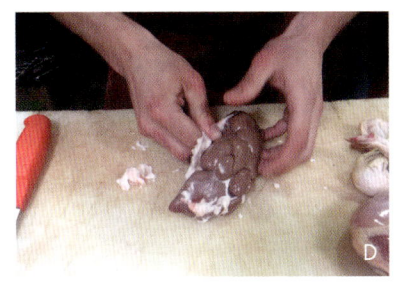

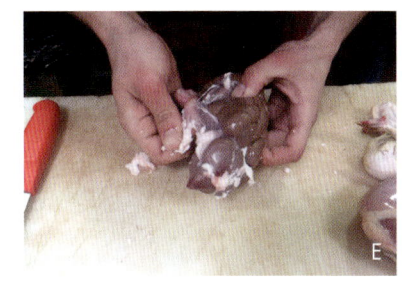

OFFAL AND FATS – *LES ABATS ET LES GRAISSES*

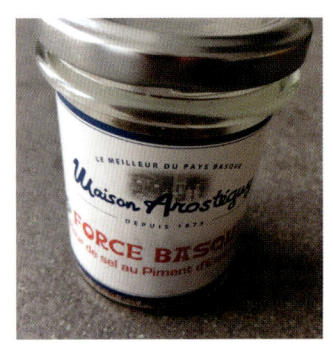

Piment d'Espelette Mixture

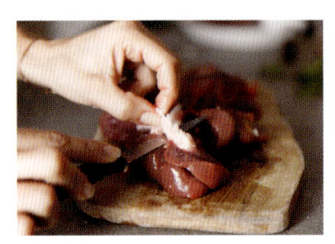

Remove White Membrane

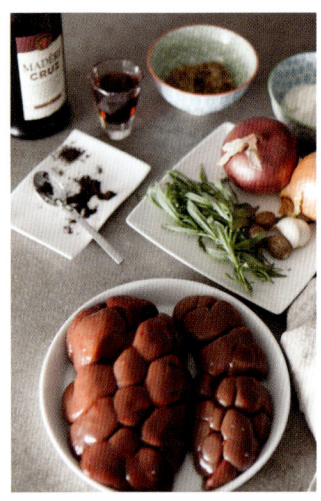

Raw Veal Kidneys and Ingredients

2 veal kidneys (1.8 to 2 pounds, or 800 to 900 g)

2 tablespoons olive oil or tallow

1 to 2 garlic cloves, minced

2 onions (red and yellow), finely chopped

4 tablespoons Madeira

3 tablespoons sour cream (*crème fraîche*)

3 tablespoons Old-Fashioned or Dijon mustard

Several sprigs of fresh tarragon, stemmed and chopped

1 teaspoon powdered vanilla

Pinch of nutmeg

2 pinches of fine salt, or sea salt and *piment d'Espelette* mixture, shown here

Pinch of ground pepper

Remove the white membrane inside each kidney using a paring knife, as shown here, left.

Slice the kidneys into 1-inch (2.5 cm) thick slices. Heat a cast-iron pot or pan over medium-high heat, and add one tablespoon of olive oil (or tallow) to the pan. Sauté the kidney slices for one minute on each side and set aside in a bowl.

Meanwhile, heat the other tablespoon of olive oil (or tallow) in the same or another pan or pot over medium to medium-high heat, add the garlic and onions to the pot, and sauté them for several minutes until the onions turn translucent.

Reduce the heat to medium or medium-low, and stir in the Madeira, followed by the sour cream, then the mustard and chopped tarragon leaves. Mix well with a wooden spoon before adding the kidney pieces. Make sure the kidneys are covered in sauce. Stir in the vanilla, nutmeg, salt, and pepper, reduce the heat to medium low or low, and cover the pot. Allow to simmer for 25 to 30 minutes, stirring a couple of times during cooking.

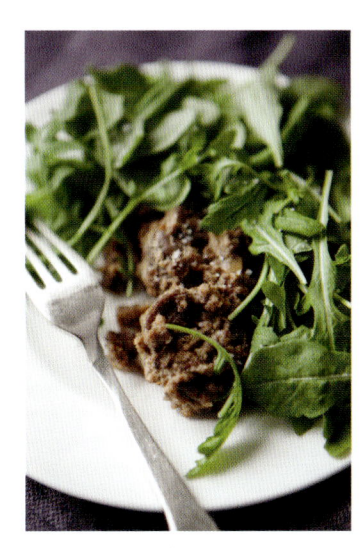

Veal Kidneys with Coconut Cream

VARIATIONS This recipe can also be made with a combination of equal parts veal sweetbreads and veal kidneys, as both go well in this sauce. Can you make the sauce for veal kidneys with coconut cream instead of sour cream and forego the alcohol? Oh yes! Here is the mini recipe: Swap out the Madeira for white wine vinegar, swap out the sour cream for coconut cream, add four tablespoons of water to the sauce (more if you prefer a sauce that is not as thick as the coconut cream, as shown here), and follow the recipe as described above. (As it turns out, chicken livers in this sauce are also delicious!) Wine pairing tip with this? Oh yes! I have had veal kidney in this sauce with a velvety Saint-Joseph, an appellation of the Northern Rhône Valley, and a wine whose nose of pepper and dark cherry goes very well with the vanilla and creaminess of the sauce. One such wine I can recommend is the organic Saint-Joseph Rouge from Cave de Tain, it is well-structured and "only" 12.5% alcohol. Oh, and this wine goes swimmingly with 100% organic dark chocolate!

WINE PAIRING TIP Enjoy a few sips of the Madeira or Porto you used for the sauce. Rébecca and I shared a refreshing, dry white Bordeaux from the Entre-Deux-Mers appellation. To match the creamy richness of this dish, sommelière Annabelle recommends red wines that are fruity and structured, many from Bordeaux, all of which are rich and complex, such as a Côtes de Bordeaux, a Lalande de Pomerol, a Pomerol, a Moulis-en-Médoc, a Pessac-Léognan, a Saint Emilion, a Saint-Estèphe, or a Saint-Julien. From the French Southwest, Annabelle suggests a Gaillac with rounded tannins that is made from a majority of Syrah (providing spice), Braucol, Duras, and Fer Savadou, with a minority of Bordeaux grapes (Cabernet Franc, Cabernet Sauvignon, Merlot), providing structure. Further afield, Annabelle suggests a robust Cornas from the Northern Rhône Valley, whose meaning in Celtic is "burned earth;" an herbaceous and leathery Fitou from Languedoc-Roussillon; a light- to medium-bodied, herbal and fruity Chinon, made almost exclusively from the Cabernet Franc grape, from the Loire Valley; a smooth Burgundy Volnay Pinot Noir, with notes of prune and spice, hailing from the Southern Côte d'Or's Côte de Beaune; or a richly-colored Vougeot, with notes of black currant and cherry, hailing from Burgundy's Northern Côte d'Or's Côte de Nuits.

VEAL KIDNEYS WITH PICKLED PEARS
Rognons de Veau, Pickles de Poires

Season Late Summer through early Spring   **Serves** 4
Cooking Time 35 minutes for the pickled pears, about 14 minutes for the veal kidneys
Chilling Time 12 hours for the pickled pears

My "offal" buddy and former neighbor in Bordeaux, Rébecca Pinsolle, and I adapted this recipe from one of my favorite French cookbooks, *Morceaux Choisis*, by Parisian butcher Hugo Desnoyer. The original recipe calls for flour, eggs, and bread crumbs, but we removed these and found that the salted kidneys went well on their own with the pickled pears, without the extra dressing and hassle. In France, pears are in season August through March, but veal kidneys may be eaten year-round. If pears are out of season, try cooking the kidneys as described below, but serve them with **Onion Marmalade** (page 411). Like sweetbreads, veal kidneys are generally soaked in water (or buttermilk) ahead of time. To prepare veal (or beef) kidneys for cooking, submerge them in water for an hour to remove residual blood. They may also be soaked in buttermilk for between one and four hours to tenderize them and reduce the strong kidney odor. You can ask your butcher to prepare the kidneys for you, but if not, use a sharp knife to cut out the largest portion of white nerve tissue on the inside of each kidney without cutting the kidney into pieces. You may choose to remove the thin outer membrane around the kidney lobe, but it can be left intact so that the kidney does not fall apart during the cooking process. The bits of white fat on the kidney may be used as cooking fat for the kidney.

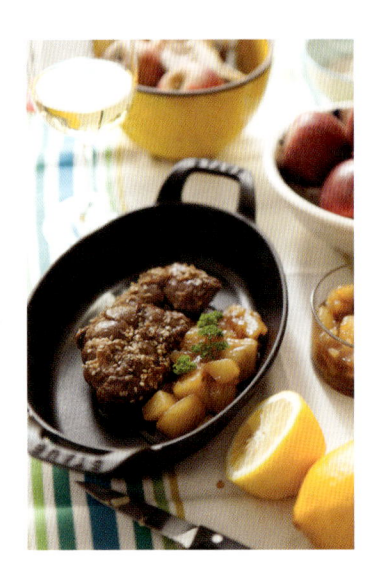

FOR THE PICKLED PEARS

14 ounces (400 g) firm pears, peeled and cubed

2/5 cup (95 ml) raspberry or cider vinegar

½ cup (110 g) brown cane sugar or honey

¼-inch (0.6 cm) piece of fresh ginger

Zest of half a lemon

1 cinnamon stick

1 allspice berry or a small pinch of allspice

1 clove

FOR THE KIDNEYS

2 veal (or beef) kidneys

Sea salt and pepper to taste, or a sea salt and *piment d'Espelette* mixture

4 ounces (115 g) chestnut flour

3 tablespoons sesame seeds

2 tablespoons tallow or olive oil

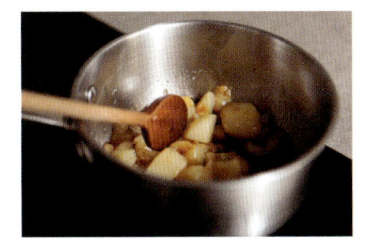

Place all the ingredients for the sauce except the pears into a saucepan over medium-high heat; bring to a brief boil. Reduce the heat, and simmer on low for 15 minutes. Add the pears, and allow to cook for 20 minutes, stirring occasionally until the pears are tender but not falling apart. Refrigerate for 12 hours or overnight to "pickle" them. Remove the pears from the liquid if it is very runny, otherwise leave them in the "syrup." Allow them to reach room temperature before serving, or reheat them, if desired.

Season the kidneys with the salt and pepper, roll them in the chestnut flour (photo A), and sprinkle on the sesame seeds (photo B). Or add the sesame seeds once the kidneys are in the pan. Melt the tallow in a pan over medium heat, and cook both sides of the kidneys for about seven minutes on each side until cooked through, but still a bit rosy on the inside.

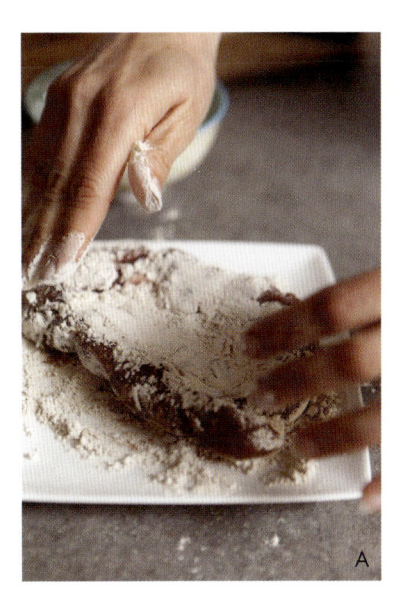

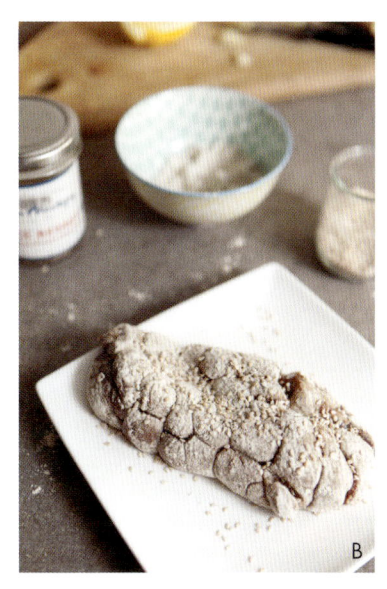

Cut the kidneys into slices if desired, or leave whole and serve them alongside the room-temperature pickled pears.

VARIATIONS The basic preparation of the veal kidneys, minus the sesame seeds, may be done while also adding a tablespoonful of **Old-Fashioned Mustard** (page 410), as in the recipe for **Lamb Kidneys with Old-Fashioned Mustard** (page 252).

WINE PAIRING TIP To complement the ginger, pickled pears, and sesame in this recipe, sommelière Annabelle recommends a vivacious, dry, and lightly fruity white wine, such as one from the Jura region of France. To play up the allspice, cinnamon, and clove, try pairing this dish with a sweet white wine, such as a Barsac or Sauternes from Bordeaux or a Jurançon from the Pyrénées.

VEAL LIVER
Foie de Veau

Season Year-round **Preparation Time** None
Cooking Time 10 to 12 minutes **Serves** 1 to 2

Liver is perhaps the most nutrient-dense food we can consume; liver from a healthy, grass-fed, grass-finished animal, that is. This classic French recipe, combined with **French Green Peas** (page 450), comes from a grandmother named Gaby, a native of the Bordeaux area. She is the paternal grandmother of my ever-patient friend Chef Frédéric, who demonstrated these recipes for me in my kitchen in Bordeaux. Chef Fréd worked in several well-known Parisian restaurants before returning to his native region of Bordeaux about 12 years ago. He was teaching cooking lessons at *Ateliers des Chefs* in Bordeaux when I met him, and now he has a thriving food truck business of his own, "Truck de Chef." This recipe may be paired with other seasonal vegetables of your choice instead of peas. I love to pair it with a slice of lard-soaked baked sweet potato. The recipe employs a particular famous red wine vinegar (*vinaigre de Banyuls*) from France's southern region of Roussillon, a sweet wine made primarily from the Grenache Noir grape, offering a heady sweet flavor to the vinegar.

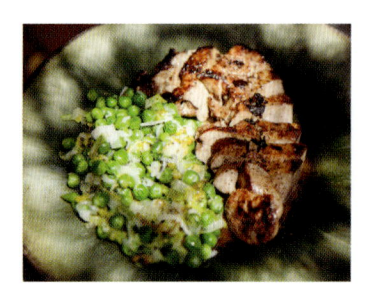

1 tablespoon butter

1 thick piece of veal liver

Fine sea salt

Red wine vinegar

Melt the butter in a pan over medium-high heat. Salt one side of the liver and place it salt-side down in the pan. Sprinkle salt on the side facing up. After a few minutes when the bottom has browned, turn the liver over. Baste the liver several times with the melted butter using a spoon to keep the butter from burning, and continue to cook on the second side for several minutes.

Remove the liver from the pan if you prefer it less cooked, or allow it to continue cooking for several minutes. Once the liver is cooked through, transfer it to a plate and cut it into several slices. Add the vinegar to the pan to create a sauce. Spoon this sauce onto the sliced pieces of liver and serve hot, next to the green peas, baked sweet potato slice, or other seasonal vegetables.

VARIATIONS For extra fat, top the liver with extra butter, ghee, duck fat, or lard, and garnish with fleur de sel. I tend to cut veal liver in thin slices before cooking, to make sure it is cooked through. And I also reduce the heat from medium-high to medium after the initial sear in the pan on the first side to avoid burning the delicate veal. I also tend to use more fat in which to sauté the liver. I usually cook veal liver in coconut oil without vinegar, as I like the mild coconut flavor. Duck fat turns out to be an excellent fat as well in which to cook veal liver. Try sprinkling a handful of **Grilled Pine Nuts** (page 50) over the liver for a bit of salty crunch. In the photo shown here, alongside the liver I have sautéed shallots, which add a bit of sweetness to the dish.

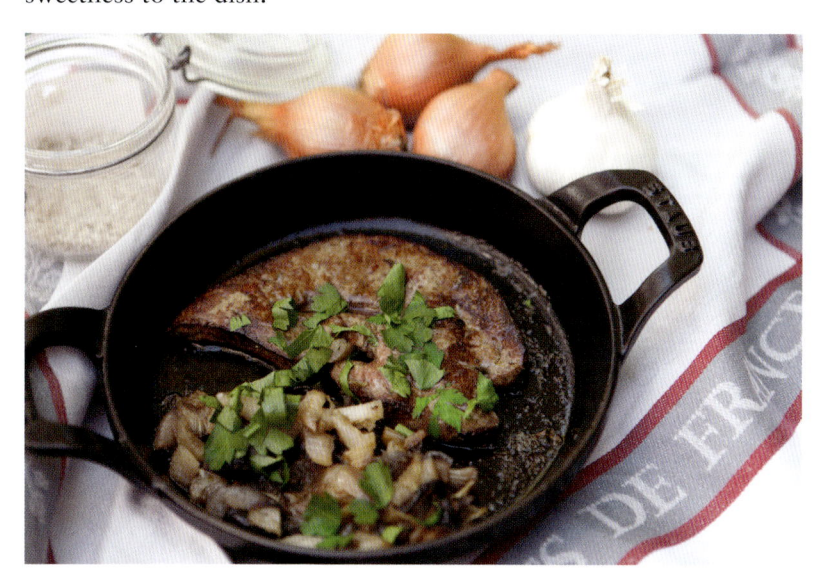

WINE PAIRING TIP I have had veal liver cooked in tallow and duck fat paired with an organic and fruity Côtes du Rhône. Whether you cook the veal liver in butter and vinegar or in coconut oil, restaurateur Annabelle recommends red wines that are rounded and fruity, with well-blended, soft tannins such as an aromatic, medium-bodied Marcillac from the French Southwest made from the Basque Fer Savadou grape and offering notes of pepper and red fruits; a delicately floral Bordeaux Clairet; an elegant Pinot Noir from Chambolle-Musigny in Northern Burgundy's Côte de Nuits, with notes of red fruits when young and notes of prune, truffle, or undergrowth when aged; a leathery and spiced Languedoc made from a blend of Grenache, Mourvèdre, and Syrah grapes; or a warming, earthy Tavel rosé, with notes of almonds and stone fruits.

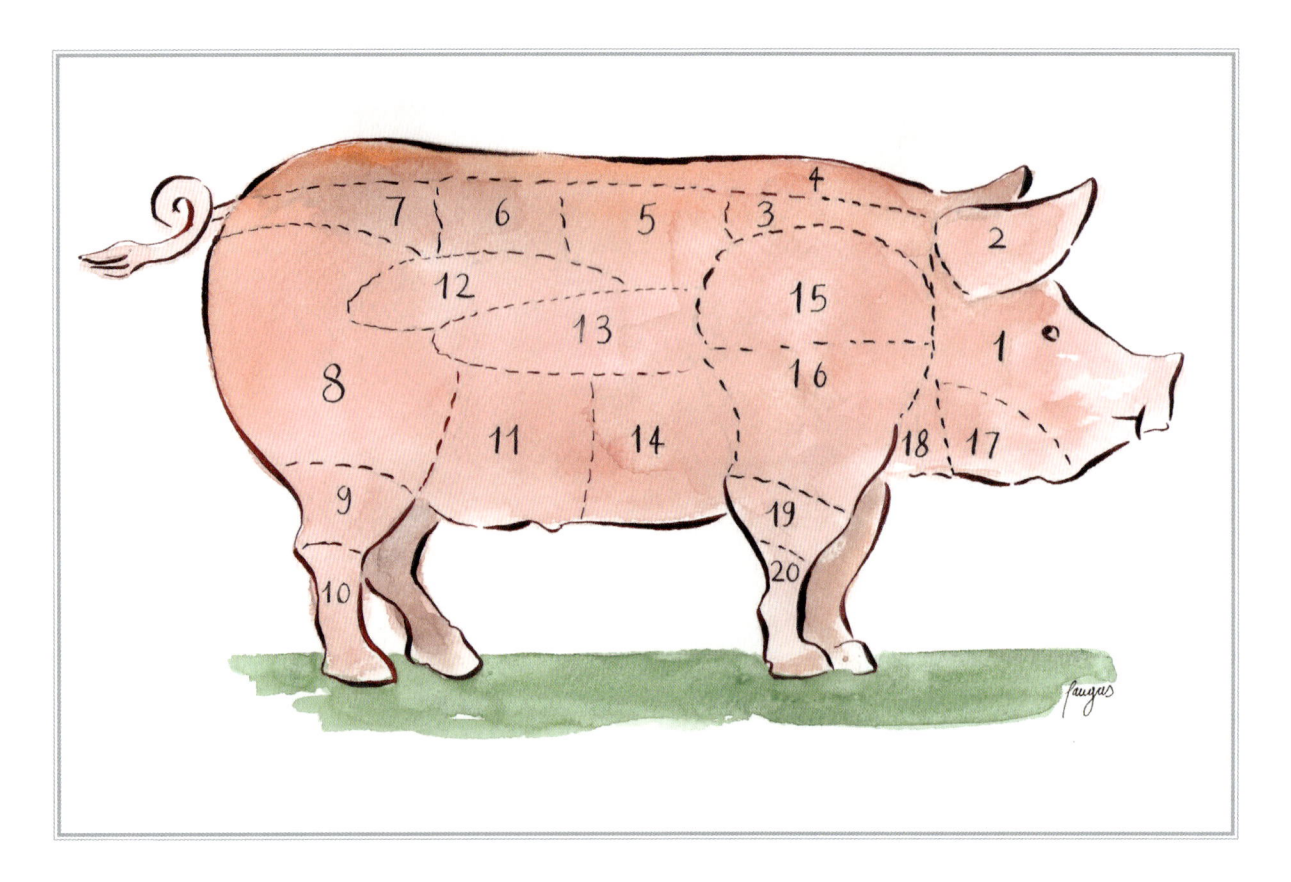

PORK – L'PORC
DIAGRAM KEY

1. Head – *Tête* (Use: Stew)
2. Ear – *Oreille* (Use: Sauté, Stew)
3. Shoulder – *Échine* (Use: Ground, Roast, Stew, Terrine)
4. Back Fat or Fat Back – *Bardière* or *Lard* (Use: Render)
5. Rib Rack – *Carré de Côtes* (Use: Boneless Roast Chops, Cutlets, Rack Roast)
6. Loin Rack – *Carré Filet* (Use: Boneless Roast, Chops, Cutlets, Rack Roast)
7. Saddle – *Pointe de Filet* (Use: Roast, Stew)
8. Ham – *Jambon* (Use: Cure, Cutlets, Roast, Sauté)
9. Hind Shank – *Jambonneau Arrière* or *Jarret Arrière* (Use: Stew)
10. Trotter (Pig's Foot) – *Pied* (Use: Stew)
11. Belly – *Poitrine* (Use: Bacon, Ribs, Roast, Stew)
12. Tenderloin – *Filet Mignon* (Use: Roast, Stew)
13. Spare Ribs – *Travers* (Use: Ribs, Rack Roast)
14. Fore Flank or Fore Ribs – *Plat de Côtes* (Use: Ribs)
15. Boston Butt or Shoulder Butt or Upper Shoulder – *Palette* (Use: Roast, Stew)
16. Picnic Ham or Lower Shoulder – *Épaule* (Use: Ground, Roast)
17. Cheek or Jowel – *Joue* (Use: Stew)
18. Neck – *Gorge* (Use: Terrine)
19. Fore Shank – *Jambonneau Avant* or *Jarret Avant* (Use: Stew)
20. Trotter (Pig's Foot) – *Pied* (Use: Stew)

PORK
Le Porc

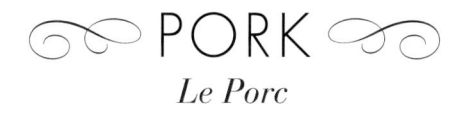

Bacon-Wrapped Prunes – *Pruneaux au Lard Fumé* 287

Basque Grandmother's Pâté – *Pâté d'Amatxi* 288

Honey-Glazed Pork Belly – *Poitrine de Porc Laquée* 290

Oven Bacon Strips – *Tranches de Poitrine Fumée au Four* 292

Pan-Fried Smoked Pork – *Bacon Fumé à la Poêle* 293

Pork Belly Pâté – *Pâté de la Carbonnade de Porc* 294

Pork Knuckle with Sauerkraut – *Jarret de Porc à la Choucroute* 297

Pork Loin Wrapped in Country Ham – *Filet Mignon au Jambon de Pays* 299

Pork Meatballs – *Boulettes au Porc* 301

Pork Roast with Herbes de Provence – *Rôti de Porc aux Herbes de Provence* 305

Pork Roast Stuffed with Prunes and Tied – *Rôti de Porc aux Pruneaux à la Ficelle* 308

Pork Shoulder Cooked in Fat – *Confit de Porc Échine* 311

Pyrénées Country Pâté – *Terrine de Campagne des Pyrénées* 314

Rack of Pork in Crusted Salt, Ginger, and Garlic – *Carré de Cochon en Croûte de Sel, Gingimbre et à l'Ail* 317

Rosemary Pork Ribs – *Coustellous au Romarin* 319

Salted Pork with Lentils – *Petit Salé aux Lentilles* 321

Sautéed Pork with Prunes – *Sauté de Porc aux Pruneaux* 324

Stuffed Cabbage Leaves – *Feuilles de Chou Farcies* 326

Morning Sausage Patties 327

Stuffed Whole Cabbage – *Chou Farci Entier* 328

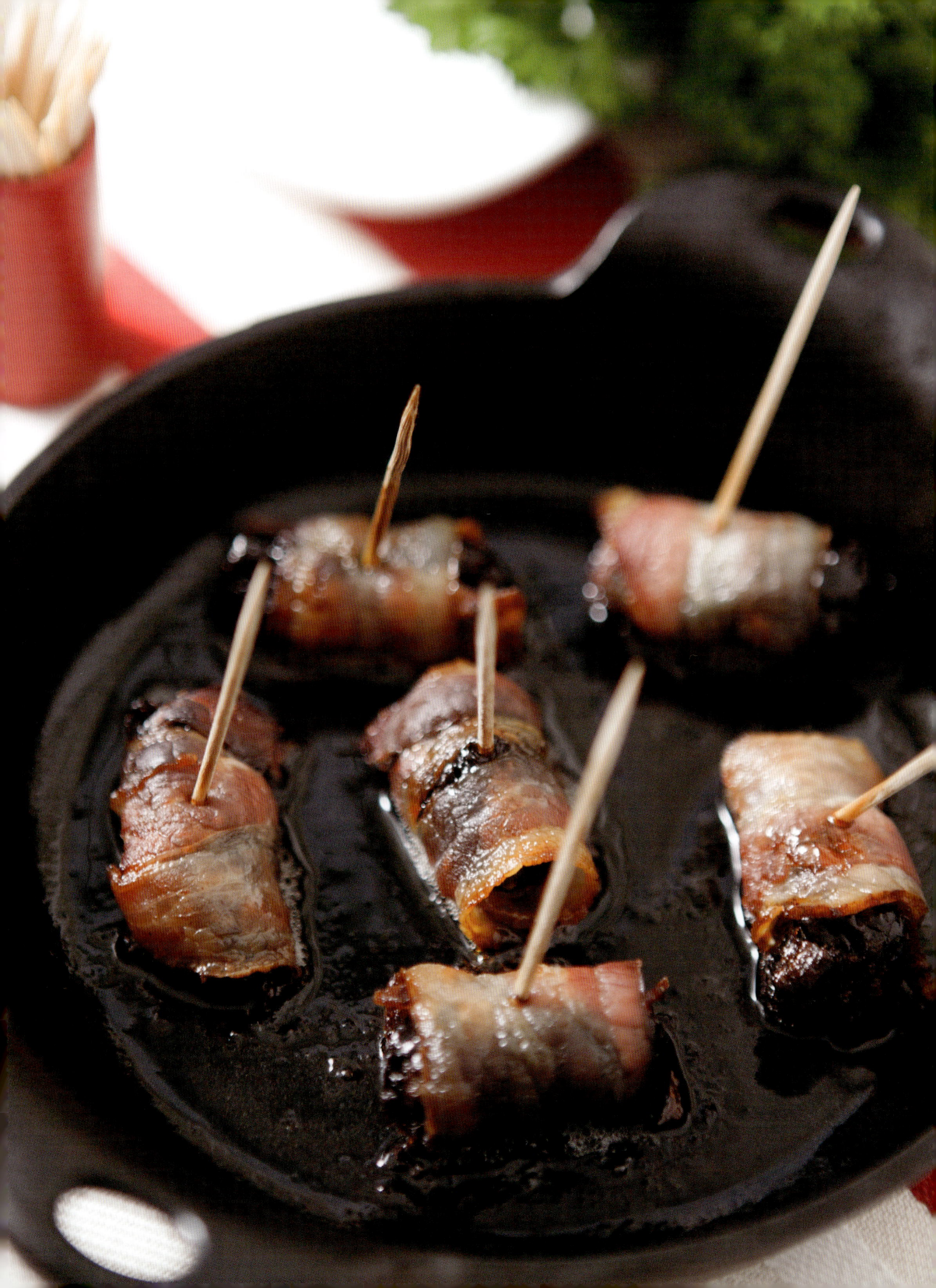

BACON-WRAPPED PRUNES
Pruneaux au Lard Fumé

Season Prunes (dried plums) are available year-round   **Preparation Time** 5 minutes   **Cooking Time** 10 minutes   **Serves** 4 to 5

This was the first appetizer served at the first apéritif we attended after moving to Bordeaux. It was in Saint Emilion at Château Guadet, the home of Guy-Pétrus and Catherine Lignac, with whom I would later make the famous traditional French dish **Braised Veal Stew – *Blanquette de Veau*** (page 422). France's prune capital happens to be in the Southwest around the town of Agen. *Pruneaux d'Agen* are plump, juicy, and reputable. In and around the town of Agen, prunes are dried, remoistened, and even stuffed in a variety of ways. People are plumb crazy about Agen prunes! The combination of prune and bacon is almost too good. It's a match made in heaven, and it's so easy to prepare. But watch out, they are also easy to overeat. This recipe really is best as an appetizer (*amuse-bouche*), or else dessert (and though that would not be very French, the French, being so accommodating, would probably forgive you for your deviation in etiquette).

6 Strips bacon

12 Prunes

12 toothpicks

Preheat the oven to 356°F (180°C). Cut bacon strips in half to make 12 pieces of equal length. Wrap each piece around a prune, place in a casserole dish, and secure with a toothpick.

Heat in the oven for 10 minutes, or until the bacon is golden brown, and serve immediately.

> **WINE PAIRING TIP** At Château Guadet, we had our prunes and bacon with the house wine, a Merlot-dominated, organic Château Guadet. You could also try similar medium-tannic Bordeaux Right Bank wines from Blaye, Bourg, Fronsac, St. Emilion, Castillon, Pomerol, or else a white Pinot Gris from Alsace, with notes of pear, apple, lemon-lime, or stone fruit, or sip on a vanilla-spiced Armagnac (lower in alcohol than its cousin, Cognac) from Gascony (the name of the region south and east of Bordeaux called by this name up until the French Revolution and sometimes still used today). A sparkling wine is always welcome with appetizers. Otherwise, go crazy with the matching pruney notes of a Southwest Cahors, made from Malbec grapes (also known as Côt), or else a full-bodied Banyuls sweet red wine with notes of baked prune and spiced fruit from Languedoc. Continue with these wines if going on to the next course, which could be beef or lamb, for example.

BASQUE GRANDMOTHER'S PÂTÉ
Pâté d'Amatxi

Season Year-round **Preparation Time** 60 minutes
Cooking Time 30 minutes **Makes** about 4 pounds (2 kg) of pâté

My friend, the butcher-chef-charcutier Florent Carriquiry, was born in Bayonne and grew up deep in Basque country at the foot of the Pyrénées. His paternal grandmother, Maria, still lives in the Basque countryside. This is Maria's pâté recipe, a living testament to authentic Basque cooking. We modified the recipe to remove the wheat in the form of bread by leaving out the bread entirely and adding an egg, and wheat in the form of flour by replacing it with chestnut flour and doubling the quantity of the flour. It is difficult to "deface" original recipes that have been handed down, but in certain cases, one can modify and achieve a tasty result that gives homage to the spirit of the original recipe. The quantity in this recipe fills about 3 or 4 pâté receptacles (*terrines*) that are about the size of a loaf of bread. (*Terrine* is also the name for a chunkier style of pâté.) You can easily cut the recipe in half, but I prefer to make more and then freeze half for a time when I need it. Pâtés are usually served cold and may be served year-round. They are usually a refreshing first course (*entrée*), but they can be eaten at any mealtime as the main dish (*plat*).

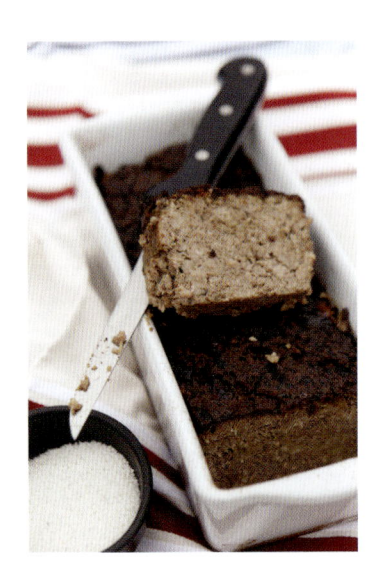

2 tablespoons duck fat

1 tablespoon sea salt

5 ounces (150 g) shallots, minced

14 ounces (400 g) chicken livers, cut in quarters

2 pounds (900 g) fresh pork belly, cubed

3 eggs

3 tablespoons or 2 ounces (60 g) chestnut flour

½ teaspoon ground white pepper (*poivre blanc moulu*)

¼ teaspoon *piment d'Espelette*

1 teaspoon powdered garlic (*ail poudré*) or fresh garlic, ground to a paste

¼ teaspoon ground nutmeg (*muscade*)

Half a bunch of parsley, stems removed, leaves minced

⅓ cup (75 g) pear brandy (*eau de vie de poire*) or white wine

⅝ cup (150 g) milk

Optional: Chilled bone broth gelatin

Preheat the oven to 395°F (200°C). Heat the duck fat in a frying pan over medium-high. Add salt, shallots, and livers, stir once, then allow the ingredients to caramelize and brown in the pan for 10 to 15 minutes over medium heat, stirring only once or twice more during that time.

Meanwhile, run the pork belly through a food processor to obtain a mousse-like texture. In a large bowl, using a wooden spoon, mix the pork belly, eggs, flour, and spices.

Return to the frying pan after 10 to 15 minutes to stir in the parsley. Add the brandy and use a wooden spoon to scrape (*déglacer*) the sugars and proteins stuck to the pan into a medium-sized bowl. Allow the liver mixture to cool, and then run it through the food processor, along with the milk, for a mousse-like texture.

Add the liver mixture to the bowl containing the pork belly mixture and stir together with a wooden spoon. Fill molds with the combined pâté mixture, flattening the top to remove air bubbles inside the mixture. Place the molds onto a tray with high edges into the oven and add room temperature (or hot) water to the tray, without getting water into the molds. This method is called a *bain-marie*, which allows the water to heat the molds but keeps the pâté mixture from getting too hot as it cooks in the molds in the oven.

After 30 minutes, turn the temperature down to 320°F (160°C) and allow to cook for one more hour.

Remove the molds from the tray in the oven carefully and allow them to cool. If desired, smooth chilled bone broth gelatin over the molds while they are still warm, or else heated bone broth if the molds have cooled off, in order to help preserve the untouched pâté for a longer period of time. The pâté will last 10 to 15 days in the refrigerator. Freeze what you will not consume within that time, though be aware that this will change the taste and texture slightly. To me, the convenience of having an extra portion ready when needed in the freezer overrides these minor changes. You can also cut the pâté into individual portions for freezing and thawing as needed. This is especially helpful for those who eat small portions or who have histamine intolerance and are required to freeze rather than refrigerate their leftovers.

Serve with raw vegetables, **Oven-Baked Beet Chips** (page 457) or other roasted veggie chips, or with **Seedy Crackers** (page 501) or other homemade grain-free crackers or grain-free flat-bread.

> WINE PAIRING TIP An accompanying sip or two of the same pear brandy is a possible choice, whereby the ingredient is also the drink, or else a regional pairing from the Basque country, such as a Txakoli, a white wine with low alcohol content but crisp acidity and "almost sparkling" qualities from the Spanish side of the Basque country. Or else try a white Irouléguy from the French side of Basque country, with notes of tropical fruits and refreshing acidity, or else a fruity but tannic red Irouléguy, preferably one that has aged several years, having allowed for the tannins to settle down.

Chef's Tip
Astuce du Chef

You can also sauté the livers whole, but cutting them into smaller cubes augments the surface of contact with the pan during cooking, which in turn increases the caramelization, or browning of the sugars, and the Maillard reaction, the browning of amino acids in the ingredients as they cook, which means a sweeter, more complex taste to the finished product.

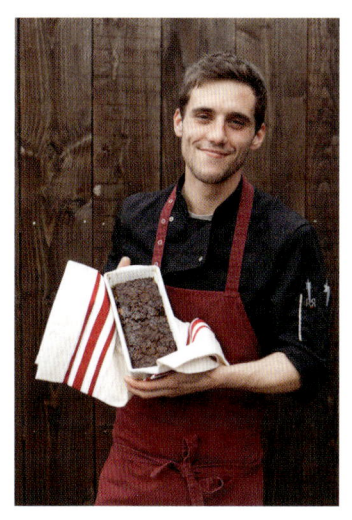

Florent Carriquiry

HONEY-GLAZED PORK BELLY
Poitrine de Porc Laquée

Season Year-round   **Preparation Time** 30 minutes
Cooking Time 45 minutes   **Serves** 6

This recipe was inspired by one of my favorite French cookbooks, *Viandes*, by Jean-François Mallet, who is both a chef and photographer. I have modified the recipe, replacing and adding ingredients, but the basic idea is there for a sweet-and-sour style pork. This recipe is the only one in this book using tamari (Japanese fermented soy sauce) as an ingredient. It is difficult find non-GMO soy products these days, but organic, gluten-free tamari sauce made from non-GMO soybeans is available if you search for it. It adds "umami," savory flavorful delight, to the dish.

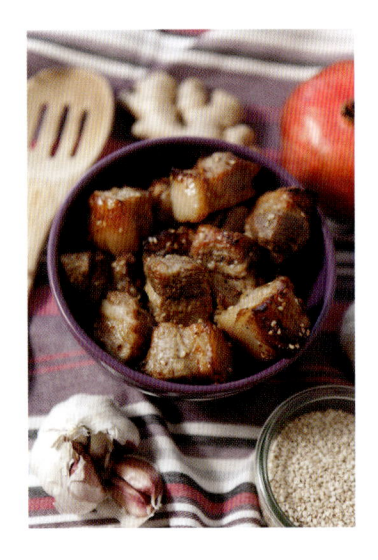

1.8 to 2 pounds (800 to 900 g) pork belly, chopped into 2- to 3-inch (5 to 7.5 cm) cubes

¼ teaspoon allspice

¼ teaspoon coriander

1 tablespoon freshly grated ginger

1 tablespoon garlic, minced

2 pinches of coarse sea salt (*gros sel de mer*)

2 tablespoons olive oil (or sesame oil)

1 teaspoon apple cider vinegar

1 tablespoon tamari

2 tablespoons raw honey

2 tablespoons sesame seeds

2 pinches of ground pepper

Reminder: A pinch (*une pincée*) is using three fingers! For fine salt, pepper, and spices, this turns out to be slightly less than ⅛ teaspoon (0.5 ml). For coarse salt, it's slightly more.

Mix together all the ingredients, including the pork, in a large bowl. Allow the meat to marinate in the refrigerator for an hour or two, or overnight if you have the time.

Preheat the oven to 350°F (175°C). Remove the meat from the refrigerator 20 minutes prior to cooking to allow it to come to room temperature for even cooking. Arrange the pieces in one layer in a large casserole dish and place into the oven for 45 minutes, stirring every 15 minutes to keep the top edges of the pieces of meat from burning and to cook the meat evenly.

VARIATIONS The honey in this dish is a key ingredient, but it can be replaced with smaller amounts of monk fruit or stevia for those with very sensitive blood-sugar responses. Actually, the honey (or sweetener), and the vinegar, can be left entirely out of the dish, and it still tastes great! Unprocessed, raw honey is one of France's most magnificent products and can be found at markets, *épiceries* (gourmet shops), and organic stores. It comes in many varieties, each of which is delicious in its own way. In this dish, the subtle honey flavors are overtaken by the tamari and vinegar, but the sweetness remains. If histamine intolerance is an issue, then you can replace the raw honey with pasteurized honey or maple syrup, replace the vinegar with half the amount of lemon or lime juice, and augment the salt to your tastes if removing the tamari sauce. If you end up with extra sauce in the casserole dish, use the sauce the next time you sauté a piece of beef or veal liver. The sauce will upgrade the taste of the liver and help you finish up that delicious sauce!

WINE PAIRING TIP I have had this dish with a young, fruity red Saumur-Champigny from the central part of the Loire Valley, made predominantly with Cabernet Franc, which gives fruity aromas while not being too tannic, and is medium-bodied to go with the sweetly flavored and ginger-infused pork. It is a sheer delight when you find a good pairing, and this was one of those times! My wine course classmate and organic wine aficionado, Vy Nguyen, suggests a light or medium-bodied red wine from the Loire or Burgundy so as to not overpower the flavors in the recipe. More specifically, she recommends an easy-to-drink, organic red Côtes de Bourg from the Bordeaux region made by Château Grand Launey. Similarly, my DUAD wine course classmate and former restaurant owner and cellar master Annabelle Nicolle-Beaufils suggests pairing this pork dish with low-tannic rosés: a Côtes de Roussillon from Languedoc-Roussillon or a Tavel from southern Rhône, said to have been a favorite of French monarch Louis XIV, the "Sun King," who made his home at the Palace of Versailles outside Paris in the late 1600s.

OVEN BACON STRIPS
Tranches de Poitrine Fumée au Four

Season Every season is the season for bacon! **Preparation Time** None
Cooking Time 9 to 14 minutes **Serves** 4

Who doesn't love bacon? As long as it is in stock in my refrigerator, I serve it almost every morning for breakfast. My children used to call it "ba-*gone*," because it is usually gone before I can get any. (Now it's *not cool* anymore to call it that.) But we do still eat bacon on most mornings.

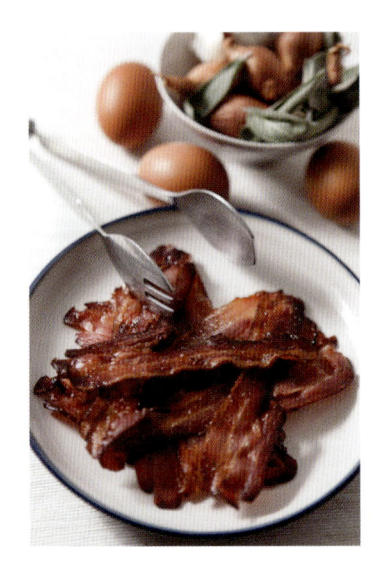

8 to 12 Strips of bacon (12 thin strips of bacon weigh about 5 ounces or 150 g)

Preheat the oven to 365°F (185°C). Lay strips of bacon in a rectangular glass pan or a tray and place in the oven. Check at the 9-minute mark for "doneness." (The lower the sides of your baking tray or dish, the more evenly and potentially more quickly the bacon will cook.) Leave in a few minutes longer if you like browner bacon. Serve with eggs or really anything, any time of day!

WINE PAIRING TIP Try a fruit-forward Beaujolais, a light-bodied Gamay from the Loire, or a rosé from Bordeaux, Languedoc-Roussillon or Provence. One in particular, recommended by my organic wine connoisseur friend and wine tasting instructor, Vy Nguyen, would be the fleshy, red-fruity organic rosé "L du Château Lavergne Dulong." None of these wines will overpower the pork with high acidity or tannins, but rather support its flavors.

I often poach eggs and then pour the warm bacon grease over my eggs for added fat. Otherwise, using a spatula to scrape it out once the pan has cooled, I save the bacon fat in a dedicated dish for use on sweet potatoes or any vegetable or meat that needs an extra splash of fat and flavor.

PAN-FRIED SMOKED PORK
Bacon Fumé à la Poêle

Season Year-round   **Preparation Time** None
Cooking Time 2 Minutes   **Serves** 4

Bacon Fumé is what we call Canadian (or Canadian-style) bacon in the U.S., a smoked (or sometimes "uncured") ham from the loin (*côtes filet*). I serve this as an alternative breakfast meat every now and then when we run out of regular bacon. This cut comes from the loin section (*carré côtes* or *côtes filet*) of the pig.

8 slices Canadian bacon or smoked pork

1 teaspoon lard or bacon fat

Melt the fat in a large skillet, add the bacon slices, turning after one minute. Cook one minute on the other side. Serve with eggs, vegetables, salad, bone broth, or more bacon!

> **WINE PAIRING TIP** If you are looking for a wine pairing with this for breakfast, then you should book your trip to France sooner than you had planned. I don't have alcohol with breakfast, but Champagne is what comes to mind for this recipe. If you are having this dish for lunch, then try an Alsatian Pinot Gris, with notes of apricot, beeswax, dried fruit, and smoke, or a floral and peachy Pinot Blanc, also from Alsace.

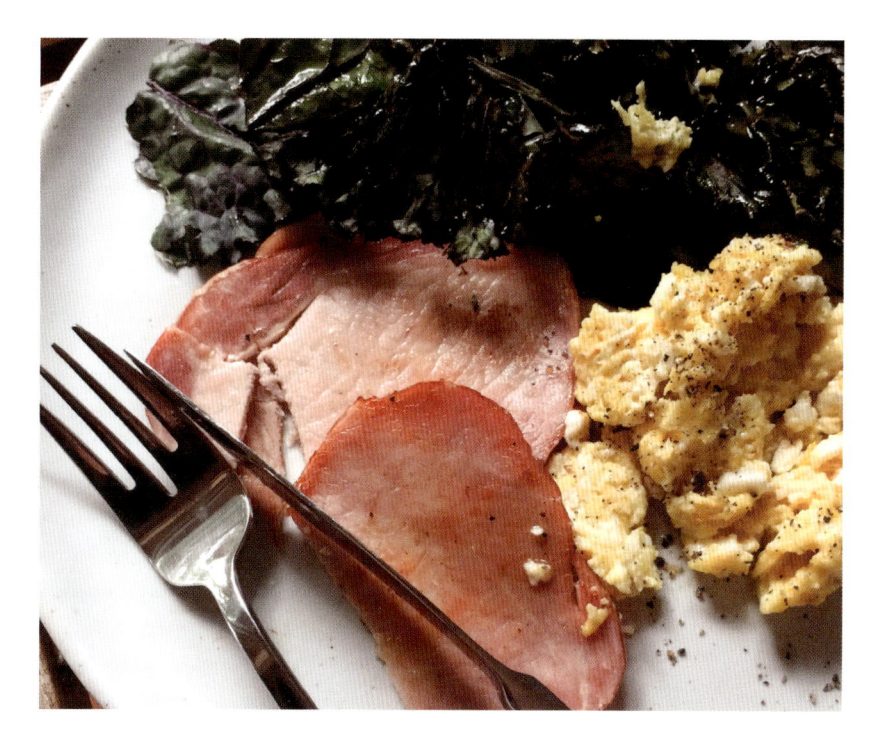

PORK BELLY PÂTÉ
Pâté de la Carbonnade de Porc

Season Year-round   **Preparation Time** 25 minutes
Cooking Time 1 hour and 20 to 30 minutes   **Serves** 6

This is my attempt at a pâté including liver but excluding dairy, as much as I love cream. If you have pork belly and are not making bacon out of it, then a pâté is a good next choice for this fatty cut of pork. (Or else try **Honey Glazed Pork Belly**, page 290.) The word "carbonnade" comes from *charbonné*, an old word for "cooked over carbon" (*le charbon*), a process we now call grilling, *griller*. Pork belly was often considered grill meat, and therefore was called *la carbonnade* when grilled. Other names are *levure* or *grillade*, but the overall butchery term for this part of the pig is *poitrine*, which we call pork "belly." The chicken livers add flavor and density to the pâté, while the eggs help bind the pâté.

1.1 pounds (500 g) chicken livers (*foies de volailles*)

1.2 pounds (550 g) pork belly, cut in chunks

2 ounces or ⅓ cup (50 g) shallots (about 3 medium-sized shallots), minced

A little less than 1 ounce, (20 g) spring or green onion, finely chopped

½ ounce (18 g) parsley, minced

1 teaspoon pepper

2 teaspoons fine sea salt

¼ cup dry white wine (see wine pairing tip below)

2 eggs, whisked together

1 tablespoon thyme

Lard or ghee (for greasing the jars)

Coarse sea salt, for garnish

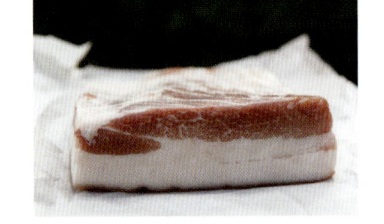

Raw Pork Belly

Grind the livers, pork belly, shallots, green onion, and parsley together in batches in a food processor, then mix together well with a wooden spatula in a large bowl with the remaining ingredients.

Grease the jars or receptacles (*terrines*) for your pâté with lard or ghee. Fill them ¾ of the way with the liver and pork mixture. You can cook the jars of pâté either at 340°F (170°C) for about 55 minutes covered (check with a thermometer that the middle of the pâté has reached 175°F – 80°C), or else, in a bain-marie (pour hot or boiling water into a tray larger than the jars or receptacle to about ⅓ the height of the jars and cook uncovered at 375°F – 190°C) for 1 hour, then cover and continue to cook 20 to 30 minutes, especially if you are using one large receptacle. ▶

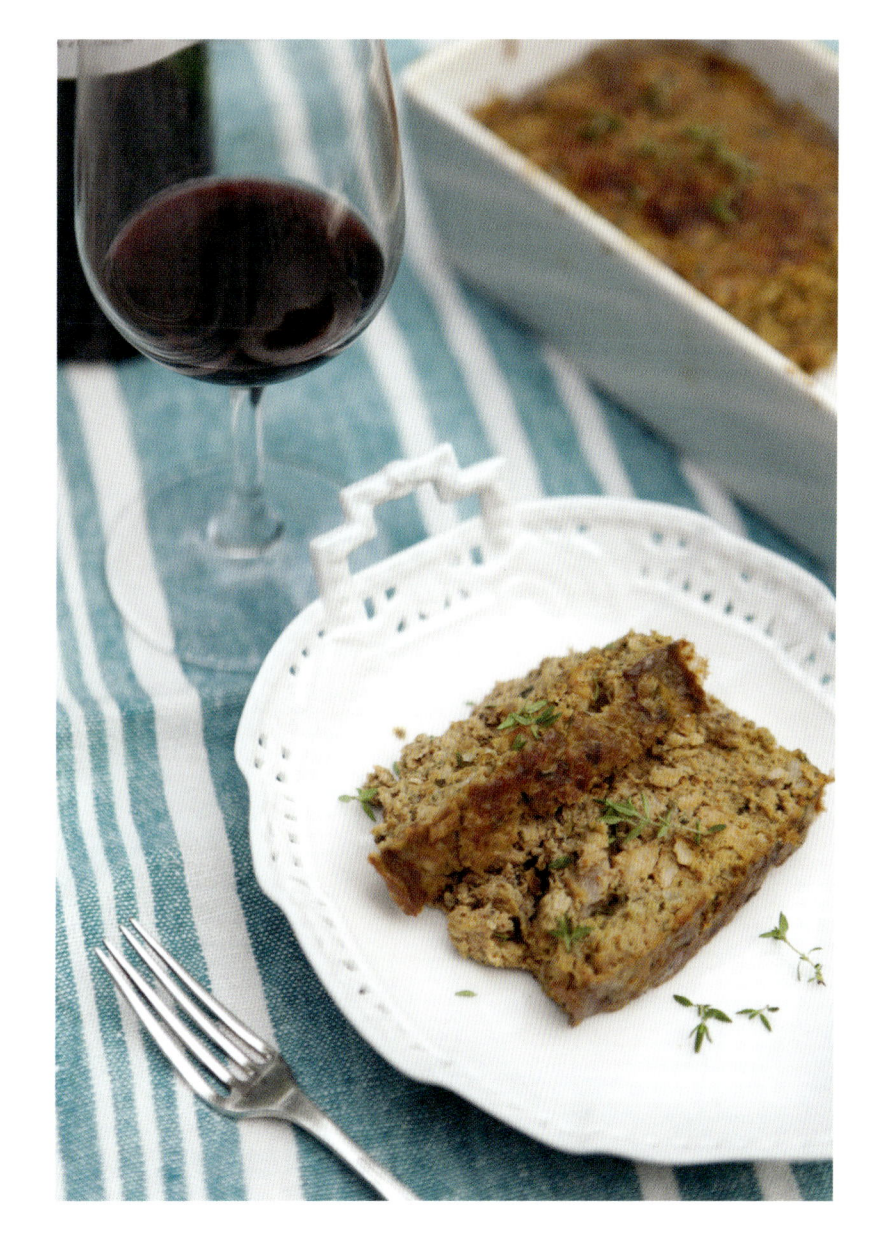

VARIATIONS If you are looking for a touch of sweetness, you can always try adding in several chopped dried figs or prunes during the food processor stage so that they are well incorporated into the mixture. You might also try adding ⅓ cup (75 ml) of Cognac or Armagnac.

Garnish with coarse sea salt. Serve on grain-free **Seedy Crackers** (page 501) or on **Oven-Baked Beet Chips** (page 457).

WINE PAIRING TIP With white wine as an ingredient, drink the rest of that wine, choosing perhaps a white Burgundy Chardonnay, a Bordeaux sweet wine, or a crisp Bordeaux Entre-Deux-Mers. Or else try a fruity majority-Merlot blend from Castillon – Côtes de Bordeaux, such as the organic and flavorful Colombre Peyrou from Château Peyrou, which I have paired with this pâté. Another option, neither all red nor all white, would be a rosé from Corsica, Languedoc-Roussillon or Provence.

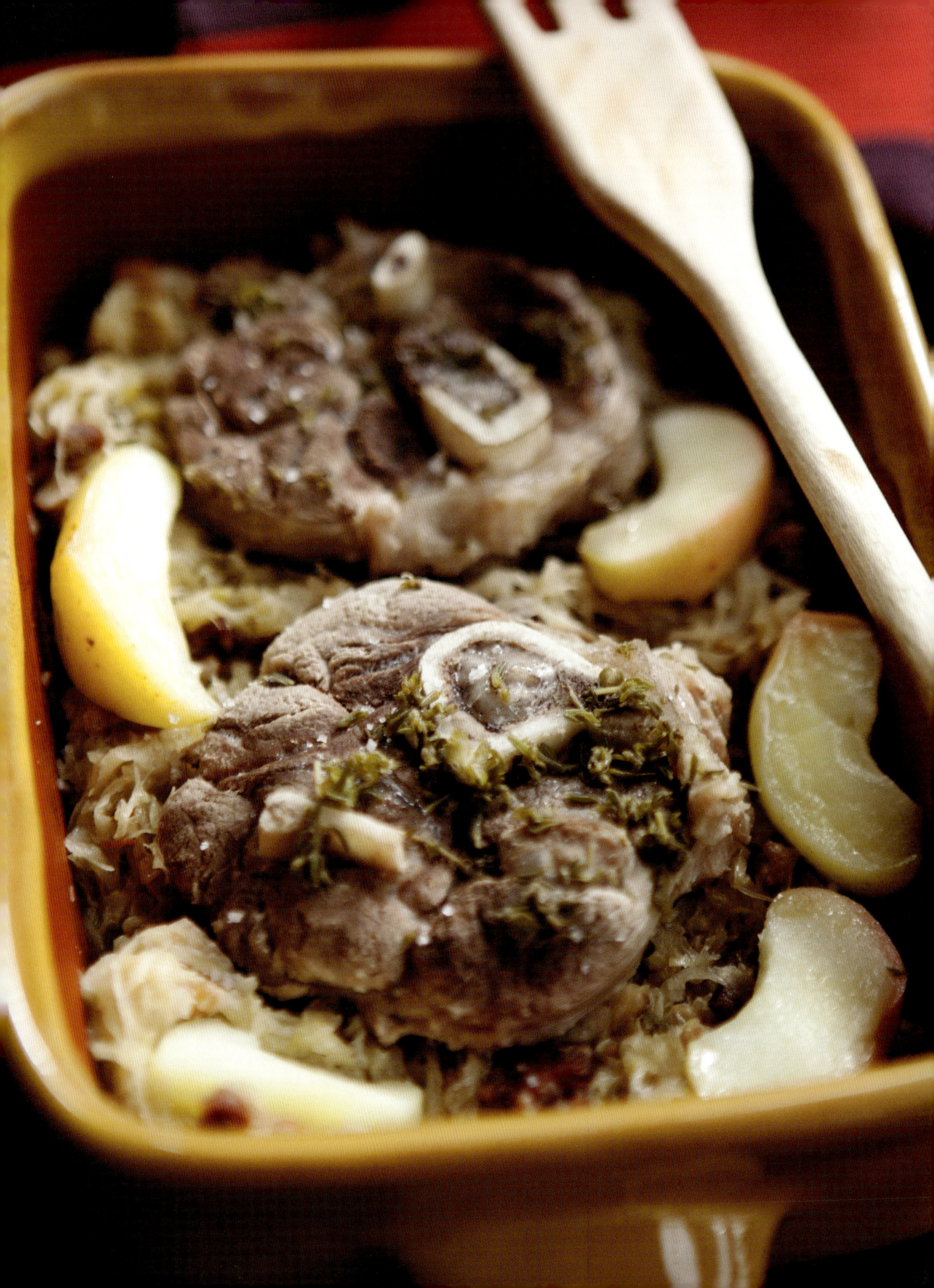

PORK KNUCKLE WITH SAUERKRAUT
Jarret de Porc à la Choucroute

Season Year-round, but usually Autumn, Winter, and Spring **Preparation Time** 5 minutes
Cooking Time 10 to 12 minutes for the apples and bacon bits, 45 minutes for the pork knuckle **Serves** 3 to 4

This is another recipe inspired by one of my favorite French cookbooks, *Viandes* by Jean-F Mallet. Again, I have swapped out certain ingredients and amounts, but this is a basic Alsatian-style recipe for pork and sauerkraut. What I do like about his recipe is Mallet's use of apples. I have reduced the number of apples to just enough to add some flavor to the dish. They can be omitted if desired, as can the walnuts, which I have added for flavor and texture. More options are listed under Variations. *Fleur de sel* is used in this and many recipes in *The Bordeaux Kitchen*. It is the top layer of salt in a sea salt bed, the "upper crust" of sea salt, which makes for a crunchy yet not too salty flavor as garnish for sweet and savory dishes. You may want to cook extra apple slices in butter to make a simple dessert everyone will love! Add cinnamon, delicious!

4 pork knuckles (*jarrets de porc*), about 1.5 pounds (680 g)

3 pinches of sea salt

2 bay leaves

2 sprigs of thyme

4 ounces (115 g) bacon pieces (*lardons*)

⅓ cup (50 g) butter (or ghee)

2 apples, peeled if desired, and sliced

½ cup (75 g) walnuts, chopped

2 cups (475 g) sauerkraut (raw if possible, to keep the enzymes and good bacteria intact)

4 pepper corns

4 juniper berries

Fleur de Sel, for garnish

Place the pork knuckles into a cast-iron pot, along with two pinches of salt, bay leaves, and thyme. Cover with hot water, allow to boil, then lower the heat to a simmer for 45 minutes.

Meanwhile, sauté the *lardons* in a small pan over medium-high heat until they are browned. Try not to eat them all right from the pan! Concurrently, melt butter in a large pan over medium heat, add apple slices. Add a pinch of salt, and stir them in the butter for 10 to 12 minutes. ▶

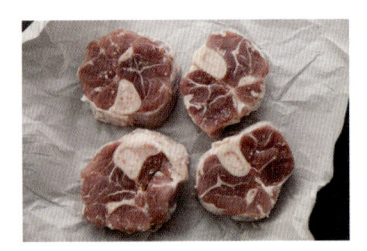

Raw Pork Knuckle

Remove the apples and set aside. Add the walnuts, stirring them into the butter remaining in the pan; allow them to sauté over medium heat for five minutes. Add sauerkraut, peppercorns, juniper berries, and *lardons*, and stir everything for a few minutes to heat them up.

Remove the pork knuckles from their pot. Keep the liquid for stock. Place each pork knuckle in a dish, add sauerkraut, and apples. Garnish with *Fleur de Sel*.

VARIATIONS For a true Alsatian *choucroute*, you could add a glass of Riesling or other dry Alsatian wine to the sauerkraut mixture as well as some pork rind or a handful of chopped smoked bacon (*lardons*) along with a variety of sausages from your local organic butcher, making sure they are fresh, without unwanted additives. Fry these up in lard or duck or goose fat in a separate pan until they are cooked through, and add them, along with any extra fat, to the heated sauerkraut along with the pork knuckle. This will increase the number of servings as well as the variety of flavors on your plate.

WINE PAIRING TIP My wine course classmate, sommelière, and former restaurateur Annabelle Nicolle-Beaufils suggests, and I concur, that the obvious pairing here would be a regional one: a citrusy, flinty, and floral Riesling, a peachy and floral Pinot Blanc, or a Sylvaner, with notes of citrus and cut grass, or other dry white wine from Alsace, where sauerkraut is a staple. Get ready to hook arms with your neighbor at the table and sing and sway with delight!

PORK LOIN WRAPPED IN COUNTRY HAM
Filet Mignon au Jambon de Pays

Season Year-round **Preparation Time** 10 to 15 minutes
Cooking Time 40 to 45 minutes **Serves** 4

This recipe was inspired by my apprenticeship at the butcher shop in Bordeaux as well as by one of my top two French cookbooks, *Viandes*, by Jean-Francois Mallet, a photographer and writer who interviewed a number of butchers for his book. Mallet uses country ham (*jambon de pays*), shown below, which is essentially dry-cured (*cru* or *sec*), as opposed to boiled ham (*cuit*), and he uses sage, which I have married with pork dishes as well—it is a delectable match. At the butcher's, I learned that you can decorate your pork with more pork! Besides *jambon de pays* (which also means cured ham "made in France," to distinguish it from other varieties cured in other countries, like *Coppa* from Corsica or Italy, *Prosciutto di Parma* from Italy, or *Jamón Serrano* from Spain), you can also employ the famous Southwest cured ham from the town of Bayonne, *Jambon de Bayonne*, or else *jambon cru*, *jambon sec*, or smoked bacon (*lard fumé*) or salt pork belly (*poitrine sèche*); so many choices! The main idea is that you are adding flavor, fat, and protection to the otherwise lean pork loin. The photo shows a pork loin cut into four pieces wrapped in *jambon de pays*, but not wrapped in butcher's string, though tying up the pieces is always an option that makes a fine presentation for guests.

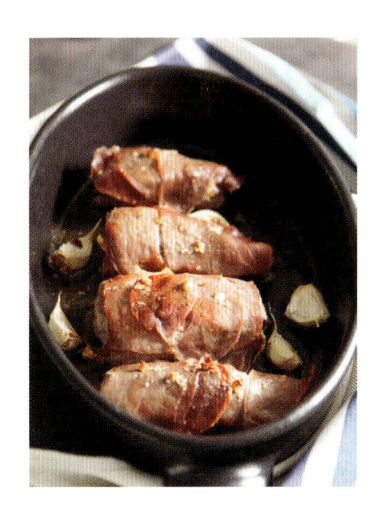

1.4 pounds (630 g) pork loin

4 to 6 sprigs of thyme

Pinch of *herbes de Provence*

4 to 6 slices of cured ham or 6 to 8 bacon strips, enough of either to cover entire pork loin

2 pinches of coarse sea salt

3 garlic cloves, minced, plus several unpeeled (*en chemise*) garlic cloves to roast in the pan

Optional: Olive oil for drizzling on top

Preheat the oven to 395°F (200°C). Lay the thyme sprigs lengthwise on the pork loin. Cut the loin into smaller pieces if you need to fit them into a particular pan, or leave it as one piece. Sprinkle the pork loin with the *herbes de Provence*. Place the cured ham slices or bacon strips next to each other along the pork loin crosswise. If you are so inclined, tie the ham to the pork loin using butcher's string. Sprinkle coarse sea salt and half of the minced garlic (and/or sage leaves or other herbs you might want to add) into an oven-safe pan. Lay the pork loin in the pan and sprinkle the remaining sea salt and minced garlic (and/or herbs) on top. At this point, you may wish to drizzle a bit of olive oil over the pork loin, for added flavor and fat. ▶

Place in the oven and, after 5 minutes, reduce the temperature to 365°F (185°C). Cook for 35 to 40 more minutes. Serve with roasted vegetables and/or potatoes.

VARIATIONS You can add potatoes to roast with the dish, or, as alluded to above, add 1 teaspoon dried or fresh minced rosemary, 2 to 3 sprigs of thyme, or 2 tablespoons sage leaves. If you adore butter, you can place small pats of butter on the pork loin before covering it with the ham or bacon. If you are in a hurry, you can cook the pork loin for only 20 minutes at 395°F (200°C), but preheat to 430°F (220°C) then turn down the heat immediately after placing the pork loin in the oven. Check with a thermometer after 20 minutes to make sure the internal temperature of the pork loin has reached about 170°F (77°C).

WINE PAIRING TIP If you are using *Jambon de Bayonne*, I would suggest going with a regional pairing from the Southwest, such as a white, slightly sparkling Basque Txakoli (pronounced TCHA-ko-lee), or a tangy white or even rosé Irouléguy (prounounced ee-ROO-lay-ghee), but try these wines even if you don't use *Jambon de Bayonne* for the sheer discovery of them! Try sommelière Annabelle's recommendation to pair this dish with fruity and "approachable" (not very tannic or structured) red or white wines, such as a red Graves from Bordeaux, a red from the Rhône Valley, a suave Pinot Noir from Alsace, with notes of dark berries, or a white Savannières, made from Chenin Blanc grapes in the Central Loire Valley, with notes of beeswax, chamomile, and straw.

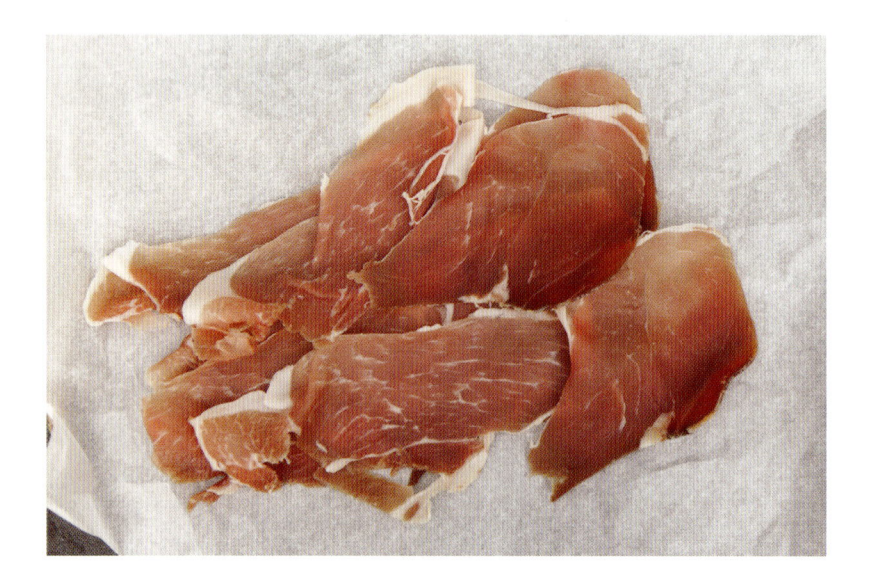

PORK MEATBALLS
Boulettes au Porc

Season Year-round **Preparation Time** 20 (more, depending on how many ingredients you add and need to prep) **Cooking Time** 30 minutes **Serves** 6

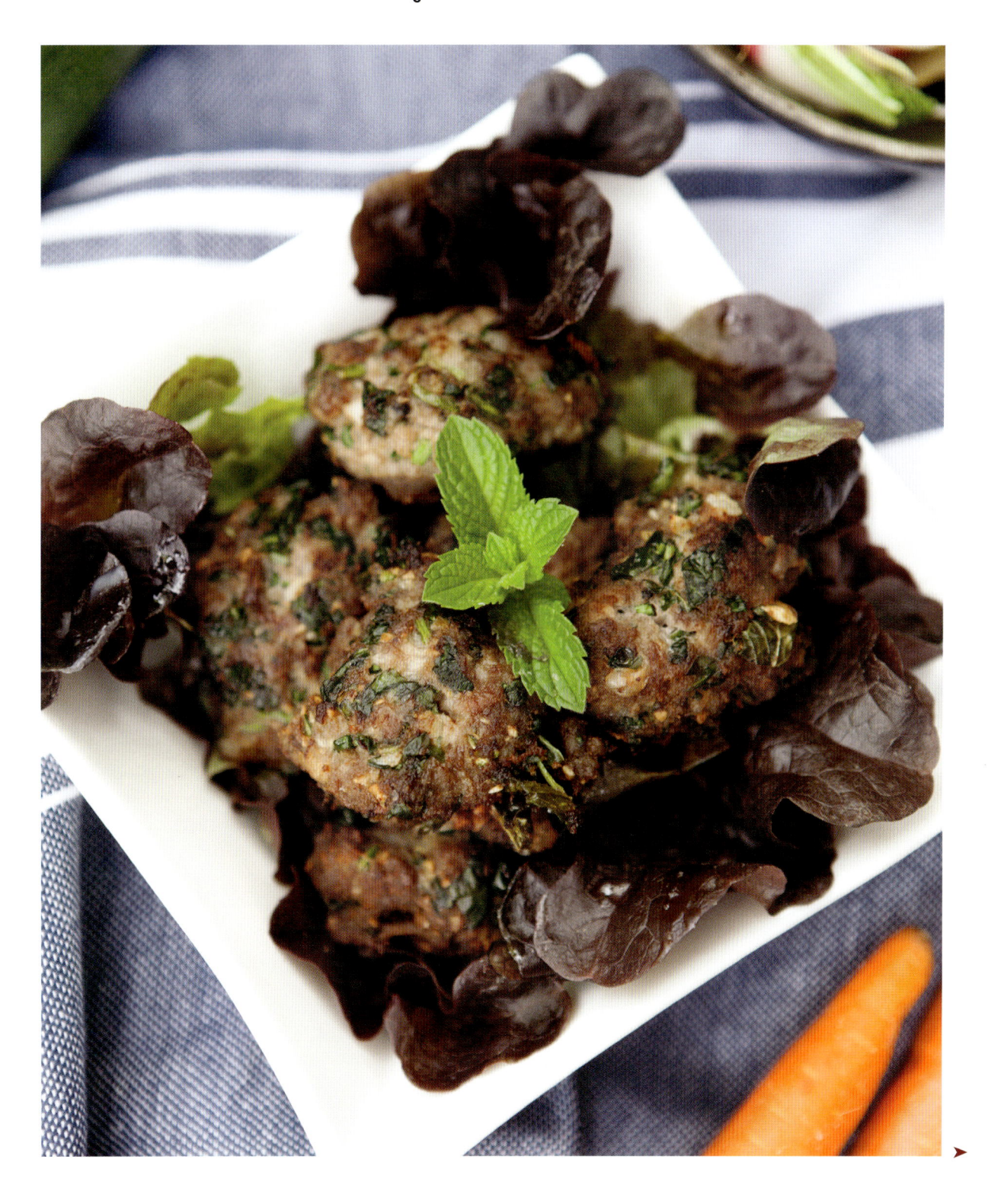

These are fun to make if you like to mix things, and children can help mix and make the meatballs. Everybody loves them, and they make a great appetizer (*amuse-bouche*) or first course (*entrée*). It's the kind of thing to which you can add your favorite ingredients. I make some plain for the kids and make the rest with whatever I have in the refrigerator. The trick is to use lots of fat so the *boulettes* stick less to the pan and soak up the fat, making them juicy, delicious, and nutrient dense. These meatballs are easy to make in large batches and then freeze for later for a quick snack or meal when you are in a pinch. Best is to thaw overnight, but if there is no time, you can generally place them in the oven at 365°F (185°C) and heat them up for 10 to 12 minutes. Store in glass containers. They are usually easy to remove if you only need a few at a time. The recipe photo opposite shows the fancier version of pork meatballs that my children don't like. They like the plain kind (no parsley, for crying out loud!), shown on the next page.

Reminder:
A pinch (*une pincée*) is using three fingers!

2.2 pounds (1 kg) pork shoulder (*échine*), ground

3 cloves garlic, minced

2 pinches of fine salt

2 pinches of pepper

Parsley, finely chopped

5 tablespoons lard or duck fat

OPTIONAL INGREDIENTS (SOME OF WHICH ARE SEASONAL)

3.5 to 7 ounces (100 to 200 g) pork liver, ground (to increase the nutritional density without affecting the taste)

3.5 to 7 ounces (100 to 200 g) veal liver, ground

Egg (for binding purposes, but not required)

Curcumin, fresh or in turmeric powder form

Zucchini, grated

Carrots, grated

Your favorite hard cheese (such as aged goat—*chèvre*, Comté, Gruyère, or Parmesan)

Spring onions, finely chopped

Cilantro, finely chopped

Shallots, minced

Collagen powder

Curry powder

Cayenne pepper

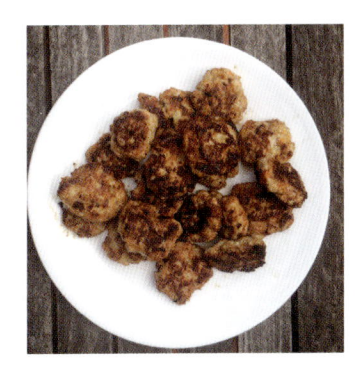

Mix all ingredients together. (When adding the optional ingredients, I eyeball it based on how much I like that ingredient or how much of it I have.) Make uniform, tablespoon-sized meatballs that are slightly flattened (*aplati*) to ensure faster, even cooking throughout the meatball.

Melt the lard or duck fat in a large pan over medium-high heat. Place the meatballs in the pan, giving each some space around it to properly brown without being crowded (cook the meatballs in batches if necessary). Cook about five to seven minutes on each side. Cut one meatball in half to see whether it is cooked through. Add more fat if necessary to keep the meatballs from burning.

Drizzle with olive oil or serve with a dipping sauce such as **Barbeque Sauce** (page 389), **Tangy Tartar Sauce** (page 414), or **Onion Marmalade** (page 411). Serve with a sauce as an appetizer or with a salad as a meal.

WINE PAIRING TIP I served this dish as an appetizer (*amuse-bouche*) during several gatherings with my wine class pals. Here are the wines they suggest to pair that will not overpower the delicate tastes of the meatballs: Organic wine connoisseur Vy Nguyen suggests a Merlot-dominated Côtes de Bourg from Bordeaux, less tannic than the neighboring Pomerol and St. Emilion wines, specifically the Clos du Mounat, an organic wine. Another good friend and sommelière Natalia Youreva recommends an elegant, well-balanced blend of Grenache, Mouvèdre, and Syrah from Les Baux de Provence, a village in the Alpilles hills of Provence. Specifically, Natalia recommends the Domaine de Lauzières, a biodynamic and organic winegrower, who also happens to produce a lovely organic Provençale olive oil. Malika Faytout, whose Château Lescaneaut in Castillon went organic in 2008 and was certified in 2012, proposes a white Savagnin from the Arbois appellation in the Jura, such as Domaine de Saint-Pierre, which delivers high-quality organic and biodynamic wines, and whose 2015 harvest (*cru*) has a medium acidity, and notes of apple, pear, and popcorn.

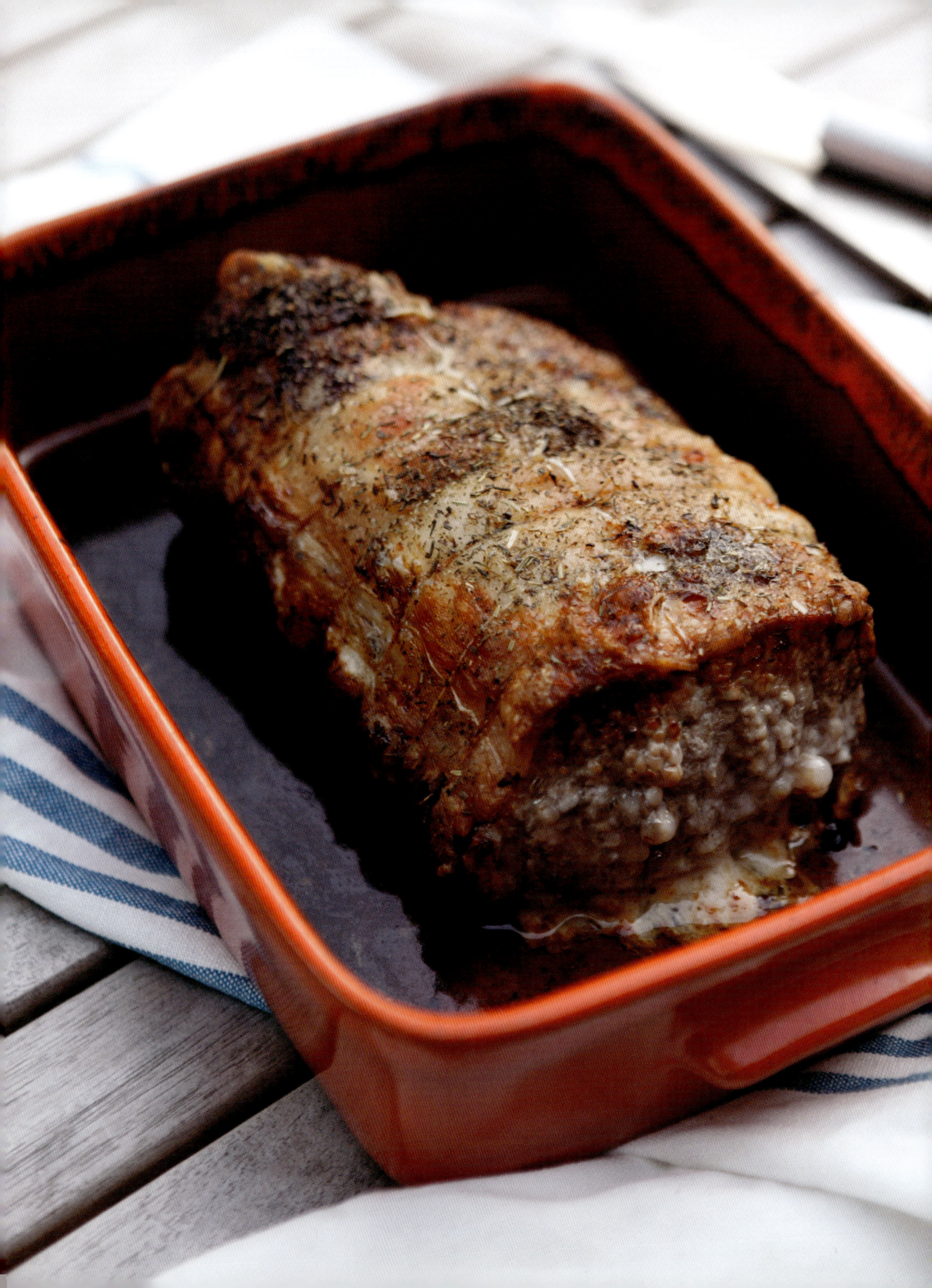

PORK ROAST WITH *HERBES DE PROVENCE*
Rôti de Porc aux Herbes de Provence

Seaso: Year-round   **Preparation Time** Less than 5 minutes
Cooking Time 1 hour   **Serves** 5 to 6

This recipe is a kid-pleaser and the easiest one in my repertoire. When you know you won't have any time for prep work, but you are at home to allow for the cooking time, this is the go-to recipe. If you generally count on a minimum of 5 to 7 ounces (150 to 200 g) per adult, a 1-kilogram piece of meat (2.2 pounds) will feed five to six people, or else a family of four with leftovers for one or both parents' lunches the next day! If you are used to smaller portions, then this size will last you longer. (Freeze leftovers if you are histamine-intolerant—histamine growth on meats halts in the freezer, but continues in the refrigerator.) The cut of meat can come from one of several parts of the pig, but most commonly pork loin (*carré côtes, côtes filet or pointe de filet*), tenderloin (*filet mignon*), or the ham (*jambon* or *pointe*) or shoulder (*côtes échine* or *épaule*), the fattiest cut. (Cooking the tenderloin, the most tender of the cuts and often the least fatty, requires less time, so check at 45 minutes.) According to *Atelier des Chefs* in Bordeaux where I took several cooking classes (see their cooking temperatures tableau on page 307), pork is cooked "medium" (*à point*) from 149°F (65°C), shown in the pork roast photo below (A), up to "well done" (*bien cuit*) at 176°F (80°C).

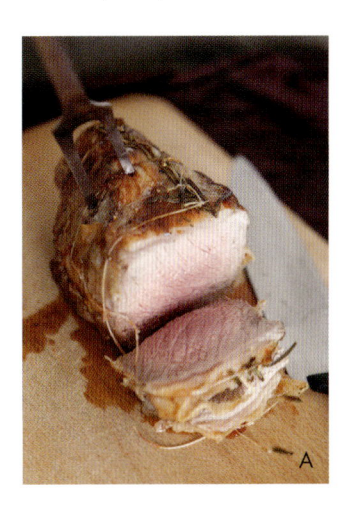

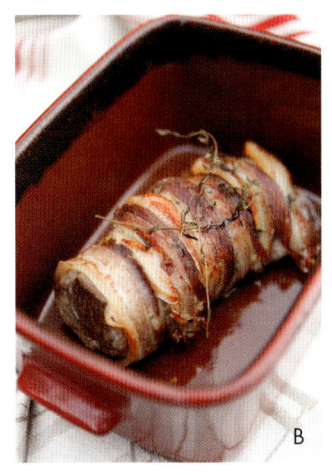

The recipe photo on the previous page shows a boneless pork loin roast that had enough fat surrounding it that it required only tying (*ficeler*) with butcher's string (*la ficelle*). Please refer to the photo tutorial on **How to Tie a Roast (without Stuffing or Barding)** on page 82 to see how this particular roast was tied. You may choose to stuff (*farcir*), wrap, or "bard" (*barder*) your roast with strips of fatback lard or bacon (*barder*) and then tie it. If you wish to stuff or wrap your roast before tying it (the pork roast shown in photo B is wrapped in bacon), please refer to the photo tutorial on **How to Stuff, Wrap, and Tie a Roast** on page 83. You may wrap and tie a roast using these steps without stuffing it; just skip the stuffing steps and begin by wrapping the roast in bacon or slices of fat or else just tying the whole roast, for a neat and tidy look and to keep the roast from changing shape as it heats in the oven. Wrapping in bacon or lard and using butcher's string adds 10 to 15 minutes to the preparation time, or less, as you become more adept at this. You may remove the string before slicing the roast to avoid pieces of string attached to the slices.

Herbes de Provence

Herbes de Provence is a traditional combination of four herbs: savory (a kind of wild basil), oregano, thyme, and rosemary, but also sometimes marjoram (*marjolaine*). It is used in many recipes and is an easy (if sometimes overused) tool to flavor a recipe. It goes with pretty much all meats and white fish. ➤

Reminder:
A pinch (*une pincée*) is using three fingers!

Pork Shoulder Roast

4 tablespoons olive oil

2.2 pounds (1 kg) pork meat

2 pinches of coarse sea salt

2 teaspoons *herbes de Provence*

Optional: Pinch of pepper

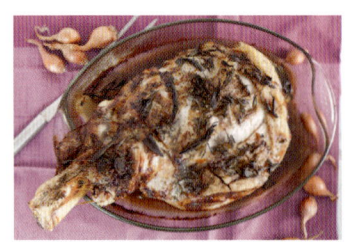

Preheat the oven to 185°C (365°F). Place the pork into a casserole dish that is the approximate length of the piece of pork. Pour the olive oil over and under the pork. Sprinkle sea salt and *herbes de Provence* (and optional pepper) on and under the meat. Place in the oven and cook for one hour. Check that the roast's internal temperature has reached 167°F to 176°F (75°C to 80°C). That's it!

VARIATIONS If you happen to have fresh rosemary, thyme, sage, or any of the ingredients that go into *herbes de Provence*, you may place entire sprigs beneath and on top of the roast (as shown here with this bone-in pork shoulder roast). I do this with chicken and beef roasts sometimes as well, and/or I chop them up and sprinkle them on top. To make an extra-flavorful sauce, place several thinly sliced onions and a few peeled garlic cloves around the roast in the dish before it goes into the oven. The cooking process caramelizes the onions and mixes the fats and juices to create a delectable sauce for the meat. You can also pour half a glass of Muscadet wine from the Nantais region of the Loire Valley (made from the Melon de Bourgogne grape, with apple, citrus, and pear aromas) over the pork before adding the other ingredients. Enjoy the rest of the bottle with the meal!

WINE PAIRING TIP I have had this dish with a light-bodied, low-alcohol, and fruity Bourgeuil from the Loire Valley as well as a full-bodied, refreshing Pouilly-Fuissé Chardonnay from the southern Mâconnais region of Burgundy. My friend, DUAD wine course graduate and Bordeaux Wine School instructor Ilona Guitz, proposes for this dish a rosé in warmer months or a red with a lighter tannic structure and subtle "animal" aromas, such as a Bordeaux Supérieur, or else a Listrac or Moulis from the Médoc. From their time aging in barrels, these also lend subdued smoky notes to the pairing.

Meat Temperatures at Atelier des Chefs, Bordeaux

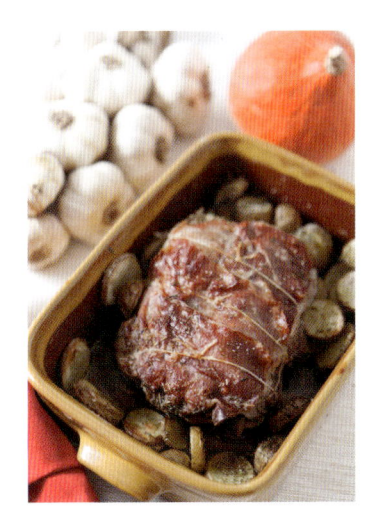

Degrees of Doneness for Pork
Températures de Cuisson à Coeur or *Stades de Cuisson Pour le Porc*

Medium Rare: 145°F to 148°F (63°C to 64°C)

Medium – *À point:* 149°F to 160°F (65°C to 71°C)

Well Done – *Bien Cuit:* 170°F to 176°F (77°C to 80°C).

Butcher's Tip
Astuce du Boucher

Cook roasts for about 15 minutes per 1.1 pounds (500 g), thicker roasts for about 20 minutes per 1.1 pounds (500 g)

PORK – LE PORC

PORK ROAST STUFFED WITH PRUNES AND TIED
Rôti de Porc aux Pruneaux à la Ficelle

Season Year-round   **Preparation Time** 15 minutes (Using butcher's string adds 10 to 15 minutes or less, as you become more adept at tying the string.)   **Cooking Time** 1 hour to 1 hour and 15 minutes   **Serves** 5 to 6

This is an eye-pleasing dish, taught to me by Basque butcher Florent Carriquiry in Bordeaux. It is a lovely roast to make for guests or when you have a bit of time, as the stuffing, bacon-layering, and tying are extra steps, and you will need butcher's string/cooking twine. (Tying is not absolutely necessary, but it does hold the prunes and bacon in place and make for a pretty package.) Kids and adults alike love the melty prunes (a native fruit of the Southwest) inside and the crunchy bacon outside (the Basques use a lot of bacon and charcuterie). The slicing, stuffing, and tying will take more time than a simple pork roast, but it makes for a very nice-looking package and a delicious meal. Again, like other pork roasts, the cut of meat can come from one of several parts of the pig, but most commonly pork loin (*carré côtes, côtes filet* or *pointe de filet*), the ham (*jambon* or *pointe*) or shoulder (*côtes échine* or *épaule*), the fattiest cut (and shown in the recipe photo opposite), or even the tenderloin (*filet mignon*). This recipe is another kid-pleaser, as they like the sweet, melty prunes inside their slice of pork.

2.2 pounds (1 kg) pork roast meat

10 to 12 prunes

Optional: Pinch of fine sea salt

Optional: 4 tablespoons olive oil

Fleur de sel or coarse sea salt, for garnish

Preheat the oven to 185°C (365°F). Slice into the meat lengthwise, cutting it sandwich-style, leaving the two pieces connected) and stuff the roast with a line of prunes. Sprinkle a pinch of salt along the line of prunes (optional). Close up the "sandwich" of prune-stuffed meat and use butcher's thread to hold the two haves and prunes in place, lining strips of bacon prunes on top, if desired, and topping the bacon with a line of prunes down the middle of the top of the roast. Tie up the roast. For further instructions on how to stuff, wrap, and tie up a roast, follow the steps in the photo tutorial on **How to Stuff, Wrap, and Tie a Roast** on page 83.

For added flavor and fat, pour olive oil in a casserole dish the approximate size of the piece of pork, place the meat in the dish, and pour olive oil over the meat.

Place your masterpiece into the oven and cook for one hour to one hour and 15 minutes, depending on its size and your oven. Check the roast at about 50 minutes if you are unsure about the "doneness" (*la cuisson*) of the center of the roast, which should reach about 170°F (70°C). Cook an additional 10 to 25 minutes if needed.

Allow the roast to rest for 10 minutes before carving into slices. Cut and remove the strings before slicing, and garnish the slices with coarse sea salt or *fleur de sel*. Serve with roasted or sautéed vegetables or salad.

> WINE PAIRING TIP For a Southwest pairing with the prunes, try a red, medium-bodied Buzet from the Southwest. Otherwise try a red Côte Chalonnaise, made from the Pinot Noir grape in central Burgundy, with notes of red and black berries and undergrowth, or else a cherry-flavored Sancerre Rouge (also a Pinot Noir) or a more tannic and berry Chinon Rouge, both from the Loire Valley. See **Sautéed Pork with Prunes** on page 325 and **Bacon-Wrapped Prunes** on page 287 for more wine pairing ideas.

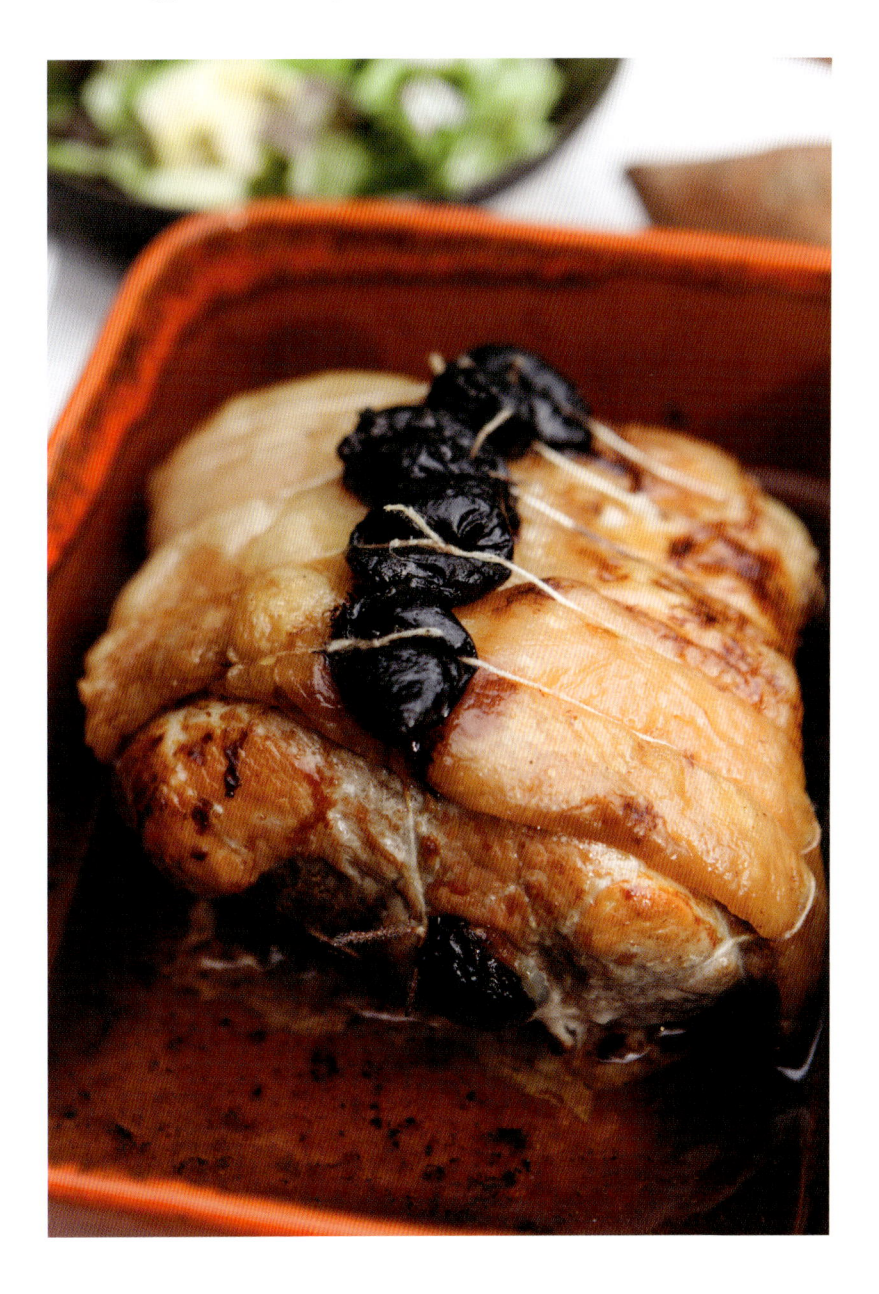

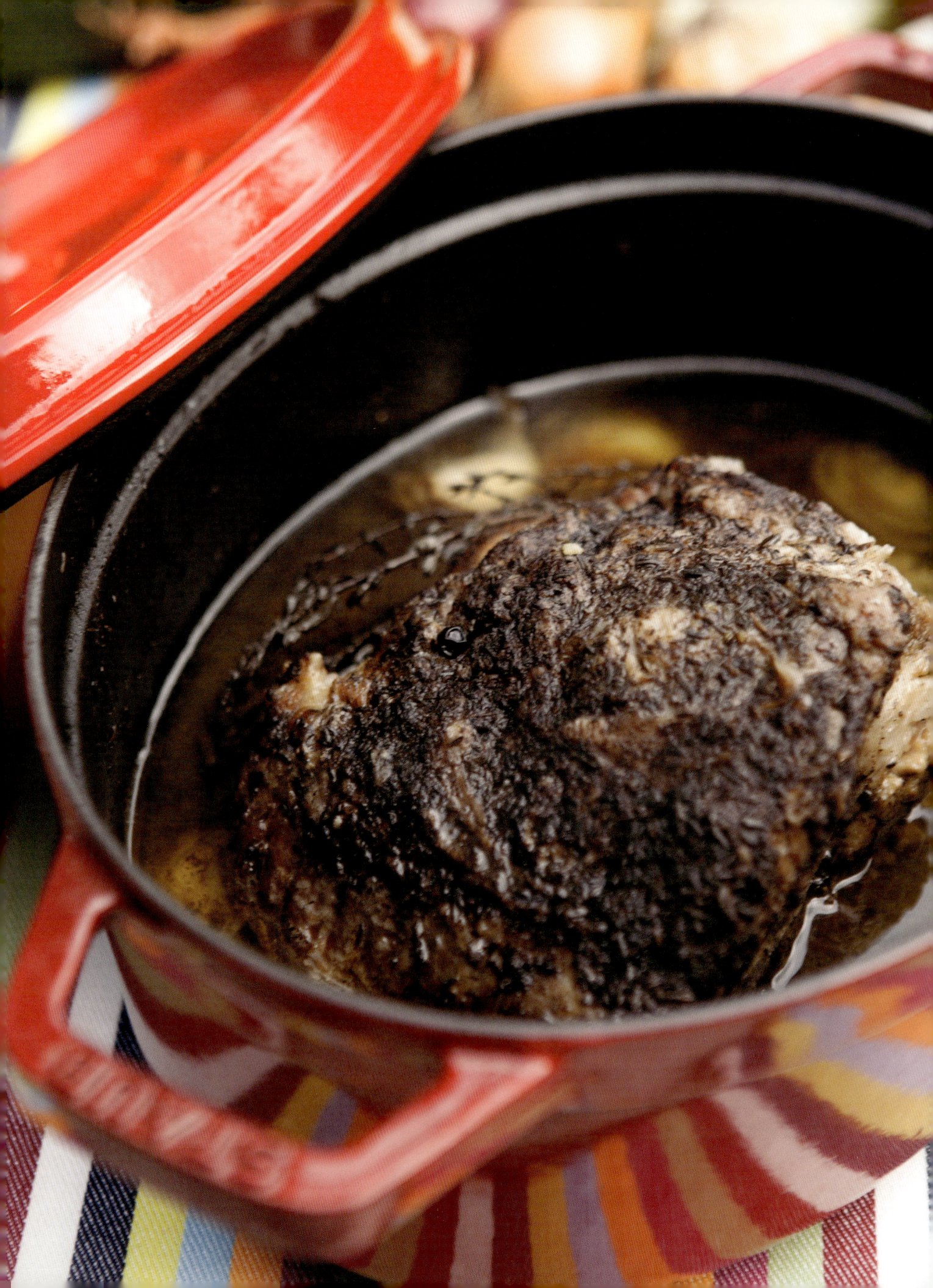

PORK SHOULDER COOKED IN FAT
Confit de Porc Échine

Season Year-round   **Preparation Time** 5 to 10 minutes, marinate overnight
Cooking Time 1.5 hours minimum, up to 4 or 5 hours   **Serves** 8 to 10

This is one of my favorite dishes. It is easy to prepare ahead of time, though in a pinch, I have skipped the marination time, browned the pork, and added the spices right before the slow-cooking process. It comes out just fine, tasty, and tender. You may allow it to cook up to five hours on the stove, and the meat just melts in your mouth. This is the French answer to pulled pork. All in all, there are many ways to make this dish in terms of time, fat used, and aromatics (*les aromates*) added. This shoulder cut is located alongside the first five ribs of the pig and is the fattiest cut on the pig. This is a slow-cooking dish, which renders this already fatty cut of meat very tender. Basque butcher-chef-charcutier Florent Carriquiry revealed his ingredients for this dish to me, and used for this version of the recipe. This became an instant favorite in my family due to the sweetness imparted by the combination of spices, flavor, and fat. A cooking time of three or more hours is best. A general rule of thumb I learned from Florent is that a pork shoulder needs to cook for 15 minutes per pound (about 500 g), though check your meat's internal temperature for the "doneness" you are looking for. The French tend to eat their meats rarer than Americans.

If you have leftovers, it not only makes a great lunch or dinner the next day, but you will see how the fat has risen to the top of the dish in which you have stored your leftover pork shoulder, and how beneath the layer of fat there is a flavorful, gelatinized broth. If you do not use all of this fat and broth for your pork leftovers, you may drink it as a broth or add it to vegetables or other dishes where you might need a stock or a sauce to spruce up the flavor. You can also use leftover fat to cook other vegetables or to scramble eggs. After the long cooking time, this fat becomes very aromatic.

2.2 pounds (1 kg) pork shoulder (*échine de porc*)

3 pinches of coarse sea salt (*gros sel de mer*)

2 bay leaves (*feuilles de laurier*)

6 juniper berries (*baies de genévrier*)

2 to 3 cloves (*clous de girofle*) or 1 pinch of powdered clove—this step is optional, as children do not always like clove

2 pinches of ground pepper

2 pinches of ground nutmeg (*muscade*)

3 pinches of thyme dried or fresh (I used dry in the photo)

3 to 5 cloves of garlic, unpeeled (*en chemise*, literally, "in its shirt") and crushed

4 tablespoons, plus 3 tablespoons lard

ADDITIONAL SPICING OPTIONS

1 teaspoon fresh or powdered ginger (*gingembre*)

1 teaspoon cinnamon (*cannelle*)

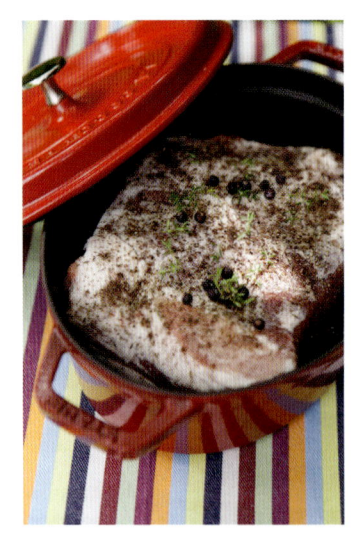

Raw Pork Shoulder with Aromatics

Chef's Tip
Astuce du Chef
Chef Florent suggests peeling the crushed garlic and rolling it in salt and pepper as a way to infuse the dish with these flavors.

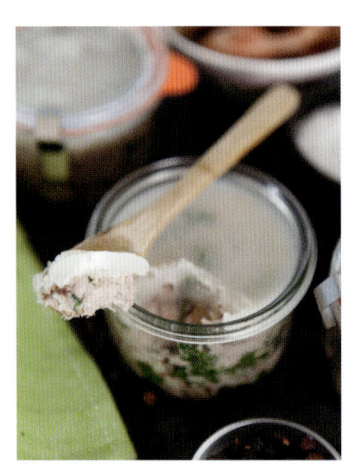

Pork Meat Pâté

Combine all the ingredients except the lard in a large cast-iron pot the night before. (I have done this one and two nights in advance.) This allows the pork to marinate in the aromatic herbs and spices.

The next day, remove the meat, spices, bay leaves, and garlic from the pot and pour the liquid that has collected from the meat into a cup. (These will all be added back to the pot after the meat has been browned separately in the pot).

Melt the lard in the pot over medium-high heat. Brown the meat on each side for several minutes. Use a splatter screen, as the moisture from the meat will cause the fat to spit. Add the spices back to the pot as well as the liquid in the cup and two pinches of salt. Turn down the heat to medium low and cover the pot securely to lock in the moisture.

At this point you have the option of either adding three tablespoons more lard or adding up to about 1.5 cups (350 ml) more lard, or at least enough so that about one third of the pork is submerged in the fat. The greater amount of fat allows more of the meat to be really cooked in the fat and is an added bonus but not absolutely necessary. Cook for one and a half to three hours on low.

Serve with root vegetables roasted in olive oil, chards sautéed in duck fat (**Sautéed Swiss Chard** – page 474), or leeks with cubed bacon (*lardons*), a green salad, and a baked sweet potato or **Sarlat Sautéed Potatoes** (page 468). Or serve **Fennel with Red Onion** (page 445) on the side (May through November for fennel). In the spring, eat this dish with green or white asparagus.

Pork Meat Pâté
Rillettes de Porc
If you cook the meat for four hours or beyond, you will have such a tender roast that you can make *Rillettes de Porc*, which is simply jarred pulled pork preserved in fat. Place cooled chunks of meat in a jar or single-serving jars, mix in chopped parsley if desired, and press down with the back of a spoon and flatten all around, leaving a half-inch of room at the top, adding salt and pepper on top, as desired. Melt lard in a pan or in the oven, and pour it over the meat in the jars, covering the meat. Seal and refrigerate, eating over the course of a week, or freeze. Serve room temperature or warmed. Eat by the spoon or spread on **Seedy Crackers** (page 501) or on **Oven-Baked Beet Chips** (page 457). To up the excitement of this otherwise very simple meat pâté, serve it as an appetizer with a rich Pinot Meunier (or other) Champagne. See the following wine pairings for other suggestions. ➤

VARIATIONS Butchers like remaining true to the meat being cooked and using the corresponding fat, but will also vary the fats to make for slightly different flavor combinations. Instead of using lard, you can also use the venerable duck fat for the subtle, delicious complexity of flavors that it brings to any dish, including this one. I have also used this recipe with beef roasts from the chuck (*basses côtes*) or plate (*plats-de-côtes*) parts of the cow, using tallow as the fat, including the ginger and cinnamon, and employing white pepper for a subtle change of flavor. My cooking times have ranged from 2 hours and 20 minutes to 5 hours, defined by when I remember to put the roast in the pot! Serve with **Onion Marmalade** (page 411). Pair the beef with a medium-bodied, fruity Grenache wine from Languedoc, or a spicy Syrah from the Rhône Valley.

WINE PAIRING TIP Serve the pork shoulder (or the *rillettes de porc*, as mentioned above) with a sweet wine to enhance the sweetness of the dish, or else a dry white from Alsace, Entre-Deux-Mers in Bordeaux, Burgundy, or Jura to cut the sweetness a bit and lend acidity to the dish, or else a light-to-medium-bodied red, such as a Pinot Noir from Burgundy or the Jura, so as to not overpower the delicious flavors of the pork. With a pork dish like this full of spices, my friend, wine consultant, and teacher, Ilona Guitz recommends southern French wines with their own potent balsamic (woody, tree resin) aromas and spices, such as reds from Languedoc-Roussillon, in particular the appellation of Corbières, whose main grape variety is Carignan N, or else, for those inclined to drink a wine from Bordeaux, she would advise an organic and biodynamic wine from the Côtes de Bourg appellation—lower in tannins than other Bordeaux appellations: Les Demoiselles de Falfas, the second wine of Château Falfas, where Merlot is the dominant grape, followed by the other grapes of the well-known Bordeaux blend: Cabernet Sauvignon, Cabernet Franc, and Malbec. This recipe is one for which Ilona would also recommend a Bordeaux Sauternes sweet wine. To go with the subtley spiced and tender pork meat, also try red wines that are fruity, fleshy, and/or supple: a supple Minervois from Western Languedoc; a fresh and aromatic Lirac from the Central Rhône Valley, with notes of black and red fruits, leather, scrub (*garrigue*), and spice, thanks to the many grape varieties used in the blend; or a fresh and elegant Côtes du Rhône Villages, with notes of ripe fruits and spice, also blended from many grape varieties.

PYRÉNÉES COUNTRY PÂTÉ
Terrine de Campagne des Pyrénées

Season Year-round   **Preparation Time** 45 minutes   **Makes** 4 to 6 jars, depending on jar size
Cooking Time About 40 minutes for smaller jars (10 ounces or 300 g), 65 minutes for larger jars (18 ounces or 500 g)

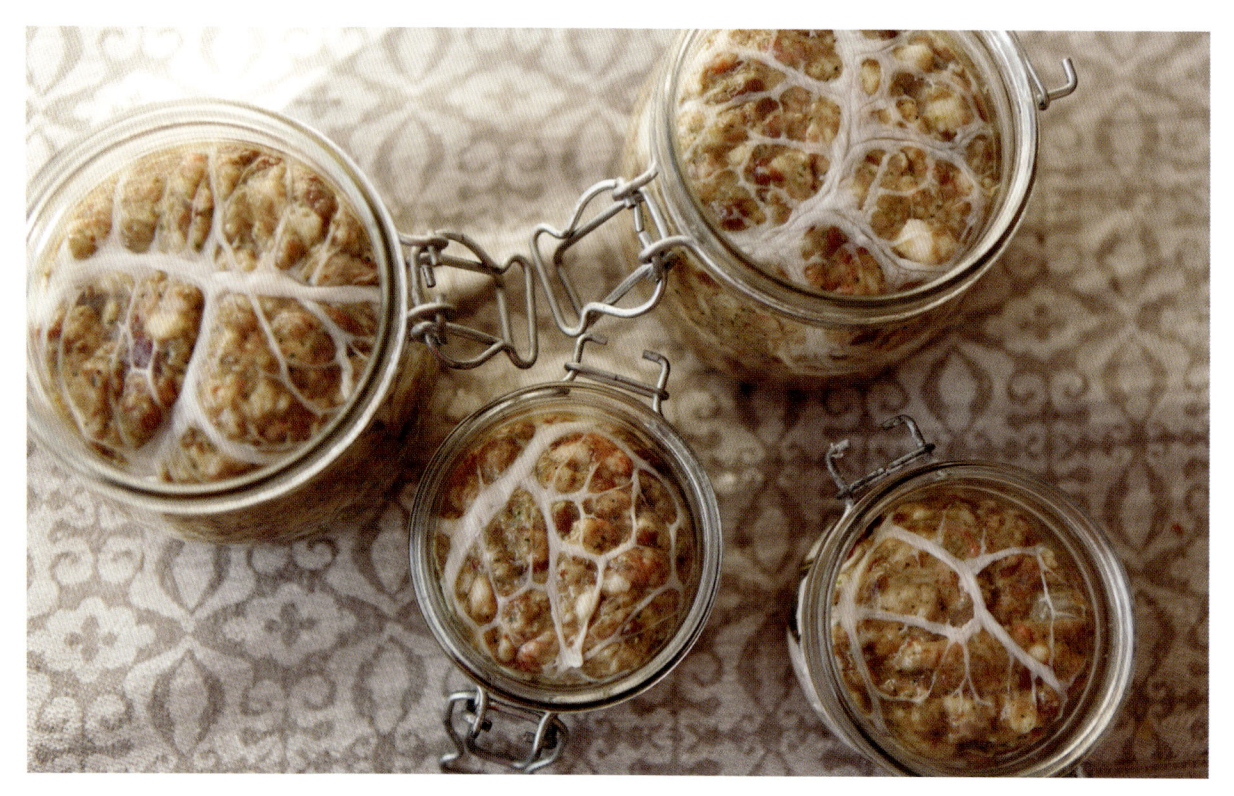

This is a classic, economical, everyday "village" pâté that one eats with one's family (*en famille*). Pâtés have a high fat content and tend to be of a smooth consistency, as opposed to *terrines*, which usually contain larger chunks of meat. *Terrine* is also the name of the ceramic, clay, glass, or porcelain dish in which pâtés and terrines are made. Traditionally, terrines are oval or rectangular in shape. Often a pâté will also contain Cognac or Armagnac, a brandy from the French Southwest. Pâtés often contain mushrooms. This particular recipe contains neither alcohol nor mushrooms, but there is room for experimentation! For those with allergies to fungus and mold, however, this is the gold standard. This recipe comes from Chef Frédéric's grandmother who lived in the Pyrénées. Every family has their own basic recipe from which one can then modify by adding their favorite ingredients. This recipe calls for pork caul (*la crépine*), which is the sheath of fat that looks like webbing and envelopes the viscera of the pig and is good for keeping ground ingredients together in a variety of meat preparations. Do not worry if you cannot obtain this, just go without. Often, a pâté will be three parts pork to one part other meat. Here, the meats are all from pork. This recipe calls for pork neck (*gorge de porc*), but pork shoulder (*échine de porc*) may be substituted. Both are fatty, flavorful cuts of pork. The most precise way to cook a pâté is to use a thermometer to assure each one has reached 175°F (80°C). Pâtés can be eaten year-round, though strictly speaking, parsley, a key flavoring ingredient in this recipe, is in season April through November. Parsley comes in two main kinds: "flat" (*persil plat*) or "curly" (*persil frisé*). Otherwise, the recipe ingredients can be found year-round. Slices of pâté or terrine make a great snack or appetizer and are generally chilled like cold cuts.

Chef's Tip
Astuce du Chef
Keep the parsley stems (*les tiges*) for bone broth or to make a "garnished bouquet" (*bouquet garni*), a mini bouquet of fresh or dried thyme, laurel leaf, parsley, and leek greens, which you can use in other recipes.

1.8 pounds or 28 ounces (800 g) pork neck (*gorge de porc*), sliced

10 ounces (300 g) pork liver (*foie de porc*), sliced

1 garlic clove (*gousse d'ail*)

½ onion, chopped into two pieces

5 branches flat parsley (*persil plat*), stems removed (*éffeuiller le persil*)

7 tablespoons fresh heavy cream (*crème fluide*)

3 eggs

1 tablespoon fine sea salt (*sel de mer fin*)

2 teaspoons ground pepper (*poivre*)

Optional: 14 ounces or 1.7 cups (400 g) pork caul (*crépine*)

Fleur de sel, for garnish

Preheat the oven to 320°F (160°C). Pass the slices of pork neck and liver, garlic cloves, and onion pieces through a meat grinder (*hachoir*) (photo A), or cut big pieces into smaller cubes to run in batches briefly through a food processor, until you have a ground consistency to the meat mixture (*le haché*) (photo B).

Mix the parsley leaves with the cream. Run the cream, eggs, pepper, and salt through a blender (*un blendeur* or *un robot*) for 30 seconds (photo C). Pour the egg and cream mixture over the ground meat mixture and stir together by hand until the ingredients are blended (photo D).

Fill clean jars (*terrines*) with the ground mixture, but leave a good margin at the top (do not overfill as the level will rise a bit during cooking). Wipe the tops clean (photo E). ➤

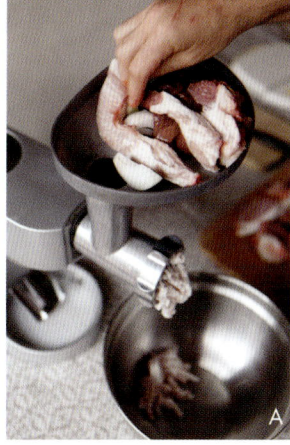

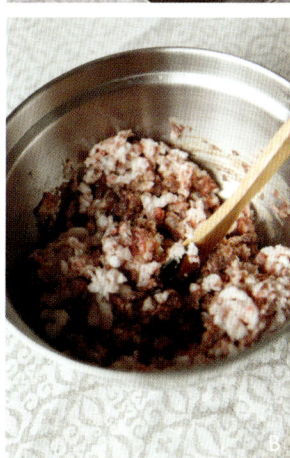

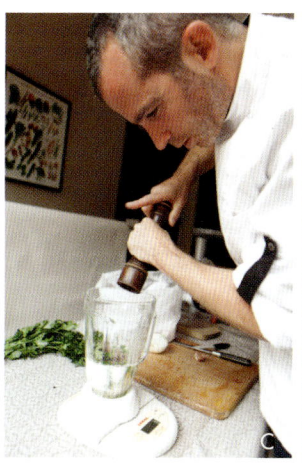

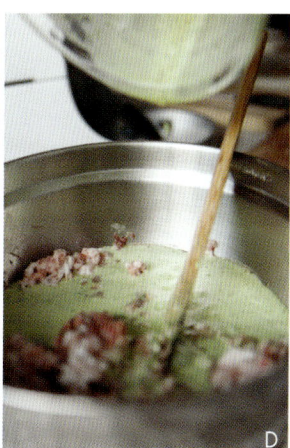

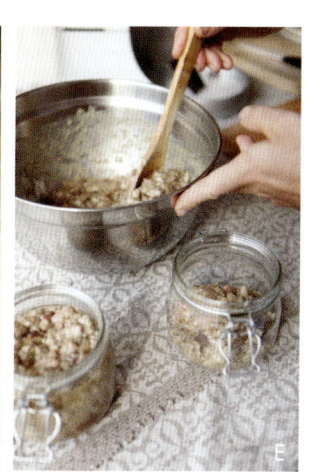

PORK – LE PORC

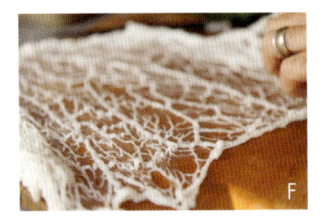

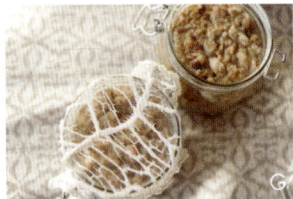

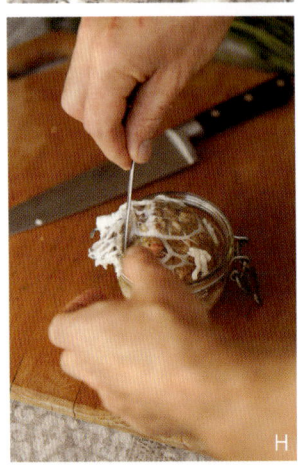

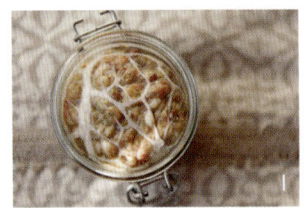

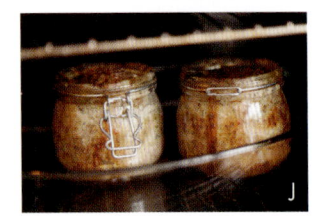

Wash the pork caul several times in a bowl with cold water, like you would wash salad or spinach leaves, to cleanse and whiten the color of the pork caul. Spread the pork caul onto a clean surface (photo F). Cut pieces of pork caul that are a bit larger than the openings of the jars you are using. Place a piece of trimmed pork caul lightly over the filled jar (photo G). Using the flat end of a fork or spoon or a dull knife, gently tuck the edges into the sides of the jar around the top of the pâté, all the way to the bottom of the jar if the piece is large enough (photo H). Repeat this for each jar until each jar is covered in caul (photo I).

Cook the filled jars uncovered in the oven, checking their temperature after the first 30 minutes (photo J).

As each jar reaches 175°F (80°C), remove it from the oven. Depending on the jar size this will take from 30 to 45 minutes. Do not cover the jars right away unless you want to sterilize them. Cover the jars after they have come down to about room temperature. The pâté lasts 12 days if not sterilized. Sterilize the jars ahead of time for longer keeping if desired. To sterilize the jars, cover them in a pot of cold water and boil gently for 45 minutes.

Wait at least two days for the flavor to set in before eating the pâté. Garnish with *fleur de sel* before serving.

> WINE PAIRING TIP Enjoy with a few sips of brandy or Armagnac, or else a light-bodied red Bourgeuil from the Loire Valley, a subtly aromatic Pinot Gris from Alsace, a medium-bodied chardonnay from Burgundy, or a low-tannic, floral and grape Brouilly or Côte de Brouilly made from Gamay Noir, from the Beaujolais region. Restaurateur Annabelle Nicolle-Beaufils recommends fruity and spicy red medium-bodied wines, such as one from the Bordeaux Supérieur appellation, or a Marcillac, made from the tannic grape Fer, in the Aveyron region at the easternmost edges of Southwestern France, or else similarly structured reds such as a Beaujolais, a Côtes-de-Provence, a Grenache-heavy Languedoc, or a Lirac from the Rhône Valley, said to be a favored wine of French monarchs Henry IV and Louis XIV.

RACK OF PORK IN CRUSTED SALT, GINGER, AND GARLIC
Carré de Cochon en Croûte de Sel, Gingimbre et à l'Ail

Season Year-round, but especially good in cold weather

Preparation Time 10 minutes, plus 1 hour or more, or overnight, to marinate   **Cooking Time** 2 hours   **Serves** 12

This recipe was inspired by one of my favorite French cookbooks, *Morceaux Choisis* ("Chosen Pieces") by Parisian butcher Hugo Desnoyer, whose work I admire. His recipe calls for over a kilogram of large grain salt (*gros sel*), which would form the crust, later to be removed. But I can't bear losing any meat or salt, therefore, when I first made this recipe, I used only one-tenth the amount of salt, and even that was too much. I have cut the salt again by half, and that is easier on the taste buds. However, the combination of salt, garlic, and ginger is always a winner, especially when warding off colds in the winter. This recipe can be cut in half if you do not have many people to feed or if you do not want leftovers, however, this is a great dish to have around to reheat for a few more meals or freeze for an easy reheat at a later date. ➤

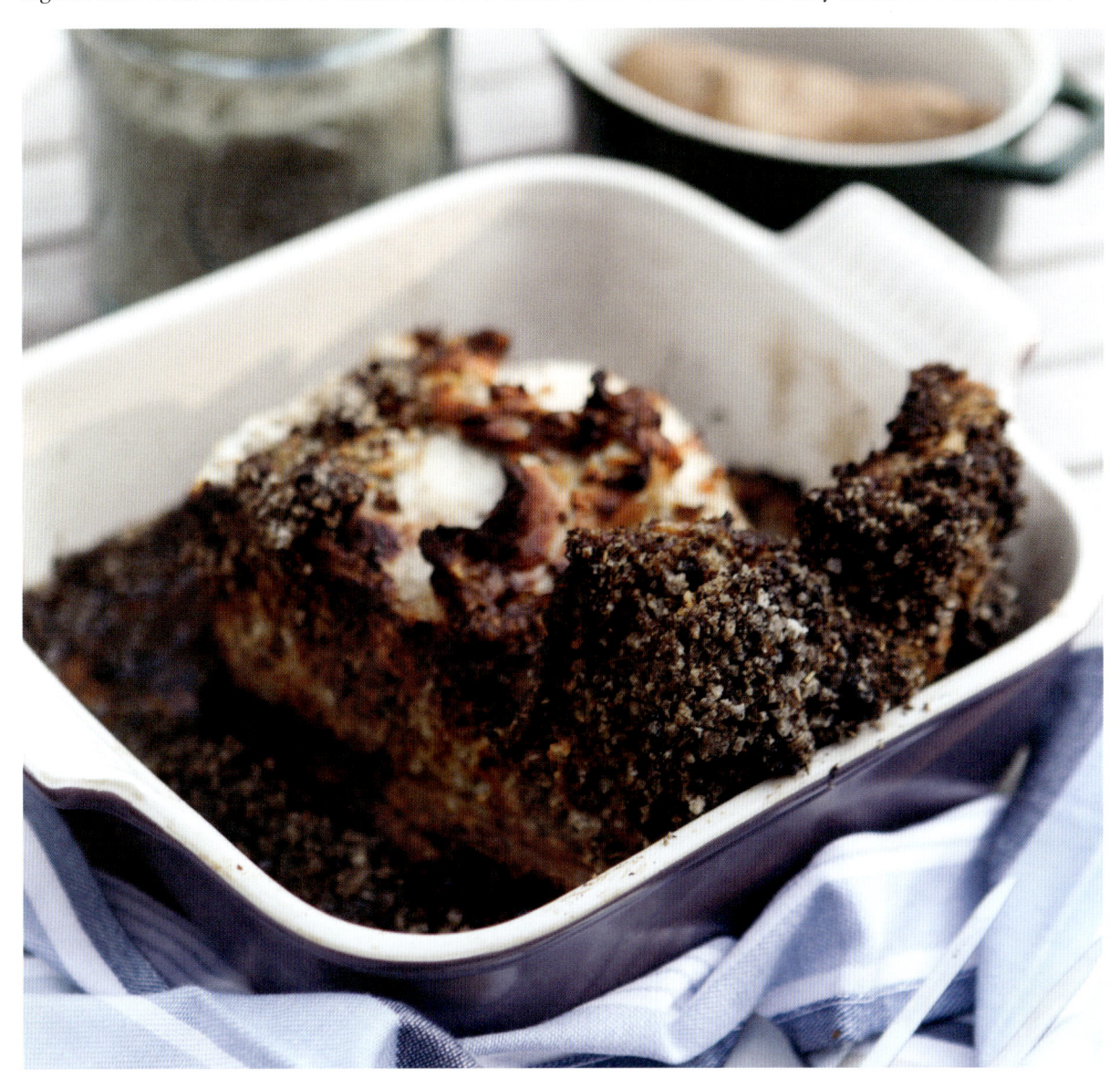

1.8 ounces or ¼ cup (50 g) ginger, minced

6 cloves garlic, minced

6 tablespoon olive oil

3 pounds (1.3 kg) rack of pork (*carré de cochon*)

2 pinches of ground pepper

2 tablespoons *herbes de Provence*

1.8 ounces or ¼ cup (50 g) large grain sea salt (*gros sel de mer*)

Mix the ginger, garlic and oil in a bowl. Make an incision along the bones in order to stuff the meat with the ginger, garlic, and oil mixture. Rub the remaining mixture around the entire piece of meat and sprinkle on ground pepper. Allow the meat to marinate for an hour or even overnight in the refrigerator in a covered container. (I use glass—no plastic wrap! No need for extra chemicals to enter your food). Remove the meat from the refrigerator about an hour before cooking to allow the meat to come to room temperature for even cooking.

Preheat the oven to 300°F (150°C). Mix the *herbes de Provence* with the sea salt in a separate bowl. Use your hands or the back of a spoon to pat or smear (*badigeonner*) the spice and salt mixture onto all sides of the meat, including the bottom. Place the meat in a casserole dish and allow it to cook for two hours.

After removing the meat from the oven, let it "rest" for 5 to 10 minutes before carving so that the juices are retained in the meat and do not seep out. Remove the bones and cut the meat into slices. Serve with roasted vegetables.

> **WINE PAIRING TIP** My DUAD wine course classmate Delphine Dentraygues, a Parisian perfumer transplanted to the wine world of Bordeaux, recommends a crisp Sancerre Rouge, fragrant with berries, made from the Pinot Noir grape in the Loire Valley, or a red Gigondas from the Southern Rhône Valley. Often providing comic relief during our more serious lectures and tastings, my classmate Laeticia Ouspointour suggests one of her own family's organic wines, a red Le Château Vieux Mougnac in the Bordeaux Supérieur appellation, especially the 2012, which is acidic and fruity. I have had this wine and agree with her recommendation. Because of the spicy ginger and strong aromatics of this dish, it can also be served with a sweet Sauternes or Barsac from Bordeaux, or else a sweet Jurançon from the Southwest; this way you have a built-in dessert!

ROSEMARY PORK RIBS
Coustellous au Romarin

Season Year-round   **Preparation Time** 5 to 10 minutes
Cooking Time 35 minutes   **Serves** 4 (3 to 4 ribs per person)

This recipe is so easy but so good every time. Children love nibbling on spare ribs (*coustellous* or *coustelous* as they are called in the French Southwest, or else *coustons* or *travers de porc* in the rest of France). These ribs are great finger food, good for exercising your jaws (these ribs do not fall off the bone as slow-cooker ribs do), but they are very flavorful thanks to all the fat, and they are a great way to cover your face in rosemary. My younger daughter can put away four or five of these ribs at a time. I try to get as many as I can from the butcher, as they are also easy to reheat. The pig has 26 ribs, 13 per side, ranging in length from two to three inches (5 cm to 8 cm) to six to seven inches (15 cm to 18 cm). I will usually make a batch of about 12 to 16 ribs, either cutting them myself or having the butcher cut the racks into individual ribs for me. In restaurants they are served in racks, I prefer cooking the already cut ribs so that I do not have to fiddle around with cutting hot ribs for the family. The aromas of garlic and rosemary will fill the house and make everybody hungry!

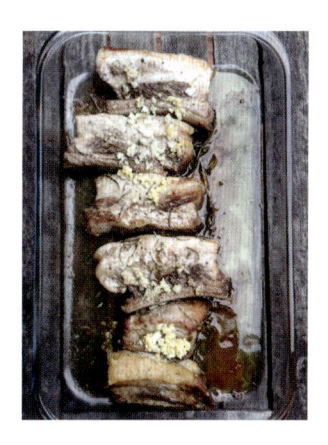

12 to 14 pork "spare" ribs

2 to 3 tablespoons olive oil

1 tablespoon garlic, minced

1 tablespoon rosemary, fresh or dried and minced

2 pinches of coarse sea salt

Preheat oven to 365°F (185°C). Rub the ingredients on the ribs beginning with the oil. (This can be done the night before, several hours before, or minutes before cooking.) Instead of rubbing, you can also just throw the ribs in a bowl, toss in the ingredients, and mix around with your hands until the ribs (and your hands) are covered in the marinade.

Lay the ribs side by side in a large casserole dish. Place in the oven and cook for 35 minutes. Serve with any vegetable. ➤

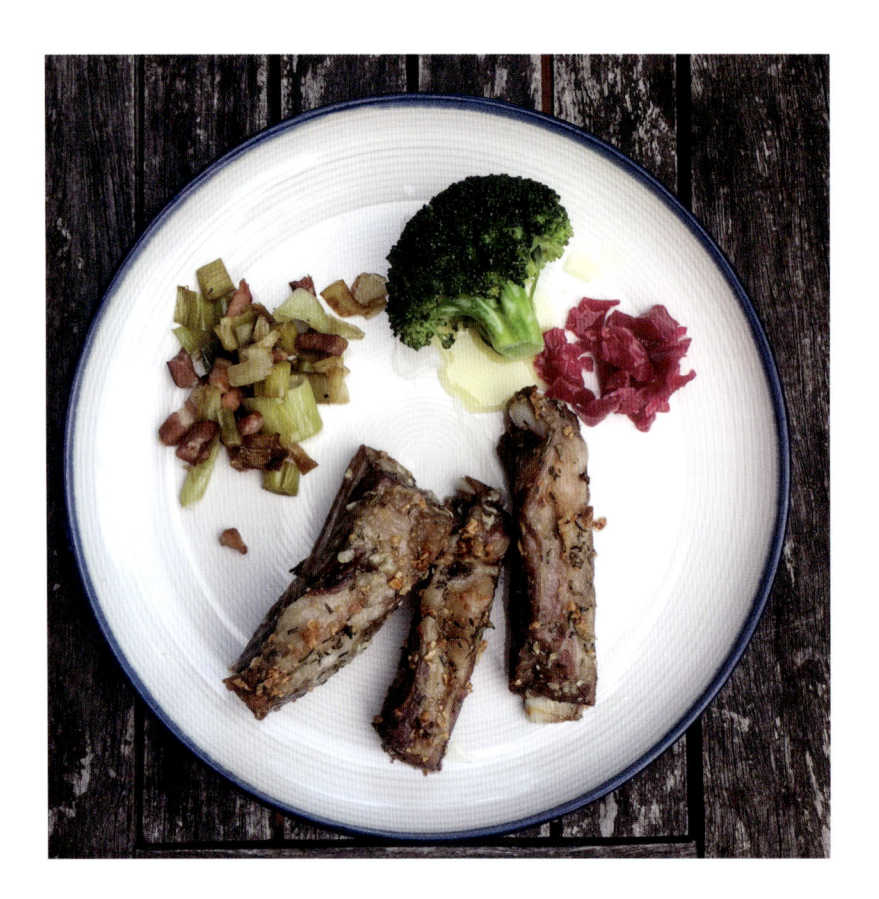

VARIATIONS For a "low and slow" cooking variant, bake the ribs in the oven for four hours at 230°F (110°C).

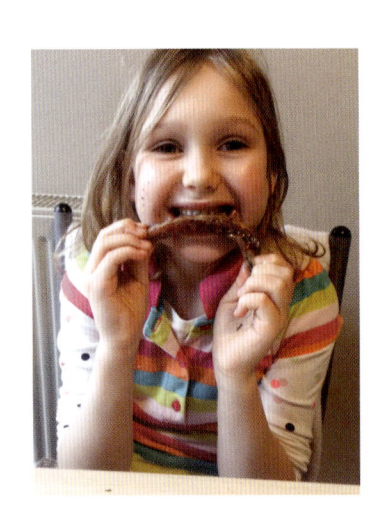

WINE PAIRING TIP I have tried this dish with a southern Côtes-du-Rhône blend of Grenache, Syrah, Cinsault, and Mourvèdre grapes from the Gigondas appellation, which is fruity but also brings spicy notes to the meal. I have also had this dish with a red Graves from Bordeaux, namely, Clos Floridene, produced by my wine professor and his family. We never tasted it in class, but I discovered it at the one-Michelin-star Le St. James cooking school *Côté Cours*, where I took a few classes. This wine is almost 50-50 Cabernet Sauvignon and Merlot, with a bit of Cabernet Franc. There are notes of black currant, licorice, and smoke, and it has a smooth tannic structure. A balanced wine, true to its legendary producer, Denis Dubourdieu. According to the Burgundy wine website Bourgogne (www.bourgogne-wines.com), an Irancy Pinot Noir from Northern Burgundy matches the rich flavors of the ribs with the wine's powerful aromas and tannins.

THE BORDEAUX KITCHEN

SALTED PORK WITH LENTILS
Petit Salé aux Lentilles

Season Year-round   **Serves** 5 to 6, depending on how much each person fills up on lentils vs. meat
Preparation Time Start soaking lentils two to three days in advance of serving this dish. The pork is desalinated for 2 hours, boiled, then simmered for 2 hours, creating a gelatinous broth, and refrigerated 1 day in advance of cooking with lentils and serving. Otherwise, prep time is 5 minutes to cut the carrots and peel the onion.   **Cooking Time** 1 hour

Lentils come up every now and then in a French dish, and this is one of the most common. I first saw this recipe in one of my favorite cookbooks, that of *Morceaux Choisis*, by French butcher Hugo Desnoyer. The French traditionally have used *Lentilles vertes de Puy*, French green Puy lentils, but any dark or green lentil will do. Lentils have proteins and other potentially useful nutrients, but they also have their drawbacks for those who are sensitive to their anti-nutrients, namely their phytates, for example. These can be reduced by soaking and sprouting the lentils.[1] This dish uses salted pork, which is pork salted in brine for one to two days and is sometimes obtainable from a butcher, but if you cannot find salted pork, or do not want to brine it yourself, regular pieces of pork and extra salt to taste will do. A small warning: this dish has so many steps and must be started 2 to 3 days in advance, I almost did not include it. But for those who would like to have lentils, this is one way to reduce the phytates and have lentils in a traditional French dish. This dish also uses carrots. No need to peel them, this is a rustic dish. In fact, I never peel my carrots, including when we are eating them raw.

2 cups green lentils

1 salted ham hock (*jambonneau demi-sel*), about 1 pound (450 g)

½ rack of salted spare ribs (*travers de porc demi-sel*), about 1.4 pounds (650 g)

1.3 ounces (550 g) upper front leg or lower shoulder (*palette de pork*), salted or unsalted

1 red or white onion, stuck (*piqué*) with 3 cloves (*clous de girofle*)

7 black peppercorns

1 sprig of thyme

4 sprigs of parsley

10 ounces carrots (300 g) or 4 medium carrots, quartered and cut into 2-inch (5 cm) pieces

Day 1: Soak the lentils in filtered, cold water for 24 hours.

Day 2: Drain the lentils in a metal colander, where you can leave them another 24 hours to allow them to begin to sprout. Stir them around in the colander with your hand over the course of the day to air them and spread around the moisture at the bottom of the colander. (Supposedly, you can sprout them for up to 3 days, I just do it for one day.) ➤

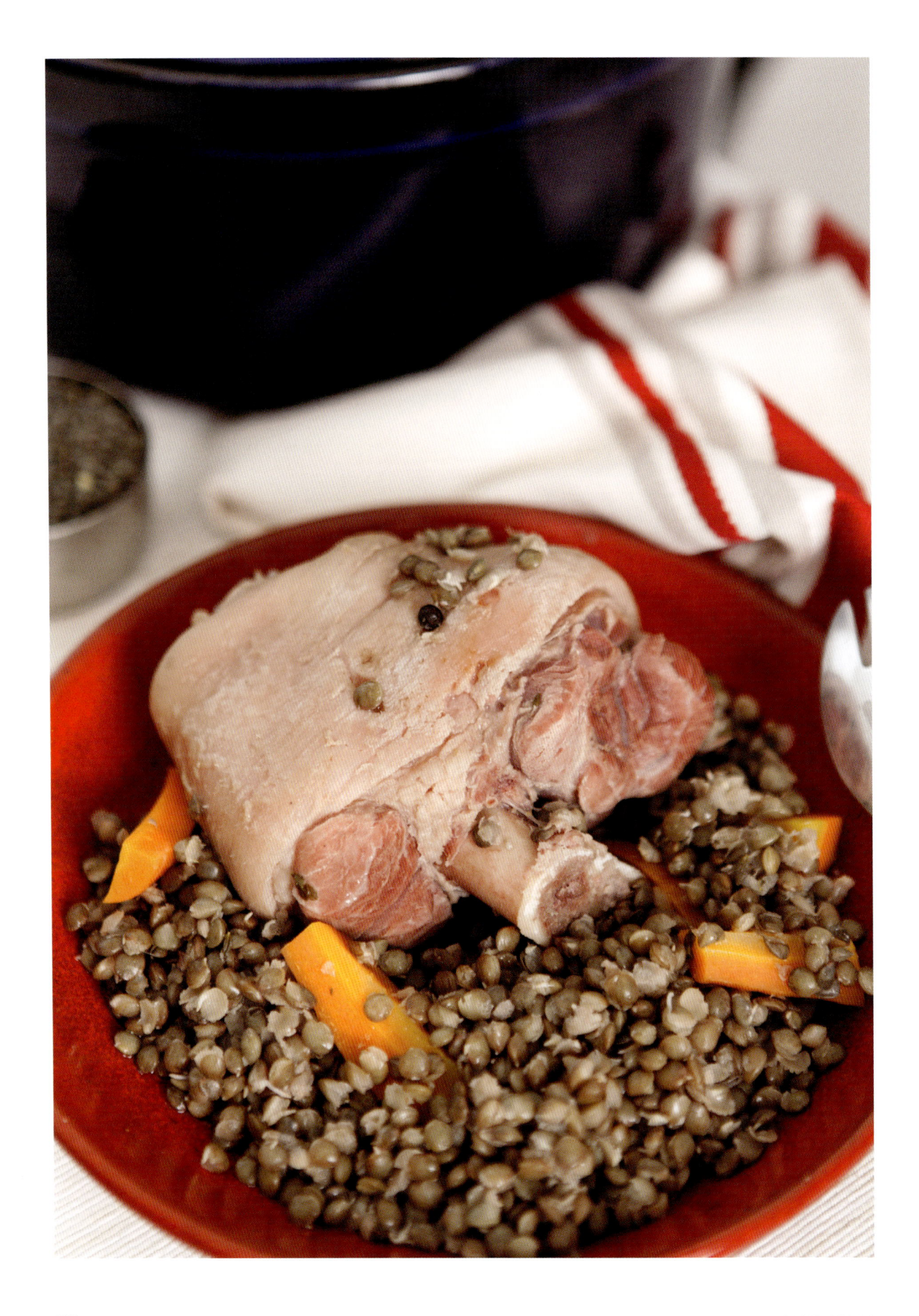

Meanwhile, submerge the salted pork pieces in cold water in a large bowl for two hours, changing the water twice. (There is no need to soak unsalted pork pieces.) Remove the pork from the bowl, place it in a large cast-iron pot (*cocotte*), and add the onion, peppercorns, thyme, and parsley. Cover with water and bring to a boil. Turn the heat down to medium-low and allow to simmer for two hours. (This process draws some gelatin and flavor from the meat, herbs, and spices, as in a stock.) After two hours, remove from heat, allow to cool, and place in the refrigerator overnight.

Day 3: Place the sprouted lentils in a pot, cover them with water, and boil on medium heat for 15 minutes. Turn off the heat and allow the lentils to sit in the water for 15 minutes. Drain the lentils in a colander. Remove the pot of pork and stock from the refrigerator. (Modern day recipes will tell you to skim off the fat. Do not do this, this is perfectly good, flavorful fat! It's like taking the eggs out of Béarnaise sauce. You just can't do it.) Add the lentils to the pot containing the pork and stock, and add the carrots. Bring to a boil, then turn down the heat to medium and allow the pot to simmer for 40 minutes, uncovered, to allow some of the bouillon water to boil off.

If your pieces of pork were not salted, then you will need to adjust the salt by tasting the bouillon and lentil mixture and adding salt, if desired. After so much cooking, the pork pieces can be easily cut and divided into individual servings. Serve the pork in bowls with the lentils and broth.

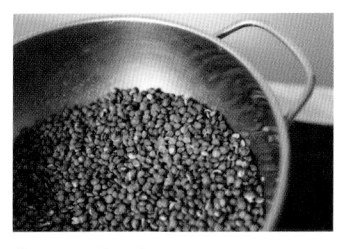

Sprouting Lentils

> WINE PAIRING TIP For a Southwest pairing, try a dry white Pyrénées Jurançon or a floral and citrus Pacherenc-du-Vic-Bilh from Gascony. (One of the most famous Gascons is the Comte D'Artagnan, on whose life 19th Century French writer Alexandre Dumas' 1844 fictional work, *The Three Musketeers*, was loosely based.) Other wines to try would be medium-bodied, moderately structured reds from around France: Beaujolais, Burgundy, Languedoc-Roussillon, Provence, or the Rhône Valley.

SAUTÉED PORK WITH PRUNES
Sauté de Porc aux Pruneaux

Season Year-round   **Preparation Time** 10 to 15 minutes
Cooking Time 30 minutes to brown the bacon and pork, 1 hour and 30 minutes to simmer the entire dish   **Serves** 4

While working at the butcher shop, I learned about the value-added option the butchers offered their clients by creating a stir-fry (*sauté*), an uncooked combination of chopped meat vegetables using extra meat, cut from nobler cuts and roasts, that customers would only have to throw in the pan and cook up quickly (*à la minute*), such as a *sauté de boeuf*, *sauté de volaille*, or *sauté de veau*. This *sauté de porc* is a butcher's delight, using cured bacon pieces (*lardons*), any kind of pork meat chopped into cubes or bite-sized pieces, and the versatile prune, a local product of the region around the French Southwest town of Agen (*Pruneaux d'Agen*), and a dried fruit which goes so well with pork.

VARIATIONS For extra pizzazz, brown a chopped carrot with the shallots and/or a handful of sprouted pine nuts, or else you can replace the prunes with apricots, in which case try a wine pairing of a Muscat de Rivesaltes from Languedoc-Roussillon, but just a small amount, as this is a fortified sweet wine (*vin doux naturel*, a wine mixed with grape must to stop the fermentation and retain the natural sugars), with a high alcohol and sugar content.

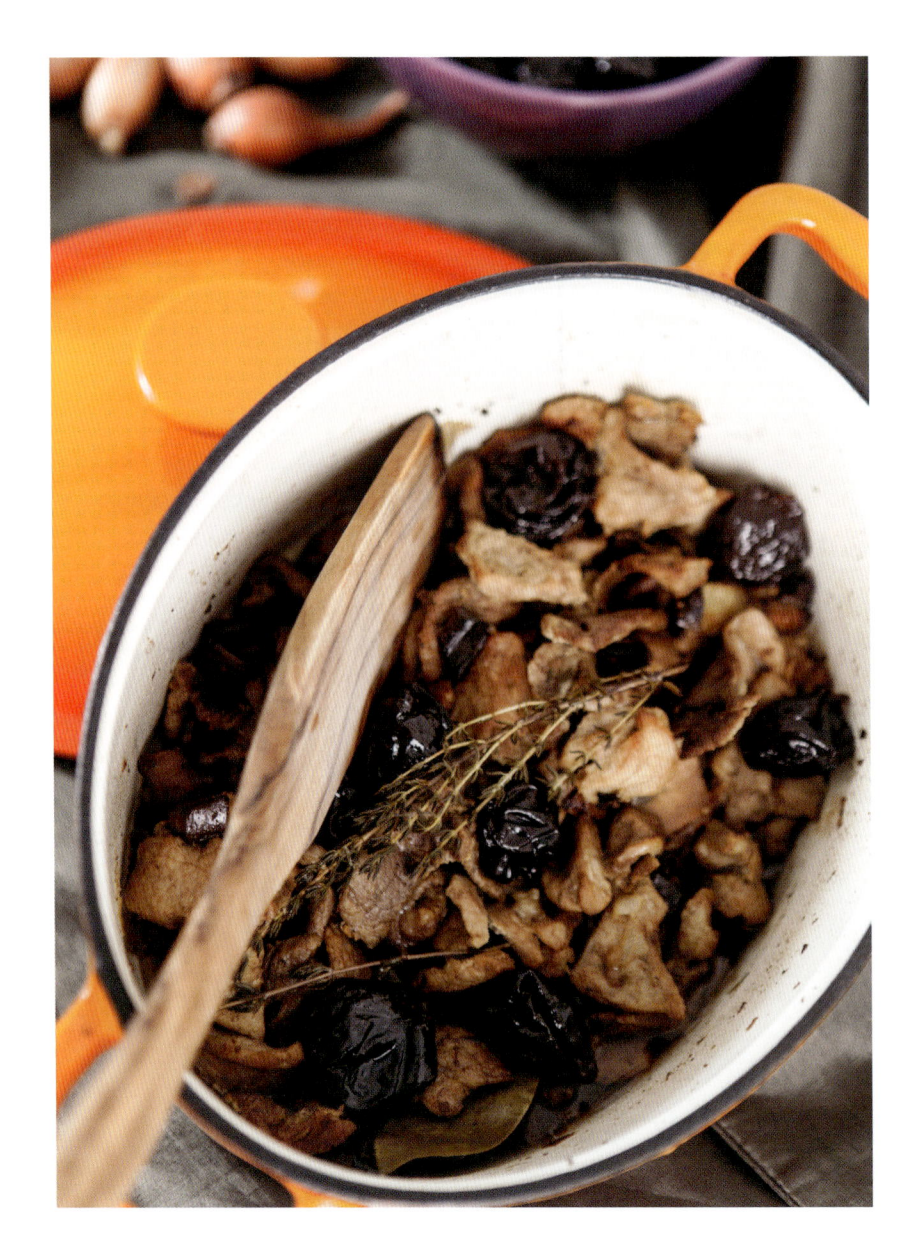

3 ounces (85 g) cured pork belly cut in small cubes or rectangular pieces (*lardons*)

3 to 4 tablespoons lard for the pork, 1 teaspoon for the *lardons*, 1 teaspoon lard (or butter) for the shallots

1.1 pounds (500 g) pork meat, cut into bite-sized pieces or cubed

3 pinches of fine salt

3 ounces (85 g) shallots, minced

1 bay leaf

2 to 3 sprigs of thyme, fresh or dried

8 prunes

¾ cups (180 ml) water or stock

Brown the *lardons* in a small pan over medium-high heat with one teaspoon of lard (the extra fat helps keep them from burning) for five to ten minutes, depending on how browned you like them. I like them nicely browned like bacon. They will cook further with the pork later.

Melt two tablespoons of lard in a cast-iron pot (*cocotte*) over medium-high heat and brown the pork meat in batches (with a pinch of salt for each batch), removing and setting aside the batches of pork in a bowl. After the pork is finished browning, add the shallots and brown them in lard or butter for three to four minutes before adding the pork back into the pot. Stir for a couple of minutes, turn down the heat to medium, and add in the *lardons*, the bay leaf, thyme, prunes, and water. Cover and simmer on low for one and a half hours.

> WINE PAIRING TIP Pair this pork and prunes dish regionally with a tannic, colorful, and acidic Madiran from the Southwest, or try a Saumur Champigny or other less tannic, but fruity and medium-structured reds from the Loire Valley to support the prune flavors. Or else, to offset the fruitiness of the prunes, Restaurateur Annabelle Nicolle-Beaufils suggests pairing this dish with powerful dry white wines, such as a Côtes-du-Lubéron from the southernmost region of the Rhône Valley, a Coteaux-du-Cap-Corse from the island of Corsica, a floral Côtes-du-Rhône Villages, or a structured and flavorful Languedoc (formerly called Coteaux-du-Langeudoc).

STUFFED CABBAGE LEAVES
Feuilles de Chou Farcies

Season Year-round, but most often a meal for Autumn or Winter   **Preparation Time** 25 minutes   **Cooking Time** 1 hour   **Serves** 4 to 5

Similar to the **Stuffed Whole Cabbage** next in this chapter, this recipe simplifies the number of ingredients. However, the stuffing is wrapped by individual cabbage leaves, rather than stuffing a whole cabbage. This is a slightly quicker version to prep than the traditional stuffed cabbage recipe but has just as long a cooking time to ensure the pork is cooked through. This recipe makes for easy-to-store portions at about one cabbage leaf per person.

4 pinches of salt, plus more to taste

6 leaves of Savoy cabbage

1.1 pound (500 g) ground pork

2 pinches of nutmeg

1 teaspoon thyme

Pinch of pepper

3 tablespoons butter, cut into small chunks (or 3 tablespoons olive oil)

Add a pinch of salt to a pot of water and bring to a boil. Place the cabbage leaves into the boiling water and blanche (*blanchir*) for one minute. Remove the leaves and place them into ice water for 5 minutes. Remove the leaves from the ice water and cut out two inches (5 cm) of the thickest part of the stem.

Preheat the oven to 320°F (160°C). Use your hands to mix the ground pork with the nutmeg, thyme, pepper, and 3 pinches of salt in a bowl.

Wrap each leaf around a handful of pork and place in one or more casserole dishes. Should you run out of cabbage leaves to stuff, fill single-serve oven-safe dishes (*mini-cocottes*), as shown in the recipe photo on the next page.

Distribute the chunks of butter onto each stuffed leaf (or pour on the olive oil). Sprinkle with salt and pepper. Cover the dish with parchment paper (or foil, but do not allow the foil to touch the food to avoid heated aluminum transfer to the food), to keep the leaves from burning. Cook for one hour. Serve with roasted or sautéed vegetables.

MORNING SAUSAGE PATTIES

Essentially containing the same ingredients as the stuffed cabbage leaves, minus the thyme, you can make delicious sausage patties for a morning (or any time of day) meal that are also easy to freeze and easy to cook.

1.1 pounds (500 g) ground pork

3 pinches of sea salt

2 pinches of nutmeg

Pinch of pepper

3 tablespoons butter, lard, or olive oil

Mix the salt, nutmeg, and pepper with the ground pork and form flattened, palm-sized patties. Melt the fat over medium-high heat in a pan and cook the patties for 15 minutes, turning occasionally to make sure both sides are cooked through. Serve with vegetables, salad, and/or eggs.

VARIATIONS If you love garlic and onion, add a few minced garlic cloves or a small, minced onion to the ground pork mixture after sautéing them for a few minutes in butter or lard. This dish can be made with ground turkey instead of ground pork, in which case you could sauté three small onions and four garlic cloves, all minced, in one tablespoon duck fat or lard, and add it to 2.2 pounds (1 kg) of ground turkey along with one egg (optional), 10 fresh minced sage leaves, a small handful of chopped parsley, and salt and pepper to taste, and wrap it up in 10 to12 cabbage leaves, as described above. You can also place the mixture into meatloaf pans for a meatloaf. Makes 10 servings.

WINE PAIRING TIP Sommelière Annabelle recommends a range of low- to medium-bodied reds and whites from around France, including a low-tannin red Beaujolais, a rich and aromatic white from Touraine in the central Loire Valley, a crisp white Sancerre from the upper Loire Valley, a citrusy and peachy Saint-Bris made from Sauvignon Blanc, or an aromatic and fruity Irancy Pinot Noir, both from Northern Burgundy. Also have a look at the **Stuffed Whole Cabbage** wine pairing suggestions on page 330.

PORK – LE PORC

STUFFED WHOLE CABBAGE
Chou Farci Entier

Season Winter   **Preparation Time** 35 minutes
Cooking Time 1 hour   **Serves** 6

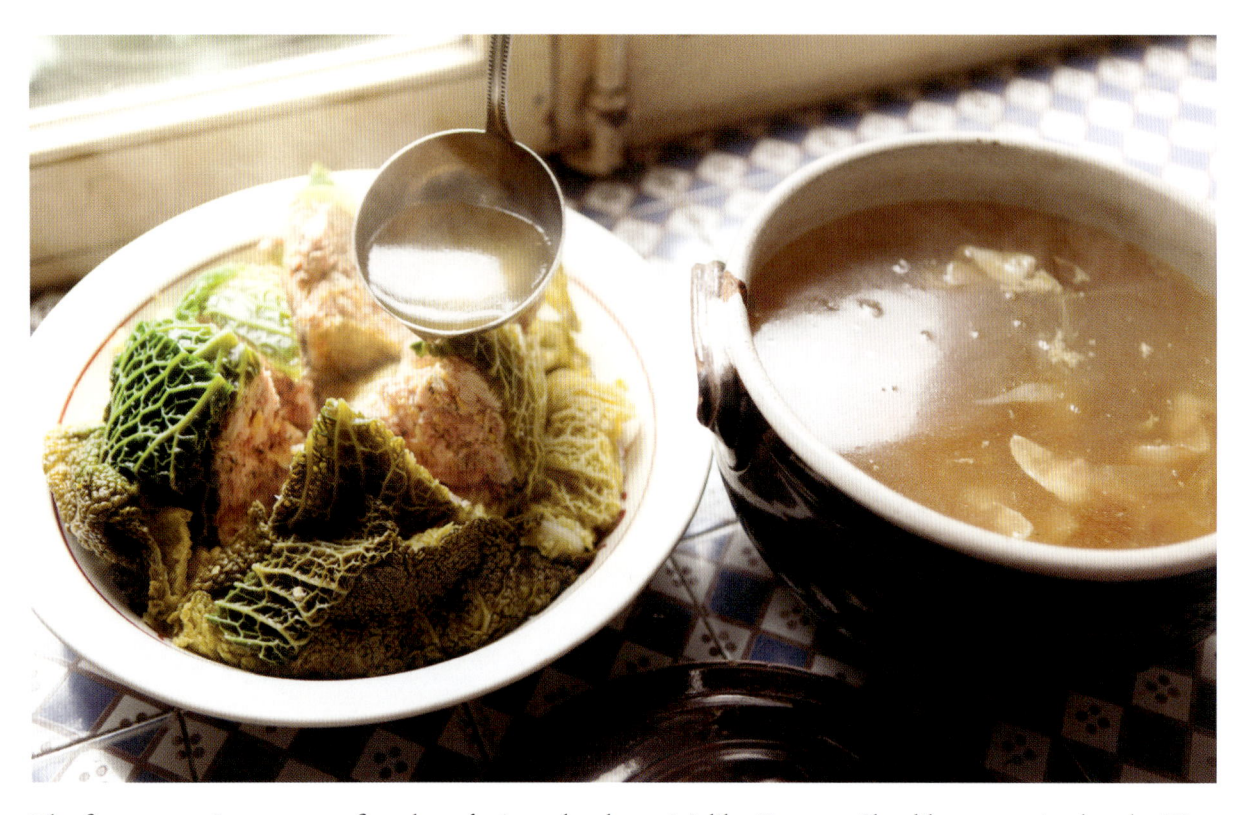

The first person I met on my first day of wine school was Malika Faytout. She, like me, arrived early. We are the type who, out of anxiety (me) and respect and enthusiasm (both of us), like to sit in the front row of the class. We became known as the "front row girls" (*les fayottes*), a kind of "goody two-shoes." I was there to learn about how to taste wine; she was there to learn how to run her family's wine business. We spent the academic year sitting next to each other in class, and she helped me prepare for the final exam with her brilliance and patience. She also supplied me with pen and paper on several occasions when I forgot to bring them to class. Malika's family vineyard is situated in Castillon, along the Dordogne River and next to the more famous wine appellation of St. Emilion. While St. Emilion wines can be very serious and are highly sought-after, Castillon wines are their lesser known cousin, well worth your attention, and similar in their blend of a majority of fruity Merlot, mixed with Cabernet Sauvignon and Cabernet Franc.

This wintery recipe, which we made in January, calls for a pinch of "four spices" (*quatre épices*), a blend of spices often used in French cuisine and consisting of ground clove, ginger, nutmeg, and pepper (white, black, or both). Use a bit of each if you do not have this blend already combined. This stuffed cabbage recipe, whose main meat components are pork and chicken, is an old family winter dish passed down through generations. Her father, François, joined us in the cooking to make sure we were preparing the dish properly. He also proudly pulled all sorts of treasures out of the cupboards, including an antique wooden-handled butcher's cleaver (shown on the next page) and a serving bowl from 1846 (shown above, right) that was given as a gift to Malika's great grandmother on her wedding day and with which we served the broth from this recipe. Now *that's* ancestral!

1 head Savoy cabbage

Pinch of fine sea salt

½ cup (100 g) plus 2 strips uncooked bacon or pork belly (*ventrèche fraîche*), ground or finely chopped

1 cup (200 g) ground pork (*porc haché*)

2 chicken breasts (*blanc de poulet*), ground

1 cup (200 g) veal, ground

2 eggs to bind the stuffing

Handful of parsley, chopped

1 piece of cheesecloth large enough to tie around the entire cabbage

Pinch of "four spices" (*quatre épices*)

2 to 3 medium carrots, chopped into large chunks

1 onion, quartered

1 teaspoon butter

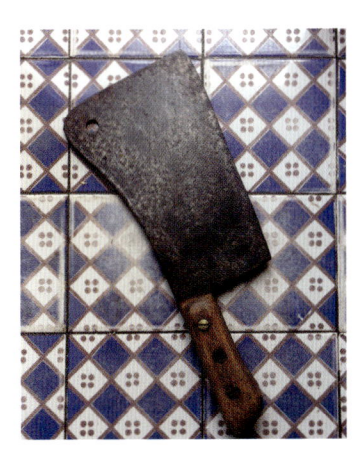

Bring a large pot of salted water to boil. Chop off the core of the cabbage sticking out at the bottom and the outer coarsest leaves. When the water boils, submerge the entire cabbage in the pot and allow to boil gently for about 5 minutes to blanche (*blanchir*) the leaves and remove the bitterness of the cabbage (*enlever l'amertume*).

Meanwhile, using your hands, mix the pork belly (saving 2 strips to add later to flavor the broth), ground pork, ground chicken breast, and ground veal in a large bowl with two eggs, parsley, four spices, and sea salt.

Remove the blanched cabbage from the boiling water and drain it upside down in a sieve over the sink so that the water between the leaves drips out.

Place into boiling water the carrots, onion, and two strips of pork belly (collectively called *la garniture*—they form the flavors for the soup base), along with a knob (*une noisette*) of butter, about a teaspoon, to make the broth (*le jus*) in which the stuffed cabbage will cook for one hour. ➤

Pull the leaves off the cabbage one by one. Cut away the thickest part of the stem of each leaf using a paring knife (photo A). The core and stems can be used for soup stock at a later time, while the small, innermost light green leaves may be chopped and added to the ground meat stuffing.

Place each leaf, as if reconstructing the cabbage, onto a cheesecloth (photo B).

Place the mixed ground meats into the center of the cabbage and close each leaf around the center to reconstruct the cabbage into a nice package (photos C & D).

Tie the top edges of the cheesecloth at the top with butcher's twine and place the cabbage package into the boiling pot (photos E & F). Partially cover the pot and allow the submerged cabbage to boil gently for one hour on medium or medium-low heat.

Carefully remove the cooked cabbage with the help of a large slotted spoon and place it onto a baking dish (photo G). Untie the twine and open the cheesecloth (photo H).

Place the cabbage onto a wide serving dish and cut into slices like a pie (photos I & J).

Serve with a side salad, boiled or baked potatoes, or roasted vegetables. We had the **Beet, Blood Orange, Walnut, and Goat Cheese Salad** as our colorful side dish (page 438).

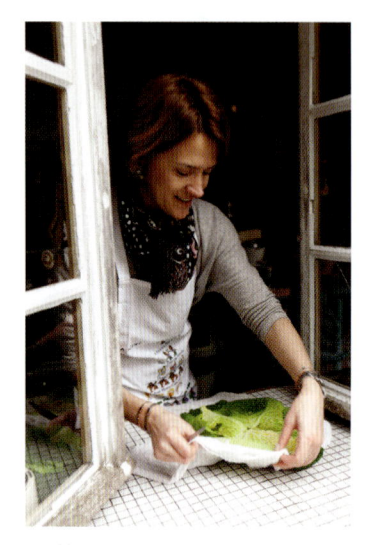

Malika Faytout

> WINE PAIRING TIP We had the house wine, Château Lescaneaut's organic 2012 Castillon – Côtes de Bordeaux. Malika also suggests another organic Castillon – Côtes de Bordeaux: La Cuvée Mouna from Château Franc-La Fleur en Castillon-Côtes de Bordeaux, which is organic, 100% Merlot, with notes of cherry, fruit, and licorice. Malika also recommends the expressive and sensual wines from Castillon made by the biodynamic winemaker Thierry Valade of Château Puy-Arnaud. Meanwhile, restaurateur Annabelle recommends a few interesting whites to go with this traditional fare: a white Beaujolais Villages Chardonnay; a Sancerre Sauvignon Blanc from the Loire Valley, offering notes of acacia, citrus, and mint; or a citrus and floral Sauvignon Blanc from Saint-Bris, not far from the town of Chablis in Burgundy.

PORK – LE PORC 331

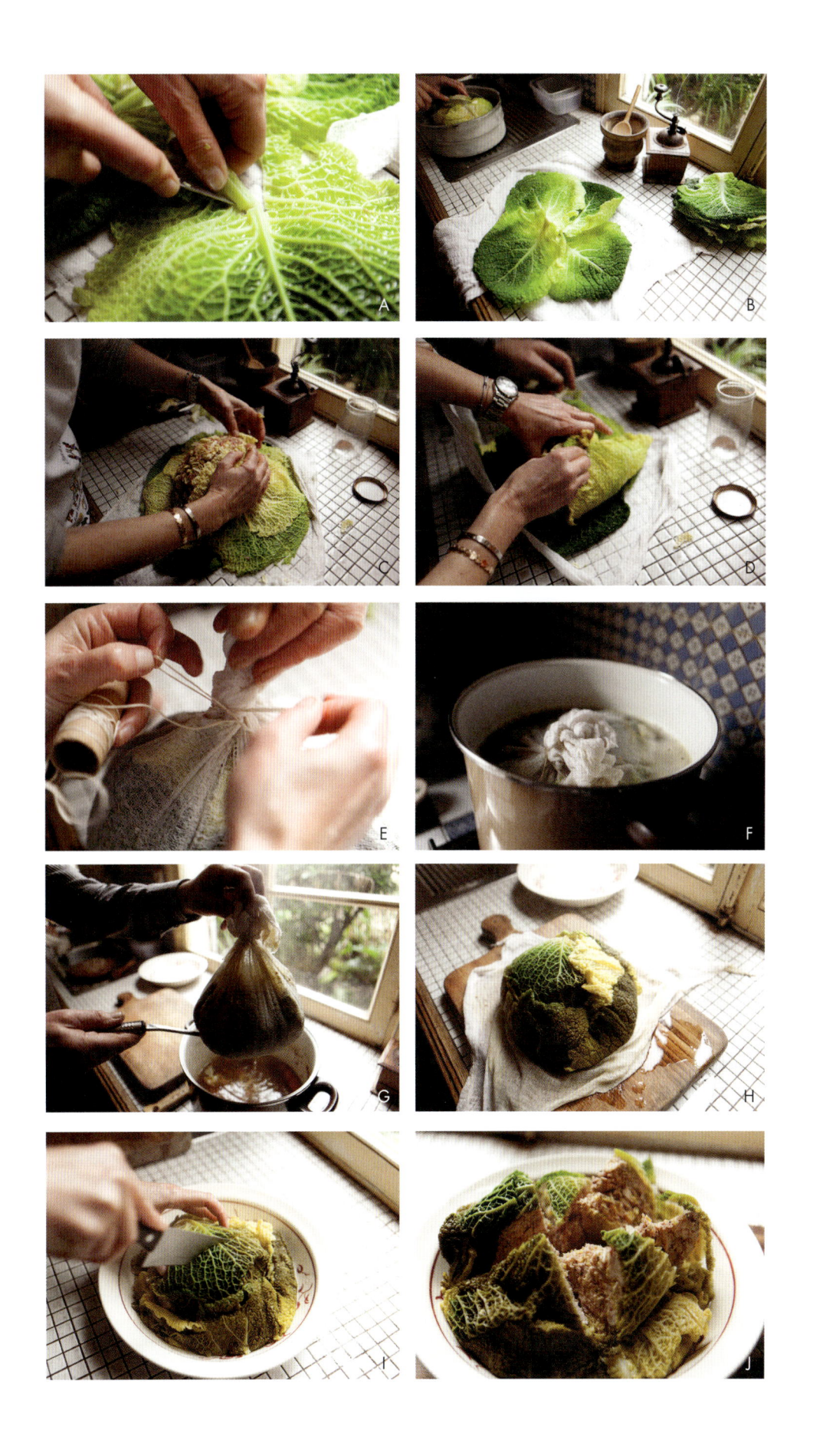

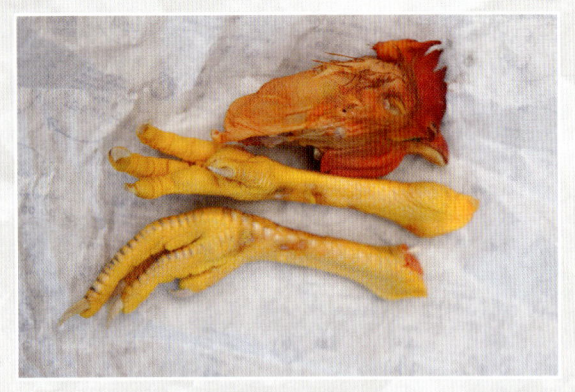

Chicken Head and Feet – *Tête et Pattes de Poulet*

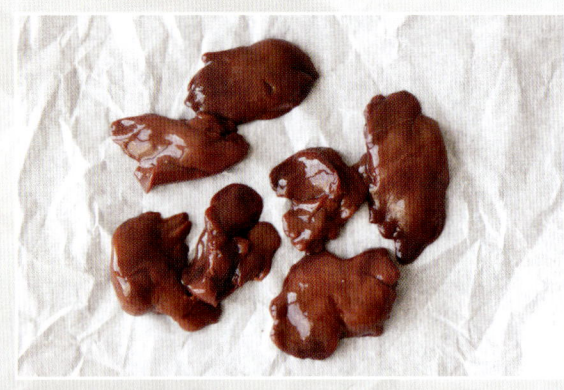

Chicken Livers – *Foies de Volaille*

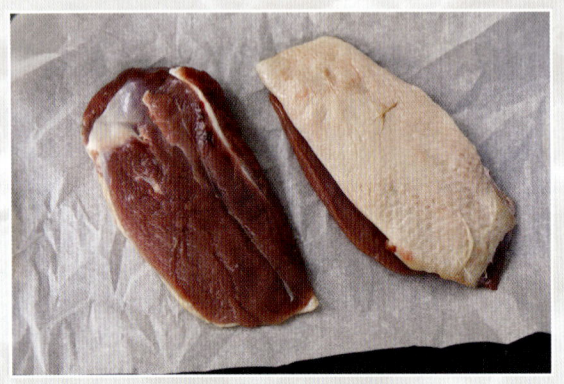

Duck Breast – *Magret de Canard*

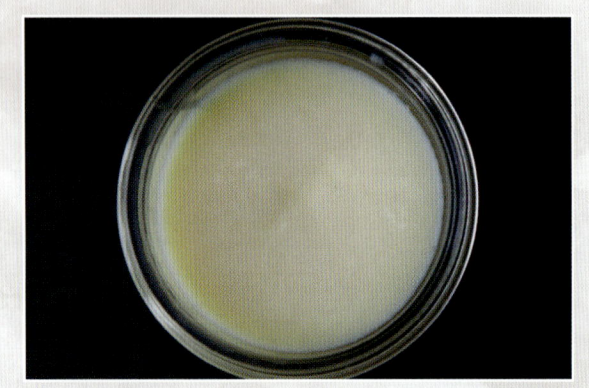

Duck Fat – *Graisse de Canard*

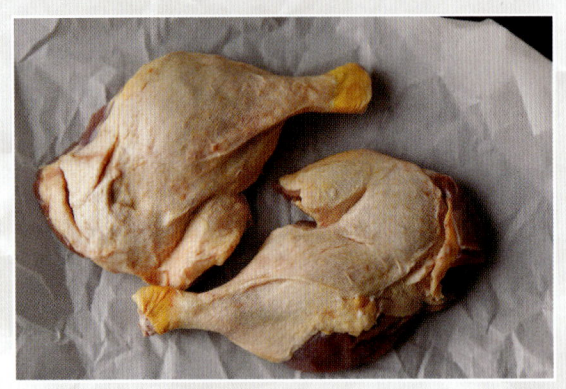

Duck Legs – *Cuisses de Canard*

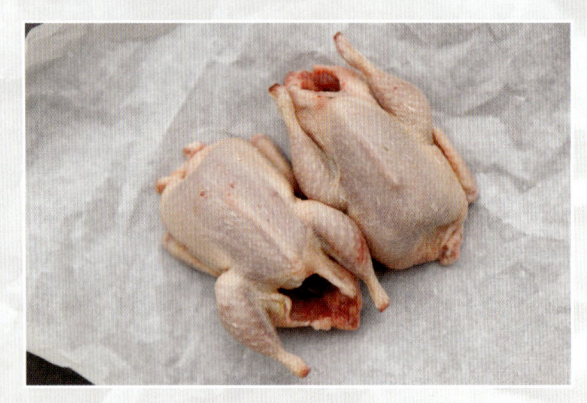

Quail – *Cailles*

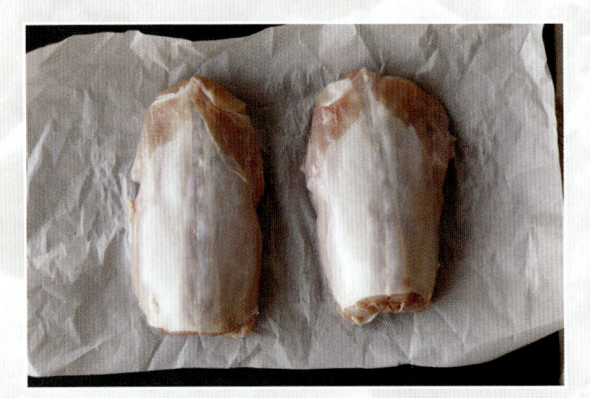

Rabbit Saddle – *Selle de Lapin*

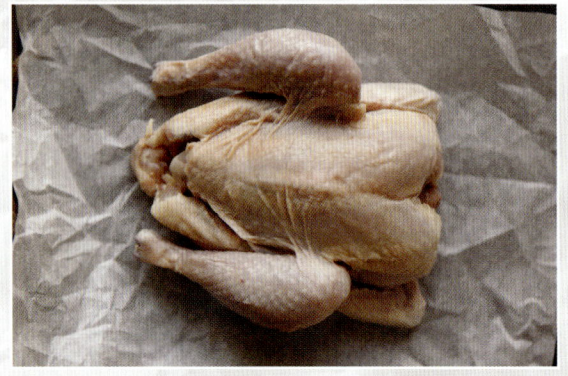

Whole Chicken – *Poulet Entier*

POULTRY, EGGS, AND RABBIT
La Volaille, les Oeufs, et Le Lapin

Basque Chicken – *Poulet Basquaise* 334

How to Butcher a Chicken..336

Béarnaise Garbure Soup – *La Garbure Béarnaise*..338

Chicken Cordon Bleu – *Cordon Bleu au Poulet* 341

Chicken in Wine Sauce "Coq au Vin" – *Coq au Vin* 345

Omelet with Herbs – *Omelette aux Fines Herbes* 349

Orange Duck Breast – *Magret de Canard à l'Orange* 351

Oven Roasted Duck Legs – *Cuisses de Canard au Four*...355

Preserved Duck Legs – *Cuisses de Canard Confites* 357

       Duck Rinds – *Grattons de Canard*..359

Pyrénées Farm Scrambled Eggs – *Oeufs Brouillés des Pyrénées* 360

Rabbit Stew with Onions and Duck Fat Potatoes – *Lapin aux Oignons et Pommes de Terre à la Graisse de Canard* 363

Stuffed Quail – *Cailles Farcies* 366

Stuffed Rabbit Saddle – *Râble de Lapin Farci* 368

Turkey Ragout – *Ragoût de Dinde*..370

Whole Roast Chicken with Herbes de Provence – *Poulet Rôti aux Herbes de Provence*.......373

Whole Stuffed Duck – *Canard Entier Farci* 375

Whole Stuffed Holiday Goose – *Oie Farcie pour les Fêtes* 377

BASQUE CHICKEN
Poulet Basquaise

Season Early-Summer through mid-Autumn   **Preparation Time** 50 minutes
Cooking Time 1 hour 15 minutes   **Serves** 4 to 5

Poulet basquaise is a traditional braised (browned and then slow-cooked) chicken dish from the French Basque country in Southwestern France. It has several steps, one of which is to cut the chicken into eight pieces. (See the photo tutorial on **How to Butcher a Chicken** on page 336.) As in many slow-cooked recipes, an aromatic "garnished bouquet" (*bouquet garni*) is employed in this recipe. A *bouquet garni* is a small bundle of aromatic herbs, usually comprised of a bay leaf, a green piece of leek sheath, a few sprigs of parsley, and a few sprigs of thyme (it may also include rosemary or savory), tied together with string, as shown in the recipe photo, or in a cheese cloth. Tomatoes in France are in season May through October, and bell peppers are in season June through October.

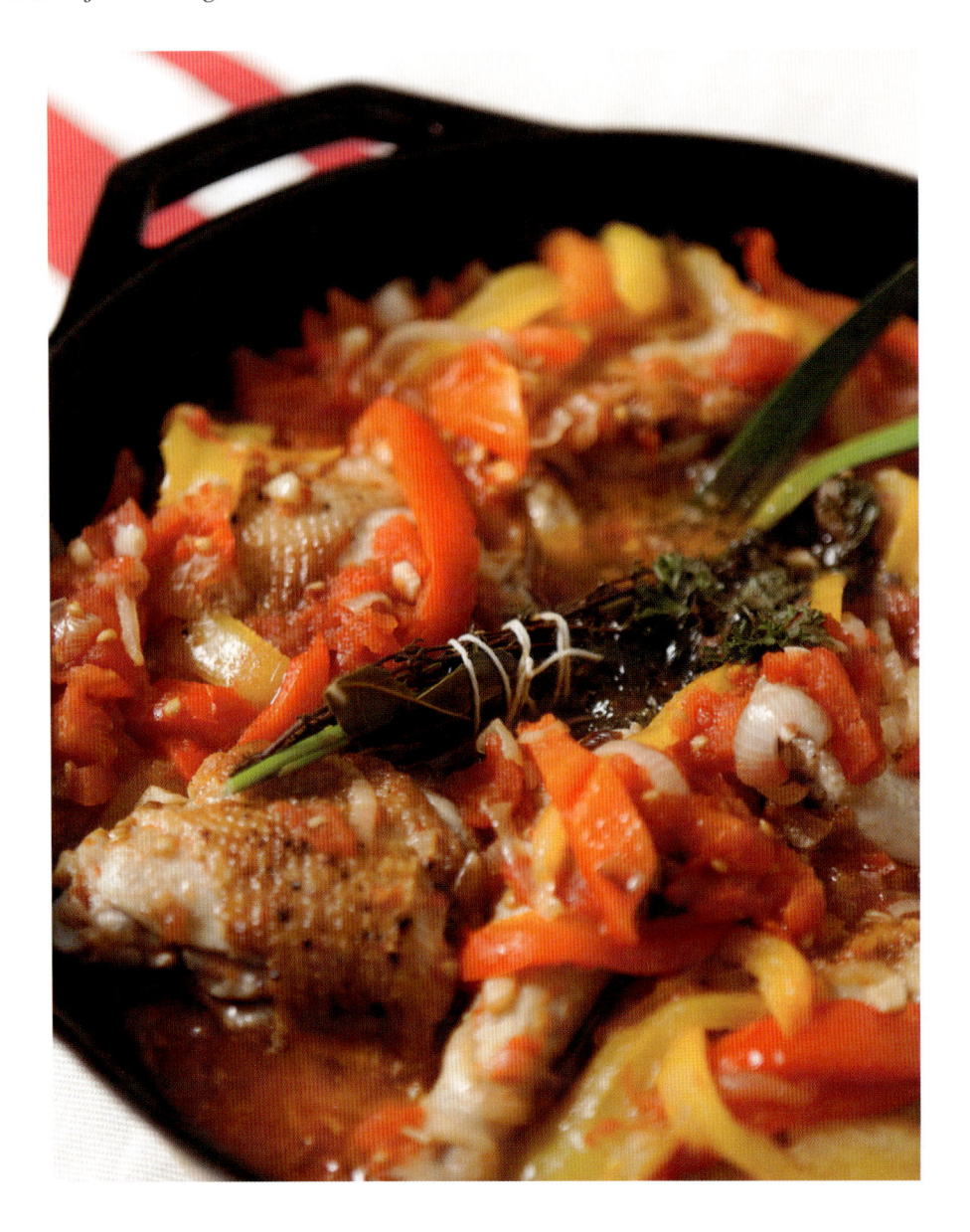

How to Blanche a Tomato

Bring a pot of water to boil with a pinch of salt. Boil the tomatoes for 30 to 60 seconds. Remove them from the water, briefly run under cool water, and peel the skin with a paring knife.

2 large bell peppers, halved and seeded

4 tablespoons duck fat or lard

Pinch of fine sea salt

3 garlic cloves, minced

4 onions (or 3 onions and 1 shallot), halved and sliced

4 tomatoes, blanched (see sidebar), peeled and chopped

Fine salt and ground pepper, for seasoning

1 chicken, cut into 8 pieces

Bouquet garni

½ cup (120 ml) dry white wine

Sea salt

Preheat the oven to 375°F (190°C). Place the peppers in an oven-safe dish and roast in the oven for 20 minutes to soften the outer skin. Peel the skin and cut into thin strips (*lamelles*).

Melt two tablespoons duck fat or lard in a large cast-iron or stainless-steel skillet over medium heat, add a pinch of salt, and sauté the garlic and onions for several minutes until the onions turn translucent. Add the roasted peppers and sauté the vegetables another five minutes. Add the tomatoes. Cover and simmer on low heat for about 10 minutes.

Season each piece of chicken with salt and pepper. Melt two tablespoons of duck fat or lard in another pan or a cast-iron pot over medium-high to high heat. Sauté the pieces, skin side down first, for five to seven minutes on each side until golden brown and crispy. Add these to the vegetables. Add the *bouquet garni* and the wine. Reduce the heat to medium-low, cover, and cook for about 35 minutes.

> WINE PAIRING TIP For a regional pairing, try a fresh and floral white or an aromatic and lively (*nerveux*—meaning having crisp acidity and sweetness) rosé Irouléguy from the Basque country. Also from the French Southwest are a Sauvignon Blanc and Sémillon blend such as a floral and crisp Côtes-de-Duras, or a Graves de Vayres, with floral, fruity, and boxwood (*buis*) aromas from Bordeaux's Entre-Deux-Mers appellation. I have used a Sauvignon Blanc from IGP (a geographic region whose agricultural production is regulated by the French government) Pays D'Oc from Languedoc-Roussillon for the recipe, drinking the rest with the meal. Also from Languedoc, try a Grenache and Syrah-based Cabardès, with notes of prune, spice, and vanilla.

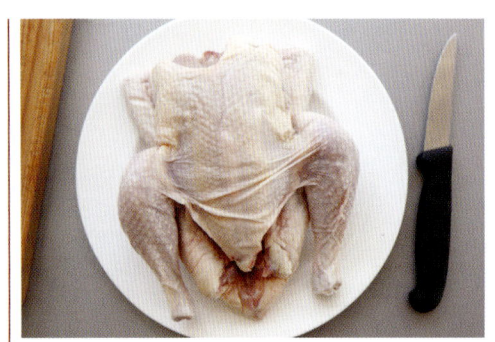

How to Butcher a Chicken

In this series of photos, my husband Toby was the model and had never butchered a chicken before. With some coaching from me and patience on his part, he butchered the chicken while I instructed and photographed his work. A professional butcher may have done a more precise job than we did and in less time, but like anything else, one's skills improve with practice.

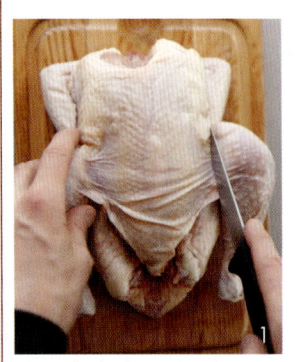

1. Place the knife on the skin between the breast and the thigh.

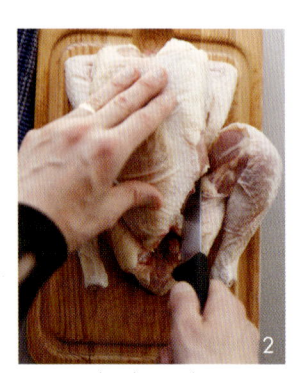

2. Cut into the skin and downward until you hit the bone.

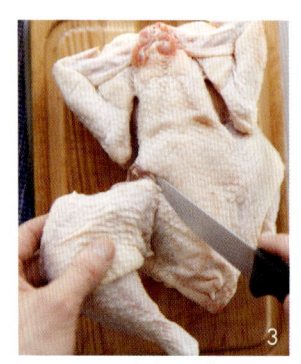

3. Sometimes it helps to flip the chicken over and rotate the leg backward (toward you) until you hear it snap.

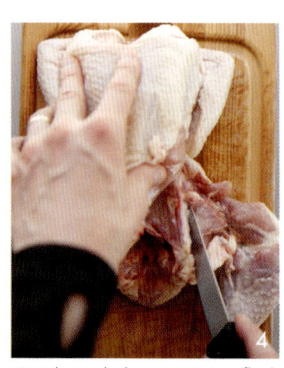

4. Cut through the remaining flesh and around the joint.

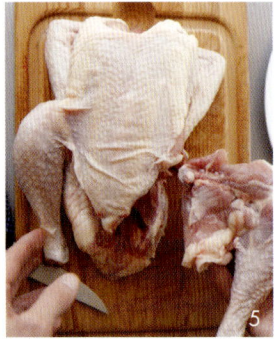

5. Separate the leg from the carcass.

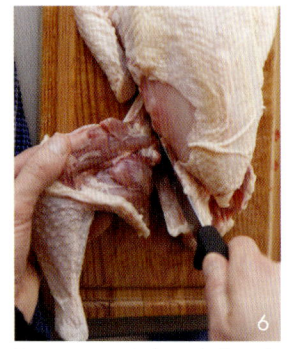

6. Repeat steps 1 through 5 on the other side to separate the leg from the carcass.

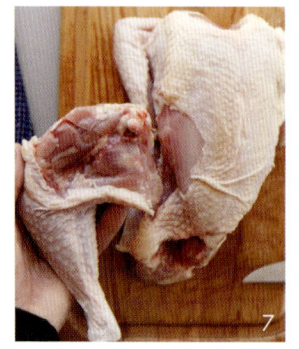

8. To remove the breast and wing, begin in the middle at the top of the breast on either side of the breastbone.

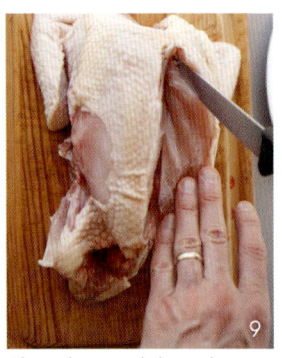

9. Slice along and down the breastbone, following it closely so as to cut away as much breast meat as possible.

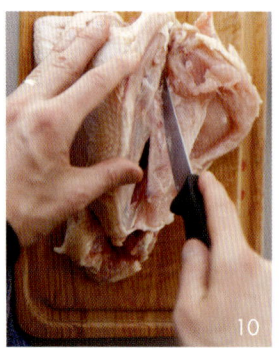

10. Cut along the bottom of the carcass to separate the breast (with the wing still attached).

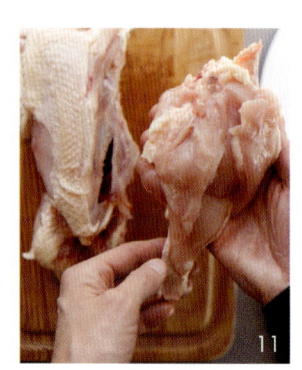

336   THE BORDEAUX KITCHEN

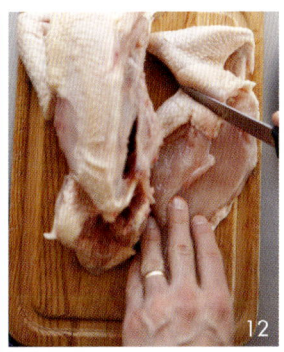

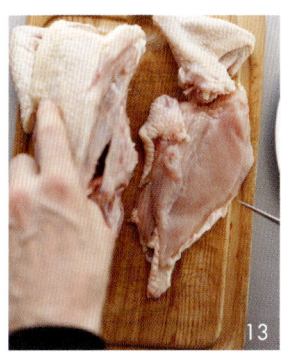

12. Cut the breast meat away from the wing joint and separate the breast from the wing.

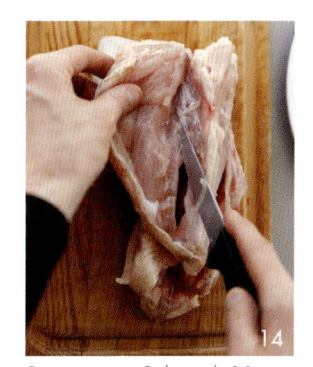

14. Repeat steps 8 through 11 to remove the other breast and wing.

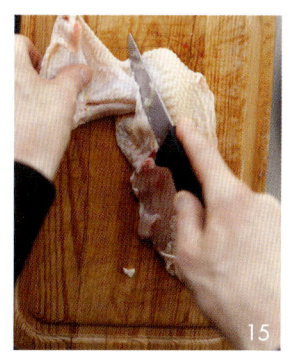

15. Separate the breast from the wing at the wing joint.

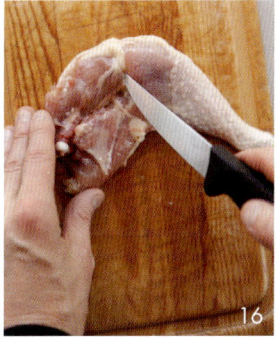

16. To separate the thigh from the drumstick, find the joint. (A line of fat marks the link between the muscles, where the tip of the knife is pointing.)

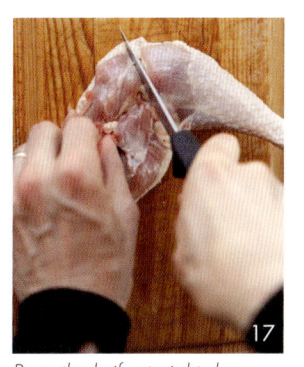

17. Press the knife straight down through the center of the joint, where it should be easy to cut through.

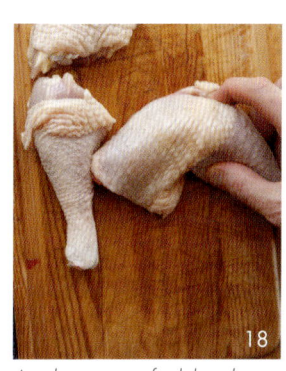

18. Another way to find the place to sever the thigh from the drumstick is to feel for the joint with your index finger.

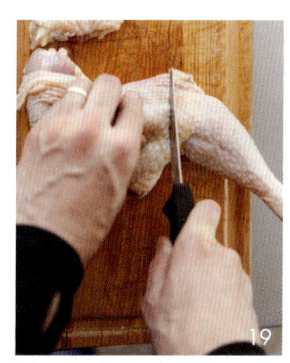

19. Place the knife above that spot and cut straight down.

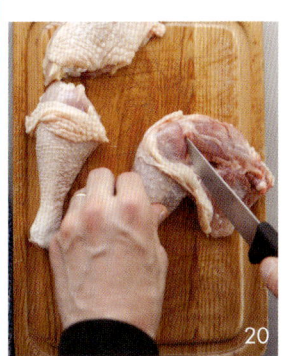

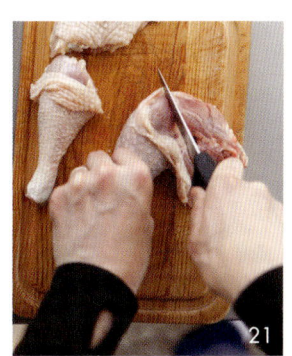

20–21. If that trick doesn't work, flip the drumstick over again, find the line of fat again, and cut through the joint.

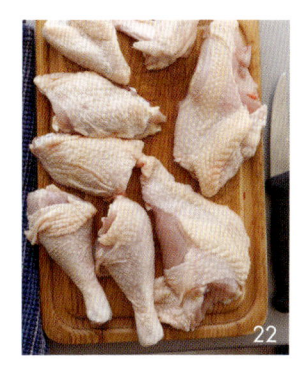

22. You now have 8 pieces ready for such recipes as **Coq au Vin** (page 345), **Basque Chicken** (page 334), or **Chicken with Herbes de Provence** (page 373), with chicken pieces instead of a whole chicken. Plus, you have the carcass, which can be roasted and then used in **Bone Broth** (page 394), **Chicken Stock** (page 417), or **White (or Light) Stock** (page 398).

POULTRY, EGGS, AND RABBIT – *LA VOLAILLE, LES OEUFS ET LE LAPIN*

BÉARNAISE GARBURE SOUP
La Garbure Béarnaise

Season Late Autumn and Winter   **Preparation Time** 15 minutes
Cooking Time 2 hours 20 minutes   **Serves** 4

La Garbure Béarnaise, also known as *La Soupe des Pyrénées Atlantiques,* was a traditional, everyday meal for the Gascons, people from the Basque and surrounding regions of Southwestern France, reaching almost to Toulouse and parts of northern Spain. The words Basque and Gascon are derived from Vascones and Wasconia, the words used to refer to the people and region, respectively, during the Middle Ages. The *garbure* varied from family to family, as most ancestral recipes do. It followed the rhythm of the seasons and was adaptable to what was available in the garden or the "salting room" (*saloir*). Preserved (*confit*) meats such as duck legs (*confit de cuisses canard,* or *confit de canard*) and duck wings (*confit de manchons*) are usually used in this dish, as they become more tender over time in their preserved state (see page 357). The white beans (*haricots blancs*) used in this dish should be soaked in filtered water overnight (or up to 24 hours) and then thoroughly rinsed to reduce their phytic acid and lectin content[1,2] and to soften them up. (The white beans may be cooked separately in salted water for about two hours prior to being added to the *garbure*, in order to soften them further and make them easier to digest.[3]) The original recipe calls for duck stock (*bouillon de canard*), using duck only, to keep the flavors homogenous (see details in the **White Poultry Stock** recipe on page 417). Chicken or poultry stock, however, may be used instead. Make (or thaw) the stock ahead of time.

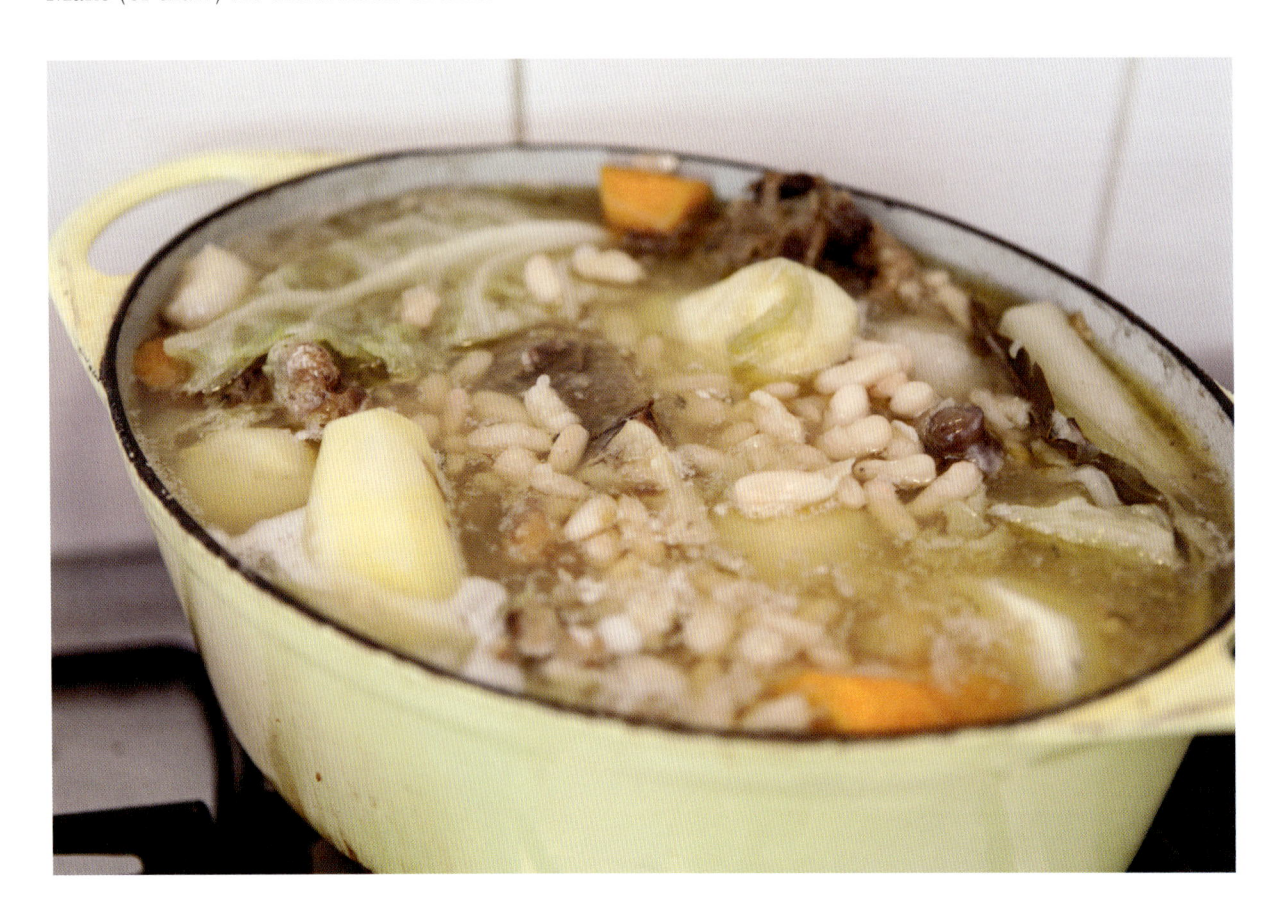

1 tablespoon duck fat

2 onions, chopped

3 pinches of fine salt

2 cups (475 ml) duck stock (or poultry stock)

5 carrots, chopped into 1-inch rounds (*rondelles*)

3 leeks (*poireaux*), chopped into 1-inch (2.5 cm) rounds

6 or 7 turnips (*navets*), quartered

1 sprig of thyme

1 small cabbage (*chou*), cut into quarters

1 ham hock (*os de jambon*)

2 duck legs (*confit de canard*) or 4 duck wings (*confit de manchons*)

5 small potatoes, halved

1¼ cups (300 ml) or 10 ounces (285 g) white beans (*haricots blancs*), soaked overnight

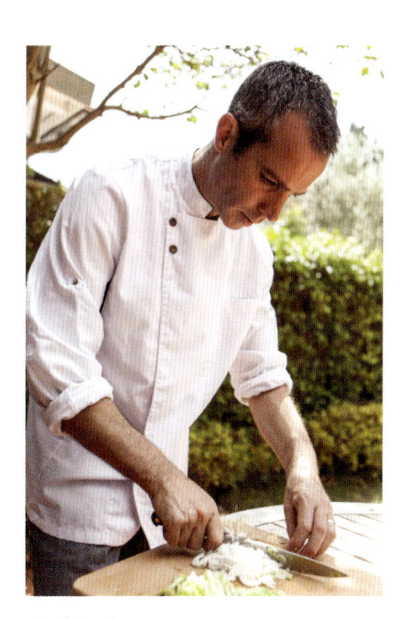

Chef Frédéric

Melt the duck fat over medium-high heat in a cast-iron pot. Add the onions and salt, and brown the onions, stirring occasionally, for several minutes.

Add the duck stock to the onions in the pot. Combine the carrots, leeks, turnips, thyme, cabbage, and ham hock, and bring to a boil.

Reduce the heat and simmer for a minimum of two hours. After the first 45 minutes, remove the cover to evaporate some of the liquid. Continue to simmer.

After 1-½ hours of simmering, divide each duck leg into two pieces, one half per person, or one wing per person, and add these to the pot. Add the white beans and potatoes and cook an additional 30 minutes, for a total of two hours of cooking.

Serve hot in a bowl with a side salad.

VARIATIONS To increase the fat content, start with more duck fat in the beginning (two or three tablespoons). Some Béarnese add a half a glass of red wine to their soup bowl to make a soup with wine added (*faire chabrol*, also called *chalorot* or *chabrot*, depending on the region), thought to be fortifying to one's health (see page 560). This soup is served as a "reinforcement" food in autumn and winter.

POULTRY, EGGS, AND RABBIT – *LA VOLAILLE, LES OEUFS ET LE LAPIN*

Garbure vs. Cassoulet

Garbure is similar to *cassoulet* because of the slow cooking technique and the inclusion of pork and white beans in the ingredients. In a *cassoulet*, however, there are usually pork sausages and a meat such as mutton in the dish instead of duck, as *cassoulet* originates further East, from Toulouse where pork is perhaps more frequently incorporated into regional dishes than duck. This *Garbure* recipe calls for ham hock (*os de jambon*), the bottom part of the pork leg (*la crosse*). Its purpose is to add aroma and flavor (*parfumer*), and not much meat (*viande*) on the bone is needed. Much like the **Pot-au-Feu** (page 123), the *garbure* is served in the form of a soup (*potage*) or as a main course, as plated vegetables and meats served to bolster the mountain shepherds. This particular version of *garbure* comes from Chef Frédéric's father's restaurant refuge (*chalet auberge*), "La Caverne," which operated in the late 1990s and early 2000s in the Vallée d'Ossau in the Pyrénnées.

WINE PAIRING TIP My wine course classmate and former restaurant owner Annabelle Nicolle-Beaufils recommends dry, full-bodied red wines. For a regional pairing from the Southwest, she suggests an herby and spiced Cahors with notes of cherry made from the Malbec grape (known locally as *Côt* or *Auxerrois*), or a classic Gascon pairing of a rich Madiran, made from the tannic Tannat grape, or a hearty Cabernet Sauvignon-heavy Médoc. From other regions, Annabelle proposes a spiced Côtes du Rhône Villages from the Southern Rhône Valley, made from 50% Grenache grapes and a combination of Mourvèdre and spicy Syrah, or else a bold Côtes du Roussillon Villages, made from the Carignan, Grenache, and Syrah grapes from Northern Roussillon, just South of the Languedoc part of the Languedoc-Roussillon region.

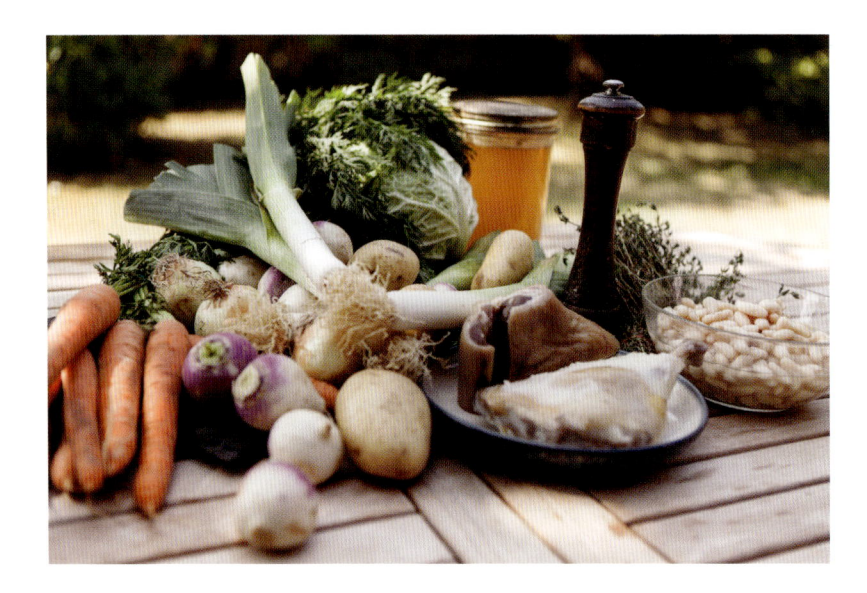

CHICKEN CORDON BLEU
Cordon Bleu au Poulet

Season Year-round   **Preparation Time** 15 minutes
Cooking Time 8 to 10 minutes   **Serves** 2

The *Cordon Bleu* is originally the name for a blue ribbon given to individuals inducted into knighthood in the late 1500s by Henri III of France, but more recently has been used for dishes and chefs of superior quality and capability. Perhaps the most famous cooking school in the world is *Le Cordon Bleu* in Paris, where Julia Child studied in the 1950s. Chicken Cordon Bleu as a dish actually originated in Switzerland, where it is called *Schnitzel Cordon Bleu*. Another variant of the Cordon Bleu dish is Veal Cordon Bleu, in which a slice of veal is pounded thin and wrapped around slices of ham and cheese. This Cordon Bleu recipe was first demonstrated to me by Chef Frédéric, whom I originally met at Bordeaux's cooking school, *Atelier des Chefs*. Chef Frédéric is a natural teacher and is always willing to show me how to do even the most basic of dishes. Chicken Cordon Bleu is a butterflied breast of chicken (sliced almost all the way through the middle and laid open like a book), then stuffed with a slice of ham and a slice of cheese and then pan-fried in flour and bread crumbs. I do not use bread crumbs, only chestnut flour. (Walnut or coconut flour may also be used.) The cheese used is usually a hard, strong-flavored cheese, such as Gruyère or Cantal. For children or those who do not like strong cheeses, a milder cheese may be used, such as Swiss cheese (*Emmental*) or Mozzarella. (I used Emmental in the recipe photo and the step-by-step photos.) You may also make **Turkey Cordon Bleu** using butterflied turkey breast, or else even more simplified, turkey breast steaks. (See Variations and photo at end of this recipe.)

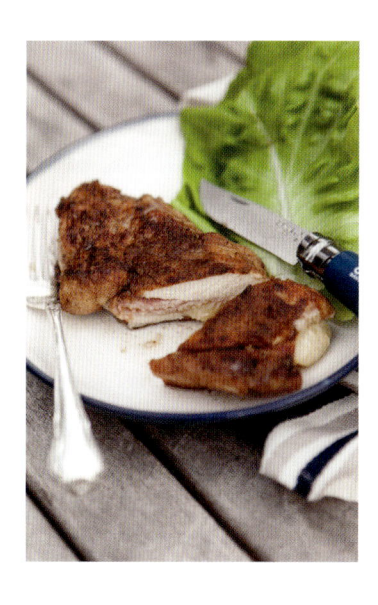

2 boneless, skinless chicken breasts

2 slices of ham

2 to 4 slices of cheese

1 egg, raw, yolk and white whisked together on a plate

2 tablespoons chestnut flour

Fine sea salt, for seasoning

2 teaspoons duck fat or lard

POULTRY, EGGS, AND RABBIT – *LA VOLAILLE, LES OEUFS ET LE LAPIN*

342 THE BORDEAUX KITCHEN

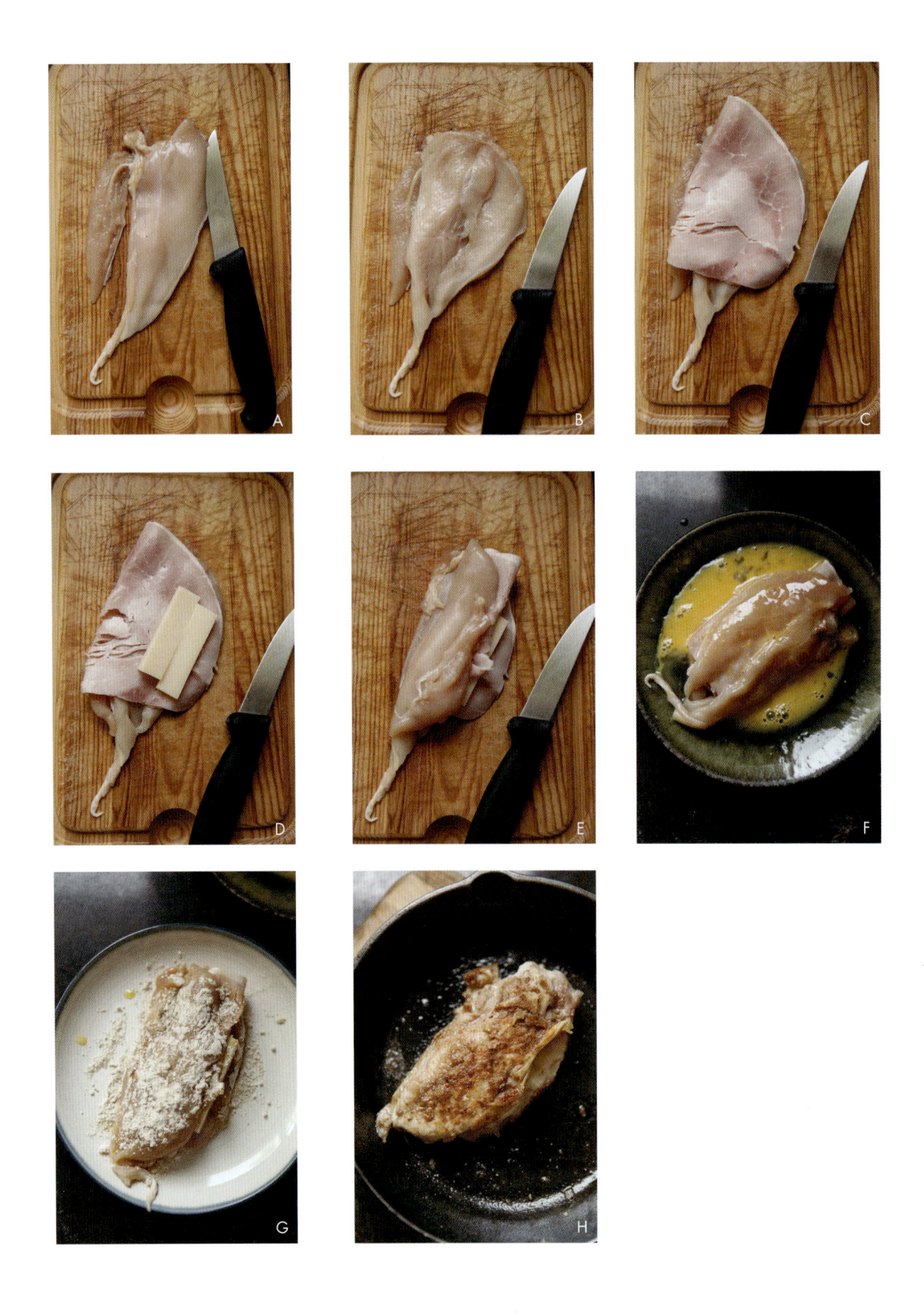

Chef Frédéric demonstrated this recipe as well as the **Omelet with Herbs** (page 349) from his then new fandango food truck in Bordeaux, "Truck de Chef." He actually designed the interior to fit his needs and says that after having done so, he realizes the tweaks he would make on his next truck. He's got it down to the placement of decoration, toothpicks, cabinet drawers and handles, grilling options, light, water, electricity, cooking, and utensil placement. He even has outdoor dining equipment for the clientele who prefer to eat "on location" (*sur place*) rather than take away their lunch.

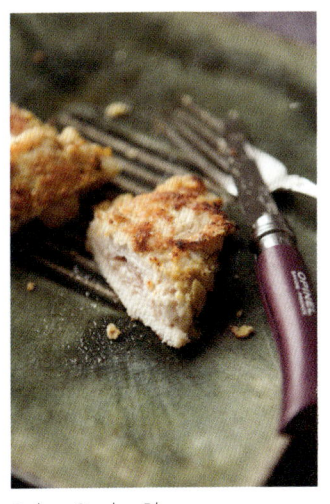

Turkey Cordon Bleu

Butterfly each chicken breast by slicing through the width of the breast and opening it like a book (photos A and B). Fold a piece of ham and lay it across each chicken breast (photo C). Cover one half of the breast with a slice or two of cheese (photo D). Close the breast like a book (photo E). Roll both sides of each breast in the raw egg (photo F), then in the flour (photo G). Season each side with salt.

Melt the duck fat or lard in a medium skillet over medium heat for four to five minutes on each side (photo H). (Chestnut flour burns easily, therefore it is better to cook slowly and a few minutes longer than quickly over high heat.)

VARIATIONS Using coconut flour in lieu of chestnut flour makes a Chicken or Turkey Cordon Bleu taste like chicken or turkey nuggets. (In this case, coconut oil can also be used for flavoring the "nuggets.") Kids love this. **Turkey Cordon Bleu** can be made from butterflied turkey breast or thin turkey breast steaks. For about a pound (500 g) of turkey breast steaks (about 4 steaks), you will need ¼ cup chestnut flour (or coconut flour, as shown in the Turkey Cordon Bleu photo), one egg, a pinch of salt, and one-and-a-half tablespoons or more of duck fat, lard, or coconut oil. (Coconut flour absorbs fat, so you may need additional fat if using coconut flour.) Butterfly slices of turkey breast as described above for the chicken breast. If the steaks or butterflied turkey breasts are thick, they may need additional time (10 to 15 minutes) in the oven (set at 365°F or 185°C) to cook through. Try this recipe using thin veal and chestnut flour for a **Veal Cordon Bleu**.

WINE PAIRING TIP Restaurateur Annabelle suggests crisp and flavorful white wines, strong enough to hold their own but not overly oaked so as to overtake the flavors of the Cordon Bleu: a floral and acacia Mâcon chardonnay from Southern Burgundy; an almond, apple, and flinty chardonnay from Auxey-Duresses in Burgundy's Côte de Beaune; or an aromatic Patrimonio, with intense notes of white flowers and exotic fruits, from the island of Corsica. Crisp and flavorful whites from Bordeaux could include a citrus and mango Bordeaux Blanc from the Graves region (which I have paired with both Chicken *and* Turkey Cordon Bleu, as the wine magnifies the flavors of both itself and the dish), a lemony-crisp Blayes-Côtes de Bordeaux, or else a fresh Bourg, Côtes de Bourg, or Francs-Côtes de Bordeaux. I have also paired an aromatic provençale rosé from Côtes de Provence with the Turkey Cordon Bleu—a lovely combination.

POULTRY, EGGS, AND RABBIT – *LA VOLAILLE, LES OEUFS ET LE LAPIN*

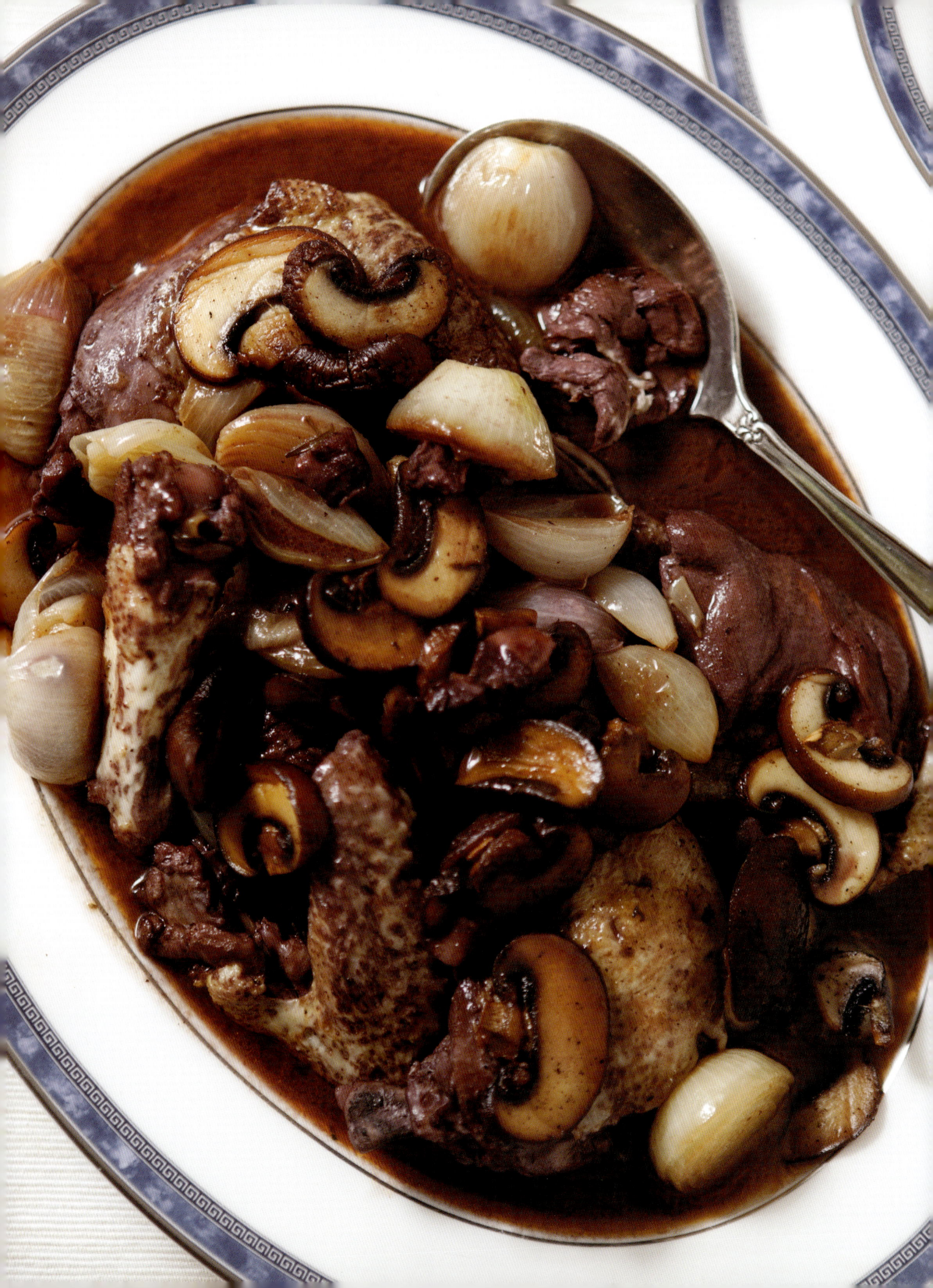

CHICKEN IN WINE SAUCE "COQ AU VIN"
Coq au Vin

Season Mid-Autumn through late Spring   **Preparation Time** 1 hour
Cooking Time 1 hour 30 minutes   **Serves** 5

This recipe wins the prize for the highest number of steps, but that does not make it impossible to do. For this recipe, I referred to Julia Child's recipe in her book, *Mastering the Art of French Cooking*, because it was one of the first recipes she demonstrated in her cooking shows and I wanted a version of this recipe that was authentic but made in a way that was straightforward. This is the not the kind of recipe you do for everyday meals, simply because of the various parts that add up to a long time commitment (unless you are the kind of cook who has chicken stock brewing and a continuous supply of sautéed mushrooms and braised onions when you need them; the best restaurants definitely have this capacity). As a result, this is a recipe with other recipes within it, **White Stock** (page 398) or **Veal Stock** (page 415), brown-braised onions, and butter sautéed mushrooms. This recipe, if done all at once from onions to mushrooms to chicken including all the prep work, takes me two and a half hours (actually three due to half an hour of interruptions from children, which is part of the reality of being a mom). It is a recipe with such complexity of flavor that it really is amazing, and you will wow your friends and guests. In the end however, it's still just chicken dressed up in a sauce. Veal or beef seem more rewarding in terms of matching the intensity of flavor between meat and sauce. But that's why we have **Beef Burgundy** (page 109) and veal stews! As in many traditional French recipes, a "garnished bouquet" (*bouquet garni*) is used here which may be comprised of four to six parsley sprigs, one to two small thyme sprigs, one small bay leaf, a piece of leek, and sometimes parsley, all tied with a string or inside a cheese cloth. The common mushroom "Agaricus Bisporus" (*Champignon de Paris*) used in this recipe is in season October through May. A thick slab of bacon is called for in this recipe because of the flavor it provides. In France, bacon is sold with the rind on. Remove the rind from the slab of bacon and save it as an ingredient for your next round of stock or bone broth. The bacon must be cut into ½- to 1-inch strips (*lardons*), or else take 4 ounces of thinly-sliced bacon and cut them into small pieces. For this recipe, the chicken carcass must be cut down into six pieces: two wings, two legs, two breasts. (See the photo tutorial on **How to Butcher a Chicken** on page 336.) This recipe also calls for **Brown Stock**, which you will find on page 397.

FOR THE ONIONS (50 TO 60 MINUTES)

1½ tablespoons butter

1½ tablespoons duck fat

10.5 ounces (300 g) small onions (or shallots), halved

Bouquet garni

½ cup (120 ml) veal or white stock

Pinch of salt

Pinch of pepper

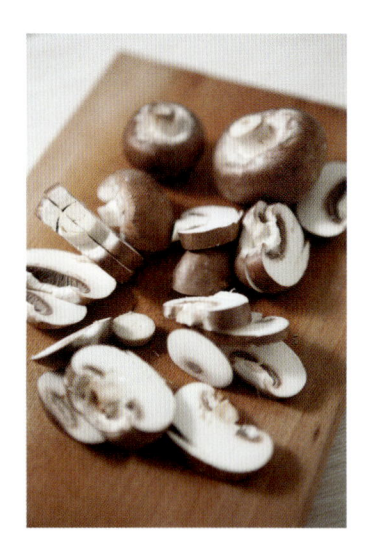

FOR THE MUSHROOMS (15 MINUTES)

2 tablespoons butter

1 tablespoon duck fat

Up to half a pound (140 g to 225 g) mushrooms, sliced

FOR THE REST OF THE COQ AU VIN

2 tablespoons butter

4-ounce (115 g) slab of bacon, cut into ½- to 1-inch (1.25 cm to 2.5 cm) strips (*lardons*)

2½ to 3 pounds (1 to 1.5 kg) chicken, cut into 6 pieces

Fine salt and ground pepper, for seasoning

¼ cup (60 ml) cognac

3 cups (750 ml) of a young, full-bodied red wine (see Wine Pairing Tip below)

1 to 2 cups (240 to 475 ml) brown stock (chicken or veal)

1½ teaspoons tomato paste

1 bay leaf

2 garlic cloves, peeled and crushed

Pinch of salt

Salt and pepper for seasoning

3 tablespoons chestnut flour

2 tablespoons butter, softened

Parsley, for garnish

For the onions, melt the butter and duck fat in a medium stainless-steel pan or cast-iron pot over medium heat. Add the onions and sauté them for about 10 minutes. Add the *bouquet garni*, veal or white stock, salt, and pepper. Cover and simmer on low for 40 to 50 minutes.

For the mushrooms, melt the butter and fat in a large skillet or pan over medium-high heat until foamy, then add mushrooms without crowding the pan. If necessary, do the browning in batches. Brown on each side for a few minutes, allowing each side to turn a nice golden, slightly crispy brown. Sliding the pan back and forth will make the mushrooms slide around and remain covered in the butter. As soon as the mushrooms are browned on both sides, remove them from the pan and set aside in a bowl. This process takes about 15 minutes. You now have sautéed mushrooms. (The mushrooms may be prepared in this way as a side dish for other meals as well.)

For the rest of the *Coq au Vin*, melt two tablespoons of butter in a cast-iron pot over medium heat and brown the *lardons* slowly for about 10 minutes or until nicely caramelized. Remove the bacon from the pot and set aside.

Brown the chicken on both sides for two minutes each side in the pot, starting with the skin side first. Allow enough room for each piece to have space in the pot, browning in batches if necessary.

Salt and pepper the chicken. Return the bacon to the pot. Cover and cook on medium heat for 10 minutes turning the chicken once.

Pour the cognac in the pan and remove the pan from the vent and heat. Quickly but carefully put a lit match or butane kitchen torch near the edge of the pan to flambé the chicken. (I let the match drop in and get it out later.) Shake the pan back and forth carefully, while the flames are burning to distribute the burning Cognac. If the flames seem to be taking too long to die down (it should only take a few seconds), you can briefly cover the pot with a lid.

Pour in the wine. (Chill the rest of the wine in the fridge for a half a glass to enjoy during the meal. As I have mentioned before, often a cook will buy two bottles of the same wine, one for cooking and one to drink with the meal!) Add the brown stock, tomato paste, bay leaf, garlic, and salt. Cover and simmer on medium-low for 25 to 30 minutes.

Transfer the chicken to a separate bowl. Add salt and pepper if needed to the remaining liquid in the pan and boil rapidly, reducing the liquid by a little less than half (making about 2-½ cups, about 600 ml, of liquid.) This takes about five minutes. Remove from heat and discard the bay leaf.

In a small bowl, blend three tablespoons of chestnut flour with two tablespoons of soft butter with a spatula. Beat the butter and flour paste into the liquid with a wire whisk. Bring to a simmer for a minute or two. With chestnut flour, the sauce does not thicken like wheat flour might, but it does give the sauce a bit more of an unctuous quality than without it. Add the sautéed mushrooms and onions to the sauce and allow them to warm up for a few minutes in the pot.

Serve the chicken, covered with the sauce on a platter, garnished with parsley. *Coq au Vin* is traditionally served with parsley potatoes, but you can also try buttered peas or other vegetables of your choice, possibly just steamed or buttered, as the sauce is rich enough in flavor and fat to coat any accompanying vegetables. ➤

Leftover Sauce

You may have quite a bit of sauce left over, and like any leftover sauce, I recommend you save it and use it for another meal or freeze it. In the case of leftover *Coq au Vin* sauce, I might recommend beginning the recipe with more chicken (such as using two small chickens or 10 to 12 pieces of chicken total) or roasting plain chicken and adding the sauce to it for a quick meal in this unctuous sauce that seems to gain in complexity of flavor by the day. It may sound like heresy to some, but the chicken is almost too plain (and scant) to warrant such a regal sauce. I have added the leftover sauce to pieces of stewed lamb meat, and the combination is extraordinary! I think lamb, beef, veal, even perhaps duck would be a better match for such a rich, complex sauce. Something to experiment with!

WINE PAIRING TIP In *Mastering the Art of French Cooking*, Julia Child recommends both making *and* serving this dish with a young, full-bodied red wine, such as Beaujolais, Burgundy, Côtes du Rhône, or Italian Chianti. Child mentions that this dish can also be made using the white wine Riesling, made in Alsace (and in Germany), in which case the dish would be called *Coq au Riesling* and could be served with a bottle of Riesling. For a Southwestern pairing, sommelière Annabelle recommends a tannic, fleshy, and richly pigmented Southwestern Cahors, with notes of red and black fruits and flavors of licorice. Otherwise, she suggests a rich Faugères with notes of vanilla and toast from Languedoc-Roussillon, or a full-bodied Châteauneuf-du-Pape or a powerful Hermitage, both from the Rhône Valley. From Burgundy, Annabelle suggests a fleshy Gevrey-Chambertin, with notes of red fruits, which is from the Côte de Nuits, Burgundy's northern half of the Côte d'Or (meaning "Golden Slope") region, or a Pommard, with notes of berries, cherries, and plums from the Côte de Beaune, Burgundy's southern half of its Côte d'Or.

OMELET WITH HERBS
Omelette aux Fines Herbes

Season Spring for the scallions, otherwise year-round   **Preparation Time** 5 minutes
Cooking Time 8 to 10 minutes   **Serves** 1

This is a standard omelet that appears on most French café menus along with the *Croque Monsieur* (crunchy toast with ham and cheese) or the *Croque Madame* (crunchy toast with ham, cheese, and an egg on top). For the herb, my friend, Chef Fréd, and I used *l'oignon aillé*, a very aromatic (*très parfumé*) cross between a scallion or green onion (*oignon vert*) and garlic (*l'ail*), a variety local to Bordeaux in the spring, shown below. Scallions and other in-season herbs and vegetables may be used as desired. Spring is the season for scallions and some herbs, but these may be chopped and frozen for use throughout the year. If you have an indoor herb garden, so much the better for fresh herbs! ➤

This method of making an omelet is the French standard, shown to me by Chef Frédéric who says that omelets are served *baveuse*, literally "drooling," in France, *not* well done like we often serve in the U.S. Overcooking the eggs ruins the flavor, and the French are used to the runny texture. So, if you order an omelet in France, remember it will be runnier than what you may be used to. Otherwise, this recipe will get you used to the runny style. (For those afraid of raw eggs, beware. Pregnant and nursing women might want to avoid this type of omelet if they are concerned about bacterial issues with raw eggs.) *Piment d'Espelette*, the dried red sweet chili powder, is called for in this recipe and is a typical Basque condiment used in the French Southwest. Chef Frédéric is the one who showed me that a "pinch" of salt means two fingers and your thumb, reaching into a small bowl of salt and then sprinkling this over the food. It is actually a good, consistent, and tactile measure and better way to use salt than a salt shaker or grinder with which you cannot *feel* the salt (or pepper or spice) in your hands.

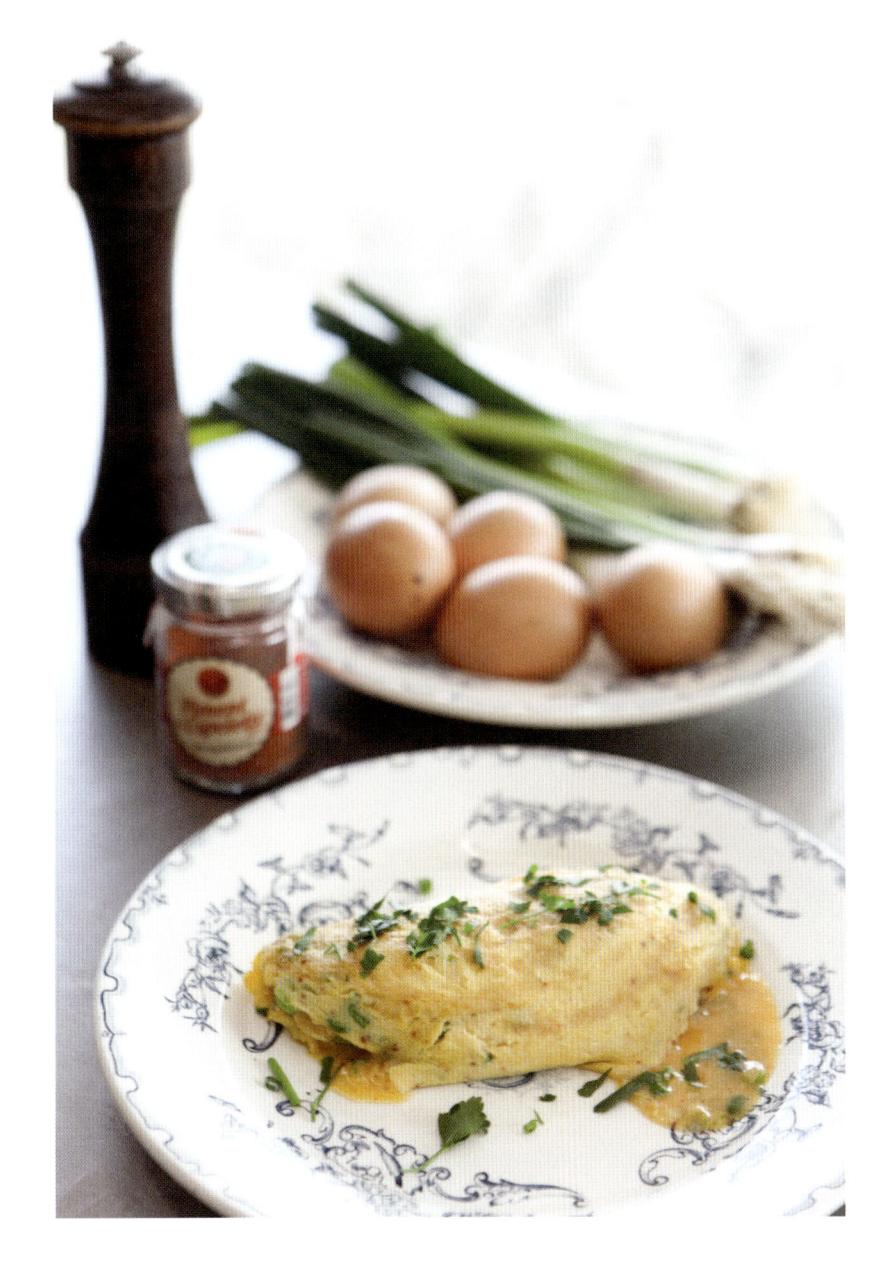

POULTRY, EGGS, AND RABBIT – *LA VOLAILLE, LES OEUFS ET LE LAPIN*

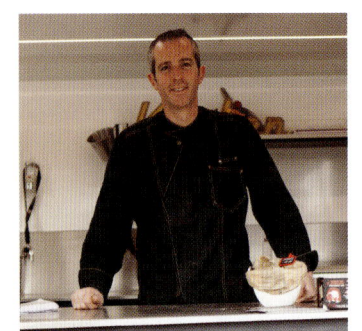

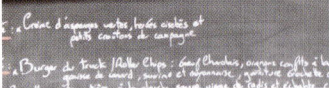

Chef's Tip
Astuce du Chef

To finely chop an herb or a scallion (or anything, for that matter), the fingers holding down the herb should be curved, like fingers on piano keys, to form a wall alongside of which the knife moves and is guided, so as to avoid being cut, as Chef Frédéric demonstrates here.

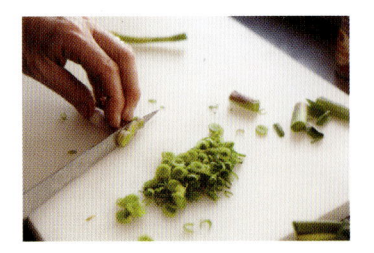

Tilting the Pan

1 tablespoon olive oil or butter

Several sprigs of chives or one or two green onions (green part only), finely chopped *(ciselés)*

3 medium eggs

Pinch of fine salt

Pepper to taste

Optional: *piment d'Espelette* to taste and for color

Optional: cheese and/or ham

Heat the olive oil or melt the butter in a small pan over medium-high heat. Add the herbs and sauté them for three or four minutes until just colored (*coloré*).

Crack the eggs into a bowl and whisk them together, not too much (*ne fouetter pas trop*). Add the salt, pepper, and optional *piment d'Espelette*. Combine (*mélanger*) the eggs into the herbs in the pan like scrambled eggs, then let the eggs sit on the heat for several minutes until the bottom of the omelet solidifies. The surface will still be runny.

At this point, you can add in cheese and/or ham as a variation. Fold the omelet in half. Tilt the pan toward yourself and tap the handle so that the underside of the omelet slides forward beneath the omelet surface (a very handy but technical chef technique for an omelet, as depicted in the photo below). Roll the omelet onto itself again to make a kind of burrito effect. *Voilà*!

Variations The French love their truffles, a tablespoon of which, chopped and white or black, can be added per four eggs (about two teaspoons for a three-egg omelet), plus a dollop of sour cream (*crème fraîche*).

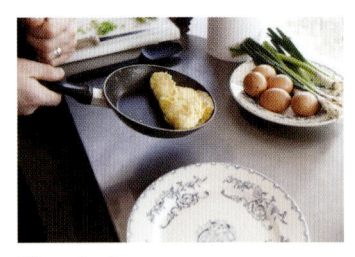

Wine Pairing Tip If this is breakfast, try a Champagne or other white or rosé sparkling wine, or a fruity chardonnay from Burgundy or the Loire Valley. Otherwise, Restaurateur Annabelle recommends oaked red wines with body, such as a Médoc Cru Bourgeois from Bordeaux's "Left Bank" region, or a powerful and dark Cornas, with notes of blackberry, dark cherry, and spice, made uniquely from the Syrah grape in the Rhône Valley, or else a spiced and elegant Côtes du Rhône Villages.

ORANGE DUCK BREAST
Magret de Canard à l'Orange

Season Autumn through Spring   **Preparation Time** 15 minutes
Cooking Time 25 to 30 minutes   **Serves** 4 to 5

This was one of the very first dishes I learned from Chef Frédéric while he was an instructor at *Atelier des Chefs* in Bordeaux. Headquartered in Paris, *Atelier des Chefs* has a network of ateliers throughout France, with cooking classes conducted in French and short tutorials online. If you can keep up with the French, the classes are fun to attend and a great way to learn basic and more complicated techniques. The most famous fatty duck breasts in France come from the Moulard duck from Gascony in France's Southwest. The breed is endowed with large thighs as well, used in duck leg recipes (see pages 355 and 357). Muscovy duck breasts, with a thinner layer of fat, may also be used for their rich, meaty flavor. Both types of duck are available in the U.S. from D'Artagnan at www.dartagnan.com, a company run by Ariane Daguin, a chef herself and daughter of the famed Gascon two-Michelin-starred chef André Daguin.

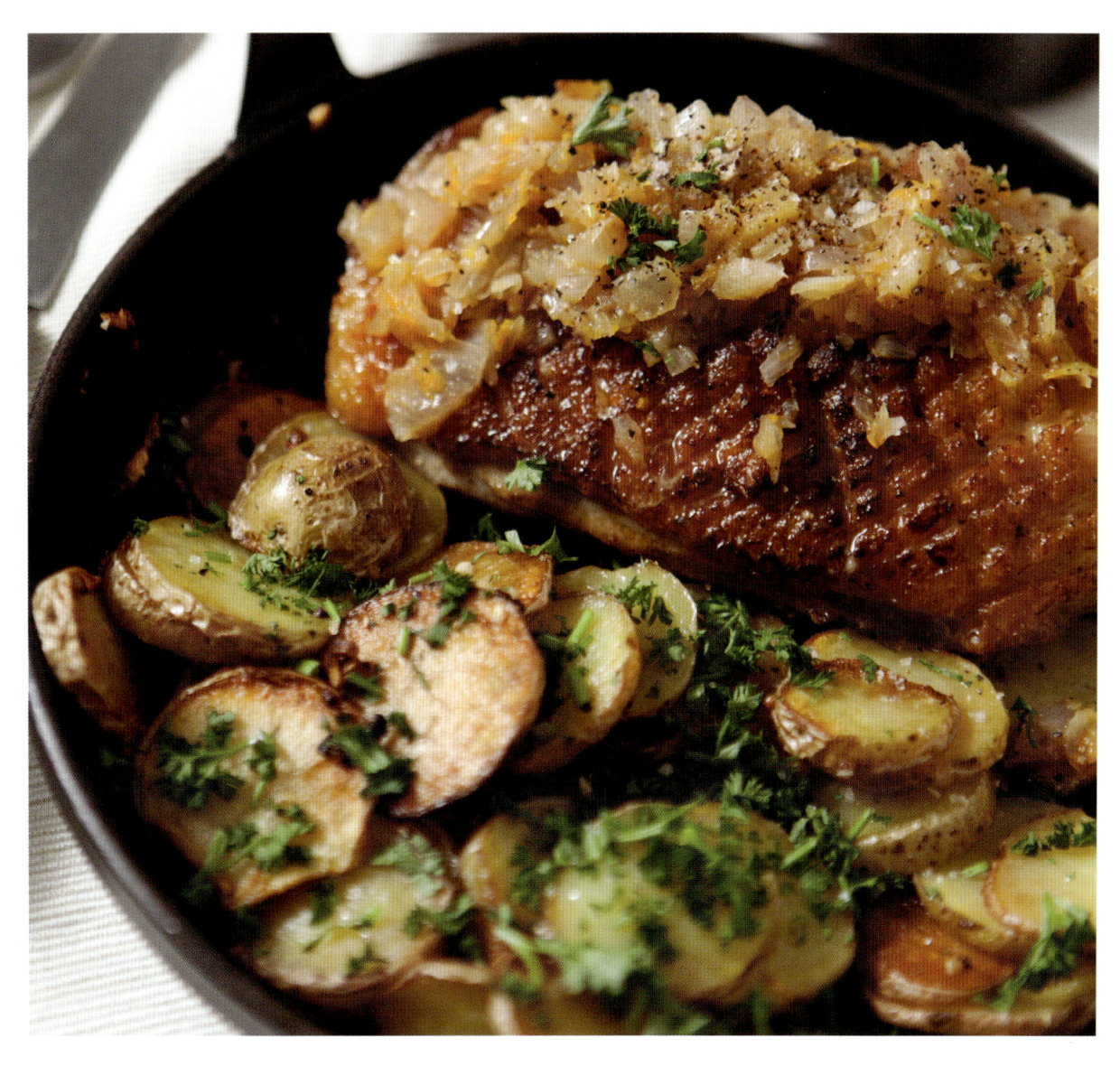

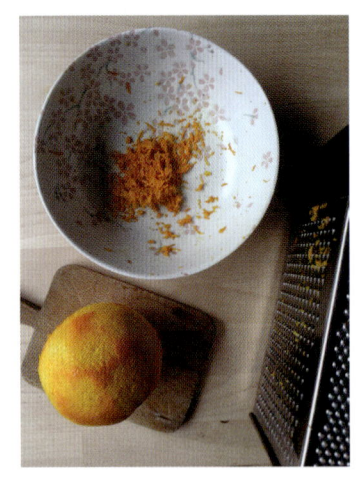

Grated Orange Peel

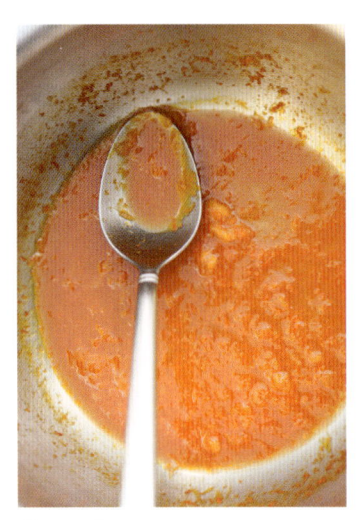

Orange Sauce

3 duck breasts, scored

Fine salt and ground pepper for seasoning

5 to 6 shallots, minced

Optional: 1 tablespoon balsamic vinegar

Pinch of fine salt

Zest of one orange or blood orange, grated

Juice of one orange (including the pulp)

Optional: 1 to 2 tablespoons honey

Handful of parsley, minced, for garnish

Heat a large cast-iron or stainless-steel skillet or pan over high heat. Season the fatty side of each duck breast with salt and pepper. Allow the skillet to become hot. (Sprinkle a few drops of water into the pan. If the droplets sizzle, the pan is hot enough.) Place the duck breasts into the pan fat side down and season the top side with salt and pepper. Cover with a mesh splatter screen. Allow the duck breasts to cook for six to 10 minutes until nicely browned and caramelized. Reduce the heat to medium-high after the first few minutes before turning each breast over with stainless-steel tongs or a long cooking fork.

Preheat the oven to 365°F (185°C). Allow the duck breasts to cook for another six to 10 minutes on the second side, then place them into an oven-safe dish, fat side up. Place into the oven for eight to 10 minutes to finish off the cooking, if you prefer not to eat the duck rare on the inside. Check the duck breasts with a meat thermometer or cut into one after about eight minutes to see how cooked it is.[5] At 10 minutes in the preheated oven, I have found that thick duck breasts will reach 150°F (about 66°C), medium to medium well, and still be delectably juicy.

Reduce the heat beneath the pan to medium or medium-low and stir the shallots and optional vinegar into the liquid duck fat remaining in the pan from the duck breasts. The shallots will soak up the fat and deglaze the pan. Stir in a pinch of fine salt.

Reduce the heat to low after about three minutes. Stir in the orange rind, orange juice, and optional honey, and allow the sauce to thicken for several minutes, stirring occasionally, while the duck breasts are in the oven.

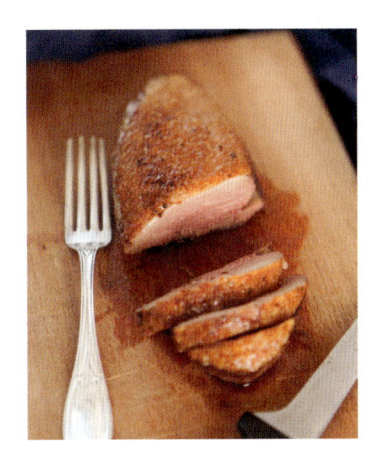

Serve the duck breast whole on a plate or in slices (as shown here), garnished with the orange shallot sauce and minced parsley with a side of **Sarlat Sautéed Potatoes** (page 468), as shown in the main recipe photo. Another option is to serve the duck with a dollop of **Homemade Plum Preserves** (page 63) or **Orange Plum Sauce** (page 412).

VARIATIONS For the shallot and orange sauce, a glass of wine or else a half cup of **Brown Stock** (page 397) may also be added to deglaze the pan. Reduce the sauce over medium heat for several minutes before serving over the duck breast.

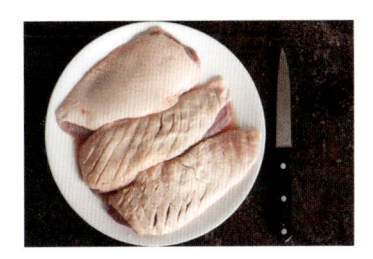

I have included in this recipe optional honey and vinegar, which is how I was taught at *Atelier des Chefs*. You may or may not wish to use them. The vinegar lends a savory tang to the shallots in the duck fat and makes this part of the dish worthy of its own food group, it's so good! The amount of orange juice used in the recipe may also be reduced if desired. This recipe can be used for a young female duck (*canette*) as well: the *canette* breast is smaller, carries less fat, and can be more tender. A regular duck breast weighs between 12 and 13 ounces (between 340 g and 360 g). Unlike chicken, duck is a red meat and therefore can be eaten rarer.[4] To make the duck breasts look pretty and to keep them from curling under the heat, score the duck breasts in a crisscrossed pattern, as shown in the photo here, in which the top breast is unscored, the middle breast is scored one way, and the bottom breast is scored both ways in a crisscross pattern.

WINE PAIRING TIP As this is a typical dish from the French Southwest, I would suggest a regional pairing of a red Bergerac, similar to the Bordeaux blend of Cabernet Franc, Cabernet Sauvignon, and Merlot. A tannic Madiran from the Southwest will also hold up well to the robust flavors of the duck breast. I have also paired this dish with a Ventoux from the Southern Rhône Valley, which carries sufficient tannins and density of flavor to match the robustness of the duck. In *Mastering the Art of French Cooking*, Julia Child recommends with this classic dish a Bordeaux Médoc or else a chilled white Burgundy, such as a Mersault from the Côte D'Or, or a Montrachet or Corton-Charlemagne from the Côte de Beaune. Andrew Dornenberg and Karen Page, in their book, *What to Drink with What You Eat*, recommend Gewürtztraminer, Riesling, or Pinot Noir,[6] which come from the Alsace and Burgundy regions, respectively, and most famously. I highly recommend Child's book as a premier reference on all things French cuisine in English and Dornenberg and Page's book as an inspiring reference on food and wine pairings.

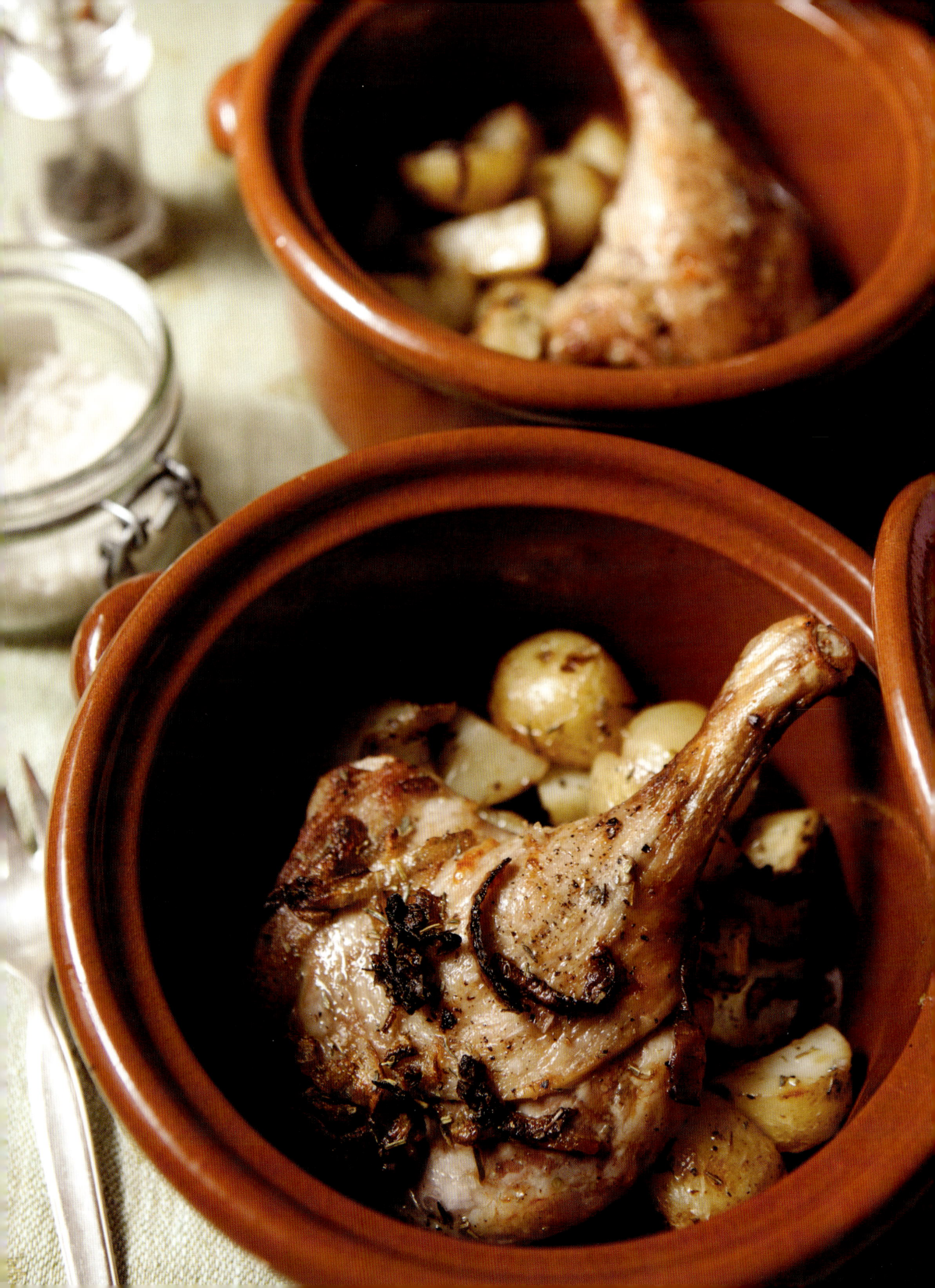

OVEN ROASTED DUCK LEGS
Cuisses de Canard au Four

Season Year-round **Preparation Time** 35 minutes
Cooking Time 10 to 12 minutes in the pan, then 20 to 30 minutes in the oven **Serves** 6

Duck legs can be eaten fresh or after they have been "preserved in fat" (*confit*). This recipe shows you how to prepare them fresh. See the recipe for **Preserved Duck Legs** on page 357 on how to preserve them yourself. Duck legs are more expensive when bought *confit*, as this process takes extra effort and time. The preservation in fat confers a tenderness to the duck meat, which is chewier when cooked fresh. When you do cook fresh duck legs, using a steel-mesh splatter screen over the pan will help keep hot duck fat from getting all over you, your stove, and your kitchen wall. (A simple mesh splatter screen is best, as the thicker, tighter, "odor-reducing" carbon screens are so thick that they do not allow moisture to escape, forcing it to condense and drip back onto the meat, causing more spitting and steaming the top side of the meat before it's had a chance to brown.)

6 fresh duck legs

Fine salt and ground pepper, for seasoning

2 tablespoons duck fat

2 onions, halved and finely sliced

14 garlic cloves, peeled and crushed

16 small potatoes, quartered

4 pinches of *herbes de Provence*

4 pinches of coarse sea salt

2 pinches of ground pepper

Preheat the oven to 365°F (185°C). Season each duck leg with salt and pepper. Melt a tablespoon of duck fat over medium-high heat, and place three legs, fattiest side down. Allow to brown on this side for five to six minutes, caramelizing the skin. This browning gives flavor and crispiness to the skin. Turn down the heat one notch if the pan begins to smoke. Remember the splatter screen, as the fat will spit.

Turn the legs in the pan, allowing the other side to brown, and add half of the chopped onion, crushed garlic, and quartered potatoes. Sprinkle two pinches of salt, two pinches of *herbes de Provence*, and one pinch of pepper over the duck legs and vegetables. Cook for another five to six minutes, stirring the vegetables a bit in the pan. Transfer all the contents of the pan to a large casserole dish (or into individual oven-safe clay pots) and set aside. ▶

Herbes de Provence

This recipe calls for *herbes de Provence*, a combination of herbs that may include thyme, rosemary, savory, oregano, hyssop, marjoram, parsley. If you do not have *herbes de Provence*, put it on your shopping list, as it's a very handy seasoning mixture to have on hand. Use what you have in your spice rack in the meantime.

Melt another tablespoon of duck fat in the pan and repeat the browning process with the other three legs, adding the remaining onion, garlic, and potatoes, *herbes de Provence*, salt, and pepper after the legs have been turned onto the second side. Transfer these to the large casserole dish or into individual clay pots.

Place the casserole dish (or clay pots) into the oven and cook for 20 to 30 minutes, depending on how well-done you would like the legs. Serve the duck legs with the accompanying vegetables on a plate or in the individual clay pots. Serve with a salad or sautéed or roasted vegetables.

WINE PAIRING TIP According to the very helpful French website Le Guide Hachette des Vins (www.Hachette-vins.com), preserved (*confit*) duck or goose go well with wines that are fleshy (like biting into a ripe fruit), with soft, melty, and rounded tannins, just like the melt-in-your-mouth style of preserved fowl meats. Whether you are using fresh or preserved duck legs, the softness and richness of the wine should go well with both styles. Hachette's suggestions include the flavorful Southwest reds of Cahors and Madiran, as well as Languedoc's Corbières, Minervois, and Cabardès. See also the wine pairing recommendations for **Preserved Duck Legs** (page 358).

PRESERVED DUCK LEGS
Cuisses de Canard Confites

Season Autumn and Winter   **Preparation Time** 30 minutes (plus optional storage overnight)
Cooking Time 1 hour 30 minutes   **Serves** 6

My friend and trained chef, Dewey Markham, Jr., a transplanted New Yorker who has made his home and is raising his family in Bordeaux, does not consider himself a chef, but simply "someone who applies heat to food." His modesty hides a wealth of culinary knowledge he has practiced over several decades. He explained to me that the French word *confire* means to preserve. Therefore, *confit* means preserved, as in fruit preserves (*confiture*). In the case of duck legs, these are preserved in duck fat in a process that goes back centuries in which the fat is the preserving agent. All you needed was fat, glass, or clay containers or pots and space in a cool, dark cellar. (For information on how to render duck fat, see page 266.) It takes about one to one-and-a-half hours to render two to four pounds (one to two kg) of duck fat, which results in duck rinds, like cracklings resulting from rendering pork or beef fat. (See the recipe in the sidebar on page 359 for further use of **Duck Rinds**.) Once preserved, duck legs are the kind of thing one has in storage to pull out in case of emergency, when a market or grocery run did not materialize. Preserved duck legs are easily heated in a pan in some of the fat in which they were preserved. They are more tender than fresh duck legs and cook more quickly, as they have been pre-cooked.

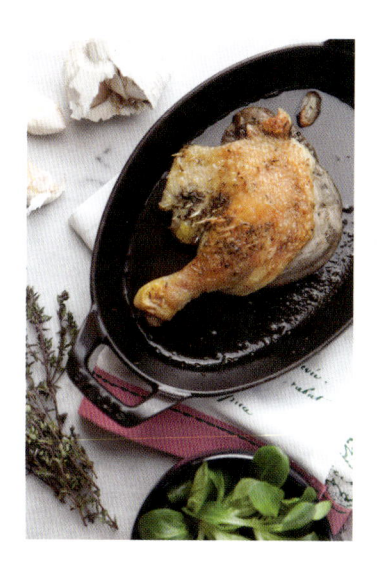

6 raw duck legs

Several tablespoons coarse sea salt

4 garlic cloves, peeled and crushed

1 teaspoon ground pepper

1 tablespoon thyme, plus several sprigs

4.4 pounds (2 kg) rendered duck fat

Rub each leg with salt. The coarse salt crystals break into the flesh in minute lacerations that help drain the moisture from the meat, preventing moisture-loving bacteria from having a chance to grow. Rub the garlic over both sides of each leg. Then rub the ground pepper and thyme into each leg.

Press each leg into the remaining salt, pepper, and thyme. To maximize moisture release, place the legs meat side down (instead of skin side down) into a platter to drain excess moisture from the legs overnight in the refrigerator. This increases your chances of a better *confit* than cooking the duck leg right away, though this overnight step, in theory, can be skipped. ➤

POULTRY, EGGS, AND RABBIT – *LA VOLAILLE, LES OEUFS ET LE LAPIN*

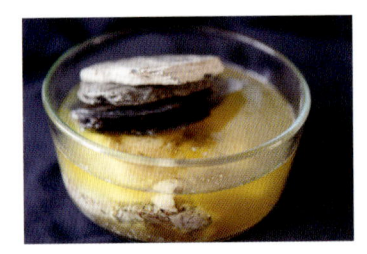

Preserved Duck Leg in Liquid Fat Under Slate

In much of France, but especially in the Southwest, in particular in the *Périgord* region, preserving duck legs has traditionally been a common and practical method of preserving food for the winter. As I have found out, however, it is not as easy as it seems, as I have ended up with rotting duck legs when air bubbles are trapped between the meat and the fat. My answer to that is storing the legs in the refrigerator, allowing them to "cure" in the fat for several days or up to two weeks, before frying or roasting and eating them, to avoid spoilage.

Melt the duck fat over low heat in a large cast-iron pot. Brush off the excess salt from each leg and place them in three pairs, meat sides facing each other into a pot just large enough to fit the duck legs. Add the sprigs of thyme and garlic and cover the legs in duck fat. It helps to place a weight over the duck legs, such as a pan cover or other heavy flat object. (In the Pyrénées, they use flat slate pieces from the mountains, otherwise used for roof tiles, to keep the duck legs submerged in the fat, as shown in the photo on the left.) Cover the pot and simmer on low (do not bring to a boil) on the stove, or place in the oven uncovered at 320°F (160°C) for up to 40 minutes. (Dewey only cooks them on the stove for 15 to 20 minutes, so as not to overcook and toughen up the meat). Check once during cooking to ensure that all legs are covered in fat, turning them if necessary. According to Dewey, the ideal way to determine doneness of the duck legs is to stick a skewer in the thickest part of the thigh and see if the juices run clear. If they are clear, the meat is cooked through. If not, continue to simmer for 10 to 15 minutes and check again.

Once the legs are ready, place them into sterilized (by oven heat or by boiling) mason jars (two per jar, for example), other glass containers, or pots, and allow to cool before covering with a weight. When packing the legs into jars, they should fit tightly into the container. Air bubbles must not be present, as these will allow for bacteria to "breathe" and invade the meat. The legs must be packed in tightly, submerged in adequate fat. This helps ensure a successful preservation process.

Dewey allows the legs to "age" in the fat for four to five months in a cool, dark place such as his cellar, after which time the texture of the meat should have softened and taken on more flavor. If you have kept them in the refrigerator for only a week or two, they may not be as tender, but it's better than losing the duck legs altogether to deterioration. Either way, you will be happy to have the duck legs on hand for an easy meal.

When you remove the duck legs from their preserving jars days, weeks, or months later, place them in the oven for eight to 10 minutes at 365°F (185°C) or else fry them up in a frying pan for several minutes on each side. Reuse any excess duck fat to sauté or roast in-season vegetables, or else use the fat to make **Sarlat Sautéed Potatoes** (see page 468), which are served with preserved duck legs, particularly in the Périgord region of the French Southwest.

> **WINE PAIRING TIP** Dewey and I shared a Pinot Noir from Burgundy when we sat down to our duck legs, brought up from his cellar. Sommelière Annabelle suggests dry and powerful reds, such as the Southwestern Cahors or Madiran. Otherwise, she recommends several reds from the Rhône Valley: a robust Cornas, an elegant Côtes du Rhône Village, a fruity Gigondas, a densely flavored Plan de Dieu, or a peppery and spiced Saint-Joseph. ➤

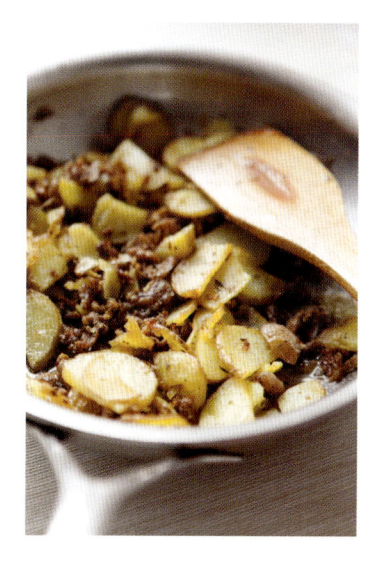

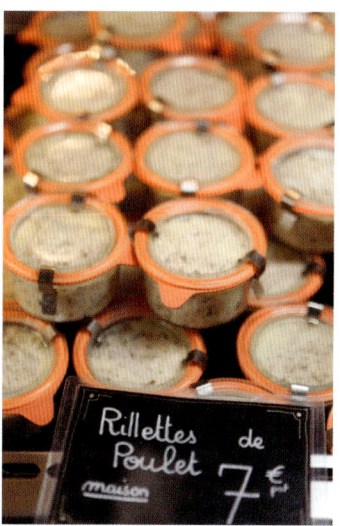

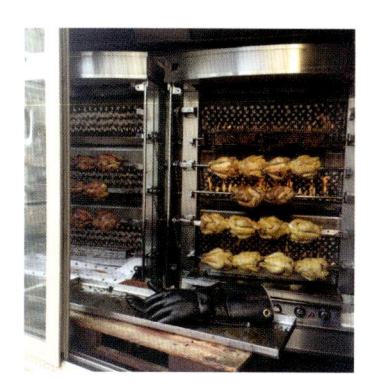

Duck Rinds
Grattons de Canard

For an added bonus after making preserved duck legs and rendered duck fat, you will have duck rinds (*grattons* or *grillons de canard*). Scrape (*gratter*) the bottom of the pot where the duck legs simmered and add any meat or scraps (*rillettes*), if you obtained the duck legs from whole duck carcasses, or else from any fat you have rendered. You may have to do several batches of duck legs, as most people do when they are going through the trouble in the first place to preserve duck legs and duck parts, to get enough duck rinds (*grattons*). Add salt, pepper, allspice (*quatre épices*), crushed garlic, and thyme to a pan along with half a cup of white wine and allow to simmer for one and a half hours, stirring occasionally. Drain (but keep!) the excess fat. Dewey runs the duck rinds through a food processor briefly to chop them finer (but not to a purée) to make them more spreadable and better suited to use as a filling in omelets and stuffings. Spoon the duck rind mixture into sterilized jars. The *grattons* can be used as a spread or eaten by the spoonful. Another option is to drain off or scoop out with a ladle the excess fat when you heat the duck rinds and save this fat for other dishes, while continuing to cook the rinds over medium heat. They will continue to lose fat into the pan. You can sauté some sliced potatoes, a shallot, and several garlic cloves along with salt, thyme, and rosemary to make a duck rind and potato dish that is crunchy, fatty, and irresistible, as shown here in the pan. See also page 198 on using duck rinds in **Duck Parmentier**. If you have a lot of chicken leftovers, (which somehow no one usually does, unless they are in the business of roasting lots of chickens at once, like *Le Poulailler d'Augustin* in Bordeaux) they can be used to make chicken meat pâté (*rillettes de poulet*), shown here, neatly packaged in little picnic-sized glass jars.

POULTRY, EGGS, AND RABBIT – *LA VOLAILLE, LES OEUFS ET LE LAPIN*

PYRÉNÉES FARM SCRAMBLED EGGS
Oeufs Brouillés des Pyrénées

Season Year-round   **Preparation Time** 5 minutes
Cooking Time 7 minutes   **Serves** 1

This recipe is for a hearty, farm-fresh breakfast of scrambled eggs, home-cured bacon cut into small pieces (*lardons*), and potatoes, inspired by ingredients frequently used in the French Southwest. Bayonne ham (*Jambon de Bayonne*) cut into pieces is a well-suited replacement for the bacon and needs a much shorter time if any at all to fry up before adding the eggs. The potatoes used are either already baked, boiled, or sautéed. This is a nice way to use those starchy leftovers. If you need more fat to cover the potatoes, use two or three tablespoons of fat instead of just one.

1 tablespoon duck fat, lard, or butter

Large handful of *lardons* or 3 to 4 strips of bacon, chopped

3 eggs

Several pieces of baked, boiled, or sautéed potatoes

2 tablespoons parsley, minced

Pinch of *fleur de sel*

Pinch of pepper

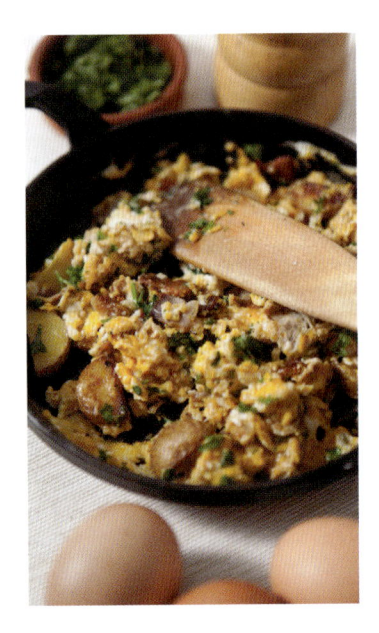

Melt the fat in a pan over medium heat and brown the *lardons* for several minutes until they are crispy, stirring them occasionally. Mix the eggs together in a small bowl then pour them into the pan, using a flat, wooden spatula to mix the eggs and the *lardons*. Stir in the potatoes, parsley, salt, and pepper, and remove from heat. Serve topped with extra fat, if desired.

VARIATIONS Sauté a small minced onion along with several strips of bell pepper and a section of tomato to make Gascon "piperade" style scrambled eggs, garnished with *piment d'Espelette*.

WINE PAIRING TIP Try a dry white or rosé champagne if this is breakfast. See also the wine pairing tips for **Omelet with Fine Herbs** on page 350.

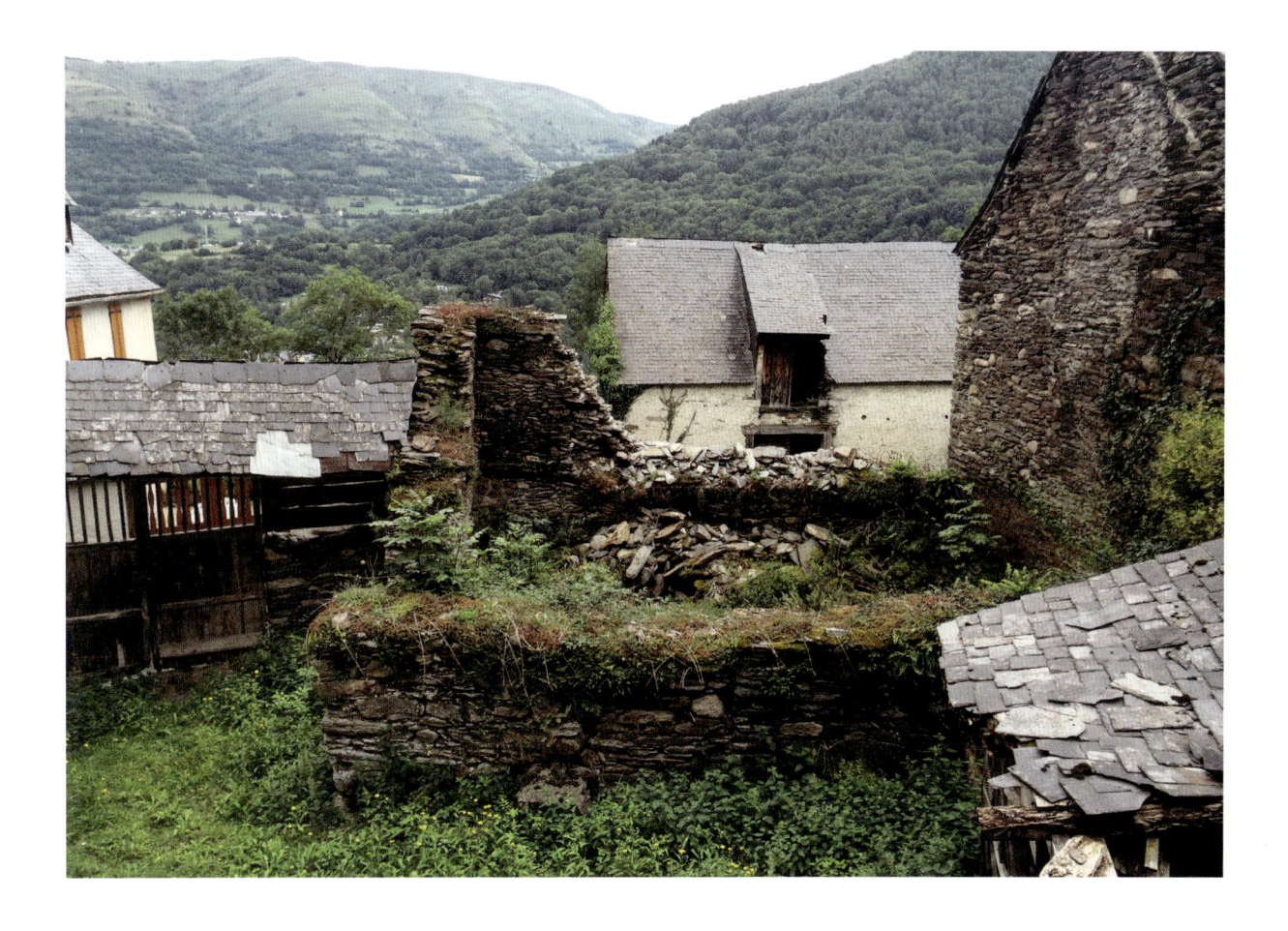

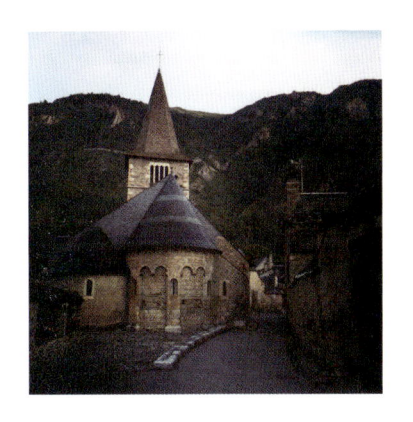

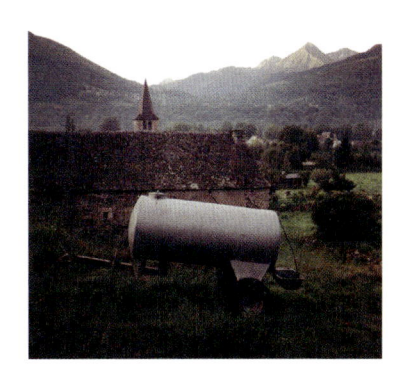

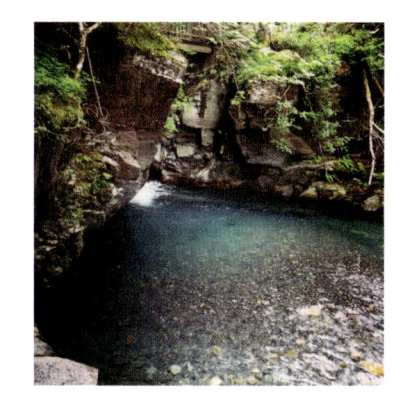

POULTRY, EGGS, AND RABBIT – *LA VOLAILLE, LES OEUFS ET LE LAPIN*

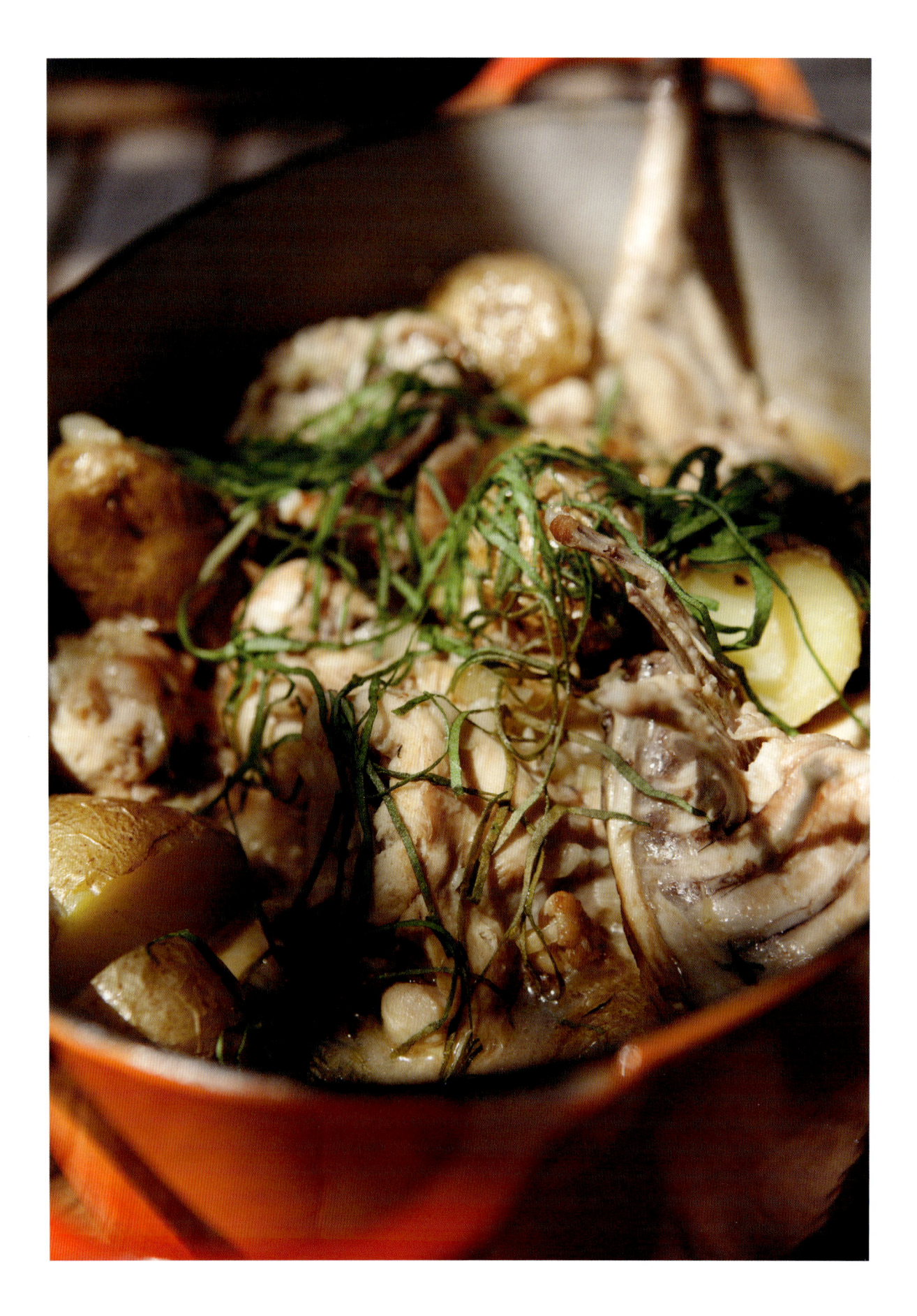

RABBIT STEW WITH ONIONS AND DUCK FAT POTATOES
Lapin aux Oignons et Pommes de Terre à la Graisse de Canard

Season Year-round   **Preparation Time** 15 minutes   **Cooking Time** 1 hour (15 minutes to brown the rabbit pieces, 40 to 45 minutes to stew, 20 to 25 minutes for the potatoes while the rabbit stews)   **Serves** 5 to 6

This was the first recipe Chef Frédéric and I made together at my house at the very beginning of this cookbook project in the summer of 2014 when I began photographing in addition to collecting ideas, which I had been doing since late 2013. Chef Frédéric was kind enough to take the chance that it would be worthwhile for him to spend his morning cooking with me, a novice. I had previously taken classes with him at *Atelier des Chefs* in Bordeaux, and he saw that I was serious about learning. This was also the moment when I heard Chef Fréd's simple culinary philosophy: The cook's job is to work with each fresh ingredient in such a way as to bring out the best of its qualities. Each ingredient gets its due (*on travaille chaque produit*).

This Southwestern French recipe comes from Gaby, Chef Frédéric's paternal grandmother, born in 1921 in Libourne, in the Bordeaux region. This is a fine example of a recipe composed of perfectly matched and inextricably linked ingredients: the rabbit, the aromatics, the stock, and the "side" (*garniture*) of potatoes boiled in duck fat. Even after being boiled in duck fat, the potatoes do not taste overly fatty to the uninitiated. And they can be prepared separately as a side dish anytime, as well, though salt should be added. They are melt-in-your-mouth delicious! Adding bitter and acidic greens at the end as a garnish to this rabbit dish counters the smooth, sweet texture and flavor of the potatoes cooked in duck fat. ➤

FOR THE RABBIT STEW (COOKING TIME: 15 MINUTES FOR BROWNING, 40 TO 45 MINUTES FOR THE STEWING)

1 tablespoon duck fat

1 rabbit, chopped into 8 pieces, plus the liver and kidneys

2 pinches of fine salt

1 onion, chopped

2 sprigs of thyme

Bay leaf

2 cups (475 ml) **White Poultry Stock** (page 417)

Handful of sorrel (*oseille*) or other bitter green, shredded, for garnish

Today rabbit is not as commonly eaten as it once was in the United States, but it is still prepared in many households in France. Chop the rabbit into medium-sized pieces (not including the head, which can go into a bone broth) as you would butcher a chicken into six or eight pieces for the **Chicken in Wine Sauce "Coq au Vin"** (page 345), separating wing, thigh, and breast. In the rabbit's case, separate the four legs, dividing the back into two pieces crosswise, and the ribs also crosswise into two pieces, or have a butcher do this for you. Keep the kidney and liver for this dish. As with many French recipes where "browning" the meat or vegetables is involved, you have what is called the Maillard reaction (see the Chef's Tip at the end of this recipe), **White Poultry Stock** (page 417), and slow-cooking, three secrets to French cooking that, when combined, produce some of the most flavorful dishes that are not necessarily difficult to make.

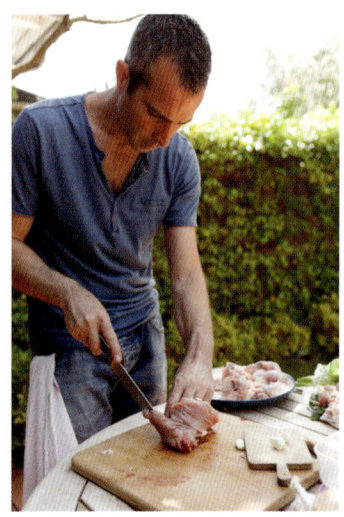

Chef Frédéric Cutting Rabbit Pieces

FOR THE POTATOES (COOKING TIME: 20 MINUTES)

6 to 8 small local heirloom potatoes (*rattes* or *grenailles*), unpeeled

Several garlic cloves, unpeeled (*en chemise*)

Bay leaf

A few sprigs of fresh thyme

About 2 cups (475 ml) duck fat, liquid or softened at room temperature

Melt the duck fat in a cast-iron pot over high heat and place about four to five pieces of rabbit into the pot, or what will fit with some room around each piece in the pot. The idea is to caramelize the rabbit pieces for flavor and a caramel color. Sprinkle a pinch of salt over the pieces and turn them after a few minutes of browning. Set aside the first batch of browned rabbit pieces in a large bowl. Add the second batch of pieces, including the liver and kidneys and another pinch of salt. Brown and turn after several minutes to brown the other side. Transfer the second batch of browned rabbit pieces to the large bowl.

Using the same pot on high heat (*à feu vif*), deglaze the meat juices (*déglacer les sucs*) stuck to the bottom of the pan by adding the onions—the water from the onions will perform the deglazing action. Add the sprigs of thyme and the bay leaf. After a few minutes you will hear the sizzling of the onion pieces, at which point you add the poultry stock (*bouillon de volaille*). Chicken stock may be substituted.

Reduce the heat to medium-low and transfer all the rabbit pieces back to the pot. Allow to simmer lightly (*mijoter*), uncovered, for 40 to 45 minutes.

Combine the potatoes, garlic, bay leaf, and thyme in a small pot over medium-low to low heat. Pour in enough duck fat (which becomes liquid at room temperature) to cover the potatoes. Do not cover the pot, as the condensed water on the underside of the lid will drip back into the pot and cause the oil to spit, which can splatter on you and any bystanders when the lid is lifted. Using a fork, check the tenderness of the potatoes after 20 minutes. Remove the potatoes and the garlic cloves from the fat and set them aside.

Once the rabbit has finished cooking, transfer the garlic and potatoes to the pot with the rabbit and turn off the heat. Garnish (*garnir*) with shredded sorrel (*oseille*) or lettuce and serve warm in a bowl.

Chef's Tip
Astuce du Chef

Do not chop the onion too finely. The onion's sugars will help bind the sauce, so that there is no need for flour. The sticking of the juices is called the "Maillard reaction" *(la réaction Maillard)*, named after French chemist Louis-Camille Maillard who, in 1912, observed the effect of amino acids and sugars in food browning or coloring when heated, adding to the complexity of aromas and flavors in what is called non-enzymatic glycation. This browning technique is one of the secrets to flavor in French cuisine. Similarly, our cells undergo a "browning" glycation process as well. There is indeed a tradeoff between cooking and caramelizing food and eating food raw or only steamed without much flavor. Browning food may seem an unnecessary health risk to some, because of the glycation of sugars, but browning meats and vegetables is, as I have said before, one of the keys to flavor in French cooking.

VARIATIONS To augment the fat content of the dish, drizzle some hot duck fat from the potatoes over each serving bowl. Try swapping out the potatoes and cooking a chopped sweet potato or tubers instead in the duck fat. This dish is often also cooked with about 2 cups (475 ml) of chopped cabbage, plus four to six cloves stuck in a small peeled onion, to keep from "losing" the cloves in the soup.

WINE PAIRING TIP For rabbit dishes, sommelière Annabelle recommends fresh and full white wines (see the wine pairing suggestions for **Stuffed Rabbit Saddle** on page 369), fruity and flavorful (*gourmand*) red wines, or spiced and fleshy (*charnus*) red wines. For pairings with these types of red wines, Annabelle suggests a low-tannin, fresh Touraine, with notes of cherry and plum, a supple, light to medium-bodied Saumur, or a medium-bodied, crisp Bourgueil, all three of which hail from the Loire Valley. From other regions, Annabelle proposes such wines as a warm, fruity, and spicy Côtes du Rhône; a fragrant and much-loved Châteauneuf-du-Pape, assembled from numerous grape varieties in an area cultivated by Papal sovereigns since the 1100s; a Fitou from Languedoc, made from a majority of the Carignan and Grenache grapes, followed by Syrah and Mourvèdre, with herbaceous and leathery aromas, black fruits and spice; or a Côtes de Roussillon, made with the same grapes, with notes of fresh red and black fruits and spice. For a Southwestern paring she recommends full-bodied reds from Cahors, Madiran or Bordeaux's Médoc region.

STUFFED QUAIL
Cailles Farcies

Season Year-round   **Preparation Time** 1 to 2 hours or overnight to marinate the raisins, 15 minutes to stuff the birds   **Cooking Time** 35 minutes   **Serves** 4 to 5

Quail (*caille*) is a small bird prepared as an occasional special treat in France. My friend Edouard at the rotisserie restaurant *Le Poulailler d'Augustin* in Bordeaux demonstrated the entire process of dressing quail, from chopping off the head to removing the entrails. Usually, you will receive a quail carcass already plucked, entrails removed, and ready for stuffing and cooking. The general serving size is one quail per person, but my husband can easily put away two if he is hungry enough. In this recipe, the quail are stuffed with one to two prunes per bird and one to two teaspoons of marinated raisins per bird. The raisins are marinated for one to two hours, or overnight, in Grand Marnier, a French, orange-flavored liqueur made from Cognac. Though it looks like a white meat, quail has gamier flavors than chicken.

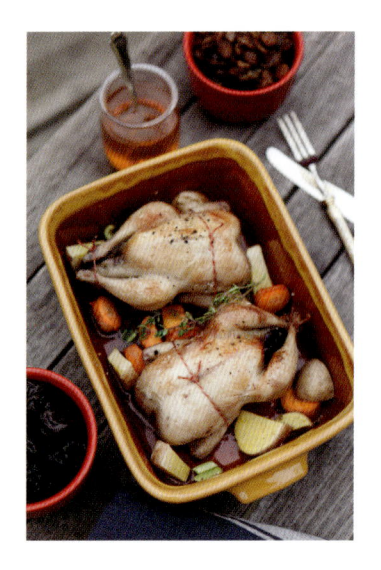

10 teaspoons raisins (about ½ cup or 120 ml), marinated ¼ cup (60 ml) Grand Marnier

5 quail

5 to 10 prunes

5 tablespoons olive oil

Fine salt and ground pepper, for seasoning

Marinate the raisins one to two hours or overnight in the Grand Marnier. Preheat the oven to 365°F (185°C). Stuff each quail with raisins, leaving room for one or two prunes at the end to "plug up" the opening.

Place the quail in one or more oven-safe dishes and drizzle the olive oil over each quail. Season the quail with salt and pepper and cook in the oven for about 35 minutes.

VARIATIONS You might consider adding diced carrots, potatoes, and celery. (These need to be chopped small enough—in half-inch or 1.25 cm cubes—to be able to cook in half an hour.) If you have larger chunks of vegetables, these will be less cooked (*al dente*). Add about five minutes to the cooking time with the added vegetables.

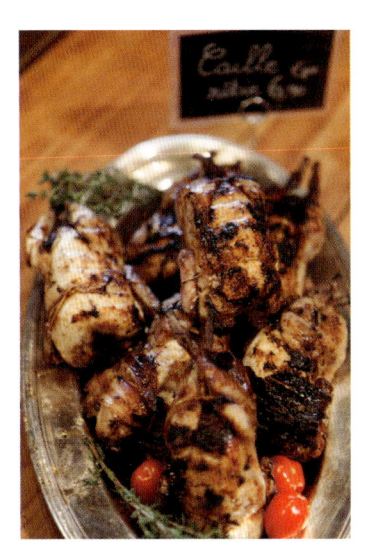

Edouard's Stuffed, Roasted Quail

WINE PAIRING TIP Having a bit of a Provençale bent, *Le Poulailler d'Augustin* sells a lot of rosé from Provence to go with their roasted birds. To go with the gaminess of the quail, Annabelle recommends red wines that are fleshy (like biting into a fresh, ripe fruit) and supple. For regional Southwest pairings try a supple and fruity Bergerac, containing a "Bordeaux blend" of Cabernet Sauvignon and Merlot; a rich and structured Madiran, made from the tannic Tannat grape; or a fruity Tursan made with the Cabernet Franc and Tannat grapes. For wines outside the French Southwest, Annabelle suggests a number of options: a Moulin-à-Vent, with notes of animal, cherry, faded rose, and spice, or a Brouilly with rounded tannins and notes of raspberry and violet, both made from the Gamay grape in the Beaujolais region; a Beaune Pinot Noir, with robust tannins and notes of red and black fruits, from the Côte de Beaune, the southern half of Burgundy's Côte d'Or ("Golden Slope"), or an aromatic Chambolle Musigny with notes of red berries from the northern half of Burgundy's Côte d'Or; a Côtes du Roussillon Villages, with notes of blackberry, raspberry, and spice; a Rhône Valley Vacqueyras, made with at least 50% Grenache grapes, with notes of red berries, licorice, and spice; a fresh Collioure from Roussillon, with notes of black and red berries, scrub bush, and vanilla; or else a robust Corbières, with a nose of ripe berries and thyme, a berry-nosed Fitou, a berry, floral, and cacao Minervois, a Pic-Saint-Loup or other Languedoc red (formerly known as Coteaux du Languedoc), with notes of red and black berries, licorice, and spice.

STUFFED RABBIT SADDLE
Râble de Lapin Farci

Season Year-round   **Preparation Time** 45 minutes
Cooking Time 30 minutes   **Serves** 2 to 4

Rabbit saddle (*râble de lapin*) is the back of the rabbit, the most "prized" piece of the rabbit. If large enough, the saddle may be divided into four smaller pieces, stuffed, wrapped or "barded" in strips of fatback lard, and tied. The best is to ask a butcher to sell you the strips of lard, as he has the proper slicing equipment. In order to be "stuffed," the saddle must be deboned. It's a tricky business removing the backbone and rib cage from the meat, and it's easy to sever the saddle piece.[7] If the saddle is large enough, however, it will be cut anyway to make two separate pieces, one on each side of the backbone, which can then be cut in half yet again to make four pieces. If the rabbit is not sizeable enough, a second rabbit saddle will be needed. The deboned saddle, cut in half or into four pieces is "stuffable," not unlike the **Stuffed Veal Cutlets** (page 427). The filling or "stuffing" is a *mousseline* (a sauce enriched with cream) that is combined with chicken breast, but the Basques will stuff their rabbit with chopped squid (*chipirons*), clams (*palourdes*), and local Bayonne ham (*jambon de Bayonne*). In this recipe, I have employed whole-fat coconut milk instead of whole cream or sour cream (*crème fraîche*) for a dairy-free version, but of course dairy is used in France for the filling. Butcher's string, or "cooking string" is used to secure the fatback lard strips around the rabbit saddle. This recipe is more work than simpler dishes because of the stuffing, "barding," and tying, but it is a delicious way to eat rabbit and makes for a lovely, if rustic, presentation for guests (as in the recipe photo).

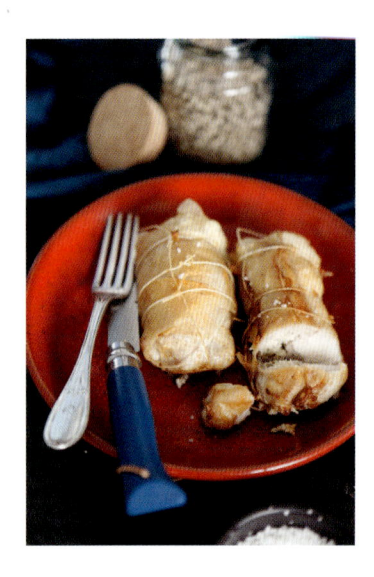

FOR THE MOUSSELINE FILLING

1 egg (yolk and white whisked together)

2 chicken breasts (about 5.7 ounces or 160 g), skin removed and ground

3 tablespoons whole fat coconut milk

Pinch of ground white pepper

Pinch of ground nutmeg

Pinch of fine salt

1 large shallot (about 1.8 ounces or 50 g), minced

FOR THE RABBIT

Mousseline filling

1 large rabbit saddle, deboned and cut into 4 pieces (or 2 small saddles, deboned and cut in half)

8 to 12 thin strips of fatback lard

1 tablespoon duck fat or lard

Pinch of fine salt

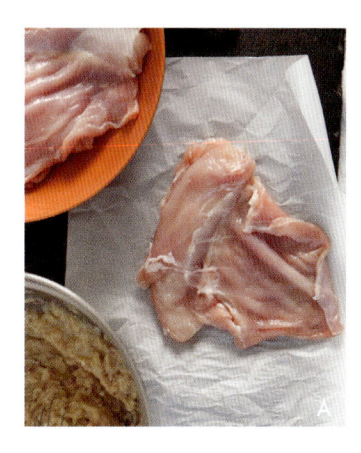

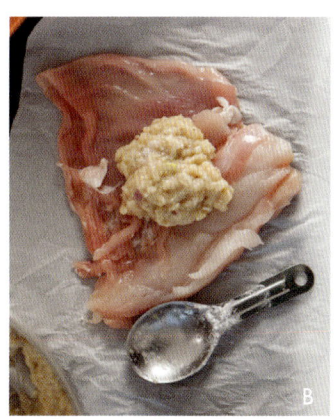

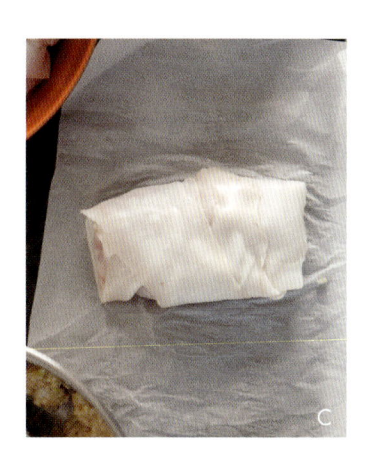

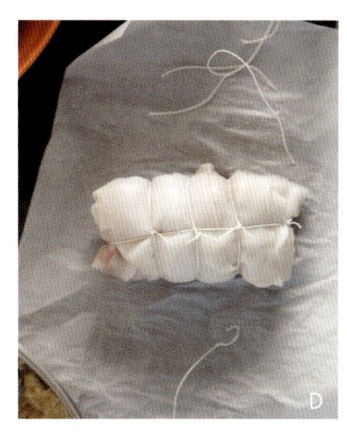

Preheat the oven to 350°F (175°C). Using a whisk, combine all the ingredients for the *mousseline* in a bowl and mix well.

Spread out each piece of the rabbit saddle on a flat surface (photo A). Place two tablespoons of filling into the middle of each piece of meat (photo B). Roll up the saddle like a sausage. (If you end up with several tablespoons of *mousseline* filling left over, they can be incorporated into scrambled eggs.)

Using one or more strips of lard, wrap a layer of lard around each rolled up rabbit saddle (photo C). Secure the lard, tying the rolled up and wrapped (or "barded") saddle pieces using butcher's string (photo D).

Melt the fat over medium-high to high heat in a cast-iron pot large enough to fit the four wrapped saddle pieces. Sprinkle a pinch of fine salt into the pot and brown the saddle pieces for about two minutes on each side. Use a splatter screen as the fat will splatter somewhat from the pot.

Place the pot, uncovered, into the oven, and allow to roast for 30 minutes. Covering the pot will steam (*étouffer*) the rabbit saddle, which is also a possibility, but I prefer the slight crispiness of the outer layer of lard when roasted uncovered. Serve with or without the sauce (*fond de poêlage*) in the pot drizzled over each saddle piece.

VARIATIONS You can additionally stuff the saddle with parsley or other herbs, bacon pieces (*lardons*), and/or garlic.

WINE PAIRING TIP Sommelière Annabelle recommends fresh and full-bodied white wines to go with this delicately-flavored dish. From Bordeaux, she suggests pairing a crisp Entre-Deux-Mers, an elegant Graves or a citrus, floral, and lightly fruity Côtes de Blaye. Otherwise, she suggests a medium-bodied fruity and spiced white Saint-Joseph from the Rhône Valley, or a flinty Loire Valley Pouilly-Fumé or a floral Saumur, with notes of peach and pear, also from the Loire Valley and known for its wines since the Middle Ages. Annabelle also proposes a number of red wines, such as a Pinot Noir from Alsace with notes of black fruits, leather, and vanilla, an elegant Chiroubles, with notes of raspberry and strawberry, made from the Gamay Noir grape in Beaujolais, or a fruity Chinon Rouge from the Central Loire Valley, with notes of red and dark berries and even pencil shavings (*retaille de crayon*), a signature scent of the Cabernet France grape, the predominant grape in this wine. See also the wine pairing suggestions for **Rabbit Stew with Onions and Duck Fat Potatoes** on page 365.

TURKEY RAGOUT
Ragoût de Dinde

Season Year-round   **Preparation Time** 35 minutes   **Cooking Time** 1 hour and 15 minutes to 2 hours   **Serves** 6

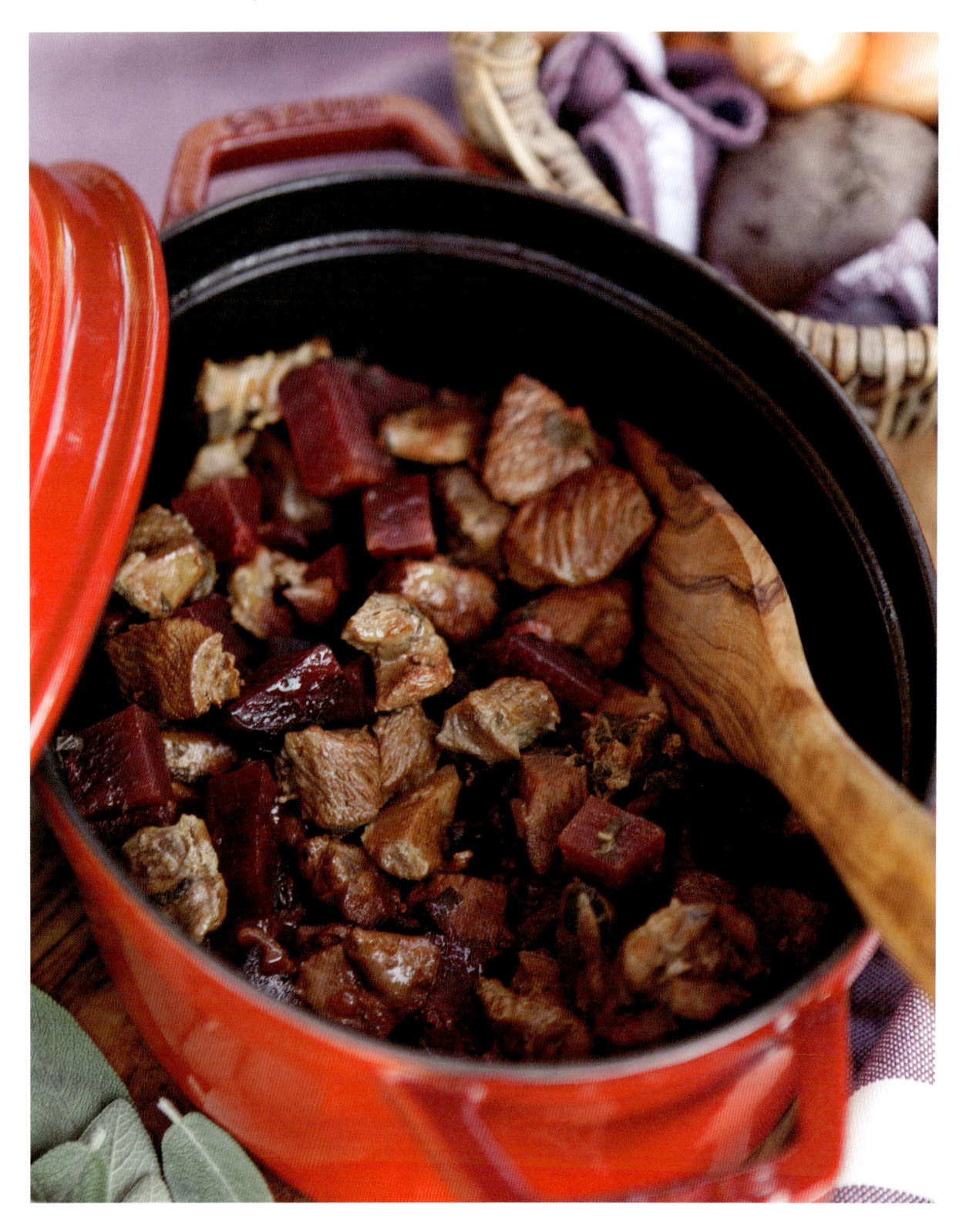

Browning and slow-cooking the meat are again the keys to flavor in this recipe, as with most of the other stews in *The Bordeaux Kitchen*. The fresh sage adds that dimension that only fresh herbs can add. Beets are in season in France from May through October but are available already cooked and preserved in jars as well. I remove the stem and any gnarly, stringy roots but keep the rest of the skin on for the nutrients and microbiota in the skin, but many people prefer peeling them. If you use cooked beets, add them in during the last 15 minutes of cooking. Vegetables other than beets may be substituted, such as carrots, potatoes, or other root vegetables.

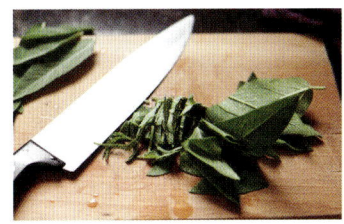

Freshly Chopped Sage Leaves

2.2 pounds (1 kg) turkey meat, cut in 1-inch (2.5 cm) cubes

3 tablespoons lard or duck fat

4 pinches of fine salt

2 small onions (about 4 ounces or 110 g), halved and sliced

3 to 4 tablespoons fresh sage, chopped

2 to 3 small raw beets (about 10 to 12 ounces or 285 g to 340 g), chopped into bite-size pieces

½ cup (120 ml) water

Divide the turkey meat into three batches. Melt one tablespoon of fat in a large pan over medium-high heat and brown each batch of cubed meat for two to three minutes on each side, sprinkling each batch of meat with a pinch of salt. Transfer each batch to a large bowl before starting on the next batch.

Add the onions with the last batch of meat to brown the onions as well. Add the sage, beets, and another pinch of salt, and transfer the other browned meat pieces back into the pot. Add the water, bring to a boil, then cover and reduce the heat to medium-low or low. Allow to simmer for a minimum of one hour and 15 minutes before serving. At two hours the meat is guaranteed tender.

Serve in bowls as is or with a dollop of sour cream (*crème fraîche*) for added creaminess and to accent the flavor of the onions.

WINE PAIRING TIP Try a dry white with structure and character. The French wine website PlatsNetVins (www.platsnetvins.com) suggests white wines of this type from Languedoc-Roussillon, Provence, the Rhône Valley, and the Southwest, and rosés from Bordeaux, Languedoc-Roussillon, Provence, and the Rhône Valley. I have paired this dish with a floral and fruity, organic Côtes de Provence rosé (a blend of Grenache, Cinsault, and Syrah) from the Domaine de la Grande Pallière. The balance of acidity and sweetness of the rosé along with its aromatic freshness delicately underscores the flavors of this dish on the palate.

POULTRY, EGGS, AND RABBIT – *LA VOLAILLE, LES OEUFS ET LE LAPIN*

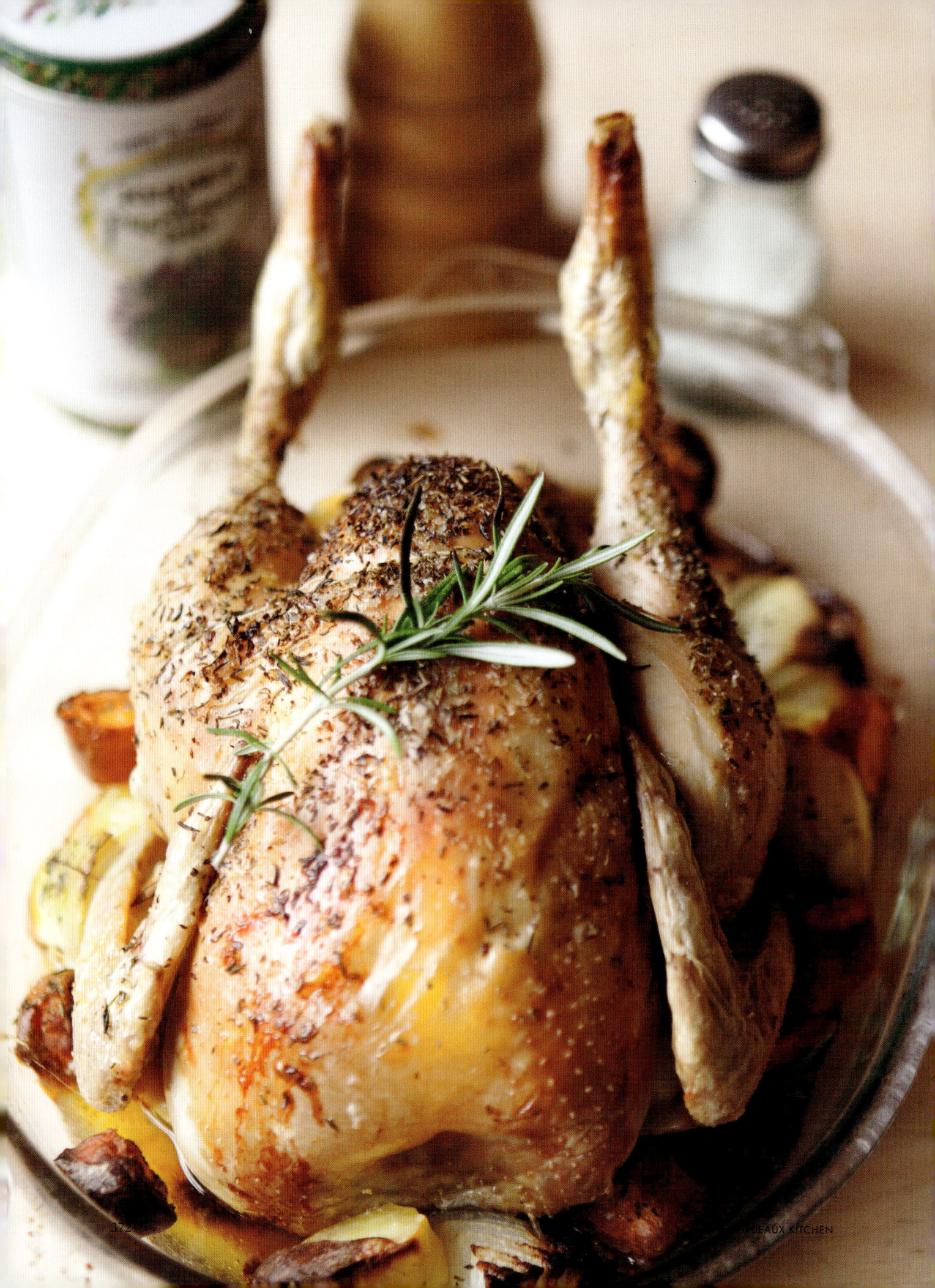

WHOLE ROAST CHICKEN WITH *HERBES DE PROVENCE*
Poulet Rôti aux Herbes de Provence

Season Year-round   **Preparation Time** 5 to 10 minutes
Cooking Time 45 minutes to 1 hour and 10 minutes   **Serves** 4 to 5

This recipe is so easy and can be dressed down or up, depending on what you have in your refrigerator and pantry. This recipe came about after our move to Bordeaux, out of my own need for an easy, tasty recipe that was economical (buying a whole chicken is less expensive than buying it cut up), and that I could make without really needing to do any thinking or preparation. *Herbes de Provence* is a mix of dried herbs, usually including thyme, rosemary, savory and oregano. It is a magical combination that can be used in many meat and vegetable dishes and can really save the day, if it's not overused. Vegetables such as carrots, onions, potatoes, squash, and zucchini can be roasted in the casserole dish along with the chicken for a one-dish meal. And after you have finished eating the meat from the carcass, you can use the carcass to make your next **Brown Poultry Stock** (see explanation in **White Poultry Stock** on page 417), **Bone Broth** (page 394), or **White (or Light) Stock** (page 398).

To extract maximum flavor, the garlic cloves are smashed in this recipe. Use the flat surface of a butcher knife to smash each clove in its skin. The skin is easily removed but can also be left on if you are in a hurry, as the garlic flavor will infuse into the dish.

1 whole chicken (internal organs removed)

1 carrot, chopped

1 onion, chopped

5 garlic cloves, smashed

Optional: Several potatoes, chopped

5 tablespoons olive oil

2 pinches of coarse sea salt

Optional: 1 to 2 pinches of ground pepper

1 tablespoon *herbes de Provence*

Extra sea salt and pepper to taste

The larger the chicken and the more accompanying vegetables or items stuffed into the chicken, the longer it will take to cook.[8] Sometimes I will roast two chickens simultaneously, so as to have leftovers. According to *Atelier des Chefs*, chicken is cooked when it has reached an internal temperature of 176°F to 185°F (80°C to 85°C); other sources say 165°F (75°C).[9] My little meat thermometer says 180°F (82°C) for poultry, so I generally go with that. Place the thermometer in the center of the thigh for a temperature reading.

Preheat the oven to 365°F (185°C). Place the chicken in an oven-safe dish with sides two to three inches (5 cm to 8 cm) high. Place the carrot, onion, and garlic around and inside the chicken. Place the optional potatoes into the dish around the chicken.

Cover everything with generous amounts of olive oil (or butter, ghee, or coconut oil), and sprinkle the salt, pepper if desired, and *herbes de Provence* over the vegetables and chicken. Place in the oven and allow to cook for up to one hour and 10 minutes. While the chicken cooks, you can prepare a variety of other vegetable side dishes (and/or dessert!)

Check one of the thighs with a meat thermometer at 45 minutes to see if the chicken has cooked through. If not, continue cooking and check again after another 10 to 15 minutes. Season with extra salt and pepper if desired. Serve with the roasted vegetables and a side salad.

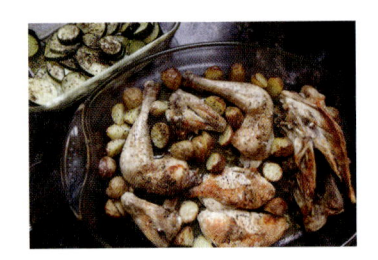

VARIATIONS Add chopped potatoes covered in salt, oil, and herbs to the pan with the chicken for an easy side dish; roast in the oven all together for about one hour. See page 336 for a photo tutorial on **How to Butcher a Chicken**.

WINE PAIRING TIP For a regional pairing from the French Southwest, sommelière Annabelle recommends a fruity white IGP Côtes de Gascogne ("geographically protected" in Europe: *Indication Géographique Protégée*), made primarily from Colombard and Ugni Blanc, the same grapes used in Armagnac in the same region. Among other whites, she proposes a crisp Vouvray Sec with notes of apple, citrus and peach or a neighboring Montlouis-sur-Loire, with notes of almond, flowers and verbena, both wines from the Loire Valley and made from the Chenin Blanc grape, also known as "Pineau de la Loire." As for red wines, Annabelle suggests ones that are fresh and fruity and not overly oaked (generally having too strong coconut or vanilla aromas): an Alsatian Pinot Noir, with notes of dark fruits; a Beaujolais-Villages, with melty tannins and notes of raspberry and strawberry; a medium-bodied Languedoc (formerly known as Coteaux-du-Languedoc); an herbaceous Chinon from the Loire Valley; a powerful, spiced and well-structured Bandol from Provence; or a medium-bodied, warming and spiced Côtes du Rhône.

WHOLE STUFFED DUCK
Canard Entier Farci

Season Autumn and Winter   **Preparation Time** 10 minutes
Cooking Time 2 hours 45 minutes   **Serves** 8

Whole Stuffed Duck is a holiday kind of meal, but it's so good, I wonder why I don't cook it at other times as well. And for a family of four, the leftovers are generous. Since duck is a "red" meat, it can be cooked rarer than chicken. A duck weighing 6.6 pounds (3 kg) takes about two hours and 45 minutes to cook through. A smaller duck might take less time to roast, and a larger duck might need more time.

1 duck (internal organs removed)

1 tablespoon *fleur de sel* or coarse sea salt

1 tablespoon fresh or dried thyme

1 carrot, chopped

1 onion, chopped

3 bay leaves

1 clementine, peeled and segments separated

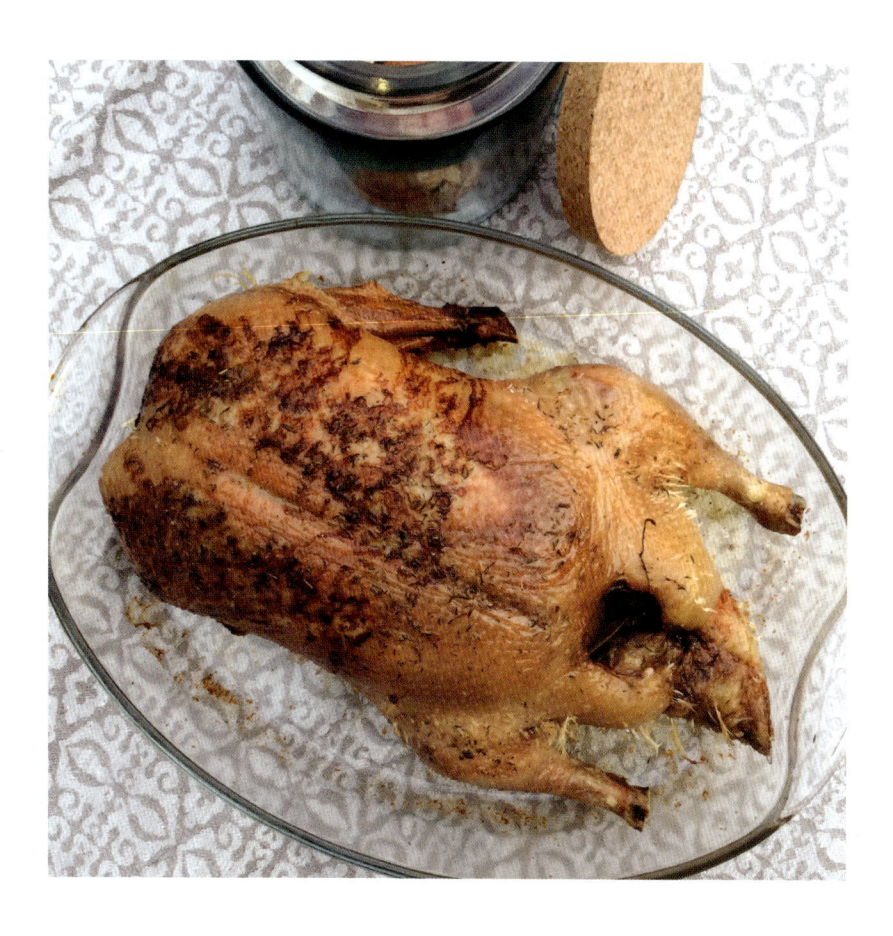

Preheat the oven to 395°F (200°C). Rub the duck with the salt and thyme. Stuff the duck with the carrot, onion, bay leaves, and clementine. Place the duck in a large oven-safe dish and cook uncovered in the oven for 10 minutes before reducing the heat to 365°F (185°C). The initial higher heat will help brown the skin. Cook uncovered for another 50 minutes.

After the first hour of cooking, use a large spoon to baste the duck with some of the liquid fat from the bottom of the pan. Feel free to spoon out more fat to use for sautéing accompanying vegetables or to make **Sarlat Sautéed Potatoes** (see page 468). Reduce the heat slightly to 355°F (about 180°C).

Check the internal temperature of the meat after two hours of cooking by placing a meat thermometer into one of the thighs. Baste the duck again with the liquid fat from the bottom of the pan.

Once the duck has finished roasting, carve and serve with the liquid fat drizzled over each serving. Serve with accompanying vegetables and homemade cranberry sauce or **Orange Plum Sauce** (page 412).

VARIATIONS For the stuffing, add ½ cup chopped, blanched almonds or almond flour mixed in a food processor with the duck's liver, heart, and kidneys, along with two tablespoons of *fromage blanc* (a fresh white cow's cheese, similar to cream cheese or ricotta) or sour cream (*crème fraîche*) and two shallots.

> WINE PAIRING TIP For a traditional, Southwestern pairing with the duck, go with a Madiran, with notes of raspberry and juniper berries, or a full-bodied Cahors. or try a fresh and aromatic Lirac, with notes of black and red fruits and leather, from the Southern Rhône Valley. See also the wine pairing suggestions for the **Preserved Duck Legs** (page 358).

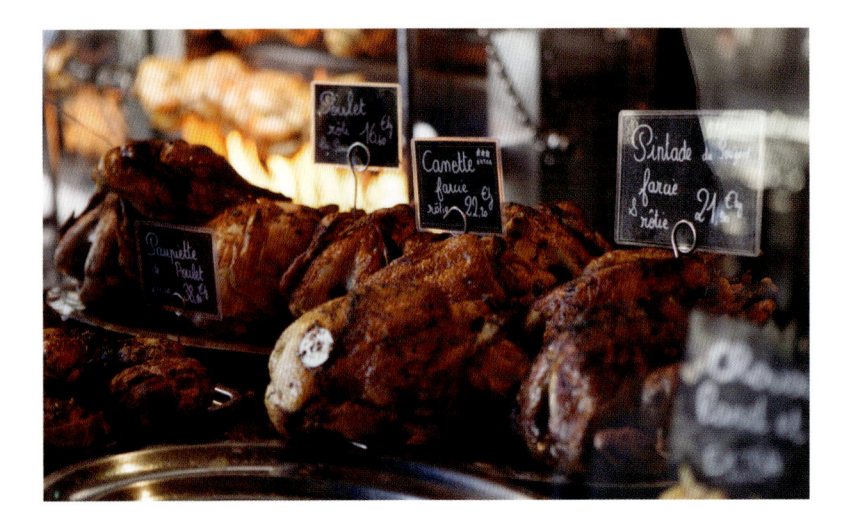

WHOLE STUFFED HOLIDAY GOOSE
Oie Farcie pour les Fêtes

Season Autumn and Winter **Preparation Time** 10 minutes
Cooking Time 2.5 to 3 hours **Serves** 8 to 10

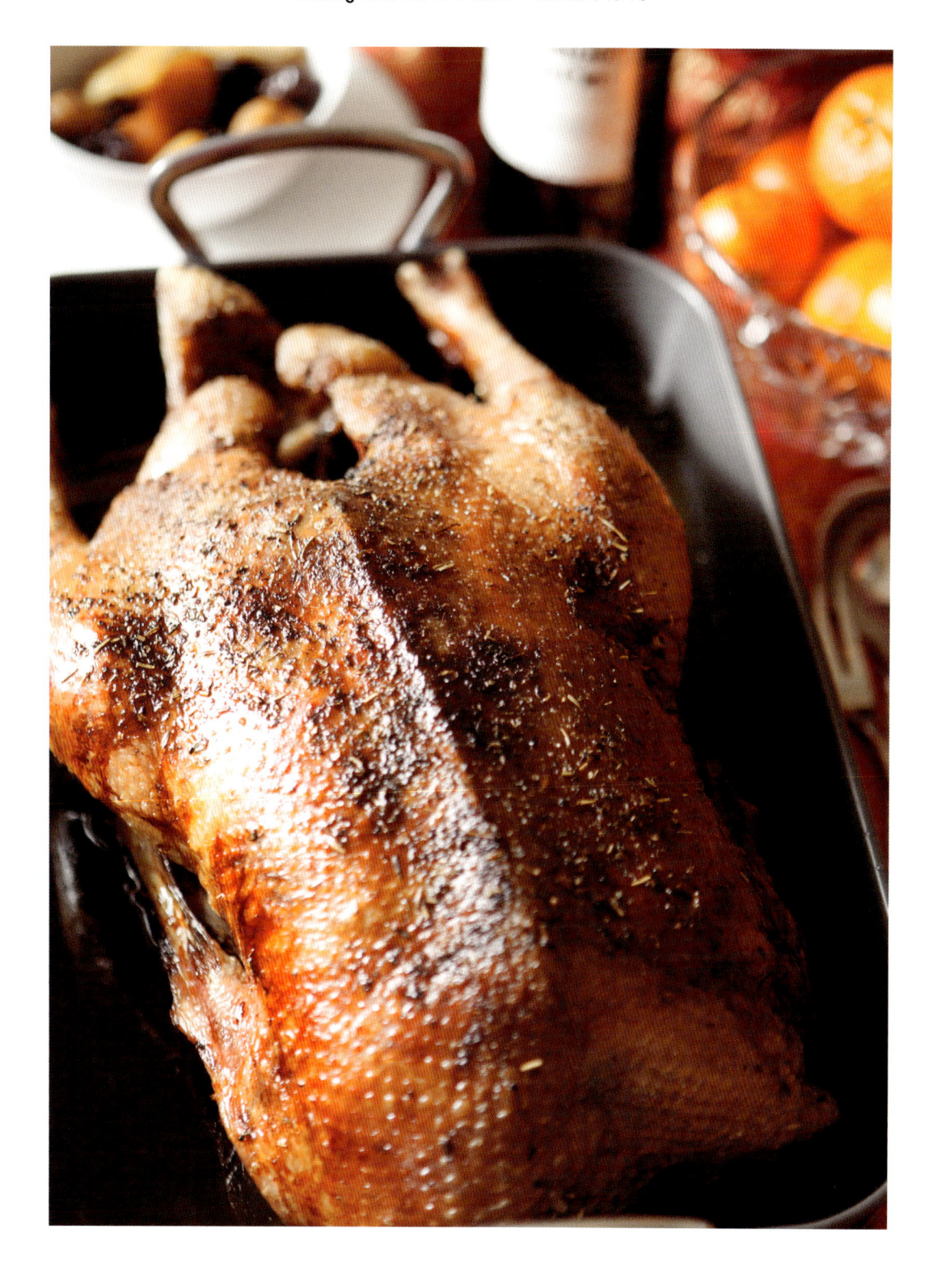

Like the **Whole Stuffed Duck** (page 375), whole goose is a nice meal around the winter holidays when we really crave the fat. Below is one way to stuff a goose, but other cooks might add chestnuts, shallots and/or ground pork, and other spices.

8 to 10 pound (3.6 kg to 4.5 kg) goose

2 tablespoons coarse sea salt

1 to 2 clementines, peeled and segments separated

2 to 3 small onions, halved

2 to 3 bay leaves

Several sprigs of thyme

Several sprigs of rosemary

Handful of sage leaves

Preheat the oven to 395°F (400°C). Rub the goose with one tablespoon of coarse sea salt. Stuff the goose with the clementines, onions, herbs, and remaining salt and place the goose in a large oven-safe dish. Place in the oven uncovered and allow to roast for up to three hours, basting it in its own juices and fat with a spoon every half hour. As with **Whole Stuffed Duck**, feel free to spoon out some fat to use for sautéing accompanying vegetables or to make **Sarlat Sautéed Potatoes** (page 468).

After the first hour of cooking, reduce the heat to 350°F (175°C) for the remaining time. Check the internal temperature of the meat after two and a half hours of cooking by placing a meat thermometer into one of the thighs. Continue to baste the goose with the liquid fat in the bottom of the pan.

Once the goose has finished roasting, carve and serve with the liquid fat drizzled over each serving. Serve with dried fruit, red cabbage sauerkraut, boiled potatoes with parsley, roasted Brussel sprouts, or other roasted vegetables.

> WINE PAIRING TIP I have paired the goose with a full-bodied red Cahors, or try a Madiran, both from the Southwest. See also the wine pairing suggestions for **Whole Stuffed Duck** (page 376) and **Preserved Duck Legs** (page 358).

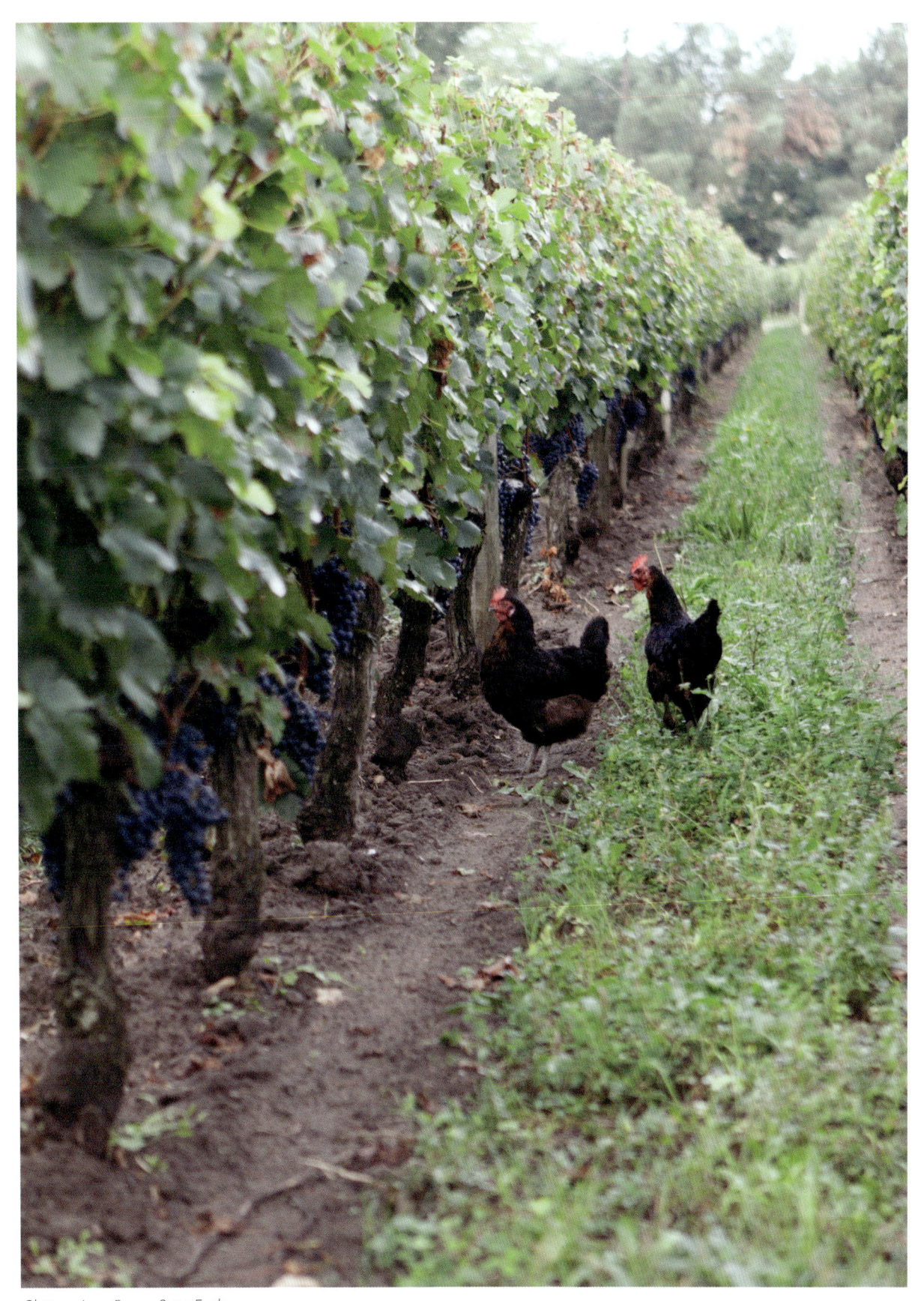

Château Jean Faure, Saint Emilion

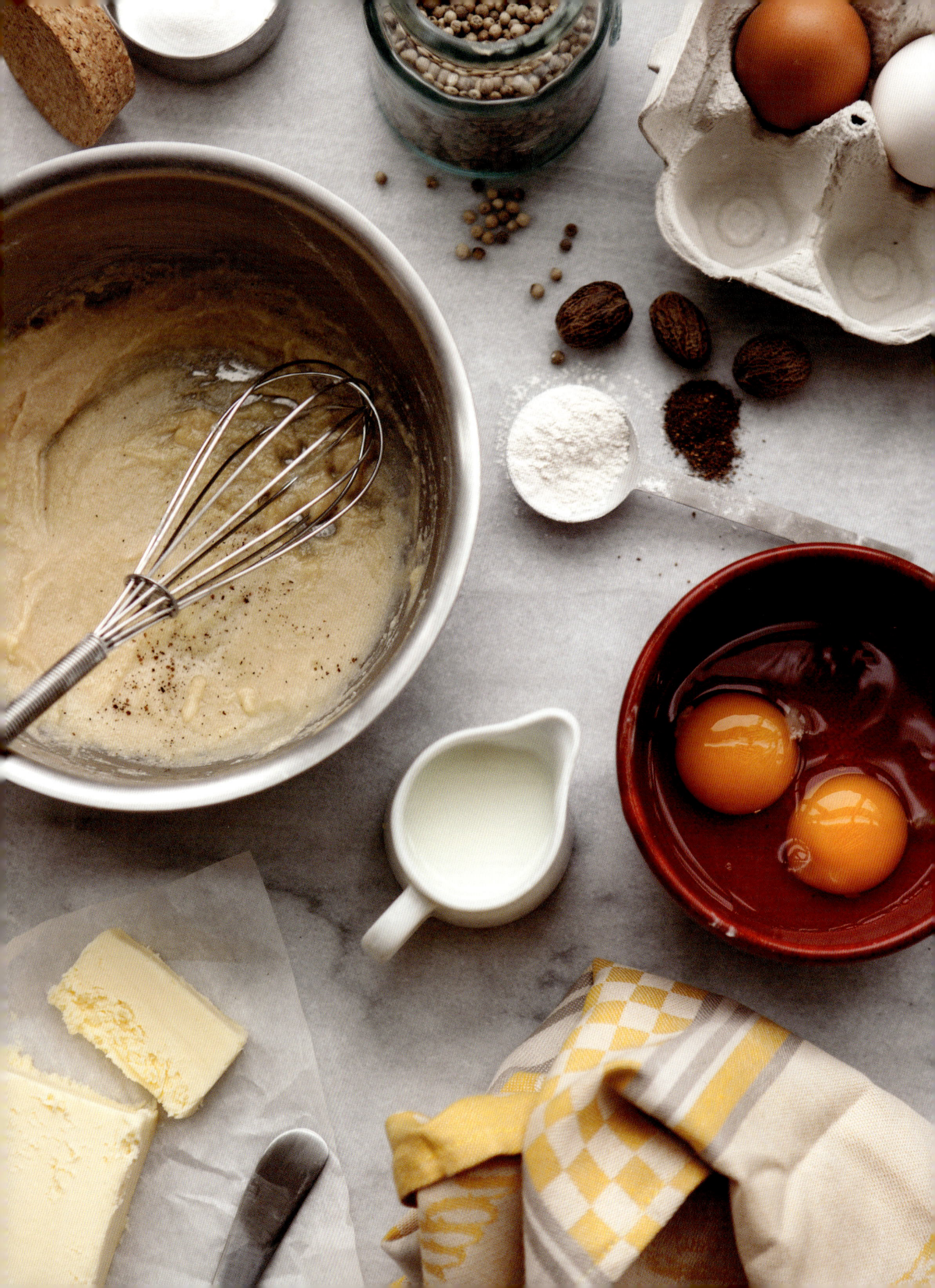

STOCKS AND SAUCES
Les Fonds, Bouillons, et Sauces

Allemande Sauce – *Sauce Allemande* 384

Anchovy Sauce – *Sauce aux Anchois* 386

Barbeque Sauce – *Sauce à Barbeque* 389

Béarnaise Sauce – *Sauce Béarnaise* 391

Béchamel Sauce – *Sauce Béchamel* 392

Bone Broth – *Le Bouillon* 394

Brown Roux and White Roux – *Roux Brun et Roux Blanc* 397

Brown Stock and White (or Light) Stock – *Fond Brun et Fond Blanc* 398

Crab Sauce – *Sauce aux Crabes* 400

Cream Sauce (Supreme Sauce) – *Sauce Velouté à la Crème (Sauce Suprême)* 402

Fish Stock – *Fumet de Poisson* 403

Hollandaise Sauce – *Sauce Hollandaise* 404

Homemade Mayonnaise – *Mayonnaise Fait Maison* 406

Mornay Cheese Sauce – *Sauce Mornay* 407

Niçoise Vinaigrette – *Vinaigrette Niçoise* 409

Old-Fashioned Mustard – *Moutarde à l'Ancienne* 410

Onion Marmalade – *Confiture d'Oignons* 411

Orange Plum Sauce – *Sauce aux Prunes à l'Orange* 412

Shallot and Vinegar Dip for Oysters – *Vinaigre aux Echalotes pour les Huîtres* 413

Simple Vinaigrette – *Une Vinaigrette Simple* 413

Tangy Seafood and Salad Dressing (Tartar Sauce) – *Sauce Rémoulade* 414

Veal Stock – *Fond de Veau* 415

White Poultry Stock – *Bouillon de Volaille or Fond Blanc de Volaille* 417

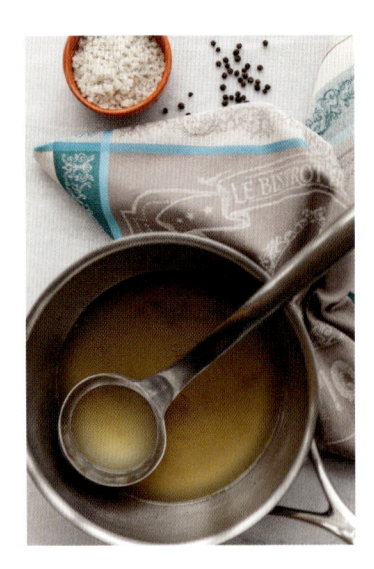

Another secret to French cooking is the use of stocks (*fonds*) and "bone broths" in sauces, purées, vegetable dishes, and as soup bases. Broths without meat are called bouillons, but so are broths with some meat in them. Bouillons are often served as a first course (*entrée*) which comes from the French word to enter (*entrer*). For some strange reason in the U.S., we call the main course an "entrée." Don't make this mistake in France. On a menu, *Les Entrées* are the appetizers, or the first course, while the main course, or second course, is called *un plat*. On a menu, "main courses" will read *Les Plats*.

As mentioned in the timeline "Selected Highlights of Food Culture in France and the United States" (page 13), the first restaurant opened in Paris in 1765, where a "restorative" broth or soup (*bouillon*) was served at tables for the first time. In Germany as early as 1870, this "strengthening brew" (*Kraftbrühe*) showed up in a bouillon cube cookbook, several decades after the science of transforming meats into bouillon cubes had been developed by French chemists Antoine-Augustin Parmentier (see recipes carrying his name on pages 137 and 197) and Joseph Louis Proust.[1] The word "strengthening" is the key here, as the broth or stock serve as foundations for one's health and the flavor of a dish.

Often you will find stock or broth recipes recommending you to skim off the fat. I never do this. The fat on the surface of a stock or broth comprises much of the nutritional value and flavor! Can you imagine hungry and hardworking peasants in France siphoning off fat from their nourishing broths and discarding it? Nevertheless, French cookbooks I have combed through dating from the 1300s through the 1900s will recommend skimming off (*écumer*) the fat and impurities. I'm not convinced, as the added nutrient value and satiety are undeniable to me now. Revisionist French cookbooks from the 1980s, reinterpreting French recipes from the past several hundred years, also recommend discarding the fat, and chefs in France continue to do this. These are clear signs to me that our modern societies developed an unnecessary fear of fat, the "impure," and the "carnal," associating these with sinfulness, death, and decay. The low-fat, fat-phobic spell under which we have functioned in recent decades continues and causes us to see the past through this distorted lens.[2]

I present you with some full-fat broths, stocks, and grain-free sauces to use in your healthy cooking.

382

Béchamel Sauce ›

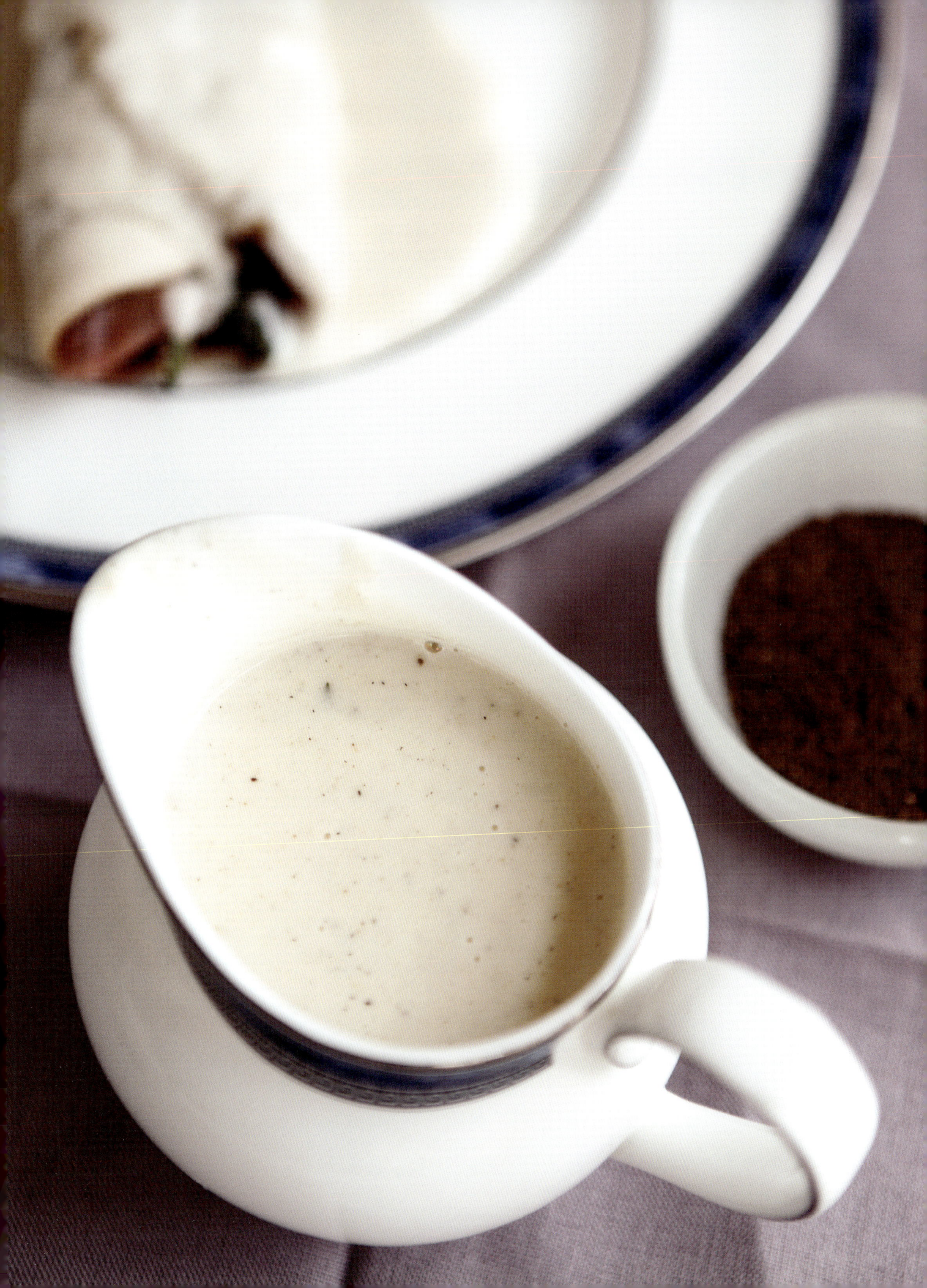

ALLEMANDE SAUCE
Sauce Allemande

Cooking Time 20 minutes   **Makes** 2 cups

"Allemande" in French means "German." Allemande sauce was allegedly renamed by the early 20th century Parisian chef Auguste Escoffier as *Sauce Parisienne* after World War I. Allemande sauce is a "white sauce" (*sauce blanche*) or "blonde sauce" (*sauce blonde*). According to *Larousse Gastronomique*, this sauce is also a "bound (with flour) sauce" (*velouté lié*), a thick sauce (*velouté épais*), and a "compounded sauce" (*sauce composée*).[3] A *velouté* is a creamy sauce, but it can also refer to a thickened soup. Soup *veloutés* are made from a base of chicken stock (*fond de volaille*), fish stock (*fumet de poisson*), or light or white stock (*fond blanc*), enriched either with cream or with a "white roux" (*roux blanc*)—a paste of butter and flour. Sauce *veloutés* are made similarly, or else with milk instead of stock. (One white *velouté* sauce enriched with cream is called **Sauce Velouté à la Crème (Sauce Suprême)** and can be found on page 402.) For the white *velouté* sauces, such as the Allemande Sauce, I have used cassava flour[4] to replace wheat flour, but feel free to experiment with others. In Julia Child's Allemande sauce, she enriches it with *both* egg yolk *and* cream,[5] while other recipes use *either* egg yolk *or* cream. Extra butter, added before serving, is optional. You will find recipes for all of the sauces mentioned later in this section. Now that you know the lingo, no waiter can get saucy with you when you see any of these on a menu!

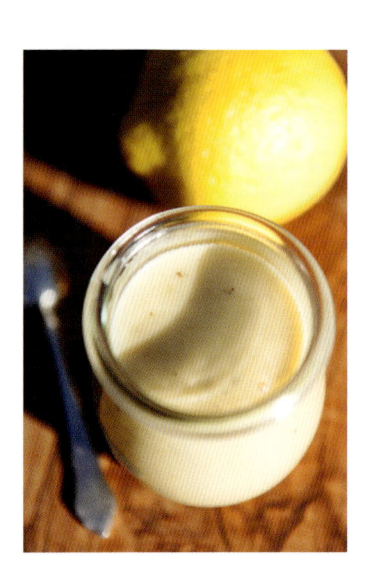

5 tablespoons cassava flour

3 tablespoons butter (or ghee)

1.5 cups (360 ml) **White (or Light) Stock** (page 399)

2 egg yolks

½ cup (120 ml) heavy cream

2 pinches of white pepper

3 pinches of fine salt

Optional: Pinch of nutmeg

Optional: 1 squeeze of lemon juice

Optional: liquid cream

Optional: 1 to 2 tablespoons butter

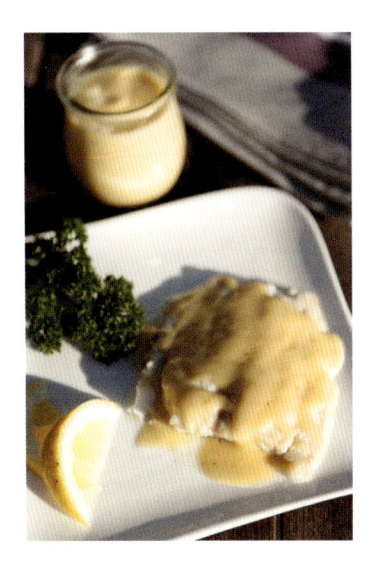

First make the roux, which is a paste of butter and flour. (See page 397 for instructions on how to make a **White Roux**.)

Add the stock to the roux. Combine the egg yolk and cream in a large bowl. Add the white stock and roux sauce slowly to the egg yolk and cream mixture, drawing figure eights with the whisk almost continuously. Once well blended, return the mixture to the pan. Bring to a boil for one minute over medium heat. Strain the sauce in a fine mesh strainer if desired. (I don't bother.)

Simmer over low heat for about 10 minutes until the sauce is thick enough to coat the back of a spoon. Stir in the white pepper, salt, optional pinch of nutmeg, and optional squeeze of lemon juice. If the sauce is too thick, the sauce may be diluted with extra liquid cream.

Keep warm until served. Another optional step is to mix in one or two more tablespoons of butter just before serving, to add to the sauce's unctuous texture. Allemande sauce is indeed thick and white and is traditionally served over eggs, meats, offal, poached chicken, or vegetables. When made with fish stock, Allemande sauce is served over fish, but I have made this sauce with chicken stock and served it over white fish (as shown here), and even over veal liver. It's a great way to add fat to a low-fat fish. This sauce may be frozen for later use.

ANCHOVY SAUCE
Sauce aux Anchois

Season Year-round   **Preparation Time** 5 minutes
Cooking Time 15 minutes   **Serves** 4

Anchovies "melted" into a sauce came into French cooking in the second half of the Sixteenth Century[6] and is evidenced by the 1651 publication of Pierre Francois La Varenne's *Le Cuisinier François*.[7] Anchovy sauce is supposedly the secret sauce used at a restaurant in Bordeaux called *Entrecôte*, where people line up outside for two different dinner seatings, and with one thing on the menu: beef rib-eye steak (*entrecôte*) with sauce, plus a glass of red wine. The anchovies impart a salty (rather than fishy) element to the sauce, and they are small oily fish (high in omega-3 fatty acids) and good for us to eat![8] For this sauce, you can use the fillets or whole anchovies. Whole is best—nose-to-tail—to respect the entire animal. But you can chop off the heads and tails if you wish. Fresh is best, but otherwise, try to find them preserved in the highest quality olive oil in glass jars or tins. When you drain the anchovies, catch the oil in which they are preserved and measure out the three tablespoons (listed below), adding additional olive oil from a bottle as needed for the recipe. Use high-quality, organic wine vinegar, or else use your own homemade vinegar from leftover wine. (For homemade vinegar, use two parts wine to one part "live" vinegar, or a vinegar "mother," as your starter culture. It takes two or three months for the wine to ferment to achieve a tart vinegar.[9])

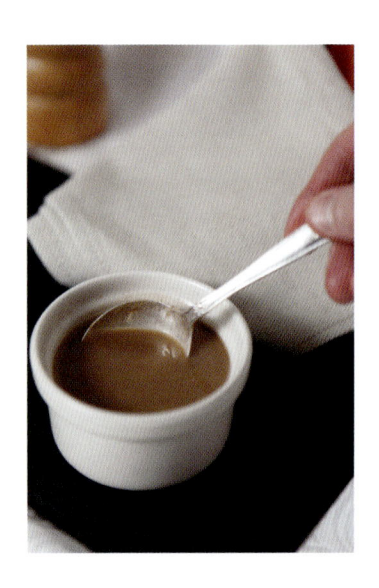

12 anchovies, drained (catch the oil) and chopped

2 garlic cloves, minced

3 tablespoons olive oil

2 tablespoons white wine vinegar

3 tablespoons water

4 tablespoons butter

Combine the anchovies, garlic, and oil with a whisk in a thick saucepan and boil gently on medium heat, stirring occasionally, until the anchovies fall apart and take on a creamy consistency. Add the vinegar and allow the sauce to reduce by a third on a gentle boil, stirring occasionally. Add the water and bring to a boil again.

Remove from heat and whisk in the butter in small chunks, stirring the sauce until it thickens. Serve over thin or regular beef steaks, as shown here, as well as over "thick cut" beef steaks (*pavés*), or else over other red or white meats.

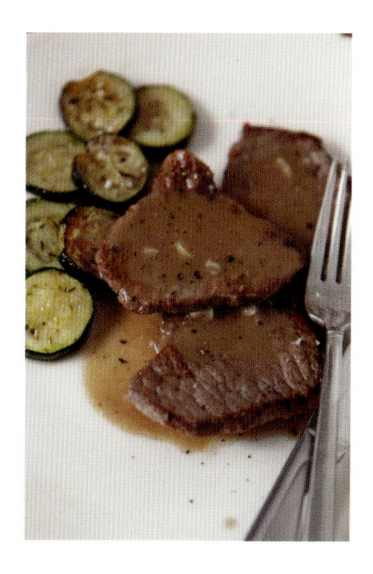

VARIATIONS The following ingredients may also be added: one to two tablespoons whole cream, one egg yolk, lemon juice to replace the vinegar, one teaspoon of chopped fresh rosemary, or, as La Varenne did in the mid-1600s, add a pinch of nutmeg and use the sauce over fried or scrambled eggs.

WINE PAIRING TIP When serving this sauce over beef, try pairing it with a medium or full-bodied red wine from Bordeaux or from the Rhône Valley.

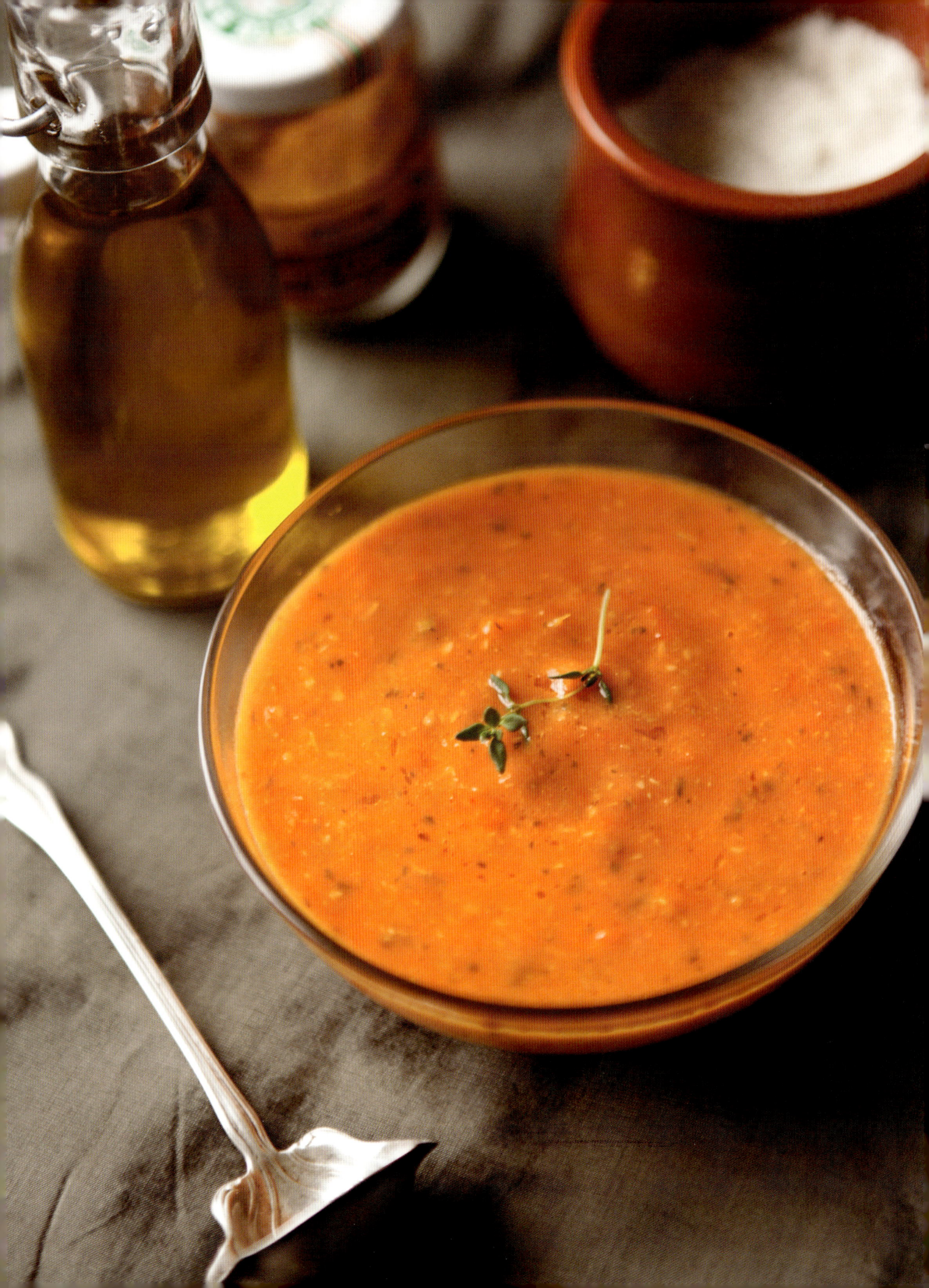

BARBEQUE SAUCE
Sauce à Barbeque

Season Summer   **Preparation Time** 10 to 15 minutes
Cooking Time 30 minutes to roast the garlic   **Serves** 8 (Makes about 1 cup or 240 ml)

Rather than relying on bottled high fructose corn syrup, here is a BBQ sauce to go with any grilled steak or meat. As I am lazy, I do not bother peeling off the skin from the tomatoes. I find the skin and seeds just add to the texture of the sauce. You can place the tomatoes in boiling water for about 30 to 60 seconds, remove them with a slotted spoon, and easily pull off the skin (*monder*). This recipe calls for roasted garlic, which is easy to make but needs a half hour to roast in the oven before making this sauce.

1 garlic bulb, roasted then peeled

18 to 20 summer cherry tomatoes (orange, red, or yellow), diced

1 teaspoon honey

4 tablespoons olive oil

2 teaspoons white wine or cider vinegar

2 teaspoons fresh thyme, minced

Dash of *piment d'Espelette* or paprika

2 pinches of fine sea salt

2 pinches of ground pepper

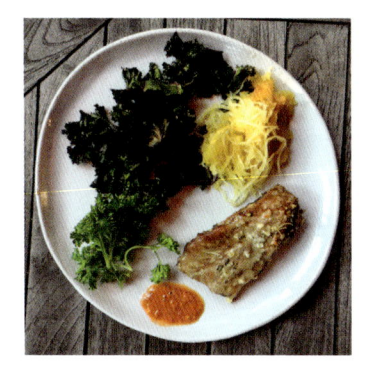

Preheat the oven to 365°F (185°C). Place half a garlic bulb in the oven. You can wrap it in parchment or foil, although this is not absolutely necessary. Allow to roast for 30 minutes.

Peel the roasted garlic and combine it with the remaining ingredients in a thick saucepan. Simmer on medium heat for 15 minutes, stirring occasionally and until warmed through. Remove from heat and stir in the honey. Allow to cool before serving. Purée in a blender, or with an immersion blender, for a smooth consistency. Or if you prefer, leave the BBQ sauce "chunky."

Serve over meat, on the side, or in a little ramekin or sauce dish.

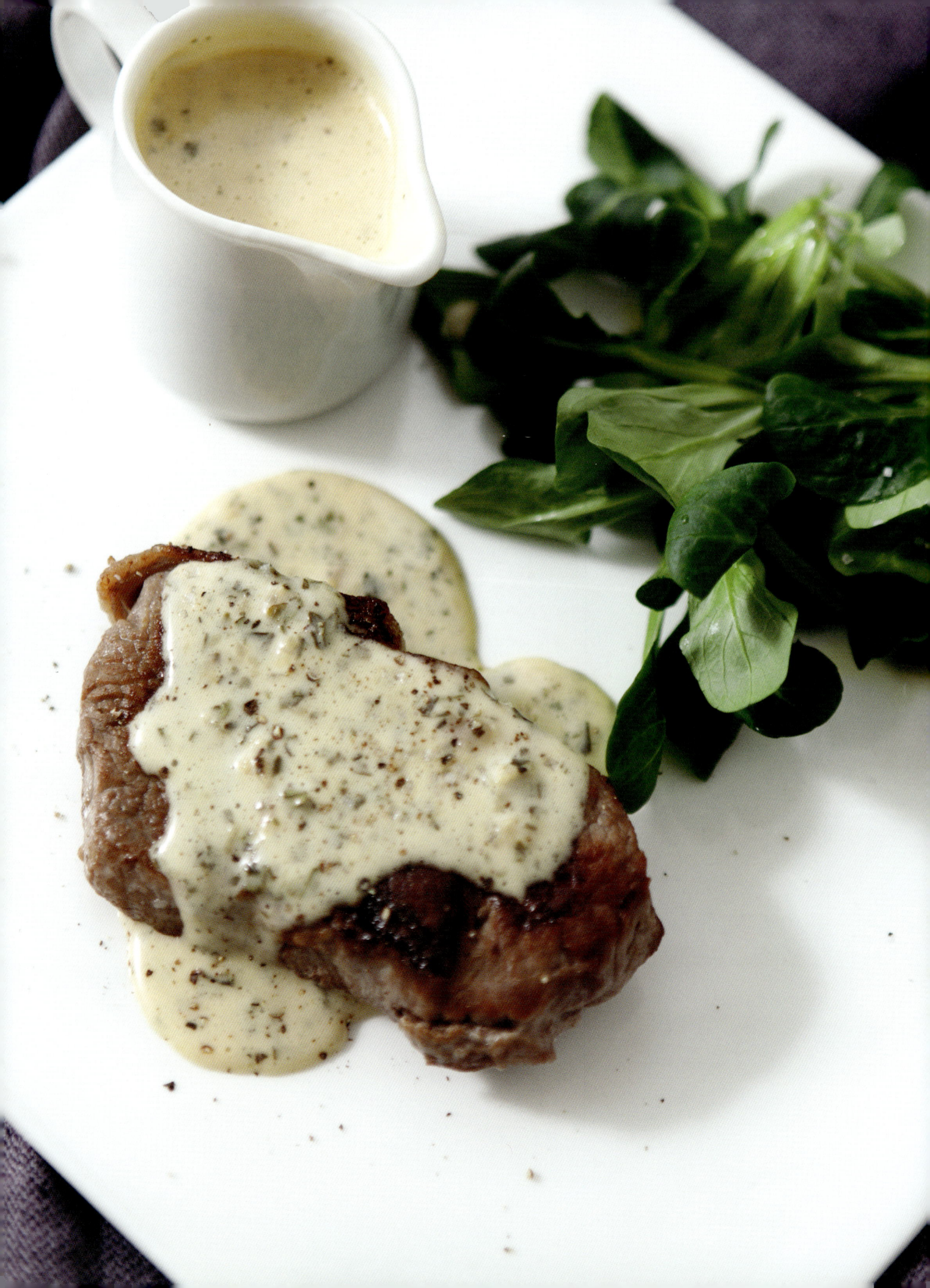

BÉARNAISE SAUCE
Sauce Béarnaise

Season Spring for fresh tarragon, or year-round using dried tarragon   **Preparation Time** 15 minutes   **Cooking Time** 30 to 35 minutes   **Serves** 6

The use of sauces in cooking has been traced back to Roman times, when Apicius, a Roman gourmand, wrote about the art of cooking.[10] Today, French sauces are famous the world over. If done well, they lend extra flavor (and fat) to any dish. Béarnaise sauce is a "sabayon sauce" (*sauce sabayon*). Originally an Italian term, *zabaglione* or *zabaione*, a sabayon sauce is a moussy mixture of egg yolks and dry or sweet wines used as the base of some sauces and desserts. Béarnaise sauce originates from the region around Béarn in France's Southwest, the region's capital being Pau, a jumping off point for skiing and hiking in the beautiful Pyrénées mountains. This sauce can be used liberally on grilled fish and meats. Some people use it on breaded fish, or as a stand-in for mayonnaise. It may be served warm or at room temperature. Pictured here with the Béarnaise Sauce is a rib-eye (*entrecôte*) steak, pan-grilled using two tablespoons of tallow and one teaspoon of ghee and seared for two to three minutes on each side. This sauce may be frozen, then thawed again when needed.

5 tablespoons white wine

3 tablespoons white wine vinegar

1 large or 2 small (1.8 ounces or 50 g) shallots, finely minced

3 tablespoons tarragon (*estragon*) fresh or dried, minced

2 pinches of fine salt

2 egg yolks

2/3 cup (160 g) butter, chopped into ½-inch (1.25 cm) chunks

Pinch of white pepper

Combine the wine, vinegar, shallot, two tablespoons of the tarragon and a pinch of salt in a thick saucepan and bring to a boil. Cook on medium-high for seven to 10 minutes to reduce the liquid a little bit. Set aside from heat to cool for 10 to 15 minutes.

Whisk the egg yolks into the sauce for about a minute, until well incorporated. Place the pan over low or medium-low heat and stir continuously with the whisk in figure eights (the infinity symbol, it may indeed feel like you are stirring for infinity) for five to seven minutes. Allow the sauce to foam up for several minutes, but stop at 149°F (65°C) maximum. (Keep a digital thermometer probe in the sauce as you heat it.)

Add the butter, chunk by chunk, while stirring. Add another pinch of salt, the pepper, and the remaining tarragon. Serve warm over meats and fish.

BÉCHAMEL SAUCE
Sauce Béchamel

Season Year-round   **Preparation Time** None   **Cooking Time** 15 minutes   **Serves** 6 to 7

This sauce bears the name of Louis de Béchameil, marquis de Nointel (1630-1703), the chief steward (*maitre de l'hotel*) of French King Louis XIV, though the recipe was already in existence (using bread crumbs) in the 1651 publication of *Le Cuisinier François* by Pierre François La Varenne (1618-1678). Béchamel sauce, a *velouté* sauce made with cream, fish stock, or chicken stock, much like *Sauce Suprême*, or *Velouté à la Crème*, is made nowadays from a *roux blanc*, a mixture of melted butter and flour which forms the basis for white sauces (*sauces blanches*), often with added milk. Though this recipe is grain-free, employing cassava (yucca root) flour instead of the "usual" wheat flour, it is still high in carbohydrates. A little sauce can go a long way, especially if adequately salted and spiced. Sauces are a messy business, especially if you drop the whisk. Wear an apron. (Ghee was used in the recipe photo.)

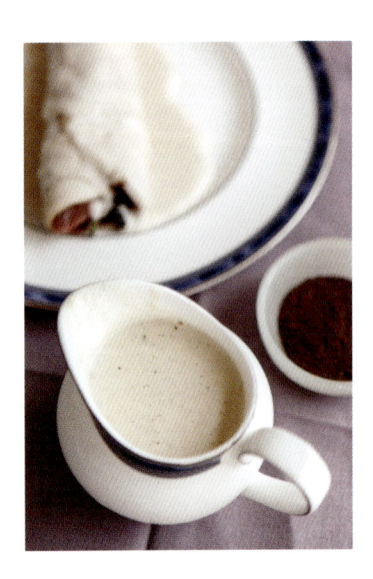

FOR THE ROUX

3 tablespoons butter or ghee

5 tablespoons cassava flour

FOR THE REST OF THE SAUCE

2 cups (about ½ L) milk

Optional: *Bouquet garni*

3 pinches of fine salt

Pinch of ground white pepper

Optional: Pinch of ground nutmeg

Garnished Bouquet
Bouquet Garni

Reminder: A *bouquet garni* is a small bundle of aromatic herbs in a combination which may be comprised of laurel (bay) leaves, thyme, leek and rosemary, parsley or savory tied together in a small bundle with string or in cheese cloth.

Begin by making the *roux*. Melt the butter in a thick saucepan over medium-low or low heat. When the butter begins to bubble, add the flour in one go, whisking and blending well for three to five minutes until you have reached a somewhat sandy and moussy consistency, and before the sauce begins turning brown. If the roux turns brown, it is called a "brown roux" (*roux brun*), instead of what we need in this recipe, which is a "white roux" (*roux blanc*). (Refer to **Brown Roux and White Roux – *Roux Brun et Roux Blanc*** on page 397). Because cassava flour has no gluten, the roux is runnier than with wheat four. (Nevertheless, it will thicken if chilled and reheated. Leftover sauce is thick and still delicious.)

For the rest of the sauce making, whisk in the cold milk, bit by bit (several tablespoons at a time) to the warm roux over medium heat. Each splash of milk needs to heat to a gentle boil while being stirred

Chef's Tip
Astuce du Chef

According to Julia Child in *Mastering the Art of French Cooking*, should the sauce become lumpy, continue to stir and heat it a bit more for a few minutes and pass it through a fine mesh sieve. Sauce can be thinned with cream, milk, or stock, one spoonful at a time, until the desired consistency is reached. Sauce can be thickened by boiling it down for a few minutes over medium-high heat or by adding a tablespoon or two of **White Roux** (a paste of flour and butter, page 399) and mixing this in over medium-high heat for a minute.

before the next splash is added. According to *Atelier des Chefs*, a French cooking website and school, the secret to a successful Béchamel sauce is the difference in temperature between the warmed roux and the cold milk. If your roux is cold, then the milk must be heated. After all the milk has been combined, add the optional "garnished bouquet" (*bouquet garni*) for added flavor, decrease the heat again to low, and continue stirring occasionally for about 10 minutes until the sauce begins to thicken and has taken on a smooth consistency. Remove from heat. Remove the *bouquet garni*, and season the sauce with salt, pepper, and optional nutmeg. For a smaller batch of sauce, use three tablespoons of flour and two tablespoons of butter, and less milk.

Serve warm over fish, veal, chicken, or vegetables, or, in spring, over asparagus and ham wrapped in crêpes (as shown). (See page 503 on how to make **Sweet and Savory Crêpes**.)

VARIATIONS In modern recipes, there is no egg yolk or vinegar, as in the original recipe by La Varenne. His recipe also contains no flour because it is the egg that is charged with binding the sauce (*un oeuf pour lier la sauce*).[11] Therefore, you might experiment with this version without the flour. In other renditions, ½ cup of white wine may be slowly added to the sauce after the milk has been incorporated. Julia Child gives the option of replacing the milk with light or "white" stock.[12] (See **Brown Stock and White Stock** on page 398.)

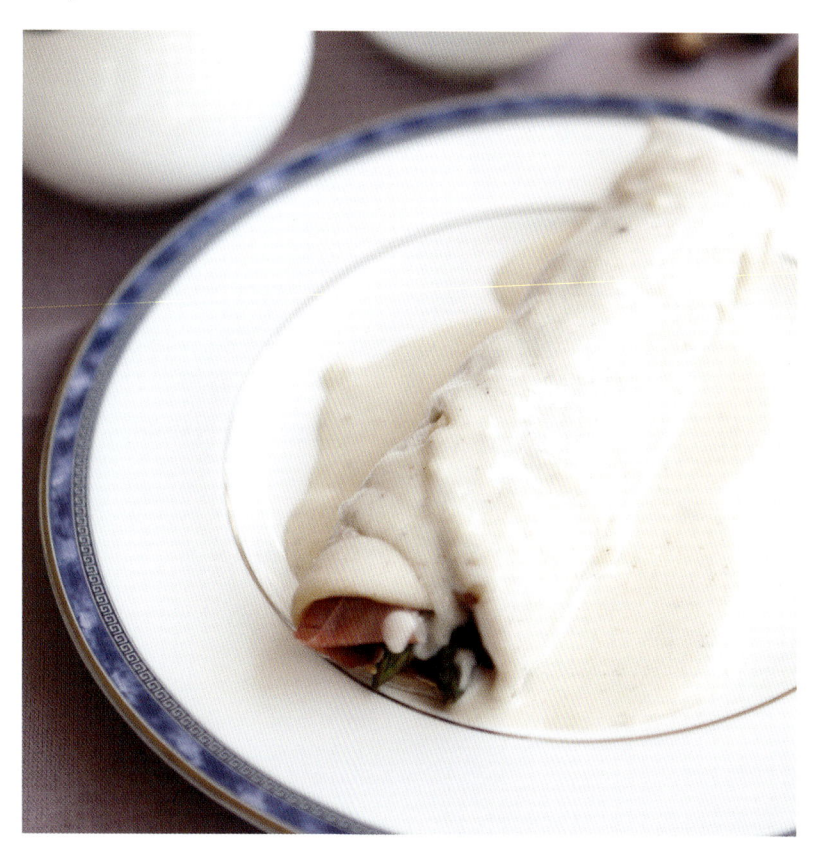

Béchamel Crêpe

STOCKS AND SAUCES – *LES FONDS, BOUILLONS, ET SAUCES*

BONE BROTH
Le Bouillon

Season Year-round   **Preparation Time** 5 minutes   **Cooking Time** 2 hours minimum, all day if possible

Bone broth is very popular among those following an ancestral diet. Bone broth is made by cooking bones for up to 24 hours, although some people even cook their broth up to 48 hours. I usually cook my broths from first thing in the morning to last thing at night. Then, when I'm tired and impatient, I have to fill glass Pyrex containers with the precious liquid. But it is worth the extra bit of trouble, and actually, bone broth is no trouble. It's worth the extra bit of work at the end of the day, as it is a healing "witch's brew." Throw in whatever you have in terms of bones if you are not aiming for a specific flavor or type of stock, such as lamb stock (using primarily lamb bones), **Veal Stock** (page 415), or duck stock (find under **White Poultry Stock** page 417). Broths are tremendous for the gut, but they can also be problematic: knuckle joints in broth can be high in FODMAPs, and broth can be high in histamines and arginine. In this case, some people prefer **Fish Stock** (see page 403) or they use marine collagen. That said, bone broth is high in the amino acid glycine, which balances out the methionine we obtain from eating muscle meats.[13] The savory flavor of bone broths is much enhanced if the bones have been roasted first. A general rule of thumb is to roast previously unroasted bones (such as those you could procure from a butcher) for about half an hour in the oven at 395°F (200°C).

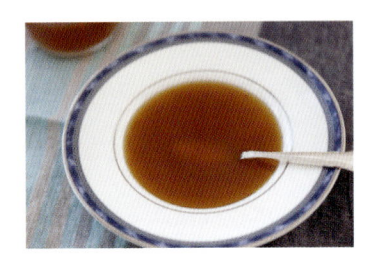

SOME COMBINATION OF THE FOLLOWING INGREDIENTS IS WHAT I USUALLY PUT INTO A POT OF BONE BROTH:

Garnished bouquet (*bouquet garni*)

Roasted chicken carcasses (roasting them first adds to the flavor)

Roasted chicken feet (feet have lots of collagen)

Leftover bones from lamb cutlets, bone-in steaks, and pork chops

Leftover bones from rib meals and bone-in roasts

Pork (including pig tails) or beef bones from a butchered piece of meat that will fit in the pot (roasting them first adds flavor)

Uncooked, cured pork rind (*bout de poitrine séchée* or *bout de ventrèche séchée*)

Poultry necks and gizzards (save the hearts and livers for sautéing separately or for a pâté; roast the necks for extra flavor)

Onions, Carrots, Garlic, chopped

Celery stalks

Ends of leeks, white or green

Sprigs of rosemary and thyme

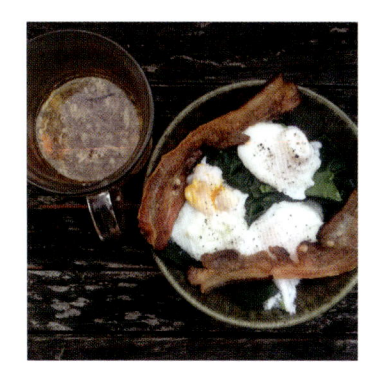

A few pinches of course sea salt (I like my broths on the saltier, more flavorful side)

2 to 3 tablespoons apple cider vinegar (to help draw out minerals from the bones and add a tinge of flavor)

1 or 2 bay leaves

Sea vegetables (such as *dulse, kombu, nori,* or *wakame*)

Combine the ingredients that you have on hand and would like to incorporate into your broth and cover with water. Bring to a boil, then cover and turn down to a simmer for the entire day. Stir every now and then. The soup will fill the house with the aroma of lunch the whole day. No siphoning off the fat here, for that is what gives the broth so much of its flavor and richness. Be careful when sipping a mug of piping hot broth, as that layer of fat that covers the water also retains the heat, just like fat does on an animal. By ladling the soup after cooking into containers, you can easily spot and remove bones as you go, rather than filter the soup, but you may use a sieve to remove unwanted sprigs and bits. If the broth is to become part of a sauce, you can filter out the pieces for visual homogeneity, otherwise, keep all the good stuff in there! Also, you can pick off some of the meat that comes off easily from the bones if you have a few minutes of extra time and patience. If you can tolerate butter or ghee (or coconut, olive oil, or even extra duck fat or lard), you can add these to your broth before drinking. Don't forget to add an extra pinch of coarse sea salt to your mug of broth for a delightful, savory experience. My favorite breakfast (shown above) consists of a cup of bone broth alongside poached eggs over spinach or lettuce with bacon or chicken livers!

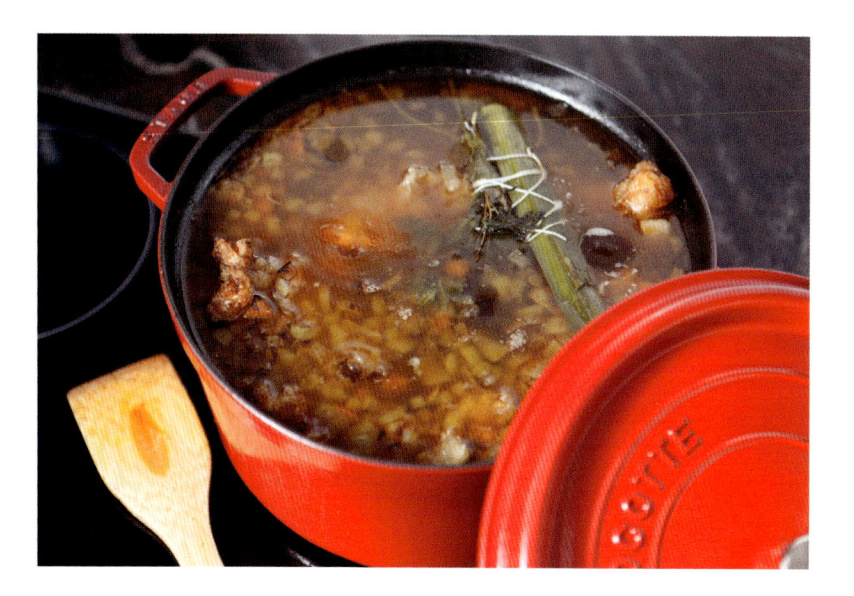

STOCKS AND SAUCES – *LES FONDS, BOUILLONS, ET SAUCES*

Freezing Vegetable Leftovers for Use in Stock

One easy technique I learned both from Mark Sisson's blog, *Mark's Daily Apple* (www.marksdailyapple.com), and from legendary French chef Jacques Pépin cooking with Julia Child in her *Cooking in Concert* series for PBS,[14] is to collect vegetable leftovers in the freezer. When you are ready to make a stock, pull them out of the freezer and throw them in the stock. As a result, my small European freezer is literally popping with celery, chard and kale stalks, carrot and leek ends, and parsley stems. I generally try to sequester them into paper bags, so that they don't come raining down on me every time I open the overhead freezer door.

Soupy Vocabulary Explained

In French, *bouillon* is the catchall phrase for a stock or soup broth. The way Chef Jean-Luc explained the progression of "reduction" stages or thicknesses of the broth (from watery to thick enough to cut into gelatinous cubes) and vocabulary goes as follows:

Réduction – The transformation of a *bouillon* into *glace*:

Bouillon – Watery broth

Fond – More concentrated broth or stock base

Demi-Glace – Gelatinous but not solid

Glace – Solid gelatin

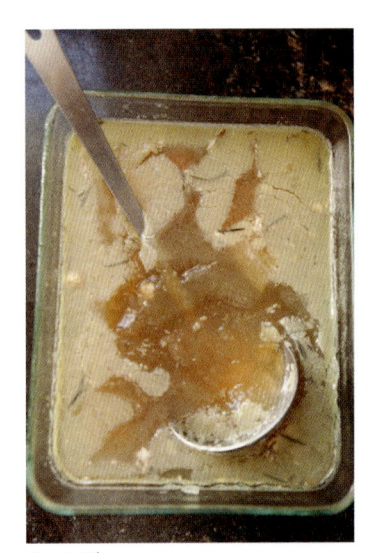

Demi-Glace

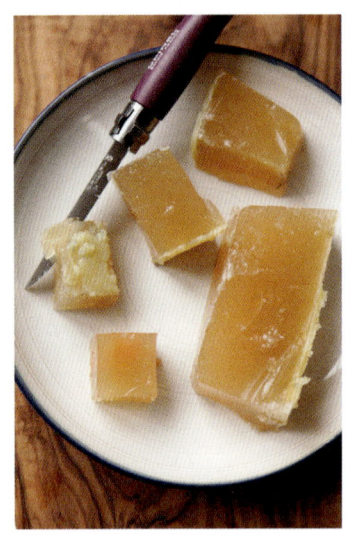

Glace

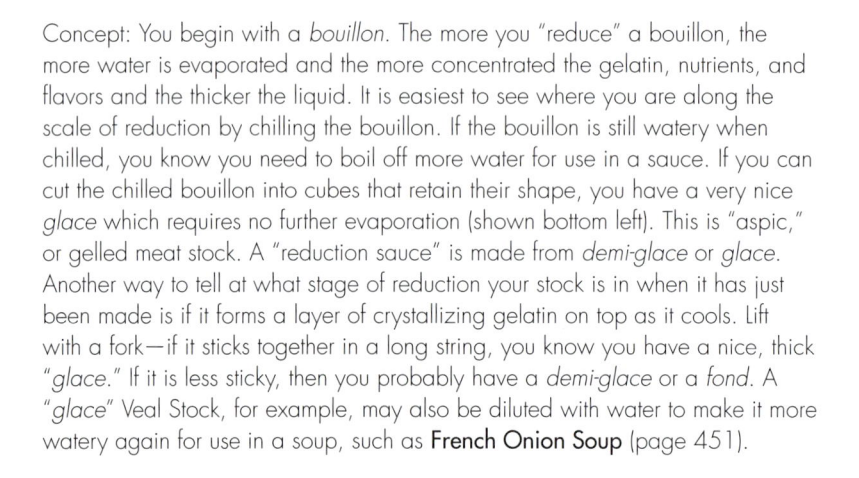

Concept: You begin with a *bouillon*. The more you "reduce" a bouillon, the more water is evaporated and the more concentrated the gelatin, nutrients, and flavors and the thicker the liquid. It is easiest to see where you are along the scale of reduction by chilling the bouillon. If the bouillon is still watery when chilled, you know you need to boil off more water for use in a sauce. If you can cut the chilled bouillon into cubes that retain their shape, you have a very nice *glace* which requires no further evaporation (shown bottom left). This is "aspic," or gelled meat stock. A "reduction sauce" is made from *demi-glace* or *glace*. Another way to tell at what stage of reduction your stock is in when it has just been made is if it forms a layer of crystallizing gelatin on top as it cools. Lift with a fork—if it sticks together in a long string, you know you have a nice, thick "*glace*." If it is less sticky, then you probably have a *demi-glace* or a *fond*. A "*glace*" Veal Stock, for example, may also be diluted with water to make it more watery again for use in a soup, such as **French Onion Soup** (page 451).

Just for clarification purposes, a "clarified" soup (*consommé*) is a stock with the fat (*la graisse*, from which the English word for grease developed) and nutrients (so-called "impurities") removed using protein-binding egg whites (much like the process of "fining" wine, the clarification and removal of dead yeast cells and debris out of wine) and straining the stock. Again, this "clarification" to me assumes that there is an inherent impurity in meat and fat which should be removed if one is *fearful* of these things. Instead, I would argue that we *need* all the proteins and fats in the stock. These are some of the key restorative elements of stock, along with the hydration from the water, and therefore they must not be filtered out. A bright, clear consommé might be needed for a chef's special artistic creation, but for home cooking, nutrient density is the goal.

BROWN ROUX AND WHITE ROUX
Roux Brun et Roux Blanc

Season Year-round   **Preparation Time** None   **Cooking Time** 3 to 5 minutes   **Makes** about ½ cup (125 ml) roux

A *roux* is a mixture of melted butter and flour that forms the basis for white sauces (*sauces blanches*). Although this recipe is grain-free, employing cassava (yucca root) flour instead of the "usual" wheat flour, it is still high in carbohydrates. A little sauce can go a long way, especially if adequately salted and spiced.

3 tablespoons butter

5 tablespoons cassava flour

Melt the butter in a thick saucepan on medium-low or low heat. When the butter begins to bubble, add the flour in one go, whisking and blending well for three to five minutes until you have reached a somewhat sandy and moussy consistency, but before the sauce begins turning brown. If the roux turns brown, it is called a "brown roux" (*roux brun*). Before it turns brown, it is a "white roux" (*roux blanc*). Because cassava flour has no gluten, the roux is runnier than when made with wheat flour. Use roux in sauces such as **Allemande Sauce** (page 384), **Béchamel Sauce** (page 392), and **Cream Sauce** (page 402).

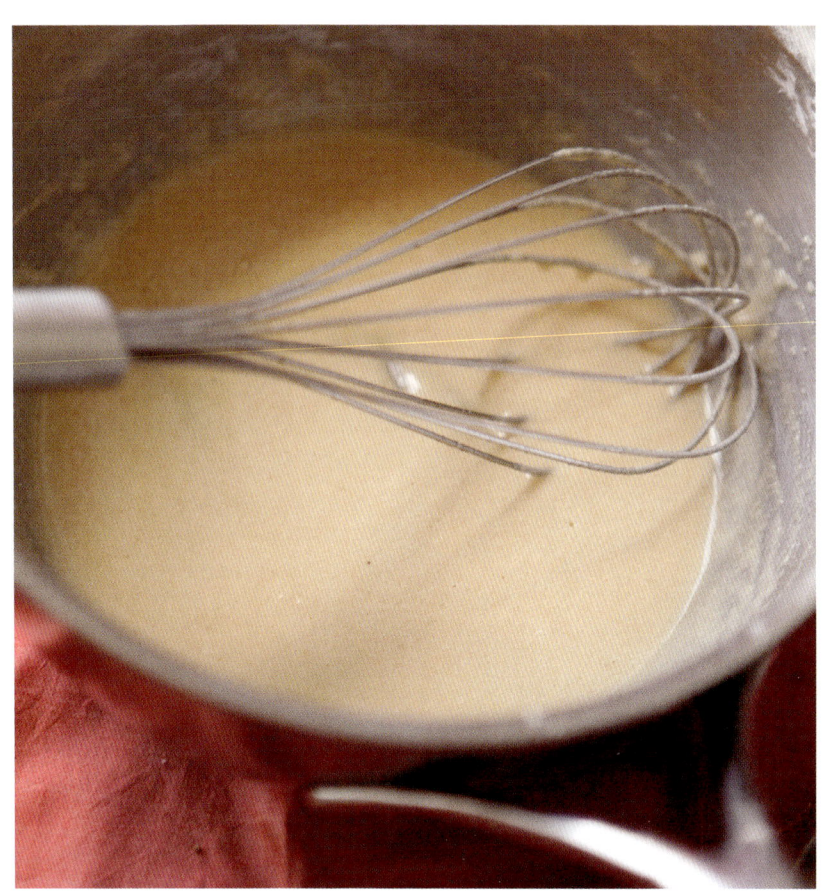

STOCKS AND SAUCES – *LES FONDS, BOUILLONS, ET SAUCES*

BROWN STOCK AND WHITE (OR LIGHT) STOCK
Fond Brun et Fond Blanc

Season Year-round   **Preparation Time** 5 minutes   **Cooking Time** 2 hours minimum, all day if possible

Both Brown and White (or Light) Stocks are essentially simplified **Veal Stock** (page 415). Brown stock (*fond brun*) employs *both* veal meat *and* bones, while white or light stock, shown in the recipe photo on the next page uses chicken bones *and/or* giblets and veal bones or veal knuckle (*jarret de veau*), but *no* veal meat, which colors the stock. Brown Poultry Stock (*fond brun de volaille*) and White Poultry Stock (*fond blanc de volaille*) differ in that the Brown Poultry Stock contains poultry meat and bones browned in a pan before cooking, which changes both color and flavor. White Poultry Stock contains bones and meat either raw or roasted, but *not* browned in a pan. Following are recipes for both Brown and White Stocks. See **White Poultry Stock** on page 417 for information about chicken stock. Chicken giblets include the gizzard (stomach muscle), heart, liver, and neck. I do not put heart or liver into my stocks because I cook those separately (see **Chicken Hearts with Garlic and Parsley** on page 230 and **Chicken Livers with Bacon** on page 236). Whenever I make a stock or broth of any kind, I begin in the morning and allow it to simmer until the evening, thereby maximizing the nutrients extracted from the bones.

BROWN STOCK

2.2 pounds (1 kg) veal meat and bones, browned

8 cups (2 liters) water

Parsley stems

Carrot, chopped

2 small yellow onions (about 2 ounces or 60 g), chopped

1 to 2 celery stalks

Bouquet garni

4 pinches of coarse salt

Combine all the ingredients for the Brown Stock in a stock pot, bring to a boil. Cover the pot and reduce the heat to low. Allow to simmer for at least two hours, all day if possible. For **Brown Poultry Stock**, use only poultry meat and bones (see page 417). Brown them over medium-high heat for 10 to 15 minutes in a pan before combining into the stock.

WHITE (OR LIGHT) STOCK

2.2 pounds (1 kg) chicken and veal bones

Optional: Handful of chicken giblets

8 cups (2 L) water

Parsley stems

Carrot, chopped

2 small yellow onions (about 2 ounces or 60 g), chopped

1 to 2 celery stalks

Bouquet garni

4 pinches of coarse salt

Combine all the ingredients for the **White Stock** in a stock pot and bring to a boil. Cover the pot and reduce the heat to low. Allow to simmer for at least two hours, all day if possible. For **White Poultry Stock** (see page 417), you would use only poultry meat and bones, either raw or roasted, such as from a **Whole Roast Chicken** (page 373), **Whole Stuffed Duck** (page 375), or **Whole Stuffed Holiday Goose** (page 377).

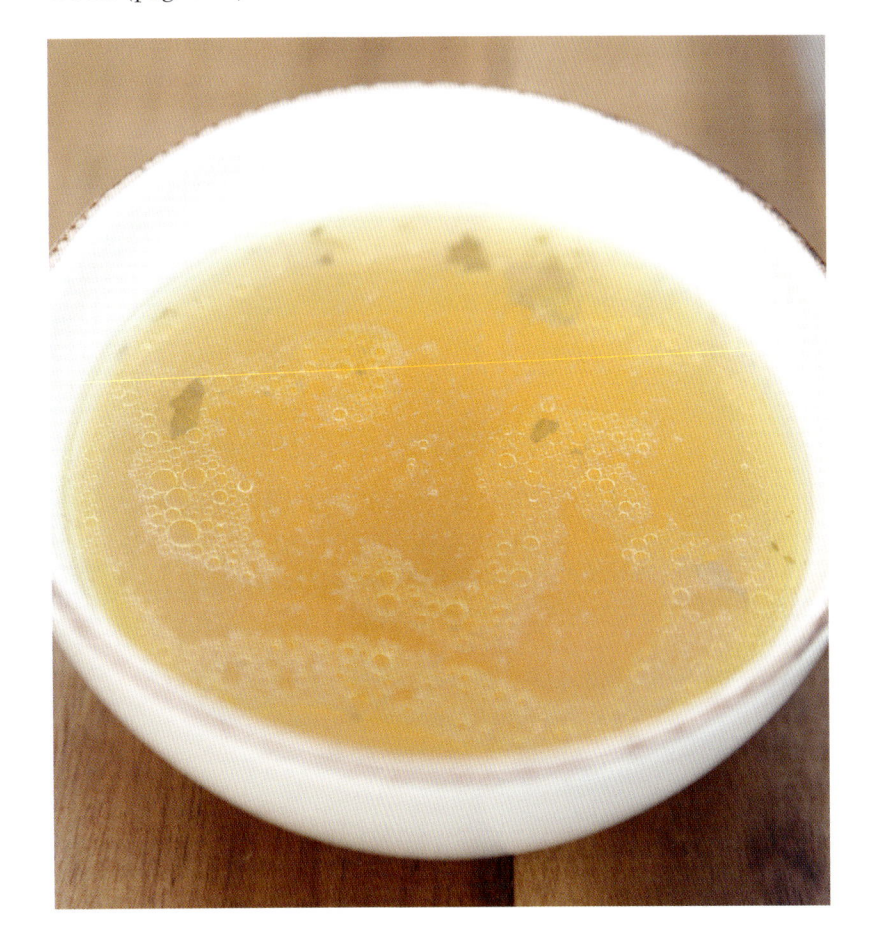

CRAB SAUCE
Sauce aux Crabes

Season Late Spring through early Autumn   **Preparation Time** 30 minutes
Cooking Time 30 minutes   **Serves** 4

Chef Célia of one-Michelin-star restaurant and hotel Le Saint James showed me this sauce, which goes with her grandmother VonVon's **Chicken Liver Cake with Crab Sauce** (page 233). Crayfish (crawfish) may be used instead of the river crabs, which are quite small in size. The small crustaceans give the sauce a distinct flavor when combined with the white wine and Armagnac liquor. Because of the techniques used to make this recipe, it's usually the kind of thing one orders in a high-end French restaurant, but you can make it at home if you have the crabs or crayfish. River crabs (shown on the next page) are in season May through August, while crayfish are in season May through September. In Lyon, this sauce is also eaten with quenelles, a doughy, oversized gnocchi made with flour, eggs, and Gruyère cheese.

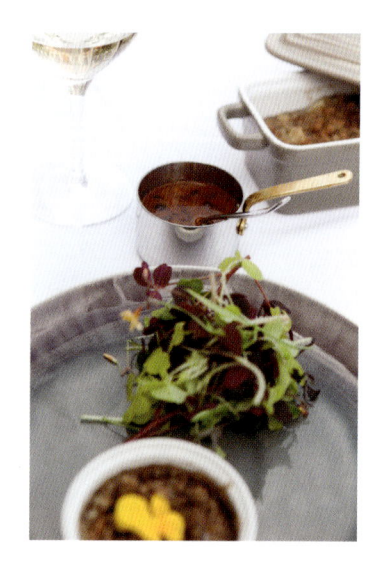

2 tablespoons olive oil

5 small lake or river crabs (or crayfish), live or freshly caught

1 tablespoon butter

½ medium onion, diced

1 garlic clove, minced

1 sprig of thyme

3 tablespoons Armagnac

5 ounces or ⅗ cup (140 ml) white wine

1 teaspoon tomato concentrate

2 tablespoons water

4 tomatoes, peeled, seeds removed, and chopped

2 tablespoons black or green olives, pitted

Fleur de sel, for garnish

Heat a sauce pot over high heat and add the oil. (Use a pot with thick sides for making sauces, so that you are less likely to burn the sauce.) When the oil is heated, add the crabs (or crayfish) and allow them to change color (photo A). Smash the crabs in the pot (photo B) with a flat-ended mallet (*maillet*); the mallet handle has to be long enough. Otherwise, use a flat-ended baton the length of a rolling pin (*bâton cuisine*). (Apologies for the violence, but please keep in mind that this is a typical method for making seafood bisques and sauces, especially at a restaurant that uses fresh ingredients when you have your lobster or seafood bisque. Compare this to an industrial-scale canned bisque operation and this individual scale will seem much less horrifying. It's nose-to-tail eating, very fresh, and not industrially refined, not that it's necessarily enjoyable to watch or do.)

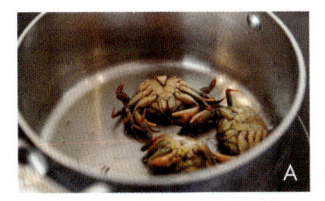

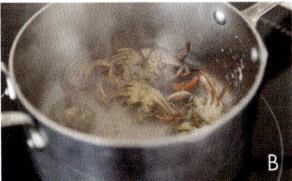

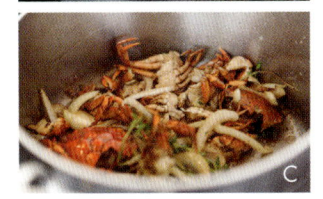

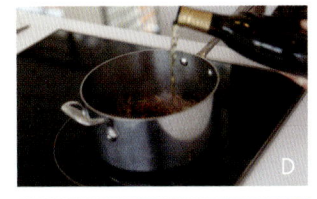

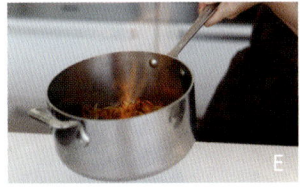

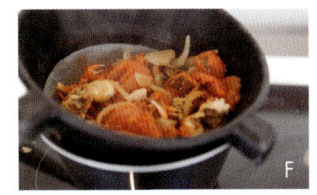

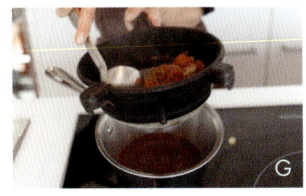

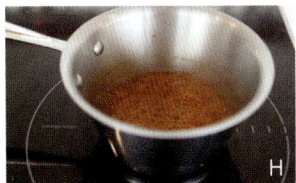

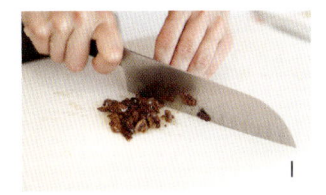

Add the butter, onion, garlic, thyme (photo C), and Armagnac (photo D). Remove from ventilation. Carefully light a match or a torch and hold it at the rim of the pan, pulling away as the alcohol catches fire to *flamber* the sauce (photo E). Shake the pan until the flames subside and turn the heat down to medium.

Add the wine and stir for two minutes before adding the tomato concentrate, the two tablespoons of water, and the tomatoes. Allow to reduce, uncovered, at a lively boil for about 20 minutes, stirring occasionally. Strain through a sieve (photo F), pressing the vegetables and crab pieces using the bottom of a ladle (photo G) for a smooth consistency to the sauce. Bring the sauce again to a rolling boil for a minute or two (photo H) while you chop the olives (photo I).

In a small bowl, mix the sauce with the olives and garnish with *fleur de sel*.

Serve with any liver pâté, but especially with the **Chicken Liver Cake with Crab Sauce** (page 233).

> WINE PAIRING TIP Try pairing this sauce with crisp, unoaked white wines: a citrusy Alsatian Riesling; a fresh Chablis from Burgundy, a mineraly Sancerre, made from the Sauvignon Blanc grape, from the Loire Valley. For a regional French Southwest dry white pairing, try a crisp Entre-Deux-Mers, a rich Pessac-Léognan or Graves, all from the Bordeaux region, or a light, floral and fruity Southwest Côtes de Duras, using the same grapes as the Bordeaux whites. See also the wine pairing suggestions for the **Chicken Liver Cake with Crab Sauce** (page 235).

STOCKS AND SAUCES – *LES FONDS, BOUILLONS, ET SAUCES*

CREAM SAUCE (SUPREME SAUCE)
Sauce Velouté à la Crème (Sauce Suprême)

Season Year-round   **Preparation Time** None   **Cooking Time** 12 to 15 minutes
Makes about 2 cups (500 ml) of sauce

Also called *Sauce Suprême*, this extra creamy white sauce is described as a "bound (with flour), velvety sauce" (*sauce veloutée liée*) or a "composed sauce" (*sauce composée*), made from a base of cream and **Béchamel Sauce** (a combination of butter, flour, and milk, see page 392, or **White Poultry Stock**, page 417). There is no egg yolk added to this sauce, but there is always the option of incorporating one to two tablespoons of butter just prior to serving to add to the unctuous texture of the sauce.

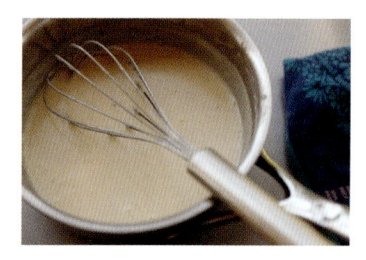

3 tablespoons butter

3 tablespoons cassava flour

1.5 cups (375 ml) cold milk or cold **White Poultry Stock** (page 417)

3 pinches of salt

Pinch of white pepper

Squeeze of one small lemon slice

½ cup (125 ml) whole cream

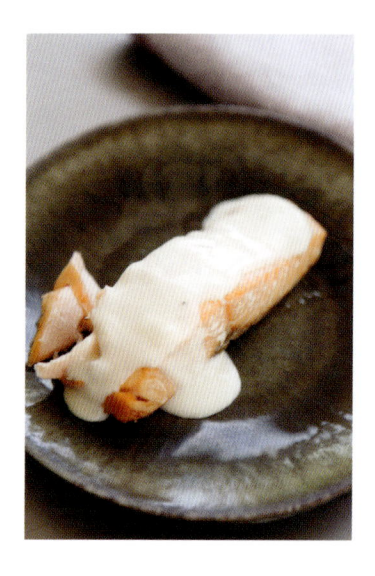

Melt the butter in a thick saucepan over medium-low heat. Add the flour in one go, whisk it together with the butter, and heat on low for 3 minutes. This is your "white roux."

Add the cold milk, bit by bit, using a whisk and stirring continuously. Once the milk is incorporated, heat the mixture to a boil over medium-high heat. Boil for one minute, stirring vigorously in figure eights. Add the salt, pepper, and lemon juice. This is your Béchamel sauce.

Using the whisk, beat the cream into the sauce in spoonfuls, slowly dribbling into the pan over medium-low heat. Stir for two minutes over the heat. Your creamy sauce has now been elevated to supremely creamy! Keep warm until served. If not served immediately, Julia Child recommends pouring a thin layer of milk or melted butter over the top of the sauce in the pan to keep a layer of skin from forming on the surface.[15]

Serve over eggs, poultry, offal, and vegetables. I have served this sauce over salmon, as shown here, a rich and delicious combination.

FISH STOCK
Fumet de Poisson

Season Year-round   **Preparation Time** 5 minutes
Cooking Time 30 to 45 minutes

This basic stock is easy to make with leftover fish bones. It can be frozen for future use if you cannot consume it all immediately.

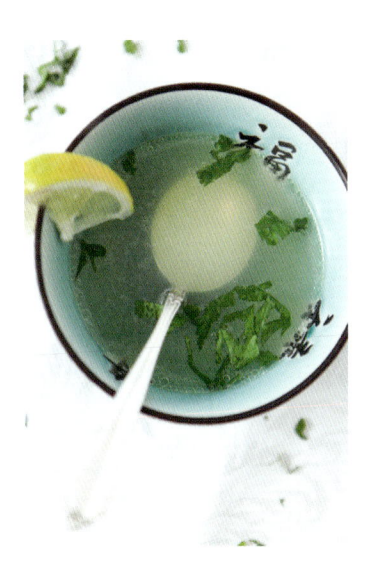

Fish bones

Parsley, basil, or cilantro stalks

Sea salt to taste

Optional: Gelatin powder

Optional Ingredients: *Dulse, kombu, wakame,* or other sea vegetable, leftover vegetable broth from steaming or boiling vegetables, celery stalks, lemon juice, mushroom parings, clove of garlic

Place ingredients in a pot and cover with water. (If you only have a few bones, it will make a small amount of stock.) Bring to a boil, then cover the pot and cook on low. Add gelatin powder if desired to make it more gelatinous. One option from the cookbook from the early 1700s, *Le Cuisinier Roïal et Bourgeois*, by François Massialot, recommends adding a glass of white wine to fish stock. Consume within 24 hours or freeze.

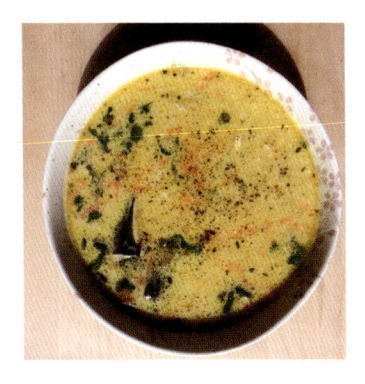

VARIATIONS   Add the Asian spice galangal, lemongrass, and coconut milk and you have yourself a delicious South Asian fish soup (shown here, left).

STOCKS AND SAUCES – *LES FONDS, BOUILLONS, ET SAUCES*

HOLLANDAISE SAUCE
Sauce Hollandaise

Season Year-round   **Preparation Time** 15 minutes (to clarify the butter)
Cooking Time 5 to 7 Minutes   **Makes** about 6 Servings

While this sauce may have originated in the Netherlands, the French have upheld it as one of the major sauces in French cuisine since at least the 1600s. With his 1651 publication of *Le Cuisinier françois*, Pierre François La Varenne has since been considered the father of French classical cooking. He cooked for French royalty along with other chefs, many of them from Italy, whose cooking had influenced French royal cooking thanks to the Renaissance originating there.[16] Before it was known as "Hollandaise" sauce, La Varenne called it "white sauce" (*sauce blanche*) and used it over asparagus, employing a bit of vinegar and nutmeg.[17] Similar to Béarnaise, this sauce is a heated, emulsified sauce, in which eggs and butter are combined for an irresistible richness. In France its primary use is as a sauce over steamed springtime white asparagus, but it can be eaten with other dishes as well, as noted below. Chef Frédéric, my patient instructor, while showing me this recipe also showed me how to clarify butter (see next page). But ghee, itself a kind of clarified butter, could also be used. Lillet blanc, a white wine-based *apéritif* originating from the Bordeaux region, may replace the water.

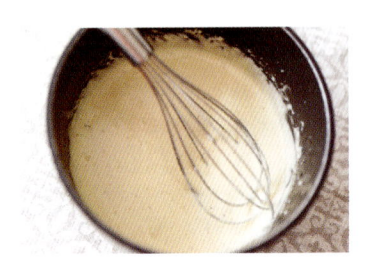

3 egg yolks (*jaunes d'ouef*)

3.5 tablespoons water (or Lillet blanc)

1 cup (240 g) unsalted butter (*beurre doux*), clarified (*clarifié*)

1 teaspoon lemon juice (*jus de citron*)

Fine salt (*sel fin*)

Pepper (*poivre*)

Optional: Pinch of ground nutmeg

Whisk the yolks together with the water (or Lillet blanc) in a saucepan continuously (*tout le temps*) over medium heat to make a moussy *sabayon* (originally an Italian style dessert cream, *zabaglione*, made with whipped eggs and sugar). Turn down the heat to low (*feu doux*), do not boil the sauce, and add the clarified butter slowly with a ladle (or in small chunks if it is solidified). Whisk in the lemon juice, salt, pepper, and optional nutmeg.

Serve the Hollandaise Sauce over plain chicken and fish dishes (as they definitely need the extra fat!), steamed springtime asparagus or over other vegetables, or, as in "Eggs Benedict," over poached eggs and Canadian bacon or ham.

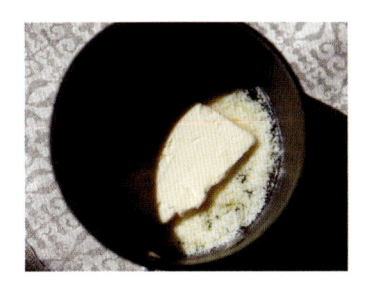

Clarified Butter
Beurre Clarifié

In France, butter is either salted (*demi-sel*) or unsalted (*doux*) and is often sold as a 250g stick of butter (*une plaque de beurre*), 16 tablespoons, or two sticks, of butter. You can transform a whole stick of butter into clarified butter and store what you do not use or make only as much as you need immediately. *Beurre clarifié* is clarified butter, which can be made by gently (*tout doucement*) melting (*faire fondre*) the butter in a saucepan or the oven until liquified. The butter will separate into three parts. Skim off the mousse on top. Spoon the clarified butter out and into a glass jar or container for storage or directly into the recipe you are making. What has settled to the bottom is the whey (*le petit lait*), which you don't use here, though it may be used for other things. The French often use whey in marinades and ragouts or to make baked goods like sweet *crêpes* or savory pancakes (*galettes*). See page 503 for grain-free **Sweet and Savory Crêpes**. Ghee is made similarly but essentially cooks longer and tends to have a nuttier, more concentrated flavor.

VARIATIONS You can replace the lemon juice with one teaspoon of white wine vinegar, à La Varenne. To make a whipped cream sauce called *Sauce Chantilly*, also called "muslin sauce" (*Sauce Mousseline*), fold in ½ cup whipped cream into the Hollandaise Sauce immediately before serving. This thick and creamy sauce is typically used over fish and boiled vegetables.

WINE PAIRING TIP If white Lillet is in the sauce, try pairing this sauce with the Lillet. Otherwise, try white wines with lots of character to match the sauce, such as a fresh and full-bodied Pinot Auxerrois (or Auxerrois Blanc) from Alsace; a fresh and richly-flavored Chablis from Burgundy; a nutty and flowery Chardonnay-based white from the Côtes du Jura; or a white Bugey, with notes of flowers and grilled nuts, from the Savoie-Bugey region. From the Loire Valley, try an aromatic Quincy from the Central Loire Valley, with notes of blackcurrant buds and citrus, or a famous Pouilly-Fumé, made with the Sauvignon Blanc grape, with notes of green apple and flint, or a citrus, floral, and mineral Reuilly.

HOMEMADE MAYONNAISE
Mayonnaise Fait Maison

Season Year-round   **Preparation Time** None   **Mixing Time** 5 to 10 minutes
Makes about ½ cup (about 120 ml) mayonnaise

Emulsions, in which we attempt to bind opposing elements, like oil and water, are by nature temporary. Patience is the key in making mayonnaise. This recipe was demonstrated by my friend Stephen Davis, as it is one of the ingredients for his tartar sauce: **Tangy Seafood and Salad Dressing (Tartar Sauce)**, page 414. Wear an apron!

1 egg at room temperature

½ cup (120 ml) olive oil (or avocado oil, or a mix of olive and avocado oils)

Salt and pepper to taste

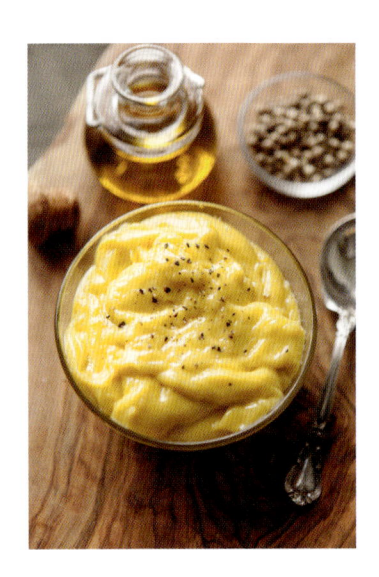

Separate the yolk from the white and put the yolk into a small mixing bowl. (Discard the white or save it for a multi-egg omelet or other recipe requiring egg white.) Very slowly, drop-by-drop at first, drip the oil into the bowl with the yolk while whisking. Once it begins to thicken and bind, you can begin to add more oil at a time. A hand mixer may be used as well. (Again, patience is the key here! If the egg and oil do not emulsify, try again by using another egg yolk. Then pour the first mixture slowly into the egg yolk. At the end, slowly add another ½ cup of olive oil.) The mayonnaise will keep for up to one week in the refrigerator. Remember that this is raw egg yolk. The egg white can be used in another recipe in which it is needed to bread something, such as **Breaded Veal Sweetbreads "Meunière"** (page 227).

Adjust the seasoning with salt and pepper. If you like a bit more tang to your mayo, you can add a teaspoon of white wine vinegar or apple cider vinegar or a ½ teaspoon lemon juice. Some recipes call for a teaspoon or even a tablespoon of mustard as well. Experiment!

MORNAY CHEESE SAUCE
Sauce Mornay

Season Year-round **Preparation Time** 5 minutes
Cooking Time 10 minutes **Makes** about 1.5 cups (360 ml)

This dairy-laden sauce layers fat upon fat using cream, egg yolk, butter, and cheese. This sauce was first served in the 1840s at the restaurant *Le Grand Véfour*, which was located at the Palais Royal in Paris. It was eventually named after a certain Comte de Mornay. The "heaviness" and complexity of the sauce was one of the hallmarks of *la cuisine bourgeoise* of post-Revolutionary France, when a higher standard of living had been achieved by the French population.

The Mornay Cheese Sauce uses **Béchamel Sauce** (page 392) as its base, with cheese and cream added, according to *Larousse Gastronomique*. In lieu of the cream, a few spoonfuls of fish stock may be added (for use as a sauce on fish) or chicken stock (for use as a sauce on meat or vegetables) may be added, according to Charles Ranhofer's 1920 publication of *The Epicurean*. More recent Mornay recipes even add an egg yolk, as in this recipe. The recipe photo shows Mornay Sauce made with Cream Sauce (see Variations below) and Emmental cheese, but no additional butter.

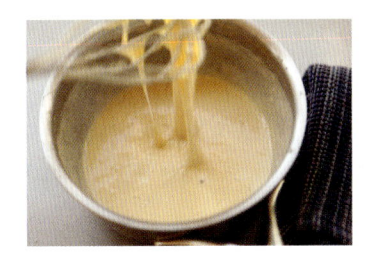

1 cup (240 ml) **Béchamel Sauce** (page 392)

½ cup cream (120 ml), or 5 tablespoons fish stock or chicken stock

Optional: 1 egg yolk

⅓ cup (75 ml) grated Emmental, Gruyère, or Parmesan cheese

Pinch of fine salt

Optional: 1 tablespoon butter

Warm the Béchamel Sauce over medium-low heat, and whisk in the cream (or stock). Whisk in the egg yolk now, if you are adding one. Continue using the whisk to incorporate the grated cheese into the sauce, making figure eights in the sauce with the whisk. Bring the sauce briefly to a boil over medium heat. Remove from heat and stir until smooth (about two minutes). Season with a pinch of salt. Stir in the optional tablespoon of butter. Another optional step, which Julia Child recommends for sauces in *Mastering the Art of French Cooking*, is to add a teaspoon of butter on the surface of the sauce as it cools to keep it from forming a hard crust.

This sauce may be served as is or gratinated in the oven (cooked until the sauce bubbles on top) over eggs, fish, poultry, veal, or vegetables. (If gratinating, Julia Child recommends not adding the extra butter at the end, which might separate from and pool above the sauce.) I have served this rich sauce over asparagus (as shown on the next page), broccoli, and salmon.

VARIATIONS Instead of Béchamel Sauce, you can instead use the even richer **Cream Sauce** (page 402), which is made using Béchamel Sauce along with extra milk and cream. Just add the optional egg yolk (for richness and extra fat) and the grated cheese, salt, and optional butter.

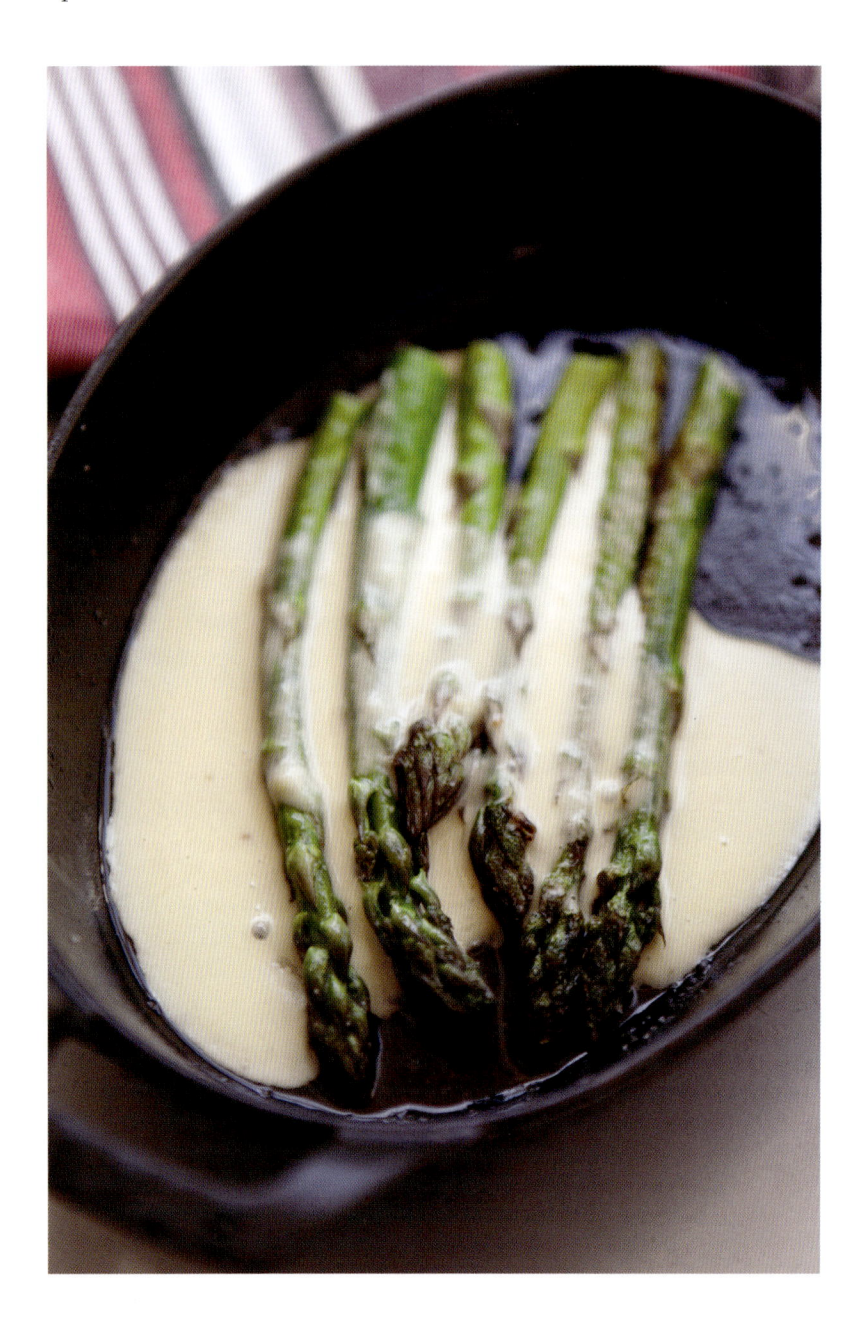

NIÇOISE VINAIGRETTE
Vinaigrette Niçoise

Season Year-round   **Mixing Time** Less than 5 minutes   **Serves** 2

Authentic, simple, and thick, this vinaigrette recipe comes from my friend Joelle Luson, a native of the French Mediterranean city of Nice. Use dried parsley and basil if you do not have them freshly available.

1 teaspoon Dijon or **Old-Fashioned Mustard** (page 410)

1 tablespoon lemon juice or vinegar

3 tablespoons olive oil

Handful of flat parsley, minced

Five small basil leaves, minced

Salt and pepper to taste

Mix ingredients together in a small bowl and serve over a **Traditional Salad from Nice** (page 476), or liven up a simple green salad.

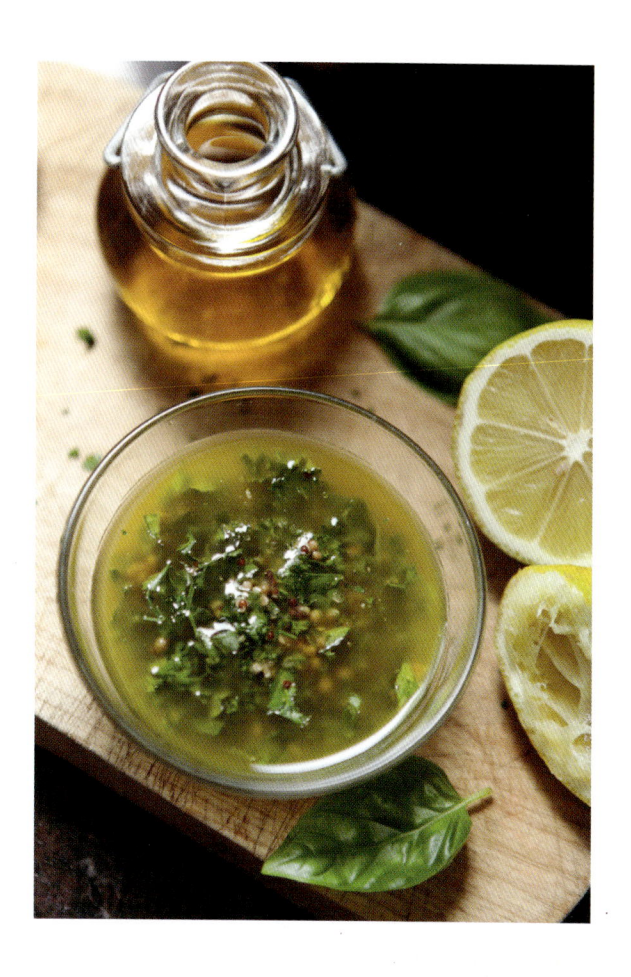

OLD-FASHIONED MUSTARD
Moutarde à l'Ancienne

Preparation Time 1 hour to roast garlic, 24 hours to soak mustard seeds   **Mixing Time** Less than 5 minutes
Makes about 2-½ cups (600 ml) mustard

Old-Fashioned Mustard is the kind of traditional mustard that is grainy (*en grain*), as it is made from mustard seeds, which come in different colors. For this traditional recipe, shown to me by my friend, Stephen Davis, mix equal parts brown seeds with yellow seeds. Dijon mustard is said to originate from the wine-producing region of Burgundy, whose capital is the city of Dijon. Dijon mustard was traditionally made with verjuice (*verjus*), meaning "green grape," a juice extracted from unripened grapes and used in mustard like vinegar.

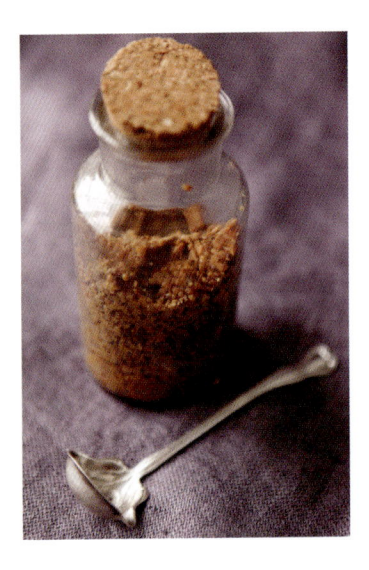

- 2 cups (500 ml) dry mustard seeds (or more if you fancy making a larger batch)
- 1 cup (240 ml) apple cider vinegar
- 1 cup (240 ml) room temperature water
- 1 tablespoon fine sea salt
- 4 cloves garlic, roasted (see Roasting Garlic note in the sidebar)
- 2 tablespoons maple syrup or honey

Pour the mustard seeds, vinegar, water, and salt into a large mixing bowl and mix together. Allow the seeds to soak for 24 hours, stirring every now and then until all the vinegar and water is absorbed by the mustard seeds.

In a blender, mix *half* of the mustard grain mix, peeled roasted garlic cloves, and maple syrup into a fine paste. Stir this mixture into the other half of the whole grain mix to give it the old fashioned grainy mustard look. Transfer the mustard into clean jars. Mustard will keep for up to a year in the pantry or longer in the refrigerator. For a creamier version, blend the entire batch.

Roasting Garlic

Roast garlic by wrapping it in parchment paper or foil and baking it in the oven for 30 minutes at 365°F (185°C). Roasted garlic also makes a great condiment for grilled or roasted meats and vegetables.

ONION MARMALADE
Confiture d'Oignons

Season Year-round   **Preparation Time** 15 minutes
Cooking Time 1 hour   **Makes** 1.5 cups (350 ml) of preserves

Onion Marmalade is a Southwestern condiment often used for duck, pâtés, or cold meats but is also delicious on warmed dishes. Its sweetness and tang make it very easy to overeat. Some recipes call for cardamom or balsamic vinegar.

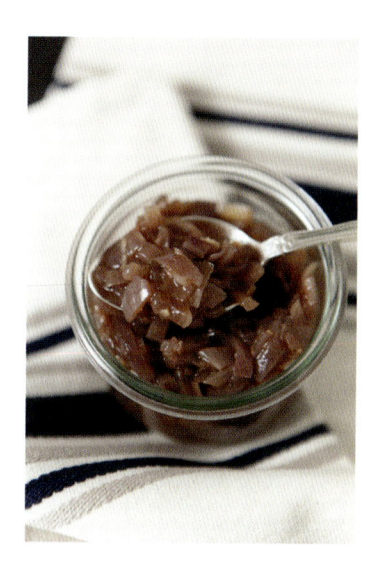

1.1 pounds (500 g) red onions, finely chopped

3 tablespoons olive oil

1 tablespoon raw honey

2 tablespoons white wine vinegar

Pinch of fine sea salt

¼ teaspoon cinnamon

1 teaspoon grated ginger

Stir the onions and olive oil in a large pan over medium heat until warmed, then reduce the heat to low and stir in the honey. Here I used a dark honey, "heather" (*bruyère*). Cover the pan, allowing the onions to slowly caramelize over 45 (up to 75) minutes. Deglaze the pieces stuck to the bottom of the pan with the vinegar, and add the salt, cinnamon, and ginger. Cover again and cook for an additional 10 minutes on low. Allow the marmalade to cool to room temperature.

Serve a dollop of the marmalade with liver pâté, *foie gras*, or hot or cold meats. Store up to two weeks in the refrigerator or freeze in small quantities for future use.

ORANGE PLUM SAUCE
Sauce aux Prunes à l'Orange

Season Winter through early Spring **Preparation Time** 5 minutes
Cooking Time 10 to 15 minutes **Makes** 4 to 6 small servings

This sauce is the perfect accompaniment (*accompagnement*) to **Orange Duck Breast** (page 351), with or without the shallots listed in that recipe. This recipe calls for **Homemade Plum Preserves** (page 63), but you can also cook down a few jarred or fresh, chopped plums for 20 to 30 minutes in a pot, and use those for this sauce.

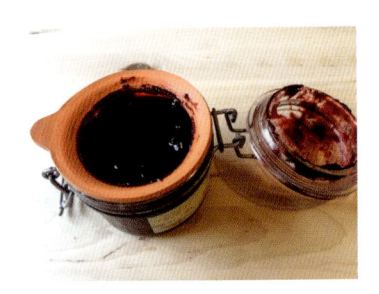

Juice of one orange (or 2 to 3 clementines)

½ teaspoon zest of orange (or clementine)

4 tablespoons plum preserves

Optional: Dash of *fleur de sel*

Combine the juice and zest in a small pot over medium to medium-high heat and reduce the juice by about half or two-thirds for 8 to 10 minutes, stirring occasionally. Stir in the plum preserves until heated.

Mix with sautéed shallots or serve as a separate sauce alongside the shallot sauce. Remove from heat and spoon over a serving of duck leg or breast or serve a dollop on the side on each plate. Garnish with a few grains of *fleur de sel*.

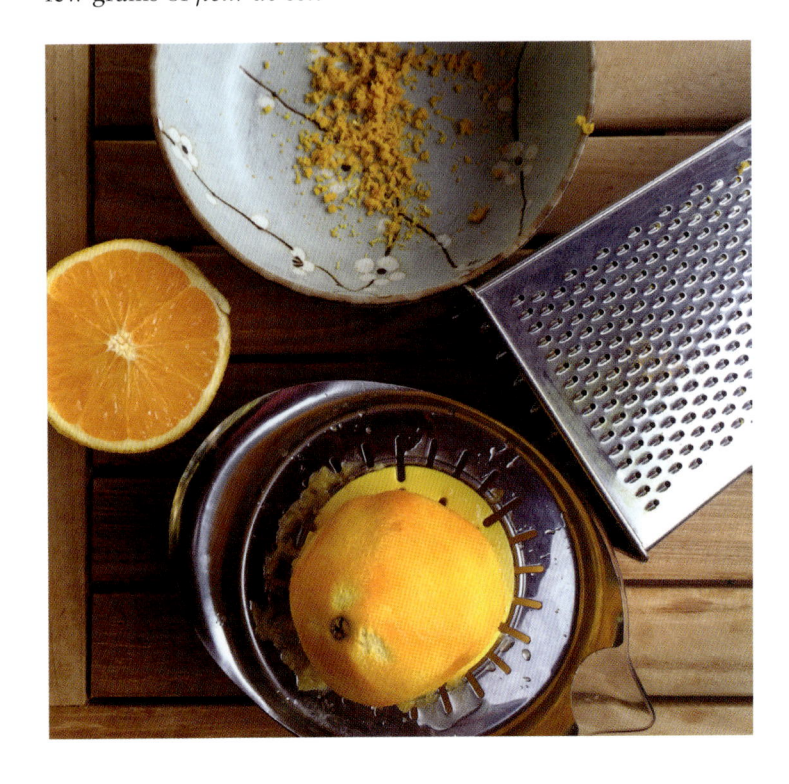

SHALLOT AND VINEGAR DIP FOR OYSTERS
Vinaigre aux Echalotes pour les Huîtres

Season Fall through Spring, when oysters are generally eaten
Preparation Time Less than 5 minutes   **Serves** 4

This tangy sauce goes beautifully with raw oysters. It is served *de rigeur* in the French Southwest when eating raw oysters.

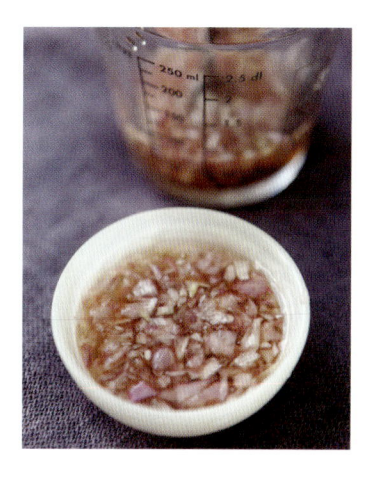

3 ounces (100 ml) white wine vinegar

2 shallots, finely minced

Mix the vinegar and shallots in a bowl and pour into small dipping bowls for each person.

SIMPLE VINAIGRETTE
Une Vinaigrette Simple

Season Year-round   **Mixing Time** Less than 5 minutes   **Serves** 2

This is a simple vinaigrette from my lovely friend Joelle Luson. It's as easy as 1, 2, 3! This recipe calls for mustard. You can use **Old-Fashioned Mustard** (page 410). The recipe photo below shows vinaigrette with balsamic vinegar, but use your favorite vinegar if it's not balsamic.

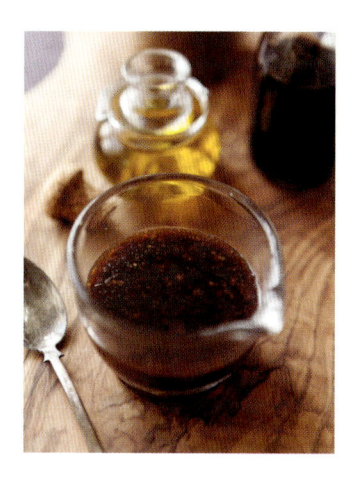

1 tablespoon mustard

2 tablespoons balsamic vinegar

Salt and pepper to taste

3 tablespoons olive oil

Combine the mustard, vinegar, salt, and pepper. Whisk in the olive oil.

VARIATIONS Try adding one teaspoon honey, a pinch of ground clove, and/or one teaspoon of lemon juice.

STOCKS AND SAUCES – *LES FONDS, BOUILLONS, ET SAUCES*

TANGY SEAFOOD AND SALAD DRESSING (TARTAR SAUCE)
Sauce Rémoulade

Season Year-round   **Preparation Time** Less than 5 minutes   **Makes** about ⅓ cup (80 ml)

This recipe is from my good friend Stephen Davis, a long-time resident of France (Montpellier and Bordeaux), who uses this recipe as the foundation for his **Spreadable Fish Paste** recipe (page 186). This recipe makes about five tablespoons of tartar sauce, probably enough for 4 people as a condiment, or else just the right amount to go into the fish paste recipe.

1 garlic clove, grated

3 to 4 tablespoons **Homemade Mayonnaise** (page 406)

1 tablespoon **Old-Fashioned Mustard** (page 410)

2 teaspoons lemon juice

Salt and pepper to taste

Whisk all the ingredients together in a measuring cup or small mixing bowl. Use as a salad dressing or in the **Spreadable Fish Paste** (page 186).

VARIATIONS You can also add one to two teaspoons minced tarragon, and/or two to three minced anchovy fillets, or a teaspoon of anchovy juice or liquid from a sardine can, for extra flavor.

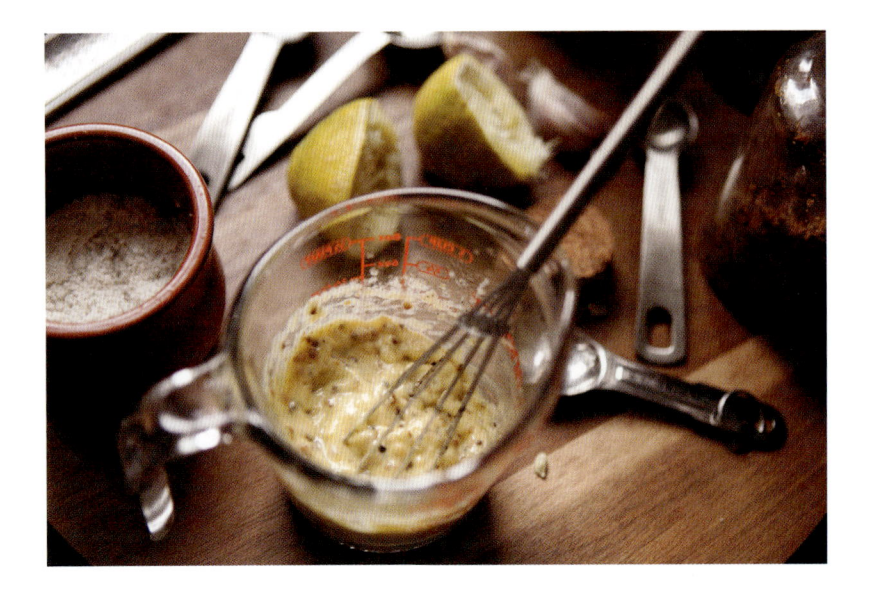

VEAL STOCK
Fond de Veau

Season Year-round
Preparation Time 30 to 90 minutes to roast the bones, 40 minutes to prep and brown the meat and vegetables
Cooking Time 4 hours   **Makes** about 6 cups (1.5 L) of stock, plus about 1 cup for stew

My friend Chef Jean-Luc Beaufils kindly shared his professional chef's version of this much-used stock in French cuisine. Veal Stock has a distinct flavor, stronger than a chicken or other meat stock, thanks to the strong flavors of the veal (marrow) bones, feet, and meat. It becomes very gelatinous and can be slice into cubes that keep their shape when it's chilled. The meat used for this stock may come from a variety of cuts used for stew meat, such as the breast (*poitrine*), flank (*flanchet*), neck (*collet* or *collier*), or shoulder (*épaule*). The veal is easy to cut into small cubes if the meat is partially frozen, as shown. If you have only veal bones, but no veal feet, that's okay, too. You can just add about 10 more ounces (285 g) of meat and bone. This recipe requires that you roast the veal bones (and foot) in the oven first, for half an hour for fresh or thawed bones, or for one and a half hours if the bones are frozen. This will add to your total cooking time. There is no call for salt or pepper in this recipe as it is a reduced stock to be used as a base for other recipes, which will be salted and peppered as necessary later. Veal Stock is often used as a base for **French Onion Soup** (page 451). After the initial four hours of cooking, the stock can be cooked additionally, uncovered, to reduce and concentrate it until the desired consistency is achieved.

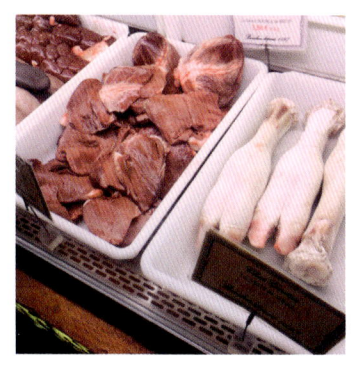

Beef Heart (left), Calf's Foot (right)

2.2 pounds (1 kg) calf's leg or knuckle bones, chopped into 3 or 4 large pieces

1 calf's foot

2.2 pounds (1 kg) veal breast, diced into ½-inch (1.25 cm) cubes

2 tablespoons tallow

2 large carrots (about 6.5 ounces or 185 g), diced

1 onion or 2 shallots (about 3 ounces or 85 g), diced

½ cup (120 ml) water

Bouquet garni

1 garlic clove, crushed

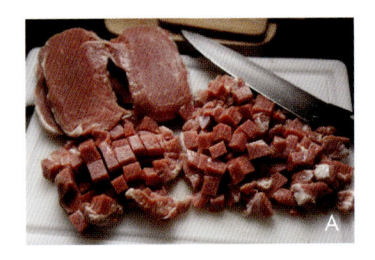

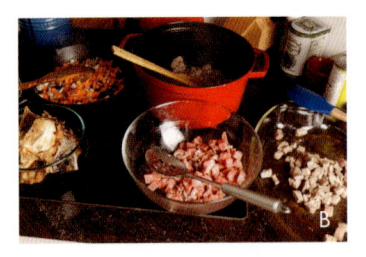

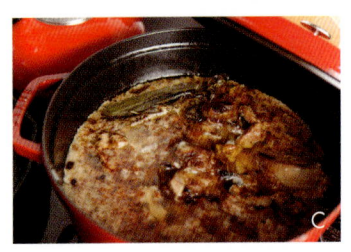

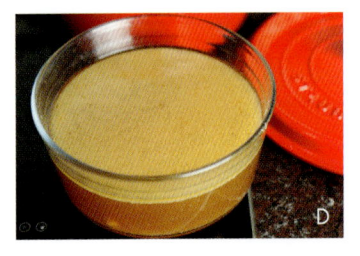

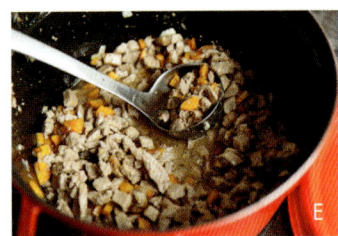

Preheat the oven to betwen 400°F and 430°F (200°C to 220°C). Place the veal (and foot) bones in a large casserole dish. Roast the bones in the oven for half an hour (or 1.5 hours if the bones are frozen).

Set the bones aside in a bowl and pour the liquid fat rendered from the roasted bones into a large cast-iron pot, also called a *marmite*. Brown the veal breast pieces (in batches) on high heat using this fat.

As each batch of meat is browned, place the meat temporarily back into the casserole dish. This process can take 15 to 20 minutes (photo B).

Meanwhile, melt the tallow in a pan over medium-high to medium heat and brown the carrots and onion (or shallots) for about 10 minutes. Set aside for the moment.

After browning all the meat, deglaze the juices and solids stuck to the bottom of the pot with the half cup of water, scraping the pot with a flat-ended wooden spatula. Place the roasted bones into the pot. Add the meat back to the pot, along with the browned carrots and onion (or shallots), *bouquet garni*, and crushed garlic, and cover the ingredients with water (photo C).

Bring the pot to a boil, cover, and allow to gurgle on low (*mijoter*) for about four hours. Strain out the ingredients with a slotted spoon and reduce the remaining liquid to the desired consistency. Again, many chefs will skim off the fat, I never do (photo D)—that's the tastiest part!

Discard the bones and the *bouquet garni* and save a bit of the liquid for the remaining meat and vegetables, which will make for a delicious, hearty veal stew (photo E). Remember to add salt to the meat for the stew, as this will release its savory flavors.

Use the Veal Stock in recipes such as **French Onion Soup** (page 451) or as a base for other soups, sauces, or gravies.

VARIATIONS You may add celery, clove, tomato sauce, and/or red wine, but this recipe as it is here is the real deal.

WHITE POULTRY STOCK
Bouillon de Volaille or Fond Blanc de Volaille

Season Year-round   **Preparation Time** None   **Cooking Time** 45 minutes minimum

According to my friend, Chef Frédéric, poultry stock is the kitchen's trash can, *la poubelle de la cuisine*, because you can throw into it all the discarded ends (*les parures* or *les bouts*) of vegetables like onion, leek, carrot, turnip. Nothing is wasted. Poultry stock can be a mix of poultry, or made of only chicken bones or duck bones, and so on, depending on what you have and what your goal is. Using only duck bones in the stock when making **Béarnaise Garbure Soup** (page 338), for example, which calls for duck and makes a duck stock (*bouillon de canard*), keeps "like with like," a homogenous taste combination of stock and meat. Chef Frédéric's stock calls for wings, as these have lots of cartilage and flavor, but you can use other bones from the bird as well if you have them. A chicken stock will have only chicken parts in it (carcass, bone, feet, head, organs). If you wanted to make this a Brown Poultry Stock, you would brown the chicken meat and bones in a pan in butter or fat. Roasting the bones darkens the stock and also alters/enhances the flavor. A mild stock is one like this White Poultry Stock, in which the bones are left unroasted and boiled directly.

Incidentally, this poultry stock is close to the gut-healing stocks Dr. Natasha Campbell-McBride advocates in her *Gut and Psychology Syndrome* (GAPS) book for children and adults.[18] Combining collagenous meats and bones, such as whole chicken (particularly gentle on the stomach), beef oxtail, leg meat, and marrow bones, and boiling these for three to four hours (less time than bone broth, therefore fewer brain-inflaming histamines and glutamates) without vegetables or herbs but with mineral salt (sea or ancient sea salts), provides a healing elixir for all ages. The French seem to have known this for centuries, as they were the first to give these broths a name and sell them in restaurants as *bouillon*.

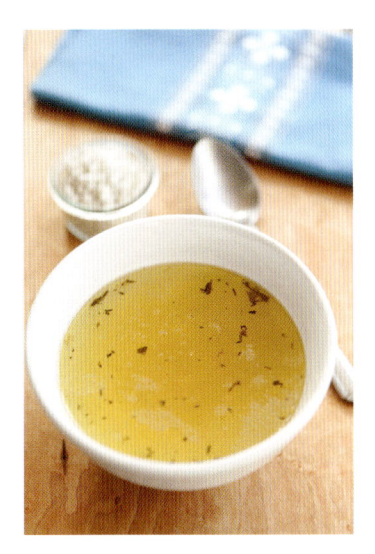

Bits and ends of vegetables on hand

1.1 pounds (500 g) wings (*ailerons*) or other poultry bones

Bay leaf

Several sprigs of thyme

2 to 4 cups (½ to 1 liter) water

Heat a saucepan on medium-high heat. Place all the vegetable ends into the pan and stir them for several minutes without browning (*sans coloration*) the vegetables. The heat will cause the vegetables to "sweat" (*faire suer*), reducing their water content (*enlever l'eau*) and gaining in flavor (*gagner le goût*). Add the wings (and any other chicken bones you would like to add), the bay leaf, and thyme, and cover the ingredients with between 2 and 4 cups water. Bring to a boil, then reduce heat and cover, allowing to simmer for a minimum of 45 minutes, longer if you have the time. If desired, you can pass the stock through a sieve to filter out the small pieces of vegetable ends. Enjoy the stock on its own by sipping a cup of it, or use it as a base for other soups, stews, or sauces.

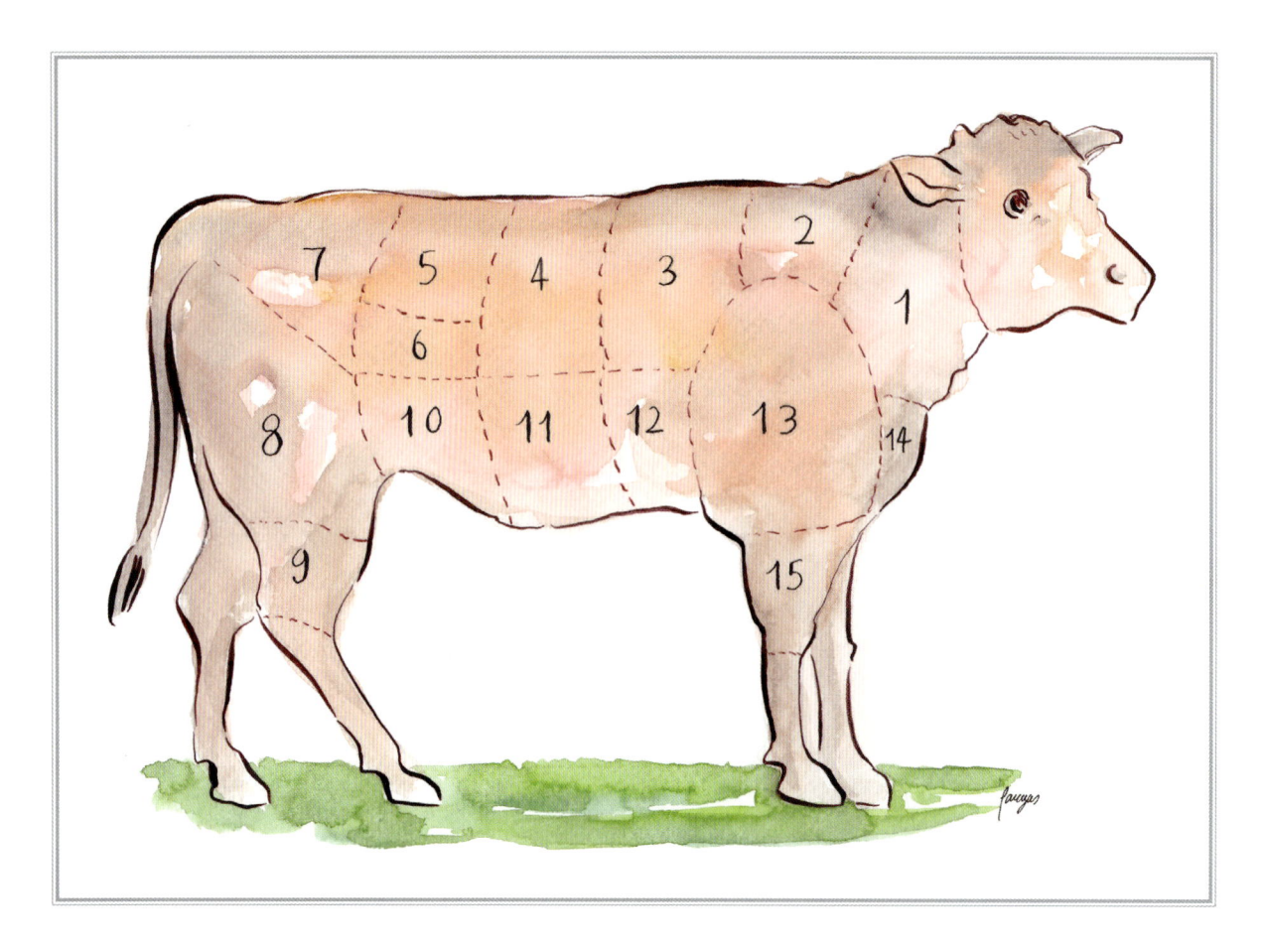

VEAL – *LE VEAU*
DIAGRAM KEY

1. Blade (Neck) – *Collet* or *Collier* (Use: Ground, Roast, Stew)
2. Rib – *Côte Découverte* (Use: Chop, Roast, Sauté, Stew)
3. Rib – *Côtes Secondes* (Use: Chop, Roast, Sauté, Stew)
4. Loin – *Côtes Premières* (Use: Chop, Roast)
5. Sirloin or Strip Loin – *Longe* and *Côte Filet* (Use: Roast, Steak)
6. Tenderloin – *Filet* (Roast)
7. Rump – *Quasi* (Use: Cutlets, Roast, Stew)
8. Round and Top Round – *Noix, Sous-Noix* and *Noix Patissière* (Use: Cutlets, Roast, Steak, Tartare)
9. Hind Shank or Hind Knuckle – *Jarret Arrière* (Use: Marrow, Stew)
10. Flank – *Flanchet* (Use: Cutlets, Ground, Stew)
11. Breast (Plate) – *Tendron* (Use: Ground, Stew)
12. Breast – *Poitrine* (Use: Ground, Roast, Sauté)
13. Shoulder – *Épaule* (Use: Cutlets, Ground, Roast, Sauté, Stew, Tartare)
14. Breast – *Poitrine* (Use: Ground, Roast, Sauté)
15. Fore Shank or Fore Knuckle – *Jarret Avant* – (Use: Marrow, Stew)

VEAL
Le Veau

Basque Veal with Peppers – *Axoa* 420

Braised Veal Stew – *Blanquette de Veau* 422

Braised Veal Shanks – *Osso Bucco (Jarret de Veau)* 425

Stuffed Veal Cutlets – *Paupiettes de Veau* 427

Veal Tagine Stew – *Tajine de Veau* 431

Veal Tartare – *Tartare de Veau* 433

BASQUE VEAL WITH PEPPERS
Axoa

Season Autumn and Winter   **Preparation Time** 35 minutes
Cooking Time 1 hour 30 minutes   **Serves** 8 to 9

Axoa is a traditional everyday Basque dish using their beloved sweet chili peppers (*les piments d'Espelette*) in both fresh and powdered form. Pronounced "atch-wa," the name *Axoa* actually comes from the French word, *haché*, meaning ground, as in ground veal. While you may not necessarily have *piment d'Espelette* on hand (though it is available from various vendors on Amazon at reasonable prices, for example), and you can technically go without it, for the Basques, this ingredient is essential to the dish, making it the authentic *Axoa*. (Nightshades are in heavy use here. Skip this recipe for now if you are on an Autoimmune Paleo diet.) This recipe calls for veal chuck roast, either from the neck (*collier*) or the shoulder (*épaule*), though ground veal from other parts of the animal may be substituted (or even ground beef or pork, but the traditional recipe calls for veal). Butcher Florent Carriquiry suggests *macreuse*, from the shoulder. Veal that is milk-fed (up to about six months) has a pinker tint to it than veal that has begun to eat grass. A calf is considered "veal" (*veau*) between six months up to 24 months.

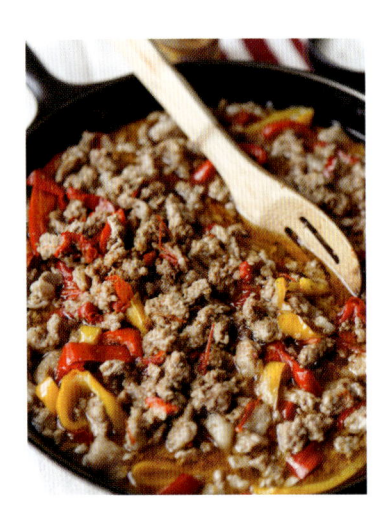

3 tablespoons duck fat

4 garlic cloves, minced

1 onion, diced

2 sweet red or green chilies (about 10 ounces or 290 g), seeds removed and julienned (sliced in long strips)

2 small bell peppers (about 10 ounces or 290 g), seeds removed and julienned

3.3 pounds (1.5 kg) veal chuck roast, ground or diced

5 small sprigs of fresh thyme, stemmed or 1 teaspoon dried thyme

3 tablespoons olive oil

1 bay leaf

4 pinches of fine sea salt

2/3 cup (160 ml) water

Optional: 1 to 2 pinches of *piment d'Espelette*, for color

Melt the duck fat over medium-high heat in a large skillet (for which you have a lid) or a cast-iron pot. Add the garlic, onion, chilies, and bell peppers, and allow them to soften for 15 minutes, stirring frequently.

Combine the veal chuck roast, thyme, olive oil, bay leaf, and salt in the pan with the vegetables, stirring frequently for about 10 minutes. Add the water and reduce the heat to medium-low or low. Cover and allow to simmer for 45 minutes.

Remove the cover and allow to continue simmering for another 20 minutes, thereby allowing some of the liquid to evaporate.

Garnish with the (optional) *piment d'Espelette*. Serve over plain boiled potatoes, rice, or roasted root vegetables.

VARIATIONS To "sweeten" the dish, Florent recommends adding another diced onion or two and allowing them to caramelize (cook longer and slowly) before adding the meat. The secrets to this dish, according to his Basque grandmother (*amatxi*) Maria, are to deglaze the vegetables with 1¼ cups (300 ml) apple cider vinegar (or less if you prefer), and a few spoonfuls of **Veal Stock** (page 415) or other meat stock, then remove the vegetables, brown the meat, and add the vegetables back in. Along with the meat, she also adds a slice of diced Bayonne ham (*Jambon de Bayonne*) or dried ham (*jambon seché*), cured for at least 18 months, for flavor, of course!

WINE PAIRING TIP Pair this very regional dish with a crisp Basque cider (*cidre* in French, or *Sagarno* in Basque) made from local Basque region apples, or else try a wine from the Southwest: a Béarnese rich red Madiran, a tannic red or tangy white Basque Irouléguy, or a nearly-sparkling white Txakoli from the Northwest French Basque region, or a fruity and spicy Rioja or a Txakolina (also called Chacolí) from the Spanish Basque region. Because the Basque country extends from Southwestern France into Northern Spain, the Basques (*Euskadi*) prefer describing the Basque country regional divide as that of the North (*Ipareta*) and the South (*Egoalda*). I have also paired this dish with a Bordeaux rosé, namely Clarendelle, a refreshing and velvety rosé with notes of strawberry and red currant from Clarence Dillon Wines, inspired by Château Haut-Brion, a top-notch "First Growth Bordeaux" (Premiers Crus) from the Graves Pessac-Léognan appellation.

BRAISED VEAL STEW
Blanquette de Veau

Season Year-round   **Preparation Time** 25 minutes
Cooking Time 2 hours minimum, up to three hours   **Serves** 6, at about 7 ounces (200 g) veal per person

This classic dish requires a cast-iron pot with a cover. I was shown this dish by my "adopted French mother," Catherine Lignac, of Château Guadet in St. Emilion. Hers was the first family we befriended upon moving to Bordeaux, and whether they liked it or not, I became immediately attached! Catherine is an exquisite cook from the coastal Landes department in Southwestern France. Château Guadet happens to have one of the best real underground limestone cellars which has been in use for centuries and is viewable during their wine tasting visits. Catherine and her husband, Guy-Pétrus Lignac, run the business side of the château, while Vincent, also a University of Bordeaux DUAD graduate from the 2000's and best taster (*dégustateur*) in his class, runs the organic vineyard operations. I have had the distinct pleasure and honor to capture their vineyard in photographs through each season over 3 years (see pages 523–525 in the Wine chapter), and thereby have also been able to sample Catherine's delicious cooking at lunchtimes as a (sometimes self-invited) guest. They have become my adopted French parents whom I adore!

The original recipe actually calls for flour, as in most versions of **Beef Burgundy** (see page 109 for *The Bordeaux Kitchen* version), but Catherine has never used flour in her recipe, and the dish is nevertheless a family favorite in her household. Usually, the "common mushroom," or *Basidiomycete* (*Champignon de Paris*), is used in the *Blanquette de Veau*. Omit the mushrooms if you have allergies to molds and fungi. This recipe serves as an everyday foundation for the *gourmand*, but it can be "dressed up" (*habillé*) for festive occasions with other ingredients as desired, particularly seasonal vegetables.

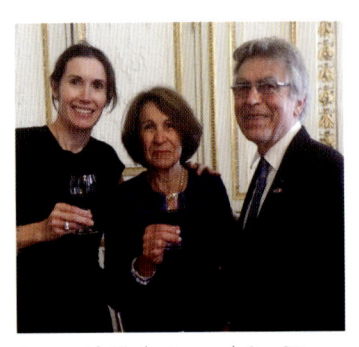

Tania with Catherine and Guy-Pétrus Lignac

In French cooking, 1 teaspoon (5 g) of butter is called *une noisette*, not to be confused with the color butter is given when it begins caramelizing in the pan, obtaining a hazelnut color and flavor (*beurre noisette*).

1 tablespoon olive oil or tallow

1 teaspoon butter, plus 1 tablespoon

2.6 pounds (1.2 kg) veal, cut in cubes of 1 to 2 inches (2.5 to 5 cm)

6 small veal marrow bones (1 per person), for flavor and nutrients

Bouquet garni

Pinch of salt

2 cups (300 g) onions, finely sliced lengthwise

2 cups (150 g) mushrooms, cut in slices

2 tablespoons rich sour cream (*crème fraîche épaisse*)

1 egg yolk

½ lemon, juiced

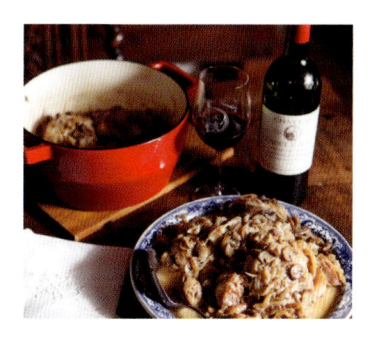

The veal used for this dish traditionally comes from the front of the animal, where it puts most of its weight when nursing or bending down to eat grass: the shoulder (*épaule*), neck or "blade" (*collier* or *collet*), or breast (*tendron*, *flanchet* or *poitrine*). As a result, these cuts require longer cooking, but other cuts such as shank (*gîte*) will do as well. The *blanquette* is a dish that can be made with other "white meats" such as chicken, pork, rabbit, or turkey, but veal is the most common.

Heat the oil and one teaspoon of butter in the iron pot over medium-high heat. Place each piece of meat, one by one, in the pot and brown (*revenir* or *saisir*) all sides. Next add the bones, *bouquet garni*, and salt. Cover the pot securely and allow the meat to simmer on low (*mijoter*) in its own juices for at least two hours, more if you have time. If you do not have a real cast-iron pot or a crock pot with a tight-sealing lid, then add half a cup to a cup of water at this stage to avoid accidental burning of the meat.

Separately, brown the mushrooms and onions with one tablespoon of butter. Add these 10 minutes before turning off the stove. Moments before serving, place the meat and vegetables into a dish, leaving some sauce in the pot. Stir the sour cream into the sauce in the pot with the egg yolk and the lemon juice, and then ladle the creamy sauce onto the meat and vegetables.

VARIATIONS Like many French traditional dishes, so many variations on this classic exist, depending on the occasion and season. Here are some ingredient variations suggested by my lovely friend, Joelle Luson from Nice: carrots cut in circular slices or rounds (*rondelles*); an onion cut in half with a clove stuck into each half; a celery branch; a pinch of nutmeg; a leek cut into rounds; and mushrooms first sautéed in a pan with butter. Pepper to taste can be added to the pot, as well as a cup or more of water, depending on how much liquid is desired. Extra cream and one or two yolks, chopped parsley, and crushed garlic may be whisked into the sauce at the end instead of the sour cream, with a dash of lemon juice whisked in just before serving. Again, it all depends on your tastes, habits, and what is in stock in your pantry!

WINE PAIRING TIP We paired this meal with Château Guadet's Grand Cru Classé ("Classified Superior") de St. Emilion, a fruity but tannic, delicious, and elegant wine that is 60-80% Merlot and 20-40% Cabernet Sauvignon, depending on the year. Over the past several years, I have tried many a Château Guadet vintage (*millésime*), and every time it's like coming home. My DUAD wine course friend and French restaurateur Annabelle Nicolle-Beaufils suggests delicate white wines that are rounded with a full mouthfeel to be able to stand up to the creaminess and flavor of this dish, such as a Pessac-Léognan or an Entre-Deux-Mers from Bordeaux, a crisp, aromatic Sauvignon Blanc from Sancerre or Reuilly in the Loire Valley, or else a Chardonnay from Burgundy's Côte Chalonnaise or Mâconnais regions. For red wines, she suggests ones lighter to medium in tannins and structure, such as those from Graves or Côtes-de-Blaye from Bordeaux, or a red Sancerre Rouge from the Loire Valley.

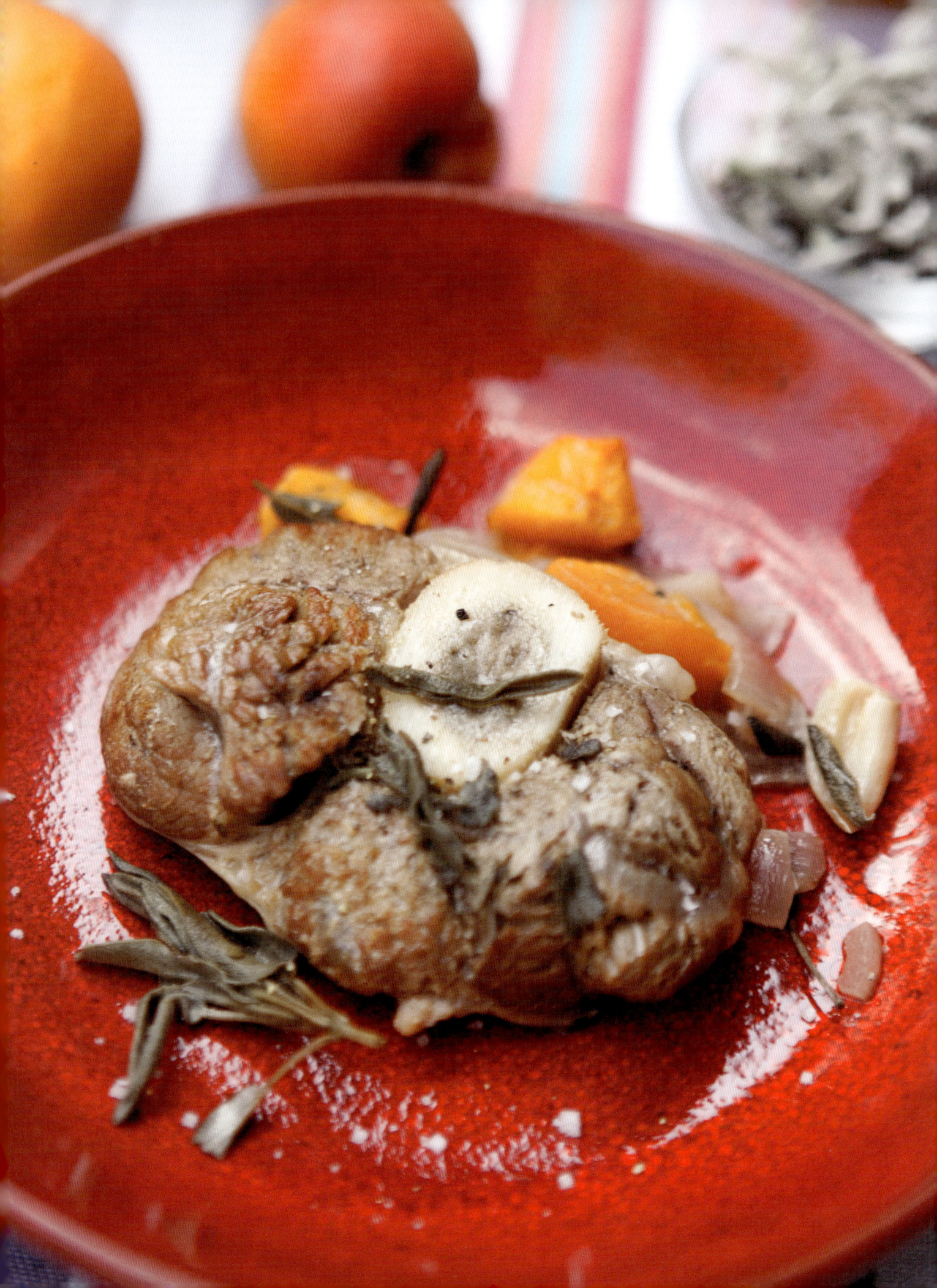

BRAISED VEAL SHANKS
Osso Bucco (Jarret de Veau)

Season Year-round   **Preparation Time** 20 minutes
Cooking Time 1.5 hours minimum   **Serves** 2 to 3

Originating from Milan, Italy, this dish is well known throughout France and makes good use of the veal shank (*le jarret* or *la gîte*), which otherwise might sadly go unused or unnoticed. Coming from the shank (leg, below the shoulder), this cut does not have much fat but does have tough meat and collagen that require long cooking to extract all the goodness from the meat and the bone. Veal shanks are usually sliced into steaks of one to one and a half inches (2.5 cm to about 4 cm) in thickness. Braising is the process of browning a meat first, then slow cooking it in broth, water, or wine.

During my apprenticeship at the butcher shop in Bordeaux, a new young butcher, Damien Denis, was brought on, and when I bought veal shanks from him to make *Osso Bucco*, he suggested that I throw in some apricots to add to the richness and sweetness of the dish. Apricots are in season in July and August. If you would like to add apricot but fresh ones are not in season, try adding one or two chopped dried apricots.

1 tablespoon duck fat

Fine salt for seasoning

10 to 12 ounces (300 g to 350 g) veal shank

1 to 2 small red onions (2 ounces or 60 g), diced

5 small garlic cloves, halved, green germ removed

1 fresh apricot (2.5 ounces or 75 g), chopped

1 tablespoon sage, chopped

1 cup water

1 tablespoon butter (or ghee)

Fleur de sel and pepper, for garnish

Melt the duck fat over high heat in a medium cast-iron pot. Salt both sides of each slice of shank, then brown each side in the pot for two minutes per side. Add the onion, garlic, apricot, sage, and water. Bring briefly to a boil, cover the pot and reduce the heat to medium-low or low, allowing to cook for one and a half hours.

During the last five minutes, add the butter to the pot. Garnish with *fleur de sel* and freshly ground pepper. Serve with boiled potatoes or roasted or sautéed vegetables. Don't forget to eat the nutritious and delicately-flavored bone marrow with a small spoon. With extra salt, it has a mild but distinctive flavor. Add the leftover bones to a stock.

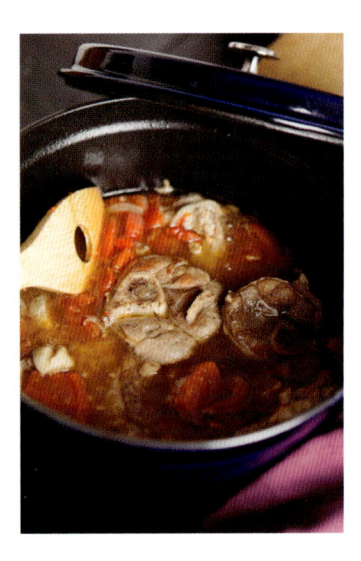

VARIATIONS In one of French chef Jacques Pépin's television appearances with Julia Child in 1994, they cook *osso bucco*. Pépin adds orange and lemon peel (not unlike **Beef Stew with Orange** on page 151) and then garnishes the dish with chopped parsley and chives and a bit of chopped fresh tomato. Pépin serves the dish over rice. You may also wish to replace half of the water with a half-cup of white wine. Veal stock may also be used in lieu of water to augment the flavor and collagen content of the dish. For a big batch (3 pounds, about 1.4 kg, or 6 veal shanks) that feeds five people, slightly more than one shank each, I have used two tablespoons of duck fat or tallow to brown the shanks. Then I added three chopped onions or shallots, 10 garlic cloves, 3 chopped dried apricots, two or three tablespoons of fresh sage, 1.5 cups (355 ml) of water, and two tablespoons of butter (or ghee) and cooked it for *two* hours. Don't like the apricots? Leave them out. I have also tried only adding shallots and carrots (like **Simplest Beef Stew** on page 153), and it tastes great, too, especially when left to cook slowly in the pot for 3 hours! Pork knuckle (*jarret de porc*) may be prepared similarly, shown here with several chopped fresh tomatoes added.

WINE PAIRING TIP With the apricots in the dish, a *Bordelais* might advise a Bordeaux dessert wine coming from Barsac or Sauternes, with their own sweet notes of beeswax, honey, preserved and dried fruits, and vanilla. I have had this dish with a low-tannin, organic "Terra Amata" Châteauneuf-du-Pape, with notes of citrus, red fruit, oak, and spice from the Rhône Valley. Restaurateur Annabelle recommends either a sweet and lively white Premières-Côtes-de-Bordeaux, with notes of acacia, peach, or vanilla, or else she suggests a range of red wines, from supple to powerful, including a Côtes-du-Rhône-Villages or a full-flavored Gigondas, both from the Southern Rhône Valley, or else a Patrimonio from Corsica, with aromas of dark fruits and vanilla. She also recommends several reds from Languedoc-Roussillon, such as a medium-bodied, medium-tannic Corbières or Fitou, both herby with notes of leather, a rich Faugères, or an aromatic Saint-Chinian.

STUFFED VEAL CUTLETS
Paupiettes de Veau

Season Year-round   **Preparation Time** 1 hour
Cooking Time 6 minutes to brown, about 25 minutes in oven   **Serves** 5 to 6

The word *paupiette* comes from the word *papillote*, meaning envelope or wrapper. Paupiettes were first served at royal tables in the 1700s and became part of *la cuisine bourgeoise* and a favorite in restaurants in the 1800s.[1] In the North of France, the paupiette is known as a "bird without a head" (*oiseau sans tête*). In Provence it is called a "lark without a head" (*alouette sans tête*). In Gascony, part of the French Southwest, this dish was called *Côtelettes de Veau en Papillotes* in which pork "more fat than lean" (*plus gras que maigre*) was called for along with shallots, parsley, and pepper in the 1864 edition of the cookbook *Le Cuisinier Gascon*, compiled as a select representation of the colorful and flavorful food of Gascony,[2] a large swath of land in the French Southwest.

Paupiettes de Veau is another dish that, like barding a roast (wrapping in bacon or fatback) requires extra time and effort, which is great for entertaining guests but can be less practical for everyday meals, unless you make a bunch ahead and freeze them. This is decidedly an American preoccupation, freezing portions for future thawing and eating, not a French one. The French either make their own fresh food, or else they buy frozen foods already prepared. Fresh cilantro (whose peak is June through August) is used in this recipe, but parsley may also be used. If you have an indoor or greenhouse herb garden and adequate sun and moisture, you can harvest your cilantro year-round.[3]

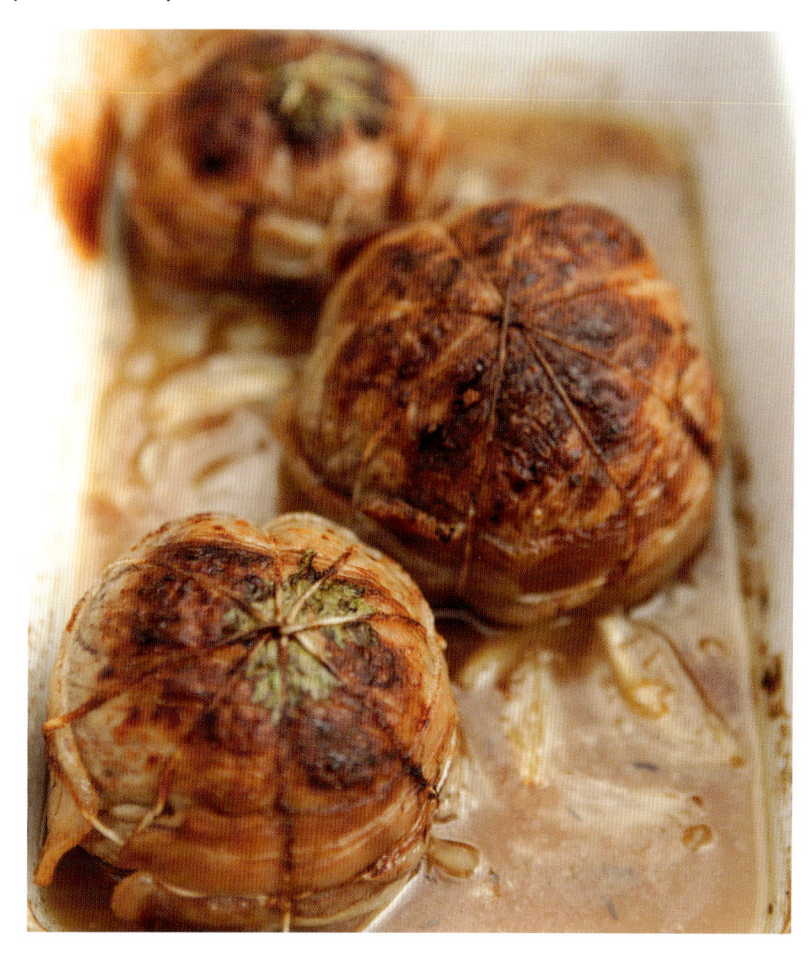

French butchers pride themselves on adding value to a product by turning something like a simple slice of veal (photo A), or veal cutlet (*escalope*), into a neat little, value-added package. I learned how to make these from my friend, Basque butcher Florent Carriquiry, at the butcher shop in Bordeaux where I apprenticed, and also from my friend Chef Edouard Remont at Le Poulailler d'Augustin, a specialty poultry vendor in Bordeaux just a few blocks from where we lived. The veal cutlet generally comes from the tender "rump" (*quasi*) or "round" (*noix*) from the back of the animal or the loin (*longe*, *filet*, or *faux filet*) from the midsection of the animal. The cut of pork usually used for the stuffing is from the fatty shoulder cut (*échine*), sometimes referred to as "Boston Butt," even though technically the meat is from the front shoulder of the animal. Veal, shall we say, is a cut above beef, in that it is more tender, younger, and thus more expensive. This recipe calls for the use of **Veal Stock** (page 415), but any meat stock or bone broth will do.

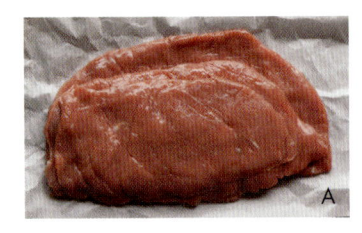

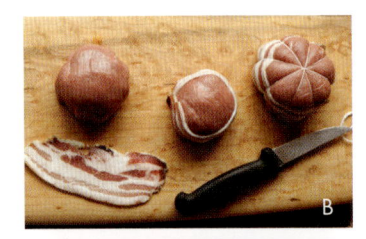

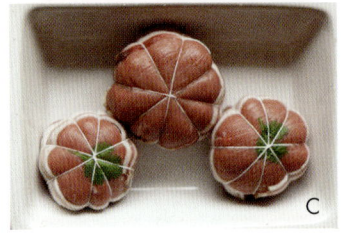

14 ounces (400 g) pork shoulder, ground

2 to 3 teaspoons fresh cilantro, minced

2 garlic cloves, minced, plus 5 or 6 whole leaves for decoration

2 pinches of fine salt

10 to 12 ounces (300 g to 350 g) veal cutlets (about 5 or 6 cutlets)

5 to 6 bacon slices

1 tablespoon bacon fat, lard, or tallow

6 tablespoons veal stock or bone broth

1 shallot, minced

In a large bowl, combine the pork, cilantro, garlic, and salt with your hands until well mixed. Flatten (*aplatir*) the veal cutlets using the bottom of a small, heavy pan if you do not have a flat meat pounder or tenderizer.

Form a ball using a small handful of pork filling and place in the middle of a cutlet. Envelope the cutlet around the ball of pork and place the smooth, most presentable side of the *paupiette* up.

Wrap a slice of bacon around the circumference of each paupiette. If you need two slices to go all the way around, you can overlap the edges of the bacon over each other. Place a cilantro leaf on top of each paupiette for decoration.

Using butcher's string, secure the bacon around the circumference of the veal ball and tie the rest of the ball by encircling it with the string, using the cilantro leaf on top as the midpoint for crossing over the string like the ribbon around a package, tying top to bottom and turning the paupiette a few degrees until you have a nice pattern around it with the string. (Photo B shows the paupiette tying process from left to right; photo C shows the paupiettes before they are browned.)

Preheat the oven to 395°F (200°C). Melt the tablespoon of fat in a large cast-iron pot or pan over high heat and brown the top and bottom of the paupiettes for two to three minutes on each side.

Spoon the veal stock or bone broth over the paupiettes in the pan and distribute the minced shallot around the bottom of the pan (not on top of the paupiettes).

Cook in the oven for about 25 minutes. Serve with roasted or sautéed vegetables.

Chef's Tip
Astuce du Chef
My friend Chef Edouard suggests slapping each slice of bacon lightly against a cutting board or flat surface to elongate the piece of bacon to make it fit all the way around the veal ball.

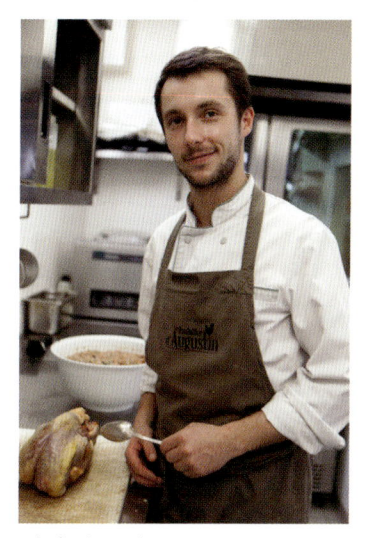

Chef Edouard

VARIATIONS Paupiettes can be stuffed with leftover meat, fish, game, or offal and can be basted in butter in addition to the veal stock. Chef Edouard showed me how to make *paupiettes de volaille* using chicken breast, which he stuffed with two proprietary blends: one using *herbes de Provence*, mustard, sun-dried tomatoes, and tomato paste, shown below, roasted and ready to eat, and one using ground pork, parsley, and spices. Both types of paupiettes are then wrapped in pork caul (*crépine*), the web-like pork fat used to hold meatballs, paupiettes, or pâtés together.

WINE PAIRING TIP For this mixed meat dish, restaurateur Annabelle recommends either white or red wines. She suggests white wines that are supple and rounded, such as a Ventoux "blanc," with notes of citrus or acacia, from the Southeastern Rhône Valley, or a white Côtes de Provence with notes of citrus, pine, and thyme. For red wines, she proposes reds that are refreshing with silky tannins or that come from the South (*méridionale*), such as a red Côtes de Provence, with notes of red fruits, bay leaf, and thyme, a Costières de Nimes, with notes of red fruit and dark berries from the Southeastern Rhône Valley, or else a medium-bodied Pinot Noir from Alsace (locally known as "Klevner") or from the Loire Valley, such as one from Anjou or Touraine.

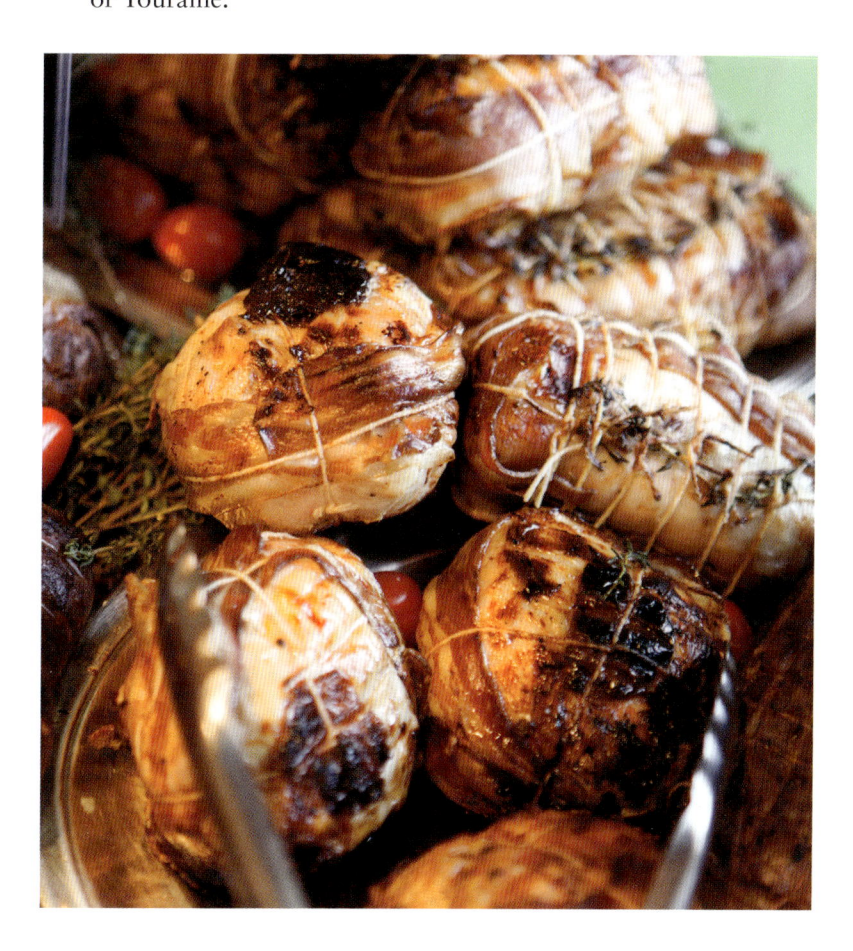

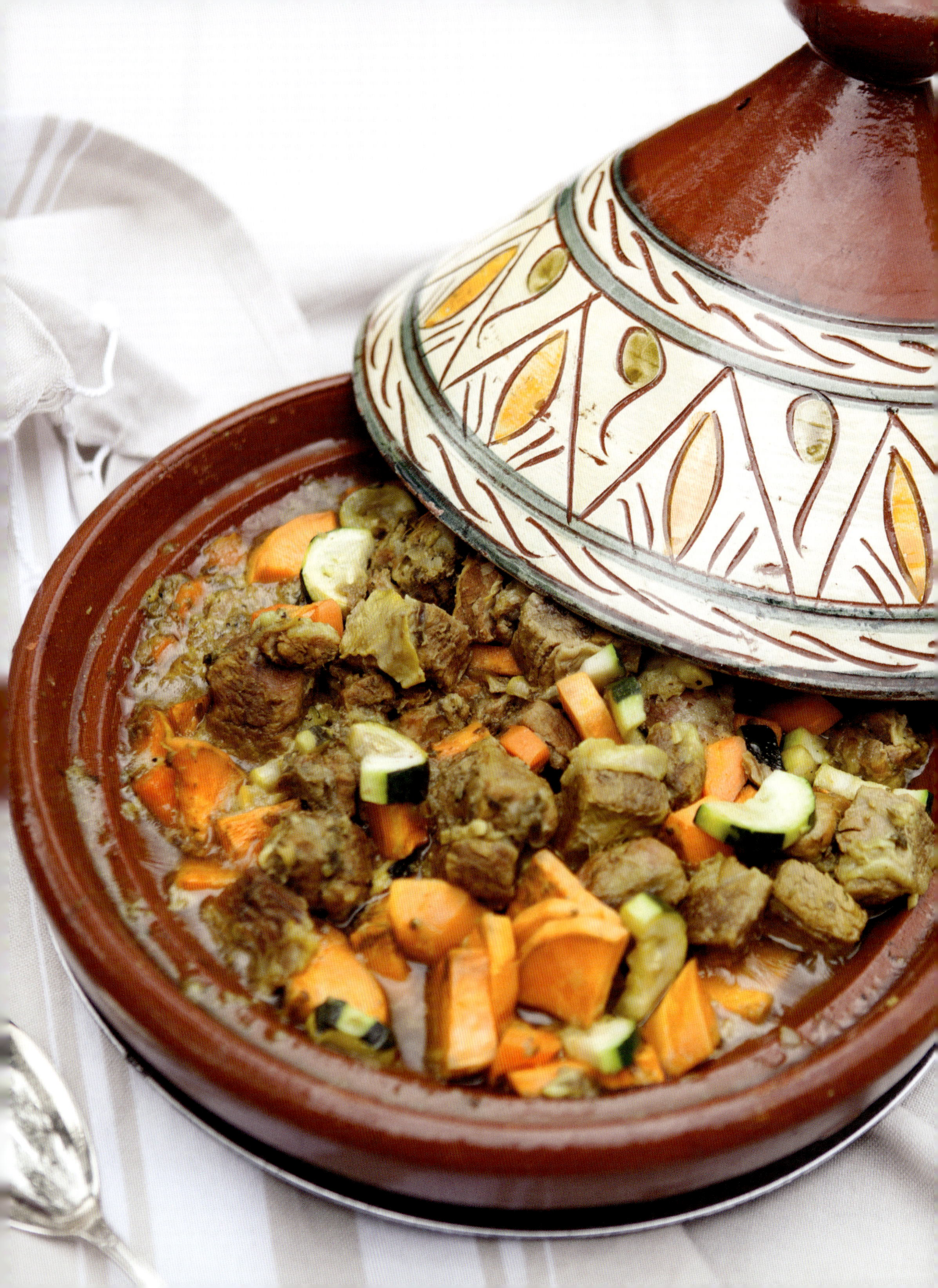

VEAL TAGINE STEW
Tajine de Veau

Season Year-round **Preparation Time** 20 minutes
Cooking Time 1½ hours minimum **Serves** 6

My French-Moroccan friend, Bouchra, cooked this recipe with me in a real clay dish made in El Saouira, Morocco, not far from her birthplace. She was 8 years old when she moved to France but has returned to Morocco many times since then, keeping up the culinary traditions of her native Morocco in France. In her kind manner, she presented me with this tagine clay pot in which we had cooked the meal together as a symbol of friendship.

For this slow-cooked stew, any of the following slow-cooking meats may be used: brisket (*poitrine*), chuck (*collet* and *épaule*), round (*rond de gîte*), rump (*rumsteck*), and plate (*tendron* or *poitrine*).

1 tablespoon beef or veal tallow

2.2 pounds (1 kg) veal meat, cubed in 1-inch (2.5 cm) cubes chuck roast

1 onion, peeled and minced

3 cloves garlic, peeled and minced

2 tablespoons olive oil

1 teaspoon coriander powder or a small handful of fresh cilantro, minced

Small handful of parsley, minced

1 teaspoon fine sea salt

½ teaspoon ground pepper

2 teaspoons fresh ginger, minced

½ teaspoon turmeric powder (or fresh grated curcumin)

4 cups (1 L) water

Optional: Pinch of saffron

1 carrot, chopped into ½-inch cubes

1 medium sweet potato, cut into 1-inch cubes

1 zucchini, cut into semi-circles

Melt the tallow in a cast-iron pot and brown the meat, onion, and garlic over medium-high to high heat. Reduce the heat to medium, and add the olive oil, coriander, parsley salt, and pepper and allow to cook for several minutes. Add the ginger and turmeric, reducing the heat to medium-low, and allow to simmer for several minutes. Add the water and the optional pinch of saffron, and simmer again for several minutes.

Transfer the contents of the pot to a tagine pot (or else leave everything in the cast-iron pot if you do not have a tagine pot) and use a metal tagine grill underneath the tagine pot to reduce the risk of the clay cracking from the heat of the gas or grill stovetop. Begin heating the clay pot on low heat for several minutes.

Add the carrot, turning up the heat to medium, and allow to boil. Add the sweet potatoes and zucchini after 10 to 15 minutes, as they take a bit less time to cook. Simmer for another hour and check the vegetables to make sure they are cooked through. Serve hot in a bowl.

> **WINE PAIRING TIP** The Moroccans would probably finish this dish off with a mint tea made from real mint leaves along with honey. For pairing this dish with wine, try a Burgundy Pinot Noir from the Côte de Nuits, such as a Vougeot, with notes of red and black fruits, or a Chambolle-Musigny with notes of violet, red fruits, and prunes, or else try a full-bodied, floral, and vegetal Volnay from Burgundy's Côte de Beaune.
>
> Restaurateur Annabelle suggests fleshy, full-flavored, and spicy red wines to match the spices of this dish: a Beaujolais Morgon, smelling of *kirsch* and ripe stone fruits; a Corsican Patrimonio, with notes of black currant, spice, and vanilla; a medium-bodied, majority-Syrah Minervois with notes of black currant, cinnamon, and vanilla from Languedoc Roussillon; or a soft, fresh and floral Lirac with notes of red fruits and almond from the Southern Rhône Valley.

VEAL TARTARE
Tartare de Veau

Season Late Spring through early Autumn   **Preparation Time** 25 minutes
Serves 2

The word "tartare" comes from "Tatar," an Islamic people spread across Eastern Europe, Turkey, Russia, China and Central Asia in the 1600s, who were confused with the Cossacks of Central Asia, Russia, and Ukraine from about the same time period. (The Cossacks were groups of self-governing, tribal, and militarized people known for their fierceness of character and for purportedly riding horseback with raw meat beneath their saddles to drain the blood from the meat.) For the unindoctrinated, eating raw meat can seem a scary concept, invoking fears of parasites and bacteria. In France, *tartares* are commonly served in restaurants, prepared by chefs who know how to handle raw meat, and can be made from raw beef, veal, or, yes, horse meat. If you are buying it yourself, you must have a trusted butcher to guide you. Eating ground veal or beef out of a package is not the idea here. This recipe requires a tender piece, such as a cut from the sirloin called *merlan* or another tender muscle near the shoulder area called *la surprise*, interior muscles which are untouched by outside bacteria. The *merlan* muscle (shown on the next page), is named in French after the fish they call *merlan*, the whiting or merling, similar to cod or pollock. The secret to a "*bon tartare,*" other than fresh raw meat, is the texture of the *finely minced* ingredients. Veal tartare can be served as an appetizer (*une entrée*) or a main course (*un plat*) and is eaten most frequently during the summer months. Again, buy raw meat only from a trusted source to avoid bacterial contamination.

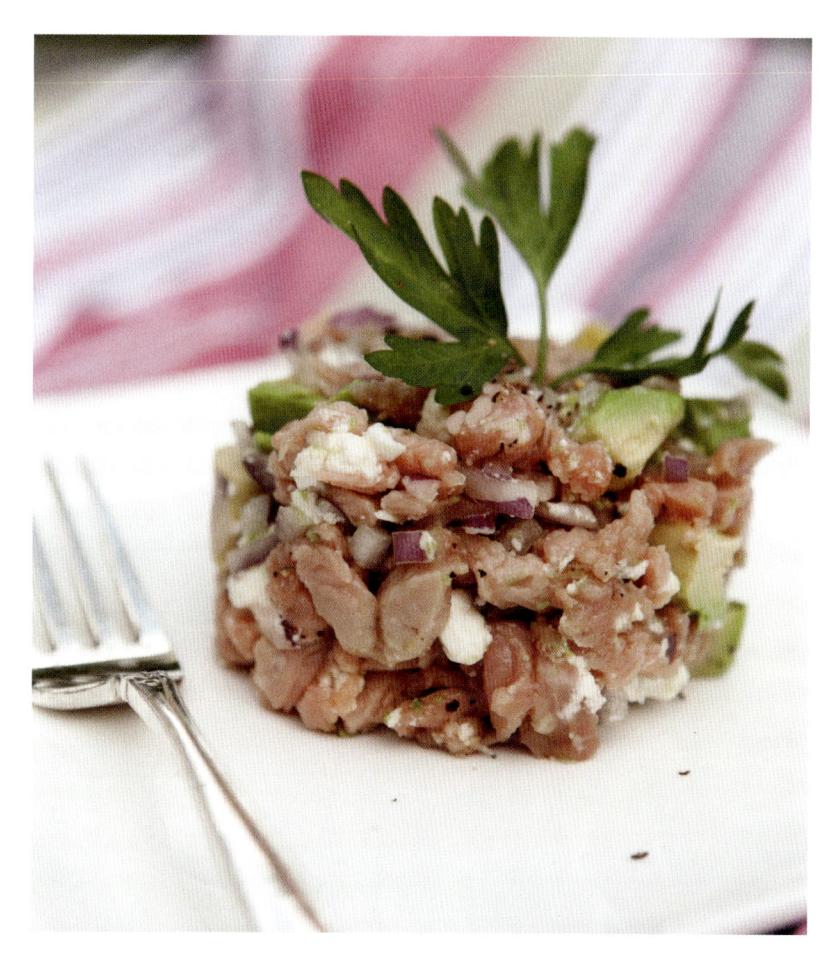

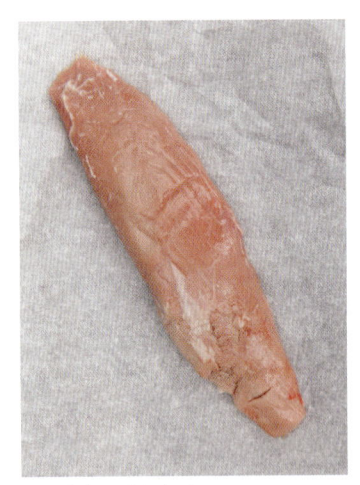

Raw Sirloin (Merlan)

8 ounces (225 g) raw veal, finely chopped (*émincé*)

½ small red onion (30 g), minced

2 pinches of fine salt

2 pinches of pepper

3 tablespoons olive oil

2 ounces (60 g) fresh goat cheese (*chèvre frais*)

1 avocado, diced

Fleur de sel, for garnish

Pepper to taste

Sprig of parsley, for garnish

VARIATIONS You may replace the grated Parmesan with another hard cheese of your choice (Cantal, Comté, Gruyère). You might also try using a different oil with this dish, such as walnut oil, as there is no cooking involved to oxidize the oil. If you are serving this dish in the spring, thinly slice asparagus lengthwise into thin pieces and brown each piece briefly in olive oil or tallow and place a few slices as garnish on the veal tartar. This is a special touch Chef Célia at the Michelin one-star Le Saint James restaurant in Bouliac outside Bordeaux showed me, and it's a winning combination. (See her grandmother's **Chicken Liver Cake** recipe on page 233.)

Place the veal into a bowl and mix in the onion, salt, pepper, and olive oil with a wooden spoon. Let stand for 10 minutes to allow the ingredients to "cook" and infuse the meat with aromas.

Gently mix in the goat cheese, and lastly the avocado. Sprinkle with *fleur de sel* and additional pepper for color and taste. Top with a sprig of parsley. Serve immediately.

WINE PAIRING TIP Try a regional pairing of this dish if you are using Comté, a fragrant and often fruity or nutty hard cheese, with a white nutty Savagnin from the Jura, Comté's region of origin. A combination of walnut oil and Savagnin will complement the dish using either goat or Comté cheese. A light-bodied Chenin Blanc, such as a Vouvray, ranging from dry (*sec*) to off-dry (*demi-sec*) to sweet (*moelleux*) with notes of acacia, apricot, and honey, from the Loire Valley pairs well with goat cheese. Or else try a crisp, aromatic white Hermitage from the Rhône Valley, with notes of acacia, almond, honey, and lemon, or a Sancerre with notes of citrus and flint from the Loire Valley. If using asparagus, pair this dish with a crisp mineral-flavored Chablis. Sommelière Annabelle recommends a dry and full-bodied white Puligny-Montrachet, with a range of notes from butter and green apple to flint, hazelnut, and honey, from the Côte de Beaune in Burgundy.

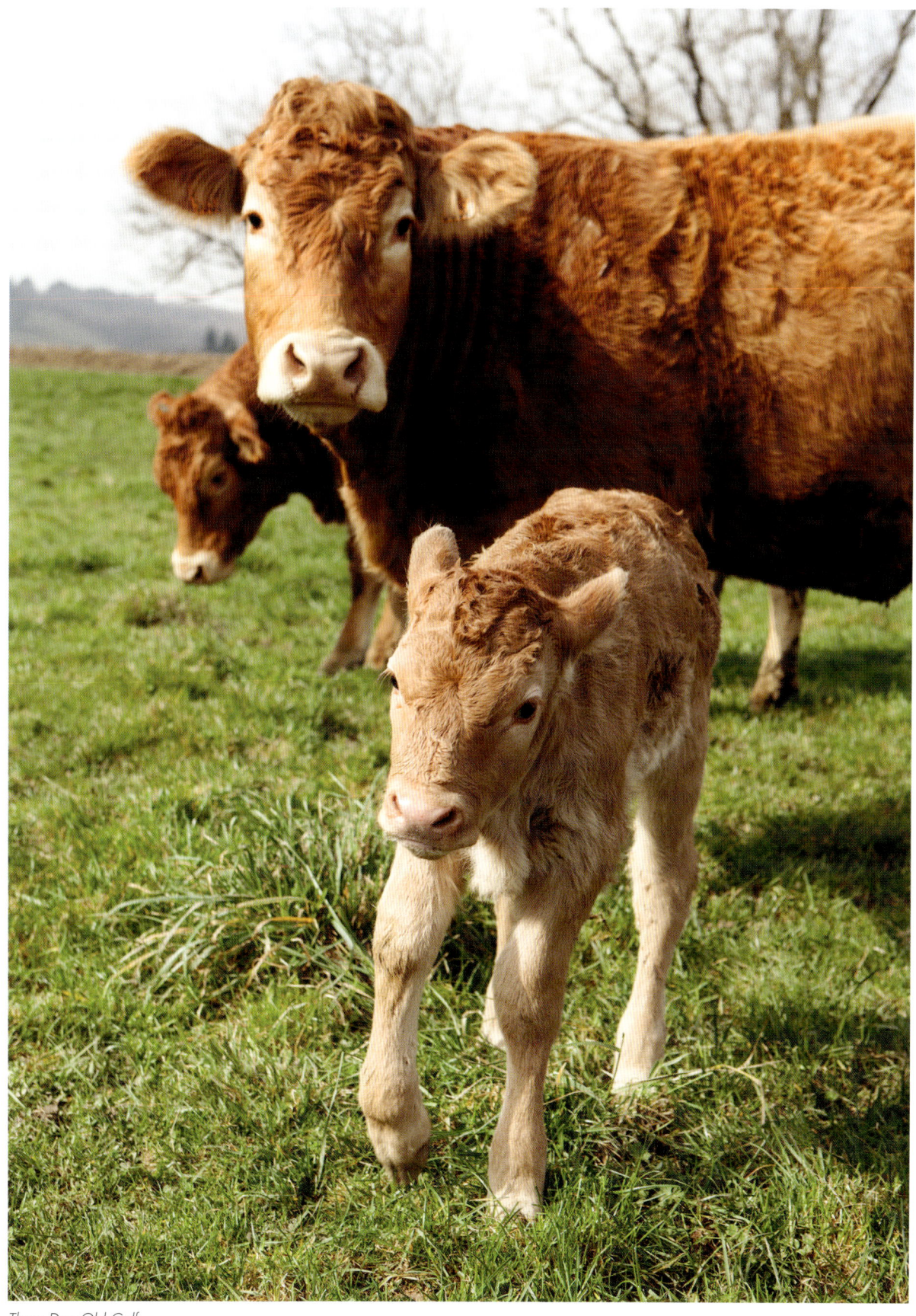

Three Day Old Calf

VEAL – *LE VEAU*

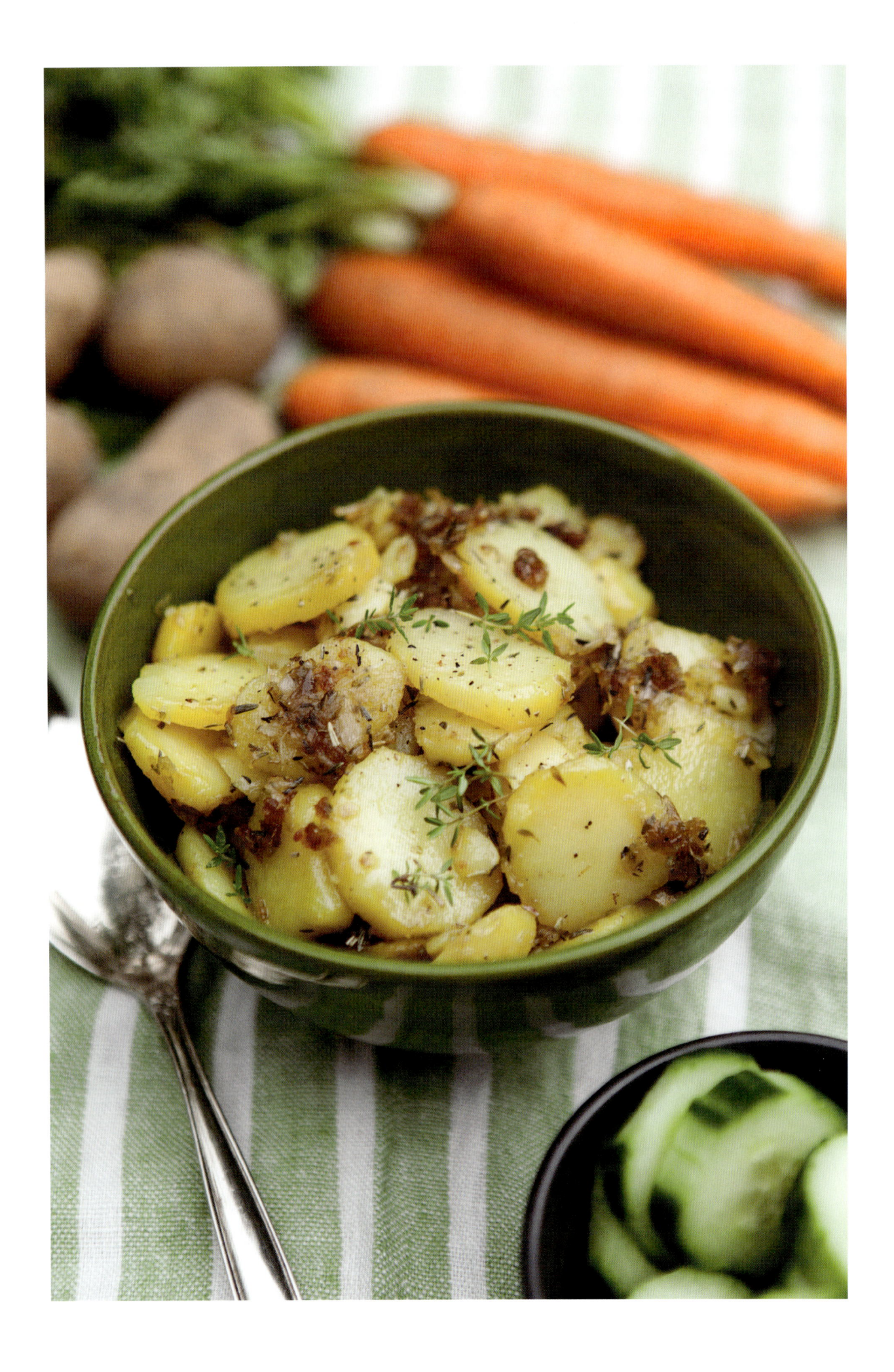

VEGETABLES
Les Légumes

Beet Salad with Blood Orange, Walnut, and Goat Cheese – *Salade de Betteraves aux Oranges Sanguines, Noix, et Chèvre* 438

Cauliflower Gratin – *Gratin de Choufleur* 439

Cauliflower "Rice" – *Riz au Chou-Fleur* 441

Celery Root Risotto – *Célerisotto* 442

Cream of Green Peas – *Crème de Petits Pois* 443

Fennel with Red Onion – *Fenouil et Onion Rouge* 445

Fermented Carrots – *Carottes Fermentées* 446

Fermented Radishes – *Radis Fermentés* 447

Field Potatoes – *Pommes de Terre des Champs* 449

French Green Peas – *Petits Pois à la Française* 450

French Onion Soup – *Soupe à l'Oignon* 451

Green Asparagus with Bacon and Hazelnuts – *Asperges aux Lardons et Noisettes* 453

Kabocha Squash and Chestnut Soup – *Velouté de Potimarron aux Chataignes* 454

Mashed Jerusalem Artichokes – *Purée de Topinambour* 456

Oven-Baked Beet Chips – *Chips de Betterave au Four* 457

Oven-Baked French Fries – *Pommes Frites au Four* 459

Oven-Baked Sweet Potatoes – *Patates Douces au Four* 460

Oven-Baked Zucchini – *Courgettes au Four* 461

Potato Gratin "Dauphinois" – *Gratin Dauphinois* 463

Pumpkin Soup – *Purée de Potiron* 464

Roasted Root Vegetables – *Légumes Racines Rôtis* 466

Roasted Summer Tomatoes with Herbs – *Tomates d'Été Rôties aux Herbes* 467

Sarlat Sautéed Potatoes – *Pommes de Terre Sarladaises* 468

Sauerkraut and Bacon – *Choucroute aux Lardons* 471

Sautéed Leeks and Bacon – *Poivrons Sautés aux Lardons* 472

Sautéed Onions – *Oignons Sautés* 474

Sautéed Swiss Chard – *Blettes Sautées* 474

Sautéed White Asparagus Slices – *Tranches Fines d'Asperges Blanches Pôelées* 475

Traditional Salad from Nice – *Salade Niçoise* 476

Vegetable "Clafoutis" – *Clafoutis aux Légumes* 479

Zucchini with Walnuts and Goat Cheese – *Courgettes aux Noix et au Fromage de Chèvre* 480

BEET SALAD WITH BLOOD ORANGE, WALNUT, AND GOAT CHEESE
Salade de Betteraves aux Oranges Sanguines, Noix et Chèvre

Season Winter **Preparation Time** 15 minutes
Cooking Time 30 minutes (for the beets) **Serves** 4

You might find several variations of this salad in a French restaurant, as it includes some favorite ingredients, most notably, the tasty combination of crunchy walnuts and goat cheese. This salad is delicious in its simplicity and is a great one for the winter when beets and oranges are readily available. My wine class comrade and cooking aficionado Malika Faytout showed me this recipe, putting her personal twist on this salad by using Valencia blood oranges, which were in season in neighboring Spain. (Any orange or grapefruit will do.) We made this salad while we were preparing the **Stuffed Whole Cabbage** (page 328) for lunch, and while "Walidia," the cat of Château Lescaneaut, also waited for her lunch.

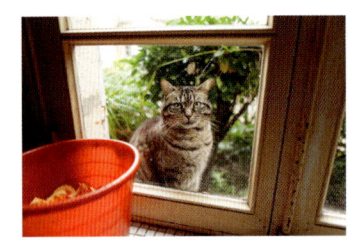

3 medium beets, peeled and boiled to tenderness (about 30 minutes)

2 blood oranges (or other orange or grapefruit)

½ cup (100 g) soft goat cheese (long, cylindrical shown in photo, *une bûche de chèvre fraîche*)

3 whole walnuts, cracked and crumbled

Olive oil to taste

Red wine vinegar to taste

Salt and pepper to taste

Slice the beets, oranges, and goat cheese and place on a serving dish. Sprinkle on the walnuts, and drizzle on the olive oil and vinegar. Add the salt and pepper. Serve as an appetizer or in lieu of a dessert.

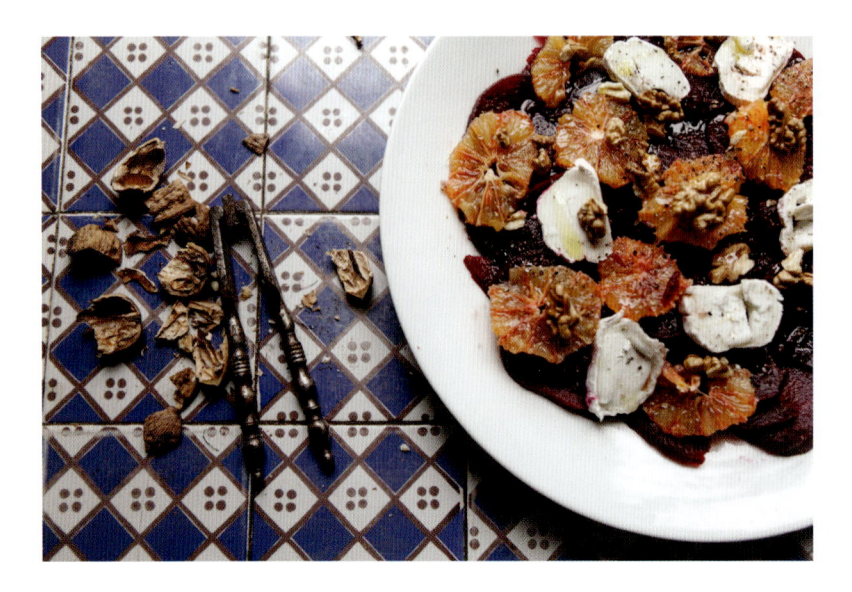

CAULIFLOWER GRATIN
Gratin de Choufleur

Season Late Spring through mid-Autumn   **Preparation Time** 20 minutes
Cooking Time 30 minutes   **Serves** 4 to 5

Au gratin means a dish has been put beneath the grill of an oven or at least baked in an oven, with some sort of topping on top, usually cheese. For this very French dish, I have gone straight to the (mostly) non-dairy, coco-nutty version. Feel free, however, to revert to the equivalent ingredients in their original, French dairy form: butter instead of ghee and coconut oil, whole milk instead of coconut milk, and lots of cheese on top. In this dish, you make a **White Roux** (page 397) by melting ghee (or butter) and mixing it with flour. You also make a **Béchamel Sauce** (page 392), in this case, using coconut milk, but again, you may use whole milk instead. For this gratin recipe, I use Gruyère cheese. If you are eating dairy-free, this step may be skipped, though the Gruyère is partly what make this dish so aromatic and flavorful. Cauliflower in France is in season May through October.

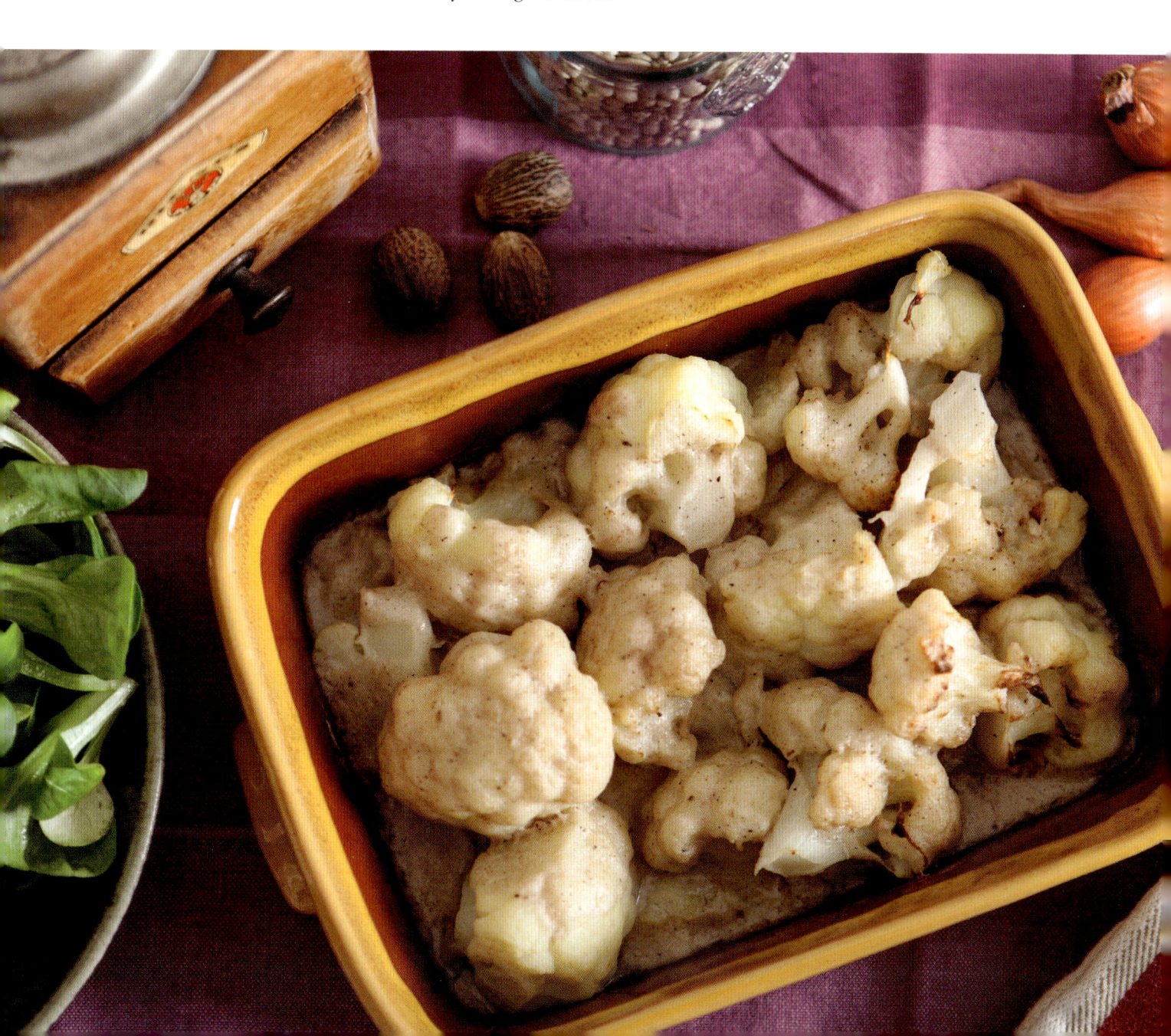

1 cauliflower (about 26 ounces or 740 g)

2 pinches of fine salt

2 tablespoons coconut oil (or ghee or butter)

1 tablespoon walnut flour (or chestnut or cassava flour)

¾ cups (175 ml) coconut milk (or whole milk)

Pinch of ground nutmeg

Pinch of ground white pepper

Optional: 3.5 ounces (100 g) Gruyère cheese, grated

Preheat the oven to 350°F (175°C). Cut off the leaves and break apart the cauliflower florets. Bring a pot of water with a pinch of salt to a boil. Boil the cauliflower florets for about seven minutes until tender. Drain off the water and place the florets into a small or medium-sized casserole dish.

In a separate pot, melt the coconut oil over medium heat and whisk in the walnut flour. Here you are making a white roux (*roux blanc*). Allow the roux to heat for one or two minutes, stirring frequently.

Stir in the coconut milk with a whisk and add the nutmeg, pepper, and a pinch of salt. Here you are making Béchamel Sauce. Allow the sauce to thicken for five minutes, stirring occasionally.

Pour the Béchamel Sauce over the cauliflower in the casserole dish. Sprinkle the optional grated cheese over the sauce and cauliflower and place in the oven. Cook for 30 minutes. Serve with grilled, roasted, or stewed meats or fish.

VARIATIONS For added fat and nutrients, like the **Potato Gratin "Dauphinois"** (page 463), you can beat an egg together with a tablespoon of sour cream (*crème fraîche*) and distribute this over the sauce and cauliflower for the last 15 minutes of cooking. Some recipes add raw minced shallots to the sauce or replace the Gruyère cheese with Roquefort cheese or aged goat cheese. Some recipes garnish with parsley after cooking, and some combine the cauliflower with chopped potatoes. Caramelized bacon pieces (*lardons*) may be sprinkled on the cauliflower for the last five minutes of cooking. Experiment to come up with your own combinations, the cauliflower takes on whatever flavors you add to it.

CAULIFLOWER "RICE"
Riz au Chou-Fleur

Season Late Spring through mid-Autumn   **Preparation Time** 10 minutes
Cooking Time 12 minutes   **Serves** 6

Every primal/paleo cook has his or her own version of cauliflower rice, a dish that steps in to fill the rice "void." My version is as follows. I prepare cauliflower for this dish by cutting off the outer green leaves, breaking off the florets, and pulsing the florets in batches through a food processor until they are small bits like rice or couscous. Mincing by hand works, too. I run the shallots and garlic together through a mini chopper to obtain very small pieces, but these can also be minced by hand with a good chef's knife. During cooking, I tend to add extra coconut oil for the flavor and extra medium-chain triglycerides (brain fuel) that coconut oil provides and for a fattier texture, which I prefer over a dry "rice." Cauliflower comes in white, yellow, and even purple (shown here, in a coated pan, before I got rid of it in favor of cast-iron and stainless-steel pans!).

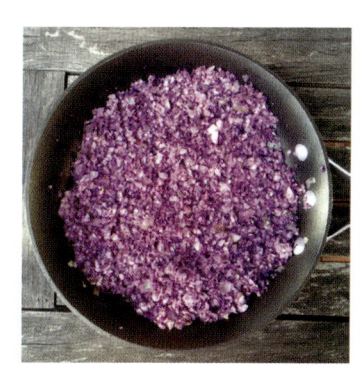

5 tablespoons coconut oil, more if desired

2 shallots, minced

4 garlic cloves, minced

3 pinches of fine salt

1 head of cauliflower, minced or pulsed in a food processor

Melt the coconut oil in a large pan over medium-high heat. Add the shallots, garlic, and salt, and sauté for five minutes until the shallots become translucent. Add the cauliflower and stir occasionally, cooking for about seven minutes. If the cauliflower seems dry, add more coconut oil.

Serve with grilled, roasted, or stewed meats or with fish.

VEGETABLES – *LES LÉGUMES*

CELERY ROOT RISOTTO
Célerisotto

Season Mid-Summer through mid-Spring   **Preparation Time** 15 minutes
Cooking Time 30 minutes   **Serves** 2 to 3

Chef Célia, instructor at *Côté Cours*, a cooking school at the one-star Michelin restaurant and hotel Saint James in Bouliac outside Bordeaux, showed me how to make this risotto style dish using celeriac or celery root (*céleri rave*). While not the "prettiest" in appearance, this knobby root vegetable effectively replaces the higher starch content of rice usually in risotto with a nutritious, lower carbohydrate and tasty side dish. In France, celery root is in season much of the year, July through April. It may be eaten raw or, as in this recipe, cooked.

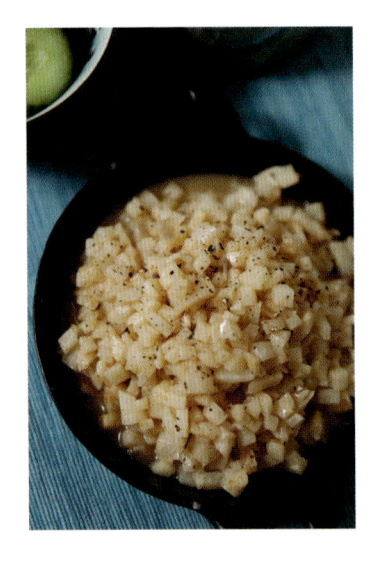

1 tablespoon duck fat

2 small shallots, minced

14 ounces (400 g) celery root, diced

2 pinches of fine salt, plus extra for seasoning

1 cup (240 g) white (or chicken) stock

Melt the fat in a saucepan on medium-high heat and sauté the shallots for a few minutes, until translucent. Add the celery root and salt and stir occasionally for 10 to 12 minutes. Stir in a cup of stock and continue cooking for 15 to 20 minutes, stirring occasionally, allowing the stock to reduce and be absorbed by the celery root. Taste the celery root to see if you like the consistency or if it is still too firm to the bite (*al dente*). Continue to cook if needed and adjust with additional salt as needed.

Serve alongside stewed, grilled, or roasted meats or fish.

CREAM OF GREEN PEAS
Crème de Petits Pois

Season Late Spring through mid-Summer **Preparation Time** 30 minutes
Chilling Time 30 minutes **Serves** 3 to 4

My chef friend and restaurateur, Chef Jean-Luc Beaufils showed me this recipe when he visited my kitchen in Bordeaux and also showed me how to flambé a steak (page 129) and how to cook pig's feet (page 259). Green peas (*petits pois*) are in season in France May through July and should be bought in their pod (*en chemise*) and then shelled. Or buy them frozen (in which case they are usually already shelled). Peas are a legume and should probably be eaten in small amounts by most people due to their lectin and phytic acid content,[1] and with lots of fat. The cream provides the fat in this recipe.

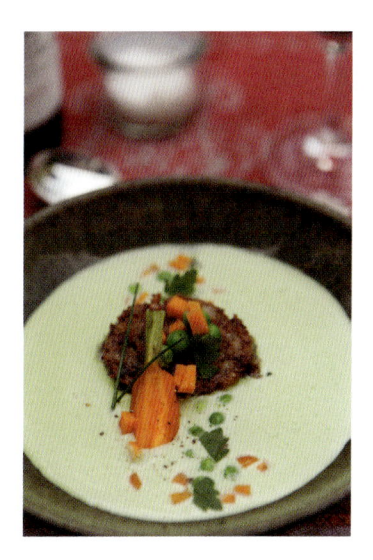

3 pinches of coarse sea salt (*gros sel*)

2.2 pounds (1 kg) green pea pods, shelled

½ carrot, diced

1 cup (about 240 ml) sour cream (*crème fraîche*) or whole cream (*crème liquide*)

Pinch of fresh or dried herbs (such as thyme or basil)

Fill a medium-sized pot with water and the salt and bring to a boil. Add the peas and allow to boil for five minutes. Remove a spoonful of peas and put them in cold water to cool them off and set their green chlorophyll color. Set these aside for decoration at the end. Transfer the rest of the peas to a blender and mix on a high setting for 45 seconds. Add three to five ounces (85 ml to 140 ml) of the salted water to the blender, depending on how thick or thin you prefer the creamed pea mixture, and mix again on high for 30 seconds.

Boil the carrot pieces for five minutes in the salted water; remove and set aside for decoration. The carrots also provide color (*couleur*) and crunch (*croquant*).

In another saucepan, bring the cream to a brief boil with one tablespoon of water so that the cream does not burn, and add a pinch of fresh or dried herbs (such as thyme or basil) to infuse into the cream. Add the herbed cream to the blender and mix again on high for 30 seconds. Pour the cream and pea mixture into a wide bowl or casserole dish to cool off rapidly (so as to maintain its color) by placing it in the refrigerator for at least 30 minutes. Serve this creamy side dish with **Pig's Feet Sliders** (page 259), as Chef Jean-Luc did, or serve with grilled beef, fish, lamb, offal, or pork.

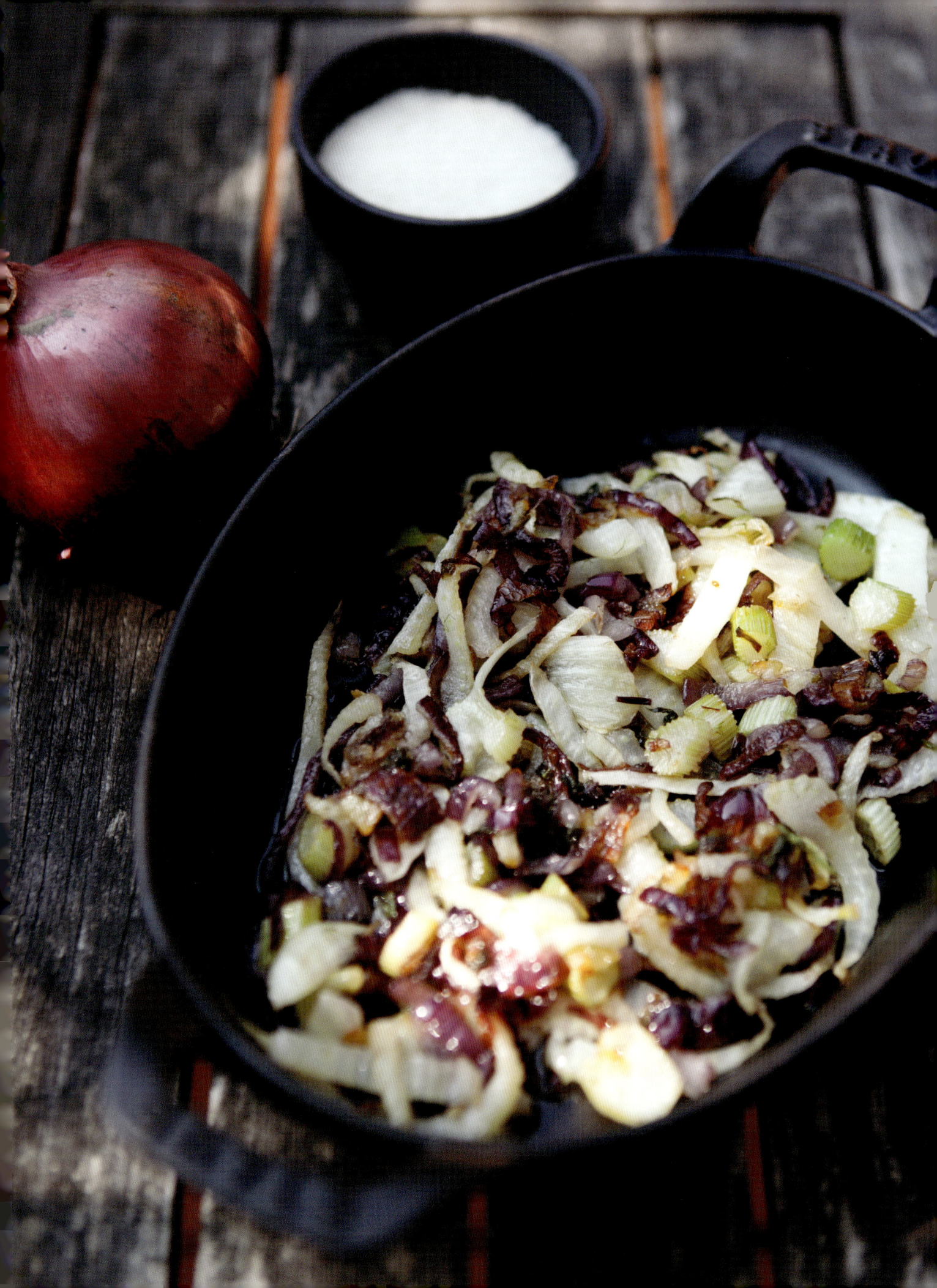

FENNEL WITH RED ONION
Fenouil et Onion Rouge

Season Spring through Autumn   **Preparation Time** 10 minutes
Cooking Time 25 minutes   **Serves** 2

I love to mix things, and one day I decided to combine two commonly used vegetables in France, fennel and red onion, to see what would happen. It turns out, that when you allow these both to caramelize together it produces a sweet and savory aromatic taste sensation that melts in your mouth. Fennel is in season May through November, while red onion is more or less available year-round. Fennel bulbs have a hard central core close to the root. I slice around the root and compost it, as it's a bit tough. I usually use ghee for this dish for its nutty flavor that adds to the flavors of the dish. This recipe is easy to double (or "guesstimate" the proportions, as many recipes are in *The Bordeaux Kitchen*); just use your largest pan for optimum caramelization of all the vegetable pieces.

3 tablespoons ghee, butter or duck fat

1 medium fennel bulb, thinly sliced

3 to 4 small red onions, halved and thinly sliced

2 pinches of fine sea salt

Melt three tablespoons of fat in a large pan over medium-high heat. Add the fennel, onions and salt. After several minutes, when the onions begin to caramelize, reduce the heat a notch to medium and allow the vegetables to brown further for about 20 more minutes, stirring occasionally.

Serve as a topping for burgers or with roasts, such as the **Beef Roast** (page 113). If you are serving a beef roast, pair it with a medium-bodied Bergerac wine from the French Southwest.

FERMENTED CARROTS
Carottes Fermentées

Season Year-round **Preparation Time** 10 minutes, Fermentation Time 7 to 8 days
Makes many small servings

The process of lacto-fermentation is simply making use of beneficial bacteria that are already present on the skin of vegetables, such as beets, cabbage, carrots, and radishes, and giving them a chance to turn the sugars in the vegetables into lactic acid, resulting in a tangy, sour taste, typical of fermented vegetables. Salt helps keep the other bacteria down while the lacto-bacillus bacteria grow.

Shred about 1 pound 5 ounces (600 g) of carrots in a food processor or cut into matchsticks. Mix two teaspoons of fine sea salt in one cup of water to make a brine. (Or mix 1 teaspoon of the salt with the carrots using your hands in a large bowl, as when making sauerkraut, and dissolve the other teaspoon of salt in the water.) Place the carrots into one or more clean glass containers. Pour the brine over the carrots and weigh the carrots down with a smaller jar containing marbles or pebbles. Allow the carrots to ferment (called malolactic fermentation, whereby bacteria convert malic acid into lactic acid), sitting on your kitchen counter for seven to eight days, then cover them and refrigerate. Their color will change a bit. Push the carrot pieces back into the brine as you dip into the jar, as they will dry out and turn grey outside of the brine. Eat a little every day or vary with other fermented vegetables daily or per meal. Lasts for about two weeks, longer if sealed and unopened.

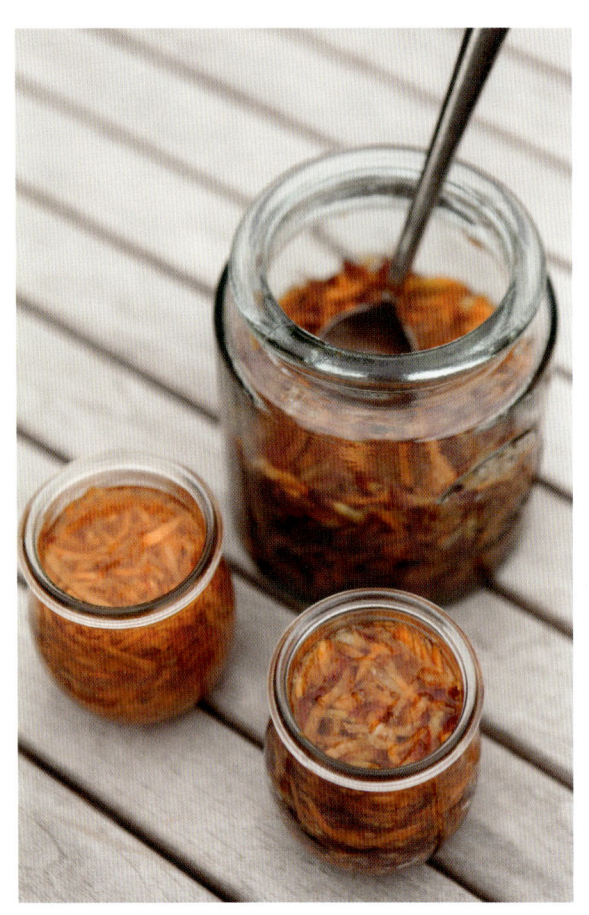

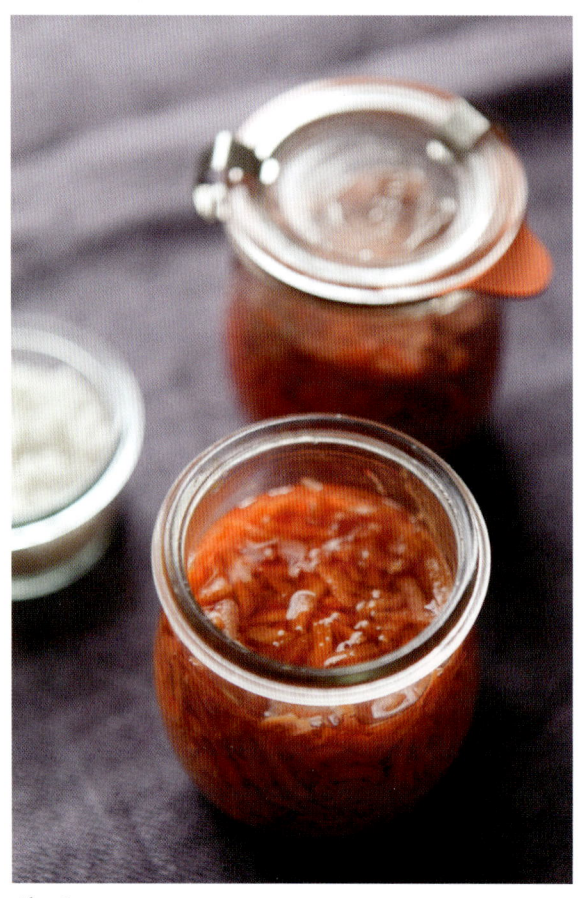

Before Fermentation

After Fermentation

FERMENTED RADISHES
Radis Fermentés

Season April through July   **Preparation Time** 10 minutes   **Fermentation Time** 7 days
Makes many small servings

I remember the jars of pickled, fermented, and canned fruits and vegetables in the cellar pantry of my aunt, Tante Doris, in Germany. They were more like specimens preserved in jars, interesting to look at, but not something as a kid I really wanted to eat. And I never thought I would ever *eat* radishes, much less *ferment* a radish. But, as I later understood, this was the traditional way of having some of these items in the winter, and I have grown to love the bitterness of fresh radishes that cut the delicious and copious amounts of olive oil I use in my salads. Fermented radishes have their own pleasant sweet-sour taste. Long-term storage involves sterilization of the jars, but for this recipe, I am simply describing an easy process for fermenting springtime radishes that you can eat over the following weeks, after only about seven to eight days of fermentation, and not necessarily for long-term storage. Radishes are in season April through July in France.

For 1.5 pounds (680 g) radishes, sliced into ¼- to ½-inch (0.6 cm to 1.25 cm) slices, make a brine of 5 teaspoons salt in two cups of warmed water. (The proportion amounts to 2 to 3 teaspoons fine salt per cup of water.) Weigh the radishes down with another jar full of marbles or pebbles, as shown, but make sure any errant radish slices sticking out of the water get pushed down beneath the surface of the liquid, unlike the two as-yet-unfermented rebel slices shown sticking up out of the liquid in the photo below, left. Allow the radishes to ferment for seven days, and then refrigerate. Their red and white colors will merge slightly to a nice pink.

Troubleshooting: Should tiny bits of mold form on the surface of the liquid, just pour them off or slough them off with a spoon, clean the jars and marbles better the next time (if they have sunken into the brine, which they might do), and/or add a bit more salt the next time. Sauté the fresh, slightly bitter radish greens on day 1 for several minutes in one tablespoon of duck fat with a pinch of salt. No waste!

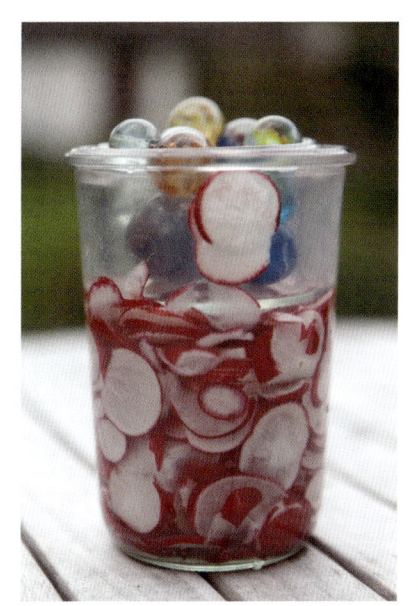

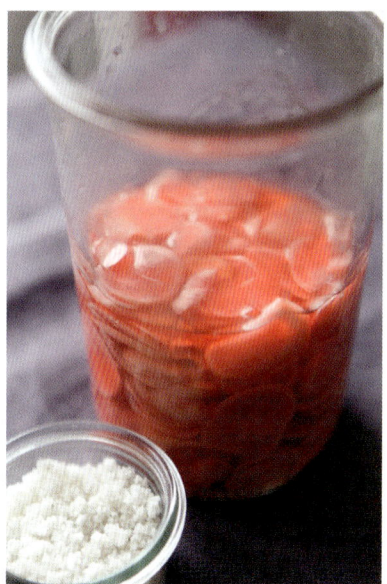

Before Fermentation

After Fermentation

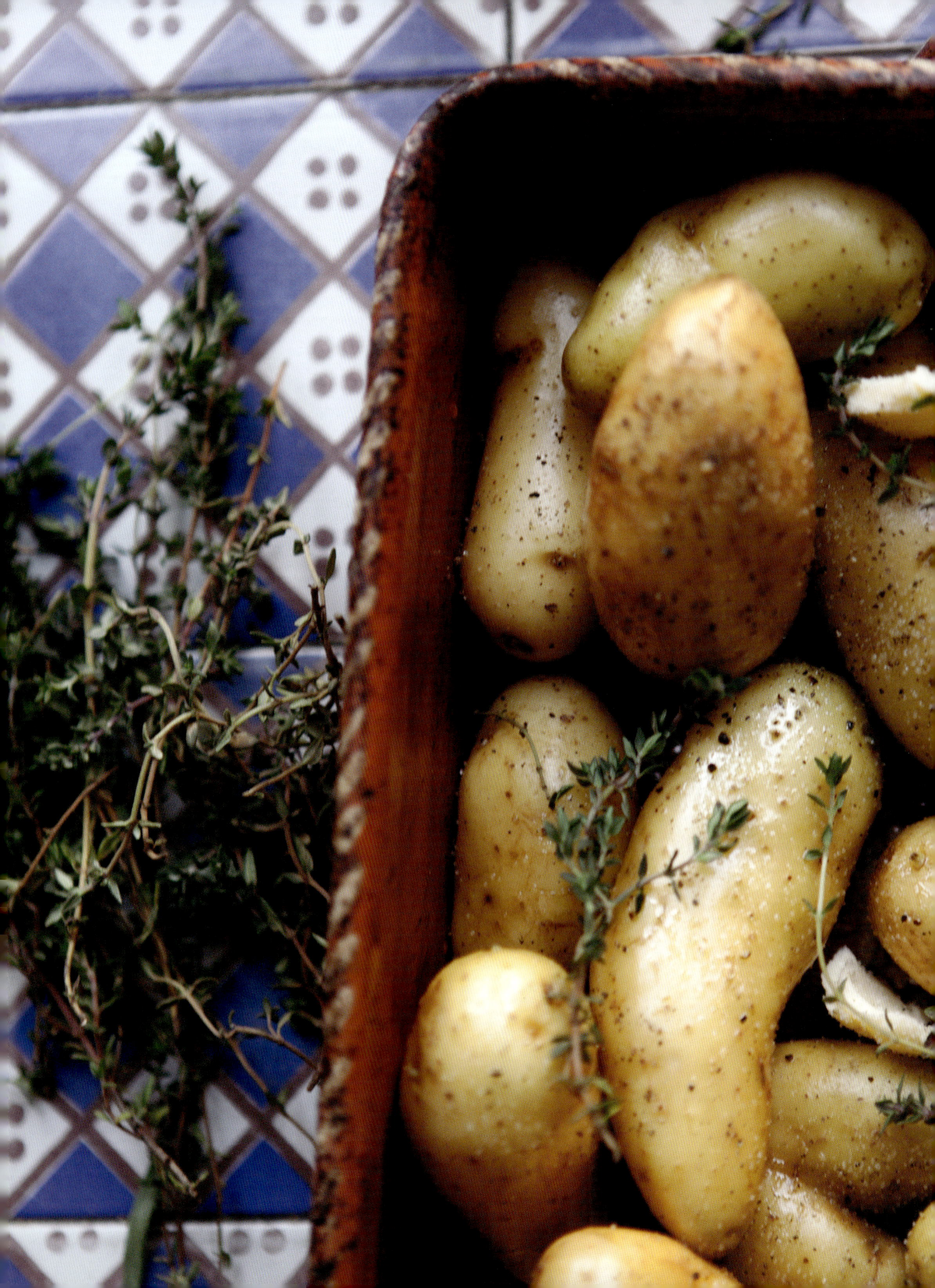

FIELD POTATOES
Pommes de Terre des Champs

Season Late Spring through Winter **Preparation Time** Less than 5 minutes
Cooking Time 45 minutes **Serves** 5 to 6

If you love potatoes and butter, this recipe is for you. It's very easy and delicious and goes with everything. My first-place-winning wine class buddy, organic winemaker, and mother of three, Malika Faytout (her last name, incidentally, can be interpreted as "Does Everything"), turned to this dish as an easy side while we were making the only slightly more involved but delicious **Herbed Rack of Lamb** (page 199). It calls for spring potatoes, but use whatever is in season, including the very cool purple potatoes (shown below), with all their health-boosting polyphenols. You don't even have to peel or cut the potatoes, this dish is so easy. Just make sure you have adequate farm fats to go with the potatoes (if not butter and olive oil, then bacon, duck or goose fat, ghee, lard, or tallow).

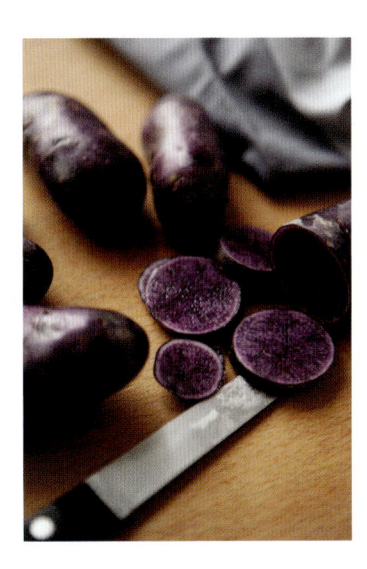

2.2 pounds (1 kg) small to medium-sized potatoes, unpeeled

3 tablespoons olive oil

3 tablespoons butter, chopped into chunks

Several sprigs of thyme

Salt and pepper to taste

Preheat the oven to 365°F (185°C). Place the potatoes in a casserole dish, distribute olive oil, butter, and thyme over the potatoes. Roast for 40 to 45 minutes. Season as desired with salt and pepper.

Serve alongside roasts, steaks, stews, or fish.

FRENCH GREEN PEAS
Petits Pois à la Française

Season Late Spring through mid-Summer **Preparation Time** 10 minutes
Cooking Time 20 minutes **Serves** 2 to 3

Spring and Summer (May through July) is the time for fresh green peas in France. Peas are a legume (containing potentially mineral-stealing lectins and phytates) and should probably be eaten in small amounts, with ample amounts of fat. Steeped in butter and stock with a bit of salt, these little, crisp, green pearls are a nice spring and summertime treat, with lots of fresh chlorophyll. This recipe was shown to me by Chef Frédéric to accompany his grandmother Gaby's classic French **Veal Liver** recipe (page 282). Although the dish itself is called "French" (*à la Française*), in a friendly nod to the English, the dish is sometimes referred to as *à l'Anglaise* when prepared without onions. The butter and stock used in this recipe serve to bind (*lier*) the peas and spring onions. The young or "sweet lettuce" (*sucrine*), in season in summer, is used here, but other lettuces may be used in its stead. Chef Frédéric calls it a delight (*un délice*)!

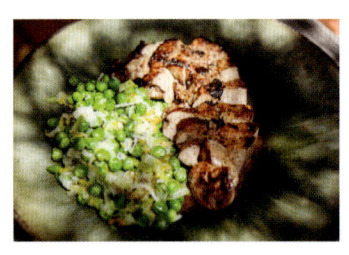

Pinch of salt

2.2 pounds (1 kg) pea pods, peas removed from the pods

1 teaspoon duck fat

Several green onions or one medium onion, minced

Sea salt

2 tablespoons butter

2 ladles of poultry stock or other stock or bone broth

Young or "sweet" lettuce, chopped

Fill a pot with water, add a pinch of salt, and bring to a boil. Add the peas and boil them for five to eight minutes over high heat. (Boil them for several minutes longer at the end of the pea-growing season, as they will be heartier and will need more cooking time.) "Shock" or quickly chill (*refroidir*) the peas in a bowl of ice water to "set" (*fixer*) the chlorophyll green color of the peas.

Melt the duck fat in another pan over medium-high heat and add the minced onions. Allow them to sizzle or "sweat" (*suer*) for several minutes. Add the salt and butter, which will help bind the stock to the onions. Add the peas and two ladles of stock. Bring to a brief boil, add the lettuce, and remove from heat.

Serve warm with **Veal Liver** (page 282) or other offal, or with roasts, grilled meats, fish, or stews.

FRENCH ONION SOUP
Soupe à l'Oignon

Season Autumn through early Spring   **Preparation Time** 20 minutes
Cooking Time 1 hour and 5 minutes   **Serves 6** (Makes 6 1-cup servings)

The secret to a rich and savory onion soup is the combination of flavors from the veal-based stock and the onions sautéed in butter. The stock used may be either **Veal Stock** (page 415) or **Brown Stock** (page 398), both made with meat and bones as their base. If you do not have four cups of either a *Glace* (solid gelatin) or a *Demi-Glace* (gelatinous but not solid) veal or brown stock, nor the time to reduce your stock down to one of these, then use instead 6 cups of a *Fond* (a more concentrated broth or stock base) or a *Bouillon* (watery stock) veal or brown stock, without adding the two cups of water as stated in the recipe. The thicker (more gelatinous) the stock, the more intense the flavor of the soup. See Variations for preparing **French Onion Soup Gratin**, which is French Onion Soup with toasted bread topped with oven-melted cheese.

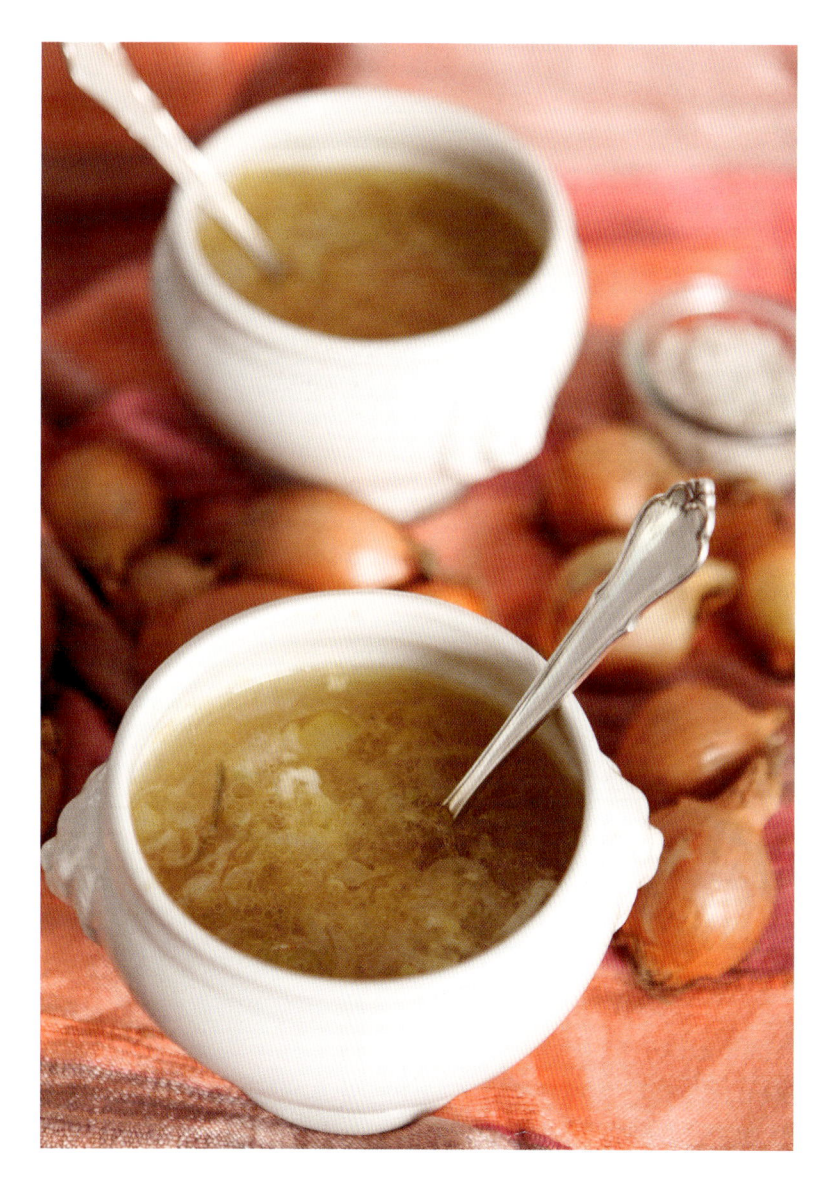

4 tablespoons ghee (or butter or lard)

1 pound (450 g) yellow onions, halved and thinly sliced

Pinch of salt

Pinch of pepper

4 cups (about 1 L) *Glace* or *Demi-Glace* **Veal Stock**

2 cups (about ½ L) water

7 ounces (200 g) Gruyère or Emmental cheese, grated

VARIATIONS **French Onion Soup Gratin** *(Soupe à l'Oignon Gratinée)* usually comes with one or two pieces of toasted bread in the bowl topped with oven-melted cheese, which is what makes the soup "gratinated" (*gratinée*). If you have grain-free bread, melt the cheese on slices of bread in the oven at 395°F (200°C) for several minutes until slightly browned on top and place the slices on the surface of the soup. Or place the bread on the surface of the soup-filled bowl, sprinkle the bread with the cheese, and heat the entire bowl in the oven for several minutes.

Melt the ghee in a cast-iron pot over medium to medium-high heat and add the onions, salt, and pepper. Allow the onions to turn translucent and brown over 25 to 30 minutes, stirring occasionally.

Add the stock and water to the pot and bring to a brief boil. Reduce the heat to medium-low, cover and allow to simmer for 25 to 30 minutes. Taste the soup, and adjust the seasoning with additional salt and pepper, if desired. Preheat the oven to 395°F (200°C). Divide the cheese among the serving bowls and heat the bowls in the oven for two minutes. Serve hot.

WINE PAIRING TIP For a French Southwest pairing, try an aromatic Bergerac, with notes of black and red currant and made from a similar blend to that of a Bordeaux, giving the wine a solid tannic structure. Try pairing a Gewürztraminer, Pinot Blanc (Klevner), or Sylvaner from Alsace, as these dry whites are typically served with sulphurous foods like cabbage and onion in Alsace. The very comprehensive and informative French vine and wine website Vin-Vigne.com (www.vin-vigne.com) offers several recommendations for French Onion Soup gratinated with Emmental cheese. For whites, among others, they suggest a floral and nutty Côtes du Jura Blanc made with the Savagnin grape, or a refreshing Côtes de Bourg, Bourg et Bourgeais from the Blaye-Bourg region of Bordeaux, with floral, grassy, and toasted (*côté grillé*) aromas. For reds, among others, they suggest a fruity and supple Beaujolais-Villages Rouge made from the Gamay Noir grape, with notes of banana and violet; an Arbois Rouge from the Jura, with notes of animal (*foxé*) and fruit; or a crisp Irancy, with notes of red and dark fruits, made from the Pinot Noir grape in Northern Burgundy.

GREEN ASPARAGUS WITH BACON AND HAZELNUTS
Asperges aux Lardons et Noisettes

Season Spring   **Preparation Time** 5 minutes   **Cooking Time** 20 minutes   **Serves** 2

Bacon is everybody's friend, including asparagus! When asparagus is in season in the spring in France, you can benefit from asparagus' healthful properties. But, one needs several ways to prepare it so as not to tire of it. Asparagus needs fat, such as that of bacon and extra virgin olive oil, as in this recipe, to be able to absorb all those nutrients. Or else it needs **Béchamel Sauce** (page 392), or at least butter. The hazelnuts, local to France, provide a nice crunch and nutty flavor in this recipe. This recipe, as many others in this book, can easily be "eyeballed," in that, you can use the ingredients in the proportions you prefer or that you have on hand.

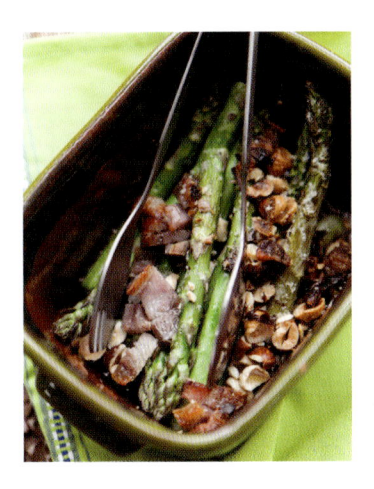

12 ounces (340 g) asparagus, bottom half snapped off

Handful (about 1 ounce or 30 g) of hazelnuts, chopped

1 ounce (30 g) bacon pieces (*lardons*)

3 tablespoons olive oil

Pinch of fine salt

Preheat the oven to 365°F (185°C). Combine the asparagus, hazelnuts, and bacon pieces in a small oven-safe dish, drizzle with the olive oil, and sprinkle on the salt. Place in the oven and roast for 20 to 25 minutes.

Chef's Tip – *Astuce du Chef*
My friend Chef Célia showed me the trick to removing the tough ends of asparagus, both green and white. Simply snap the shoot in half around the middle of its length. It makes a very satisfying snap. (Something fun for children to help with.) If it is thin and short or "young" asparagus, then just slice off the tip of the bottom end. White asparagus shoots must additionally be peeled with a peeler. I peel them first before snapping off the ends.

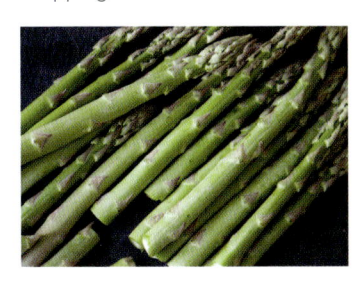

VARIATIONS Try this combination of bacon and hazelnuts with chopped Swiss chard (thick white stems removed) instead of asparagus. Brown the bacon in a pan over medium heat for five to seven minutes with a teaspoon of lard, then reduce the heat to medium-low, add the remaining ingredients and sauté them for several minutes until the chard wilts. Pecans also go well with chard cooked this way, as does duck fat. Another simple combination for roasting green asparagus in the oven involves a teaspoon of minced garlic sprinkled over the asparagus, along with olive oil and the juice from half an orange drizzled on the asparagus, topped with a pinch of fine or coarse sea salt. Brussels sprouts are also delectable with bacon, in fact pretty much the only way I like to eat them, with or without nuts. Brussels sprouts may need a full 30 minutes in the oven.

KABOCHA SQUASH AND CHESTNUT SOUP
Velouté de Potimarron aux Chataignes

Season Autumn through Winter   **Preparation Time** 20 minutes
Cooking Time 1 hour and 15 minutes to roast the squash, 10 minutes to heat the soup   **Serves** 6

Kabocha squash (*potimarron*), dark reddish-orange in color, and chestnuts (*chataignes*) seem to pop up everywhere around the Southwest in the fall. Chestnuts ripen in early autumn and are best September through December. Probably because of its rich flavor, vivid color, and symbiotic pairing with native chestnuts, the kabocha squash, originally a Japanese variety, seems to be quite popular in France. October and November are their harvest season, but because they store so well, they are a welcome dash of color and flavor during the winter months. Roasted squash is easy to make after removing the seeds and stringy pulp in the middle: just chop the kabocha into one-inch (2.5 cm) cubes and roast in the oven at 365°F (185°C) until tender, adding a pinch of fine salt and generous drizzling of olive oil. This takes about an hour: less for smaller chunks, more for larger chunks. You can just eat it like that as a side dish, even adding *herbes de Provence* or a pinch of dried thyme and extra salt. In general, squash may be roasted at 365°F (185°C) for about one hour to one hour and fifteen minutes, or until tender.

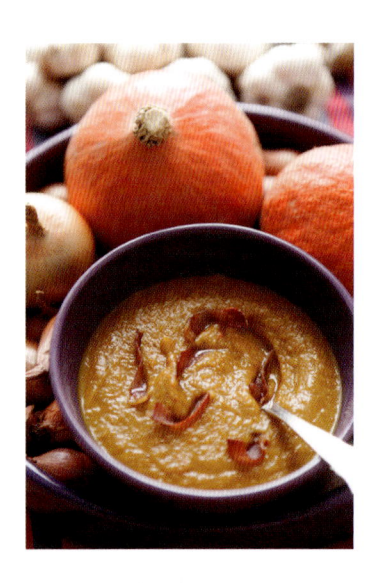

For this soup, you can roast the kabocha ahead of time, even the night before if your schedule requires, which mine often does. Chestnuts are one of the few ingredients I buy in a jar already "processed." In France, you can find them organically grown, shelled, peeled, and hermetically preserved in a glass jar or vacuum packaging, *sous vide*, without additives. Dartagnan.com sells them already cooked and vacuum packed, and I have seen them sold on Amazon. They only last several days, however, once the jar or package has been opened. Both kabocha and chestnut are vitamin-rich but very starchy and are therefore to be eaten in small quantities with adequate fats. In fact, the chestnut tree has been referred to as the "bread tree" (*l'arbre de pain*) by some in the Southwest, according to regional expert and cook Paula Wolfert in her cookbook, *The Cooking of Southwest France*. Perhaps this is why squash and chestnuts appear in the fall, to help fatten us up for the winter. This soup could be served as an appetizer (*amuse-bouche*, literally "amusement for the mouth"), if not as a modest side dish.

1 tablespoon butter or ghee

1 medium onion, minced (about 3.5 ounces or 100 g)

2 pinches of fine salt

6 ounces (170 g) chestnuts, shelled (raw or roasted)

14 ounces (400 g) roasted squash, skin on, chopped in cubes and cooled

2 cups (500 ml) poultry or other stock or bone broth

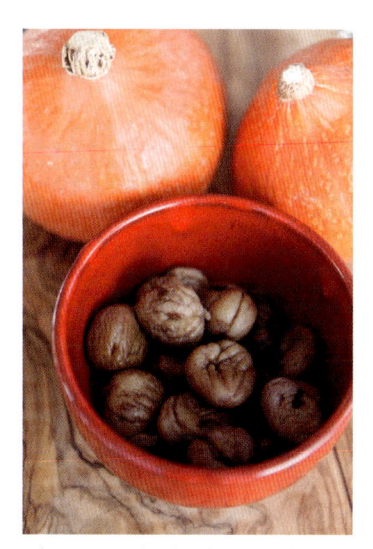

Chestnuts and Kabocha Squash

Melt the butter in a pan over medium heat. Sauté the onion with a pinch of salt for about 10 minutes until the pieces have caramelized and become translucent. Set aside in a large bowl.

Chop the chestnuts to a fine, crumbly, chunky consistency in a food processor (about 15 seconds) and add to the large bowl. Purée the squash, also for about 15 seconds in the food processor and add this to the bowl. Stir in the stock, add another pinch of salt, then blend everything once more in a blender or food processor for about 15 seconds until you achieve a smooth purée.

Heat the mixture over medium to medium-low heat in a pot for 10 minutes, stirring occasionally. To add to the fat content, melt another tablespoon of butter while heating, or stir in three tablespoons sour cream (*crème fraîche*).

Serve drizzled with olive oil and/or garnish with about two ounces (57 g) of thin strips of *Jambon de Bayonne* ham or *prosciutto* oven-dried for 10 minutes at 395°F (200°C), as shown on the previous page, or pan-fried over medium heat for several minutes, just for crispiness. Or else, just add bacon!

> WINE PAIRING TIP My Bordeaux wine tour and WSET instructor friend, Caroline Matthews, suggests that if you are offering this soup as a starter along with wine, match the soup's rich flavors with a rich white wine, such as an oak-aged Chardonnay from Burgundy, like a full-bodied, nutty and buttery Meursault from the Côte de Beaune, the Southern half of Burgundy's famous Côte d'Or (the Côte de Nuits makes up the Northern half); or a dry and complex Condrieu from the Northern Rhône, with notes of apricot, peach, and flowers, and made from the Viognier grape, which lends herbal notes including lavender and thyme.

VEGETABLES – *LES LÉGUMES*

MASHED JERUSALEM ARTICHOKES
Purée de Topinambour

Season Late Spring through early Autumn   **Preparation Time** 10 minutes
Cooking Time 15 to 20 minutes   **Serves** 3 to 4

Jerusalem artichokes (*topinambour*) are a tuber or root vegetable similar to potatoes but with more texture. They also have what is called "prebiotic fiber," essentially, food for our gut microbiota. Dr. David Perlmutter (of *Grain Brain* fame) mentions the Jerusalem artichoke as such in almost every interview he does.[2] Also known as "earth apples," Jerusalem artichokes are in season March through September and make a handy substitute for potatoes. But be forewarned, your children will notice the difference in taste, so they might reject it the first 20 times or so that you serve it. I first learned about the *topinambour* from my friend Chef Frédéric, when I took a cooking class with him in Bordeaux several years ago. This is merely one example among many, demonstrating the diversity of the French diet and the creativity and resourcefulness of French chefs to uphold the traditions of incorporating seasonal vegetables, despite the ubiquitous presence of other, perhaps more well-known foods, such as potatoes. This recipe is easy to change according to proportions: if you have more Jerusalem artichoke, simply add a bit more (or a lot more) fat and more salt.

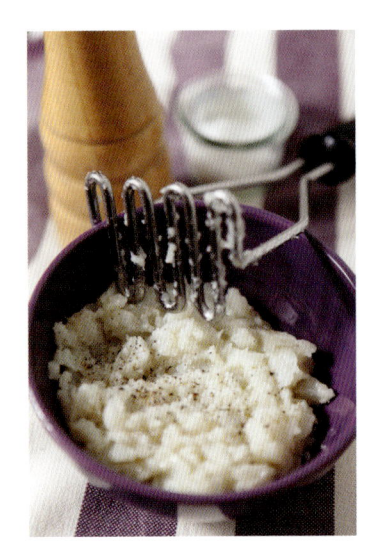

9 ounces (255 g) Jerusalem artichoke, peeled and chopped into ½-inch (1.25 cm) cubes

Fine salt

1 tablespoon butter or ghee

Fill a pot about halfway with water, add a pinch of salt, and bring to a boil. Add the Jerusalem artichoke cubes, cover, and allow to boil for 15 minutes. Drain and add one tablespoon (or more for higher fat content) of butter or ghee. Using a potato masher, mash the Jerusalem artichoke and fat together by hand until you reach the desired consistency. For a creamier texture, you can boil the Jerusalem artichokes for five more minutes and use a hand-mixer to mix it more finely than a handheld potato masher. You can also add more fat for flavor and texture.

Serve alongside stewed, grilled, roasted, or stewed meats, or fish.

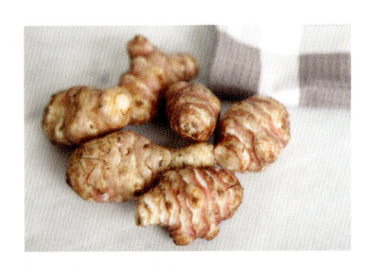

Jerusalem Artichokes

OVEN-BAKED BEET CHIPS
Chips de Betterave au Four

Season Beets: May through October, White Potatoes: May through February, Sweet Potatoes: Year-round
Preparation Time 5 to 10 minutes   **Cooking Time** 12 to 15 minutes   **Serves** 4 to 6

Beet chips are a nutrient-dense "chip" replacement using any color beet (pink, red, yellow). Beet chips are delicious on their own, but they can also be used to hold toppings such as **Turkey Liver Pâté with Figs** (page 274), **Spreadable Fish Paste** (page 186), or **Pork Meat Pâté** (page 212). The trick to beet chips is not letting them burn. The thinner the chip, the more quickly it will burn in the oven if it not rescued in time. Even with a hand grater (see photo below, top left), cutting the slices uniformly is difficult, as each slice of the beet has a different circumference. I suggest checking them after 10 to 12 minutes to see if you may already remove the thinnest and smallest before they burn, and rotate the tray while you have the oven door open.

Begin by pouring a generous amount of olive oil onto a tray or large casserole dish, then smear the olive oil evenly around the tray using one beet slice. Rub both sides of each beet slice in the olive oil and sprinkle fine sea salt on top. Bake for 12 to 15 minutes at 365°F (185°C) or at 350°F (175°C). Rotating the tray in the middle of baking can help the beets cook more evenly. Do this with slices of white or sweet potatoes as well, as shown below.

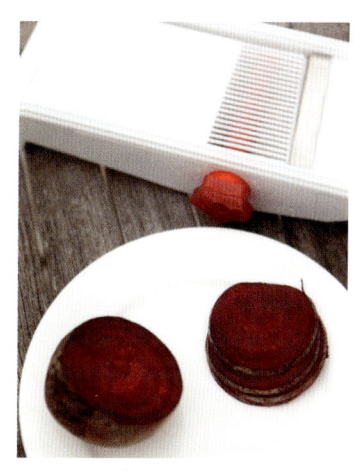

Raw Beet Chips

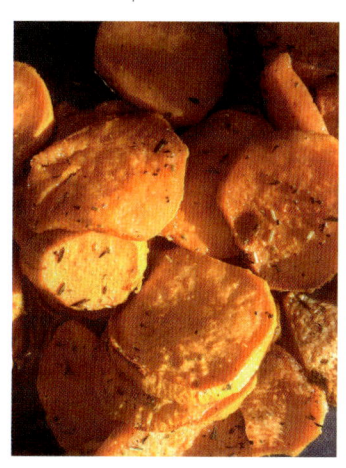

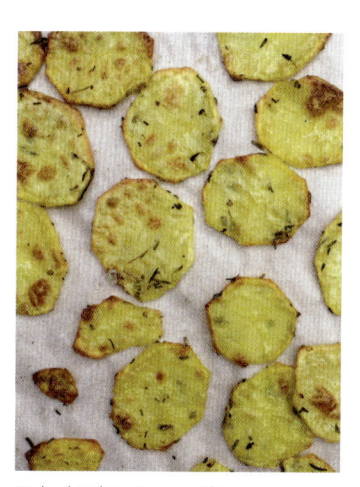

Baked White Potato Chips

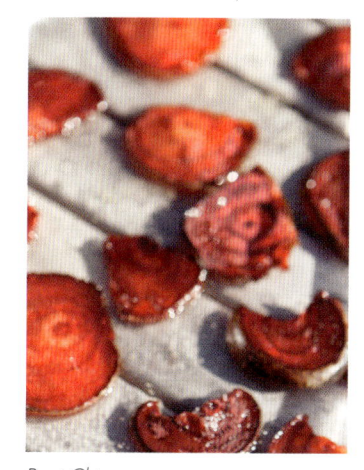

Baked Sweet Potato Chips

Beet Chips

VEGETABLES – *LES LÉGUMES*

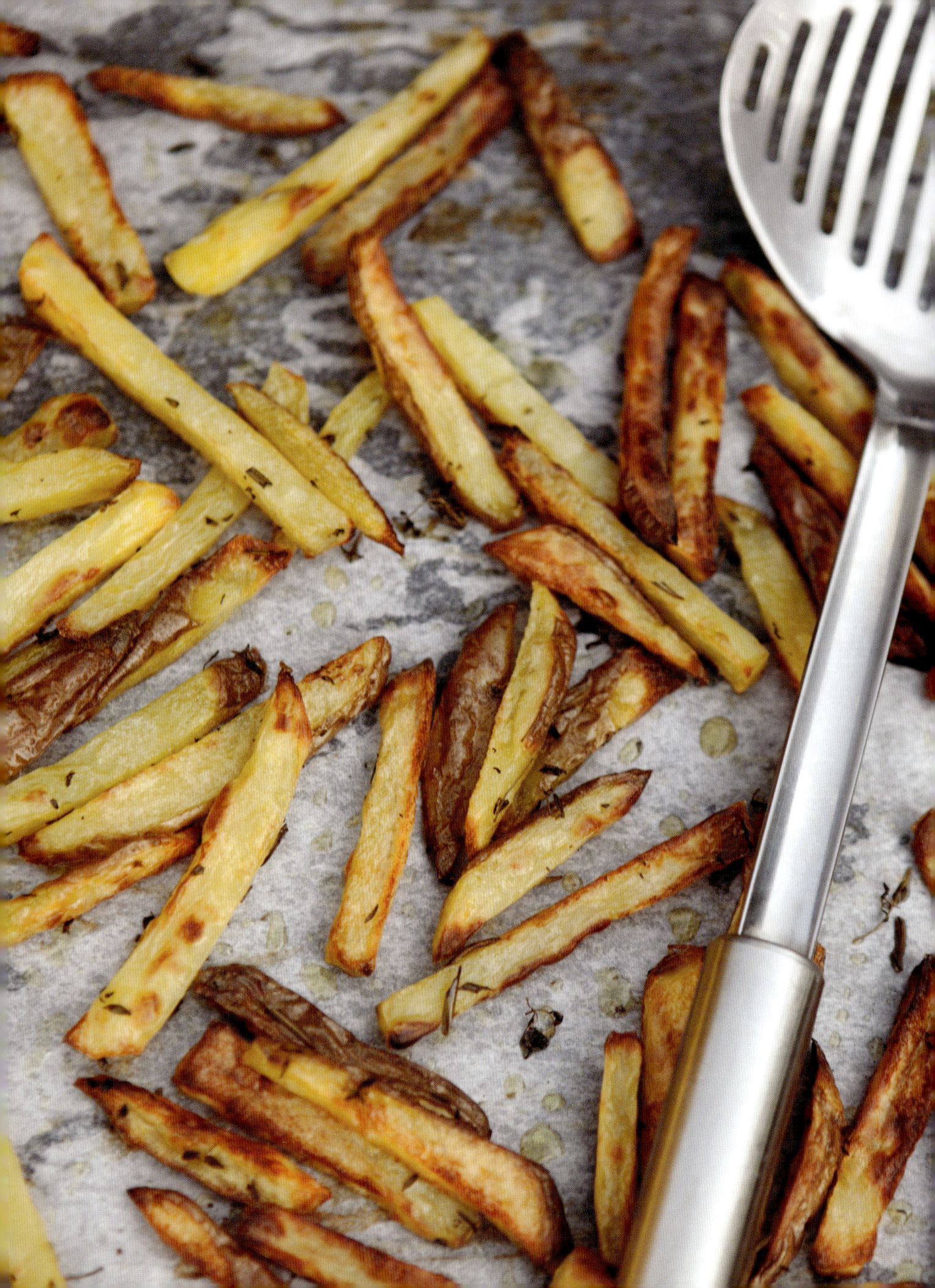

OVEN-BAKED FRENCH FRIES
Pommes Frites au Four

Season Year-round   **Preparation Time** 25 minutes
Cooking Time 25 to 30 minutes   **Serves** 6 to 8

What's a *"steak frites"* without the fries? These easy to make fries are also easy to eat—watch out or you might eat half a tray before dinner is served! In other words, don't try them until they are on your plate and you are at the table (*à table*), or their salt and crunch will lure you and all passersby (i.e., family members) toward them!

- 2.2 pounds (1 kg) potatoes
- 6 tablespoons olive oil
- 4 pinches of salt
- 1 tablespoon fresh rosemary, roughly chopped
- 1 tablespoon fresh thyme, roughly chopped

Preheat the oven to 365°F (185°C). Peel or cut out any "eyes" or other brown or green spots on the potatoes, otherwise leave the peel on. Slice the potatoes lengthwise into sticks that are about ¼-inch to ½-inch (0.6 cm to 1.25 cm) thick and resemble French fries. If you are not baking them right away, store the potato slices in water after slicing them. Drain them and dry them off with a kitchen towel (*torchon*). Otherwise, distribute the freshly-cut potato slices so that they are not overlapping among two oven trays or low-rimmed casserole dishes (the low rims aid in even baking). Drizzle the olive oil over the slices, and sprinkle them with the salt, rosemary, and thyme. Bake for 25 to 30 minutes, stirring the potatoes in their trays once or twice during baking.

Serve with steaks, roasts, or sautéed meats.

VARIATIONS If you do not have fresh rosemary or thyme, replace these with dried herbs, *herbes de Provence*, or just ground black pepper. Prepare and bake sweet potato fries similarly, or fry them in batches (so as not to crowd them in the pan) in coconut oil until cooked through.

OVEN-BAKED SWEET POTATOES
Patates Douces au Four

Season Year-round   **Preparation Time** Less than one minute
Cooking Time One hour to 70 minutes   **Serves** 6 or more

It's hard to overcook a sweet potato. It just keeps caramelizing in the oven, even after you have turned the oven off and have forgotten to remove the potatoes, which I have done on numerous occasions. In France, the organic sweet potatoes I bought came from neighboring Spain.

Preheat the oven to 395°F (200°C), poke little slits into all sides of each sweet potato, and place them in a casserole dish. Bake for 60 to 70 minutes for two to three medium-sized potatoes. This will easily serve six, at half a potato per person. If the sweet potatoes are really thick (4 inches or 10 cm in diameter or more), they might need more time; add 10 to 15 minutes to the baking time, and check if the sweet potato is a bit mushy in the middle. They are easy to reheat for 10 minutes in the oven. (I reheat almost everything for 10 to 12 minutes in oven-safe glass containers at 365°F or 185°C. No microwave needed!) Add bacon fat, butter, ghee, lard, olive oil, tallow, sea salt, cinnamon, and/or nutmeg. It's practically dessert! I eat white potatoes and sweet potatoes and other carbohydrates the way I drink wine: very slowly and deliberately and in very small quantities. It might take me several days to get through one sweet potato, and certainly through one bottle of wine. I eat chicken or veal liver twice or more weekly, and I usually have a bit of sweet potato to go with it, especially when they are in season, autumn through spring.

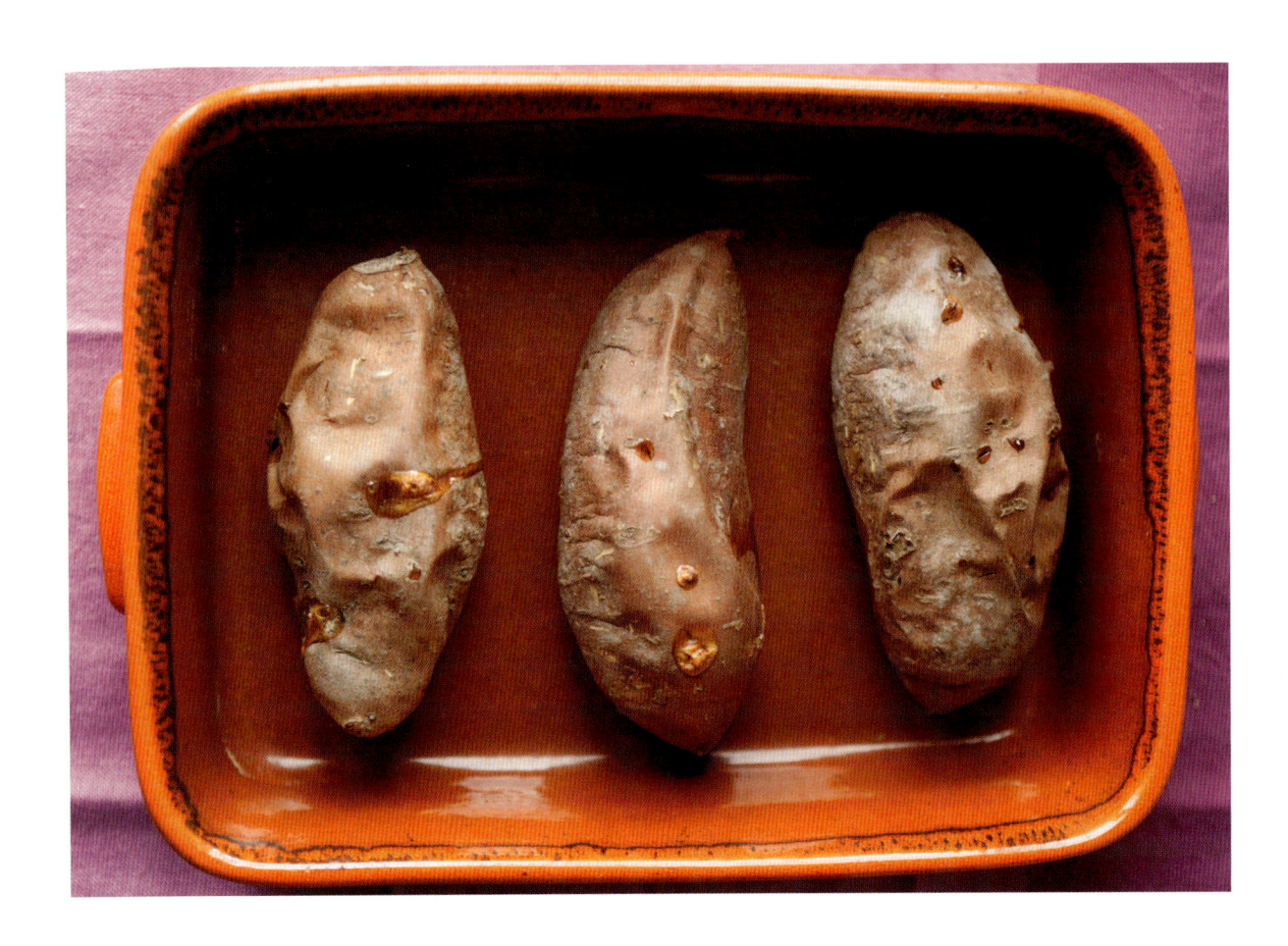

OVEN-BAKED ZUCCHINI
Courgettes au Four

Season May through October   **Preparation Time** 5 minutes
Cooking Time 30 minutes   **Serves** 4 to 5

An easy side dish, this Oven-Baked Zucchini involves very little effort. Chop a couple of zucchinis crosswise into thirds and then into quarters, lengthwise. Pour one to two tablespoons of olive oil over them in an oven-safe dish. Sprinkle on a pinch or two of salt and *herbes de Provence*. Bake in the oven at 365°F (185°C) for about 30 minutes, more if you prefer your zucchini softer. The more olive oil you add, the mushier they are likely to become from soaking in the oil. Add additional olive oil after baking to avoid mushiness. Zucchini are in season June through September. Serves 4 to 5.

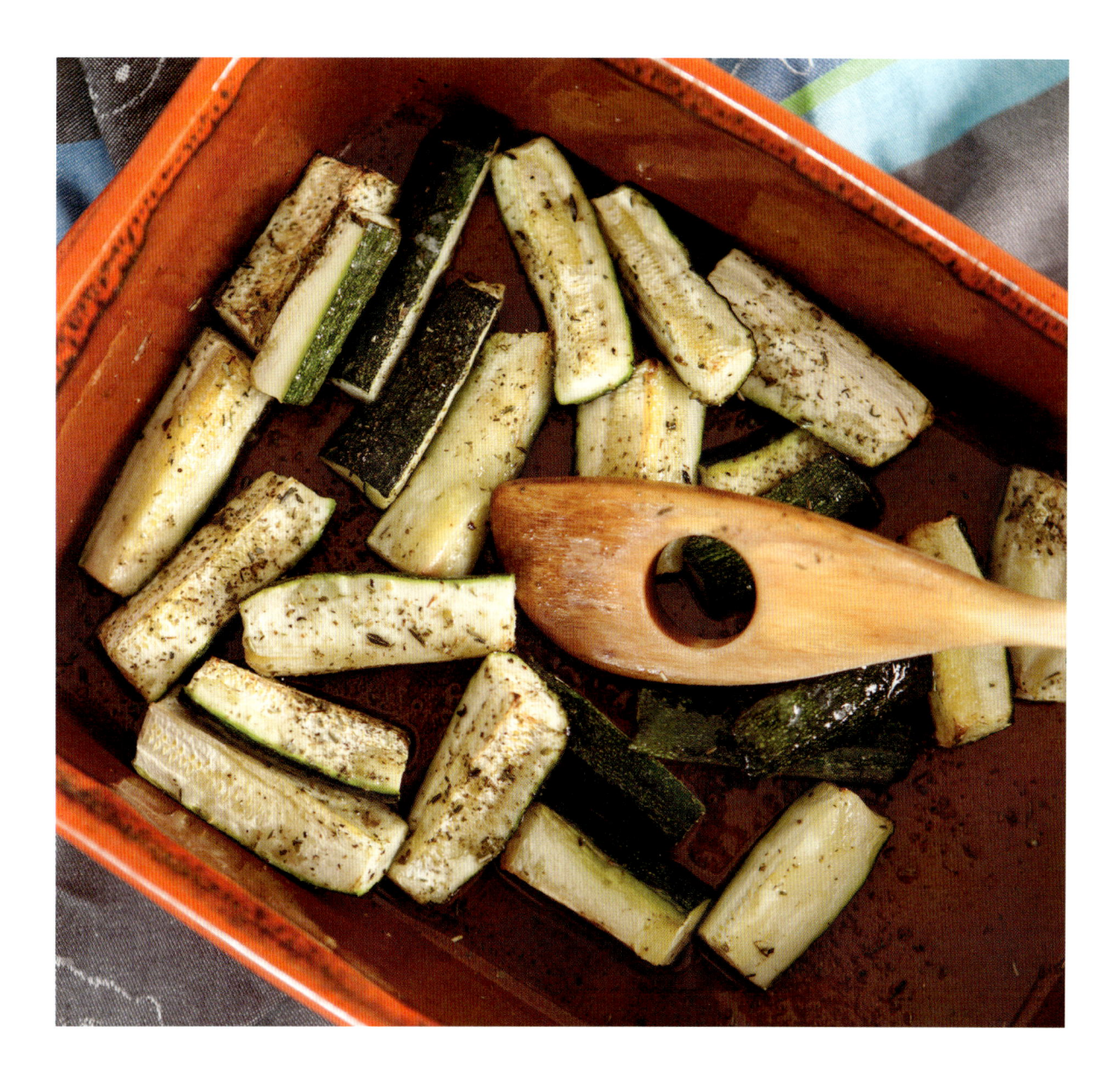

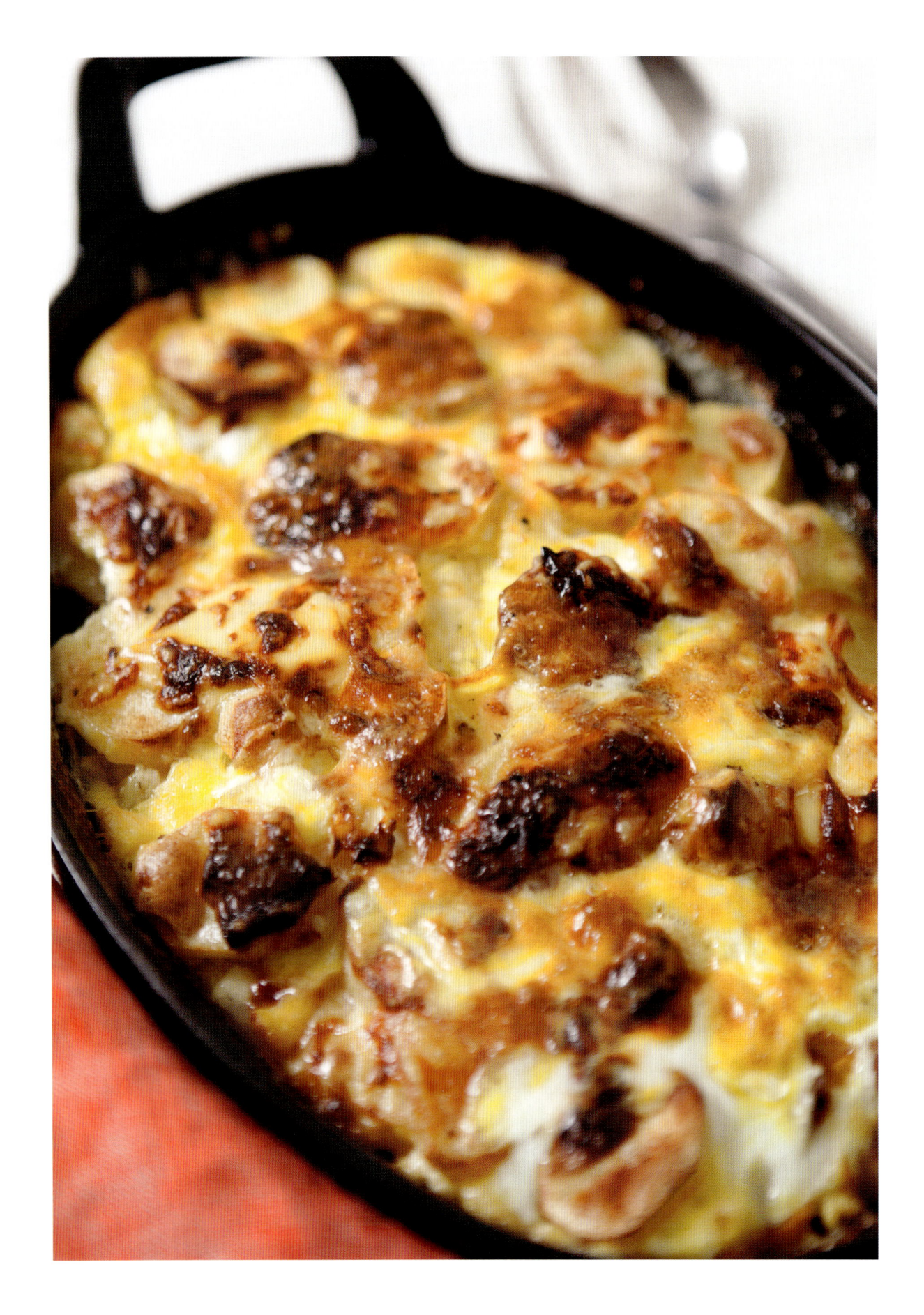

POTATO GRATIN "DAUPHINOIS"
Gratin Dauphinois

Season Late Spring through Winter   **Preparation Time** 45 minutes
Cooking Time 1 hour and 15 minutes   **Serves** 6 to 8

This dish originates from the Southeast of France and was first served alongside small fowl in the late 1700s. Born in mid-19th century France, famed Chef Auguste Escoffier added the flourish of the egg and sour cream topping to complete this dish. Escoffier updated France's traditional cuisine to *haute cuisine* and was responsible for elevating cooking to a respected profession along with publishing the definitive textbook and guide to cooking, *Le Guide Culinaire*, in 1903.

This dish is loaded with the usual high-fat ingredients of butter (*le beurre*), sour cream (*la crème fraîche*), milk (*le lait*), and cheese (*le fromage*). This recipe actually calls for Emmental (Swiss cheese), but you could also use French Gruyère or another hard cheese of your liking. You can't go wrong unless you are allergic to dairy or if the potatoes are likely to spike your blood sugar levels too much, in which case the portion can be made smaller, depending on your tolerances.

1 tablespoon butter (more if desired)

4 garlic cloves (more if desired), minced

3.3 pounds (1.5 kg) potatoes, peeled and sliced in ⅛-inch (0.3 cm) rounds (*rondelles*)

Fine salt and ground pepper, for seasoning

⅖ cup (200 ml) sour cream (*crème fraîche*)

7 ounces (200 g) Emmental cheese, grated

⅘ cup (200 ml) whole milk

1 egg

Serve with roasted vegetables and a grilled or roasted meat dish, such as leg of lamb, or a poultry or pork roast.

Preheat the oven to 365°F (185°C). Butter a casserole dish on the bottom and sides. Add extra chunks of butter to the bottom, if desired, for an extra buttery base. Sprinkle the garlic around the base of the dish. Add a layer of potato slices and sprinkle with salt and pepper. Using a spatula or the back of a spoon, spread a layer of sour cream on the potato layer. Cover the sour cream layer with a thin layer of cheese. Start again with a layer of potato slices and continue layering until you have filled the dish to about half an inch from the top of the dish, saving one tablespoon of sour cream. Finish with a layer of cheese on top. Gently pour in the milk, distributing it over the potatoes. Cook for one hour.

Beat the egg with the tablespoon of sour cream and distribute this over the potatoes at the one-hour mark. Place the casserole dish in the oven again and allow to cook for about 15 more minutes until golden brown on top.

PUMPKIN SOUP
Purée de Potiron

Season September and October   **Preparation Time** 30 minutes
Cooking Time 1 hour 15 minutes   **Serves** 8

If you have a whole pumpkin, use one half of the pumpkin for this purée and the other half for a Paleo Pumpkin Pie,[3] for example (shown below, left). Only in season September and October, pumpkins can luckily be stored whole until about December if kept cool and dry. Pumpkin and squash can also be roasted and then frozen, and some people even ferment them. Pumpkin (and butternut squash) is a useful ingredient to have on hand, not only for this soup, but also for sweet pancakes or savory fritters.

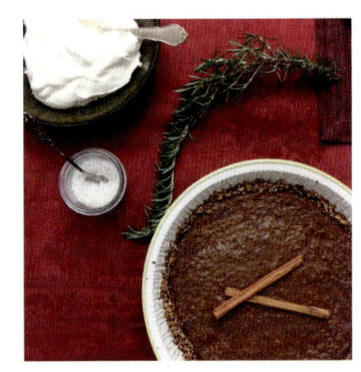

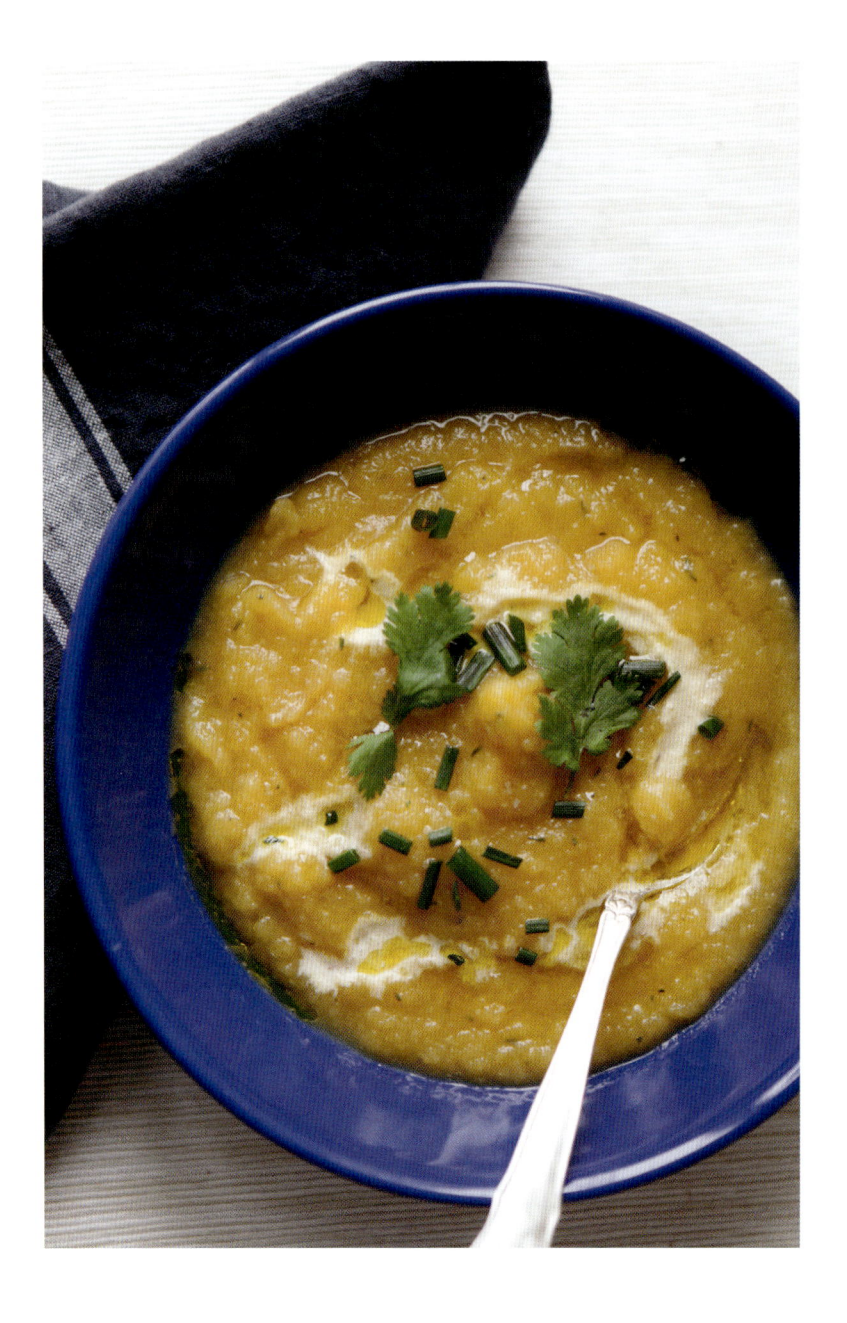

Paleo Pumpkin Pie

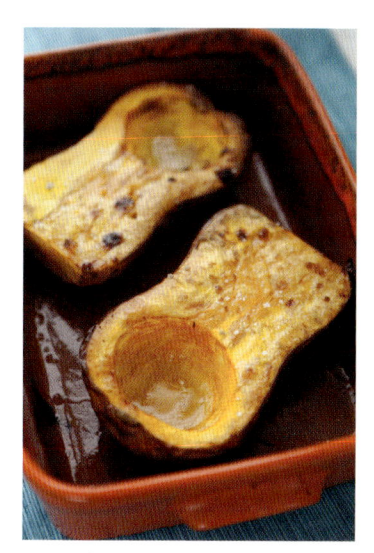

½ large pumpkin (about 5 cups, 640 g, of pumpkin flesh)

2 tablespoons olive oil, plus more to taste

4 pinches of sea salt, plus more to taste

2 tablespoon butter or ghee

2 shallots, minced

2 cloves garlic, minced

1 teaspoon fresh grated ginger

2 cups (475 ml) poultry or chicken stock (page 417)

1 teaspoon thyme, fresh or dried

Roasted Butternut Squash

Preheat the oven to 365°F (185°C). Cut the half pumpkin in half again. Drizzle the olive oil over the pumpkin pieces and sprinkle them with a pinch of salt. Roast in an oven-safe dish for 50 to 60 minutes or until soft. Follow the steps I use for roasted butternut squash (pictured).

Allow to cool. Peel off the skin with a paring knife and cut the pumpkin flesh into chunks. (Now you have roasted pumpkin and could stop here. Add *herbes de Provence*, and just eat that!)

Heat the butter in a pan and sauté the shallots and garlic with salt until the shallots become translucent.

Combine the ginger, poultry stock, and thyme with the roasted pumpkin chunks, shallots, and garlic in batches in a blender. For a thinner consistency, add ½ cup (120 ml) more stock. Cook in a pot for 15 minutes on low.

Drizzle the pumpkin purée with cream or olive oil (or both!), if desired. You may top with ground pepper, fresh herbs (such as thyme), cinnamon, nutmeg, bacon bits (*lardons*), and/or coarse salt or *fleur del sel*. Serve with **Pig's Feet Sliders** (page 259) as shown.

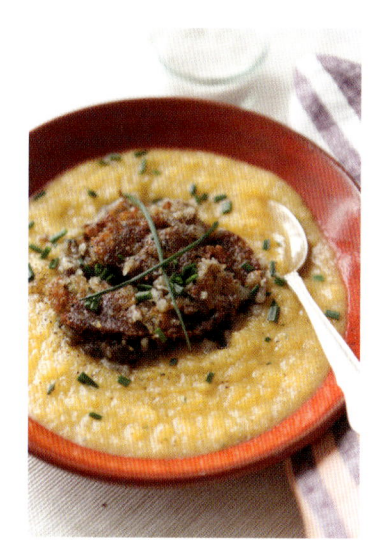

*Pumpkin Purée with **Pig's Feet Sliders***

ROASTED ROOT VEGETABLES
Légumes Racines Rôtis

Season Most Root Vegetables are Year-round   **Preparation Time** 10 minutes
Cooking Time 40 to 60 minutes   **Makes** multiple servings, depending on the number of vegetables prepared

As mentioned in Chapter 4 on the topic of "Root Vegetables in France" (page 51), the French use a variety of these in their cooking. Root vegetables of one kind or another can be found year-round. Fresh root vegetables can easily be roasted in the oven for a simple side dish by drizzling olive oil (or duck fat) over them and sprinkling dried or fresh herbs, such as rosemary or thyme, and adding some coarse salt (for crunch). For example, you could roast several chopped beets, turnips, and potatoes, as shown, for 40 minutes at 395°F (200°C) or for 50 to 60 minutes at 365°F (185°C), stirring every 10 to 15 minutes to ensure even cooking and to distribute the oil and salt among the vegetables. Root vegetables are starchy by nature, hence small portions combined with lots of fat are advised.

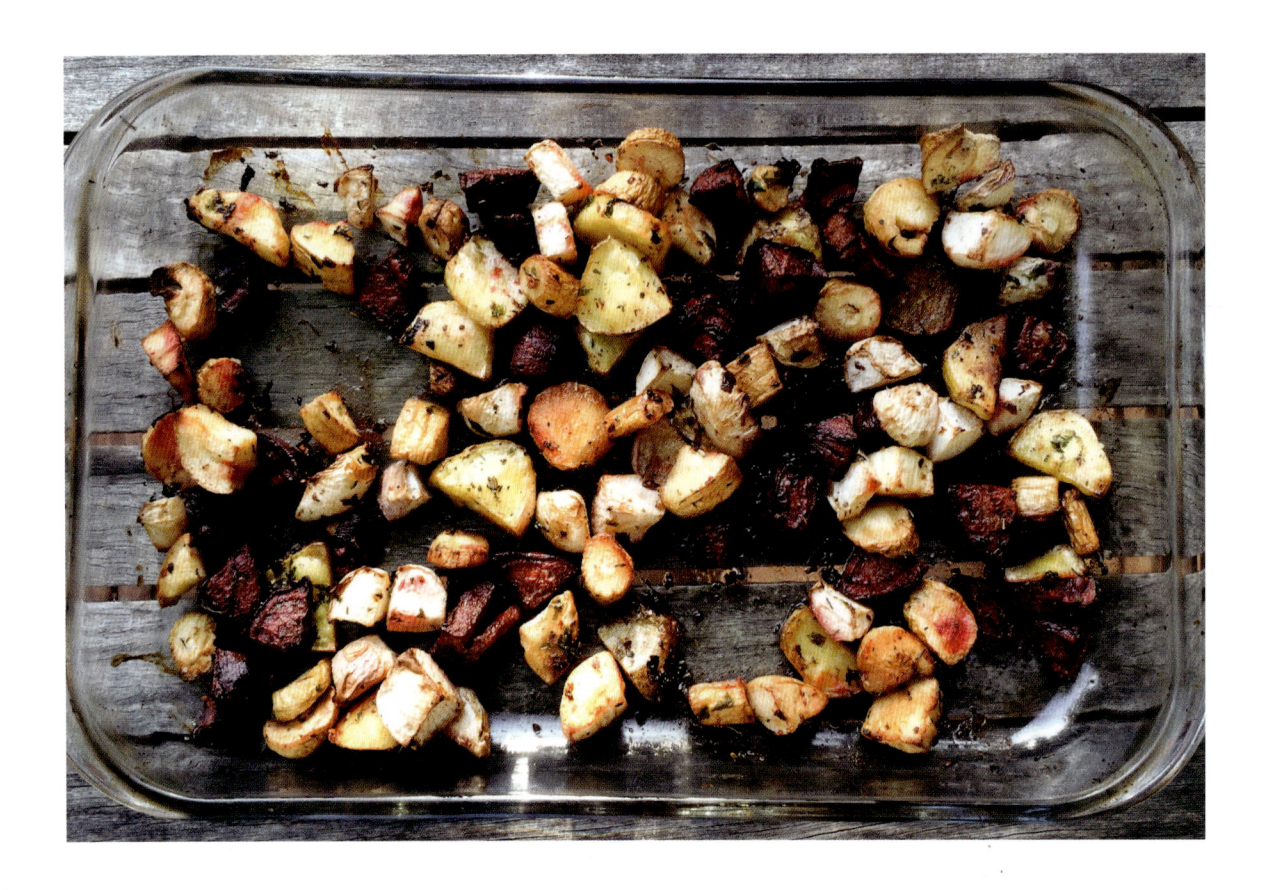

ROASTED SUMMER TOMATOES WITH HERBS
Tomates d'Été Rôties au Herbes

Season May through October   **Preparation Time** 5 to 10 minutes
Cooking Time 30 minutes   **Serves** One to two tomato halves per person

The ripest, most flavorful tomatoes are often found during the summer, though their extended growing season is May through October. As an easy, flavorful side dish, cut a few medium or large tomatoes in half, drizzle them with olive oil, and sprinkle on coarse salt and fresh, chopped herbs (such as rosemary or thyme, or *herbes de Provence*), and roast in the oven at 395°F (200°C) for 30 minutes. One ancestral technique for those sensitive to nightshade vegetables is to peel and deseed the tomatoes first. (Blanching a tomato in boiling water for 30 to 60 seconds will loosen the skin for easier peeling.)

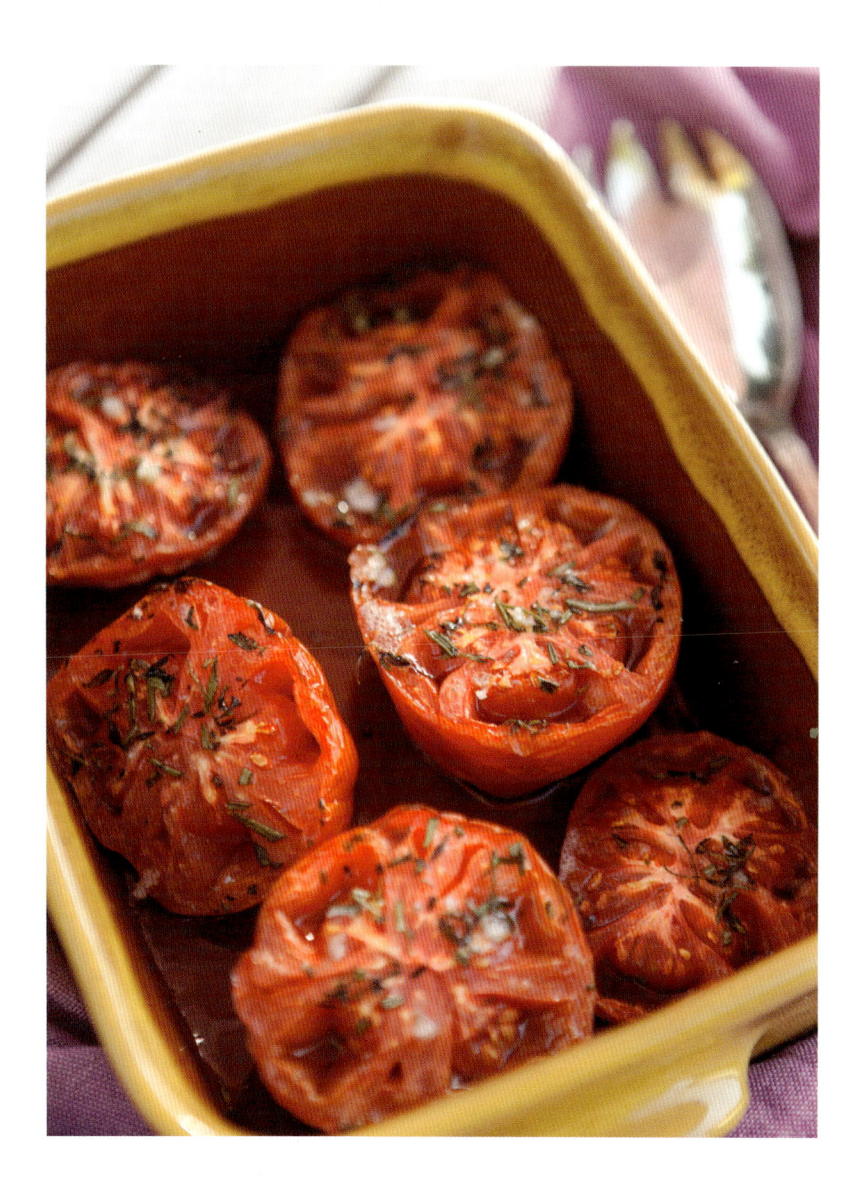

SARLAT SAUTÉED POTATOES
Pommes de Terre Sarladaises

Season Late Spring through Winter   **Preparation Time** 15 minutes
Cooking Time 30 minutes   **Serves** 6 to 8

This is one recipe I have prepared seemingly hundreds of times on the stove (or sometimes in the oven), as it goes with everything cooked in the Southwest of France, but most famously with **Preserved Duck Legs** (page 357). The recipe's origin is Sarlat, a medieval town deep in the Périgord region of the Southwest, known for its ducks (and duck fat), pork, truffles, and walnuts, and located in the district of Dordogne. Duck farming, *foie gras*, and **Sarlat Sautéed Potatoes** (*Pommes de Terre Sarladaises*) are culinary mainstays of the Périgord. In fact, in the interest of tourism and geographic distinction, the Périgord is divided into four agricultural and topographical sub-regions: Green (*Périgord Vert*, with Nontron as its capital) for its forests and vegetations; White (*Périgord Blanc*, with Périgeux as its capital) for its chalky-white earth and river-hewn cliffs; Purple (*Périgord Pourpre*, with Bergerac as its capital) for its vineyards; and Black (*Périgord Noir*, with Sarlat as its capital) for its dark oak and chestnut trees and fertile soil.[4] Incidentally, just outside Sarlat you will find Lascaux, one of the largest and most intact Paleolithic caves in France, discovered by chance in 1940 by four boys and their dog.

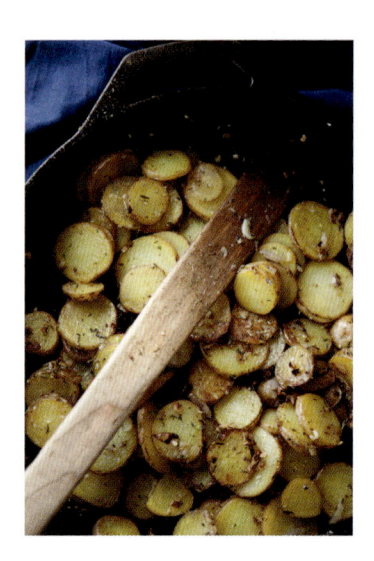

Potatoes are in season almost year-round, from May through February, and they preserve well out of season. To keep peeled potatoes from turning brown, I often submerge them in water immediately after peeling and/or cutting them. However, for this dish, I have found that the potatoes become too floppy for sautéing in the pan after being soaked in water. So, for this dish, I do not peel them, and I just try to be swift about slicing them. These potatoes may be slathered in even more duck fat, as desired. Being potatoes, they are a bit addictive. Watch your serving size, it might suddenly grow and the number of servings diminish as people come back for seconds. Kids love these potatoes, too. If you are doubling the recipe, use a separate pan for each pound (about 500 g) of potatoes, as they take longer to cook and get steamed rather than fried if they are too crowded in a pan. There are many ways to season this dish: with or without parsley, with or without pepper, etc. Onions (red or yellow) may replace the shallots if you do not have shallots on hand. Shallots have a sweeter, milder flavor than onions, which is perhaps partly why children tend to love this dish. As I have found my preferred combinations of ingredients, you, too, will find the combination that works for you based on what you have on hand in your pantry or based on your flavor preferences.

3 tablespoons duck fat

1.1 pounds (500 g) potatoes, cut into ⅛-inch (0.3 cm) slices

3 pinches of coarse sea salt

5 garlic cloves, minced

2 shallots, minced

2 tablespoons fresh thyme

Optional: 2 tablespoons olive oil

Optional: 1 tablespoon parsley, minced

Optional: 2 pinches of *herbes de Provence*

Optional: 2 pinches of ground pepper

Melt the duck fat in a large skillet over medium-high heat. Add the sliced potatoes, stirring occasionally for 7 to 10 minutes, allowing the potatoes to partially cook through (about 15 minutes) before adding the remaining ingredients. Allow another five minutes of cooking before reducing the heat to medium and cooking for another 10 to 15 minutes, stirring frequently as the ingredients stick to the bottom of the pan and caramelize. (This is where much of the flavor comes from!) The total cooking time will be about 30 minutes. Once the potatoes are cooked through, the skillet may be left on low for several minutes to keep it warm, stirring occasionally, while you finish preparing the other parts of your meal.

Serve with **Preserved Duck Legs** (page 357), chicken, hamburgers, and other red meats (grilled, roasted, or sautéed), or with fish. (The French will also serve these potatoes with trout, for example.)

VARIATIONS This recipe varies slightly in ingredients from cook to cook, with the exception of the potatoes, garlic, salt, and duck fat. The original recipes do not call for *herbes de Provence* or olive oil, as these are from the Southeast of France and this is a traditional recipe from the Southwest, in which parsley is usually used. Nevertheless, olive oil can augment the duck fat. I tend to make *pommes sarladaises* with (fresh and dried) thyme and rosemary or *herbes de Provence*, again, according to what I have available to me at the time of cooking. Some cooks add bacon pieces (*lardons*) or porcini mushrooms (*cèpes*). To make a similar dish from the Landes, a sizeable region in the French Southwest, called **Landaise Sautéed Potatoes – *Pommes de Terre à la Landaise*,** sauté diced potatoes in duck or goose fat, along with two diced onions, several pinches of salt and pepper, and then, during the last five minutes of cooking, add two handfuls of diced ham.

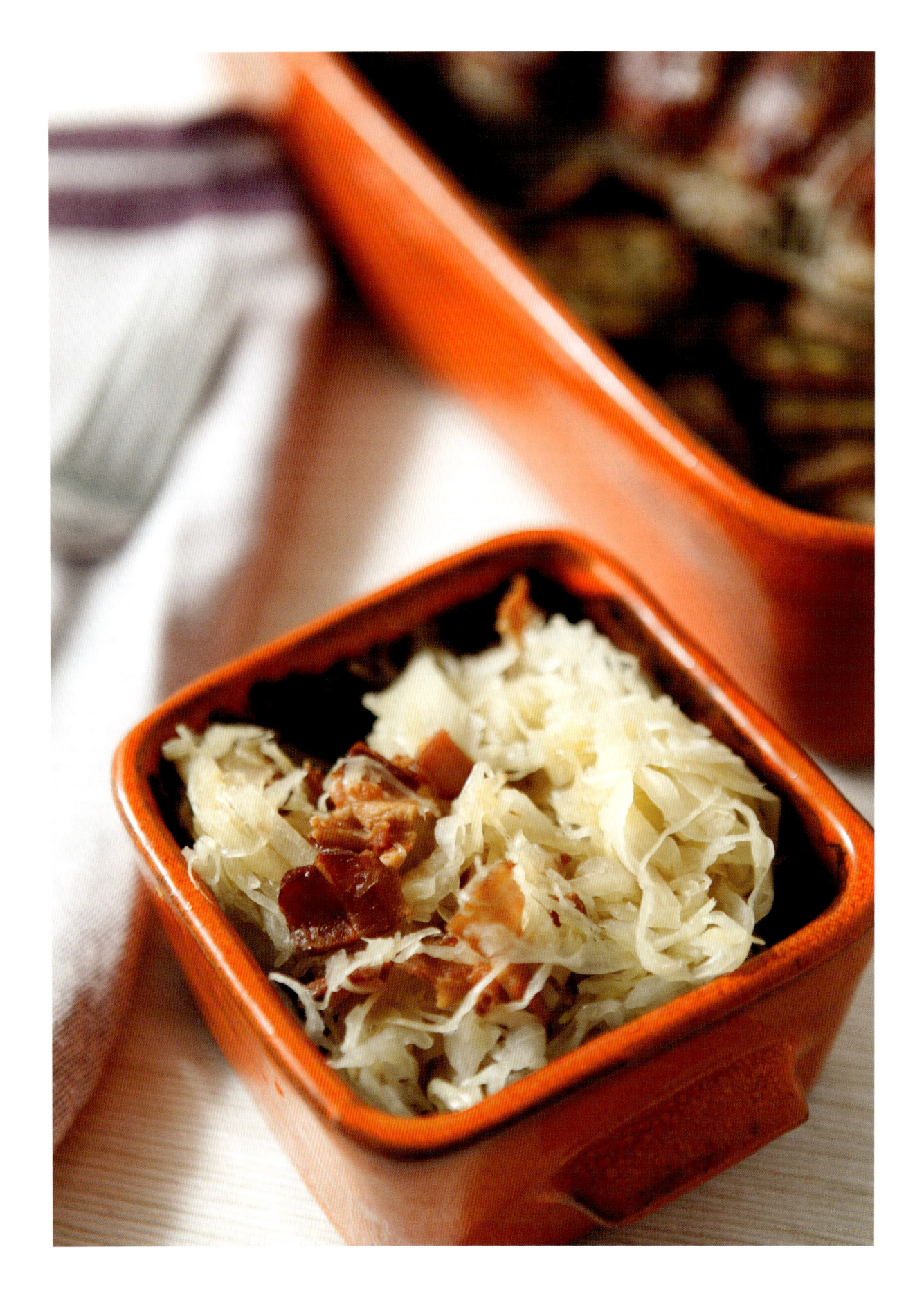

SAUERKRAUT AND BACON
Choucroute aux Lardons

Season Year-round   **Preparation** Time None
Cooking Time 10 minutes   **Makes** many small servings

Sauerkraut (*choucroute*) and bacon is an Alsatian staple side dish. You can make your own homemade sauerkraut (see page 52), which is fermented cabbage, for use in this simple dish, or buy it readymade. I sometimes buy organic sauerkraut already spiced with juniper berries and unpasteurized, but the best is always homemade.

1 tablespoon lard

4 ounces (115 g) bacon pieces (*lardons*)

1.1 pounds (500 g) raw sauerkraut

Melt the lard in a pan over medium-high heat and add the bacon pieces. Stir occasionally until all the pieces have turned the desired shade of brown and crispiness. (This might take 5 to 10 minutes.) Stir in the sauerkraut until just incorporated and turn off the heat. This will keep some of the enzymes and good bacteria intact (not fully cooked off), maintaining the beneficial bacterial integrity of the raw sauerkraut.

Serve with pork or sausages made from beef, chicken, pork, turkey, or veal.

SAUTÉED LEEKS AND BACON
Poivrons Sautés aux Lardons

Season Autumn through early Spring   **Preparation Time** Less than 5 minutes
Cooking Time 15 minutes   **Serves** 4 to 6

The French get their daily dose of sulfurous vegetables by eating a lot of onions, garlic, and leeks. These are also all FODMAPs (fermentable oligo-, di-, mono-saccharides, and polyols—essentially large, difficult carbohydrate molecules to digest), so some people need to limit these in their diet. Leek greens are part of the garnished bouquet (*bouquet garni*), a small bunch of herbs, usually tied together with a string and including leek, thyme, parsley, and a bay leaf. Here I have combined leek with bacon pieces (*lardons*), as the flavor combination is rich and savory and makes a fine accompaniment to grilled meats, roasts, white fish, or salmon. Leeks are in season September through March, therefore they are a handy staple for all those soups and slow-cooked meals through the fall and winter.

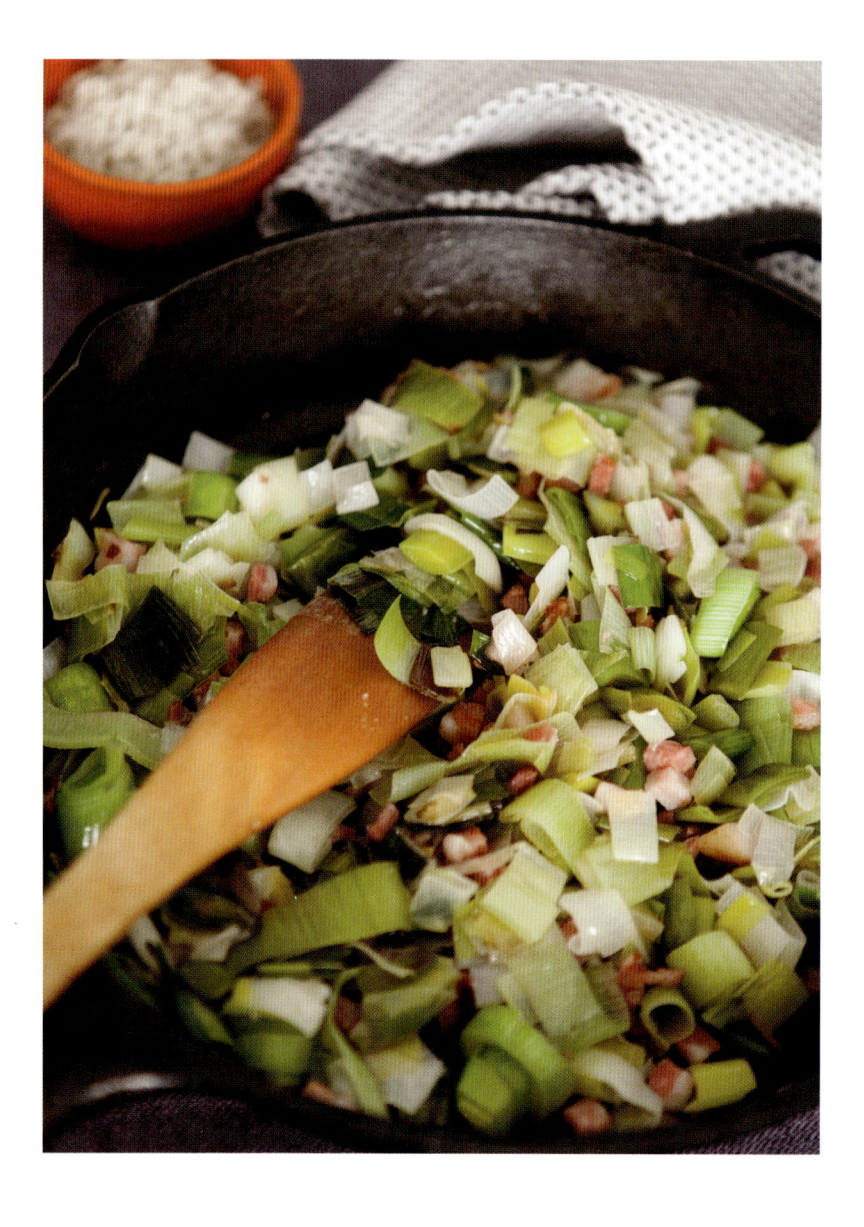

Washing Leeks

My method of washing leeks is simply to tear the outer layers open halfway and rinse out the dirt in between the layers (at about the spot where the "leaves" begin to separate and change from light green to dark green) and then run these under cold water. You can also cut the leeks at this spot and soak them in water for a few minutes, swishing them around to release the dirt stuck between the layers of "leaves" in the sheath. Either way, you usually end up chopping the leek, so looks don't matter so much. I am usually more concerned about time than appearance, unless the vegetable is having its portrait taken.

1 tablespoon lard or duck fat

1 to 2 leeks, washed and sliced into ⅓-inch to ½-inch (0.8 cm to 1.27 cm) rounds

Handful of bacon pieces (*lardons*)

Pinch of fine salt

Melt the fat in a large frying pan over medium heat, and add the leeks, bacon pieces, and salt. Stir occasionally for 15 minutes, allowing the leeks and bacon to brown, then reduce the heat. Serve with grilled meats, roasts, or fish.

VARIATIONS I have added chopped radicchio to this mix, and the fat cuts its bitterness. Chopped palm or "Lacinto" kale (*chou palmier*) may also be sautéed with *lardons* (as shown in the photo below), as can Swiss chard (see the recipe for **Sautéed Swiss Chard** on page 474), but both need less time to sauté. In the case of kale and chard, begin browning the bacon for several minutes before adding the greens. The options are many. What *doesn't* go with bacon?!

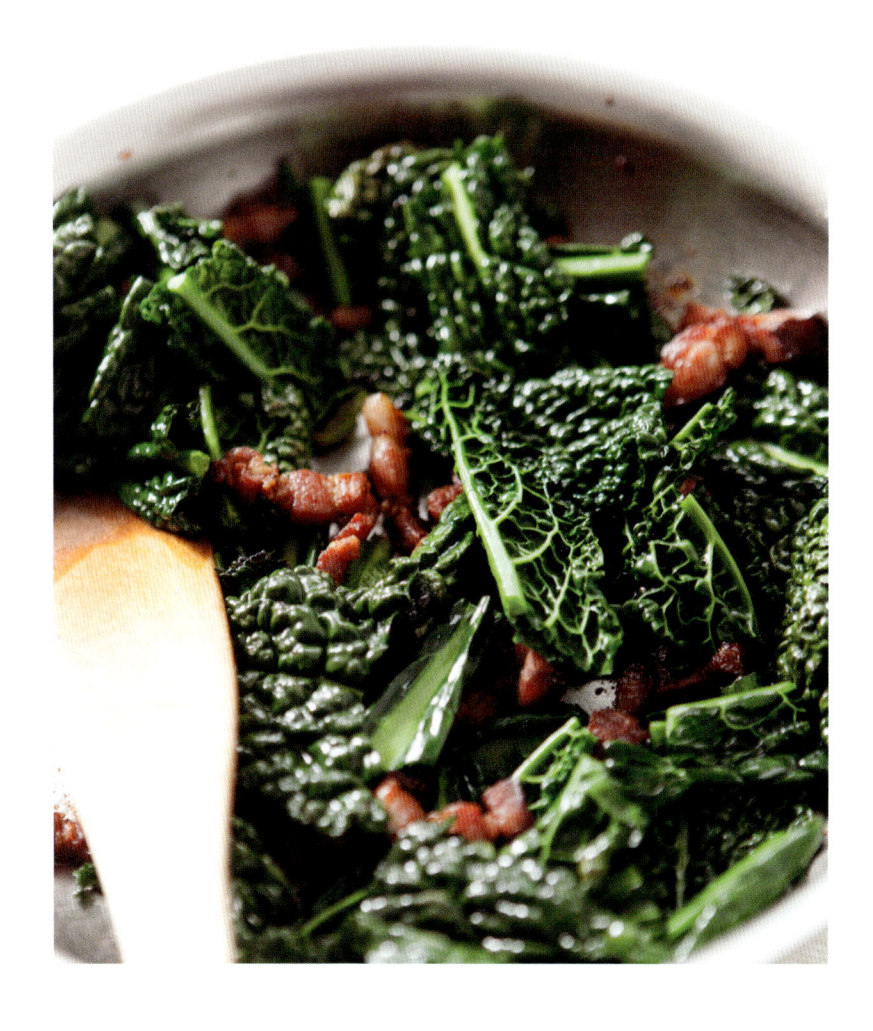

SAUTÉED ONIONS
Oignons Sautés

Season Year-round   **Preparation Time** 5 minutes   **Cooking Time** 20 minutes   **Serves** 3 to 4

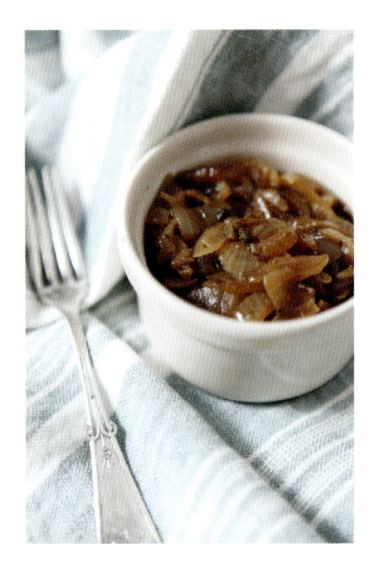

Always a welcome garnishing side dish when buttery, melt-in-your-mouth flavor is called for, **Sautéed Onions** are simple and delicious. They can be prepared as described here or as in the **Chicken in Wine Sauce "Coq Au Vin"** recipe on page 345.

2 tablespoons butter or ghee

4 onions, quartered and sliced

Melt the butter in a large pan over medium-high to high heat. Brown the onions for several minutes, then reduce the temperature to medium and continue to brown for another 10 to 15 minutes until desired softness is achieved.

Serve over steaks or roasts.

SAUTÉED SWISS CHARD
Blettes Sautées

Season April through October   **Preparation Time** Less than 5 minutes
Cooking Time 15 to 20 minutes   **Serves** 4 to 6 per bunch of chard

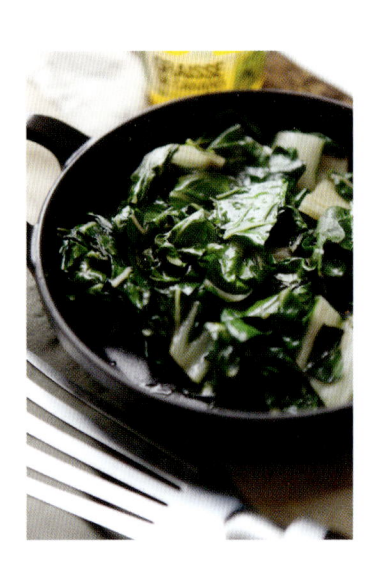

This recipe can of course be used for other types of chard, such as rainbow chard. Chard is in season April through October. I have found that sautéing chard on higher than medium heat makes the stems turn a brownish black. To avoid this, I have found that removing most of the stems and heating the chopped leaves slowly works best. If you have several vegetable sides in the making, put these on the stove first so they have a good 15 to 20 minutes to sit on medium-low on the stove. Stir them occasionally in duck fat (*graisse de canard*), as shown here, or coconut oil, until they reach the consistency you like, either just wilted and a bit crispy or completely wilted and a bit mushier (easier to digest for some people). Chop the stems into bite-size chunks and boil them separately for 25 minutes in water and/or stock. Add salt, pepper, butter, and grated cheese or a white sauce like **Béchamel Sauce** (page 292) for another tasty side dish.

SAUTÉED WHITE ASPARAGUS SLICES
Tranches Fines d'Asperges Blanches Pôelées

Season Mid-Spring through early Summer   **Preparation Time** Less than 5 minutes
Cooking Time 5 to 7 minutes   **Serves** 4 to 6

I learned this simple recipe from Chef Célia, instructor at the *Côté Cours* cooking school in Bouliac outside Bordeaux where I took several cooking classes. This "trick of the trade" was really meant as a pretty and tasty garnish for seafood or meat, with just a few slices gracing an appetizer or main dish, but more slices will make a side dish. Instead of thinly slicing the asparagus, you can also just slice the shoots in half or use green asparagus, slicing larger shoots in half lengthwise or sautéing thinner ones unsliced. White asparagus shoots must additionally be peeled with a peeler. I peel them first before snapping off the ends. Their season is short, April through June, so enjoy them while they are bountiful and at their peak (and least expensive). This recipe amounts to simply frying up asparagus, rather than steaming it, which is the only way I had known one could prepare asparagus! But where's the fat in that? Use your favorite fat, and lots of it.

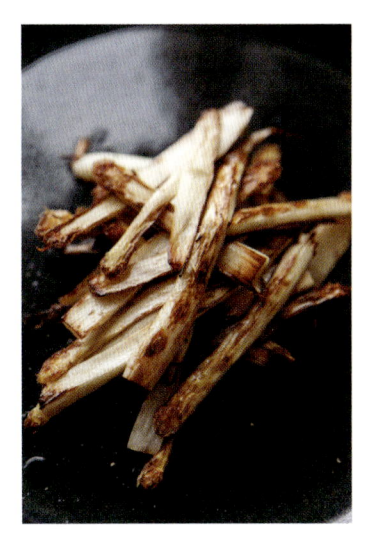

2 tablespoons duck fat or lard

1.1 pounds (500 g) white asparagus, thinly sliced, ends snapped off

Pinch of fine salt, plus extra if needed

Melt the fat in a pan over medium-high heat. Place as many slices of the asparagus flat in the pan as will fit without crowding them. If they do not all fit, sauté them in batches, sprinkling a bit of extra salt onto each batch. Sprinkle the salt over the asparagus. Flip each slice over after two or three minutes.

Serve over fish or meat dishes as garnish or as its own side dish.

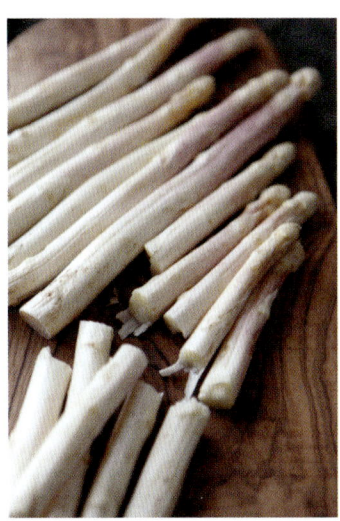

TRADITIONAL SALAD FROM NICE
Salade Niçoise

Season Late Spring through early Autumn   **Preparation Time** 15 minutes
Cooking Time 14 minutes (for hard boiled eggs), 10 minutes for softer yolks   **Serves** 4

Being from Nice, my friend Joelle could not forego the chance to show me how to make an authentic Salade Niçoise, along with a **Simple Vinaigrette** (page 413) or **Niçoise Vinaigrette** (page 409).

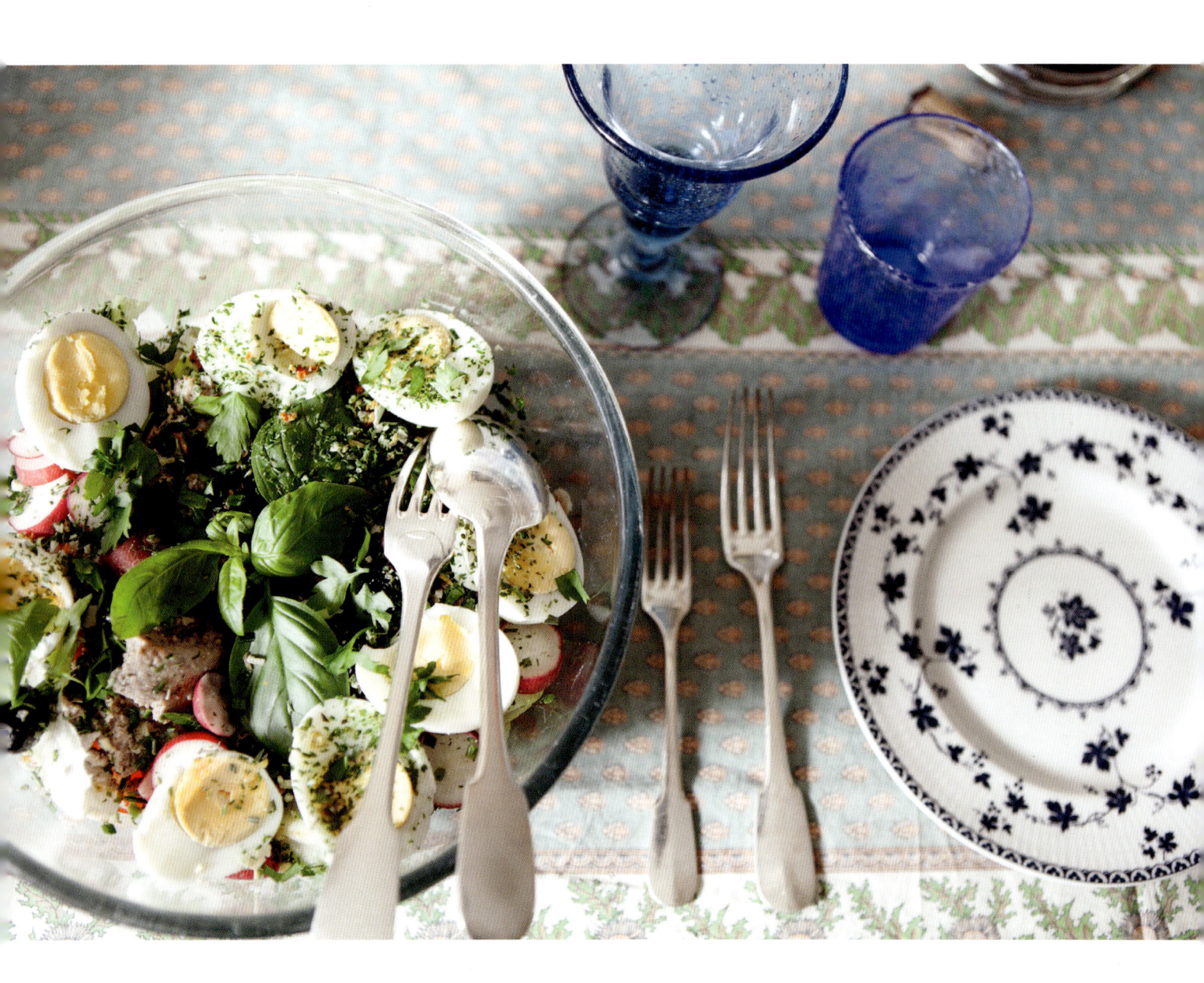

1 onion, chopped

1 to 2 garlic cloves, minced

4 to 6 large, ripe tomatoes, cut into 8 to 10 semi-circle slices

1 long or 2 short cucumbers, sliced into rounds

1 celery heart, chopped

5 radishes, finely sliced

Small handful of chives, minced

4 hard-boiled eggs, peeled and quartered or sliced

1 can of tuna (*thon*) in water or olive oil

1 can of sardines (*sardines*) in olive oil

1 green pepper, sliced into strips (*lamelles*)

1 lettuce heart or lamb's lettuce (*la mâche*)

6 to 10 black olives, originating from Nice, of course! (*bien sûr!*)

Gently mix the ingredients together in a large bowl, topping the salad with the olives. Serve with a **Simple Vinaigrette** (page 413) or a **Niçoise Vinaigrette** (page 409).

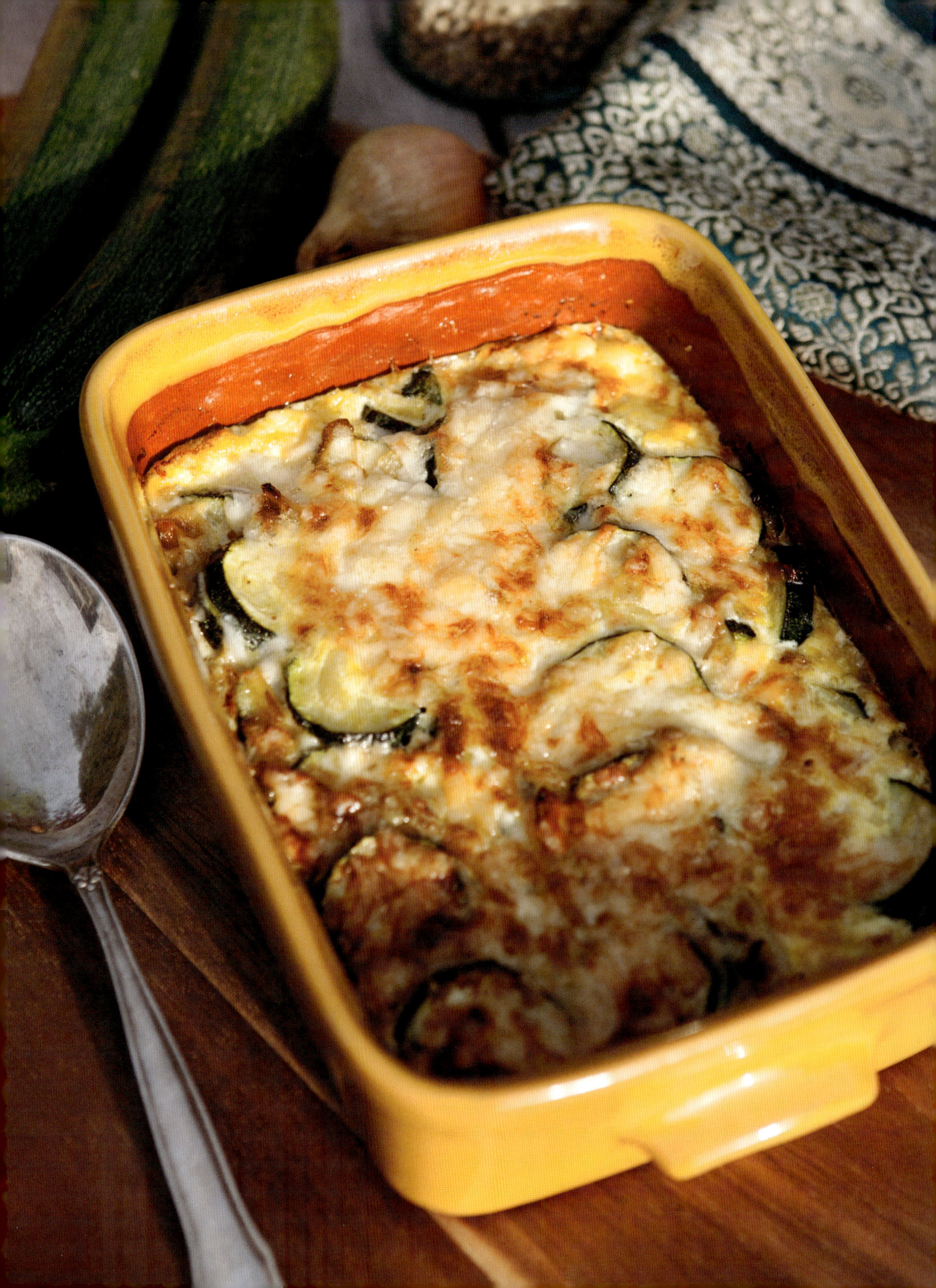

VEGETABLE "CLAFOUTIS"
Clafoutis aux Légumes

Season Depends on the choice of vegetable   **Preparation Time** 10 minutes
Cooking Time 12 to 20 minutes on the stove, plus 25 to 30 minutes in the oven   **Serves** 6 to 8

The *clafoutis* originates from the Limousin region in the French Southwest where it is made with whole, unpitted dark cherries and served as a dessert. (See **Aunt Lucie's Millas** recipe on page 484 for the dessert version of a clafoutis to which whole or chopped fruit may be added.) A vegetable clafoutis is much like an omelet, or a *frittata* (an Italian fried or baked egg dish), or a quiche without the crust. A clafoutis can be eaten at any meal as a side dish. The trick to a vegetable clafoutis is softening the vegetables in lots of butter (or ghee) in a pan before baking them in a milk and egg mixture. In this recipe, I use zucchini and onion as a typical example, but other in-season vegetables may be used instead. White pepper is used here for its herbaceous, vegetal aroma and because it blends in well with the white-colored mixture of the clafoutis. Feel free to use black pepper instead or even other powdered or ground spices of your choice, such as cayenne pepper, garlic, ginger, turmeric, etc. Zucchini is in season from June through September.

VARIATIONS To add flavor and richness to the clafoutis, sauté 3 garlic cloves along with the zucchini and onions and add two tablespoons of sour cream (*crème fraiche*) and ½ teaspoon turmeric to the milk and egg mixture. Top with ⅓ cup of a hard cheese, like Emmental or Gruyère, as shown in the photo below. Another option is to sprinkle the clafoutis with **Duck Rinds** (page 359.)

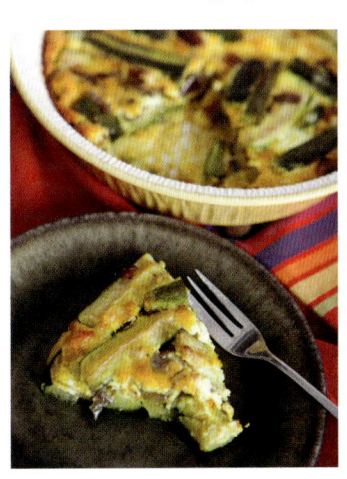

4 tablespoons butter, ghee or duck fat

2 to 3 medium zucchinis (about 1 pound or 450 g), cut into ⅓-inch rounds (0.8 cm)

2 to 4 small onions (about 5 ounces or 140 g), halved and thinly sliced

2 pinches of fine salt

3 pinches of white pepper

2 eggs

¾ cup (180 ml) whole milk

Optional: ½ cup (about 4 ounces or 110 g) grated hard cheese

Preheat the oven to 365°F (185°C). Melt three tablespoons of butter in a large frying pan over medium-high to medium heat. Stir in the zucchini, onions, salt, and pepper and sauté for 12 to 20 minutes, depending on how soft you prefer your vegetables. Transfer the sautéed vegetables to an 8- or 9-inch (20 cm to 23 cm) casserole dish.

In a separate bowl, whisk together the eggs and milk. Pour this mixture over the vegetables in the casserole dish and flatten the zucchinis in the dish so that they are mostly covered by the mixture. Optional step: Top with ½ cup grated hard cheese such as Gruyère, as shown in the main recipe photo. Bake for 25 minutes, until it is brown on top and a bit "custardy" inside. Serve alongside grilled or roasted meats.

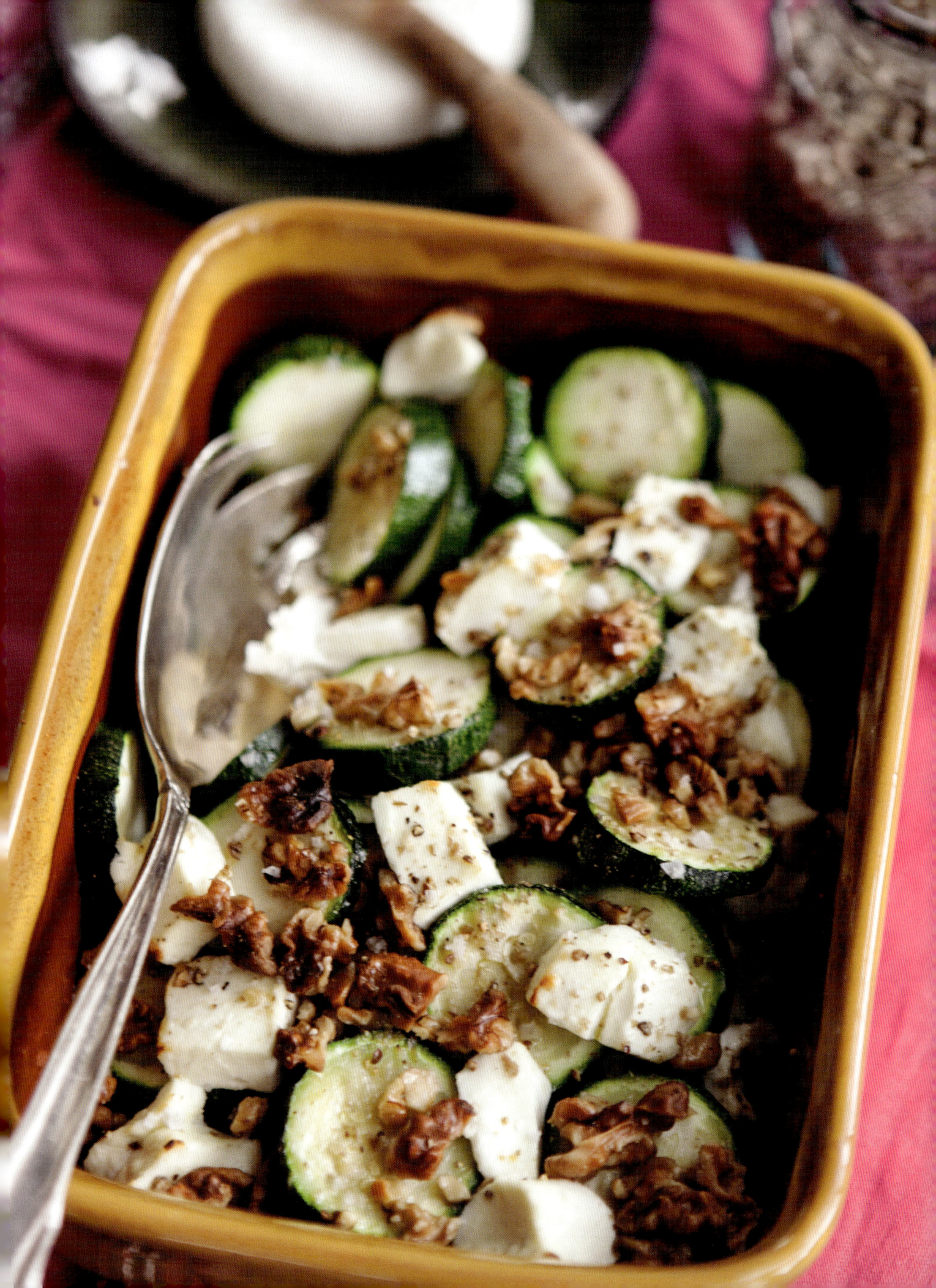

ZUCCHINI WITH WALNUTS AND GOAT CHEESE
Courgettes aux Noix et au Fromage de Chèvre

Season Mid-Summer through early Autumn **Preparation Time** 5 minutes
Cooking Time 25 to 30 minutes **Serves** 5

Zucchini is in season from June through September. Zucchini pairs well with goat (*chèvre*) cheese, fresh (*frais*) or aged (*affiné*). You could pick any *chèvre*. Aged goat cheese intensifies in flavor as it cooks, while fresh goat cheese retains its milder flavor.

- 2 zucchinis (about 14 ounces or 400 g), sliced in ¼-inch (0.6 cm) rounds
- 3.5 ounces (100 g) goat cheese, fresh or aged
- Handful of walnuts (about 1 ounce or 28 g), crumbled or coarsely chopped
- 4 tablespoons olive oil
- *Fleur de sel* to taste
- 2 pinches of coarse sea salt
- 2 pinches of white or black pepper

Preheat the oven to 365°F (185°C). Combine the ingredients in an oven-safe casserole dish. Cook for 25 to 30 minutes. The zucchini will still be *al dente*; cook longer for softer zucchini.

Serve with roast lamb, beef, or pork.

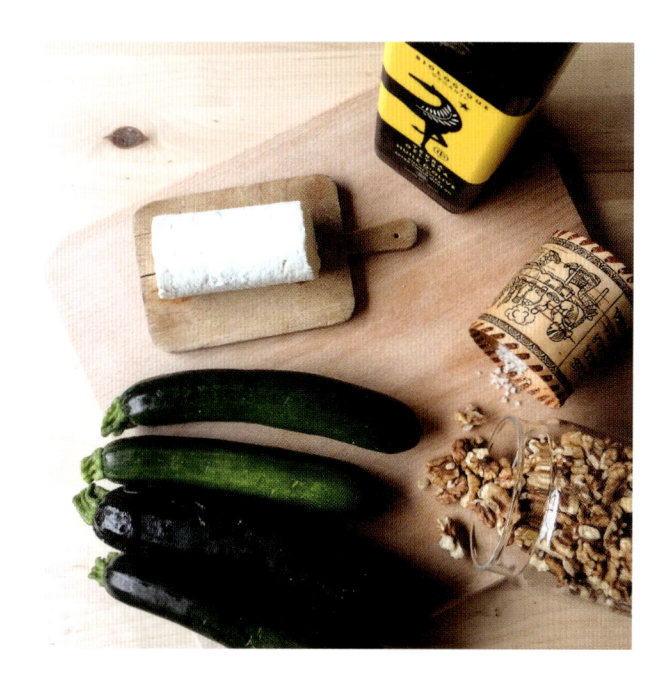

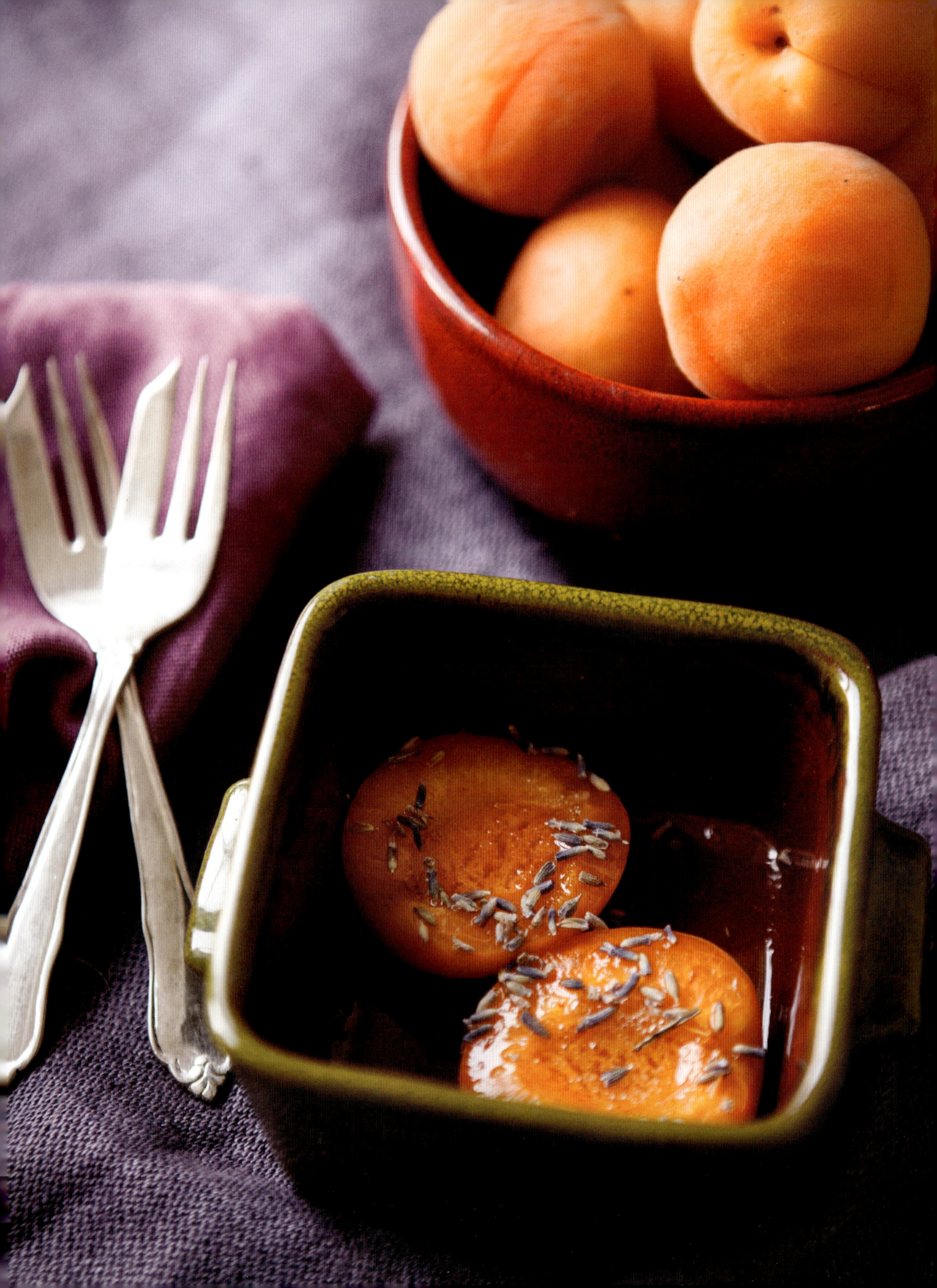

DESSERTS
Les Desserts

Aunt Lucie's Millas – *Le Millas de Tante Lucie* 484

Baked Apricot with Lavender – *Abricot Rôti au Lavendre* 486

Berry Tart – *Tarte aux Fruits des Bois* 487

Caramelized Apples – *Pommes Caramélisées* 489

Chocolate Mousse – *Mousse au Chocolat* 490

Coconut Almond Crumble with Seasonal Fruit
Le Crumble au Noix de Coco et aux Fruits de Saison 493

Custard with Seasonal Fruits – *Fromage Blanc aux Fruits de Saison* 495

Pears in Butter and Cinnamon – *Poires au Beurre Cannelle* 497

Raspberry Verbena Syrup and Gelatin – *Sirop et Gelée de Verveine à la Framboise* 499

Seedy Crackers – *Craquelins au Graines* 501

Sweet and Savory Crêpes – *Les Crêpes et les Galettes* 503

Vanilla "Burned" Cream – *Crème Brûlée à la Vanille* 505

Walnuts in Milk – *Intxaursalsa (Noix au Lait)* 509

AUNT LUCIE'S MILLAS
Le Millas de Tante Lucie

Season Year-round   **Preparation Time** 10 minutes
Cooking Time 40 to 55 minutes   **Serves** 8

My lovely wine-course classmate Malika Faytout, the epitome of a classic French mother who elegantly juggles family, career, and multi-generational cooperation, showed me this simple almond-flavored dessert, a cross between a cake and a flan (a kind of firm pudding). In France, the *millas* or *milhas* originates from the word "millet," traditionally used in this French Southwestern dish, though Tante Lucie uses wheat flour. *Millas* is also made with corn (*maïs*), as a polenta-style side dish. Millas is similar to a *clafoutis*, another dessert that is similar in consistency, but which uses pieces of fruit instead of, or in addition, to the almond flavoring. A *clafoutis* may also be made with vegetables as a savory side dish (which is more like an Italian *frittata*, as explained in Variations.)

Malika's paternal great-aunt, Tante Lucie, who was born in 1931, still makes this traditional dessert today. Malika and I made the Millas using chestnut flour (*farine de châtaigne*) instead of the usual wheat flour that Tante Lucie uses. Malika's father did not necessarily approve of this switch in ingredient, as it made the consistency a bit heavier than he is used to. But overall, everyone at lunch thought it was tasty. The recipe calls for more sugar than I would typically use in a dessert. Feel free to reduce or replace the amount of sugar with your favorite substitutes.

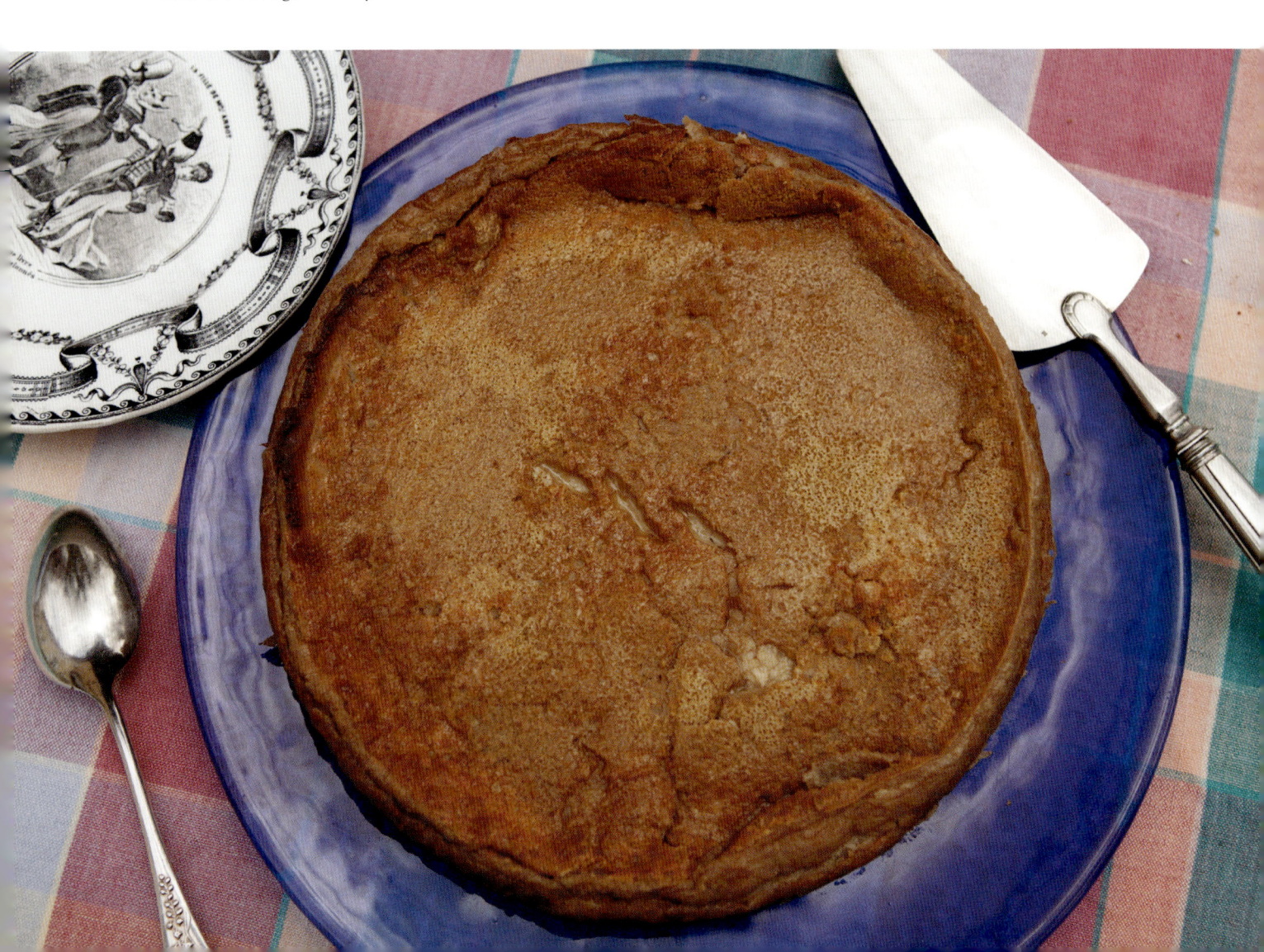

6 eggs

4 ⅕ cups or 34 ounces (1 L) whole milk

10 tablespoons (125 g) organic raw cane sugar (or other sweetener)

12 tablespoons (200 g) chestnut flour

1 teaspoon amaretto or almond extract

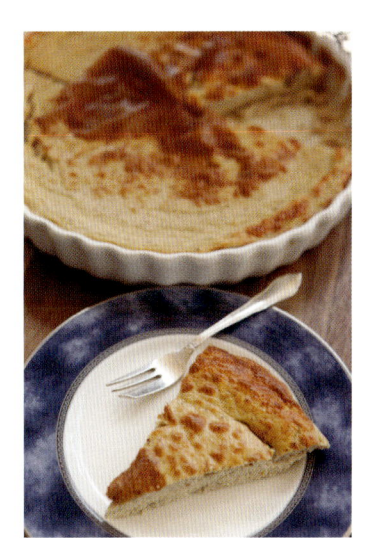

Preheat the oven to 465°F (240°C). Whisk the eggs together in a large bowl, then whisk in the milk, sugar (or sweetener of choice), flour, and amaretto or almond extract, until well blended. Pour the mixture into a round pie or quiche mold with about a 9-inch (23 cm) or 10-inch (25.5 cm) diameter, 1.5 (4 cm) to 2 inches (5 cm) in height, and place on the bottom rack in the oven. After 10 minutes, turn down the temperature to 355°F (180°C) for another 40 to 45 minutes.

Serve at room temperature plain or sprinkled with chopped nuts for crunch or a few berries for color.

VARIATIONS For a richer *millas*, you can replace a portion of the milk with whole cream. For a non-dairy version of *millas*, try using **Homemade Almond Milk** (page 48), a frequently-used ingredient in France since the Middle Ages. For the almond milk millas, shown here, use six eggs, 34 ounces (1 L) almond milk, 1 teaspoon almond extract, ½ teaspoon powdered bourbon vanilla, about 20 drops of liquid stevia, and one tablespoon powdered collagen for good measure. Bake in the oven for 10 minutes at 465°F (240°C), then for 35 more minutes at 355°F (180°C). Serve *chilled* with berries and cinnamon. You can also use full-fat coconut milk to make a millas. You can also add a cup of seasonal chopped fruit, such as apples, cherries, or pears, in which case the dessert becomes more of a *clafoutis*. Savory versions of *clafoutis* are plentiful and are much like an omelet or a *frittata* (an Italian fried or baked egg dish) or a quiche without the crust. A savory **Vegetable Clafoutis** (page 479) may be eaten at any meal.

BAKED APRICOT WITH LAVENDER
Abricot Rôti au Lavendre

Season Summer   **Preparation Time** 2 minutes
Cooking Time 10 minutes   **Serves** 1 to 2

This simple dessert is aromatic and an easy recipe to double or triple to make for guests or family members. Lavender grows in the South of France and when dried is a lovely, edible flower bud, which is also delightful as an herbal tea (infusion). Use either coconut oil (as shown here) for the fat enthusiasts or honey (as shown in the Desserts opening photo on page 482) for the sweets enthusiasts.

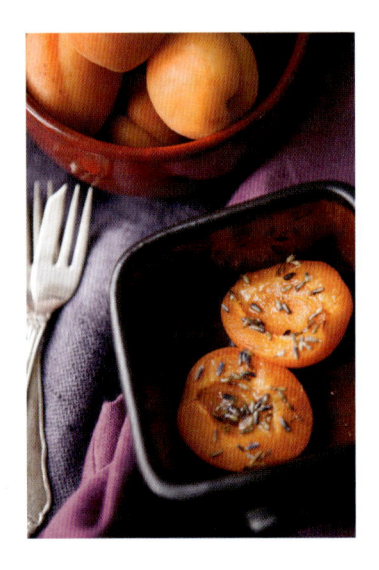

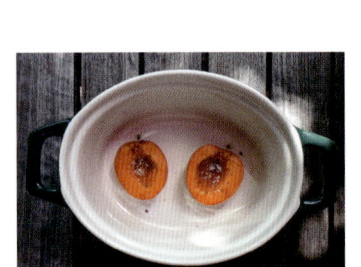

1 apricot, halved, pit removed

1 teaspoon honey or coconut oil

Pinch of dried lavender buds

Fleur de sel, for garnish

Preheat the oven to 365°F (185°C). Place the apricot halves in an oven-safe dish, and drizzle on the honey or the coconut oil. Sprinkle the lavender buds and *fleur de sel* over the apricots. Place in the oven and bake for 10 minutes. When done baking, place half an apricot on a dessert plate and serve.

VARIATIONS There is lots of room for improvisation here. You can try replacing the honey and lavender with butter and cinnamon (shown below). Don't forget the salt, as it will enhance the flavors. Another variant is to use a fresh fig with honey and cinnamon, or else plum with lavender and honey, topped with a fresh mint leaf. Another stone fruit you could use is a peach, topped with the honey and either lavender or pine nuts for some crunch. Serve a baked peach alongside **Orange Duck Breast** (page 351), omitting the orange part of the recipe.

WINE PAIRING TIP Layering sweet upon sweet is almost too much of a good thing, but if a wine is expected or desired with this dessert, then definitely go for a dessert wine such as a Bordeaux Barsac or Sauternes, with their fresh, balanced acidity and aromas of honey and apricot.

BERRY TART
Tarte aux Fruits des Bois

Season Summer **Preparation Time** 20 minutes
Cooking Time 45 minutes **Serves** 8

Summer berries are one of the joys of the season. Everybody loves a berry tart. Berries are nature's candy, so low-carb this dessert is not; there is plenty of fructose here. When served warm right after baking, this tart is actually more like a crumble, as the crust pretty much falls apart. It's a crowd-pleaser nevertheless! For a crust that hangs together a bit better, serve chilled or even the next day. I used one cup each of fresh gooseberries, raspberries, and black currants (shown in the top left photo). An optional step is to pour some warmed **Raspberry Verbena Syrup** (page 499) over the pie after it has cooled a bit for added glaze, gelatin, and sweetness (not that more sweetness is needed).

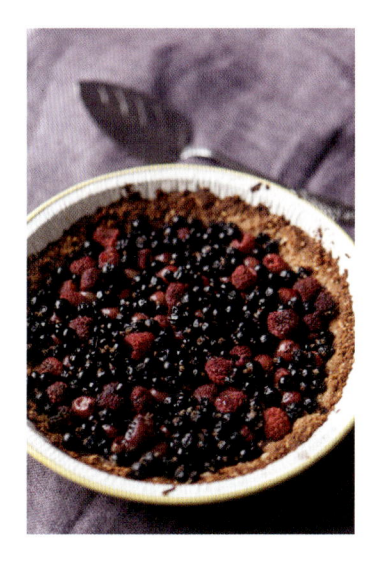

1½ cups (350 ml) coconut flour

½ cup (120 ml) almond meal

2 pinches of fine salt

10 tablespoons ghee (room temperature)

3 cups (710 ml) fresh berries

Optional: ⅓ cup (80 ml) Raspberry Verbena Syrup

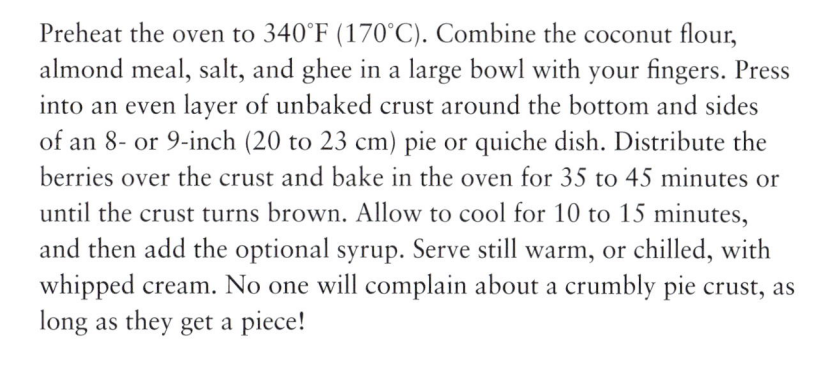

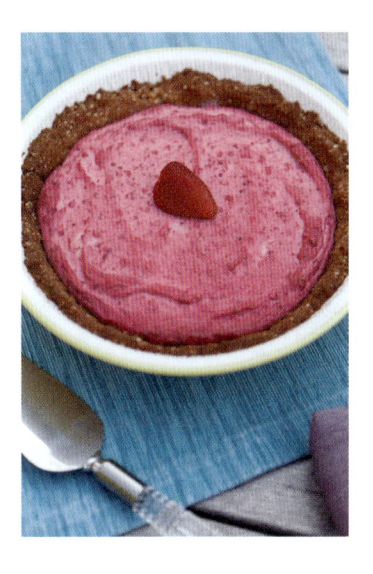

Preheat the oven to 340°F (170°C). Combine the coconut flour, almond meal, salt, and ghee in a large bowl with your fingers. Press into an even layer of unbaked crust around the bottom and sides of an 8- or 9-inch (20 to 23 cm) pie or quiche dish. Distribute the berries over the crust and bake in the oven for 35 to 45 minutes or until the crust turns brown. Allow to cool for 10 to 15 minutes, and then add the optional syrup. Serve still warm, or chilled, with whipped cream. No one will complain about a crumbly pie crust, as long as they get a piece!

VARIATIONS For a creamy berry tart, as shown bottom left, use the same crust, but bake it on its own for 15 minutes at 340°F (170°C) or until it begins to turn brown. Allow it to cool. Combine 1⅓ to 1½ cups (300 ml to 350 ml) fresh or thawed berries in a blender with 9 to 12 ounces (250 g to 350 g) mascarpone cheese (essentially a heavy, "double" cream) used in Italy in the dessert *Tiramisu*. Run through the blender for several seconds until blended. Spread out into the cooled pie crust and bake for another 15 minutes in a preheated oven at 340°F (170°C). Chill for three hours or overnight before serving. Add fresh fruit on top if desired.

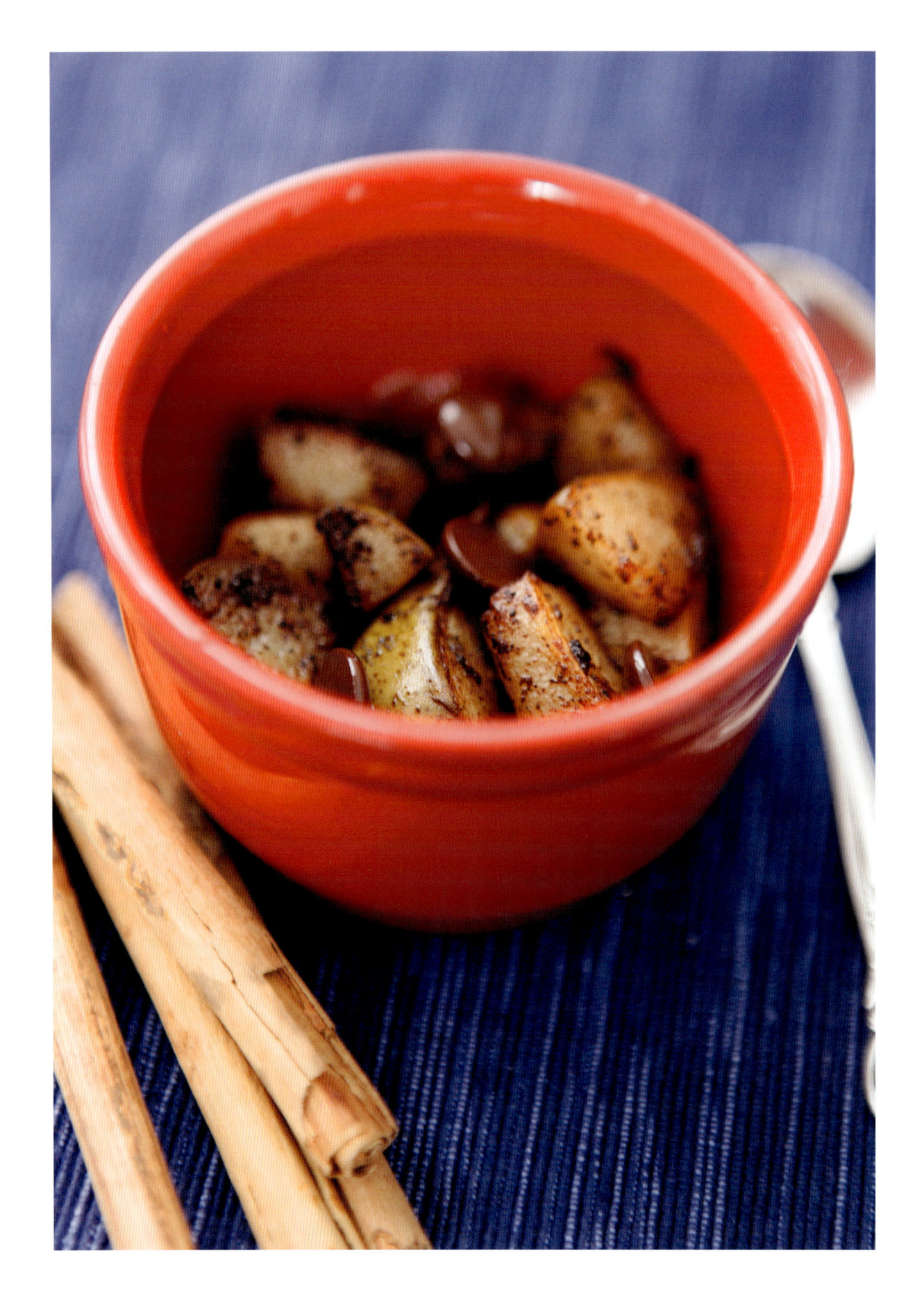

CARAMELIZED APPLES
Pommes Caramélisées

Season Mid-Summer through mid-Spring   **Preparation Time** 15 minutes
Cooking Time 25 to 30 minutes   **Serves** 4

Caramelized Apples is another easy dessert to throw together, and it's a kid-pleaser. Start cooking the apples right before you sit down to eat dinner so they will be ready for dessert time, or else start this recipe while you are sautéing something for dinner and allow the apples to stay warm and gooey in the pan until they are ready to be served, reheating briefly if necessary.

2 tablespoons butter or ghee

3 apples, peeled or unpeeled and chopped

1 orange, juiced

1 teaspoon orange zest

1 cinnamon stick or 1 teaspoon cinnamon

Optional: Handful of dark chocolate chips

Melt the butter in a medium-sized pot over medium heat. Add the apple pieces, orange juice, zest, and cinnamon. Cover and cook for 25 to 30 minutes.

Serve topped with dark chocolate chips (as shown in the recipe photo). Other toppings could include whole raw cream, whipped cream, *fleur de sel*, or some baked **Coconut Almond Crumble** (page 493), reheated and sprinkled on top. After you have emptied the pot, add some water to the pan and your favorite herbal tea, such as thyme, and allow the liquid to heat to almost a boil. Remove from heat, pour into a cup, and add honey for a delicious, deglazing, pot-cleaning tea to end your day.

CHOCOLATE MOUSSE
Mousse au Chocolat

Season Year-round (since cacao grows at the equator, every season is the season for chocolate!)
Preparation Time 20 minutes   **Chill Time** 3 hours or overnight   **Makes** 8 to 10 small portions

Who doesn't love a good chocolate mousse? Every French household has its own chocolate mousse recipe. Most chocolate mousse recipes call for more sugar. I have tried to pare down the extra sugar, as there is already some in the chocolate (unless it's 100% cocoa, which I have tried using but it is *so bitter*, I don't recommend it for a mousse). Even the staunchest, 90%-dark-chocolate-eating manly-man in your family will find it bitter. For the chocolate mousse, stick with 85% chocolate or lower. Kids tend to prefer 65% to 75%. The 85% dark chocolate is quite potent, and the amount of dessert per person required is low, just a few spoonfuls is "satiating." You can try experimenting with other sweeteners, such as honey, monk fruit sweetener (I often use Lakanto brand, a combination of monk fruit extract and erythritol), or stevia if you choose not to use raw cane or coconut sugar. Many people like to celebrate the fact that chocolate is high in tannins (polyphenols, or compounds found in plants with antioxidant effects),[1] much like red wine. And it turns out that some red wines go very well with chocolate. Attention: raw eggs are in use here. Get the freshest, highest-quality pastured eggs you can find to use in this recipe.

3½ tablespoons butter

7 ounces (200 g) dark chocolate

Optional: 1 tablespoon sugar raw cane or coconut sugar

2 pinches of fine salt

6 eggs, separated

Melt the butter and chocolate in a thick saucepan or a double boiler on medium to medium-low heat, mixing with a spatula. Remove from heat.

In a bowl, whisk the sugar and salt into the egg yolks and incorporate them gently into the chocolate butter mix using the spatula.

Beat the egg whites with a hand mixer for several minutes on high until firm. Gently incorporate a few spoonfuls of the egg whites at a time into the chocolate mix, loosening it up as you go.

Makes just under 3 cups (about 700 ml). Fill small ramekins and place in the refrigerator for several hours, and then serve chilled.

VARIATIONS Serve as is, or top with chocolate shavings, chopped nuts, *fleur de sel*, or else sprinkle on a bit of *piment d'Espelette* (powdered, sweet chili pepper) for a Basque twist. This recipe can be halved, in which case you would use 2 tablespoons butter, 3.5 ounces (100 g) chocolate, one to two teaspoons sugar (or monk fruit or several drops of stevia), three separated eggs, and one pinch of fine salt.

WINE PAIRING TIP The notes of cherry and spice and oaked vanilla flavors of a Côtes du Rhône, or the spice and dark fruits of a rustic Rasteau (made with a regulated minimum of 50% of the Carignan Noir grape and also hailing from the Rhône Valley) go well with dark chocolate, as does a medium-bodied, fruity, and citrusy Bergerac from the Southwest, where the chocolate becomes coated in the wine and just melts in fruitful delight in the mouth. Rich in alcohol and flavor, a red Banyuls from the hilly Southeastern corner of Roussillon, with its roasted notes of coffee and cooked fruits, also pairs well with dark chocolate.

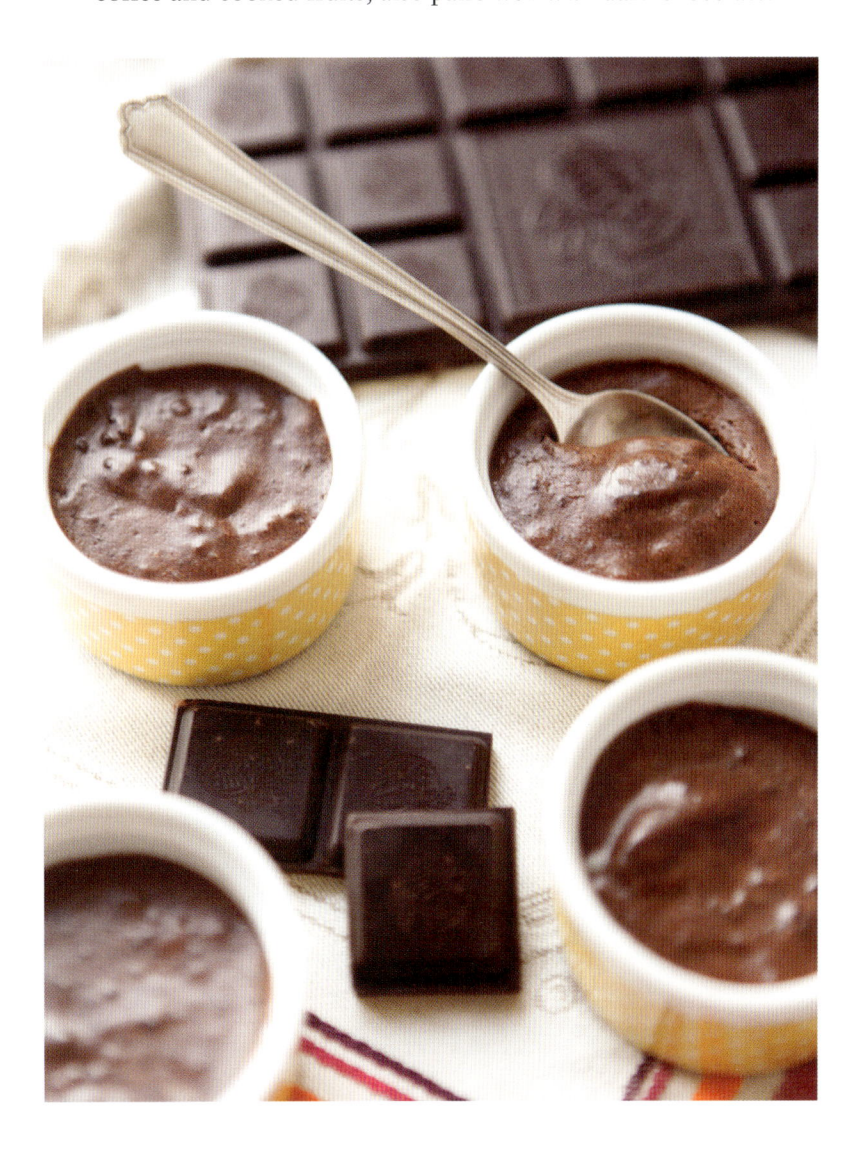

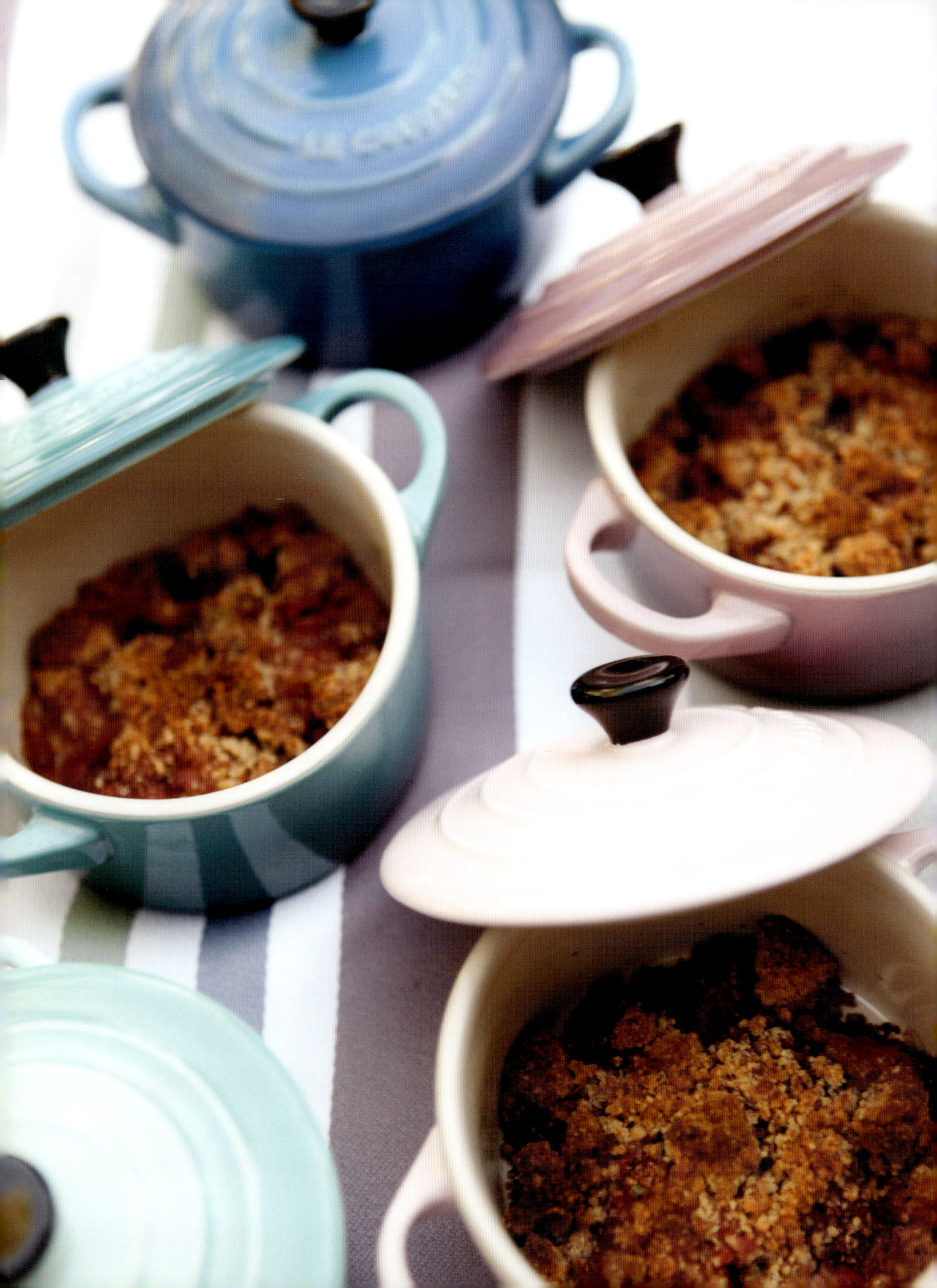

COCONUT ALMOND CRUMBLE WITH SEASONAL FRUIT
Le Crumble au Noix de Coco et aux Fruits de Saison

Season Year-round   **Preparation Time** 30 minutes
Cook Time 20 to 25 minutes   **Serves** 7 to 8

Also known as a crisp or cobbler, I learned this basic crumble recipe in Bordeaux's *Atelier des Chefs*, a group-style cooking school where you can sign up for a class and learn to cook a meal or part of a meal, or just desserts. This is a decidedly modern-day recipe originating from the United Kingdom since World War II, however, it is frequently found throughout France.

Easy and fun to make with children, this recipe falls just within the primal/paleo "guidelines." (It should be saved for special occasions, because let's face it, it is a carbohydrate bomb.) I therefore keep the portions small. The original recipe calls for regular refined flour, which can be easily substituted for with coconut flour or even cassava (yucca root) flour. As almond meal (essentially ground almonds, skin on, as opposed to almond or blanched almond flour in which the skin is removed) is already a part of this recipe, some other options for the flour substitution could be chestnut, hazelnut, macadamia, or walnut flours, each contributing its own flavor (and texture if chopped instead of ground) to the dish. Mixed berries, apples with cinnamon, and stone fruits like apricots, plums (or moist prunes), or peaches all go well with the crumble. Pears and melted dark chocolate (see More Variations at end of recipe) are another popular combination. A slightly lower "added sugar" option would be to use four teaspoons of sugar. Again, a sugar-like substance such as a monk fruit sweetener, that looks much like sugar and may be replaced in equal proportions, is a good non-glycemic substitute to obtain sweetness.

3.5 ounces (100 g) coconut flour

7 tablespoons or 3.75 ounces (100 g) unsalted butter

3.5 ounces (100 g) almond meal

8 teaspoons or 1 ounce (28 g) coconut sugar

Pinch of fine sea salt

2 cups chopped berries (200 g) (shown in the recipe photo) or fruit, fresh or frozen

Preheat the oven to 395°F (200°C). Mix the flour, butter, almond meal, sugar, and salt with the tips of your four fingers and thumb. This technique will keep you from squeezing the dough too hard while getting the dough to the right "sandy" consistency. The dough can be clumpy depending on the fineness of the flour.

If the butter becomes mushy, cool the crumble in the refrigerator for one hour or in the freezer for 20 minutes to firm up the crumble before baking it. ➤

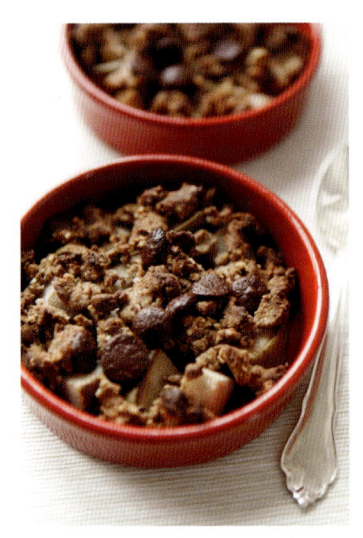

Apple Crumble with Chestnut Flour

Place chopped fruit or berries in an 8- to 10-inch oven-safe dish or into individual ramekins and sprinkle the crumble over the fruit. Bake uncovered for 15 to 20 minutes until golden brown. Serve warm as is, or with whipped cream or vanilla or coconut ice cream on the side.

VARIATIONS If you are using chestnut flour instead of coconut flour, you will probably find the clumps are bigger because the chestnut flour compacts so easily and does not produce the same sandy consistency. Shown here is an apple crumble using chestnut flour, topped with dark chocolate chips. When using chestnut flour, bake at 350°F (175°C) for 25 minutes, as chestnut flour tends to burn easily. Unbaked crumble can be frozen. The crumble can also be baked at 395°F (200°C) on its own without fruit, spread out, and uncovered on a tray for 15 to 20 minutes or until golden brown and then frozen for future use. It can then be sprinkled onto **Caramelized Apples** (page 489).

MORE VARIATIONS For a savory version of this recipe, replace the sugar with grated Gruyère or Parmesan, equating the quantity of the cheese with that of the almond meal. Make a *gratin* by sprinkling the crumble over chopped zucchini, along with goat cheese, *lardons*, and walnuts before placing in the oven. Or try, as pictured in the **Pears in Butter and Cinnamon** recipe on page 497, using ½ cup (120 ml) almond meal, ½ cup coconut flour, ½ cup butter, a pinch of fine salt, and one teaspoon monk fruit powder for two cups of pears chopped into small chunks. Makes four 4-ounce (115 g) servings, baked for 15 minutes at 375°F (190°C).

CUSTARD WITH SEASONAL FRUITS
Fromage Blanc aux Fruits de Saison

Season Year-round, using seasonal fruits   **Preparation Time** Less than 5 minutes   **Serves** 1

Fromage blanc is a white and creamy cheese falling somewhere between a custard, cottage cheese, and yogurt and can be made from cow, goat, or sheep milk. In France, *fromage blanc*, though unsweetened, tastes generally sweeter (less acid-containing) than the *fromage blanc* made in the US. If you cannot find *fromage blanc*, use whole fat plain yogurt or your favorite white, custardy cheese instead (always organic). This recipe is basically yogurt and fruits, but combined by you, rather than a factory machine. If you make your own yogurt, use that—even though the consistency might be less creamy—because after all, you made it yourself! The French usually eat *fromage blanc* plain (*nature*) or with honey or fruit if it is not being baked or whipped into another more elaborate kind of dessert or dish.

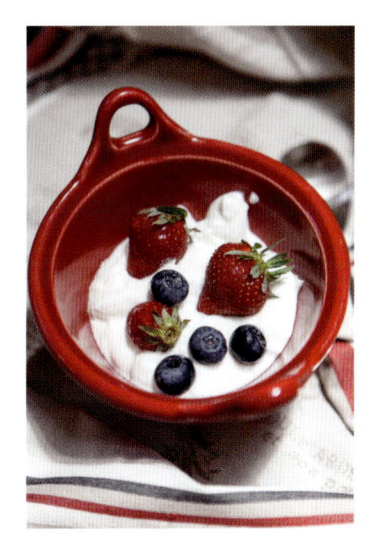

4 tablespoons *fromage blanc* or other custard or yogurt

Small handful of seasonal berries or chopped fruit

Spoon the *fromage blanc* into a dessert dish and add the fruit.

VARIATIONS Spoon the *fromage blanc* or custard into a dessert dish. Top with the berries or chopped fruit and coconut flakes. If you would like to add coconut oil to increase the fat content of the dish, melt one teaspoon to liquefy it, and then drizzle over the dessert. (Coconut oil is solid at room temperature until 76°F or 24°C, thereafter it becomes liquefied.) You may try topping with coconut flakes, cacao nibs, chia seeds, chopped nuts, cinnamon, *fleur de sel*, honey, or sprouted pumpkin or sunflower seeds.

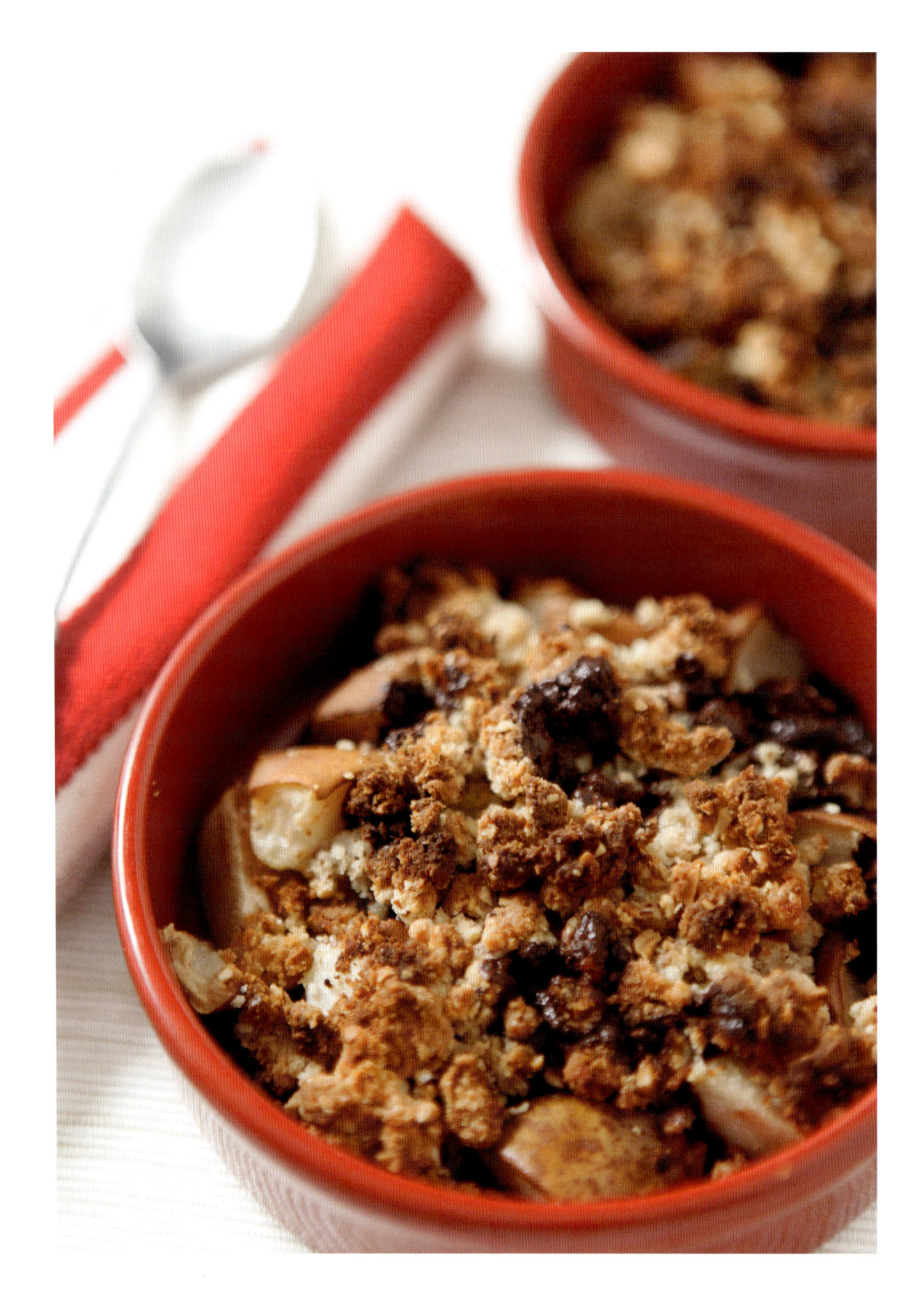

PEARS IN BUTTER AND CINNAMON
Poires au Beurre Cannelle

Season Late summer through January   **Preparation Time** 5 minutes
Cooking Time 10 to 15 minutes   **Serves** 4 to 5

Pears figure in many French recipes, and combined with butter and cinnamon, you can't go wrong. Add dark chocolate chips, and the combination is immediately addictive—careful as she goes! Usually, French dessert recipes call for peeled pears (or apples, which you could substitute in this recipe). I leave the decision as to whether the peel is desired or not up to you. Without the peel, such desserts are more "melty" (*fondant*), but with the peel you have the nutrients that go with it.

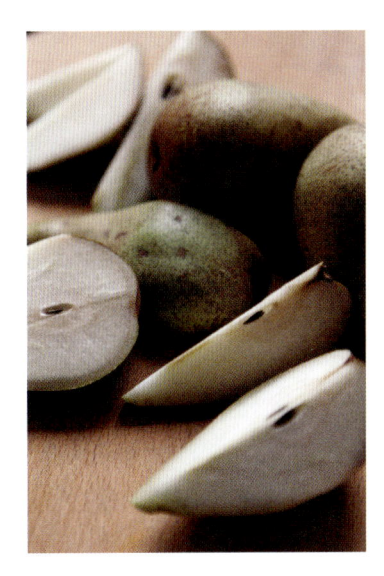

2 tablespoons butter (or ghee)

3 pears, chopped

Optional: 2 teaspoons raw cane sugar or other sweetener

1 teaspoon cinnamon (*la cannelle*)

¼ teaspoon cardamom (*la cardamome*)

⅛ teaspoon fine salt

Juice of half a lemon

Melt the butter in a medium-sized pan over medium heat and stir in the pears and the optional sugar, cinnamon, cardamom, salt, and lemon. Allow the pears to simmer and soften for 10 to 15 minutes before removing from the pan. Serve on their own or with whipped cream.

VARIATIONS Add a few bits of chocolate and **Coconut Almond Crumble** (page 493), as shown in the recipe photo. Heat in the oven for a few minutes, and you have another fruity dessert variation.

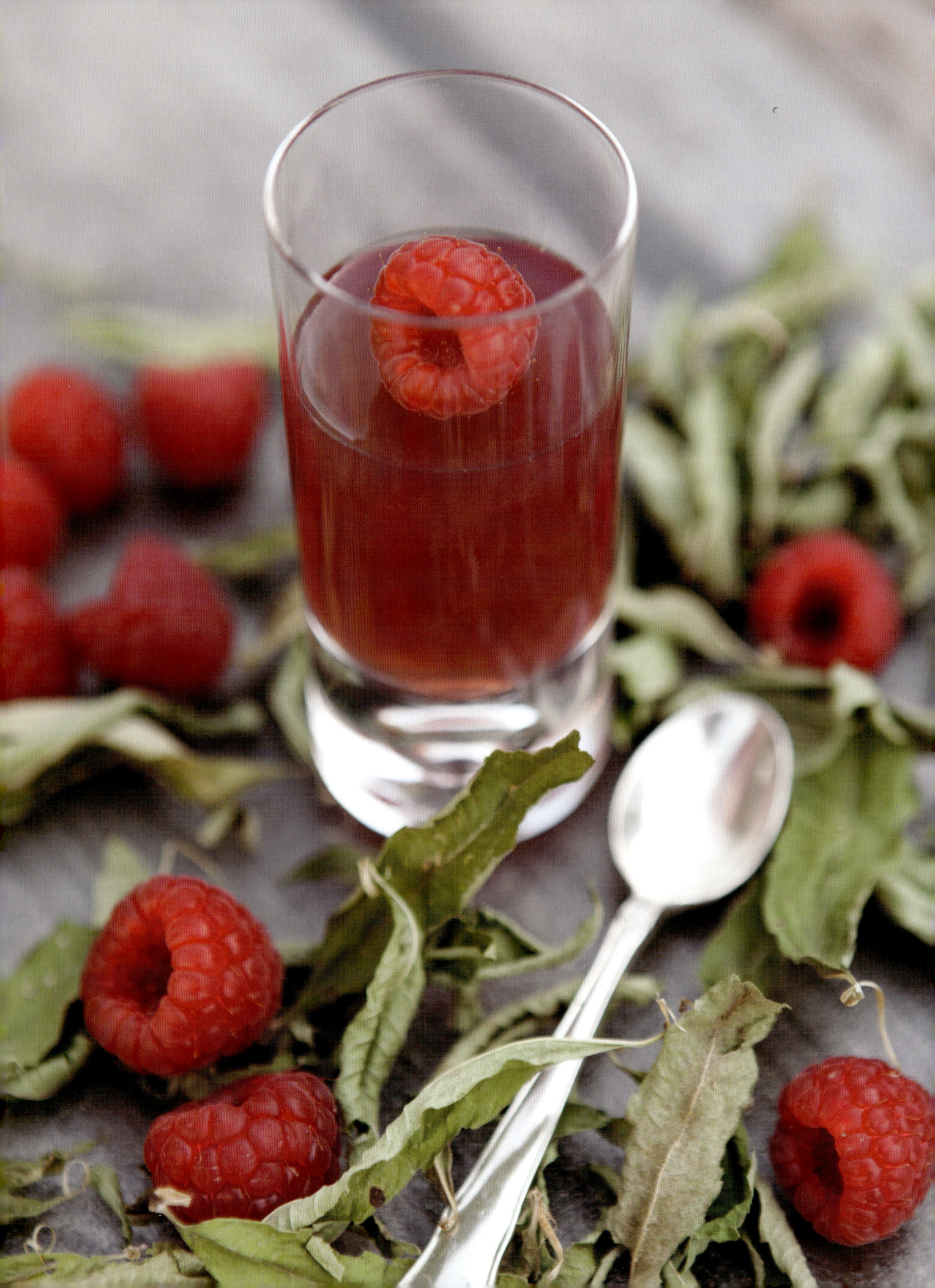

RASPBERRY VERBENA SYRUP AND GELATIN
Sirop et Gelée de Verveine à la Framboise

Season Summer through early Autumn **Preparation Time** 5 minutes
Cooking Time About 50 minutes **Makes** about 2 cups syrup

When the French drink an herbal tea (*infusion*), one of the most popular is verbena (*verveine*), perhaps for its lemony aromatic character. As a flavoring, verbena is often infused into desserts. This recipe was inspired by part of a multi-fruit dessert recipe from *Atelier des Chefs*, a French cooking school which provides recipes, videos, and explanations of French traditional and modern dishes online and in kitchen classrooms around France. For this recipe, I found that by using honey instead of the ubiquitous white sugar, and by adding gelatin, I could make a multi-use syrup *and* a gelatin, alongside the much-loved ingredients verbena and raspberries. You may replace the honey with other sweeteners, but you might need to experiment a bit to see what works best for you. To make a proper herbal tea bag, it is helpful to use a piece of cheesecloth. Fresh raspberries are in season June through September, though frozen raspberries could be used in place of fresh ones for an occasional burst of color and flavor out of season.

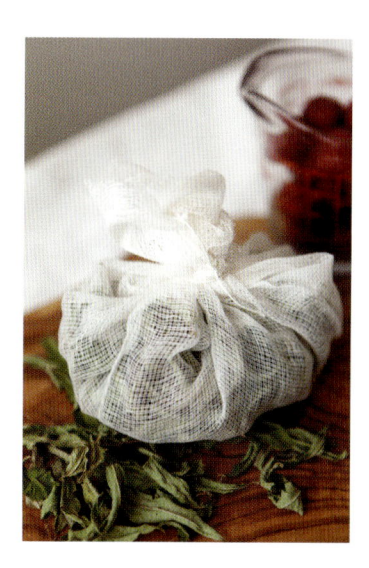

0.2 ounces (6 g) dried verbena leaves

4 cups (950 ml) water

¼ cup (60 ml) or 3 ounces (85 g) honey or other sweetener

1 cup (240 ml) or 6 ounces (170 g) fresh raspberries

⅓ cup (75 g) powdered gelatin

Cut out a square of cheesecloth about 12 inches by 12 inches (about 30 cm by 30 cm). Place the verbena leaves into a medium-sized or large bowl and use another bowl of similar or slightly smaller size to compress the leaves so that, crushed, they will fit into the middle of the cheesecloth. Gather the four corners of the cheesecloth around the verbena and tie it closed with kitchen twine.

Bring 4 cups of water (about 1 L) to a boil, place the verbena tea bag in the water along with the raspberries, and simmer on medium heat for 10 to 12 minutes.

Remove the verbena tea bag. (Put it in a teapot for a tea later on.) Continue to boil off or "reduce" (*reduire*) the liquid for 40 minutes on medium heat.

Remove the pot from heat and stir in the honey. Strain out the raspberry mush but save it to use it the same day as a topping on vanilla or coconut ice cream, to put in a shake, or to freeze for future use. ▶

DESSERTS – LES DESSERTS

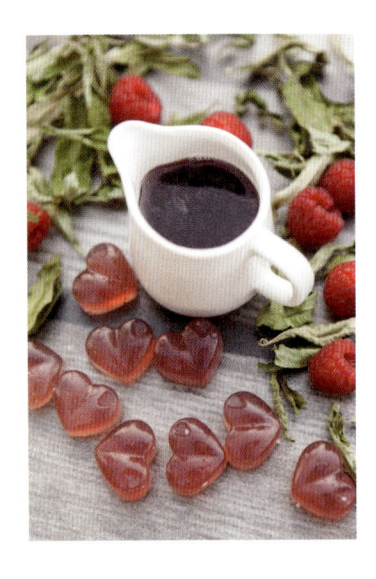

Whisk in ⅓ cup (75 g) powdered gelatin to make about two cups of syrup. Pour a small amount warmed over plain yogurt or coconut ice cream as a syrup or pour into silicone candy molds to make gummies, like the gelatin hearts shown to the left. Chill the molds in the refrigerator for at least 20 minutes before removing the gummies from the molds. Store the syrup in the refrigerator for several days or in the freezer for up to three months. Heat it gently in the oven to warm it up for use (or it will remain solid!)

VARIATIONS   For "flu-busting elderberry syrup[2] and gummies,"[3] check out Wellness Mama's excellent recipes on her website (wellnessmama.com). I feed my family both the elderberry syrup and the gummies (shown below) through the winter, which helps us avoid colds and boosts our immunity. No flu shots necessary!

WINE PAIRING TIP   Raspberries go together with champagne like strawberries and champagne. Try also a pink (*rosé*) champagne for flavor *and* color coordination.

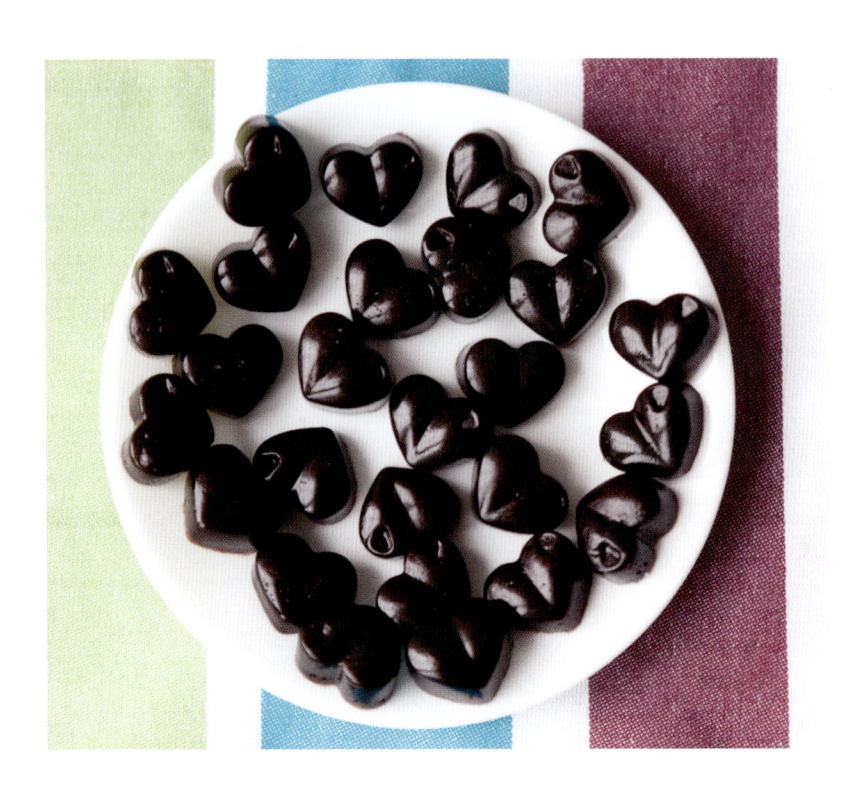

SEEDY CRACKERS
Craquelins au Graines

Season Year-round   **Preparation Time** 10 minutes
Cooking Time 30 minutes   **Serves** 8

Inspired in part by Patricia Daly and Domini Kemp's *The Ketogenic Kitchen*, as well as by six or seven other cracker and flatbread recipes (as Daly and Kemp use no flour, and the others use too much), I have developed a cracker that is palatable to my children and to all others who crunch into one. In our family, we call these "seedy crackers." While not distinctly French, these crackers are a kind of flat bread or "transitional bread" for our family (to transition from grain to grain-free) and are much better than any store-bought cracker or flat bread. They are something akin to the European grain crackers my children love, minus the grain. These crackers may be used for any of the spreadable recipes in this book, such as **Foie Gras** (page 244) or **Pork Meat Pâté** (page 312). Since my children (to my amazement) will eat crackers and liverwurst for *dessert*, I have put these crackers in the Desserts section. There are some carbohydrates in them due to the cassava flour, and they are extremely "easy" to eat, therefore, beware of over-indulging. The crackers may be refrigerated for up to a week or frozen. Thaw them out for several minutes before reheating for four minutes at 395°F (200°C) to regain their crispiness. You may want to pull out your mini chopper to reduce the size of the pumpkin and sunflower seeds a bit.

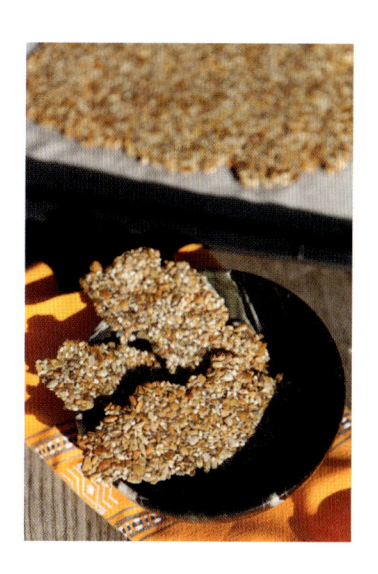

2 ounces (about 60 g) pumpkin seeds

2 ounces (about 60 g) sunflower seeds

2 ounces (about 60 g) golden flax seeds

1 ounce (about 30 g) chia seeds

1 ounce (about 30 g) sesame seeds

3 tablespoons cassava flour

1 tablespoon olive oil

4 pinches of fine salt

3 tablespoons coconut oil

¾ cup (180 ml) hot water

Preheat the oven to 320°F (160°C). Pulse the pumpkin and sunflower seeds a few times in a mini chopper to reduce them to smaller pieces. Combine all the seeds, flour, olive oil, and salt in a large bowl. Bring the water to a boil in a pot, add the coconut oil to melt it, and pour over the seed mixture in the bowl. Combine the ingredients in the bowl well with a whisk. *Note:* You can also just put the coconut oil in the bowl with all the other ingredients and pour the hot water over it all, stirring with a whisk. This is actually how I do it most of the time because then I don't have to wash another pot! ▶

Using a spatula, spread the mixture out on a flat baking pan lined with parchment paper so that it is evenly distributed and about a ¼ inch (about 0.6 cm) thick. Bake in the oven for 30 minutes. Serve with **Duck Liver Pâté** (page 242), **Pork Meat Pâté** (page 312), **Spreadable Fish Paste** (page 186), or any of the other pâtés in *The Bordeaux Kitchen*.

VARIATIONS Try adding 1 teaspoon garlic powder, 1 teaspoon dried thyme, or 1 teaspoon dried rosemary to the mixture in the bowl, and/or sprinkle coarse sea salt on top of the spread-out mixture in the pan before baking.

SWEET AND SAVORY CRÊPES
Les Crêpes et les Galettes

Season Year-round   **Preparation Time** 5 minutes
Cooking Time 1 hour 10 minutes   **Makes** 8 crêpes

Crêpes, generally made with refined white flour, are the French version of a thin pancake. *Galettes*, originating from Brittany, are the savory version of crêpes and are usually made with rustic-flavored buckwheat (*sarrasin*) flour and salted (with sea salt) butter. This recipe replaces the white flour and the buckwheat with cassava (yuca root) flour[4] for an all-purpose, sweet or savory crêpe. It's a bit of a glorified tortilla; nevertheless, when you need a crêpe, this will do the job, and the sea salt augments the flavors of the savory or sweet crêpes. This recipe also replaces the butter with ghee, which has a higher smoke point than butter and has almost all the casein removed, for those who are intolerant. Feel free to use butter or clarified butter instead. For regular butter, turn the heat down a notch so as not to burn it. In many French recipes, buckwheat flour, once mixed with all the ingredients, needs to stand and set for two hours. I have not found this step necessary when using cassava flour. The crêpes end up being large and can be split in half or quarters for those desiring to eat fewer carbohydrates.

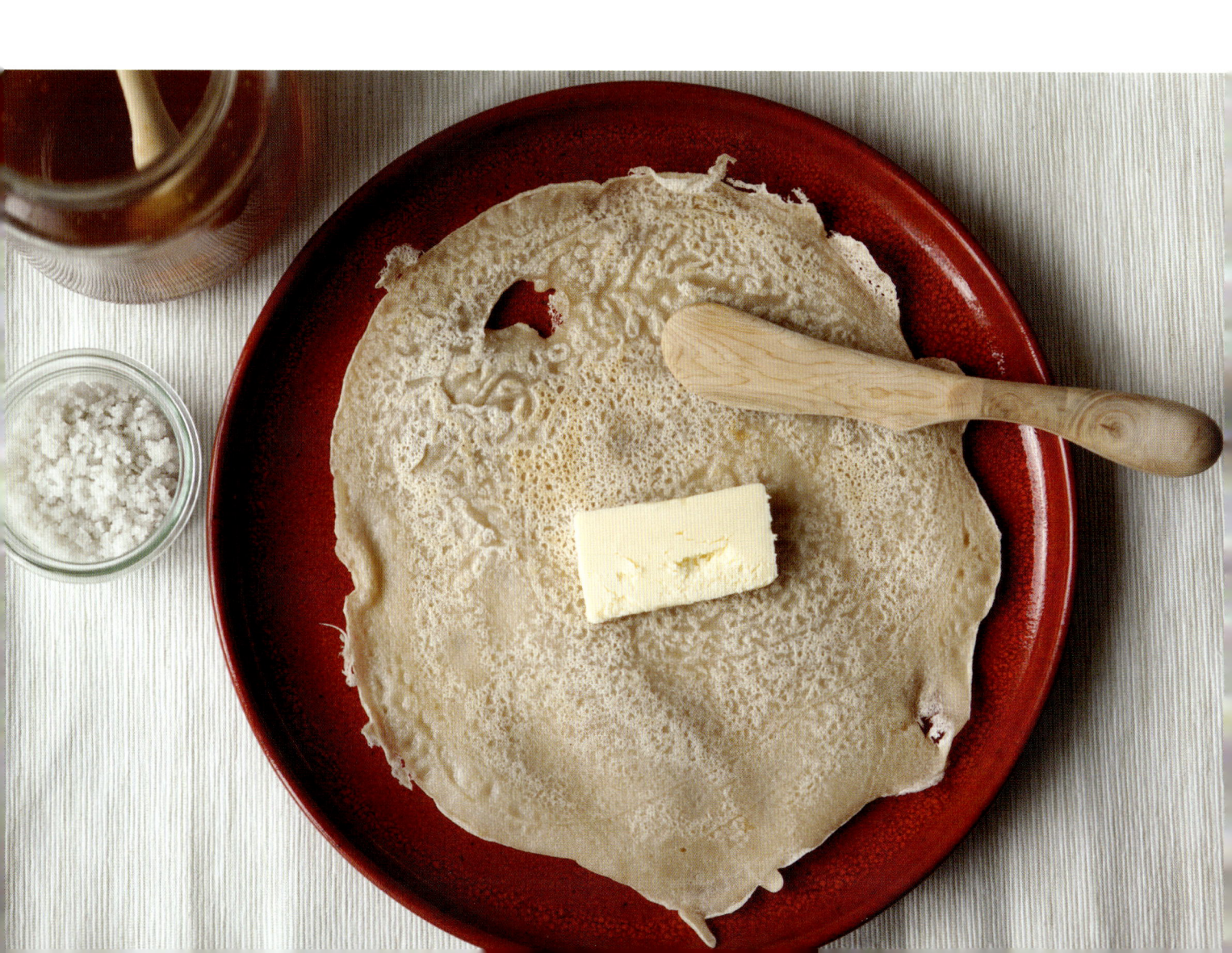

- 12 ounces (340 g) cassava flour

- 2 tablespoons arrowroot powder

- 2 teaspoons coarse sea salt (*gros sel*)

- 3 cups (about 700 ml) water

- 1 egg

- 1 tablespoon ghee, butter, or lard, plus several teaspoons more (as needed for cooking the crêpes)

In a large bowl, combine the flour, arrowroot, and salt. Whisk in 1 cup of water at a time, then whisk in the egg.

Melt the ghee in a large (11-inch or 28 cm) pan over medium to medium-high heat until it bubbles. Using a flat-ended wooden spatula, spread the ghee evenly around the pan. Pour one ladle-full (about ½ cup or 120 ml) of crêpe mixture into the hot pan. Smooth out and distribute the mixture in the pan evenly using an angled icing spatula or a wooden crêpe spreader, or else the flat end of a regular wooden spatula.

Flip the crêpe after five to six minutes and allow it to cook another three to five minutes. The first crêpe somehow always seems to take the longest. It might take 11 to 12 minutes, while the second and rest of the batch might take three to four minutes on each side. (Allowing the pan to heat sufficiently will shorten the time for the first crêpe.) To keep the crêpes from sticking to the pan, you can add one teaspoon of ghee between each or every other crêpe, as needed.

For sweet crêpes, top with butter and drizzle on a little honey or marmalade.

VARIATIONS For savory crêpes, in other words, not dessert, serve topped with butter and *fleur de sel*, or make a *Galette Breton* by topping the crêpe with ham, Gruyère, or other hard cheese and a fried egg, and pair it with cider from Brittany. In the spring, you can roll a few asparagus shoots and a piece of ham in a crêpe and serve topped with **Béchamel Sauce** (as shown on pages 392-393) or grated cheese and pair with a white Alsatian wine such as a Muscat, Pinot Gris, or Sylvaner. As anyone who has been to France knows, there are a multitude of options from which to choose when it comes to sweet and savory crêpes.

VANILLA "BURNED" CREAM
Crème Brûlée à la Vanille

Season Year-round **Preparation Time** 25 minutes **Makes** 5 to 8 servings
Cooking Time 45 minutes, plus 15 minutes to melt the sugar before serving **Chill Time** 4 hours or overnight

I suppose no cookbook of French recipes would be complete without a recipe for *crème brûlée*. *Crème brûlée* dates back to the early 1700s. This recipe calls for the use of scraped-out whole vanilla beans or powdered vanilla. You can use the scraped-out bean hulls (or whole vanilla beans) to flavor sugars or flours by simply storing the beans in the same container. You can also place the beans in a small bottle and cover them in vodka to make your own vanilla extract, which can be topped up and will last for a couple of years.

Vanilla, was used by the Aztecs and then "discovered" in the 1500s by the Spanish when exploring what is now Mexico. Vanilla has been used in France since the time of the French monarch Louis XIV in the mid-1600s. The French first cultivated vanilla in the 1830s on the French island of La Réunion (formerly called *l'île de Bourbon*). Vanilla contains vanillin, another one of those magic antioxidant plant polyphenols, and an intoxicating mix of aromas.

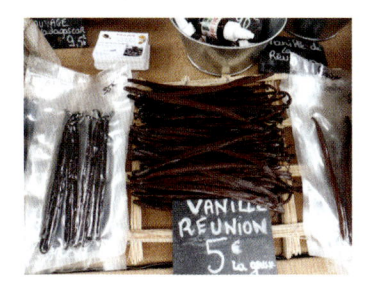

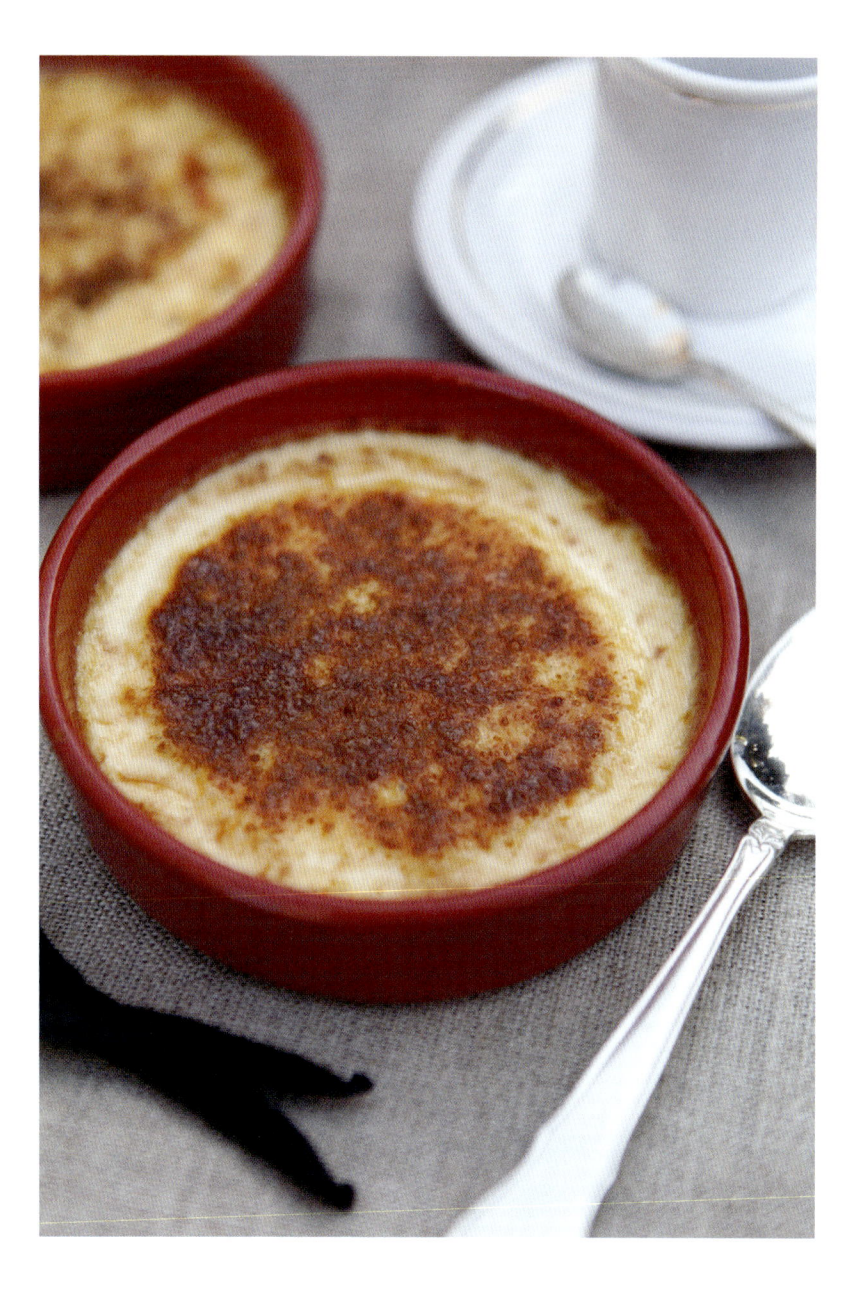

DESSERTS – *LES DESSERTS*

With regard to the original recipe, as shown to me by my friend, Chef Frédéric, this is yet another creamy French dessert made using dairy. Luckily, it is also possible to make a similar concoction using coconut milk (see Variations). You might also want to try using coconut cream or other ingredients, but this is the basic recipe, albeit with honey instead of the usual white sugar. The part that makes it "burned" is the last step, when a thin layer of sugar is caramelized by a flame or beneath the oven broiler grill. In the modern recipes for *crème brûlée*, usually a tablespoon of flour is employed, which supposedly provides the dessert with an unctuous texture. This flour-free recipe from Chef Frédéric will please any discerning gourmand. It is possible to leave the sweeteners out of the cream, or to reduce the honey to two tablespoons. Or you can experiment with a small amount of another sweetener such as stevia or monk fruit. It all depends on your sweetness threshold and blood sugar reaction. If you can handle the cream and eggs, this dessert is a classic that people will ask for again and again. I find the regular-sized five-ounce (142 ml) French ramekins for *crème brûlée* of 4.5 inches (about 11 cm) in diameter (like the ones from French manufacturer Emile Henry or Revol) to be just too much of a good thing. Therefore, I use smaller ramekins for smaller portions.

3 vanilla beans (or 1 teaspoon vanilla powder)

1 cup (240 ml) milk

1 ⅔ cups (400 ml) whole cream, chilled

¼ cup (60 ml) honey, or several drops of liquid stevia or other sweetener

6 egg yolks at room temperature

Preheat the oven to between 195°F and 210°F (90°C and 100°C). Slice the vanilla beans lengthwise down the middle and use a small paring knife to scrape out the pulp (the little black specks). Stop for a moment and enjoy that vanilla aroma—it's alluring, exotic, and delicious; no wonder it is used in so many desserts!

Heat the milk over medium heat in a thick saucepan to just under boiling, at which point you will see steam rising, at around 176°F to 180°F (80°C to 82°C). Use a cooking thermometer to determine the temperature of the milk. Remove from the heat, and whisk in the cream. In a separate bowl, mix the honey together with the yolks, and then stir this mixture into the pot.

Heat again to 180°F (82°C), stirring frequently, until you see steam rising again, and whisk in the specks of vanilla. Remove from heat. This process of heating the milk mixture twice takes approximately 10 minutes.

OPTIONAL STEP: Pass the mixture through a fine mesh strainer to filter out the largest pieces of vanilla bean that may have gotten into the mix.

Fill six to seven ramekins no more than an inch (2.5 cm) deep. Place them in the oven for 45 to 60 minutes. When the consistency is gelatinous, and the surface is a bit dry looking, remove from the oven and place in the refrigerator to cool for about four hours. (The best results are achieved by allowing the ramekins to chill in the refrigerator overnight. This is therefore a good dessert to make ahead of time, preferably the night before you plan to serve it.)

Before caramelizing, use your fingertips to sprinkle a thin layer of brown sugar or coconut sugar around the surface of each cream-filled ramekin. Gently shake and tilt the ramekin around sideways to allow the sprinkled sugar to distribute evenly on the surface without disturbing the cream. If you do not have a special butane culinary torch (*chalumeau*) to "burn" or caramelize the sugar on the surface of the cream, then preheat the oven on "broil" (to turn on the top burner or heating element) to 400°F (200°C).

Place an oven rack in the highest position in the preheated oven so the ramekins will be close to the broiler. Allow the heat from the broiler (or the culinary torch) to melt the sugars for only about two minutes.

Caramelizing the sugar in the oven does soften the *crème*. This is why restaurants prefer using a culinary torch to melt the sugars on top. It allows the cream beneath to remain cool while achieving a crunchy, sweet layer of "burned" sugar on the surface of the chilled dessert. If you do use a torch, be aware that the coconut sugar (shown on the right side in the photo below), is less refined and will therefore burn more quickly than the brown sugar (shown on the left in the same photo). This step may be skipped if you are avoiding the extra sugar, at which point it is basically a vanilla pudding, which tastes delicious, too!

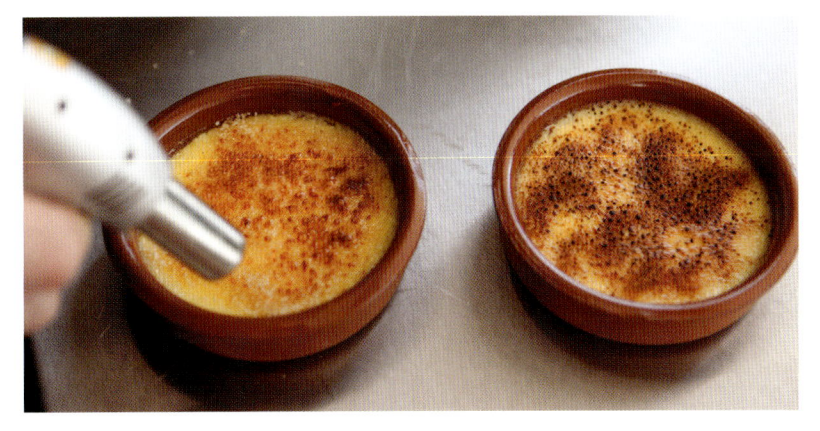

Serve at room temperature or slightly warmed. Garnish with a berry and a spearmint leaf, if desired. ➤

DESSERTS – *LES DESSERTS*

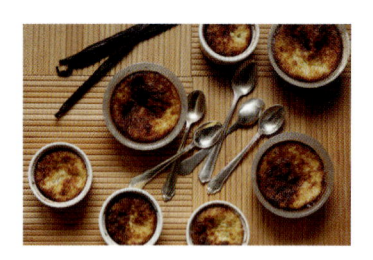

COCONUT MILK VARIATION
Use one cup of full-fat coconut milk and add two vanilla beans, cut in half. (Scoop out and use the pulp of the bean or use already scooped-out vanilla bean husks on their own, as they are still loaded with aroma and flavor even without their pulp).

Heat the coconut milk until you see steam rising, around 176°F to 180°F (80°C to 82°C), and then remove from the heat. Mix one tablespoon of honey into three yolks in a separate bowl, and then whisk this mixture into the coconut milk. Heat again to 180°F (82°C), stirring frequently. This makes about 1⅓ cups (about 300 ml) of the cream. Remove from the heat and fill about 5 small ramekins. Heat in the oven at 195°F (90°C) for 25 minutes.

Serve warm, as no additional burning is needed. The top will already be browned because the coconut milk "burns" more easily than the dairy version. If you are starting with 2 cups (475 ml) of coconut milk, use 4 eggs in the recipe. This will fill 9 to 10 small ramekins.

VARIATIONS For an extra-rich keto (low carb, high fat) custard without the *brûlée* crust, replace the milk with about ½ cup (120 ml) more cream and heat all the cream just as you would have heated the milk, and follow the recipe. The thicker cream brings out the "egginess" of the dish. Use one less egg if the egg flavor is too much, and reduce the oven time by 10 to 15 minutes. Using cream only increases the fat content and makes it easy to overcook the eggs. (Try using erythritol or monk fruit to desired sweetness, as these tend to have lower or no effect on blood sugar, or use no sweetener at all!) Makes 7 servings.

MORE VARIATIONS The original sweet (*sucré*) crème brûlée can be transformed into a savory (*salé*) dessert or appetizer (*entrée*) by leaving out the sweetener and adding in its place fine salt (and ground pepper if desired). Swap out the vanilla in this case and add a ½ teaspoon dried thyme and 7 tablespoons (100 g) fresh goat cheese (*chèvre frais*). You may still use sugar to burn the top of the *crème brûlée*. This will either increase the portion size a bit or the number of servings by one.

WINE PAIRING TIP Curious for a wine recommendation here? Most regions of France have their own regional sweet wine. An Alsatian would probably offer an aromatic, spiced, and peachy late-harvest Gewürztraminer Vendanges Tardives (from the German word for spices, *Gewürze*) while a *Bordelais* would probably suggest a Bordeaux sweet wine, like a Sauternes or a Barsac, wines teeming with apricot and honey aromas, among other sweet delicacies. Likewise, in the same vein of layering sweetness upon sweetness, a Béarnais (from the Southwest region of Béarn) might suggest a Jurançon, their sweet wine with notes of mango, or even their own late-harvest Jurançon Vendanges Tardives, with notes of beeswax and vanilla. Then there are also the dessert-style wines from Bergerac (Southwest), the Loire Valley, and Jura, and the Muscats from Langedoc-Roussillon or the Rhône Valley. When in Rome, do as the Romans do, and pair regionally. But when in Paris, a Parisian might suggest pairing your *crème brûlée* with Champagne!

WALNUTS IN MILK
Intxaursalsa (Noix au Lait)

Season Year-round (but usually enjoyed around the winter holiday season in Basque country)
Preparation Time 5 minutes   **Cooking Time** 1 hour   **Serves** 6

We end the Desserts section on a dessert with which the Basques conclude their calendar year, Walnuts in Milk. This typical walnut and coconut-infused holiday dessert is called *noix au lait* by the French and *intxaursalsa* (pronounced EEN-tcha-oor-sal-sa) or *intxaursaltsa* by the Basques and means "nut sauce." It is like a custard, or a rice pudding without the rice. Walnuts were brought by the Romans to Western Europe in the fourth century and are integral to the cooking of Southwestern France, as walnut groves abound in this part of the world. Inspired by a young Basque chef named Stéphane Garcia, whose cookbook was kindly given to me by my generous Basque friend Lilou Leonard, this recipe is a Basque standard, usually made with milk only, though I have seen versions using sour cream (*crème fraîche*) instead of the cream. Garcia's version is rich thanks to the whole cream, though in my version, I greatly reduced the amount of sweetener and added the gelatin for its healthful and congealing properties. I also have provided a variation on this dessert using coconut milk.

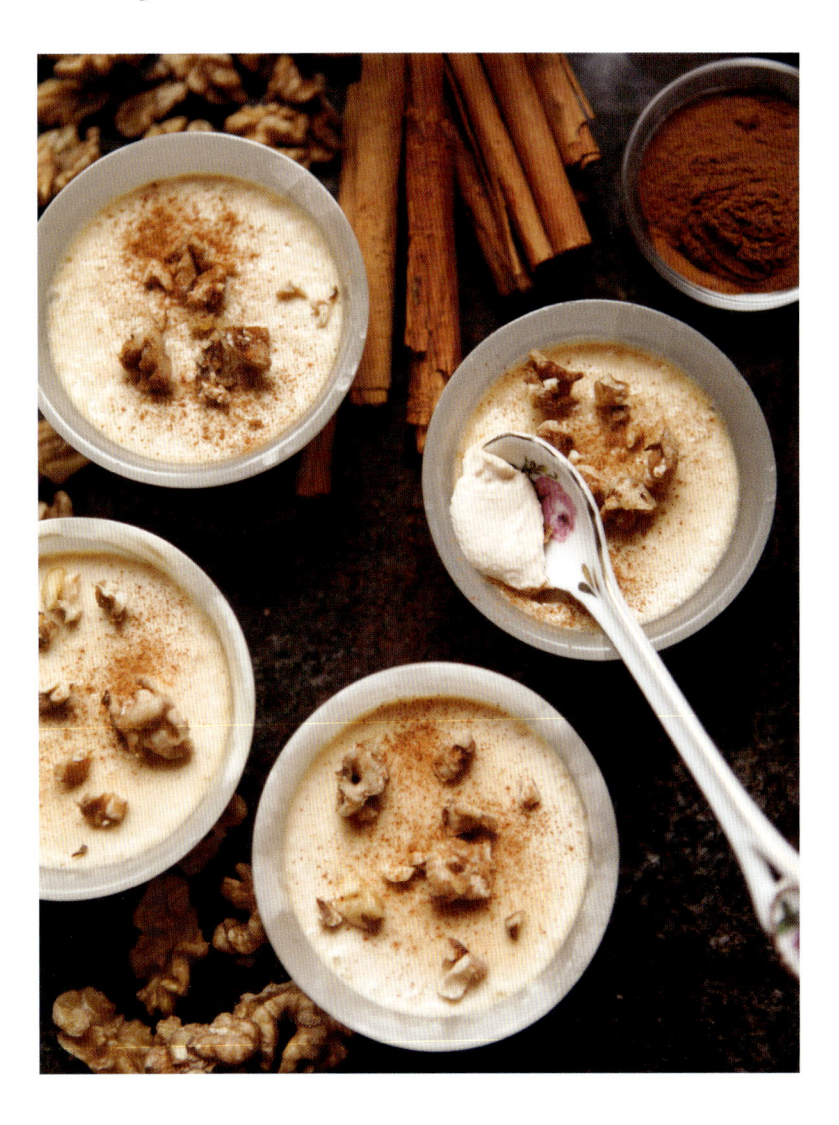

DESSERTS – *LES DESSERTS*

- 8 ounces (240 ml) whole milk
- 8 ounces (240 ml) whole cream
- 1 teaspoon raw cane or coconut sugar, or other sweetener
- 1 cinnamon stick (*baton de cannelle*)
- 3 ounces (85 g) walnuts, finely chopped
- 2 teaspoons powdered gelatin

Combine the milk and cream in a medium-sized pot over low heat. Whisk in the sugar and stir until dissolved. Add the cinnamon stick and chopped walnuts, and allow these to infuse on low heat, uncovered, for about an hour.

Pass the liquid in the pot through a sieve. (If you wish to keep the nuts in the dessert, there is no need to pass the liquid through a sieve. You might try crushing the strained walnuts into a grain-free porridge or into grain-free paleo pancakes. Make sure the consumers of the pancakes are tolerant of the residual dairy on the nuts.)

Whisk in the gelatin powder while the milk is still hot. Pour into small ramekins and allow them to set overnight in the refrigerator or cool off in the refrigerator for two hours. Makes six 1.5-ounce servings (45 ml) without the nuts, or slightly more if the nuts are included.

VARIATIONS I have also tried this dessert with coconut milk. Use one 13.5-ounce (400 ml) can, add half a can of water (200 ml), one cinnamon stick, and 2 ounces (about 60 g) of chopped walnuts. Heat on low for about 35 to 40 minutes. Add just a few grains of fine salt to enhance the flavors. I reduced the quantity of walnuts, as one of my daughters does not eat them, and proportionately, this amount of nuts is actually plenty for the dessert. Wait to add one tablespoon of raw honey (or maple syrup, monk fruit, or else a few drops of stevia) at the end of cooking. Remove from the heat and whisk in two tablespoons of gelatin. Pour into ramekins and allow them to cool. I use the brand "Natural Value" organic (unsweetened and 17% to 19% fat) coconut milk because it has no additives, unlike other brands that add guar gum, which can be irritating to the digestive tract.

WINE PAIRING TIP Ring in the holidays and new year with a slightly effervescent, dry white Txakoli from the Basque country in a regional pairing that slightly offsets yet embraces the sweetness and creaminess of the dessert. Happy New Year! *Urte Berri On!*

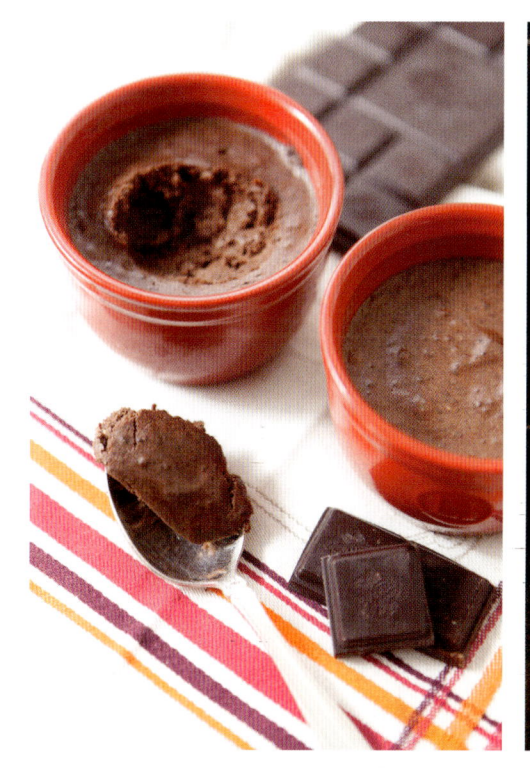

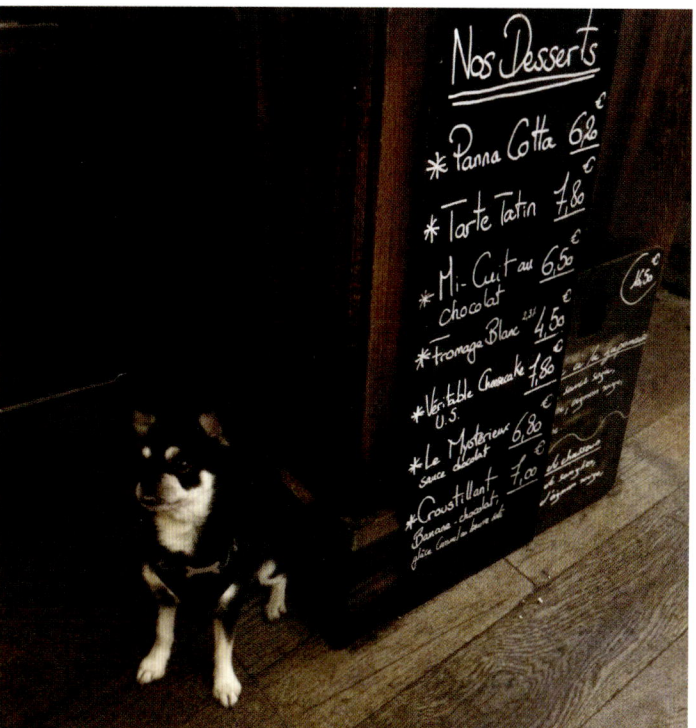

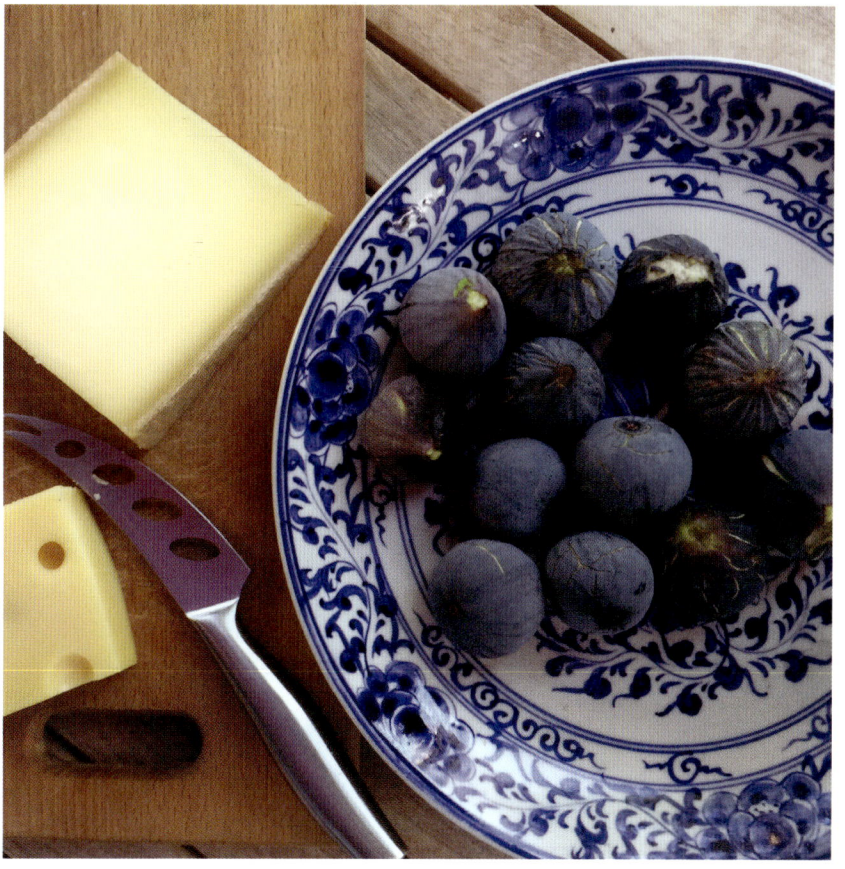

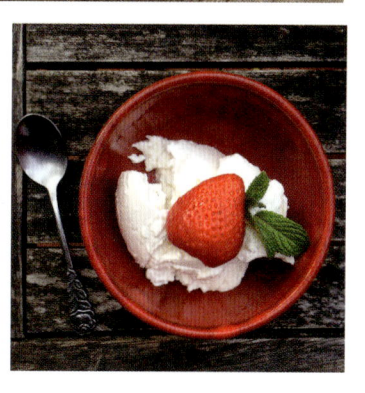

DESSERTS – *LES DESSERTS*

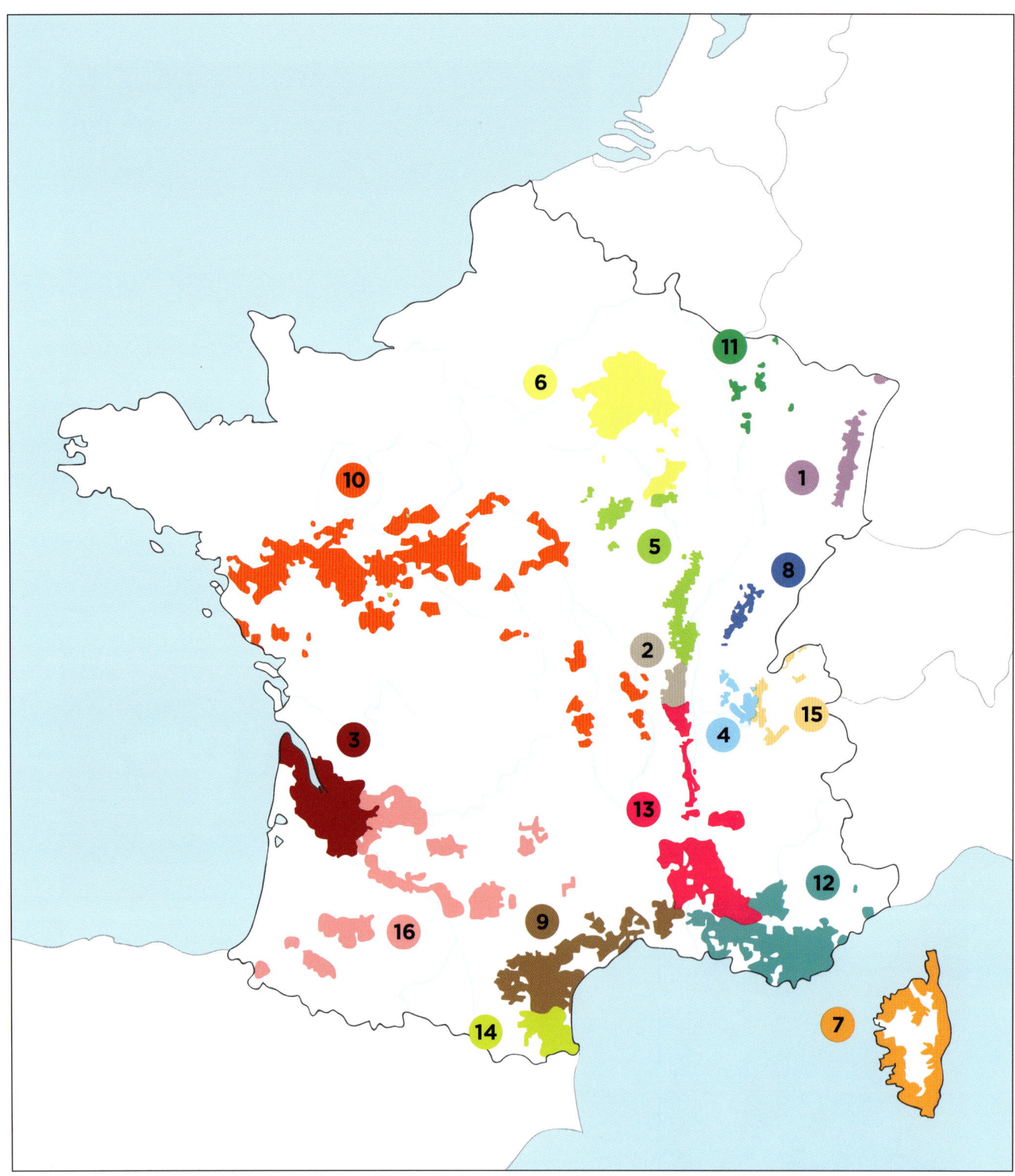

Winegrowing Regions of France – *Les Vignobles de France*

1. Alsace
2. Beaujolais
3. Bordeaux
4. Bugey
5. Burgundy – *Bourgogne*
6. Champagne
7. Corsica – *La Corse*
8. Jura
9. Languedoc
10. Loire Valley – *Val de Loire*
11. Lorraine
12. Provence
13. Rhône Valley – *Valée du Rhône*
14. Roussillon
15. Savoie
16. Southwest – *Sud Ouest*

CHAPTER 7
KNOW YOUR FRENCH WINES, HOW TO TASTE THEM, AND HOW TO PAIR THEM WITH FOOD

"Alone in the vegetable kingdom, it is the vine that gives us an understanding of the flavor of the earth."
—Colette, beloved French writer and Nobel Prize nominee in literature[1]

This chapter is dedicated to my late, highly esteemed, and decorated Oenology Professor, Denis Dubourdieu, a beloved and much sought-after wine professional who taught me and countless students and winemakers how the nuances and compromises required to make the kind of wine you would like to drink are much like those required to nurture the kind of life you would like to live. He is much missed by all who knew him.

PART I: WINE IN FRANCE, A CULTURAL INGREDIENT

Many French recipes call for wine as an ingredient in a meal, but wine really is an ingredient that intertwines, like the vines themselves, with French culture. Wine is something to be enjoyed alongside a meal, an accompaniment to the sensorial experience, if not, at times, the focus itself. When paired with an ancestral meal, wine can enhance not only the flavors of a dish, but also the social aspects of the dining experience. Wine accompanying a meal also serves as a means of slowing down to savor both the meal and the drink. Thus, tasting and drinking wine can be seen as a meditation in itself: "Drink your food and chew your wine," as they say in France.

Culinary Institute of America graduate, cook, author, photographer, wine professional, lecturer, and longtime resident of Bordeaux, Dewey Markham, Jr. realized during his first three years working in France as director of students at *L'École de Cuisine La Varenne* in the early 1990s that he was "surrounded by a culture in which wine was more than just an accompaniment to lunch and dinner; it was a natural and enriching part of daily life." The slow enjoyment of a meal paired with wine allows us to extract aromas, flavors, sensations, emotions, and later, positive memories, especially in the company of family and friends, whatever the occasion.

Every winemaker knows that wine is for drinking. It is the pursuit of pleasure for its own sake, through food and wine, and sharing the moment, that is revered in France, and certainly, in many cultures around the globe. Play for play's sake, as Mark Sisson of Primal Blueprint says. Art for art's sake, pleasure for pleasure's sake. As my friend, and organic and bio-dynamic winegrower at Château Guadet in Saint Emilion, Vincent Lignac, says, "The best wine is the one that you like *and* drink."[2] The main thing is to just try something rather than be intimidated. The joy is in the adventure, the exploration.

WINE: A SENSORY-DENSE EXPERIENCE

When we drink wine, we open our senses. We listen to the story of the wine through its color, origin, age, aromas, and taste. Regional dishes often call for regional pairings of wine and food, but there is no one right way. Balancing flavors, color, acidity, sweetness, aroma, intensity of flavor, season, time of day, and geographic origin of wine, as well as the location where the wine is being consumed, can be factors in the pairing of wine and food. Many wine blends (*assemblages*) have aromas of the things we may love to consume already: butter, coffee, chocolate, caramel, red cherries, dark berries, citrus fruits, stone fruits, apple, pear, tropical fruit, honey, nuts, spices (cinnamon, cloves, anise), even smoke (think of grilled or smoked meats). You can quench your desire for these diverse delicacies through the subtle aromas and flavors in wine. Seeking out these aromas and flavors is part of the fun and exhilaration of trying different wines. It is one of many aspects of wine that is so amazing: to think that a little fruit like the grape, fermented with care, can yield such delicious, varied, and exotic aromas from around the world, as if the grape had traveled the planet, picking up bits and pieces from Nature's vast array of fruit and plant life, before being picked at harvest time and transformed into the elixir reflecting its colors in your glass.

"One produces wine to drink at mealtime as well as to enjoy an emotion."[3]
—Eric Boissenot, Bordeaux oenologist and wine consultant.

WINE IN THE ANCESTRAL CONTEXT

Throughout our history, humans have relied on the fermentation of food and drink to aid both in preservation and digestion, and this practice continues today in many cultures around the world. While the cultivation of wine is decidedly a Neolithic activity, there is still an undeniable desire and interest among many to include it in the primal/paleo/ancestral lifestyle. Indeed, wine has accompanied French meals for centuries, as it has throughout Europe. Wine contains healthful properties, such as resveratrol and other polyphenols and even traces of vitamins as well as glutathione, which preserves the wine. But most of all, wine is something to be enjoyed alongside a meal in the company of family and friends, a complement to the sensorial experience and a means of slowing down to savor both the meal and the drink. As my friend Aline Baly of Château Coutet says, "Wine is the Kevin Bacon of industries. It's related to art, music, food, people. It links everything to everything."[4]

THE SOVEREIGNTY OF FRENCH WINE

Just as French cuisine is looked to as the premier example for cooking methodology and technique, so are French wines among the most coveted and well known, not to mention some of the most rare and expensive, most notably those from Bordeaux and Burgundy. The most refined of these wines are made from hand-picked grapes, watched over with great care throughout the year, growing in the vineyard, fermenting in the barrel, and aging in the bottle. Not to be left behind, however, are the celebrated wines from the other regions of France: Alsace, Beaujolais, Champagne, Corsica, Languedoc-Roussillon, the Loire Valley, Lorraine, the Jura, Provence, the Rhône Valley, Savoie-Bugey, and the Southwest). For details about the regions and their grape varieties, see the map of **Winegrowing Regions of France** (page 512) and the list of **Major Grape Varieties Grown in France** (page 546).

GROWING UP WITH WINE

My French friend Chef Frédéric encourages his children (and his culinary students, like me) to smell everything, from fruits to spices. Indeed, many French can be seen at the markets smelling the fruits and vegetables, cheeses, and other products they are considering for purchase and discussing these qualities with the vendors and fellow customers. The French not only allow their children to smell the wine that the adults are drinking at mealtime, but they dilute it with water for the children to sip, diluting less as the child becomes a teenager. In this way, wine (and alcohol in general) is not such an exotic, forbidden element, but rather an integral part of life and developing one's sensorial experience.

My older daughter loves to name all the fruits she smells in the aroma of wine. She does not drink it, it's too "harsh" for her, but she loves the satisfaction of pinpointing certain aromas. Before my final wine exam, my daughter and I practiced smelling aromas with *Le Nez Du Vin*, an aroma kit with 54 of the most common aromas one finds in wine, which we borrowed from my trusting friend Caroline Matthews, a wine professional, teacher, and tour guide in Bordeaux. We enjoyed trying to guess from which fruit or plant the aroma was derived. It makes for a great party game for wine enthusiasts, where one person picks a vial and everybody smells and tries to guess what it is. It's not as easy as one might think!

Americans do not tend to grow up with an emphasis on the sensorial experience of food, and certainly not of wine. If we did, we would not be as easily lured by the trappings of "modern eating," that is, the over-salted, over-sugared processed "foods" that corrupt and dull our palates. Those who *do* enjoy fresh, homegrown, homemade foods are able to sense the nuances in flavor and aroma. Anyone can do so once they release themselves from the grips of processed "foods." Unfortunately, most Americans do not grow up learning how to smell the aromas or taste the flavors of wine, because technically, drinking alcohol is not legally allowed before the age of 21. How odd and perverse it must seem to outsiders that we send our children off to war at the mild age of 18, yet do not allow them to grow up tasting the richness of wine with a meal, nor thereby pass on to them, in a relaxed family setting, the responsibility that goes with consuming alcohol.

TRAINING OUR SENSE OF SMELL

One of the visiting lecturers during my yearlong Bordeaux University "DUAD" wine course, Alexandre Schmitt, a former professional "nose" (*un nez*) from the perfume industry in Paris, admonished us to smell everything, to become aware of the scents around us and try as often as possible to describe them. By developing our olfactory sense, we would also train our brains to detect and articulate for ourselves and others the aromas in our environment, thereby training ourselves to also better describe wines. Learning to detect smells and identify their source is an important memory exercise for the brain. We all know from personal experience how a particular scent can retrieve a particular memory.

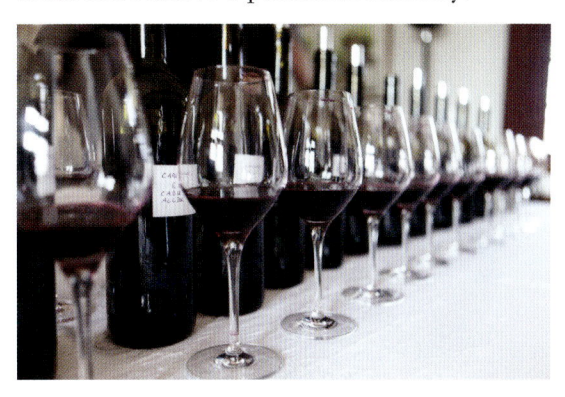

Training our brains to connect our memory to our sense of smell to enhance our ability to detect smells seems to me a form of meditation, a way of grounding our senses in the present. This is also what aromatherapy seems to support, a focus on an aroma that will help you relax, feel better, and more invigorated. Each scent or aroma seems to have a purpose. Perhaps this is why you also might feel more like having one type of wine over the other, if you have associated certain feelings or states of being to the aromas in one wine versus another.

HEALTH RISKS OF CONSUMING ALCOHOL (AND SUGAR)

Legendary Bordeaux oenologist Emile Peynaud said, "Wine, originating from live cells, contains, in diluted form, all that is necessary for life."[5] Wine indeed is composed of many substances as Peynaud notes: ethanol, methyl alcohol, glycerine (part of what gives wine its viscosity), aldehydes, amino acids, esters, cysteins, histamines, sulphites (a naturally-occurring preservative), but also traces of butyric acid, glutathione and inositol, polyphenols (like resveratrol), and other healthful vitamins and minerals.

Red wine, high in polyphenolic (plant-derived) antioxidants such as resveratrol, has been shown to have healthful properties.[6,7] Red wines from the French Southwest in particular have been shown to have high concentrations of procyanidins (polyphenols present in grape skins and seeds), contributing to the protection of blood vessels and potentially lowering blood pressure.[8] Resveratrol itself (colorless and also present in white grape skins)[9] has been shown to improve mitochondrial function,[10] and an entire book containing relevant studies has been compiled by Dr. Joseph Maroon on how resveratrol and red wine contribute to longevity.[11] Nevertheless, the health risks of over-consuming alcohol are well known: it can cause liver disease, it crosses the blood-brain barrier, and it's addictive. (These health risks seem more widely known and accepted by the public than the fact that our over-consumption of refined sugars and simple carbohydrates is also addictive and detrimental to our health.)

Interestingly, the ethanol in wine protects the wine. Pure ethanol is astringent and bitter, but becomes sweeter when diluted with water, as it is in wine. Depending on the dosage, even water and oxygen are toxic to us. Therefore, the key is to find the right balance of pleasure in the "minimum effective dose," as Primal Blueprint's Mark Sisson says. Exercise, stress, or anything else overdone can harm us.

Alcohol metabolizes as sugar in the liver and has insulinogenic, immunogenic, and addictive effects on the body, very much like sugar, especially fructose, though much of society, including me, would rather not admit it.[12] Whereas alcohol has an immediate, visible effect on our behavior and physical capacity, fructose is more chemically insidious, as the effects are not visibly obvious. Ingesting sugar causes us to become insulin resistant over time and to store fat. It also destabilizes our mood, energy levels, and gut microbiome.

(NOT) DRINKING ON THE JOB

Understanding the risks of consuming alcohol, or indeed any sugar, or refined carbohydrate, for that matter, can help us to determine our limits and a healthier intake level. (Currently, I am unable to tolerate more than a sip or two of wine. It is better for me to just sniff, swirl, sniff again, take a sip, swish, and spit once before the meal, and thereafter simply enjoy the aromas of the wine.) *Cracher* is the term for spitting out the wine. Some can do this more elegantly than others. The trick is to aim well and use the right amount of force! This is what the professionals do when tasting multiple wines a day. They must do this, or their workday would come to an intoxicated halt by 10 o'clock in the morning. More than just a few sips of wine can give some people, myself included, digestive and metabolic problems. For now, I am mostly a taster (*dégustateur*), but I am hopeful that I will tolerate more in time. While I have studied wine, I am, by no means, a wine professional or expert, but I am inspired to impart some of what I have learned in an attempt to break down some of the mysteries of French wine into an accessible language all its own. And while we need not reenact the times of our great grandparents or their French counterparts, understanding what and how they ate, drank, lived, and communed—understanding where we came from—informs who we are today.

THE GEOGRAPHY OF WINE

Around the world, wine tends to grow between the 40th and 50th parallels, in both the Northern and Southern Hemispheres, with the best wines originating nearest the 45th Parallel, a magical midpoint between the North or South Pole and the Equator.[13] This geographic positioning has to do with the amount of sun exposure and climate experienced by the grape vines, but it is up to the winegrowers to make the best of this set of advantages. By virtue of working the land, they understand the interplay between geography and climate on the soil, and indeed the microbiome of their land, and their aromatic and gustatory effects on the wines they produce, much as cheesemakers or other agricultural producers understand how the distinctiveness of their soil, animals, climate, and geography affects their produce, cheeses, or meats. This individual territorial distinction or typicity (*typicité*) is known as *terroir*.

EXPRESSION AND GEOGRAPHY

With regard to geographic positioning and wine, Axel Marchal (one of my principal professors at the Institute of the Vine and Wine at the University of Bordeaux, who now runs the yearlong "DUAD" wine course I took) points out that "very often, the most original and unique expression of a grape variety is found at the *northern* limit of its zone of maturation (the region where it matures in time for harvest before freezing or rotting), that is to say, in those places where the grape can ripen only thanks to the viticulturist's efforts combined with the right conditions of climate throughout the year. This is the case, for example, with Sancerre in the Loire Valley for the Sauvignon Blanc grape. Other examples include the Piémont wine growing region in Italy for the Nebbiolo grape, the Côtes de Nuits in Burgundy for Pinot Noir, and the Médoc region North of Bordeaux for Cabernet Sauvignon. As Denis Dubourdieu always said, the regions where the vine is too easily cultivated make for wines that are often uninteresting to taste."[14] Professor Dubourdieu also told his students that it is the very gustatory typicity or distinction of a terroir expressed in a wine and revealed with the help of the winemaker, that helps one understand a wine's true value.

APPELLATIONS OF PROTECTED ORIGINS (AOP) IN FRANCE

In order to maintain territorial integrity and quality assurance and guarantee the origin of the agricultural products from a given region in France, the AOP (*Appellation d'Origine Protégée*) label exists for France's best wines. (AOP used to be AOC—*Appellation d'Origine Contrôlée* until the European Union agricultural reforms of 2008.) The AOC/AOP label is controlled by an organization under the French Ministry of Agriculture, the INAO (*Institut National de l'Origine et de la Qualité*, previously *Institut National des Appellations d'Origine*, or INAO). Other agricultural labels such as *Label Rouge* (also given by the Ministry of Agriculture, primarily for food) each carries its own meaning and set of standards. There are more than 400 AOCs for France's wines. Winemakers can either make a wine under the rigorous and more prestigious AOC/AOP label, or else under the IGP label (*Indication Géographique Protégée*), under which wines are not allowed to be blended from across geographic zones and are made, in limited quantities, reaching a minimum alcoholic strength. The AOC/AOP system also is an official acknowledgement of the concept of terroir.

WINE GROWING AND THE IDEA OF TERROIR

The concept of *terroir* puts forth that the distinctness and flavor of an agricultural product comes from the earth, soil, climate, geography, and human practices (altogether the *terroir*) from which it originates. And for the terroir of wine, this definition includes the vine (type of grape variety) itself as well.[15] While these variable factors make it difficult to study terroir scientifically, the ultimate expression of a great terroir is undeniable to those who study, taste, and smell the difference. Some oenology experts even argue that a great terroir can only be expressed under favorable socio-economic conditions that support an orientation toward high-quality production (as compared to mass production).[16] American farmer, ecologist, and author Joel Salatin puts forth a similar argument, that the richness of a farm's bounty comes from the richness of its soil, and indeed, it's soil microbiome, and how sustainably these have been managed.

THE EXPRESSION OF TERROIR

French farmers and viticulturists alike who are focused on high quality grow their vines, produce, or livestock, or make their butter and cheese with a deep understanding of their terroir, how it has changed over the years, what grows best on their terroir, and how to best express all of these elements in their final product. The farmer understands his land and produces the best product he can given his circumstances. According to Professor Dubourdieu, the winemaker has been able to work with and overcome the handicaps and limitations of his particular terroir to create the best product he can, and this successful guidance of the terroir is another contributing factor to a wine's value. Any "foodie" or "gourmand" in the U.S., France, or elsewhere who appreciates and enjoys local or regional specialties of food or wine produced or prepared in a specific way can thus understand the value of terroir. In France, many of these terroir distinctions are regulated by governmental and certifying bodies, as mentioned previously, to maintain the integrity and value of the wine or other products made on certain terroirs.

SOIL TYPE AND WATER

French AOP wines are subject to government regulation in which no irrigation is allowed (called "dry farming"), as compared to the U.S., where in Napa Valley, for example, irrigation is allowed. Leaving the vines to their own devices forces them to expand their roots far below the surface in search of water. The depth of the vines through different soil types, along with limited water resources, for red wine vines in particular, concentrates the flavors and phenolics in the grape's energy (as opposed to diluting them in the presence of too much water). Too much "water stress" (*contrainte hydrique*), however, can be detrimental to vines. But the right amount of rainfall at the right time, particularly before the color change in the grapes (*la véraison*) is an important factor in achieving high-quality wine, albeit in limited quantities. Amazingly, the quality and type of the soils in which the vines grow (whether limestone, clay, gravel, granite, sandy, etc.) has a *direct* effect on the aromas, flavors, and textures of the resulting wines. The soil type combined with the climate and geography in which the vines grow, guided by human knowledge, all add up to the unique terroir which figures enormously in the resulting wine. This is why certain parcels of land in France yield the most globally sought-after wines.

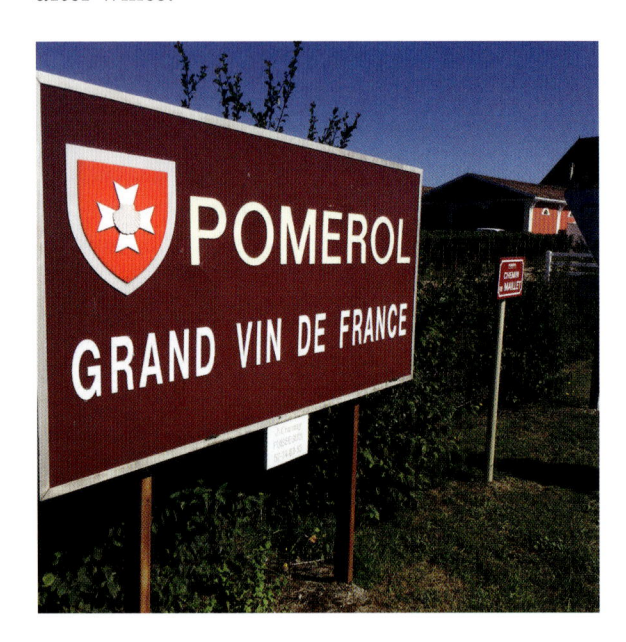

SOIL TYPES

Different types of soils create an environment in which the vine must seek water. Gravel, for example, heats up during the daytime, retaining some amount of heat past sundown, which can help grapes mature. In other soils, such as clay or silt, the water is easier to reach, and the roots need not travel as deeply. The extent to which the vine must dig deep or remain near the surface changes the resulting flavors of the wine. Certain grape varieties are better able than others to produce flavorful wines under increased severity of water restriction or water stress, such as those that must dig their roots more deeply, creating more concentrated flavors, while other varieties need more frequent hydration. Thus, we see that soil type is a major contributor to terroir. For example, the red wines of the Graves (pronounced "GRAH-v") area, south of Bordeaux—named after the gravely soils—are harmoniously balanced, with robust tannins and excellent aging potential. And the clay and limestone, clay and gravel, and sandy, clay soils of the Saint Emilion-Pomerol-Fronsac region East of Bordeaux produce smooth, powerful (tannic), and elegant wines with superior aging potential, subtle flavors, and complex aromas.

THE MICROBIOLOGY OF WINE
The alcoholic fermentation of wine is the conversion of grape juice sugars into ethyl alcohol and carbon dioxide thanks to naturally-occurring or added yeasts.[17] Fermentation is actually a continuous battle among micro-organisms, a kind of survival of the fittest. Yeast is a one-celled micro-organism, a fungus, and in wine the victor is usually of the genus *Saccharomyces cerevisiae* among the yeasts naturally present on mature grape skins. If the preferred "good" yeast strains are not nurtured and become outnumbered by other micro-organisms, bacteria, or other yeasts such as *Brettanomyces*, also present on grape skins, then the aromas and flavors of the wine can be altered, usually for the worse. Read more about this in the "Defects in Wine" section on page 538. (This is why some winemakers will add commercial yeasts to ensure the success of the "good" guys. Use of commercial yeasts is not allowed in organic and biodynamic wines.) Yeast's effectiveness at multiplying itself depends on the fluidity of the plant sterols in the cell membrane allowing nutrients in and out of its cell (depending on specific concentrations of sugar, alcohol, nitrogen, pH, hydration, among other factors), much like our own cells require the proper cell membrane fluidity (balancing cholesterol, a stiffening agent of the cell membrane,[18] and omega-3 fatty acids, which aid us in this fluidity[19]) and conditions in which to function and metabolize nutrients optimally. Temperature plays a role in the fluidity of the yeast cell membrane; therefore, the winemaker must constantly monitor the vats where fermentation occurs. Aeration is also needed at the beginning to kick-start fermentation. Incidentally, the mitochondria of yeast cells need the right conditions in which to function, just as the mitochondria in our own cells do. Indigenous yeast strains (also called "native" yeasts), naturally present on the grape skins in a given plot or parcel of a vineyard, can be selected, incubated, and employed by the winemaker in the process of fermentation of wine. Yeast naturally synthesizes and excretes glycerol proportionate to the amount of alcohol it produces. (Yeasts also excrete some sulfites naturally.) This glycerol has an effect on viscosity, or "mouthfeel," while the yeast strains have an effect on flavor and complexity on the resulting wine. Therefore, in my opinion, yeast could be added to the list of factors contributing to terroir, particularly when indigenous yeast strains are at play.

FOLLOWING NATURE'S CYCLES
When winegrowers harvest, it is not necessarily at the maximum peak of flavor of the grape, but rather at the moment when the cross-section of acidity and sweetness is at its highest, when any green, herbaceous aromas are gone and the fruity aromas are present, but the grape is not yet overripe. Every year, the anticipation of maturity in the grapes is a gamble due to the vagaries of nature, pests, and weather conditions. Environmental variability requires winegrowers to stay in tune with nature's cycles throughout the year, especially those involved in organic and biodynamic viticulture in France. Many winegrowers around France pride themselves on hand-harvesting their grapes, taking care to pick each bunch of grapes of each grape variety in each parcel of land only when it has reached its fullest potential. Some winegrowers, fewer than 1%, such as Olivier Decelle of Château Jean Faure in St. Emilion (organically certified as of 2017), have even brought back the use of horses in the vineyard in lieu of machines in order to maintain

more natural cycles and practices of soil and vine health management to their terroir. The practice of employing horses and drivers is costlier, but it exemplifies a commitment to ancestral practices and defiantly less reliance on mechanization. (See photos below.)

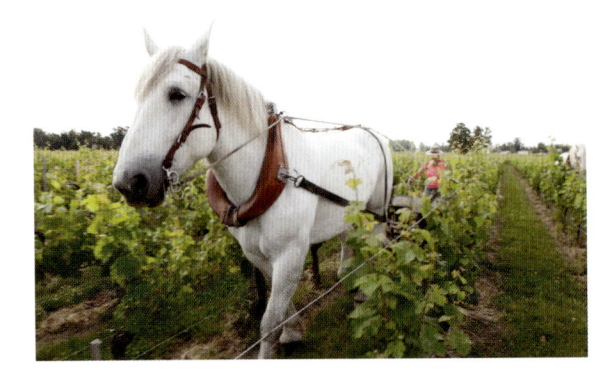

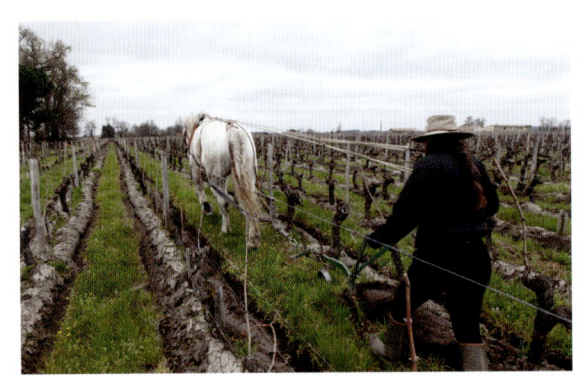

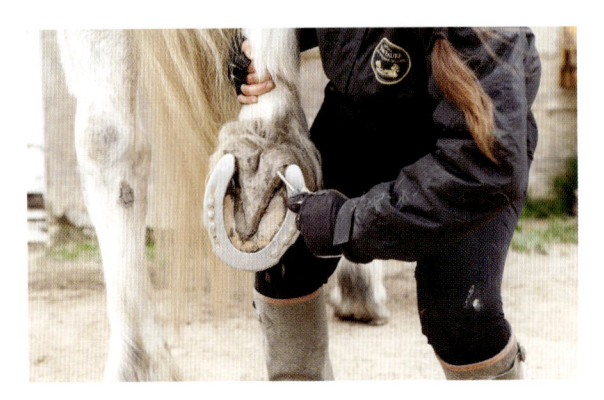

THE CASE FOR ORGANIC AND BIODYNAMIC WINES

From an ancestral perspective, the most interesting and sought-after wines are the ones originating from soils and vines that are rich in their own microbiome and indigenous yeasts. This means supporting a diverse ecosystem in and around the vines, including other existing species of flora and fauna (such as bees, birds, butterflies, and flowers), as well as the soil microbiota, without the use of GMOs, synthetic chemicals, herbicides, and fungicides. Organic and biodynamic wines must be handled by the viticulturist in the most nature-mimicking way. What's more, organic red wines have been shown to contain more antioxidant-rich polyphenols (phytochemicals, compounds found in plants, such as resveratrol) than non-organically produced wines.[20]

Organic French wines have increased in quality and diversity, according to my DUAD wine course classmate Vy Nguyen (formerly involved in a French Southwest, Aquitaine regional organic winegrowers' association, and now a viticulture consultant and instructor at the Bordeaux Wine School[21] and La Maison des Vins de Saint Emilion). She believes the advantages of drinking these wines are many: increased public awareness and support in recent years for more sustainable farming and viticulture practices in France, and by extension, the decreased use of synthetic chemicals; the public's newfound discovery of organic and biodynamic wines in general; and the fact that by definition, organic and biodynamic wines reflect their unique terroir and thereby accord value to the know-how (*savoir faire*) of the winemaker.

CERTIFIED ORGANIC FRENCH WINES

In France, certified organic (*biologique* or *bio*) wines are subject to standards set by the European Union. Grapes used for winemaking under this designation must be grown organically (without synthetic chemicals) and with only a minimum of sulfites present in the wine. The treatment and fermentation of the grapes differ from one region and winemaker to the next. But for organic wines, no sugar may be added to sweeten the deal and the addition of sulfites (which act as antioxidants and stabilizers for the wine) during fermentation is allowed only in limited quantity. Copper is one example of a naturally occurring element that organic wine producers are permitted to use, albeit in limited quantities, to combat mildew, a common problem in the vineyard. There are many uncertified organic French winegrowers who, nevertheless, follow organic viticulture, but who have not paid for or gone through the process of organic certification. In my experience in Bordeaux, in many vineyards whose terroir is highly valued to the owners and consumers, a policy of "lowest effective dose" (*lutte raisonnée*) is upheld when using pesticides and for general vineyard maintenance, regardless of whether they are designated organic or biodynamic.

Uncertified, But Terroir-Conscious

Château Haut-Bailly, located in the Pessac-Léognon region just south of Bordeaux, represents high-quality consciousness of terroir. Véronique Sanders, General Manager at Haut-Bailly since 1998 and one of the few women in Bordeaux running a large vineyard, says: "Vineyard operations at Haut-Bailly are largely traditional, with an emphasis on careful observation in the vineyard of the health of the vines, rather than a heavy reliance on technology to make our decisions. Chemical weed killers have never been used at Haut-Bailly and the grapes have always been harvested by hand. Respect for the environment means limiting the use of sprays to a strict minimum and always adapting our care of the vineyard with the least amount of intervention necessary in any given situation. 'Strict minimum' refers to the minimum quantity of chemicals needed to prevent this or that disease (in our estimation), …and we use only about 10% of the authorized quantities in our appellation."

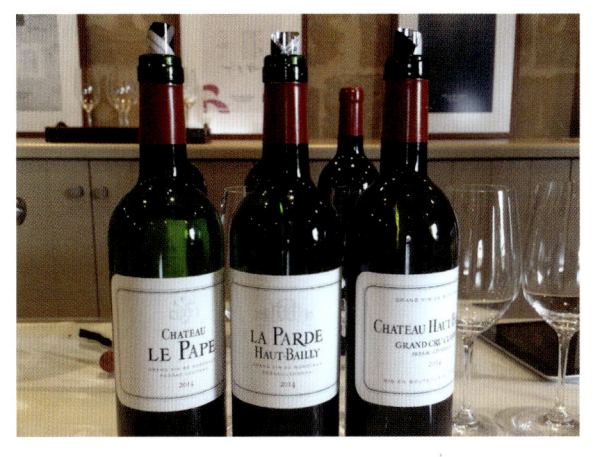

BIODYNAMIC WINES

The biodynamic (*la biodynamie*) approach to wine in France takes an even more holistic approach to the health of the vine, much like naturopathic doctors and functional medicine doctors approach the health of their patients, treating the root cause of the problem, rather than just the symptoms, as in allopathy or our modern medical paradigm. This approach to agriculture was first proposed in 1924 by Austrian philosopher Rudolf Steiner in response to growing concerns about industrial agriculture and an increasing awareness of its negative contribution to soil and ecological degradation. In the case of the vineyard, the theory is that if it is cultivated in harmony with nature, the grape will yield a greater potential. In France, both organic and biodynamic wines require certification to be labeled as such, and no GMOs or synthetic chemicals may be used. Similar natural elements, like copper, and products are allowed in both organic and biodynamic farming, but usually it is the dosages that differ. For example, according to my friend Vincent Lignac, a former graduate of the University of Bordeaux DUAD wine course, an organic winegrower can use up to 13.2 pounds (6 kg) of copper per hectare (about 2.5 acres) per year, while the limitations for a biodynamic winegrower is half that dose. Interestingly, there is no limit, nor difference in allowed doses of sulphur in the vineyard, which even Vincent finds a bit odd. Therefore, it is up to the integrity and practice of the winegrower to make the call on "chemical" usage across all types of viticulture. One biodynamic strategy Vincent uses in the vineyard is to water the vines with an "herbal tea" (*une infusion*) of nettle on his vines. The nettle tea provides nitrogen, a "good boost when the plant is young and growing," as well as iron, to facilitate the production of chlorophyll and therefore photosynthesis.[22] Nettle provides the vines with minerals, and, as it turns out, has beneficial anti-microbial properties.[23]

THE EXPRESSION OF TERROIR IN ORGANIC AND BIODYNAMIC WINES

From a biodynamic perspective, the appearance of a pathogen in the vineyard, such as a fungus, implies an imbalance in soil health, (much as pathogenic or other infections in humans signify an imbalance in the microbiota or hormonal systems in humans, from a naturopathic doctor's perspective). The holistic, biodynamic approach takes into consideration the seasonal and light and dark (solar and lunar) rhythms of nature (not dissimilar from the cycles of our own mitochondrial and circadian rhythms) for the planting, caretaking, and harvesting processes in the vineyard. Honoring this cyclical rhythm of the terroir and soil health, leads to better root health and depth, greater indigenous bacterial diversity, and healthy development of the leaves, flowers and, ultimately, the grapes. This ecosystem of nutrients conveys to the grape the unique elements of that terrain, which then yields a wine that is the true expression of the terroir. Some liken the process of biodynamic viticulture to homeopathic treatment in humans, in which very small, precise doses of elements are prescribed to promote a stronger immune system. In Vincent's experience, "the stronger the immune system, the better the quality of the fruit."

"Natural wines" are not officially a designation of wine in France, but some wines will be referred to as such. Similar to organic and biodynamic wines, natural wines respect the "natural" conditions in which the grapes have been grown. Likewise, sustainable and organic techniques are used in the vineyard, but differ slightly in the winery. Sulfites are not added (but the wine may be kept at low temperatures, without additions of yeasts or sugar, or adjustments to the acidity of the wine), and, like organic and biodynamic wines, only indigenous bacteria are used in fermentation, without fining or clarification (or *collage*, which is the removal of suspended particles in the grape must or the use of other filtration methods).

FINDING AND BUYING FRENCH ORGANIC, BIODYNAMIC, AND NATURAL WINES

While it can be challenging to find wines that are certified organic, biodynamic options, or close to it, do exist and their numbers are increasing. A few lists for organic and biodynamic wine producers exist online, but there is not yet one comprehensive site. If you ask in a wine store, however, you will usually be directed to at least a handful of organic or biodynamic wine producers. Dry Farm Wines, for example, is one such U.S. vendor of lab-tested, biodynamic, natural, and organic wines, many of which are imported from France. Some French organic, biodynamic, and natural winemakers and purveyors can be found at a number of French websites, but French language is necessary to comb through the information. Please refer to the Resources section (page 603) for lists of purveyors and winemakers of these kinds of French wines.

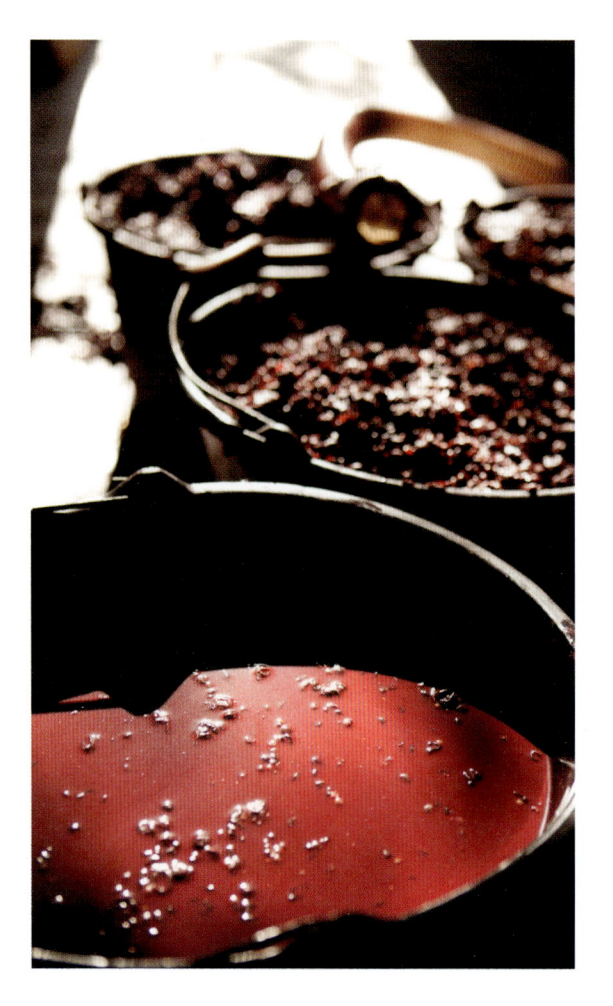

The Winemaker's Seasons: Viticulture and Winemaking Through the Year at Château Guadet with Organic Winemaker Vincent Lignac

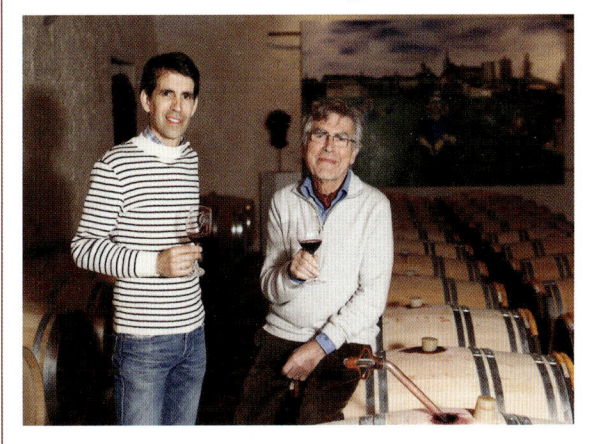

Château Guadet is an organic vineyard located in Saint Emilion, a UNESCO-protected town in the Bordeaux region receiving about one million visitors per year. Vincent Lignac and his parents, Guy-Pétrus and Catherine Lignac, run the family-operated vineyard, tours, and sales of their Grand Cru Classé wine. Vincent's approach to his wines is to allow the unique annual circumstances of his terroir to be expressed in his wines, while adhering to French organic certification standards and nurturing the vineyard and wine vat ecosystems in the most nature-mimicking way possible. The style of his wines reflects nature's work throughout the year on his predominantly Merlot and Cabernet Sauvignon grapevines.

September

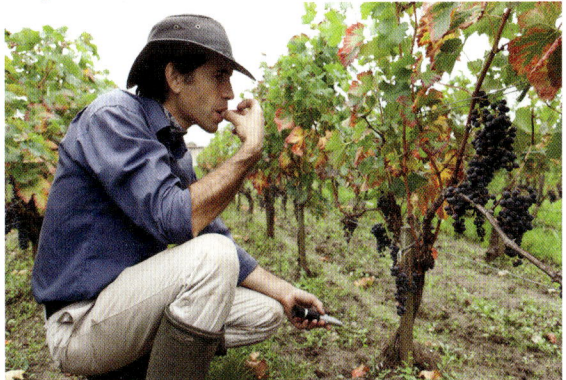

In the Vineyard – Monitoring ripening of the grapes and making decisions about oenological maturation, the optimal moment to harvest, for the best quality wine achievable, acidity balanced with sweetness, and minimal vegetal aromas (these are mostly pyrazines, smelling of green pepper). The maturity of the grape is evaluated mainly using berry tasting: skin, pulp, and seeds, as well as lab analyses as required by French law. Harvesting (*les vendanges*) may begin late-September, as it did at Château Guadet in 2015.

In the Winery – Cleaning the tanks and tools to get the winery and equipment ready for the harvest.

October

In the Vineyard – Harvesting by hand over the course of several days or weeks, depending on grape-maturity and weather.

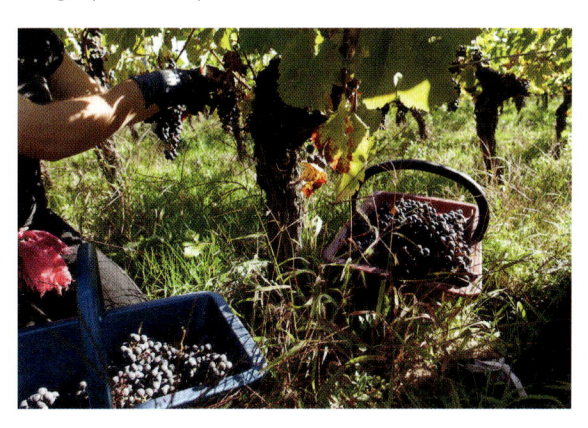

In the Winery – De-stemming and crushing of the grapes, turning over of the grapes during maceration (extracted grape juice in contact with the skins of the grapes). First fermentation, also called alcoholic fermentation, can take 20 to 40 days, monitored via tasting, at Château Guadet.

November

In the Vineyard – During the winter, the vineroots are covered with earth to protect the grafted[24] part of the vine, which is the most sensitive to frost, though winters on average have been warmer in recent years than in the past.

CHAPTER 7

523

December

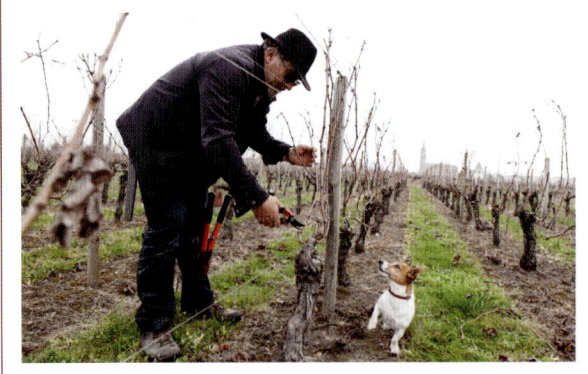

In the Vineyard – Pruning (*la taille*), which in Bordeaux vineyards usually comprises cutting off all but two branches (*Double Guyot*), or else just a single branch (*Simple Guyot*), a technique often used on Bordeaux's Right Bank (Blaye, Bourg, Castillon, St. Emilion), concentrates the plant's energy into the two branches (*baguettes*), or the one, with the most vigor. Choosing which branches to cut and which to keep is an art unto itself. One of France's champion vine pruners, Michel Duclos, shown above with his dog, pruning the vineyard of Pomerol's Château La Clémence, has shown Vincent how to prune vines. Vincent prunes his entire vineyard himself during the winter months.

January

In the Vineyard – Pruning of the vines continues.

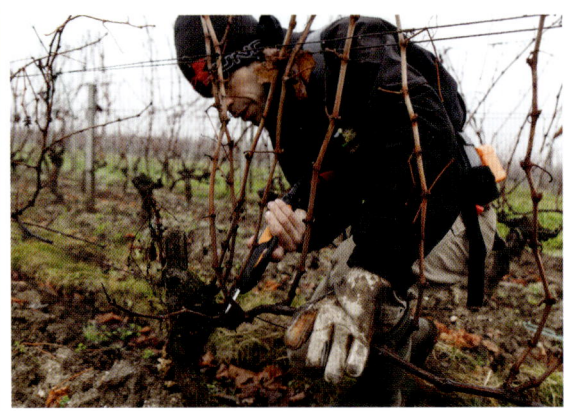

In the Winery – Secondary fermentation, also called malolactic fermentation (MLF) can take between 7 and 15 days but is usually finished within 10 days at Château Guadet. MLF is the transformation of malic acid into lactic acid and carbon dioxide by lactic acid-producing bacteria. *La Malo*, as it is fondly referred to by wine makers, is used for most red wines, many sparkling wines, and some white wines, notably Chardonnay, Pinot Gris, and Sauvignon Blanc. MLF adds complexity and flavor, lowers the wine's acidity, and increases the stability of the wine. Once it has begun, MLF goes relatively quickly, taking about 10 days. But it is sometimes hard to get started and can be delayed, beginning only in the spring or even later, especially for organic, biodynamic, and natural winemakers who are waiting for the natural selection process of the micro-organisms to occur and for the MLF to begin naturally. The wine must (fermenting grape juice) should be kept between 61°F and 68°F (16°C and 20°C). With artificially-made and implanted bacteria, MLF can be induced on the heels of alcoholic fermentation.

February

In the Vineyard – Pruning and pulling out the cut grape branches (*tirage des bois*). These cut branches or vines (*sarments de vigne*) are used for grilling many French recipes over a fire in the fall.

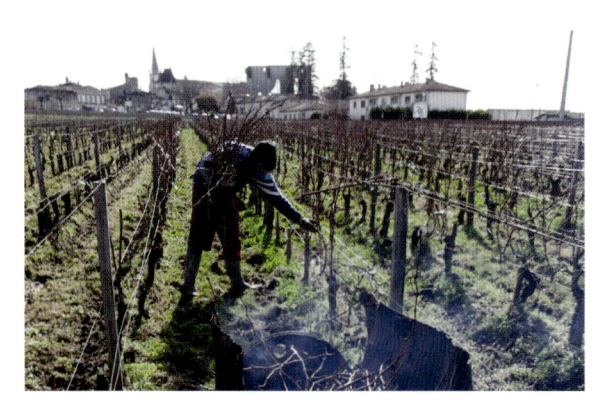

In the Winery – Racking (*soutirage*) of wine often entails using gravity and a tube to move wine from one barrel to another and to soften tannins and clarify wine by removing sediment. For biodynamically oriented wines, racking is traditionally done with the descending moon, as the deposits fall more readily to the bottom.

March

In the Vineyard – Wires are checked and tightened, while remaining vine shoots are fastened to wire (*pliage*), and the base of the vine is secured to wiring to keep aligned in its row (*calage*). Posts are fixed (*entretien du palissage*), and unneeded vines are burned (*brûlage*) to kill off unwanted microbes and diseases, while plowing loosens the soil.

In the Winery – Blending and Fining (*clarification*) sometimes with organic egg whites, although most vintners will use gelatin, an easier substance to work with. Aging in barrels. Topping up of the barrels to replace wine that has evaporated or soaked into the wood of the barrel.

April

In the Vineyard – Bud break (*débourrement*), and first young leaves. Pulling earth away from the vine roots—earth surrounding the vines is turned to give the vines room to grow. This also exposes harmful bacteria to the elements.

In the Winery – Aging in barrels. Racking (*soutirage*), another form of fining wine, that involves moving wine from one barrel into another, often using gravity alone. Topping up of barrels and tasting of wine.

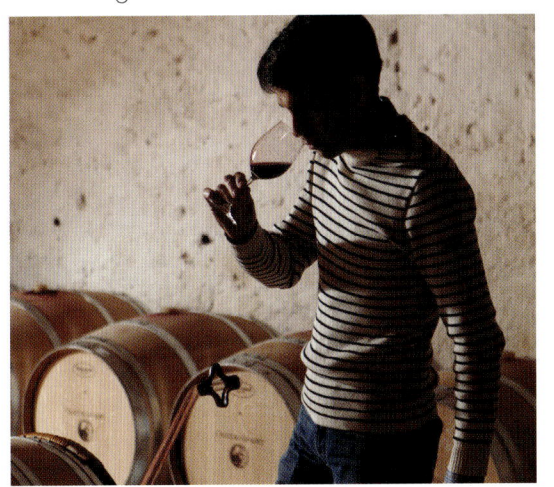

Outside the Winery – *En Primeurs* lasts for one week in Bordeaux. Winetasting professionals and journalists from around the world come to Bordeaux to see how young wines from the previous fall's harvest taste. Vincent represents Château Guadet's wines in Saint Emilion.

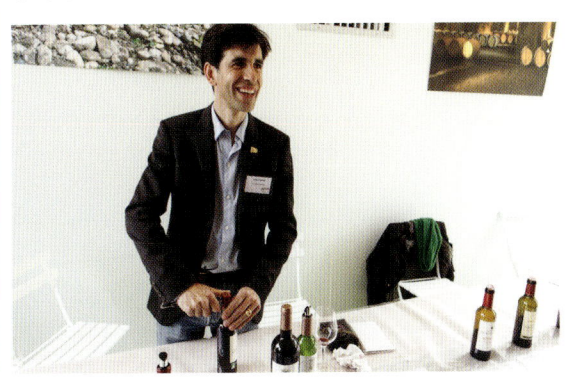

May

In the Vineyard – Removal of excess buds (*ébourgeonnage*) and unwanted vine shoots, known as desuckering (*épamprage*). Flowering (*la floraison*) begins.

In the Winery – Bottling at the end of May or in June (though it can also occur as early as April). There is normally no filtration at Château Guadet. Racking, fining, and topping up of barrels.

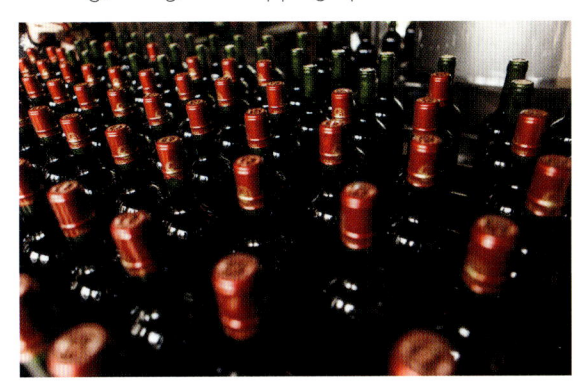

June

In the Vineyard – Flowering continues and fruit set (*la nouaison*) begins. First trimming of excess leaves on the vine root to enhance sun exposure but also to remove bacterial and parasitical access up the vine root.

In the Winery – Topping up of barrels.

July

In the Vineyard – Thinning of fruit (*éclaircissage*) to concentrate the aromas and energy into the remaining fruit on the vine. This procedure also controls the volume of the harvest. First deleafing of vines (*éffeuillage*) gives the grapes more air and sun exposure.

In the Winery – Racking, fining, and topping up of barrels.

August

In the Vineyard – First stage of ripening, which shows itself as a change in color of the grapes (*la véraison*). Green harvest (*vendanges vertes*), which is the removal of excess fruit to allow the best to grow and to concentrate the tannins and color. Second deleafing. Preparation for the next harvest.

Wines in Tune with the Seasons

An allegory for living in tune with the seasons and our ultimate dependence on nature would be winemaking's own dependence on the soil and climate throughout the year. My late wine professor, Denis Dubourdieu, perhaps the world's most prominent oenologist of his time, realized that in addition to growing the best-suited grape variety (*cultivar* or *cépage*) to a particular terroir, there were five natural, eco-physiological conditions necessary to make a great red wine in Bordeaux:

1. A rapid and precocious blossoming of the vine's flower (*floraison*), to ensure pollination during weather that is sufficiently warm and dry.

2. A rapid and precocious growth or "setting" of the fruit (*la nouaison*), for a homogenous maturity or simultaneous ripening of the grapes during weather that is sufficiently warm and dry.

3. The gradual onset of water stress or constrained hydration (*contrainte hydrique*), thanks to a warm, dry month of July, in order to slow down and then put a definitive stop to vine shoot growth during the turning or change of color (*véraison*) of the grapes. If fine weather does not come until the end of ripening, it is more beneficial to the Cabernets than to Merlot, as Cabernets ripen later than Merlot. A timely, natural constraint of hydration to the vine by the end of July keeps the grapes from growing too large and conserves the richness of their tannins.

4. The complete and homogenous maturation of the various grape varieties right up until harvest time, thanks to dry and warm (but not excessively so) weather in the months of August and September, as well as the proper management of leaf coverage and leaf removal without further growth of the vine. A combination of sun, heat, and syncopated small rains provide the right combination of hormetic stress on the vine to sustain life without drying out the vine completely.

5. Mild weather patterns (dry and medium-warm weather) during the harvest season that permit a delay in harvesting particular parcels of vines until they are adequately matured, without fear of excessive moisture that would rot the grapes or dilute their concentrations in flavor, anthocyanins, or pH (acid levels).

Successful dry white Bordeaux wines call for sweet fruity grapes in good condition with sufficient acidity and skins that are not very tannic. This balance is easy to obtain on suitable terroirs if the summer is temperate without excessive heat or drought conditions after the changing of the color of the grapes (*véraison*).[25]

THE VINTAGE EFFECT – *L'EFFET MILLÉSIME*

Since 1990, the most outstanding vintages for red wine in Bordeaux are considered to have been 1990, 2000, 2005, 2009, 2010 (less so for the Merlot grape), 2015, and 2016. But that does not mean you will like every wine you try from those years, or that other years failed. Every year has its character, its strengths and weaknesses, and it is only by trying them that you will get to know them. When choosing a wine, go with your taste buds, your heart, your mood, your budget, your health, and give what you can a try. You will learn something from each wine. The French say that if you listen to a wine, it will tell you its story.

PART II: WINE TASTING BASICS AND APPRECIATION

"Too often we eat, drink, and taste without paying any real attention to what we are tasting and smelling…during tasting… your attention needs to be focused on something specific and yet remain sufficiently flexible to notice other sensations as well. Meditation is a useful discipline in this respect."
—Emile Peynaud[26]

DISCOVERY VERSUS TASTING AND COMPARING

One of the first concepts put forth in my DUAD wine course in Bordeaux was that there is a difference between discovering a wine for the first time and tasting a wine with the goal of comparing it with others of its kind. In reality, we only can discern wines with which we are already familiar. Wine tasting is the art of reliving emotions, sentiments, and expectations that are conjured up by our previous experience with wines of the same type. In learning to taste, it is therefore primordial to memorize the overall sensations one experiences when encountering "model" or "archetype" wines of a certain category (in order to remember them and use them for comparison later). We can also be guided by friends or experienced tasters who know specifically about the category of wines in question. Too often, however, the model does not represent the category, as it constitutes an ideal esthetic, rarely encountered but always present at the origin of a specific emotion or sentiment.[27]

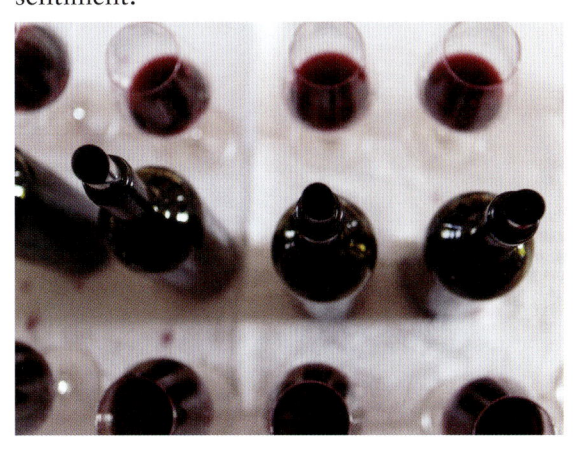

THE MODEL WINE

A useful technique taught by Professor Dubourdieu is to seek out a model or archetypical wine for a particular region or appellation to serve as a representative example of what that kind of wine should smell and taste like. By reserving this model in memory—keeping it in mind like a friend with a particular personality—you can compare other wines from that region and of this type in terms of their quality, tannic structure, flavor, aroma, and acidity. Some examples were Château Olivier for the red wines of Bordeaux's Pessac-Léognan appellation, Château Trotanoy in Bordeaux's Pomerol appellation, the Commune of Mersault for the Côtes de Beaune region, and Château Palmer for Bordeaux's Margaux appellation.

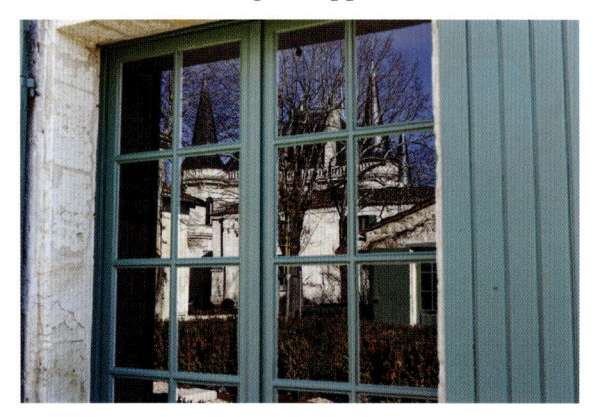

Château Palmer

The wine pairings I have suggested with the recipes in this book are intended to serve as guides. Later in this chapter, I will offer some ideas for wine-tasting theme parties, one of which has to do with acquainting oneself with the archetypical wines of a particular region. The main thing to remember is that once you have found your favorite wine of a particular type, one that "speaks" to you and arouses your senses, you will automatically refer to it later for comparisons as you go through your wine-tasting experiences.

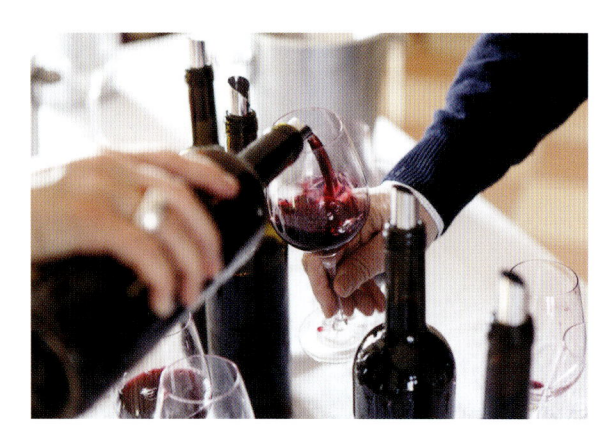

WINE DESCRIPTORS AS A COMMON LANGUAGE: THE FRENCH WAY OF DRINKING WINE

When we taste a wine, we are using multiple senses: sight, smell, touch, taste. We even use our sense of hearing when the bottle is uncorked and wine glasses are filled, we clink glasses, saying "cheers!" (or *santé!*—health) and discuss the wine over a meal or as compared to other wines. The French believe that one of the greatest pleasures, besides actually smelling and drinking wine, is to be able to share one's thoughts about the wine with one's friends and family while sharing that wine. As a result, it helps us if we have a common language to use when describing wine to each other. Many strategies exist to examine, classify and describe wines. In this section we will explore the various fascinating aspects of wine in addition to these wine tasting and appreciation strategies.

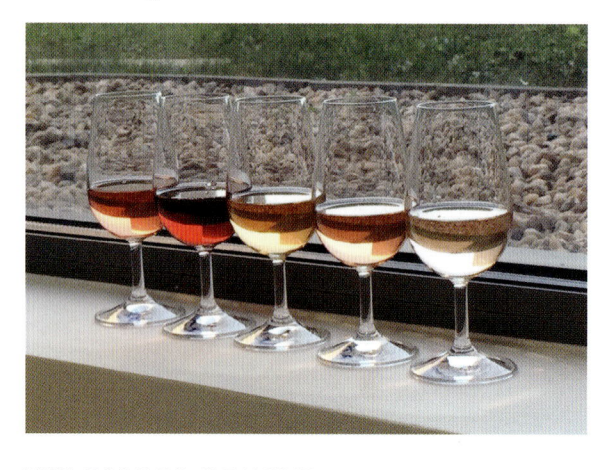

THE COLORS OF WINE

Not only are the colors of wine beautiful to behold, but the color (*la teinte* or *la robe*) of a wine can give an indication of its age. When you tilt your wine in a wine glass, you will see that the middle of the wine is more intense or dark in color than at the edges. The color glinting at the edges is the highlight, or reflection (*le reflet*), and gives you the best indication of the color and age of the wine. Generally, the more pale and less intense a wine's color, the lighter its structure.

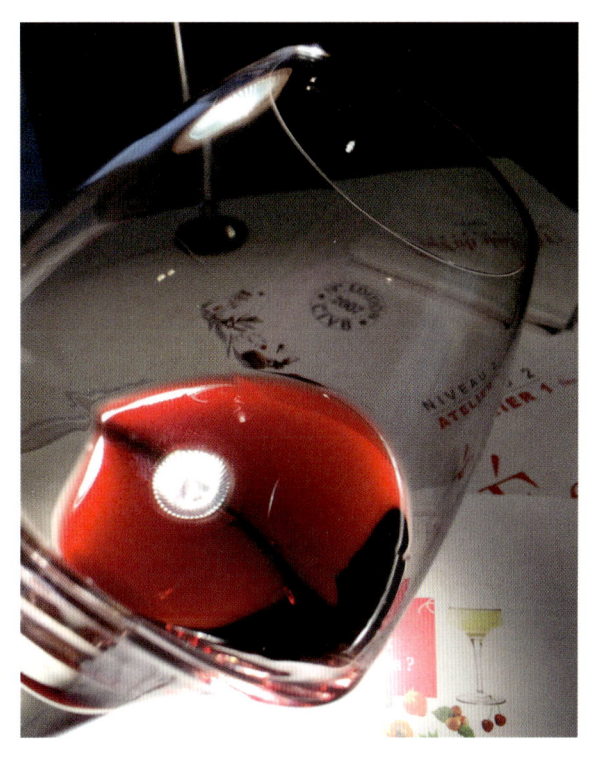

For **sweet** wines (pictured below), the colors run from a pale golden yellow in the first three years to a golden straw color for the next 4 years, bright gold yellows from seven to 14 years, and a goldenrod or even amber color beyond 15 years of age, depending on the original quality of the wine and its ability to age.

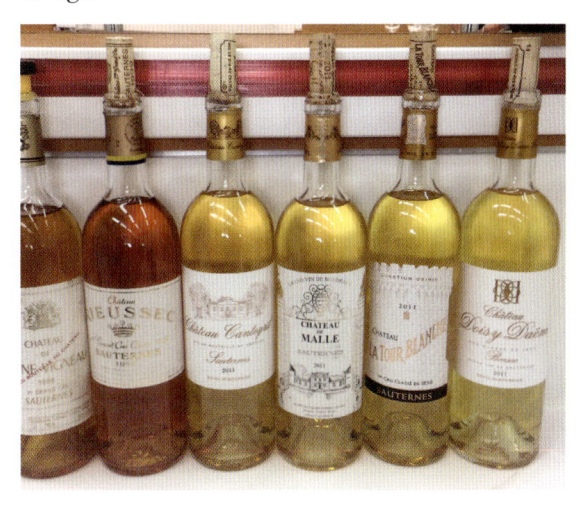

For **white** wines, the spectrum begins with a greenish yellow for young, one- to two-year-old wines. Some white wines are simply a pale yellow for about the first five years, transitioning to a pale golden yellow until year 10, after which they can take on a slightly darker yellow, straw shade.

White wines can be made from any color grape, as the grape juice is clear. Colored wines (red, rosé, clairet) obtain their color from contact with the skins in a process called maceration.

Sparkling wines retain the carbon dioxide from fermentation to make them bubbly. Only sparkling wine from AOC Champagne in France may be called Champagne, other well-known French sparkling wines include Crémant d'Alsace, Crémant de Bordeaux, and Crémant de Bourgogne. Spain produces Cava primarily in its northeastern corner, and Italy produces Moscato d'Asti in the northwest and Prosecco primarily in the northeast.

Rosé wines begin with a pink or light raspberry color during their first year or have a salmon pink color for the first five years. Thereafter, they take on a more onion skin, brownish pink. Rosé wines gain their color from brief contact with the grape skins, transferring in a matter of only a few hours a bit of color and minimal tannins.

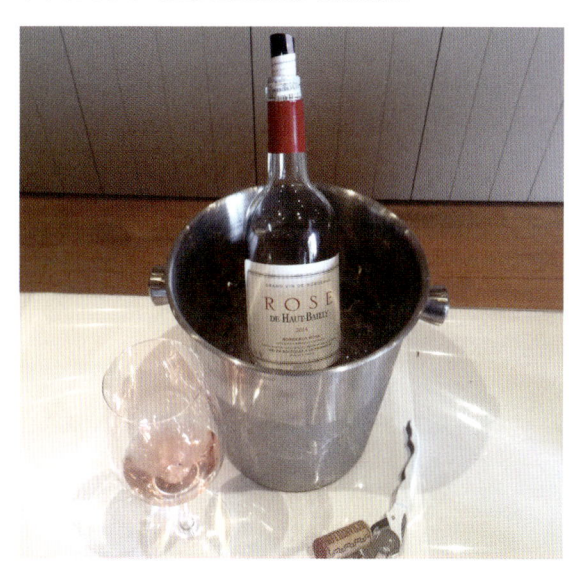

Clairet wines, unique to Bordeaux and similar to the "lighter" red wine exported to England during the Middle Ages, begin as a raspberry or cherry red for the first three years, then move on to salmon pink around

CHAPTER 7

529

three years of age and an onion skin color around five years of age, much like the rosés. ("Claret" was synonymous with "red wine from Bordeaux" in Britain.)[28]

Red wine colors are vast and beautiful and range from purples to reds as they age. Like olive oil and olives with dark skin to protect themselves from sun exposure, red grapes also contain anthocyanins, pigmented flavanoids (plant polyphenols) that contribute to flavor along with a slight astringency. They vary in color from red to blue to purple depending on pH, polyphenols with anti-oxidant properties like hydroxytyrosol, and other antioxidants—all shown to be beneficial to our bodies, as discussed previously.

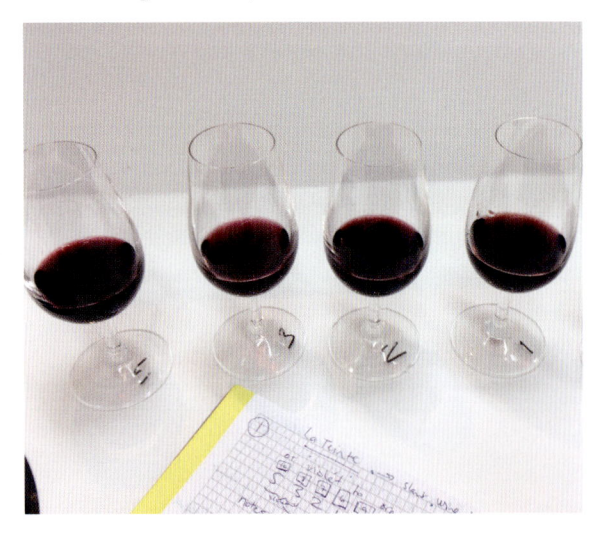

Young red wines usually begin as bright purple, and one sees this hue in Beaujolais Nouveau in its first few weeks, or during the *En Primeurs* time in the spring in Bordeaux, when all the wine buyers and brokers (négociants and courtiers) and writers flock to the region to taste the unaged wine harvested the previous fall. This is a unique moment when the Bordeaux winemakers can introduce their latest vintage to the world and receive case orders for future delivery to help continue financing their winemaking throughout the year. The wines are generally bright purple and full of tannins, which sticks to everyone's tongue, teeth, and gums. No one escapes without a purple-stained grin!

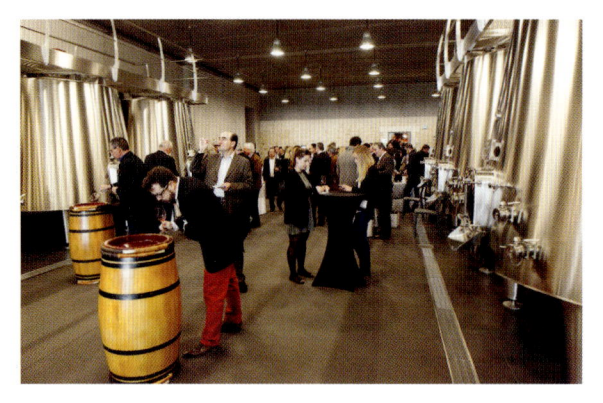

For the first one to two years, red wines are a purplish-red and move on to a ruby color up to about five years of age. As a red wine ages, its color changes from ruby to garnet to brick to a brownish amber red.

During the maceration phase of winemaking (when the grape skins and seeds, or pips, are in contact with the juice of the grapes in the initial stages of winemaking), tannins, which lend a very important gustatory element to red wines, are extracted along with the anthocyanins, which give the clairets, rosés, and red wines their initial color, but also the *intensity* or *density* of the color. Red wines spend a longer time macerating, and this is one stage during which winemaking is really an art. The tannins in red wine skins are what give that puckering feeling in the mouth. Tannins are also antioxidants and therefore help to preserve wine, which is one reason red wines tend to age better than white wines. Alcoholic fermentation, malo-lactic fermentation, and aging in barrels are other stages during which winemakers must observe, taste, and work their magic, or more precisely, allow the juices and bacteria to work *their* magic.

The **clarity** (*la limpidité*) of wine is defined by how translucent it is, which may be a factor of filtration (or lack thereof) before bottling or sudden temperature changes or other chemical changes causing particle formation during the aging process. Organic and biodynamic wines may be "cloudier" as a result of less intense or no filtration. Traditionally, egg whites were used to clarify wines, and wines were checked by candlelight for sediment as they were being clarified and "racked" or transferred from barrel to barrel. This process is ongoing in some chateaux, such as Mouton Rothschild in Bordeaux.

The **brightness** (*l'éclat*) of a wine can be an indicator of its overall health; if it is lackluster, it may have aged beyond its prime.

THE AROMAS OF WINE

Peynaud tells us in *The Taste of Wine*, "All kinds of smell are gathered together in wine in minute doses, making it a microcosm of aromas. An inspired taster is not lying when, with his eyes closed, he speaks of a whole world of scents rising from his glass."[29] To me, the aromas of wine are almost more exciting than the taste. You can smell a multitude of scents swirling a high-quality wine served at the right temperature in the right kind of glass in pleasant surroundings. Certain subtle aromas seem to vanish once the wine hits the tongue and the taste sensors take over. Aromas, like other aspects of wine, can vary in intensity from wine to wine or over time as the wine evolves, even resting in your glass or after swirling and aerating in the glass.

AROMATIC CHARACTERISTICS OF WINE

Single notes and aromas can be pinpointed and detected in wine, some more commonly than others, depending on the wine. Sometimes we just need a little help with the actual vocabulary to pinpoint what we smell. It is helpful to know exactly what aromas and flavors are possible to sense in wine, and it turns out that there are many. Everyone perceives wine differently, so there really is no right or wrong answer. What makes it more interesting is when you can name a family or category or even a specific aroma in a wine and recognize it in other wines as well. White wines tend to have certain aromas, while red wines have others. After a while, you can often tell a wine by its aromas, even if you could not see the label or even the color, in a blind tasting, for example. Certain grapes tend to have certain aromatic characteristics, but aromas are influenced by many factors and have been categorized in many ways by various people and groups over time. Certain individual items are sometimes classified into more than one category or in a different category, depending on whom you ask, but the main idea is to be able to articulate the aroma (or odor) you sense in a way that others may understand. Some of these classifications are listed below.

SCIENTIFIC AROMA CLASSIFICATION

Oenologists (wine scientists) classify aromas into three categories according to the way in which they are derived from the winemaking process: "primary aromas" (*les arômes primaires*), coming from the grape variety itself and from the terroir (including soil type, and I would argue, soil microbiome diversity), "secondary aromas" (*les arômes secondaires*), derived

The Instant Messaging of Wine

For us to be able to recognize an aroma, a series of events must occur: The molecules that waft into our nose, as we breathe in from the wine in our glass or already in our mouth, hit the olfactory mucous receptors in our nasal cavity, sending neural messages to our olfactory bulb in our forebrain. These signals set off a chain of messages to the many parts of our brain responsible for *emotion, memory, and sense of smell*: the amygdala (emotional behavior and motivation), the orbitofrontal cortex (decision-making, sensory-integration, and expectation-creating), the hippocampus (long term memory and spatial navigation), the hypothalamus (hormone-producing gland), the piriform cortex (sense of smell), and the thalamus (responsible for relaying motor and sensory signals to the cerebral cortex, the outer layer of our brain). Linked to this signaling is the visual cortex,[30] the better to *see* you with, my dear! This "instant messaging" among all these parts of our brain from the olfactory bulb is why our memory and the sense of smell and even our visual memory are so closely linked and why we can smell an aroma that made such an impression on us in the past that it will take us back to that moment emotionally and in our "mind's eye." We can use this "trick" to our advantage when trying to "learn" or memorize aromas, flavors, and wines. Repetition helps because these pathways are reinforced.

from the fermentation process, and "tertiary aromas" (*les arômes tertiaires*), acquired during the aging process.

AROMATIC FAMILIES OF WINE
Distinguished French oenologist at the University of Bordeaux and author of oenology textbooks still used today, Emile Peynaud (1912-2004), classified the aromatic characteristics of wine (including defects) into 10 groups.[31] What is so interesting to me about these aromas and defects is that they are so tied to nature, food, and the land, in impressive alignment with French culture.

Animal: Cat's urine, fish, fresh sea fish, fur, gamey, game stew, indole, meat, mouse cage, musk, sweat, venison stew, wet dog, wool fat

Balsamic: Cade oil or juniper tar, pine, pitch pine, resin, turpentine, vanilla

Chemical: Acetic acid or vinegar, alcohol, chlorine, disinfectant, graphite, hydrocarbon, iodine, medicinal, sulphur

Empyreumatic: Burnt, burnt wood, caramel, chocolate, cocoa, cooking aromas, fire, grilled, grilled almonds, gunflint, gunpowder, incense, leather, roasted coffee, rubbed flints, rubber, silex, smoked, smoky, toast, tobacco

Ethers and Odors of Fermentation: Acetone, banana, beer, butter, candle wax, cheese, cider, cow shed, diacetyl, dough, fatty acid esters, ferments, isoamyl acetate (banana oil), lactic, milk and milk products, nail varnish, pear, sackcloth, sauerkraut, soap, sour milk, stable, wheat, yeast, yogurt

Floral: blossoms of acacia, almond, apple, lemon, lime orange, peach, privet, elder, grapevine, hawthorn, sweet briar and honeysuckle,[32] carnation, chamomile, chrysanthemum, clove, floral, flowery, geranium, heather, honey, hyacinth, iris, jasmine, magnolia, marshmallow, mignonette, narcissus, pelargonium, verbena, violet

Fruit: Almond, apricot, banana, bergamot, bilberry, bitter almond, black cherry, black currants, black olive, citrus fruits, currants, dark berries, dried fig, fresh fig, golden delicious, grapefruit, green olive, hazelnut, *kirsch* (cherry brandy), melon, mirabelle, mulberry, peach, pear, pineapple, pistachio, plum, pomegranate, prune, quince, raisins, red currant, small red berries, stone fruits, strawberry, walnut, wild cherry, wild strawberry[33]

Spicy and Aromatic Spices: Aniseed, basil, camphor, cinnamon, clove, dill, fennel, garlic, ginger, green pepper, lavender, licorice, marjoram, mushroom, nutmeg, onion, oregano, pepper, peppermint, star anise, thyme, truffle, vermouth

Vegetal or Herbaceous: Aristolochia, bay leaf, black currant leaf, cabbage, cress, cut grass, dried leaves, drying vegetation, dust, earthy, French fern, French marigold, grass, green coffee beans, hay, herbaceous, herbal tea, horseradish, ivy, leaf mold, marsh, newly-mown hay, pasture, sloe, smell of greenery, tea, tobacco, tree moss, undergrowth

Wood: Acacia, bark, barrel stave, cedar, cigar box, green wood, oak, old wood, pencil shavings, *rancio* (nutty flavor peculiar to fortified wines as in Armagnac, Cognac, Madeira, and sherry)

In order to provide a language of aroma descriptors that are not subjective, numerous classifications have been created over the decades by various oenologists and perfumers. Ann Noble, Professor Emeritus of Oenology at UC Davis, created the Aroma Wheel (see diagram on next page), incorporating student and scientific feedback, in order to help people "see" the differences in wine aromas and flavors, beginning in the center with more general descriptors and moving outwards as one narrows down the specific aroma.

Richard Pfister, a Swiss perfume professional, classifies aromas similarly to Peynaud's

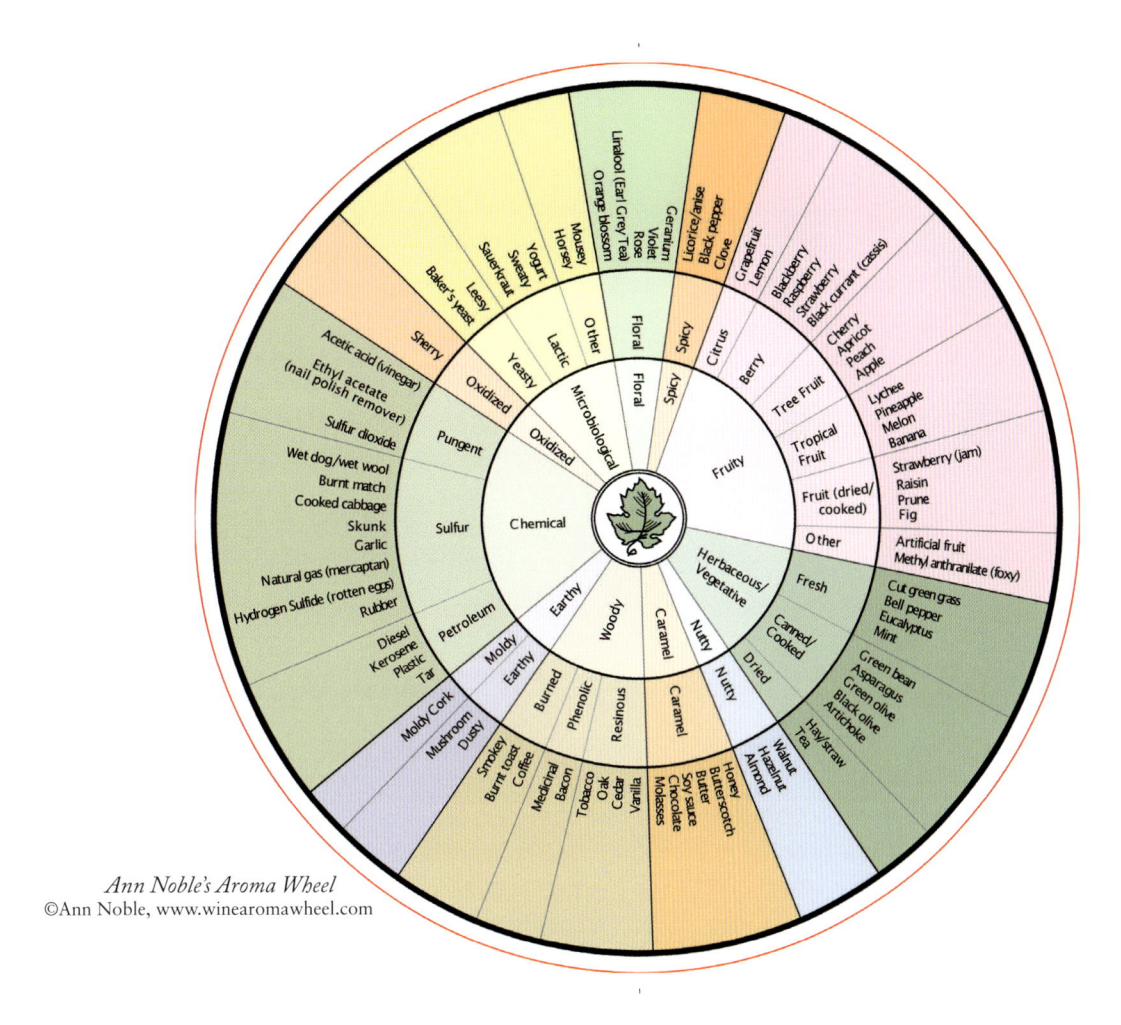

Ann Noble's Aroma Wheel
©Ann Noble, www.winearomawheel.com

classifications by family, but includes a grouping of classifications of "faults" (*défauts*) in what he calls "Oenoflair Classification."[34] The "Field of Odors" (*Champ des Odeurs*), by Jean-Noel Jaubert, is a semi-circle depiction of the range of odors as regarded in the perfume industry. Some other helpful graphics on wine aroma and flavor terminology are listed on The Guild of Sommeliers website. One graphically depicts three main chemical aromatic compounds (fruit-flower-herb, earth, and spice) and the aromas associated with them, along with the kind of molecules from which they originate.[35]

TIME IN A BOTTLE

When wine professionals speak of a wine's "bouquet," they are referring to the combination of aromas the wine has acquired during the aging process once in the bottle. As well-made wine ages, it acquires a "bouquet" of complex aromas not yet perceptible in the same wine in its younger years. The tannins in red wine settle down over time, generally becoming softer on the palate. Glutathione, an antioxidant naturally occurring in wine, helps protect wine as it ages. Though, just because a bottle has been waiting to be opened for 20 or 30 years, it does not necessarily mean it is better than it was five or 10 years ago. Each wine has its peak (*apogée*), and this is part of the discovery as well. The aging effect of time spent in a bottle changes the flavor profile and can augment the layers of complexity of a wine. Wines that are less tannic usually are consumed sooner, while tannic wines have the power to age well in the bottle. When pairing wines with food, the age of the wine is often taken into consideration, as older red or white wines tend to be smoother and subtler in flavor and texture than younger wines, which can tend to be bright, fruity, and lively on the palate.

CHAPTER 7

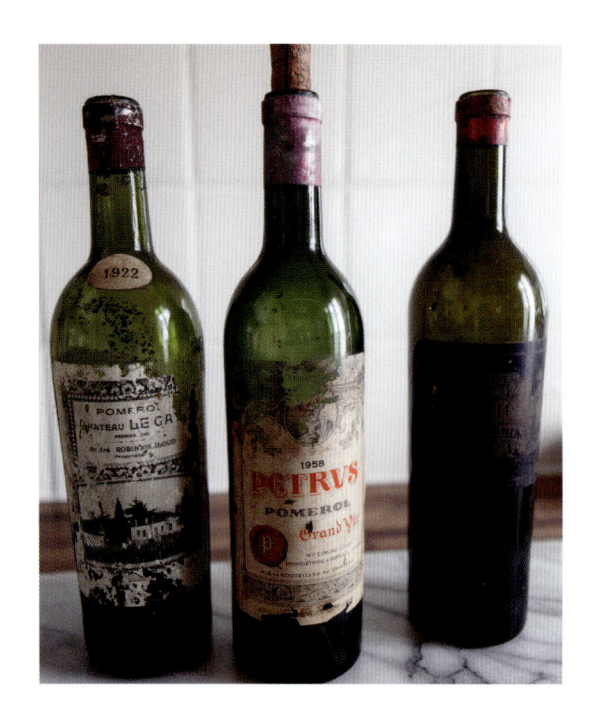

COCONUT, VANILLA, AND TOAST

Some aromas, such as vanilla and coconut or toasted notes, come from their time spent in oak barrels, which are usually some combination of used and new barrels. Wines aged in "new" or a majority of unused barrels will tend to glean oaky aromas of vanilla (usually associated with French oak) and coconut (usually associated with American oak). The amount of time spent in oak barrels (usually less than 2 years for most wines), the type of oak used, as well as the "toasting"— the use of fire to toast the wood inside each barrel as it is being made—can influence the flavors and aromas of a wine. Winegrowers even test their wine in barrels from different forests, or at least from different cooperages (barrel manufacturers), and at varying toasting levels, as the flavors from the barrels will have an impact upon the flavor of the wine. Oaking French wines can add aromas of caramel, smoke, spice, toast, and vanilla.

SOAKED IN OAK

Maturation of wine in oak barrels helps to enhance certain wines, and 100% new oak is still popular for high-end wines that benefit from this type of barrel aging (élévage *en barrique*), such as the Bordeaux Classified First Growths (*Premiers Crus Classés*) from the Bordeaux Wine Classification of 1855 of certain Bordeaux vineyards.[36] "Oaking" wine has been in practice for a long time. According to my friend Caroline Matthews, WSET level four and Bordeaux Wine School instructor, oaking wines has a positive effect on certain wines, "especially on non-Aromatic whites such as Chardonnay and Viognier, where it can add complexity and texture, and with red varieties that are naturally low in tannin (such as Merlot and Pinot Noir), where the oaking can give structure and aging potential." Oaking red wines also stabilizes their color.

Meanwhile, the practice of 200% new oak (replacing new barrels half way through aging with newer barrels), which once was popular, has now mostly stopped. Over-oaking, combined with heavy toasting can "mask the natural aromas of more aromatic varieties and therefore is less frequently used for the wines made from Riesling or Sauvignon Blanc." The practice of oaking in new barrels, with such frequency and volume, however, is a concern when it comes to sustainability.

THE FLAVORS OF WINE: HONORING TASTE AND SENSATION

Wine tasting is a sensory-dense experience, on its own or when combined with food and company. The tastes of salty, sweet, savory (*umami*, a Japanese word), bitter, and sour[37] come in different combinations in each wine, as do the sensations of astringence (dryness), tannins (puckering sensations in the mouth), and body (liquid viscosity or density). The balance of all these elements are what give a wine its *elegance*, or *finesse*, and can be achieved in virtually endless ways. This is another reason why the array of wines we can choose from is so diverse and fascinating.

In the words of my DUAD Professor, Axel Marchal,[38] the equilibrium of flavors in wine contributes to their sensorial quality. As defined by Emile Peynaud, this sensorial quality is determined by sweet and acidic flavors in white wines and by sweet, acidic and bitter flavors in red wines.[39]

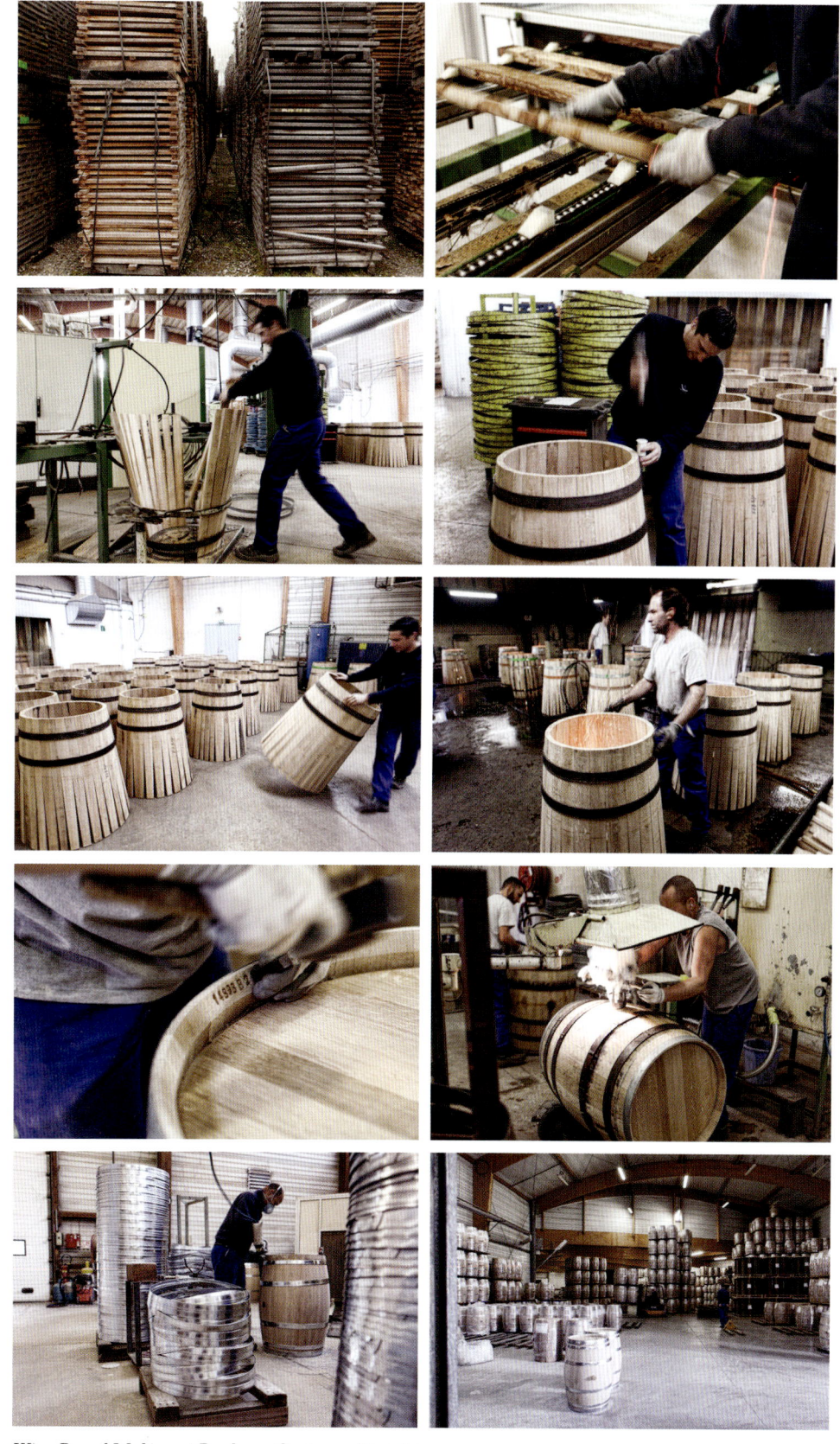

Wine Barrel Making at Bordeaux Cooperage Nadalié

CHAPTER 7

535

THE BALANCE OF A WHITE WINE

ACIDITY (Y axis)

TART, GREEN, SOUR, DRIED UP (X), THIN, HALLOW, SMALL, VERY SWEET, THICK, LIQUOREUX, UNCTUOUS, HONEYED, FULLY DEVELOPED, NERVOUS, FIRM, ACIDIC

Inner ring: SHARP, TENSE, FATTY, CLOYING, SOFT, FLAT, DRY, FRESH

Center: **BALANCED**

SWEETNESS (X axis)

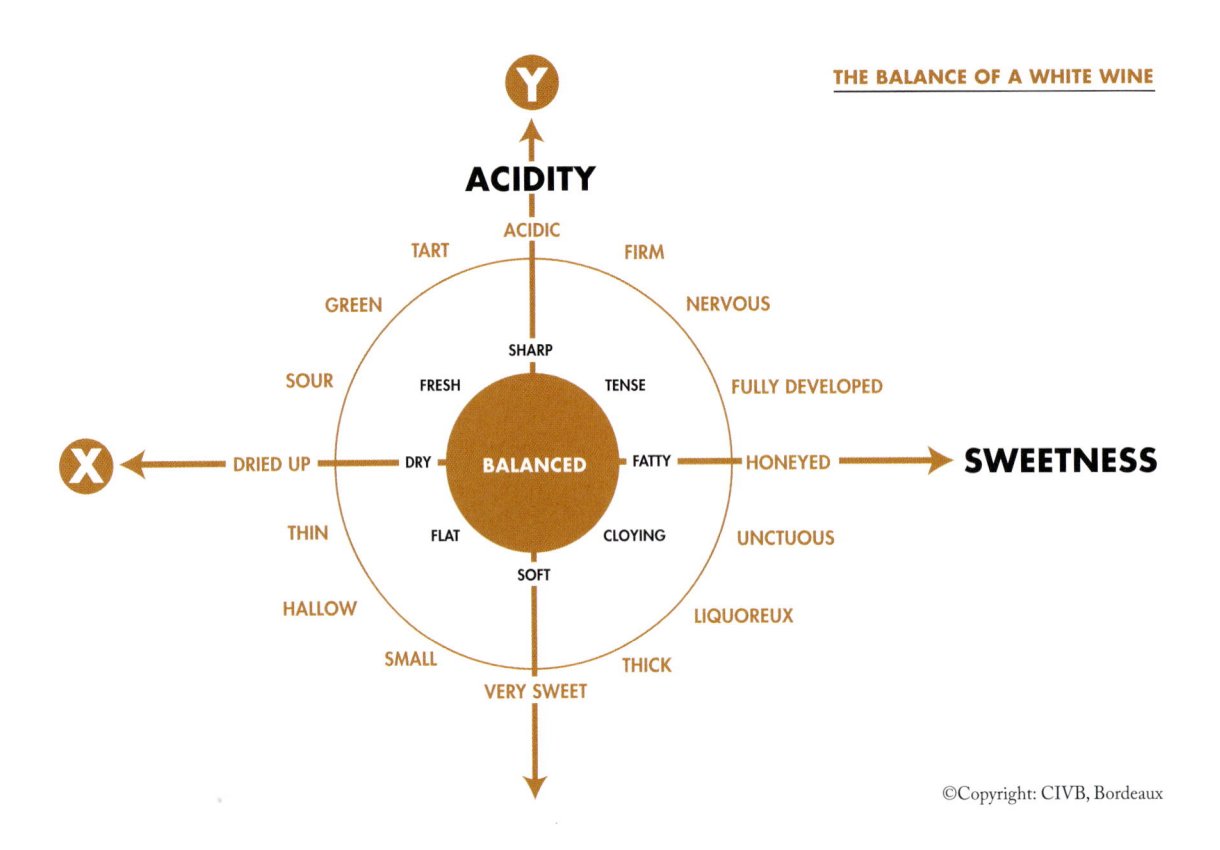

©Copyright: CIVB, Bordeaux

WHITE WINE: BALANCING SWEETNESS WITH ACIDITY

A balanced white wine is one that is both sweet and acidic (see the diagram above). The degree to which this balance varies gives a wine its character. If they were all identically balanced, wine tasting would not be interesting. Then again, a wine that is well-balanced will allow the aromas and flavors to display their full character.

In white wines, taste is characterized by an equilibrium between sweetness and acidity. Our amazing sense of taste (our taste buds) can detect myriad nuances in acidity and sweetness in wines. Over time, we can recognize certain combinations of acidity and sweetness, coupled with aromas in a wine, to be able to remember what kind of wine it is and where it is from. A white wine's flavor need not always fall in the "balanced" category. It is sometimes easier to remember a particular wine that was more tart or extra sweet rather than perfectly balanced without any outstanding characteristics, though this is always a matter of taste!

The continuum between acidity versus sweetness is laid out in an X (sweetness) to Y (acidity) graph (above) in which the upper-right-hand quadrant represents greater sweetness and higher acidity (you might find a Bordeaux Sweet, Sauternes, or Barsac, or a Jurançon from the French Southwest); the lower-right-quadrant represents higher sweetness but lower acidity (such as an Alsace Gewürtztraminer or Grüner Veltliner wine); the upper left quadrant depicts higher acidity and less sweetness (such as a dry champagne or a dry, relatively high-acid white from the Savoie); and the lower left quadrant describes wines of lower acidity and less sweetness (such as a Languedoc-Roussillon might be).[40]

SPARKLING WINES – *VINS CRÉMANTS*

Sparkling wines can be white or rosé and undergo alcoholic fermentation but no malolactic fermentation (MLF). The second alcoholic fermentation occurs in the bottle with added sugar and yeast, which creates carbon dioxide pressure in the bottle. Sparkling wines, including the famous French

Champagne, come in a range of sugar dosages. From the highest sugar content (50g/L) down to the lowest (<3g/L), their sweetness levels are respectively named: Doux, Demi-Sec, Sec, Extra Dry, Brut, Extra Brut, and Brut Nature.

SWEET WINE: BALANCING ACIDITY, ALCOHOL, AND SUGAR

Sweet wines are made in several regions around France, perhaps the most famous of which are the "Bordeaux Sweet" dessert wines. These wines are generally made in areas where the alternating morning fog and afternoon sun promote the growth of *Botrytis cinerea*, or "noble rot." This means that each grape, in a sense, becomes its own mini-barrel (*petite cuve*), in which the sugar concentrates and the water evaporates while it sits on the vine. (In Alsace, the sweet wines are called "late harvest," *vendanges tardives*, or *Spätlese* in German, but are extra sweet because of the length of time they hang on the vine, turning to raisins with concentrated sugars.) Once harvested and fermented in the larger fermenting tanks, the results are an elixir; an amber, delicious "nectar of the gods." The balance of a sweet wine is comprised of a unique blend of acidity, alcohol, and sugar. Aline Baly of Château Coutet in the Barsac appellation of Bordeaux's sweet wine producing region says that a balanced sweet wine is "where the sweetness is neither hidden nor on the forefront of the tasting experience. Of course, individual perception does play a bit of a role. We all have different sensitivities and appreciation for the three elements that contribute to the wine's equilibrium: sugar, acidity, and alcohol. Texture also influences the perception of a wine's balance." I was able to perceive the phenomenon first-hand at a laboratory tasting of 10 samples in early 2015 with Aline's uncle, Philippe Baly, at Château Coutet, in which the balance of sugar, acidity, and "bitterness" from the alcohol were composed in multiple ways as to enhance or cancel out one another while supporting complexity of aroma and texture.

RED WINE: BALANCING ACIDITY, SWEETNESS, AND TANNINS

For red wines, the balance lies between acidity, sweetness, and tannins, often characterized as bitterness (see diagram below). Most well-made red wines will fall in the "balanced" triangle, but if they fall just outside this area along one of the axes, they may be memorable or known for that particular characteristic. It is often these kinds of outlying characteristics that wine tasters will look for and be disappointed or surprised if one year it is not there as before. This is again another amazing aspect of wine, that there are always surprises as well as continuity as one gains experience. You would generally find a Bourgeuil or a Chinon from the Loire Valley further along the acidity axis than a more balanced Burgundy that might fall in the middle. You would usually find a Langueduc-Roussillon or a Côtes du Rhône wine further along the sweetness axis than other red wines, and you would typically find a Bordeaux Médoc, a Madiran, or a Cahors further along the high-tannin axis compared to other French wines.[41]

THE BALANCE OF A RED WINE

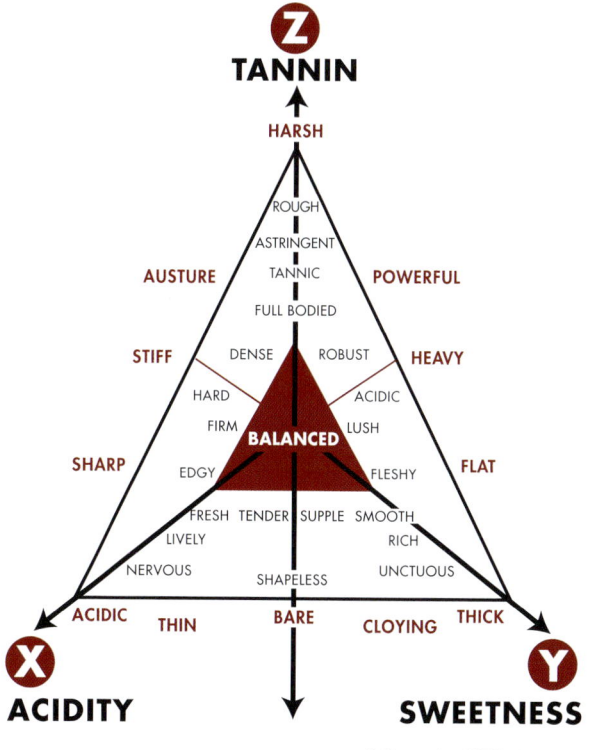

©Copyright: CIVB, Bordeaux

CHAPTER 7

537

THE BODY OF WINE - *LE CORPS DU VIN*

To me, the concept of body is one of texture or viscosity, or as my friend and wine expert Caroline Matthews says, "weight in the mouth" or "mouthfeel." The viscosity of water in one's mouth is different from that of milk, as the latter has more "body" or viscosity to it. In wine, there are differences in viscosity mostly due to the alcohol content (which is the second-most dense element in wine after water), but also from the impact and flavor it has in the mouth. Though water is technically denser than alcohol, alcohol is more viscous than water. Therefore, the higher the alcoholic content of a wine, the greater the sensation of fullness the alcohol creates in the mouth. Glycerol, created during the fermentation process also contributes to the body of wine. In red wines there is the addition of tannins that can add to the overall impression of "body" in a wine. More "body" does not necessarily mean "better," however. To me, a light-bodied wine has a light texture, is light like water, and is also lighter in color, whether in yellow hues for white wine or reddish hues for red wine. A medium-bodied wine has a more intense color, and a bit more volume and texture in the mouth. A heavy-bodied wine is denser, more viscous, usually more tannic, powerful, and intense in color and flavor. Caroline compares full-bodied wines to the weight of mango juice. "Full-bodied" can also be compared with the density of whole milk in the mouth, as opposed to the density of skim milk or water in wines that are "light-bodied."

Caroline offers two examples. A premium Bordeaux blend of Cabernet Sauvignon and Merlot is typically high in tannin and alcohol because Cabernet Sauvignon is high in tannin and Merlot is high in alcohol and also contributes tannin because of in-barrel aging. This kind of blend is therefore often full-bodied, depending on the exact blend. In comparison, a premium red Burgundy, which is predominantly Pinot Noir (a grape variety high in alcohol but naturally low in tannin), will be medium-bodied as some tannin is derived from barrel aging.[42]

DEFECTS IN WINE – *LES DÉFAUTS DU VIN*

In their training, wine professionals are taught to detect defects (*défauts*) in the wines they taste. This helps them to advise winemakers and evaluate or rank wines, as well as eliminate those that are not suitable for drinking. Usually, a defect is found in one bottle, rather than in an entire case. The wine in question is considered "corked"—contaminated by bacteria that either grows in the cork or in the wine itself, such as Brettanomyces, or "Brett," a yeast which has the unfortunate smell of a mouse cage (*souris*) or horse sweat (*cheval*). "Corked" wine may have a mildew, acetone, vinegar, or overly vegetative (green peppers) odor, or smell of other strong, volatile molecules that overwhelm the intended fruity and pleasantly aromatic molecules of the wine. Sadly, these bottles must be poured out. A sniff is usually all one needs to determine whether a wine has gone bad. While tasting a bad wine (and spitting it out) may be educational once or twice, it can ruin your palate for the remainder of the tasting, and certainly should not be swallowed. Luckily, corked wines are the exception. No one likes to lose out on the money and time spent on a bottle of wine, nor the missed pleasure of drinking it!

TASTING NOTES

When studying and tasting wines (*la dégustation*), students and professionals take notes on each wine. This forces them to really take time with the wine and get to know it. Your tasting notes, whether in your mind or on paper, can cover a variety of topics. And the more detailed you get, the more likely you are to remember the wine. Written notes are a helpful reminder, as they can help you recall the wine's color, aromas, texture, taste, and acidity. It also assists you in describing the wine to someone who has never tasted it. Taking the time to slowly and closely consider the wine in your glass is a calming aspect of the French art of eating and drinking that honors your senses and elevates your mood.

Sharing this experience with friends and family slows down time and reinforces positive associations with the occasion, as well as the special aspects of the wine.

It is one thing to open a bottle of wine over a shared meal with friends. It is another thing entirely to sit in a cubicle in a temperature and light-controlled lab in front of a sink with several glasses of wine to evaluate. In the lab, on an empty stomach, one follows a certain protocol in determining the different aspects of a wine:

Color (*La Robe*), Brightness and Clarity – Describe the color. How does it compare with other grape varieties (*cépages*) or to similar wines of its age? It helps to tip the glass, holding it over a white surface beneath bright, even lighting, to see the color of the edge of the wine (*le reflet*) as well as the depth of color, the clarity, and brilliance of the wine in order to best describe these.

1st Nose (*Premier Nez*) – What aromas do you perceive after the wine has been poured but before you disturb (swirl) it?

2nd Nose (*Deuxième Nez*) – What aromas do you perceive after swirling the wine in the glass? What is the intensity of the aromas now compared to when the wine was at rest in the glass?

1st Sip – Oxygenate by sucking in air through the mouth and out the nose for a "retronasal" or "retrolfaction" effect. This allows you to perceive aromas in the olfactory sensors in your sinus area after the wine is warmed by your mouth (as the mouth itself can only discern between acidity, bitterness, saltiness, and sweetness). Swish by allowing the wine to touch all parts of the mouth, then spit. What happens in your mouth? What aromas are the same, different, changed? Is the acidity (tartness) balanced with the sweetness?

2nd Sip – Repeat the same steps as in the first sip, but focus on the "finish," or how long the wine flavor lingers. The longer and more complex the finish, the higher the quality, and often the price, of the wine. How have the tastes changed? Is there a bitter, salty, or astringent aftertaste?

There is a lot to think about during the few seconds the wine is in your mouth and just after you spit out or swallow, as you sometimes do, at the end of the wine-tasting session. Some molecules are volatile, meaning they are easier to smell because they move around a lot. Some molecules are non-volatile and must be tasted to be properly perceived. Hence, we sniff, but also taste. In any case, every winemaker will tell you that wine is meant to be drunk and enjoyed, not only analyzed.

Some other properties to look for are the intensity, diversity, and complexity of a wine in terms of aroma, taste, and aftertaste. A wine is complex when it has a variety of aromas and flavors that appear to your senses at different moments throughout a tasting. You will even find that a wine develops or changes after several minutes of aeration. For example, after 15 or 20 minutes, a complex wine might change its aroma profile almost entirely from fruity and spicy to smoky or chocolaty. These are some of the surprises a good-quality wine can provide, and why a common language is so useful when describing wine.

I found that in groups, I could not reflect as deeply about all these things. Sometimes, or at least in the beginning, you can *taste* a few wines on your own (don't sit around drinking alone, I am not advocating that!), or with one or two interested friends and take notes as you go. Beware of "palate fatigue," in which, after trying so many wines, your palate can no longer differentiate the subtleties of the different wines. Then it is time to stop and eat, or else eat a little something between tasting several wines at a time. (This is not dissimilar to the "palate fatigue" Robb Wolf refers to in his book *Wired to Eat*, in which we become bored with the same food and tend to oscillate between salty and sweet to change up the stimuli.[43]) With practice, your palate endurance will increase as you begin to know what to expect from and look for in wine. In time, your ability to focus on certain aspects of a wine without becoming overwhelmed as you evaluate it will become more of a habit or ritual. You will develop a foundation for choosing a wine for an occasion or a meal. I grew up knowing absolutely nothing about wine but was able to begin learning more about wine than I ever thought possible, even after the age of 40.

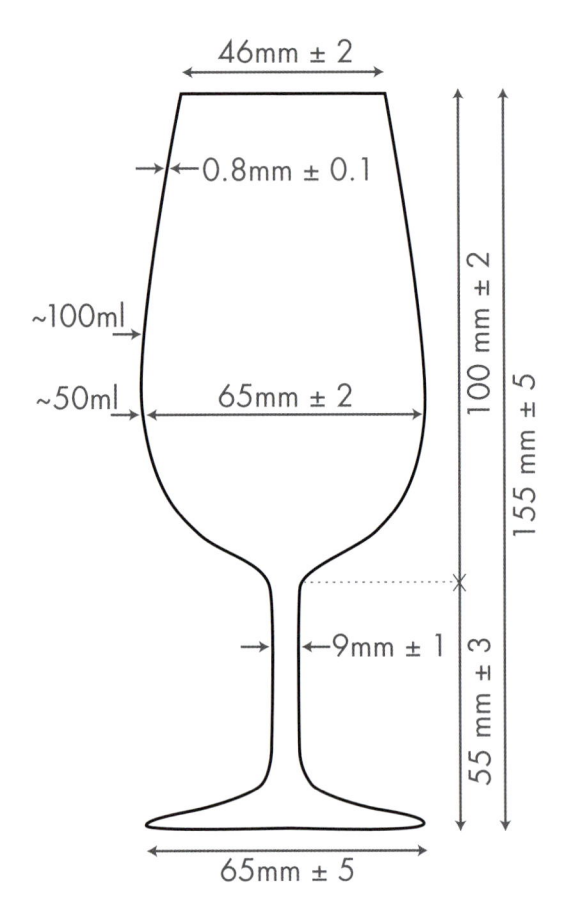

University of Bordeaux Wine Tasting Glass Size Specifications

THE WINE GLASS

I recommend using a Villeroy & Boch general wine glass that allows for good sniffing, but that is not so wide as to let out the aromatic molecules. Similar in shape to the wine glass diagram above, it stands seven inches high; the goblet itself is just under four inches from the lowest part attached to the three-inch stem to the rim; at its widest point the goblet is just under three inches and about two-and-a-quarter inches wide at the rim. This makes for easy swirling with a minimum amount of wine, and a small enough opening to trap the volatile molecules so you can sniff them before they escape the glass. On sale, mine were about $8 each. Mid-to-high range are the Rosenthal (up to $70+ per glass), Schott Zwiesel (around $50-$70 for a set of six), and Spiegelau (now owned by Riedel and $30-50 for a set of four). Riedel is the Porsche of the wine glass industry. It is light in the hand, which allows you to focus on the wine rather than the weight of the glass. After lifting one of these glasses, anything else feels clumsy. At home I stick with the Villeroy & Boch, as I am prone to breaking wine glasses while washing them, and they fit best in my budget for now. When drinking wine, hold the glass by the stem, so as not to warm up the wine with your hand.

AERATING, CARAFING, AND DECANTING WINE: WHEN AND WHY

If you think of wine as a person who ages slightly faster than the rate at which most people age, then you will understand why, when uncorking a wine, you must let it "wake up." Imagine if you were suddenly pulled out of your hibernation after a few decades of slumber, put on the table without a chance to shower and pull yourself together. You might not be able to show your true colors to a group of discerning wine drinkers in the first few minutes after being uncorked or woken up. Young, inexperienced wines require more time to aerate. They benefit from being "carafed" —poured into a carafe and exposed to oxygen. This allows the aromas to be expressed, lest the young wine seem "closed" (*fermé*) or biting, with high levels of tannins. A closed wine is one whose aromas have not had a chance to develop, probably needing more aeration and time to "open up" (*s'ouvrir*). The more tannic a wine, the longer the aeration. Most wines will benefit from being opened before drinking, anywhere from 20 to 30 minutes and even up to 45 minutes to an hour before being tasted, depending on the age of the wine. Older, mature wines will express their complexity of aromas sooner and will also oxidize sooner, therefore decanting them is possible, but preferably into a narrow decanter with a top, with less surface area exposed between the wine and the air. Once poured, older wines will develop their complexity even while in the glass. The aromas and flavors you experience after first pouring the wine may change over 20 minutes or more in the glass, bringing a new experience with each sip. This is the excitement, mystery, and appeal of drinking older wines.

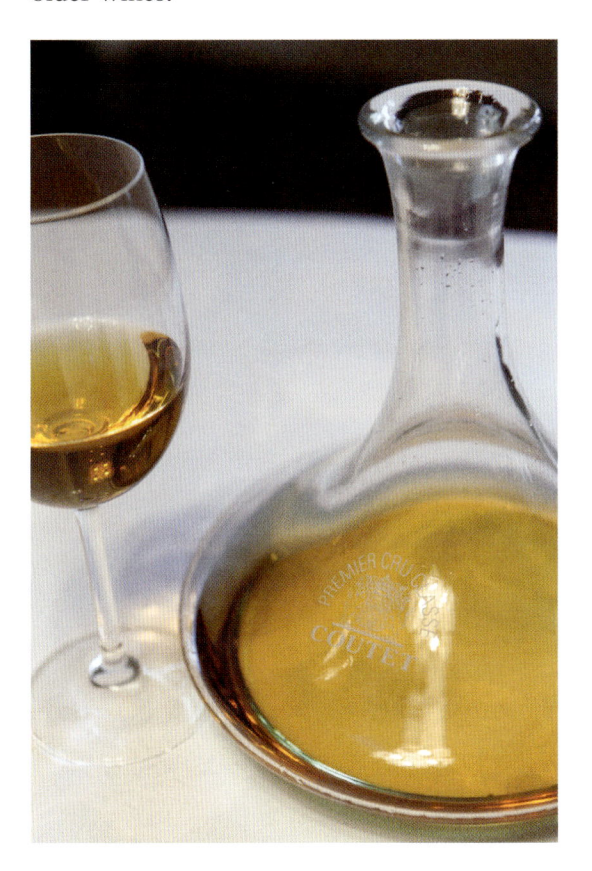

My good friend and wine professional, Dewey Markham, Jr., explains the technical differences between *carafing* and *decanting* in the following manner: "Carafing is simply transversing a wine from one container to another to give it greater exposure to air and hence improve its aromatic expression. Decanting involves separating some solid or precipitate matter from a liquid. Thus, carafing would be done to enhance the enjoyment of a white or rosé wine, which does not throw a deposit with age (lacking a significant amount of polyphenols), young red wines, in which polymerization of the polyphenols has not yet occurred, and even Champagne and other sparkling wines, which can benefit from increased aeration (I've had it done and was disabused of my skepticism). Decanting aged reds separates out the deposit from the wine; in this case the recommended equipment, in addition to the decanter itself, is a candle or other light source (or at the minimum, a bright white surface) to aid in detecting the approach of the sediment to the bottle neck. One can expect to have a certain amount of liquid left in the wine bottle, which is not the case with carafing."

SERVING TEMPERATURES

The best way to store wine long term is to keep it cooled at a constant temperature (and constant humidity, if possible), lying on its side so the cork does not dry out and allow the passage of oxidizing air. Most people don't have a limestone cellar below ground that maintains a constant humidity and temperature throughout the year. The best way to mimic this is to use a wine refrigerator. Find a size that suits your usage, small if infrequent, large if you go through more bottles per year. Otherwise, chill your wines before a meal in the refrigerator. Wine will warm up to ambient temperatures, therefore it is important to keep it chilled (or at least cool, in the case of red wine), until you actually serve it. If a wine is served too cold or too warm, it will not have the opportunity to convey its full expression to the wine taster. Rosés, clairets, young, dry white wines and sparkling wines, often served in summertime, are best if chilled to between 45°F to 52°F (7°C to 11°C). A rich and structured dry white wine or a sweet wine (*liquoreux*) is best served between 48°F to 54°F (9°C to 12°C). Young, fruity red wines in general are best at 57°F to 61°F (14°C to 16°C), or even cooler in the summer months. An older red wine is ideally served between 61°F to 65°F (16°C to 18°C).[44] In the summer, wine will warm up several degrees within minutes, which should be taken into account (thus the buckets of ice to keep wine and champagne cool).

CHAPTER 7

Ideas for Wine Tasting Parties

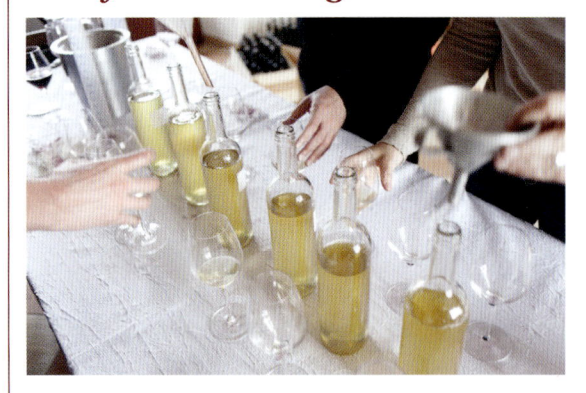

Blind Tasting: Cover the bottles in a wine sock or hide the bottles in paper bags. Try each wine, one by one, with each person giving some commentary, or pick just one to give commentary and make a guess aloud while the others guess silently.

Vertical Tasting: In a vertical tasting, the same wine is taken from multiple years and tasted for the changes due to aging and the *effet millesime*, how that year's harvest affected the wine a certain way compared to other years' harvests. Typically, one starts with the youngest wine and ends up with the oldest, which is usually the most complex in nature.

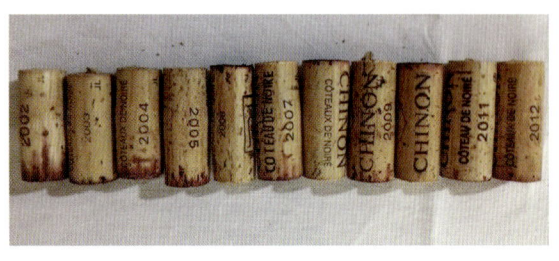

Horizontal Tasting: A horizontal tasting evaluates the styles of the same kind of wine between various producers. The wines may be only Chardonnay from Burgundy from a certain year, for example, or else a selection of Côtes du Rhône wine from across the region. Keeping certain variables consistent, such as grape variety, region or year helps keep a consistency to allow for the detection of the subtleties in wine styles between producers. In Burgundy, for example, one parcel of a vineyard will produce wine of a different character and quality than that of another parcel situated next to it, which is one reason why certain Burgundy wines are so very expensive; there are just so few bottles of each to go around.

Regional Tasting: Basically a horizontal tasting, choose several different producers of wine from a certain region, either broad or narrow. A broader regional tasting might be Médoc (called "Left Bank" wines, as they grow on the left bank of the Gironde estuary) from the Bordeaux region. A narrow selection could be from the Pomerol region of Bordeaux, which creates some of the most sought-after, flavorful wines in the world. Another regional tasting could be of white wines across the Loire Valley, or a selection, or "flight" of wines from Alsace that have distinct character but vary by grape or producer or wine style. Shown here are several different wines from the Arbois appellation of the Northern Jura, demonstrating how different wines traditionally come in different bottle shapes.

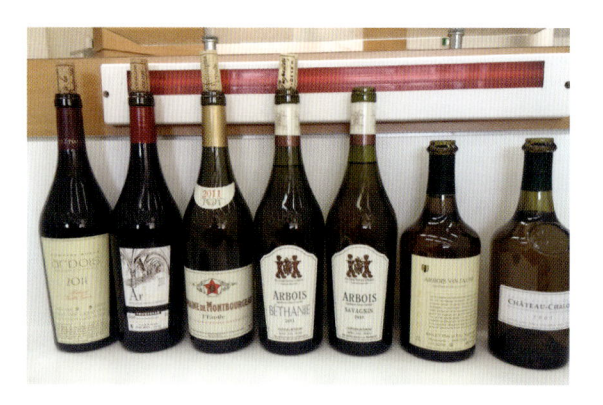

Varietal Wine Tasting: Tasting wines made from one type of grape variety (mono-varietals, *mono-cépages*), such as Cabernet Sauvignon, Chardonnay, or Merlot made in the same region in the same year.

Wine Bar Tasting: Try going to a traditional wine bar and asking about their current selection, or else try one with wine-dispensing machines where you can buy just enough wine to taste it. (Usually such establishments also serve cheese or charcuterie platters or small, tapas-style dishes.) Ask the waiter about the current assortment of their wines and what he might suggest. Wine bars often label the characteristics of a wine to give you an idea of what you might look for when tasting each one.

542   THE BORDEAUX KITCHEN

Wine Terms Reference Guide

The French language is a thing of beauty and really shines when the French use it to describe wines. One word can describe many characteristics in wine in such an elegant way that can get lost in translation. Thanks to my ever-patient friend Annabelle Nicolle-Beaufils and her lovely grasp of explaining French wine characteristics to her restaurant clientele, we have put together some basic *positive* descriptions (*assuming a good balance or equilibrium* between acidity and sweetness for white wines, and the additional balance of tannins for red wines) that come up when describing the tastes and textures of a wine, and their English translations. There is also an explanation of what's really behind the descriptions, some of which overlap, demonstrating the richness of the French language and the variety of styles people can employ in describing a wine. These may be useful to refer to when reading the Wine Pairing Tips provided with many of the recipes in this book:

Balanced Wine – *Vin Équilibré*: White wine that balances acidity with sweetness and red wine that balances acidity, sweetness, and tannins. Synonym: well-balanced (*bien équilibré*).

Bold, Powerful, or Strong Wine – *Vin Puissant*: A wine relatively high in alcohol and aromas, a noticeable and good tannic structure with lots of material to chew on in the mouth (*de la mâche/matière en bouche*). Synonym: intense.

Delicate Wine – *Vin Fin*: Subtle tannins, light to medium-bodied, well-balanced wine. Synonyms: fine, smooth, silky, suave, refined.

Dry Wine – *Vin Sec*: Higher in acidity than sweetness. Low residual sugar after fermentation. "Bone dry" connotes no residual sugar.

Fleshy or Full-Flavored Wine – *Vin Charnu*: An aromatic, dense (full-bodied), structured, and tannic wine, where the fruit flavor has been well-extracted (like biting into a ripe fruit), relatively high in alcohol and tannins, with well-balanced tannins. Synonyms: "savory" (*savoureux*) or "full-flavored."

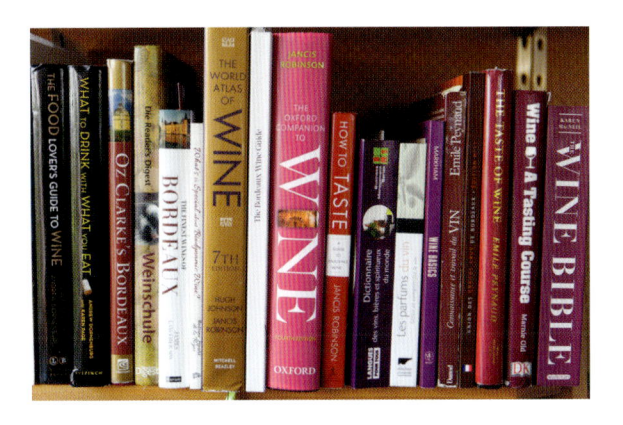

Full-Bodied Wine – *Vin Corsé*: Density similar to whole milk in terms of mouthfeel. (Alcohol is more viscous than water, therefore wines with higher alcohol content tend to have a full mouthfeel (*ample en bouche*), hence the term, "full-bodied.") In French, a full-bodied wine is also a "structured" wine. Glycerol, created during the fermentation process also contributes to the body of wine.

Intoxicating or Potent Wine – *Vin Vineux*: Wine high in alcohol and tannins (*riche en alcool et en tannins*), therefore also "full-bodied." Also described in French as "warming" (*chaud*), from the alcohol.

Light-Bodied Wine – *Vin Peu Corsé*: Density similar to water. Synonyms: soft, easy to drink.

Medium-Bodied Wine – *Vin Moyennement Corsé*: Density somewhere between water and whole milk.

Silky Tannins – *Tanins Soyeux*: Silky, suave, or subtle mouthfeel, referring to the effect of tannins in the mouth. Synonyms: soft, round or rounded tannins (*tannins ronds*), or concealed, well-blended, or "melted" tannins (*tanins fondus*).

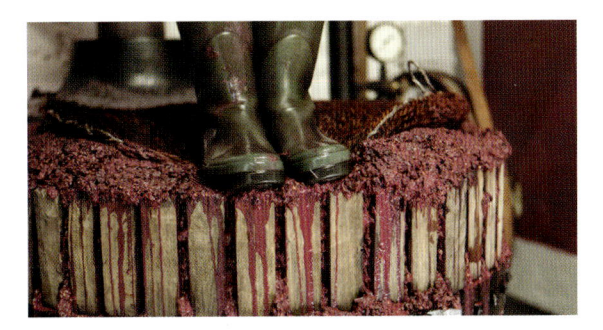

CHAPTER 7

543

Simple Wine – *Vin Léger*: A wine low in alcohol, viscosity, structure, and color, "easy to drink" (*facile à boire*), without much aromatic complexity (*complexité aromatique*) in the nose or on the palate. Low aging potential (*peu de potentiel de garde*), a wine to be drunk sooner rather than later (*à boire rapidement*). Rather than translate the word directly to "light," which in English might be taken to also mean low in calories, it is more precise to translate *léger* as "simple," as in "simple in character," or "uncomplicated," "approachable," or "soft."

Structured or Tannic Wine – *Vin Structuré* or *Vin Charpenté*: A robust wine with predominating tannins and therefore good aging potential (*bon potentiel de garde*). Structured means there is a good balance between acidity, tannin, sweetness, glycerol, and alcohol. Wines with good structure age better than those with less structure. Tannins are extracted from the skin, seeds, and stems during maceration (when they are in contact with the grape must or juice) and produce a puckering feeling in the mouth. A "structured" or "tannic" wine is essentially also a "full-bodied" wine, usually red. White wines have little or no tannins but still contain varying alcohol contents as well as glycerol, both of which contribute to body.

Supple Wine – *Vin Souple*: Supple first impression, approach, or attack in the mouth (*l'attaque en bouche*), not overly pronounced by acidity, alcohol, or tannins. A wine with low astringency (which comes from the balance of acid and tannins). Synonyms: elegant, round, or well-rounded wine (*vin rond*), where "everything is balanced and integrated" (*tout est bien équilibré et intégré*).

Sweet Wine or Dessert Wine – *Vin Doux* or *Vin Liquoreux*: Higher in sweetness than acidity.

Warm Wine – *Vin Chaleureux* – Having a warm mouthfeel or a pleasing combination of acidity, body, and flavor. Synonyms: expressive, joyous, filled with character.

Wine with High Acidity – *Vin Acidulé*: Wine with a crisp acidity that is well-balanced, just at the border of becoming too high in acidity. Acidity lends tartness and can make your mouth water. Acidity also cuts the fats and oils and balances out the sugar and alcohol. Synonyms for good acidity in wines: bright, crisp, fresh, sharp, tart, tangy.

Well-Blended Tannins – *Tanins Enrobé*: Tannins that are noticeable but well-balanced with the other aspects of the wine without overpowering them. Synonyms: finesse, subtle.

Wine with a Long or Lengthy Finish – *Vin à Finale Longue*: Aromatic persistence (*la persistence aromatique*) of a wine in the mouth after swallowing. The duration is counted in seconds (*caudalies*). The adage goes that the longer the finish, the better the wine. The delectable finish of an aged, elegant wine, whether red, white, or sweet, can haunt you for days afterward.

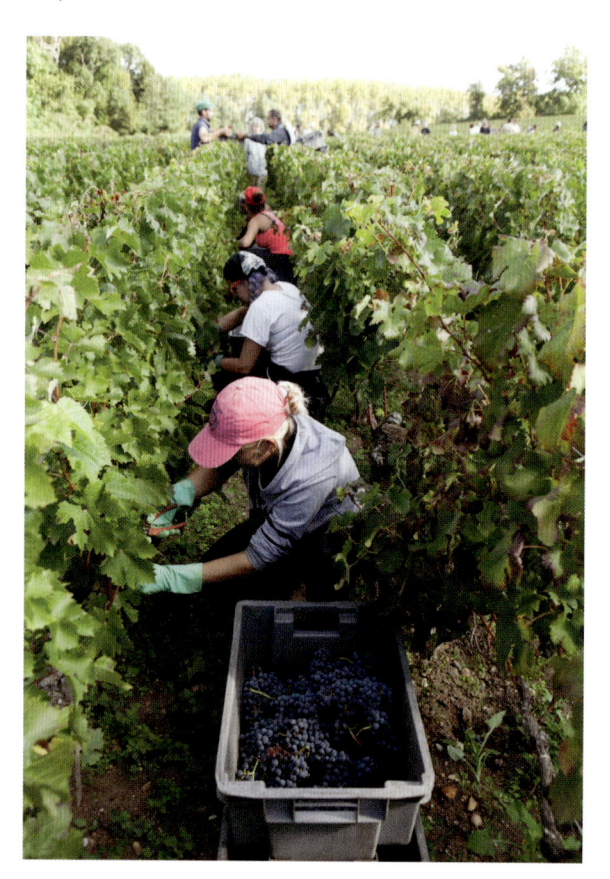

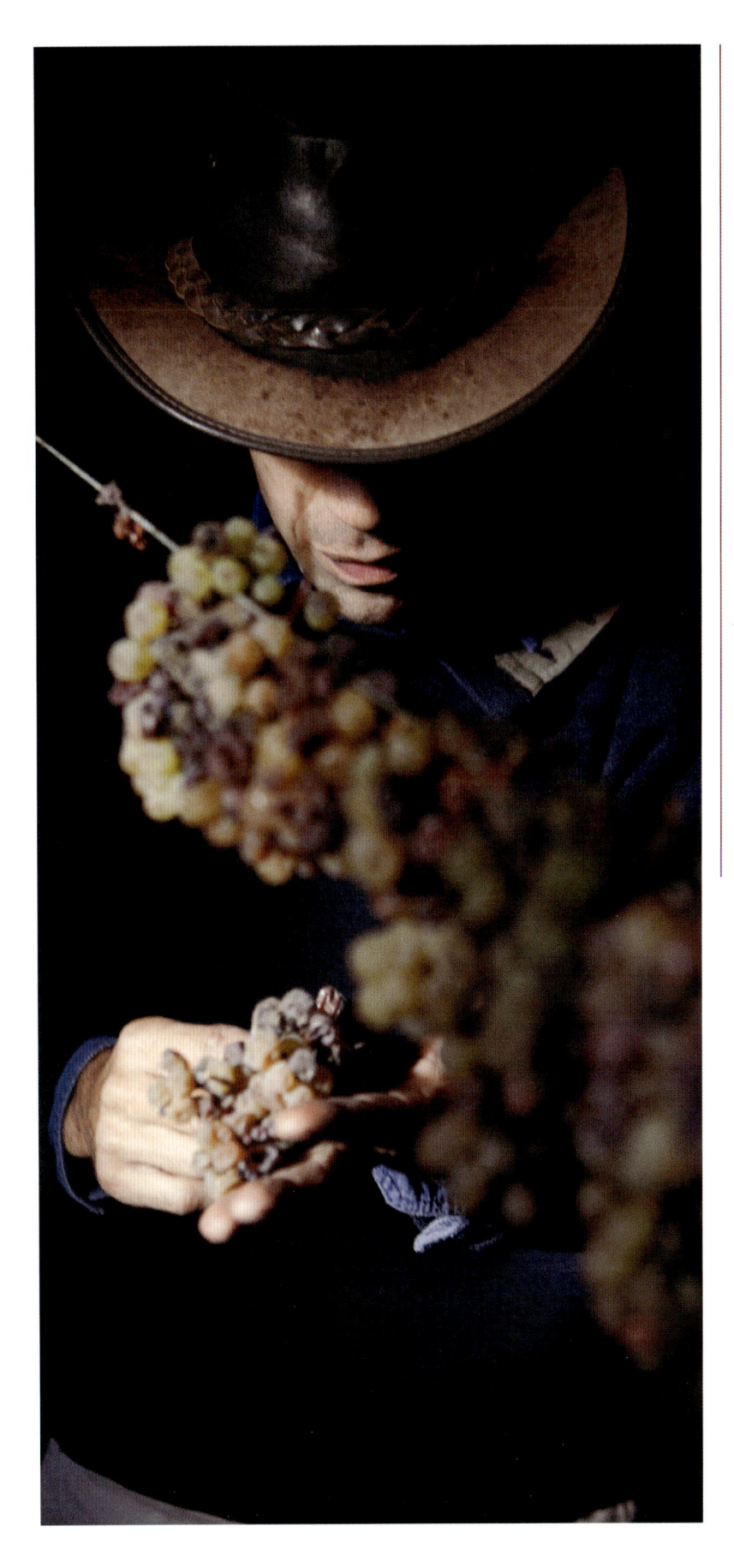

The Winegrowing Regions of France

Depending on how you divide them up, there are 16 main winegrowing regions in France. It is worth noting two regions not mentioned in the Grape Varieties section beginning on the next page: Cognac (north of Bordeaux, in the regions of Charente and Charente Maritime) where at least 90% Ugni Blanc grapes must be used and distilled to make the famous Cognac brandy, and Calvados in Normandy, which produces the Calvados apple brandy in four government-regulated appellations. All the varieties of grapes in France are from the *Vitis vinifera* species. The variation in soils and even indigenous yeasts present on the grapes in the vineyards across France allow for a multitude of flavors in each grape variety and ultimately in the wines made from them.

Major Grape Varieties Grown in France

ALSACE

Alsace, which is land that has historically passed between and been influenced by both France and Germany, lies on the border with Germany in northeastern France, nestled between the Vosges mountains and the steep granite and slate slopes of the Rhine River. Clay and limestone (or marl) soil covers the gentler slopes. Most of Alsace's wines are made from one grape variety (*monocépage*), as opposed to a blend of grapes (*assemblage*), such as is made in Bordeaux.

Alsace Red Grape Variety

Pinot Noir – Notes of blackberries, cherries, and strawberries.

Alsace White Grape Varieties

Chasselas – Originates from the Valais in Switzerland. Used as a table grape in most of France and declining in use in Alsace. Fruity and floral with good acidity. Chasselas ripens early, and its harvest date is used to help predict harvest times for other grapes around France.

Gewürztraminer – Notes of lychee, grapefruit, rose petals, and earth, with high sugar content, and low acidity.

Muscat – Crisp, fruity grape aroma, apricot, low in acidity and alcohol. Muscat wines are made here using two types of Muscat grapes, Muscat d'Alsace and Muscat d'Ottonel.

Pinot Blanc – Slight fruitiness, rose petals, good acidity, supple texture, medium to full-bodied. Also known as Klevner. Pinot Blanc is a close relative of Auxerrois, both of which form the basis for the sparkling wine of Alsace, Crémant d'Alsace. Also known as *Weissburgunder* in Germany, Pinot Blanc is cultivated widely in Italy by the name of *pinot bianco*.

Pinot Gris – A variety originating from Hungary, a country with one of the oldest traditions of winemaking. Can have subtle aromatics of spiced bread (*pain d'épices*), peaches, pears, apricots, and apple, as well as floral notes. Middle-of-the-road in dryness, and freshness (*fraîcheur*), Pinot Gris can be more sweet than acidic. Cheaper ones might have a slightly bitter aftertaste. Pinot Gris ages well, becoming more butter-and-biscuits flavored as it ages.[45] Also cultivated widely in Italy by the name *pinot grigio*.

Riesling – Notes of hydrocarbon (characteristic of this grape variety) and lemon. Fruity and tart, with some floral notes, (and sometimes coriander), this wine ages well due to its high acidity. It ranges from very dry to very sweet, and is often made into ice wine, where the grapes are allowed to freeze before harvesting in order to extract only the sweetest juices.

Sylvaner – Tart and acidic, fruity, and slightly bitter, this wine probably originated in Romania along the Danube River, but also grows on clay soils in Alsace.

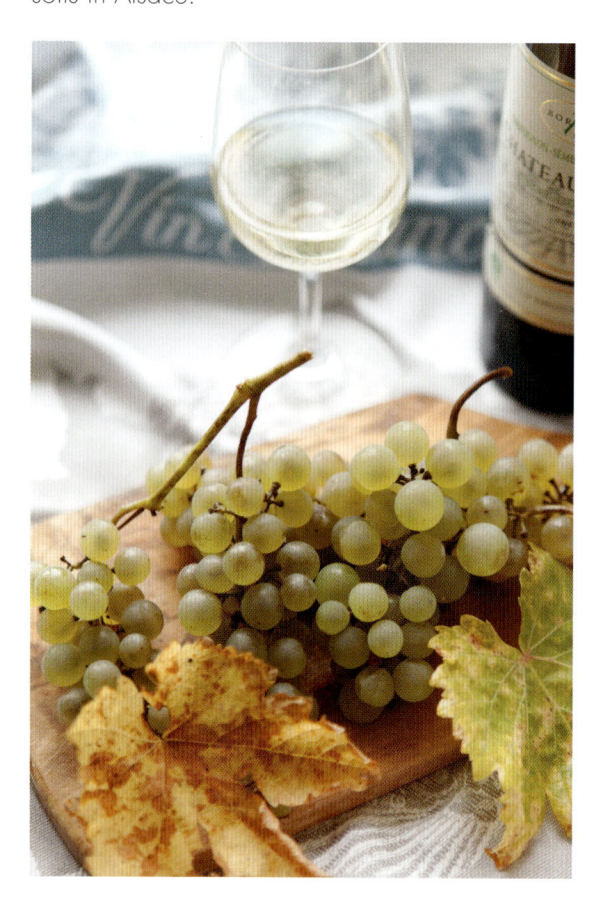

BEAUJOLAIS

Beaujolais, the southernmost region of the Burgundy wine region, and just north of the Rhône wine-growing region, is where the "natural wine" movement began in the 1960s, when some winemakers decided to make wine with less sulphur dioxide and in the more ancestral fashion of their grandparents. Most well-known abroad for Beaujolais Nouveau, a red wine meant for immediate consumption, this region also produces many other red wines, most notably the Beaujolais Crus and Beaujolais Villages, that are barrel-aged and longer lasting. A very small fraction of Beaujolais Blanc is produced from a blend of white grapes Aligoté and Chardonnay to produce fresh wines with notes of melon, pear and stone fruit.

Beaujolais Red Grape Variety
Gamay – Very fruity, notes of apple, black currant, pear, raspberry. Produces simple, approachable, light-bodied wines with low tannins and freshness. Gamay (or "Gamay Noir") goes well with fresh cheeses and charcuterie.

Beaujolais White Grape Varieties
Aligoté (see page 550)

Chardonnay (see page 550)

BORDEAUX
Bordeaux's rich tapestry of vineyards produce 15% of France's total production and 1.5% of worldwide production.[46] Thanks to economic hardship after World War II, Bordeaux wine producers were given special dispensation by the *Institut National des Appellations d'Origine* (INAO, France's governing body for protecting the geographical origin of agricultural products) to display the grape varieties on their labels.

Bordeaux wines are made from blends (*assemblage*) of two or more grape varieties with each variety of grape bringing its own qualities of aroma, structure and flavor. Bordeaux has five main regions: Côtes de Bordeaux, Entre-Deux-Mers, Graves, Médoc, Saint Emilion. Within these are over 40 appellations, including Barsac, Blaye and Blaye Côtes de Bordeaux, Bordeaux and Bordeaux Supérieur, Bordeaux and Entre-Deux-Mers Haut-Benauge, Bourg and Côtes de Bourg, Canon Fronsac, Castillon–Côtes de Bordeaux, Cérons, Côtes de Bordeaux, Côtes de Bordeaux Saint Macaire, Entre-Deux-Mers, Francs Côtes de Bordeaux, Fronsac, Graves, Graves de Vayres, Graves Supérieur, Haut-Médoc, Lalande de Pomerol, Listrac-Médoc, Loupiac, Lussac Saint Emilion, Margaux, Médoc, Montagne Saint Emilion, Moulis-Médoc, Pauillac, Pessac-Léognan, Pomerol, Premiers Côtes de Bordeaux, Puisseguin Saint Emilion, Saint Emilion, Saint Estèphe, Saint Julien, Sainte Croix Du Mont, Sainte-Foy-Bordeaux, Saint-Georges-Saint-Emilion, Sauternes. With over 28,000 winemakers, over 9,000 landowners, and over 121,000 acres of vineyards, Bordeaux produces 90% red wine, but also dry and sweet white wines, rosé wines, and a relatively small amount of clairet.

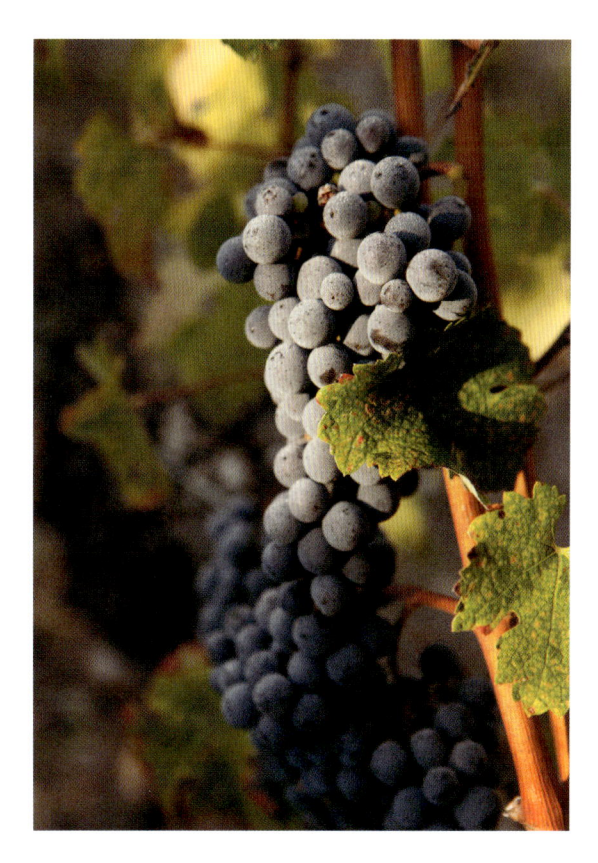

Bordeaux Red Grape Varieties
These represent about 88% of Bordeaux's vineyards.

Cabernet Franc – Mainly grown in the Libourne area near the appellations of Castillon, Pomerol and St. Emilion. Cabernet Franc is usually used to complement the Merlot grape in the blends from these vineyards to round out the tannic structure, thereby brining an "elegance" (smooth tannins) and freshness to these and to Cabernet Sauvignon-

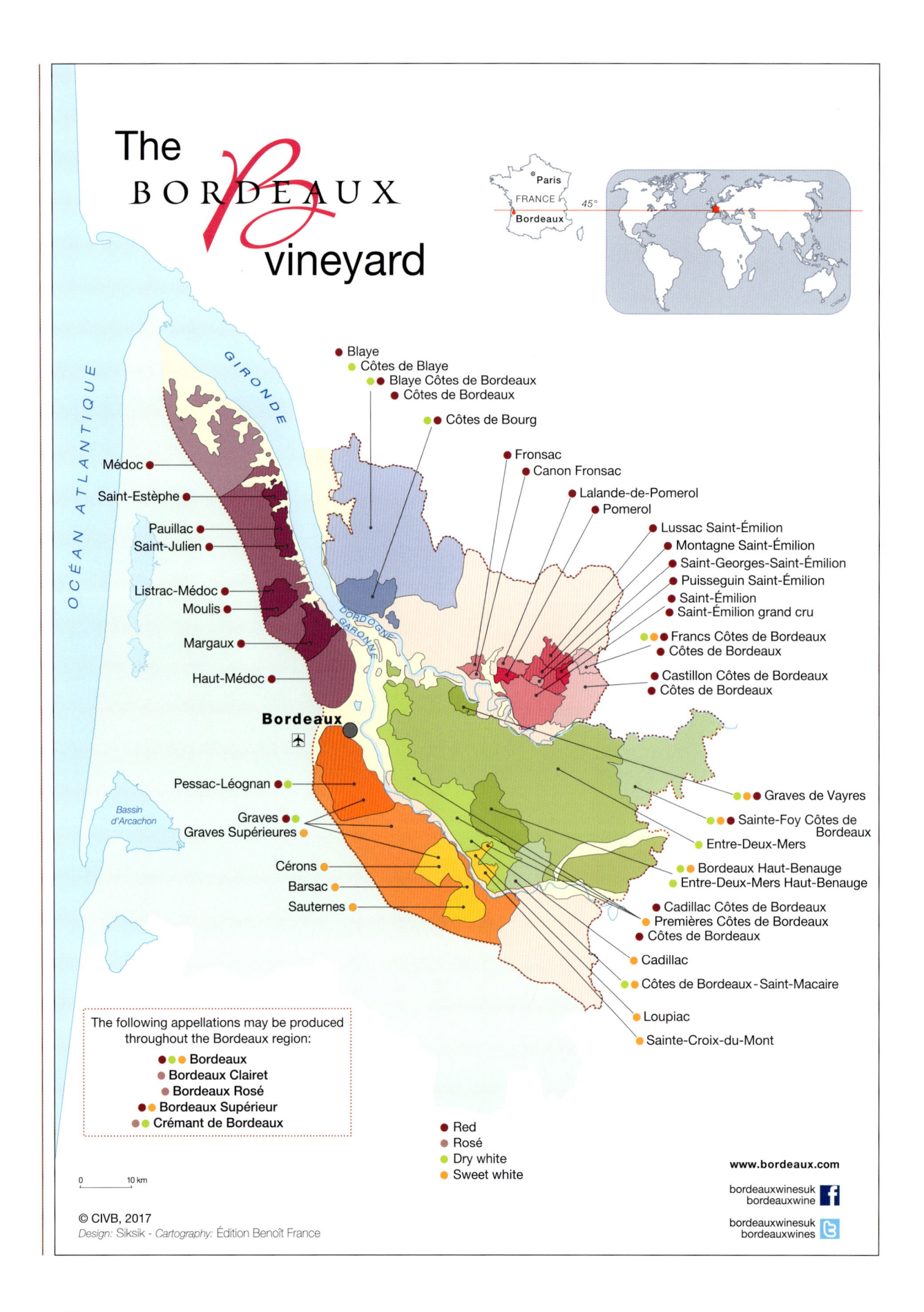

The BORDEAUX vineyard

Map legend — appellations:

- Blaye
- Côtes de Blaye
- Blaye Côtes de Bordeaux
- Côtes de Bordeaux
- Côtes de Bourg
- Fronsac
- Canon Fronsac
- Lalande-de-Pomerol
- Pomerol
- Lussac Saint-Émilion
- Montagne Saint-Émilion
- Saint-Georges-Saint-Émilion
- Puisseguin Saint-Émilion
- Saint-Émilion
- Saint-Émilion grand cru
- Francs Côtes de Bordeaux
- Côtes de Bordeaux
- Castillon Côtes de Bordeaux
- Côtes de Bordeaux
- Médoc
- Saint-Estèphe
- Pauillac
- Saint-Julien
- Listrac-Médoc
- Moulis
- Margaux
- Haut-Médoc
- Bordeaux
- Pessac-Léognan
- Graves
- Graves Supérieures
- Cérons
- Barsac
- Sauternes
- Graves de Vayres
- Sainte-Foy Côtes de Bordeaux
- Entre-Deux-Mers
- Bordeaux Haut-Benauge
- Entre-Deux-Mers Haut-Benauge
- Cadillac Côtes de Bordeaux
- Premières Côtes de Bordeaux
- Côtes de Bordeaux
- Cadillac
- Côtes de Bordeaux - Saint-Macaire
- Loupiac
- Sainte-Croix-du-Mont

The following appellations may be produced throughout the Bordeaux region:
- Bordeaux
- Bordeaux Clairet
- Bordeaux Rosé
- Bordeaux Supérieur
- Crémant de Bordeaux

Colour key:
- Red
- Rosé
- Dry white
- Sweet white

OCÉAN ATLANTIQUE — GIRONDE — DORDOGNE — GARONNE — Bassin d'Arcachon

www.bordeaux.com
bordeauxwinesuk / bordeauxwine
bordeauxwinesuk / bordeauxwines

© CIVB, 2017
Design: Siksik - Cartography: Édition Benoît France

0 10 km

548 — THE BORDEAUX KITCHEN

dominated wines, in addition to notes of raspberry and violet. Ripens later than Merlot but earlier than Cabernet Sauvignon and has a relatively higher alcohol content. Because of its light vegetal aromas, Cabernet Franc is often easily paired with vegetables.

Cabernet Sauvignon – Represents about 23% of grapes planted in Bordeaux. Originates from France and is best known in Bordeaux wines, widely planted in the Médoc and Graves regions of Bordeaux. Late ripening. Excellent tannic structure that imparts length on the palate and allows for long aging. Rich color and medium acidity. Notes of blackberry, black cherry, black currant, and licorice. More vegetal aromas give way to fruity notes as the wine matures. Harvested later than other Bordeaux grapes as it takes longer to ripen and lose its vegetal aromas. After "oaking" in new barrels, and with aging, it acquires notes of leather, mocha, and vanilla. Represents a majority percentage in many "left bank" Bordeaux blends of the Médoc.

Carmenère – Historically a more commonly planted variety of Bordeaux and considered the "grandfather" of Merlot and Cabernet Sauvignon. It now serves in less than 2% of the Bordeaux blends, bringing color, fullness (tannic structure), and notes of cedar to the blends. Needs lots of sunshine to ripen. More successful in Chile.

Malbec – Also known as "Côt." Malbec grapes produce medium- to full-bodied, darkly colored wines with relatively high alcohol and tannin levels. Notes of blackberry, cherry, chocolate, and plums. Pairs well with beef and game.

Merlot – Represents about 65% of grapes planted in Bordeaux. Notes of red fruits such as raspberry, red cherry, red currant, and strawberry. Dark fruit aromas of black cherry, fig, plum, and violet. Can have notes of prune or cooked or mashed fruits or marmalade (*fruits compotés*) in years that have had sun and heat. Supple tannins and relatively high alcohol content. The primary variety in the Bordeaux blends of the St. Emilion region, it is an early ripening grape, usually the first to be harvested in Bordeaux.

Petit Verdot – Used in blends with Merlot and Cabernet Sauvignon, adding intense color, notes of black fruit and violet, and a robust tannic structure.

Bordeaux White Grape Varieties

These represent 12% of Bordeaux's vineyards and include Colombard, Merlot Blanc, Sauvignon Gris, and Ugni Blanc, varieties that represent only 2% of Bordeaux's planted area. Among Bordeaux's sweet wines (*liquoreux*) is a blend of two to three of the grapes of Muscadelle, Sauvignon Blanc, and Sémillon, used to make wines with the aromas of ripe apricots, preserved fruits, and honey.

Muscadelle – Floral and musky notes, with low acidity. Less than 10% of Muscadelle is blended with Barsac and Sauternes sweet wines containing primarily Sauvignon Blanc and Sémillon. Muscadelle plays a greater role in the sweet wines of Loupiac and Montbazillac and is blended into the white wines of the Entre-Deux-Mers region.

Sauvignon Blanc – Notes of grapefruit, guava, mango, passion fruit, and white peach. Because of its light vegetal aromas of asparagus, ivy (*lierre*), nettle, and sometimes pyrazines (volatile molecules smelling of bell pepper, sometimes considered a fault), Sauvignon Blanc is often easily paired with vegetables. Can also have notes of coriander or cumin. Brings acidity, complexity, finesse (or subtlety) and freshness to the sweet wines. Dominant in Bordeaux white wines, it is pale yellow, with intense fruit, notes of citrus, boxwood, and even sometimes smoke.[47] Aging Sauvignon Blanc "on the lees" (*sur lie*), the dead yeast and grape sediment accumulated in the barrel, is a technique borrowed from Burgundy's process with chardonnay and further developed by my late Professor Denis Dubourdieu to achieve greater complexity of flavor and softer textures in the wine. The lees protect the wine from oxidation and help to preserve the fruity aromas.

Sémillon – Aromas of fresh hazelnut, lemon, mint, and white peach. To the dry wines, Sémillon brings notes of acacia blossoms, almond, apricot, frangipane, honey, smoke, and spiced bread (*pain d'épices*). These fragrances are enhanced by notes of dried or candied fruits thanks to the "noble rot" (*Botrytis cinerea*). Sémillon is the most important grape in the sweet wine blends due to its thin skin and the ease with which the noble rot can attack it. Sémillon wines are richly golden colored, with delicate and smooth textures in the "Bordeaux Sweet" wines.

Ugni Blanc (see page 552)

BURGUNDY – *BOURGOGNE*

Burgundy, whose wines made on sloping hills (côtes) are as famous as Bordeaux's around the world, primarily grows chardonnay, but a few others as well. Gamay and Pinot Noir were most abundantly grown here first by the Romans and spread to other regions of France by the Middle Ages. Evidence of vineyard cultivation dates back to the 4th century in Burgundy. The historically celebrated vinification and culinary practices came out of the monasteries of the Benedictine monks and the Cistercian order in this region of medieval France. (Meursault chardonnay from the Côte de Beaune is a "model" wine for a white Burgundy.) Chablis (with its notes of "flint"), Côtes de Nuits and Hautes-Côtes de Nuits (famous for its Pinot Noir reds), Côte de Beaune and Hautes-Côtes de Beaune, Côte Chalonnaise, and Mâconnais are the major regions. There are many smaller appellations that are well-known within these areas such as in Côtes de Nuits which contains Chambertin, Nuits-Saint-Georges, and La Romanée, which is only two acres (0.84 hectares). Burgundy alone has about 100 appellations.

Burgundy Red Grape Varieties

Gamay – High tannins, fresh and fruity with notes of pear, raspberry, and strawberry.

Pinot Noir – Fruity, spicy, smoky, fresh, sometimes menthol aromas. Among the highest in phenolic compounds resveratrol and anthocyanins among grapes. Dates back to the Romans, but also cultivated in French monasteries of the Middle Ages in Burgundy.

Tressot – Related to Petit Verdot, Duras, and Savagnin. Contributes color, acidity, and tannins.

Burgundy White Grape Varieties

Aligoté – Plays a key role in sparkling wines (*crémants*), dry wines with floral and herbal notes and high acidity. Notes of acacia, green apple, hazelnut, lemon, linden, and peach. Pairs well with both fresh and aged cheeses, particularly Crottin de Chavignol.[48]

Chardonnay (or "Beauois") – Full-bodied white, with notes of almond, apple, and linden. Possibly the most well-known grape variety in the world. Often "oaked" in new oak barrels to enhance its aromas and aging potential, as well as amplify the aromas of vanilla (French oak) and coconut (U.S. oak). Chardonnay is native to Burgundy, where the process of aging chardonnay wines "on the lees" (*sur lie* or *sur lies*) in the barrel (rather than filtered or "racked" into another barrel) originated. This process extracts flavor from the lees (dead yeast and grape sediment) accumulated in the barrel and adds to the wine's complexity and aging potential. This is the grape for Meursault wine from the Côte de Beaune appellation and for Chablis wines from the Chablis AOC (appellation or designation of controlled origin).

Melon de Bourgogne – High in acidity, notes of apple and citrus.

Pinot Blanc – Blended with chardonnay in Burgundy to make the Côte de Beaune Meursault wine which has buttery and nutty aromas and flavors of citrus and "minerals," thanks largely to its limestone soils.

Sauvignon Blanc – Notes ranging from almonds, apple, apricots, black currant bud, boxwood, citrus, fennel, freshly cut hay, mint, mushroom, passion fruit, straw, undergrowth, and violet.

CHAMPAGNE

Champagne's vineyard villages are divided into three types of terroirs: Grand Cru, Premier Cru, and Autres Cru. Only sparkling wines from the Champagne appellation are allowed to be called "Champagne." Champagne wines are another wine type commonly left "on the lies" (*sur lie*), giving notes of bread or toast.

Champagne Red Grape Varieties
Pinot Noir – High acidity, low tannins, aromas of black cherry, currant, and roses. Provides body and structure.

Pinot Meunier – Higher acidity than Pinot Noir but lighter in color. Aromatic and fruity.

Champagne White Grape Variety
Chardonnay – Paired with Pinot Noir to make Champagne. Provides elegance and freshness.

CORSICA – *LA CORSE*
The island of Corsica grows a wide variety of grapes, two of which are considered more local than the rest.

Corsica Red Grape Varieties
Nielluccio – Also known as Sangiovese in Italy. Solid tannic structure, high in alcohol, astringent. Fruity notes (stone fruits, marmalade, red currant), spice, and undertones of thyme.

Sciaccarello – Structured, with notes of berries.

Corsica White Grape Varieties
Vermentino – Notes of apple, apricot, chamomile, fennel, hazelnut, peach, pear, and floral notes. Can lack in acidity. Synonym for the grape variety *Malvoisie*, grown in Roussillon and Corsica.

Chardonnay (see above and page 550)

JURA
Just north of the Savoie-Bugey region, Jura wines are famous for their yellow wines (*vin jaune*) and straw wine (*vin de paille*), grapes that have been left to dry on beds of straw. There are several general appellations in Jura as well as others under the appellations of Arbois and Côtes de Jura.

Jura Red Grape Varieties
Pinot Noir (see above and page 550)

Poulsard – Very lightly colored. Used to make sparkling Jura wines. Mineral notes as well as delicate aromas of small red berries and undergrowth.

Trousseau – Intense purple color, solid tannic structure, and full-bodied. High in acidity and alcohol with notes of red fruits. A component of the *Crémant de Jura* (sparkling wine) *Macvin du Jura* and other wines.

Jura White Grape Varieties
Chardonnay (see page 550)

Savagnin – Used for *Vin de Paille*, ("straw wine") in which the grapes are dried on straw for several weeks, concentrating flavors and sugars. Also used for Jura's *Vin Jaune* (yellow wine) and used for Jura sparkling wines.

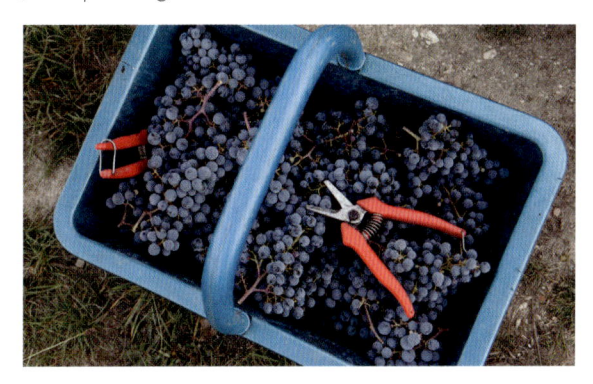

LANGUEDOC-ROUSSILLON
Located along the Eastern Edge of France's Southwest, leading to the Mediterranean Sea, Languedoc-Roussillon has almost thirty appellations producing sparkling wines, reds, and rosés. Among the appellations are Banyuls, Cabrieres, Collioure, Coteaux du Languedoc, Côtes du Roussillon, Grand Roussillon, Gres de Monpellier, La Clape, Lesquerde, Limoux, Montpeyroux, Muscat de Mireval, Picpoul de Pinet, Pic Saint-Loup, Rivesaltes, Saint-Chinian, Saint-Drezery, Saint-Jean-de-Minervois, Sommieres, Tautavel, and Terrasses du Larzac. Among the region's best vintages are 1990, 1991, 1995, 1998, 2001, 2003, 2004, 2005, 2006, 2010 and 2015.[49]

Languedoc-Roussillon Red Grape Varieties
Carignan – Good tannic structure, notes of dark berries, cherry, prunes, pepper, and herbaceous aromas.

Cinsault (see pages 553 and 554)

Grenache Noir – Notes of stewed and spiced strawberries. Used in Languedoc-Roussillon to make the red and white sweet wines (*vins doux naturels*) of Banyuls in Southern Roussillon.

Mourvèdre – High tannin levels, deep color, combined with Syrah and Grenache Noir in Langudoc-Roussillon. Notes of blackberry, black currant, pepper and touches of vegetal and leather aromas. Makes structured wines that tend to age well.

Syrah (see page 554)

Langudoc-Roussillon White Grape Varieties
Bourboulenc (see page 554)

Clairette (see page 554)

Grenache Blanc – A robust variety that can survive well in dry and rocky climates but is susceptible to "grey rot" (*la pourriture grise*) in humid conditions. Notes of apple and peach with a crisp acidity.

Macabeu – Fresh, floral, and fruity, and harvested early.

Malvoisie – Synonym for the grape variety *Vermentino*, grown in Roussillon and Corsica. Dry and acidic, flinty flavors, and makes for a straw-colored wine.

Marsanne – Associated with Roussanne. Notes of acacia, beeswax, citrus, dried nuts, honey, jasmine, licorice, truffle, and white peach.

Picpoul or Picpoul de Pinet – Also known as Piquepoul. Full-bodied with citrus aromas and high acidity. Pairs well with fish.

Roussanne (see page 555)

Ugni Blanc – Originates from Italy. Floral notes of geranium and violet. Generic grape, often distilled for use in brandies (*eau de vie*).

Viognier (see page 555)

LOIRE VALLEY – *VAL DE LOIRE*
The Loire Valley produces the third largest volume of French wine, after Bordeaux and the Rhône Valley. Among the many regions of the Loire Valley are Anjou-Saumur (with appellations such as Anjou Villages, Bonnezeaux, and Saumur-Champigny), Centre Loire (Quincy, Sancerre, Reuilly, Pouilly-Fumé, Valençay) Chenin, Haut Loire, Massif Central, the Pays Nantais (the region where Muscadet wine is made from the Melon de Bourgogne grape) in the West, "Basse Loire" or "Loire Atlantique," Touraine (Bourgueil, Cheverny, Chinon, and Vouvray, producing herbaceous whites and low-tannic, fruity reds), Sancerre (called the Tom Hanks of wine, by the Wall Street Journal writer Lettie Teague, "one that everybody loves," a wine that has famously characteristic notes of gun-flint. The Loire Valley also produces sparkling (*crémant*) and rosé regional wines. Bourgueil, made of a majority Cabernet Franc (locally called "Cabernet Breton"), with some Cabernet Sauvignon, is floral and fruity on the nose.

Loire Valley Red Grape Varieties
Cabernet Franc (see page 547)

Cabernet Sauvignon (see page 549)

Gamay (see page 547)

Grolleau – Most commonly used in production of Rosé d'Anjou. Lacking tannins, it is also susceptible to disease and not flavorful, but high-yielding.

Malbec (see page 549)

Pineau d'Aunis – Used in many Loire Valley appellations. Light-bodied, low tannins, little color but high acidity, notes of red fruits and black pepper.

Pinot Noir (see pages 550 and 551)

Loire Valley White Grape Varieties
Aligoté (see page 550)

Arbois – Also known as "Petit Pineau." Used alongside Chenin Blanc in Vouvray appellation wines. Rich in alcohol, low in acidity. Freshness with aromas of honey and pineapple.

Chardonnay (see pages 550 and 551)

Chenin Blanc – Also known as Pineau de la Loire. Used in the production of wines like Bonnezeaux and Vouvray, and used in dry, semi-dry, sparkling, and sweet white wines. Produces wines that can be light or full-bodied. Fatty texture in the mouth (*gras en bouche*). High acidity and gold color. Floral and grassy aromas. Notes of apple, grass, honey, melon, and quince.

Malvoisie (Ancenis) – Synonym for aromatic, full-bodied white grape wines using Pinot Gris, as grown in the Loire Valley. Used to label Pinot Gris sweet wines in the Valais, Switzerland, and used for Bourboulenc in Languedoc, for Clairette in Bordeaux and Savagnin in Austrian Tyrol.[50]

Melon de Bourgogne – Makes the Muscadet wines of the Nantais vineyards of the western Loire Valley, high in acidity, flavors of apple and citrus. This is another wine that is often aged "on the lees" in the barrel for added complexity of flavor.

Pinot Gris (see page 546)

Romorantin – Only planted on 60 hectares in the Cour-Cheverny appellation of the Loire. Fruity aromas of citrus, peach, pear, and notes of flint and white flowers.

Sauvignon Blanc (see page 549)

Tressalier – Good acidity and freshness, low alcohol content. Grown in the Auvergne region of the Massif Central. Used also for the *Crémant de Bourgogne* sparkling wine in Burgundy under the grape variety name of *Sacy*.

LORRAINE
Major appellations are Côtes de Meuse, Côtes de Moselle, and Côtes de Toul.

Lorraine Red Grape Variety

Pinot Noir (see pages 550 and 551)

Lorrraine Grey Grape Variety
Pinot Gris – Blended with Pinot Noir or Meunier.

Lorraine White Grape Varieties
Aligoté (see page 550)

Aubin Vert (also known as Vert Blanc) – Often blended with Auxerrois.

Auxerrois – Notes of citrus, honey, musk.

Chardonnay (see pages 550 and 551)

Pinot Blanc – Good acidity, notes of smoke and apple.

PROVENCE
The vineyards of Provence extend from inland Avignon to Nice on the Mediterranean Sea. Among the nine appellations are Bandol, Bellet, Cassis, Coteaux d'Aix en Provence, Coteaux de Pierrevert, Coteaux Varios, Côtes de Provence, (which includes the sub-appellations of Côtes de Provence Fréjus, La Londe, Pierrefeu, and Saint-Victoire), Les Baux de Provence, and Palette.

Provence Red Grape Varieties
Barbaroux – Low acidity, medium alcohol content and high likelihood for aging well. Rose colored skin. Also used as table grapes (*raisin de table*).

Calitor – Light-bodied, light in color, low in alcohol, high yielding but fast disappearing in Provence.

Cinsault – Native to Provence, brings freshness, subtlety and fruit to a blend. Used in Provence primarily for rosés.

Carignan (see page 551)

Grenache Noir (see page 554)

Mollard – Pomegranate color, fresh and light and high in acidity. Good aging potential. Aromas of black pepper, ripened red fruits, toast, vanilla.[51]

Mourvèdre – Tannic, used for the hearty, spiced Bandol wines. Brings smoothness and notes of blackberries and violet, gaining notes of cinnamon and pepper as it ages.

Syrah (see below)

Téoulier – Low acidity, medium alcohol content, and rich in color.

Tibouren – Makes lightly colored wines, with subtle berry and floral notes that should be consumed soon after being bottled.

Provence White Grape Varieties
Clairette – Aromatic with notes of white stone fruits.

Rolle (Vermentino) – Originally from Italy, aromatic, full-bodied and smooth, with notes of citrus and pear.

Sémillon (see page 549)

Ugni Blanc (see page 552)

RHÔNE VALLEY – *VALLÉE DU RHÔNE*
South of Lyon, stretching from Vienne to Arles, the Rhône Valley is made up of about twenty-six appellations, including the well-known Châteauneuf-du-Pape of southern Rhône (I'm a fan of the chocolate notes in some of these wines), and the Côte-Rôtie (literally, roasted slopes, and known for notes of black pepper, dark berries, leather and plum) of northern Rhône where primarily Syrah and Viogner are grown. Both of these appellations allow for a blend of red and white grapes, while the remaining Rhône appellations do not. Some other well-known Rhône appellations include Beaumes de Venise, Côtes du Rhône Villages, Crozes-Hermitage, Gigondas, Hermitage, Saint-Joseph, and Vacqueyras.

Rhône Valley Red Grape Varieties
Carignan (see page 551)

Cinsault – Also known as Cinqsaut and is the leading grape grown in Morocco. Yields lots of fruit, and best in dry climates, such as North Africa. Aromatic and supple, but low in tannins. Adds fragrance and lightness to blends. Part of the Southern Rhône classic blend of Grenache Noir, Mourvèdre, and Syrah.

Grenache Noir – Originates from Spain and is the second most planted grape variety in France. Grenache makes up the majority of the rosés in Southern France. Spicy pepper, white pepper aromas and coriander, floral notes, along with red fruits and raspberry, sometimes licorice as well as notes of black cherry, tobacco, or dried fig. High alcohol content and medium-bodied, with softer tannins, usually combined with full-bodied Syrah. The model Rhône appellations for Grenache are Châteauneuf-du-Pape, Gigondas and Vacqueyras.[52]

Mourvèdre – Notes of prune, blueberry, blackberry and black currant, and hints of dark chocolate. Can have notes of coriander and juniper berry. Known for its structure and intense fruit, it is combined with Grenache and Syrah to produce balanced Rhône blends. (See also Mourvèdre in Languedoc-Roussillon and Provence.)

Syrah – Also known as Shiraz, especially in the United States and Australia, it originates from Iran and has been grown in the Rhône area since Roman times. Ranges in aromas from red fruits and raspberry to dark berries and dark fruit jam (*compoté*). More floral as a young wine, when aged, it can have notes of leather, licorice, tobacco, and vanilla. Deeply colored, full-bodied, high in tannins, it adds structure to the Rhône wines, which are usually combined with Grenache and Mourvèdre in the Rhône. The northernmost Rhône Valley appellation of Côte-Rôtie is the model for Rhône Valley Syrah at its best. Syrah ages well, and therefore most prefer to drink it when aged rather than when young.

Rhône Valley White Grape Varieties
Bourboulenc – Acidic, low in alcohol, with notes of bitter almond, green apple, and floral aromas, and a slight bitterness in the finish.

Clairette – Also known as "Blanquette." Brings freshness and notes of apple, citrus, stone fruits.

Grenache Blanc – Used in famed Châteauneuf-du-Pape blends. Tendency for high alcohol and good acidity. Notes of apple and stone fruits.

Marsanne – Associated with Roussanne. Notes of acacia, beeswax, citrus, dried nuts, honey, jasmine, licorice, truffle, white peach.

Roussanne – Also known as "Bergeron." Slightly reddish skin from which it derives its name (*roux* meaning "reddish-brown" in French). Apricot, herbal, and honey aromas. Can have notes of cumin.

Viognier – Good acidity, smooth, and full-bodied. Notes of apricot, honey, lime, mango, oak, peach, pear, and tobacco.

SAVOIE-BUGEY

Bugey is part of the Auvergne-Rhône-Alpes region, situated at the foothills of the Jura mountains near Lyon, and is a very small wine producing area, but bears mentioning because it is the birthplace of the gastronome Jean Anthelme Brillat-Savarin who wrote "The Physiology of Taste" (*"La Physiologie du Goût"*)[53] in 1825. This launched a new genre, the gastronomic essay, and was one of the first to note that grains, flour, and sugar cause obesity in all animals, including humans. Savoie and Bugey each have numerous appellations.

Savoie-Bugey Red Grape Varieties

Gamay (see page 547)

Jacquère – High acidity, known for mountain freshness, and pale color. Citrus and floral notes.

Mondeuse – Usually blended with Gamay and Pinot Noir. Notes of flowers, red fruits, and spices.

Pinot Noir (see pages 550 and 551)

Poulsard – Sweet, juicy, and pale in color.

Savoie-Bugey White Grape Varieties

Altesse – Also known as "Roussette." Elegant and aromatic.

Chardonnay (see pages 550 and 551)

Chasselas (see page 546)

Roussanne (see above)

SOUTHWEST – *SUD OUEST* (EXCLUDING BORDEAUX)

There are 26 wine growing sub-regions in the French Southwest. Among them are: Armagnac, Bergerac, Cahors, Gaillac, Irouléguy (the smallest winegrowing region in France), Jurançon, and Madiran.

Armagnac – A brandy (*eau de vie*, literally water of life) of about 40% alcohol used since the Middle Ages and made in the *départements* of Gers, Landes, Lot-et-Garonne in the Southwest. It is made by distilling dry white wines, primarily from the grape varieties of Colombarde, Folle-Blanche, and Ugni Blanc.

Bergerac – Located in the beautiful Dordogne region East of Bordeaux, Bergerac encompasses nine major appellations, producing sweet and rosé wines, some dry whites and aromatic red wines blended similarly to Bordeaux's blends thanks to the similar grape varieties grown. Red grape varieties include Cabernet Franc, Cabernet Sauvignon, and Merlot, combined with Côt, Fer Servadou, or Mérille. Some Muscadelle is grown here, along with Chenin Blanc, Sauvignon Blanc, Sauvignon Gris, Sémillon, and Ugni Blanc. Flavorful sweet wines are made in the Monbazillac and Saussignac appellations. Bergerac reds can pair well with dark chocolate.

Buzet – West of the Southwestern city of Agen (famous for its prunes), the Buzet region produces mostly full-bodied red wines from Cabernet Sauvignon and Merlot grapes, similar to the wines of Bordeaux. It also produces some crisp white wines from Sauvignon Blanc, Muscadelle, and Sémillon, as in Bordeaux, along with some rosés from Cabernet Franc.

Cahors – Mostly Malbec wines are grown here, where the Malbec grape is known as *Côt* or *Auxerrois*. About 70% Malbec is complemented by Merlot and Tannat (adds color, dryness, and tannins to the wines). Cahors wines can have notes of cherry and cedar and tend to age well.

Gaillac – In the department of Tarn, north of Toulouse, red Gaillac wines are richly colored and made from blending the grapes of Cabernet Franc,

Cabernet Sauvignon, Duras (peppery notes, high tannins, and rich in alcohol), Fer Servadou, Merlot, and Syrah. The primary grapes for the white wines are Len de L'El (a low-acid, local variety), Mauzac (with apple aromas), and Muscadelle. Since Roman times, the Gaillac region has been producing a great diversity of wines.

Irouléguy – Some of the exotic sounding Basque names for the red grapes grown in the Irouléguy area (the smallest winegrowing region in France) are *Axeria* (Cabernet Franc), *Axeria Handia* (Cabernet Sauvignon), and *Bordelesa Beltza* (Tannat). And the white grapes are *Izkiriota* (Gros Manseng), *Izkiriota Ttipia* (Petit Manseng), and *Xuri Zerratia* (Courbu). Irouléguy red wines are generally fruity, full-bodied, and tannic. The whites are fragrant and high in acidity with notes of apricot and citrus.

Jurançon – The hilly, sun-kissed winegrowing region of Béarn is influenced both by oceanic and mountainous climates. It is located in the department of Pyrénées-Atlantiques, whose capital city Pau has a magnificent view of the Pyrénées and is a jumping off point for hikers and skiers alike. Grape varieties from this region are Courbu, Gros Manseng, and Petit Manseng (high acidity, notes of citrus and stone fruits), which produce some dry white wine, but mostly sweet dessert wines that age well, with notes of honey, sugared fruits, and spices.

Madiran – Madiran produces both red and white wine. The white Madiran is called Pacherenc du Vic-Bilh and is made dry and sweet (and often paired with foie gras). The more well-known red Madiran is expressive and tannic, thanks to the majority Tannat grape, and is the signature red wine from Gascony that goes well with duck and **Béarnaise Garbure Soup** (page 338). Other grape varieties in the red Madiran blend include Cabernet Sauvignon, Cabernet Franc, and Fer Savadou.

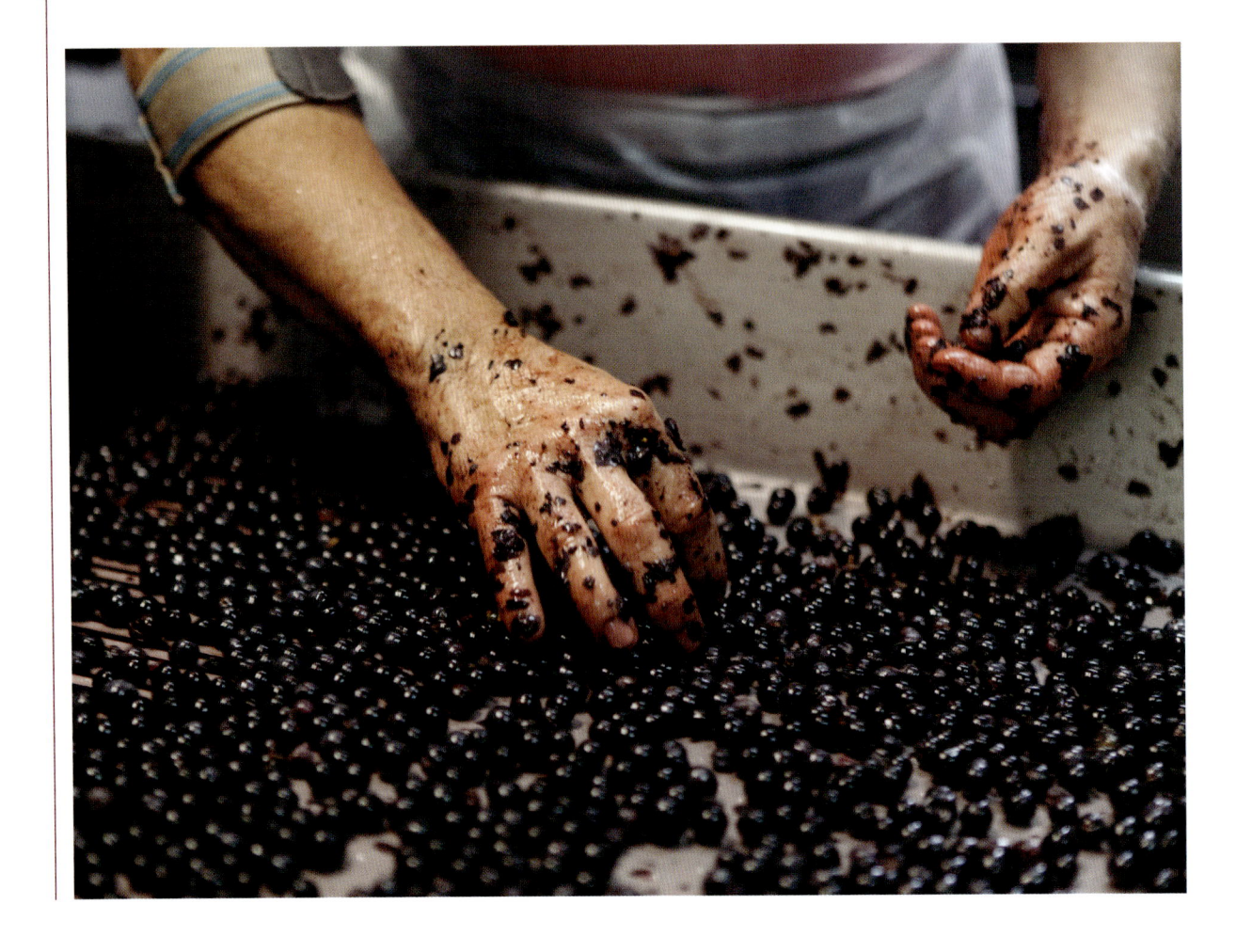

FOOD AND WINE PAIRINGS GUIDE – *ACCORDS METS & VINS*

ON THE MENU: BORDEAUX WINES

In Bordeaux, sometimes it is the food that takes a back seat to the wine. Wine takes center stage because, after all, it is *Bordeaux*. But even here it is possible to make a more reciprocal pairing or match so that one does not outshine the other, especially if the goal is to bring out the flavors of the meal. Wine can do this very well. It helps us slow down, enjoy, and digest a meal in a more relaxed manner. A good wine can bring the meal up a notch simply with its presence on the table.

WINE BEFORE DINNER – *L'APÉRITIF*

In France, alcohol, often a wine or champagne, is often served as an *apéritif*. In Bordeaux, the apéritif is often a sweet Bordeaux, from Barsac (some famous ones being Château Coutet and Château Doisy Daëne) or Sauternes (Château Rieussec and Château d'Yquem), or else a Cadillac or Monbazillac. The Bordelais also serve Champagne as an apéritif, or else red, white, or rosé wines, depending on the season, their guests' tastes, what's on the menu, and/or what they have in stock in their wine cellar (*la cave à vin*). Pineau des Charentes, also a sweet wine, originating from Charentes, north of Bordeaux, is another likely candidate for an apéritif, where Cognac, made from grapes grown in the Cognac region, also north of Bordeaux, is often served after dinner as a *digestif*. Once you have determined the menu for a dinner or an event, you can decide on the apéritif, the dinner wine or wines, and the digestif, if you are going to have all of these. In Bordeaux especially, unless it is a wine-tasting party, if wine is brought as a gift, especially from a wine maker, the hosts are not expected to open it then and there, as the wine has been disturbed in transit and should rest and be properly chilled or age further in the bottle before being consumed. It is assumed that the hosts will provide the wine based on what they are serving at the event.

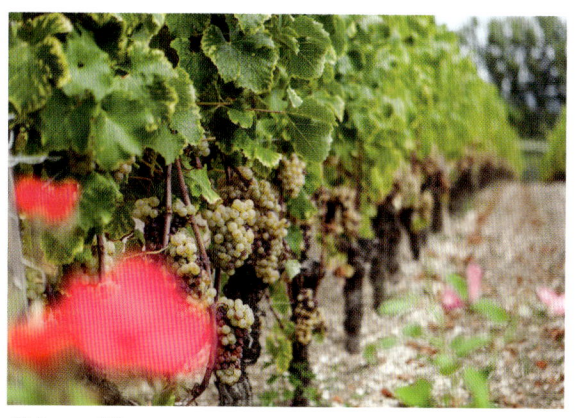

Château d'Yquem

Véronique Sanders of Chateau Haut-Bailly in Bordeaux provides a few words of wisdom on serving apéritifs and pairing wine and food: "There is nothing better than to start an apéritif with great Champagne or a Sauternes wine. Then you have to play with young and ripe vintages: You usually begin by serving the youngest vintage, moving to the more mature ones, but you can also wake up the palate with a younger wine served with cheese. Every lunch or dinner is different according to the season, the temperature, the provenance, and the age of the guests. Quality is the foundation, creativity is the key! And to quote Curnonsky, born Maurice Edmond Sailland in 1872, and the first food critic, known as the 'prince of gastronomy' (*le prince des gastronomes*): 'To host someone is to be in charge of his or her happiness.'"

QUESTIONS TO ASK YOURSELF WHEN CHOOSING A WINE TO MATCH WITH A MEAL

You may already have some favorite wines and know exactly why you like them. You may have some favorites but not know why you like them. Either way, it helps to identify what you like or dislike or find memorable about each wine. If you do not know where to start, you can ask a friend or a salesperson in a wine store. They will ask you questions similar to these to help narrow your choice:

- What is the occasion?

- Do you already have certain taste or geographic preferences?

- What is your budget?

- Is this a gift to be kept for many years or will it be consumed right away?

- What food, if any, will be served with the wine?

- What characteristics of the food are particularly interesting or dominant that you might want to accentuate using the wine?

- Who will taste the wine? Are they tolerant tasters who like strongly flavored food and drink or sensitive tasters who will appreciate subtleties in the wine?

As one who seeks out organic foods, you may also consider only organic wines, which may narrow the choices significantly—not an altogether bad thing, actually. With organic wines, you can for the most part be assured that pesticide use will be minimal, if any. Fortunately, organic vintners and vineyards are increasing (both in number and in quality), around the world.

Wine tasting and pairing as an art and science can easily overwhelm the newcomer. The key is to take the learning process one step at a time and to relax and enjoy the process. Indeed, tasting, experimenting, and sharing the experience with others is what makes food and drink, and life in general, so interesting! Incorporating some of our great-grandparents' habits and values may help us slow down and enjoy the simple moments in our own lives, especially when it comes to dining with family and friends.

According to my always-humble wine connoisseur friend, Dewey Markham, Jr., official wine pairing and wine terminology can be off-putting and distancing. "It is a matter of taste. Perfect is the enemy of the good. Everybody has their system, and not everything will go together, but that's what sommeliers have to worry about. It is not in the reach of the average wine drinker that you know so many wines, so just try to avoid the horrible ones and it'll be okay. When you go to a restaurant and look at a menu, you know what veal tastes like, so put all the ingredients together in your mind, and choose a wine based on what you know, or else feel free to ask the waiter or the sommelier, who might know whether one wine or other goes better with a certain dish."

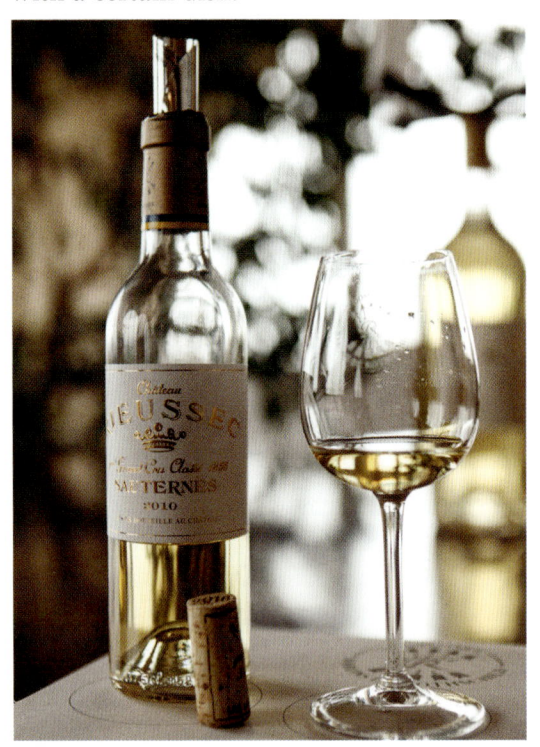

Château Rieussec, Grand Cru Classé de Sauternes

It's also worth remembering that if you do make a wine pairing "mistake," you are likely to remember it and not repeat it, one more experience under your belt about which you can feel confident! Also, you may have a bottle already opened, so even if you are having a red meat and have a bottle of white, just try it out and see if it works. I was reheating chicken livers with bacon for dinner one evening, and we had an open bottle of Chardonnay from Côtes de Jura. Because the wine, though white, was high enough in acidity, it worked to balance the strong flavors of the chicken livers.

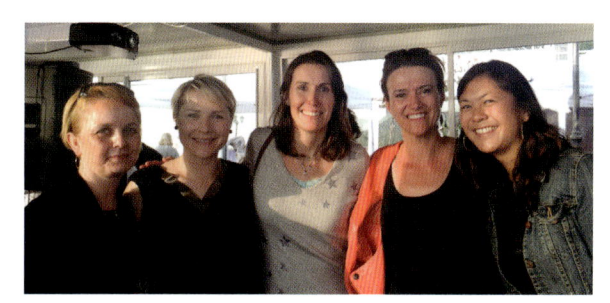

DUAD Classmates: Annabelle, Natalia, Tania, Malika, Vy

Annabelle Nicolle-Beaufils, one of my DUAD wine course classmates and a former restaurateur, kindly helped me with many of the food and wine pairings for *The Bordeaux Kitchen* and provided suggestions for some of the meat dishes, as have others wine professional friends and other of my DUAD classmates. The suggestions we have collaboratively given for recipes may be used as starting points upon which you can experiment. I recommend keeping a log of wines you have tasted, including the date, name of the wine and its year, the maker and origin, appellation, alcohol content, and any visual, olfactory, and taste descriptions you experience, or even what you eat it with. The more detail you record, the more likely you will be to remember what you have tasted and be able to recall it when referring to your notes. Following are some general concepts to consider when pairing wine and food.

BASIC RULES OF THUMB
In France, the most basic rule of thumb is pairing regional dishes with wines from the same region. Some other very basic rules of thumb would be to pair tannic, flavorful, full-bodied reds with lamb and beef; medium-tannic red wines with veal; dry white wines, rosés, and "simple" red wines, lighter in body, tannins, and overall complexity with pork; and dry and crisp white wines with fish. It is worth noting that higher levels of acidity in wine tend to cut the fats and oils in food, while also balancing out the sugar and alcohol in the wine itself. My Bordeaux winemaker friends who produce dessert wines will say that a sweet wine can probably be paired with almost any dish—appetizer, main course, or dessert! Do not feel bound by these principles, as there are countless matchings to be discovered and made!

Pairing Wine with the Texture and Intensity of the Main Dish: Grilled meat versus slow-cooked meat that melts in your mouth. Imagine these in your mouth and what kind of flavors and sensations in wine would enhance and match these main dishes. Leather, tannic, and slightly astringent goes well with steak. Suave and subtle wines enhance a slow-cooked beef or pork roast.

Balancing the Aromas and Flavors with a Dish: An example would be to pair a fruity wine to complement the fruity aromas of a pork roast stuffed with prunes. According to Caroline Matthews, it is worth noting that sweetness and savoriness, or "umami," in a dish can make a wine taste "harder" (i.e., more drying and bitter, and more acidic and less sweet and fruity). However, salt and acidity in a dish can make wine less bitter and acidic, but fruitier, sweeter, and richer, with more body.

Other guiding principles to consider are:

- balancing the acidity, sweetness, spice, or intensity of flavor with a dish

- considering the season, time of day, and geographic origin of wine, as well as location at which the wine is being consumed

- balancing the acid in the food with a higher acid wine

- balancing the sweetness in the food with a wine higher in sweetness

- cutting the sweetness or creaminess of a food with a drier wine

- cutting the bitterness of a food with a sweeter wine

Again, these guidelines are there to guide you to *your own experimentation* once you have some ideas with which to begin. Have fun and enjoy!

Sweet Wine Pairing

When asked about wine and food pairing, my friend Jane Anson, longtime writer for *Decanter* and author of several books including *Bordeaux Legends* about the "First Growths" of Bordeaux, and a recently published book on biodynamic wines said, "Some of my most interesting and enjoyable wine and food matches from Bordeaux have been with the sweet wines of Sauternes. I can remember a wonderful combination of Château Guiraud 2003 with fresh, tangy oysters from the Arcachon Bay. The salty edge to the oysters melded so beautifully with the apricot and saffron richness of a slightly older sweet wine. It was also instructive about general food and wine pairings, which is to not be constrained by what you are used to. I would definitely recommend a crisp and easy-to-drink Entre-Deux-Mers white with oysters also, but the weightier richness of a Sauternes gave a new dimension to both. That's the joy of wine—it can constantly surprise you."

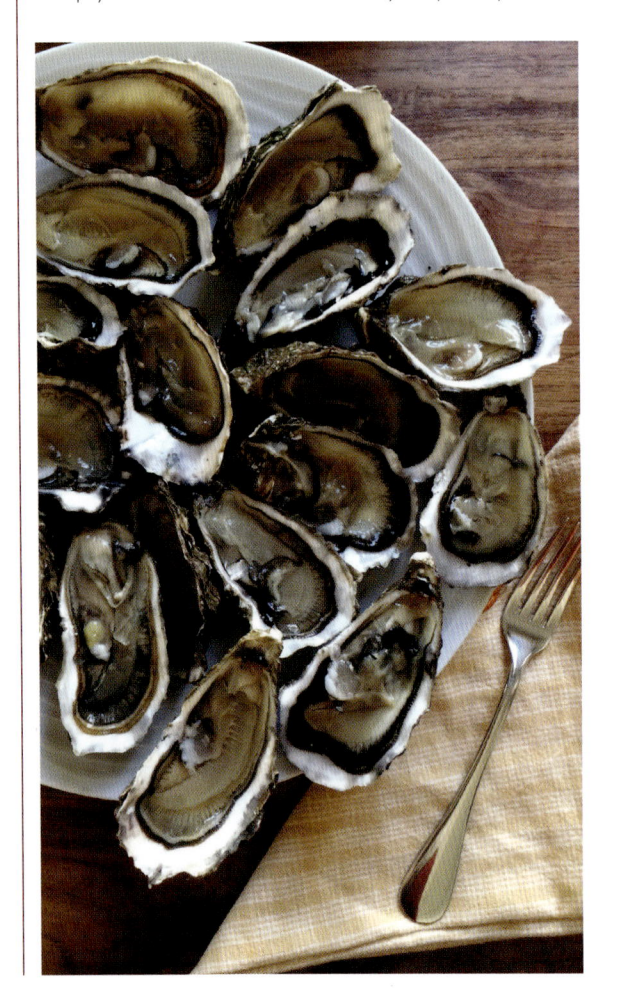

Matching Tradition and Season

One tradition that marries the season with the food and wine that is still carried out in the Bordeaux region and originating from the Périgord region nearby is that of the *faire chabrol* (also know as *chalorot* or *chabrot*), a mixing of ¼ to ½ of a glass of wine with the last sips of one's soup.

The tradition became widespread in the region by the 1800s for men working in the fields, but it was also reserved for women who had just given birth or who were lactating. For adolescents it was treated as a rite of passage to have one's first *chabrol*. It was considered a powerful medicine in itself.[54]

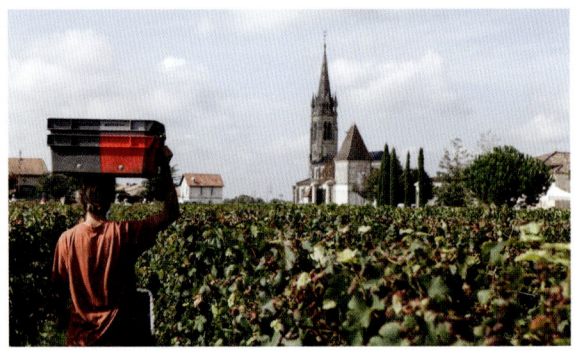

Harvest at La Fleur Pétrus, Pomerol

During harvest time at Château La Fleur Pétrus, in the celebrated Bordeaux wine region of Pomerol, the entire team, including grape pickers, lunches together. The meal always begins with a soup, the first course (*entrée*). La Fleur Pétrus family member and DUAD graduate Kelley Moueix says, "We all finish off our hot broth with a hearty *chabrol*, generally with our harvest wine (*cuvée*). Any good fruit-driven, yet lively red wine will do. The key is also in the dish: You want to have a shallow soup bowl, but surely not one with a border otherwise you send soup flying into your lap, as one traditionally finishes the soup (with the wine) by picking it up and drinking directly from the bowl. As for the soup, *chabrol* is best done with a broth soup. For us it is usually a chicken stock with simple seasonal vegetables—carrots, leeks, celery, potatoes. For the broth to be tasty, you need to cook it with some meat like chunks of ham hock." What a great way to finish off your glass! I had the pleasure of trying *chabrol* once at a La Fleur Pétrus harvest lunch, and the gesture, harvest atmosphere, and taste have stuck with me since.

How to Build a Wine Cellar with Ilona Guitz

My transplanted Belorussian friend, Ilona Guitz, after graduating from the DUAD program in 2007, created her own wine tourism enterprise and wine cellar consulting company. She teaches at the Bordeaux Wine School, organizes tasting classes, and frequently travels to Moscow, where she caters to Russian-speaking clients interested in building their own wine cellar. This is what she has to say about building your own wine collection:

"I often compare a wine cellar with a wardrobe. In the same way that we have clothing for everyday use (for going to work, shopping), we also have everyday wines. These are inexpensive, enjoyable, and not too complicated wines, just like the meals they accompany. On the weekends, we go out, or we invite friends over. We allow ourselves a bit more imagination when it comes to our clothing. We may have more time to prepare meals with carefully chosen ingredients. Therefore, we will tend to serve wines with a bit more character, with more complexity to discover and appreciate. And for special occasions, we put on our best outfits and we open our best bottles to accompany our most flavorful dishes. As far as the number of bottles in a wine cellar is concerned, that depends upon the space you have available to properly stock the wine and your habits of wine consumption. Try to evaluate the quantity consumed by month, and then annually, and by category (everyday wines, weekend wines, and special occasion wines). Then you will know how many bottles of which kind to buy and at what frequency you should buy them."

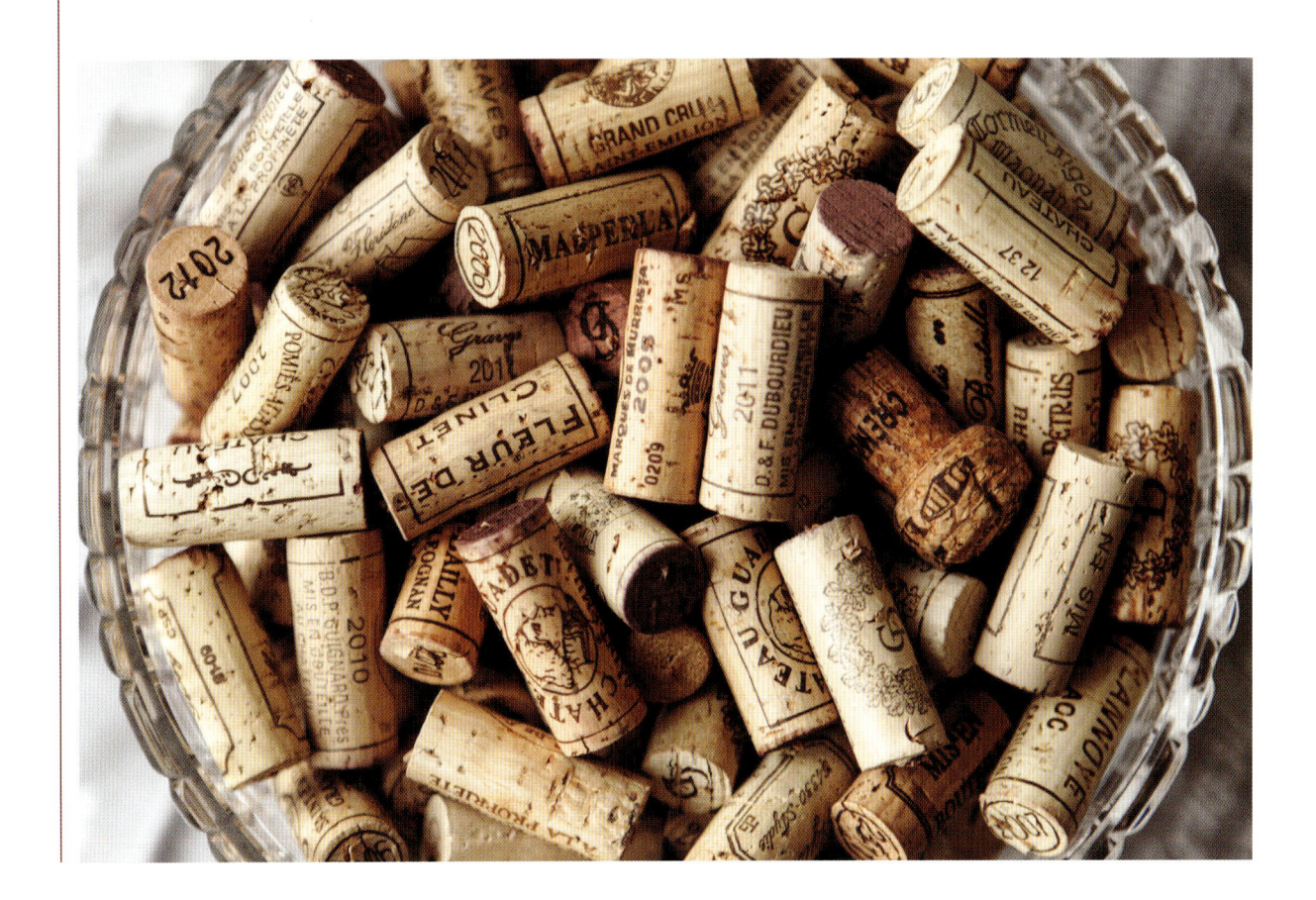

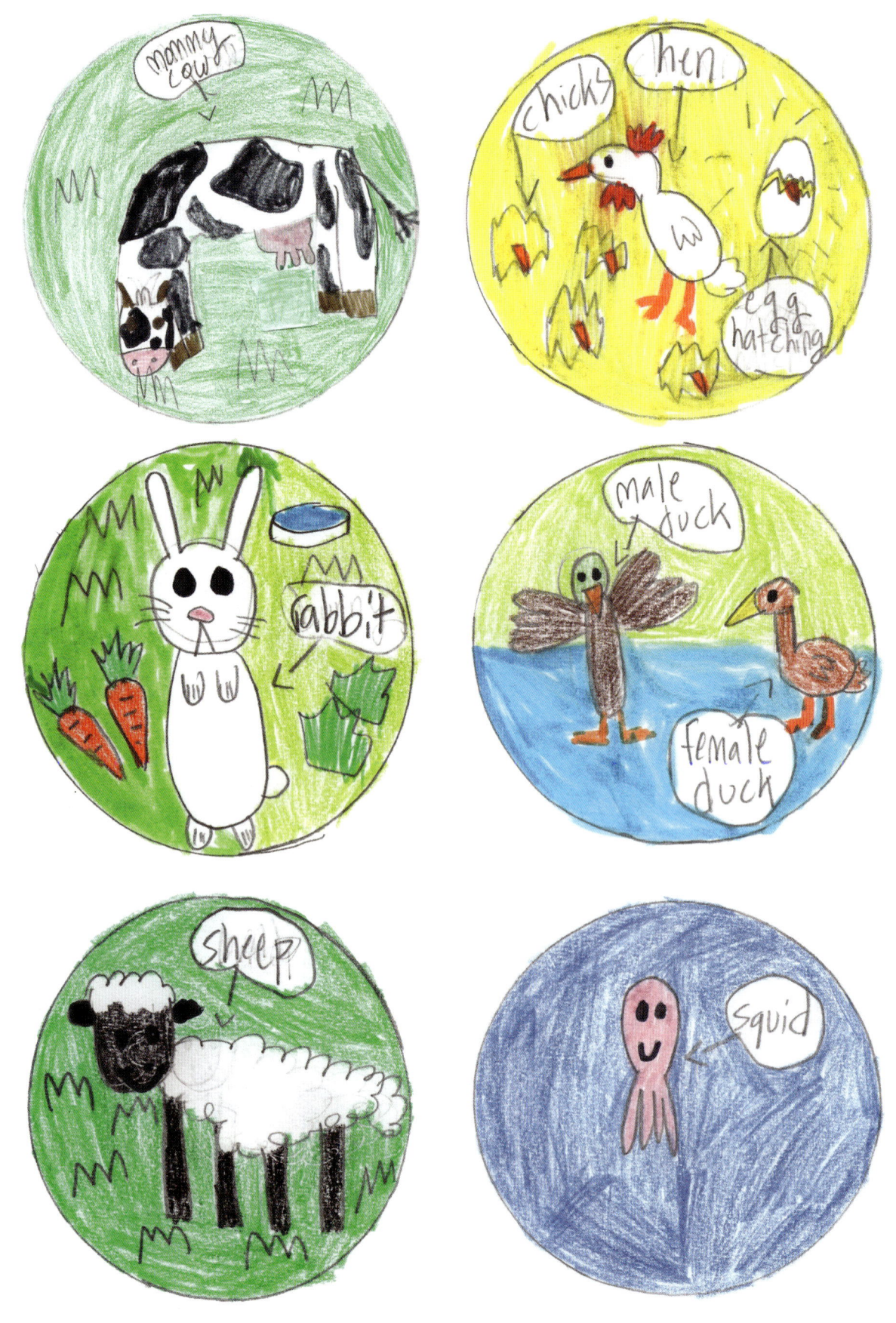

Eight Year Old's Animal Drawings

562 THE BORDEAUX KITCHEN

CHAPTER 8

LIVING WITH INTENTION, FAMILY FOOD ORGANIZATION, AND MEAL PLANNING

*"Unless someone like you cares a whole awful lot,
Nothing is going to get better. It's not."*
—Dr. Seuss, *The Lorax*

PART I: LIVING WITH INTENTION, VALUES, AND PRIORITIES

As a parent, I am naturally compelled to take care of my family and myself as best as I know how. Here I share some of our strategies on meals, screen-time, sleep, and more which have evolved over time as I have grown into this lifestyle and been influenced by the research in the paleo/primal and ancestral communities as well as French lifestyle and cooking habits. My approach continues to evolve in an attempt to *live with intention and according to our values* and is by no means the only way, nor the perfect way, but rather an example of *our* way (for now). These strategies reflect what I have learned and incorporated based on what has and what hasn't worked in the past, and what new habits are or are not working for us now. I have included here my personal experience considering family priorities, upholding the family tradition of mealtime together, along with ideas on family food organization, feeding children, the transfer of knowledge from parent to child, and some ideas on removing negative influences in the home.

THE "BALANCING" ACT

All parents want the best for their children. Isn't that why we aim to send them to the best schools and, therefore, buy houses in the best school districts and neighborhoods? We want our kids to keep up with the Jones' kids not only in terms of opportunity and skills, but also gadgets, entertainment, and fashion trends. As two-income households, we also need two cars, childcare, more stuff, and better vacations. And we end up seeking out entitlement, feeling that relaxation will come from someone else serving us, whether at a restaurant, a convenient food store, a hotel, or other place. I know because I have been there and have lived it. I also see it in our dual-income family and friends. We face a never-ending balancing act that is never really balanced, and material and career goals that are very stressful and so difficult to achieve that something always goes by the wayside, often our health.

FEEDING WITH INTENTION

I'm here to tell you that finding that perfect balance is impossible. The three words I do not like in this sentence are "perfect," "balance," and "impossible." All three words are hard to achieve in real life partly because their definitions are so elusive. I propose another way of looking at life, priorities. And juggling them. It all comes down to this: as a parent, *if you want the best for your children, feed them well.*

DISTRACTION SUBTRACTION

Valuing health and family relationships over achievement and "things" is the key here. If the foundation of your children's lives is wholesome food and regular, adequate sleep with a focus on family unity, then you build your life from there, filling in the "details." Like turning the fat-phobic food pyramid on its head, I propose turning conventional, modern life on its head. Rather than setting up your life around the 9-hour-a-day job and the daily commute and then squeezing in the rest of your life, start instead by setting up your life around family mealtime and bedtime, and then fill in the blanks. This is oversimplified and much easier said than done, but it does make us stop for a moment to consider our values and priorities. Seeing things from this perspective also helps us more readily recognize and *cut out the distractions* (such as mindless entertainment, damaging refined "foods," certain material goods, and certain social "obligations") that plague us whether we realize it or not.

CHANGING OUR MINDSET
Genuine needs like wholesome food, clean water, shelter, safety, and rest are intertwined, of course, and are the top priorities for all humans. How you arrive at each of these and under what circumstances depends on your opportunities, but also the values you recognize and adopt as yours, which may evolve over time, as you do. With this change, again easier said than done, do not blame yourself for past "mistakes" or beliefs. Turn off the tube. Ratchet down your ambition a notch to give your body, and your family, a break. Reset your goals, be grateful for the distinction you have made in this aspect of your life, and move forward. Be mindful of who you are now and what you are doing to implement positive change in your life. Once you are confident in and reminded of your true values (which are hopefully shared by your partner or spouse), you can set up your priorities and more easily manage all the rest: health care and disease management, finances, housing and car payments, aging parents, children's schedules, etc.

CHOICE
I recognize that some aspects of our lives are not easily changed. Of course, changing careers or moving out of or keeping a particular home is not always possible. (The places we have lived for the past 17 years, for example, have depended on my husband's work. Changing jobs would mean changing house, school *and* country.) What's more, in the U.S., we generally have the luxury of working and living near or with our families. Many, many people around the world and in the U.S. work "abroad," away from their families, in order to earn their living and support their families. While we may not be able to cover on a daily basis every administrative detail, along with jobs, school, exercise, pet care, grocery shopping, household maintenance, car repair, social connection, and homework help, not to mention reading, writing, meditating, or finding some sort of time for ourselves every day, we do usually have the choice to build and rely upon the foundation of our values and the priorities we set for our families. Life *is* a juggling act, there is no way around that, even without children in the household. But that is the challenge, excitement, and reality of life.

MARKET AND FARM VISITS
Our children see the care we take in procuring and preparing nutritious meals for them, though I admit that it is still much easier to go grocery shopping without them coming along. Sometimes we take them to markets (with our reusable cloth bags) or to visit farms so that they have a sense of where their food comes from. They don't always want to go at first, but once they are there, they are immediately interested. We visited Joel Salatin's Polyface Farm in the summer of 2016, and we got to meet the man himself, by lucky chance. Our meal on the car ride to Mr. Salatin's farm in Swoope, Virginia from Washington, DC was grass-fed bison burgers in thermos containers with various raw vegetables (*crudités*), a few organic corn chips, and homemade date-and-nut bars for dessert, a staple treat for school days in lieu of the processed junk surrounding us. We were excited to get to talk to Joel Salatin as well as choose from among the many types of meats and eggs his farm had for sale in their modest country store. Our children loved seeing the rabbits, pigs, and chickens and were enchanted by the chicks Joel Salatin's mother, Lucille, kindly let us observe. The girls still talk about the tiny newly-hatched chick we got to hold in our hands.

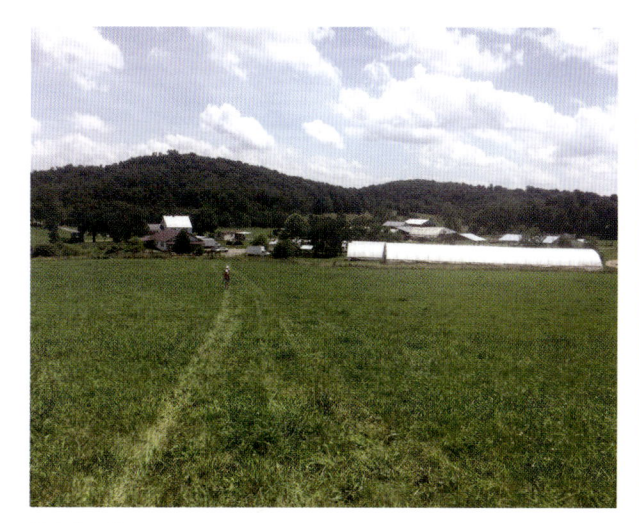

Polyface Farm

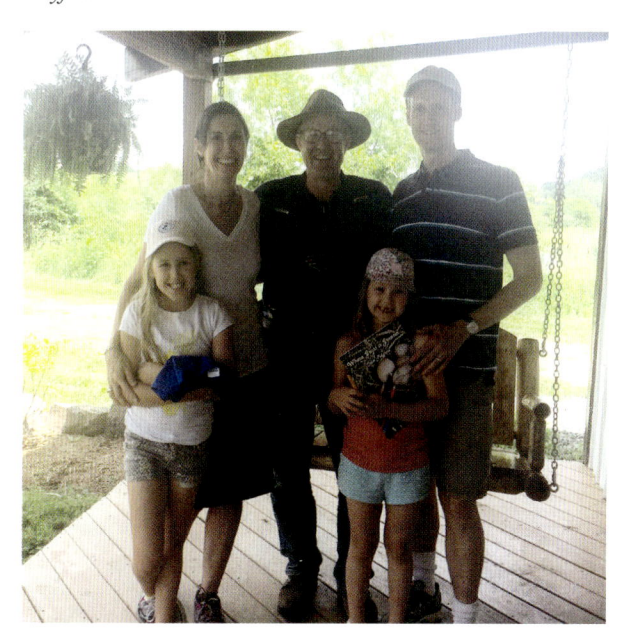

Family Portrait with Joel Salatin

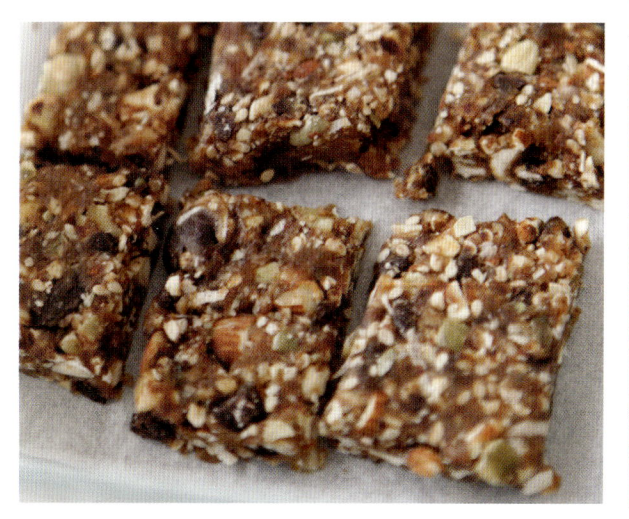

Homemade Date-and-Nut Bars

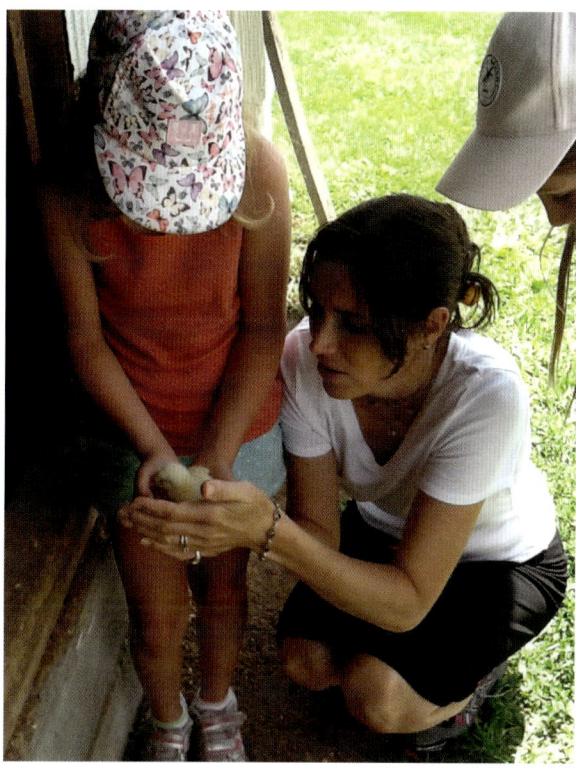

Holding the Newly-Hatched Chick

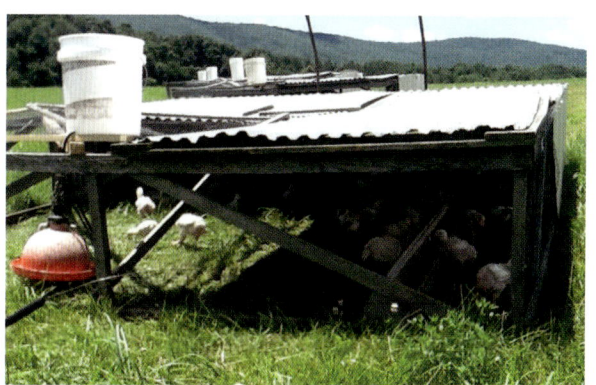

Mobil Chicken Coops at Polyface Farm

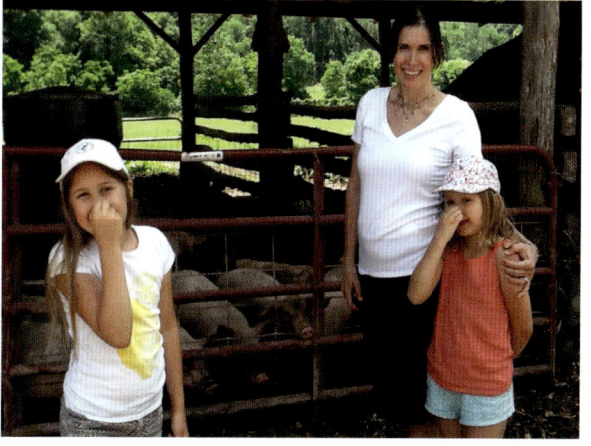

Visiting the Pig Pen

CHAPTER 8 565

In France, we have visited several farms, including a pig and sheep farm in the Basque country, and the girls still talk about the smallest of the pigs, the runt, at that farm. The more lasting effect has come from visiting the dairy goat farm outside Bordeaux, owned and operated by the Teulé family (see also page 62), with the baby goats and the most amazing fresh raw (unpasteurized) goat cheese (*faisselle*). The girls still talk about holding and feeding the baby goats, but even better, they still love to eat this kind of goat cheese topped with honey or marmalade. At markets, we encourage the girls to pick out some things they would like to eat, which usually end up being honey and marmalade!

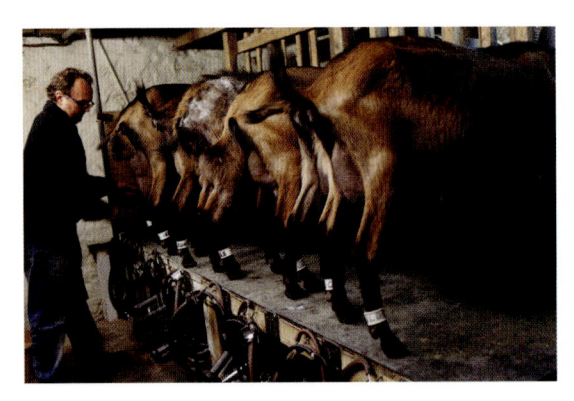

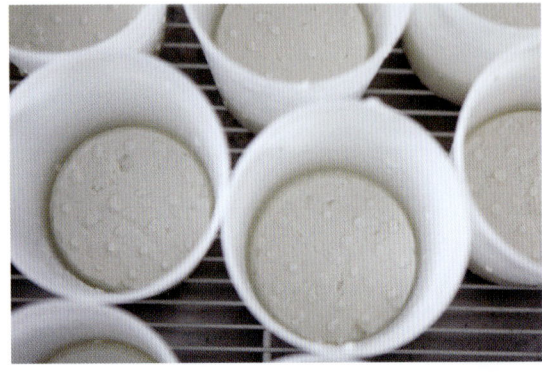

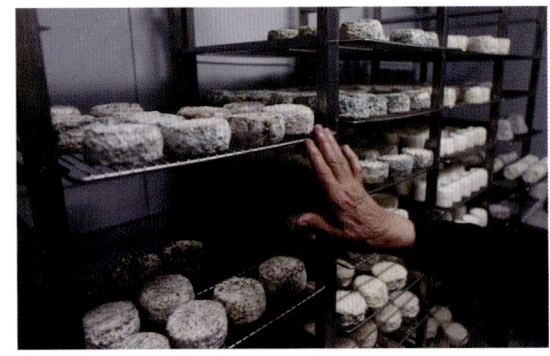

Aging Cheeses at the Teulé Goat Farm

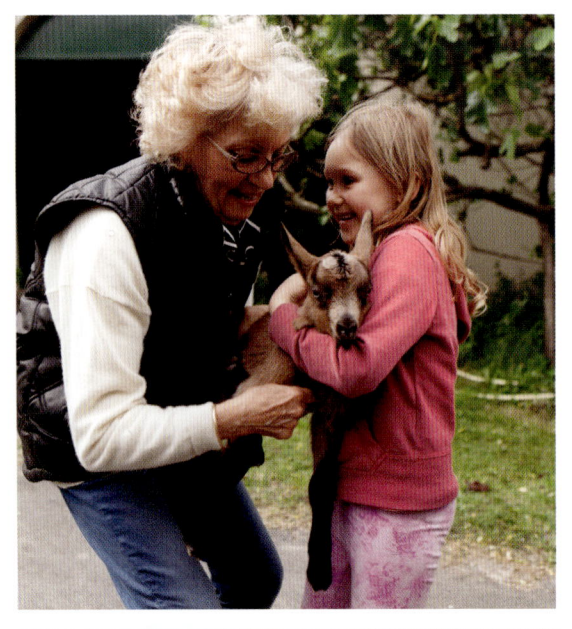

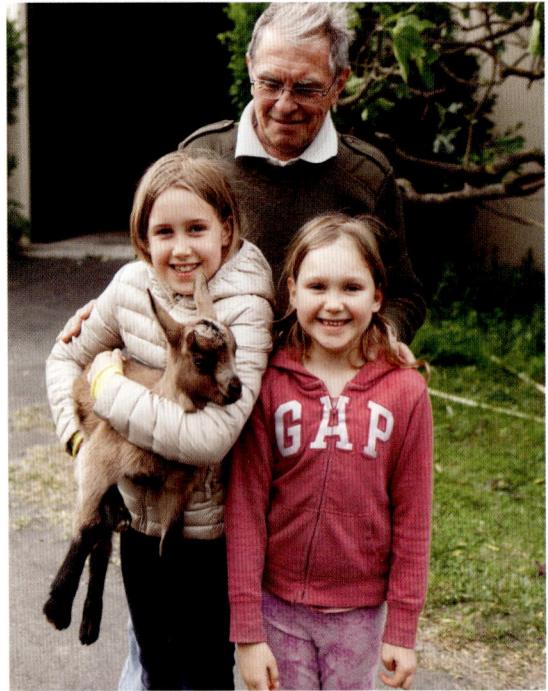

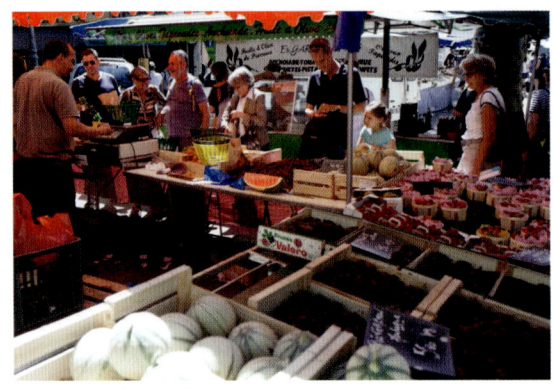

Market in Aix-en-Provence

566   THE BORDEAUX KITCHEN

THE VALUE OF SLEEP AND ROUTINES

GOOD NUTRITION AND ROUTINES SUPPORT SELF-WORTH

Involving our children in family conversations at the table keeps them from feeling left out, and therefore less rambunctious and distracted. The repetitive task of setting the table and helping in some minor way with the preparation of the meal, while tedious for me to ask of the children and for them to deliver, nevertheless builds a feeling of family teamwork, a stake in the process and therefore more interest in the outcome. Our children see how, day after day, my husband and I care enough to get up a bit earlier to prepare them a proper breakfast and make their lunches. (For me this also means going to bed earlier, relinquishing the day at 8 or 9 PM, rather than at 10 or 11 PM, or later, as I did in the past when my children were little and I was younger and uninformed. The little energy I had I burned twice as fast.) Whether children realize it or not, such a rhythm provides them with a solid foundation not only of nutrition but also of feeling cared for, and therefore it builds their self-worth. We are each "worth" the extra moments it takes to prepare a warm meal, especially our children. There is an easy analogy here: processed "food" makes for a processed self-image. If you buy into pop culture, you buy into a poor image and fast, easy "food" that doesn't make you well. If we understand that good food helps us feel healthy, then our self-worth is fostered by eating that food. As you develop an awareness about your values, which are reflected in your priorities, your intuition about what is "healthy" and worthy of eating will increase. This self-awareness, intuition with regard to priorities, and self-confidence will thus develop in your children as well and stick with them in the long run. Remember our children are always taking notes, whether they (or we) realize it or not. Teach them well: Lead them by example.

RESTING MORE

Having taken clues from our ancestors about what to do and not do and sticking to my values and priorities (and revising them along the way), I have found that we can strive to live our lives with more "balance" and less "chaos." But again, in my experience, it starts with good food (and good sleep), for parents and children. My own daily practice has included lots of rest, resting in bed for 10 to 12 hours when I can at night (especially in the winter when it is dark anyway), or at least getting to bed consistently at or before 9 PM or right after the children go to bed, and taking naps as needed, sometimes more than once in a day, some journaling, and some meditation (which usually turns into a nap.) I take Dr. Sarah Ballantyne's recent research on sleep hygiene to heart in the evenings and "go to bed."[1]

ROUTINE BEDTIMES

For children, having a regular bedtime is probably even more critical than regular meal timing. Keeping the routine of both of these, as well as daily regular bowel movements and some daily walking, play, or other exercise, are the pillars to their good health, beyond nutritious meals. We try to eat at regular times and not let bedtime get strung out too long. (Somehow, I am more efficacious at this than my husband. That must be a "tired mom" thing.) We read or talk at bedtime, and then it's lights out. "Early" bedtimes can be a source of conflict if not everyone is on board. Sometimes, bedtime is too strung out, and I'm in bed before the rest of the family, as much as I would love to squeeze more productivity out of my day, as I did, to my own detriment, in the past. I used to burn myself out, night after night, year after year, staying up late, doing my projects, whatever those were. Now I need about nine solid hours a night in bed to feel moderately refreshed in the morning. I feel like I am still making up for years of late-night wakefulness, because even nine hours is not always enough. Lights out in our household is usually between 8:00 and 8:30 PM.

Blue Light

Neurosurgeon Dr. Jack Kruse, speaking on the subject of Electron Chain Transport in the body's cells on Evan Brand's *Not Just Paleo* podcast, July 2014: "Blue light destroys DHA in the cell membranes and it destroys it in the eye, and when you destroy that you can't tell circadian signaling. You lose that ability in your central nervous system to tell light from dark, and you also lose that ability to tell seasonal changes. And that information gets directly transmitted to your mitochondria…It has major downstream effects."[10]

EMFs

According to Lloyd Burrell of ElectricSense.com, there are four categories of EMF: 1) magnetic field, 2) electric field, 3) radio frequency or "microwave" radiation, and 4) dirty electricity (irregular changes or surges in voltage). He says there are three things you can do to reduce exposure to any EMF source (cell phones, light bulbs, Wi-Fi, electronic devices, and appliances): 1) turn it off, 2) put more distance between yourself and the source, or 3) shield yourself.[11,12]

CIRCADIAN RHYTHM DISRUPTION: LEDS, BLUE LIGHT, AND EMFS

These days it is rapidly becoming harder to find the standard orange or yellow-light tungsten bulbs with manufacturers phasing them out in favor of LED (Light-Emitting Diode) light bulbs. No one notices or complains because everyone seems to think the new, electronic reliability and brightness of the LED light bulb is the cats' meow. Most light bulbs are now blue-tinted or LED, which claim to use less energy but have the capacity to stimulate our circadian rhythms and signal to our brains that it's still daylight outside.[2,3] So of course we have trouble falling asleep! Expecting to fall asleep minutes after turning off a phone or tablet screen is, unfortunately, foolish, but no electronics manufacturer will tell you so. When the sun goes down (and before it comes up), I wear my blue-blocking, orange-tinted glasses, because even the light bulbs are too searing to my eyes and I want to be able to go to sleep *and* sleep through the night.[4]

After sundown, my children are not allowed to look at screens. And if they do, it is because they have the rare homework assignment to finish, and the tablets are on "airplane mode" to reduce the EMFs (Electro-Magnetic Fields or Frequencies) being emitted from these devices. I have even requested the teachers to assign as little online homework as possible, due to the danger of EMFs negatively affecting the mitochondria in our growing children's bodies.[5,6] In early 2015 in France, a law was passed by the French National Assembly requiring that Wi-Fi routers be turned off while not in use in elementary schools and banning them altogether in nursery schools.[7] This is serious business, but widely overlooked. Children's brains are particularly susceptible to wireless radiation from Wi-Fi routers and devices (including the now ubiquitous cell phones and tablets), which they are now exposed to around the clock, at school and at home.[8,9] One solution is to keep devices off when not in use or else in "airplane mode" so that they are not sending or receiving electrical pulses. You can also use a landline phone and wired Ethernet cables instead of wireless at home. We turn off our wireless router at night, and we try to complete homework right after school. (So far, only one after-school activity once a week gets in our way of doing this.) I usually keep my cell phone on airplane mode when I am not using it during the day.

Keeping the rooms *cool* (in many European homes, the heating systems are automatically set to turn off between about midnight and 5 AM to save energy) and *dark* (with blackout curtains) helps contribute to a good sleeping environment, as does a consistent amount of sleep along with consistent bedtimes, even for adults. It is simple but hard to follow unless, like me, all that nighttime artificial light simply gives you a headache! I feel like Dracula at night or before sunrise when someone turns the light on and I cower away. This is the result of my own overuse of my body's energy reserves in the past. Now I combat artificial lighting with my blue-light blocking glasses and reduce the number of lights turned on and watts per bulb. It's okay to stop at the end of the day. In fact, you *must*. I have learned this the hard way. No one wants to hear this, of course, least of all me. And with modern-day jobs, classmates, colleagues, and deadlines to respect, it is close to impossible to find a "balance," even when those around you have also (reluctantly) shifted their lifestyle paradigm.

GOOD MORNING, SUNSHINE!

When the morning comes and the sun rises, the lights go on, the blue blockers come off, and I try to get some sunlight into my eyes for a minute or two or go for a morning walk. The winter is problematic in this way, but that is why we often feel the need to sleep more and hibernate in the winter or migrate to sunnier climates. This is the natural circadian rhythm response at which our hectic, plugged-in work and school schedules unfortunately scoff. Since getting up for school in the morning at or before 7 AM, in the dark, is really challenging for children, and for parents, who have to get up earlier, I have found that the earlier we get our kids to bed, the easier it is for them (and us) to get up in the morning.

FAMILY MEAL TIME – *A TABLE, EN FAMILLE:* **A TRADITION OF CONNECTING**

An understanding of nutrition starts in the home. Family meal-time is much more than just sitting around the table eating at the same time. It is a time to share, reflect, catch up, cut out the distractions from the day, and connect. Sharing meals means more than just eating, it means sharing life. I remember weekday breakfasts at home growing up that did not necessarily always feel rushed. We sat at the table, ate our eggs, and I'm sorry to say, our cereal, but we were together for a short while every morning. Dinners were also usually eaten together. My husband and I carry on that tradition now (minus the bread and cereal), as he grew up with this tradition as well. We usually do not let a phone call interrupt our meal, nor the television, nor other distractions, such as books, agendas, electronic devices, or toys. Mealtimes, though they can be a bit rushed, especially in the morning, are cornerstones of the day, either to begin the day feeling cared for and connected, or to end the day with collaborative reflection and a warm meal. Sometimes breakfast or dinner might be the only meal during a given day when the family is together to eat and reconnect. At the beginning of the day, we talk about who is doing what at school or work. At the end of the day, we ask each other what we did, what the good parts and bad parts were, what the challenges and learning moments were. Or else we plan a future outing or trip, or discuss certain problems, large or small, at home or at school, that need resolving. We often discuss the food and why I made this or that and how it helps us. Almost just as often, our girls roll their eyes, but I know they are listening by the comments they make about our food and how they feel. And sometimes, it's just too noisy at the table, I'm tired, and I have to tune out!

> *Eight-year-old's tableside joke:*
> "What did the pig say to the lamb? I'll meat you at the butcher shop!"
>
> *Eleven-year-old's tableside joke:*
> "Why did the tomato turn red? Because it saw the salad dressing!"

ATTITUDE OF GRATITUDE

In our family, I make the bacon and my husband prepares the eggs every morning. Of course, in other families, not everyone has the luxury of being together at the same time for breakfast. Preparing food in the morning is often a race against time, even more so if freshly-packed lunches also need preparing. It is sometimes a struggle to be on the ball every morning, but starting our day this way makes us all feel satisfied from the get-go and ready for the day's challenges. Improving self-image, participation in family mealtimes, and sharing the feeling of gratitude, along with a better understanding of where the food comes from, are all aspects supported by a family focus on nutrition in the home.

MEAL TIMING

For some adults, a warm meal in the morning is too much and they prefer a warm drink instead of food. This is something I never understood as a child, but nowadays I do like a warm cup of bone broth, usually along with my breakfast and sometimes a tea afterwards. Sometimes I am not hungry and am able to "break my fast" closer to what would be called lunchtime. This is called intermittent fasting. But I still make breakfast for my children and sit with them before they head off to school. There is a huge trend in drinking "Bulletproof Coffee," a specially formulated drink of coffee mixed with MCTs (Medium-Chain Triglycerides, an energy source easily used by our brains[13]) and other fats (e.g., grass-fed butter) to fuel the brain and improve cognitive performance. I sometimes drink this kind of coffee, and it can be useful for those who do not need or want to eat a meal in the morning. I love breakfast in the morning, though on school days it seems sometimes too early, thanks to our socially institutionalized, industrialized paradigm in which everyone must begin their day at pretty much the same early hour, even if it is the darkest and coldest of winter outside. Getting up early is great, but not when it's still dark outside during breakfast. Who wouldn't rather be sleeping? Remembering how painful it was to get up in the dark on winter mornings after a long night of homework in high school, I anticipate this kind of schedule will be just as difficult when our children are teenagers. Being the good citizen that I was, I never thought to question this late-to-bed, early-to-rise system. Many of my high-achieving high school classmates relied on caffeine in its various forms to wake up before class. Who could blame them? Now I question this "system." What are the benefits to society versus the degradation to our health from all these artificially-imposed stressors, such as early schedules and caffeine (and other beverages and drugs for boosting energy)? But I digress.

THE FAMILY MEALTIME ROUTINE

In part, the family mealtime routine also means just that, a routine: more or less constant, reliable, a start or a closure to the day. The repetition may sound monotonous, but it is the very steadiness of this routine that makes it so helpful. Lunch is at the same time every day at school, and we try to keep to our regular mealtime and bedtime schedule at home, including on the weekends, as hard as it is, with all the temptations of modern life and its activities and obligations. This means no late nights and no "pizza and movie night," which families often have. I have not yet figured out how to do this in a sustainable way, as I rarely make pizza (if so, it is still a processed, "gluten-free" mix, but still not edible to me), we don't use screens after dark, and I am proud to say that I do not even know how to turn on our television. It remains unplugged in the living room. Not relying on "news" from the television or mainstream media in general also makes us impervious to the over-dramatized, time-sucking, perpetually negative influences blasted at us by these media outlets. Our priorities remain *our* priorities. This leaves time for reading, writing, drawing, connecting with each other, going on walks together, or else time for oneself to meditate, play an instrument, or journal our gratitude (or complaints!) on paper.

BUDGET CUTS: EATING IN

In our shift to consuming almost exclusively food cooked at home, we have in the last couple of years slashed the "Eating Out" budget, shifting those monies over to the grocery budget to support the purchase of high-quality, unprocessed meats, vegetables, and other foods. I buy half a pig and debone it now myself (this takes several hours) or else have the butcher debone it for a slightly higher price per pound. This avoids the plastic-wrapped, individual-piece-of-meat expense which is invariably higher than buying a large quantity at one time. Most of the meat goes in our extra freezer (I highly recommend owning one of these) for use later as needed, while vegetables are procured every two or three days to augment the meats. I make sure I have all my fats in a row: bacon fat, butter, duck fat, ghee, lard, olive oil, tallow, rendered, stocked, ready for use.

Packing school and work lunches saves a lot of money and more importantly ensures the highest-quality lunches because *we* provide them and know every ingredient that goes into them. Our children compare their lunches with their classmates' lunches and are usually glad they have what we have packed for them. My husband is happy that he doesn't have to forage daily among local sandwich, shawarma, or pizza joints (which use vegetable oils in their "foods," no doubt, not to mention the gluten and the nutrient deficiency), spend extra money on dining out, or heat up some processed frozen meal in the microwave. Meanwhile, my husband has what he generously calls his "five-star lunches" of leftovers from the previous night's dinner of meat or fish with a variety of cooked and raw vegetables.

Going out to restaurants for both of us has become disappointing (and too late for me, especially in the winter). It's expensive, time-consuming, and often not of the high quality we had hoped for and demand of our own home cooking. Not to mention the potential for gluten exposure as well as to inflammatory industrial seed oils that we might encounter in a restaurant, even in France or elsewhere in Europe. After eating so much at home, you come to expect a certain standard of ingredients, which are questionable in most restaurants. We also end up spending a lot of time waiting around for the wait staff to *serve* us. If it isn't a really special place or occasion, it's just not worth it to us. Instead, "eating in" creates the double satisfaction of saving money and and making a high-quality meal yourself, while not wasting lots of time sitting around waiting to be *served*. The other bonus is that we feel good after a meal at home, not so, usually, after a meal at a restaurant, where we are more likely to overeat and/or choose something that we otherwise would not.

FOOD REJECTION/REINTRODUCTION STRATEGY

The inertia of good nutrition will hopefully be carried along with our children as they grow, so that they understand which foods help them and which do not. I expect them to go through phases of rejection of good nutrition, but hopefully they will have a foundation to which they will return after experimenting with all the easy-access "food" surrounding them and coping with social pressures children and modern society tend to incur on each other. If a food, such as a particular vegetable, is rejected by our children, we reintroduce it several times in the hopes that they will grow used to it. We usually ask our children to try a little bite each time. It is repetitive and sometimes quite tedious, but in theory, their curiosity will get the better of them as their palates develop.

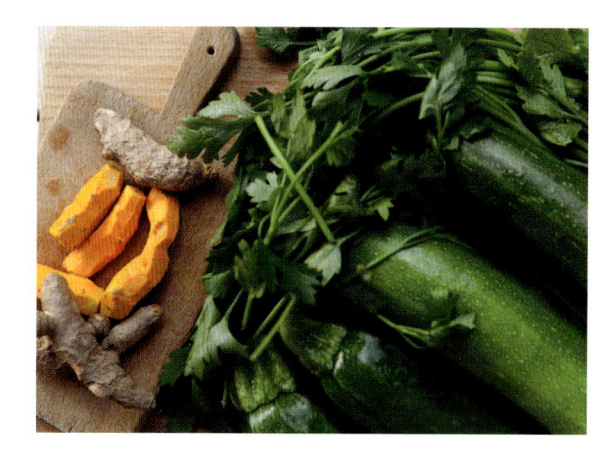

SOME CHALLENGES AND BENEFITS OF ESTABLISHING HEALTHY HABITS FOR YOUR FAMILY

LESS FAT = MORE CARBOHYDRATES

According to family physician Dr. Catherine Shanahan, "denying kids healthy fat often drives them to sugar."[14] Pediatric endocrinologist Dr. Robert Lustig says, "Sugar is the alcohol of the child."[15] I concur with both of them and would argue that this goes for all of us, children and adults, whether we like to hear it or not. I have canvassed parents and my children have asked their schoolmates what they eat for breakfast. The answer is invariably, some combination of grain, dairy, and sugar. Rarely is there much fat involved, even when it comes to the milk. Consuming low-fat pasteurized milk turns out to be foolhardy and counterproductive.[16, 17] (What a boon for dairy manufacturers to skim off the fat from their milk and put it in ice cream, as an ancillary product for those consumers who were strangely not satisfied by the fat-free milk and needed ice cream, along with its added sugars, for dessert!) Eggs are typically something saved for weekends, as are bacon and sausage. It seems to me to be a general pattern of high sugar and low nutrients, and an ingrained *fear of fat*. (See more on fat in Chapter 4.)

PICKY EATERS

It also seems to me that almost every time I speak with a parent or hear about someone's child, there is a story of past or present illness with the child, whether it is tooth decay, the need for glasses, an injury, trouble in school or behavioral issues, restlessness, lack of concentration at school or when doing homework, depression, wakefulness or trouble sleeping, an endless runny nose, recurring colds, crankiness, mysterious skin problems, or "picky eater" syndrome. I have experienced many of these myself and in my own family, but I have found that maximizing my children's nutrition by replacing the bread, cereal, and other sugars, including fruit, with nutrient-dense foods like organic meats, eggs, bacon, sausage, cheese, butter, and vegetables has helped improve such symptoms enormously. Don't get me wrong, we love berries, citrus, stone fruits, pomegranates, figs, dates, apples, pears, and bananas! They are great, but in *small* amounts, as a condiment instead of the main focus. And whenever the high-carbohydrate or refined "foods" (such as pasta, baked goods, fried fast "food," and even sugary yogurts) are reintroduced (by accident or by occasional request), the symptoms reappear. As hard as it seemed at first, we have even cut out boxed juices and those "fun" squeezable "puréed fruit" pouches, which are gratuitous, environmentally wasteful, expensive, and well-marketed single-serve sugar hits, designed to quiet down your child while you drive home from the grocery store. Weaning children from these can prove challenging at first, but the reduced sugar intake will help even out their moods, and the budgetary savings on this line item alone is significant when added up over a year.

CHILDHOOD AND DIGESTION

Several years ago, we were challenged with a chronic digestive issue in one of our children when she was in kindergarten that actually required pharmaceutical intervention because we did not know any better. We only had a small inkling to modify her diet when one astute French pediatrician asked us what our daughter ate for lunch (peanut butter and jelly on sliced bread, at the time), and suggested that we serve her a warm meal at lunch instead. I was taken aback at first, but my husband in his wisdom understood the connection immediately. Over time, the warm, more-nutritious lunches helped us eliminate the pharmaceutical intervention, but it took a year. This same daughter, now a voracious reader, notices in the Laura Ingalls Wilder *Little House on the Prairie* series (set in the 1860s) and *The Caroline Years* series (set in the 1850s) the fact that the families ate salt pork at mealtimes. My daughter also pointed out that prolific English children's book author Enid Blyton (1897-1968) published one story in 1942 that described the children's breakfasts, which included such foods as tongue or canned salmon.[18] As a mother, even when no one else wants to believe it, I can now see the difference sugar, processed chemicals, and a lack of nutrient-density can make within minutes, hours, in the night, or the following day or days. I only wish I had made this connection years earlier, when I was pregnant and addicted to sugar myself!

CONSIDER THIS
If you were to consider every ache and pain or symptom you or your child have as a form of nutrient deficiency, what would you do? What would you eat to replenish the missing nutrients? Would you grab that next bag of chips or box of cookies, or look for something truly nutrient-dense for yourself and your child? Every decision makes a difference, one way or the other.

DISEASE PREVENTION FOR THE YOUNG
It has been argued that many of our financial resources that are now going to aid *adults* in the symptom-reducing band-aid style medical paradigms of western countries are draining the coffers for the younger and future generations who need *more help earlier* with disease prevention. If policies do not reflect such a transition in the medical paradigm going forward, then it is up to us parents to support our children's welfare and prevention from disease in the first place by minimizing their toxic exposure and maximizing their nutrient exposure as they develop in front of our eyes. Let us vote with our minds, hearts, and choices. Let us vote with the future of our children and their children in mind. Let us feed them and educate them to fulfill their dreams and nourish them as generations before nourished their young, so that they may become socially intelligent, creative, healthy, loving human beings, at peace with the world around them.

SNACK TIME, AGAIN? EATING FOR OPTIMAL LEARNING
Why do children always seem to want a snack? Actually, if they have had a filling, nutrient-dense, satiating breakfast, if not of eggs and bacon, then of breakfast sausage or leftovers from dinner, then they actually don't *need* a snack or ask for one. My older daughter says that some children get to school in the mornings and say they are hungry during their first class, which is math. This is unacceptable. My daughter says many of her classmates say they eat cereal or a granola bar for breakfast. Yes, this is anecdotal, but are we paying attention as parents? After a meager breakfast, of course children are ravenous for a snack by snack time, and something quick and sugary will do to carry them just long enough until lunch time. And what of their ability to concentrate? What is particularly maddening to me is that my daughters eat a snack not because they are hungry, but because the school has built in a mid-morning snack time for all the children who are unable to focus or go without a snack until lunchtime. Then, at lunchtime, kids pull out their sandwiches, pasta, rice, and other carb-rich or carb-only lunches. Some of the bigger kids go to the local kiosk and buy themselves soda and candy bars for dessert. Giving children sweets and starchy foods only drives them to want more.[19] What are the health implications, short term and long term, on our children and their entire generation if they experience these frequent, dare I say *unnecessary*, insulin spikes from sugary snacks (and meals) throughout the day? How well are their sugar-dependent, fat-starved brains going to be able to develop? A hyper-active child, a child who cannot concentrate at school, or a child who is acting out is an undernourished child.[20] This is a real bone I have to pick with "the system" and our mindless habits, and it is something from which we must not avert our attention as parents and citizens. It is up to us "consumers" who make purchasing decisions to plow our money into local, homemade goods, or make them ourselves, and not give our money away

mindlessly to the oversized companies who are contributing to our sickness and not our health, until death do us part.

HOMEMADE IS BEST MADE
Homemade is always better, it just takes a little initiative and the right ingredients. (It also creates a lot of dirty dishes, I admit.) But homemade anything is also "quality time" that you can spend with your children. In my opinion, it is much more *patriotic* to support local home and community businesses than international "food" conglomerates that may have started as American businesses before spreading their disease-inducing tentacles across the globe. They are so oversized and successful at lobbying in Washington and the rest of the world that it is their oversized influence, not their quality or integrity, that affords them an audience of obedient lawmakers and addicted adults and children. This is not patriotic, this is bullying.

REDUCING CHEMICAL TOXINS IN THE HOME
Cleaning agents, beauty products, laundry and dish detergents often carry more than their fair share of toxins.[21,22] At home, we minimize these as much as possible, buying only unscented dish and toxic-free laundry soap and using vinegar and baking soda as our main household cleaners. We use paraben-free shampoos and conditioners, and I am in the process of moving to gluten-free bathroom products, as that darn gluten shows up in everything, with wheat in the U.S. being the cheap, glyphosate-infused commodity that it is. I never use air fresheners or dryer sheets as these contain chemicals like phthalates that linger not only in scent but in our environment and bodies. Bar soaps replace the endless pileup of plastic liquid soap containers, and antibacterial hand gel has been relegated to extreme emergency use only, as the chemicals not only dry out our skin and kill the bad germs, but they also wipe out the good microbiome on our skin, leaving us that much more susceptible to the "bad guys."

I gave up applying industrial perfume since I began studying wine several years ago, and I do not miss the frequent headaches that came along with wearing perfume. Now I can smell someone's perfume from yards away. This does not seem very natural to me that someone should leave so many chemicals in their wake when walking down the street. I have turned to essential oils for aromatherapy, lavender or pine for the bath, clary sage for the laundry, vanilla for body oil, and a mix of clove, spearmint, and cinnamon for the teeth. I have begun making my own creams with mixes of tallow, olive oil, shea butter, and beeswax, using essential oils to scent them. I always loved to mix, and still do, and this is one fun, economical, non-toxic, and useful way to mix!

SHIFTING PARENTS' FOOD PARADIGM
My sincere hope is that mothers and fathers who read this, or hear from another friend or resource other than the typical media outlets, will have the courage to make a change in their lives, to shift their paradigm just a bit by considering the nutrient-density (or lack thereof) of each food they are giving their child and its ramifications. It is a huge responsibility, more so than we realize. In fact, if I had my way, the world would have work hours reduced so that parents could focus on the *urgent* issue in their lives: the proper nutrition and nurturing of their children. It takes a lot of time, understanding, planning ahead, and energy to have enough fresh food in the house as well as the time to prepare it. It is basically a full-time job, which is why in the past, one parent, guardian or grandparent had to be home to take care of the food preparation as well as the household while others worked outside the home or on the family farm. This is the tradeoff we now make: two jobs in the family means more income and material goods, but also less time and often the need for two cars and more daycare. This tradeoff includes a greater reliance on foods prepared outside the home, factory-made instead of homemade, and quick fixes instead of long-

term, lasting, and meaningful solutions. This dire situation creates a rupture in the cycle of the passing on of knowledge about cooking, food preparation, and basic principles of living healthfully. This is happening around the modern world, including in the U.S. and France. As a modern society, we do not know how to cook anymore because we did not learn it at home or understand its significance.

BREAKING UP IS HARD TO DO

I can tell you that cutting out morning cereal is probably the hardest thing to do. My children stopped asking for it after a while, but it took months. And it is still sometimes requested, especially when those around us are having it. We all grew up with it, so changing this blind habit is difficult. But the hazardously nutrient-deficient low-fat dairy[23] (or laboratory soy milk) and sugars from industrial grains combined with added sugars and processed juices stripped of fiber is enough to keep anyone hooked for life and prone to metabolic disorders, particularly children.[24] The problem beyond the habit-forming element is that this "food" displaces the real nutrients we need. (See Chris Kresser's *The Paleo Cure*, Mark Schatzker's *The Dorito Effect,* Dr. Cate Shanahan's *Deep Nutrition*, and Robb Wolf's *Wired to Eat*.) If you are feeding your child a low-fat diet, please refer to Teicholz's excellent summary and review of the history of studies and influences that led to this unsound dietary choice, but especially Chapter 6, "How Women and Children Fare on a Low Fat Diet," in her book, *The Big Fat Surprise*.

If you turn to any of neurologist Dr. David Perlmutter's resources, whether books, website or interviews he has given, you will learn how processed "foods," gluten and glyphosate (used on corn, cotton, soy, and wheat) negatively impact our and our children's microbiome (micro-organisms in the gut) which ultimately effects their behavior (attention), neurological (cognitive) function, mitochondrial function (energy production), and levels of inflammation.[25] Our gut flora (beneficial and pathogenic bacteria, fungi, protozoa, viruses, etc.) make up 90% of the cells in our body.[26]

While it is no cure-all by any stretch, imagine if your child had liver and eggs this morning, or else the nutrient-dense leftovers from a previous meal, or a bowl of fish, like some Japanese have in the morning? (If they had grown up this way, they would not think it so strange. I eat dinner leftovers for breakfast sometimes, and in that way show my children that it's healthy and not out of the question. Well, they *do* think I'm weird sometimes, but then again, when have parents ever been *cool*? Is being "cool" our responsibility, or is feeding our children with intention?) How do you think your child would behave and perform at school after having had a nutrient-dense breakfast? Imagine the difference in ability to concentrate after eating such a meal as opposed to a "meal" of cold flakes in low-fat milk or a quick granola bar eaten on the way to school in the bus or car? This is definitely food for thought.

PART II: FAMILY FOOD ORGANIZATION AND PLANNING AHEAD

Feeding and raising children is a tall order for anyone. One "rock star" mom in this arena is Katie Wells the Wellness Mama (wellnessmama.com), a down-to-earth mother of six who also home schools her children and cooks all their meals at home, not to mention that she makes her own body care products and home remedies as well while keeping her autoimmune issues at bay through lifestyle and dietary interventions. She shares her strategies on her blog, in her book, *The Wellness Mama Cookbook*, and on her podcast, *The Healthy Moms Podcast*, and is a fantastic resource for parents seeking answers. Other powerhouse moms with great resources (books, podcasts, websites) are Sarah Ballantyne, Sarah Fragoso, Michelle Tam (of "Nom Nom Paleo" fame), and Stacy Toth. My efforts may pale in comparison, and every family is different, but with two children under the age of 13, we feed ours in the ways described in the following sections.

Lunch Prep

Cut up leftovers when they have cooled off or are cold, such as after dinner, and store them in oven-safe glass containers overnight in the refrigerator. They are easier to handle and cut when cold than when heated up in the morning before school and you are pressed for time. Heat the leftovers in the oven at the same time as the morning bacon. Use boiling water to heat the inside of thermos containers before putting the lunches into the containers and serving up the bacon for breakfast!

BREAKFAST OF CHAMPIONS

Our regular breakfasts consist of whole (sometimes raw) milk, picked up directly from a farm, bacon and eggs cooked in raw grass-fed butter. No bread, no juice, no cereal. Occasionally a small piece of fruit, a few berries, and when we have one, a slice of avocado. Every now and then we make small portions of organic oatmeal, but this has become the exception, not the norm, and we cook it with lots of unpasteurized, grass-fed butter.

LEFTOVERS FOR LUNCH

So that I do not have to cook a whole new meal for lunch, I usually pack leftovers from dinner in a thermos container for each child (and my husband), accompanied by sliced vegetables, cheese, salami and/or fruit, and a dessert of homemade organic chocolate-nut date bars or zucchini muffins, with some variants now and then. If there are not enough leftovers, I try to have organic ground beef or sausages from the butcher on hand to be able to sauté or boil up an easy lunch to pack. If only my children would eat liver! But I do sneak some liver powder into the ground beef. Working from home, I reheat leftovers as well for myself, or I make an easy organ meat that nobody else seems to want to have besides me, such as **Chicken Livers with Bacon** (page 236, my husband does like these), **Veal Sweetbreads** (page 227, he might try these), or **Poached and Sautéed Lamb Brains** (page 262, no dice!). Lunch at home on the weekends is really no different, except there is sometimes a small piece of 65% to 85% dark chocolate involved for dessert.

SNACK – *LE GOÛTER*

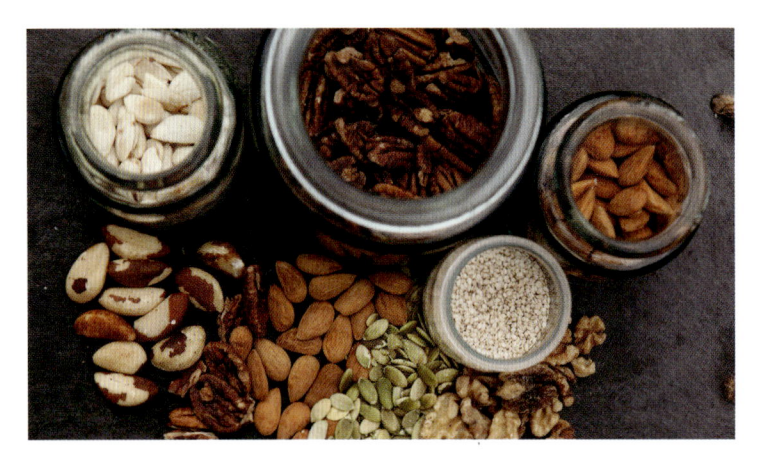

The after-school snack, called *le goûter* in French and which is almost an institution all on its own at our house (*chez nous*), is usually a combination of two or three of the following options: organic fruit, sausage, raw cheese, *nori* seaweed, peanut butter, nuts (including peanuts, which they love, but my main concern with which is the potential for mycotoxins, otherwise known as mold), or raw vegetables. I am sorry to say that the French *goûter* usually is comprised of biscuits/cookies, crackers, and chocolate, though there are certainly more "health conscious" families who refrain from processed and sugary "desserts" at snack time, though they seem to be in the minority. I understand this well because I was in the same high-carb "snack rut" myself for many years!

DINNER
Our dinners usually consist of a meat, occasionally fish (preferably wild caught), several raw and cooked vegetables accompanied by lots of sour cream (*crème fraîche*), sometimes brown or white rice or white or sweet potatoes, and dessert of fruit or plain whole-fat yogurt. If you want to obtain vitamins from vegetables, you need fat.[27] "That is why mothers in the early 20th century fed their children spoonfuls of cod liver oil. The fat from the cod liver oil is what made the spoonful of vitamins go down."[28] Sometimes my husband will make ground beef chili with red kidney beans and get help from the kids. We often eat pork or beef roasts or stews, accompanied by spoonfuls of sour cream (*crème fraîche*), as our children prefer that over most sauces. My salvation side dish is raw vegetables: carrot and celery sticks, cherry tomatoes, and cucumber slices. No cooking required! Sliced organic salami and cheese are also great on the side at any meal and as a snack.

This routine might sound repetitive and is by no means perfect, nor does it come without complaint. However, it is a good foundation for us. As long as there is no birthday party at school celebrated with a sugary, refined-grain dessert, we get through the after-school, pre-dinner hours with much success. I measure success by how much or little fighting, complaining, and whining there is after school, the kinds of stories and news our children share, and the frequency of good remarks from teachers.

We have even made fresh zucchini noodles together for dinner. For myself, I often have part of a sweet potato doused in bacon fat or lard, topped with coarse sea salt. Or else I eat squash, pumpkin, or sautéed white potatoes, usually **Sarlat Sautéed Potatoes** (page 468). I often make a salad of mixed greens, sometimes with olives, for myself and my husband. I try to introduce "new" vegetables or a salad leaf that the girls have to at least bite into, if not eat entirely. I rotate these vegetables, and now and then, there is a revelation, "Say, I *like* green kale chips!" For dessert, if it's not a small fruit, it's **Paleo Chocolate Bark** (see the sidebar on page 584), **Crème Brûlée** (page 505), **Chia Coconut Milk Pudding** (page 580), coconut milk ice cream, butter-caramelized apple slices (unpeeled), plain whole fat yogurt with honey, or liverwurst with **Seedy Crackers** (page 501).

In general, if my children have had enough sleep, time to play and explore their creativity, minimal or no screen time, and no extra sugar, we all get along. As soon as you throw an industrially manufactured "gummy" candy into the mix (whose excitatory food colorants absolutely decimate my children's good mood and mostly stable blood sugar), or a piece of sugar-laden cake, dreaded bags of laboratory-spiced tortilla chips (with their own excitatory substances), or even a croissant, the whole game changes. They become cranky, hungry, and whiny. I was like this as a child, too. In fact, I lived like that for over 40 years, in need of sugar to replace what I was *really* lacking, which was sufficient nutrients and wholesome saturated fats. To my shock, amazement, and delight, my children now willingly hand me the candy people give them, usually without sampling it, and they have begun to say things like, "I'm glad I don't have just a sandwich for lunch, I'm glad my lunch is warm."

A GRADUAL TRANSITION
If you are making a transition to less sugar and higher nutrients and satiating fats for your children, my advice would be keep it simple

and gradual. Otherwise, the process becomes overwhelming. Replacing foods gradually, one after another over time, helps everyone get used to the incremental shifts in routine. The transfer of knowledge takes time and effort, nothing like the rapid transfer of gigabytes from a computer via USB to a thumb drive that we are used to. Start with one thing, replace it, then move on to the next.

FAMILY FAVORITES

I wasn't always a good eater. My dad tells me I used to drive him and my grandfather nuts when I was little by stuffing my food into my cheeks like a squirrel. The food would stay there through an entire meal. My children don't do that, instead they just spit food out if they decide they don't want it. I'm not sure that's any better. But the longer we have been eating less of the addictive, processed "foods" and more real, homemade foods, the more my children accept both new and standby dishes that I make. Their taste buds are no longer corrupted by refined sugars, so that even at Halloween, they give me their bag of candy. I replace those kinds of candies with flu-fighting elderberry or vitamin C-rich orange flavored (from real oranges) gummies, à la wellnessmama.com,[29] or with a creamy dessert from this book, now and then. Food is not just for convenience and entertainment. Everything we eat should have a nutritional purpose.

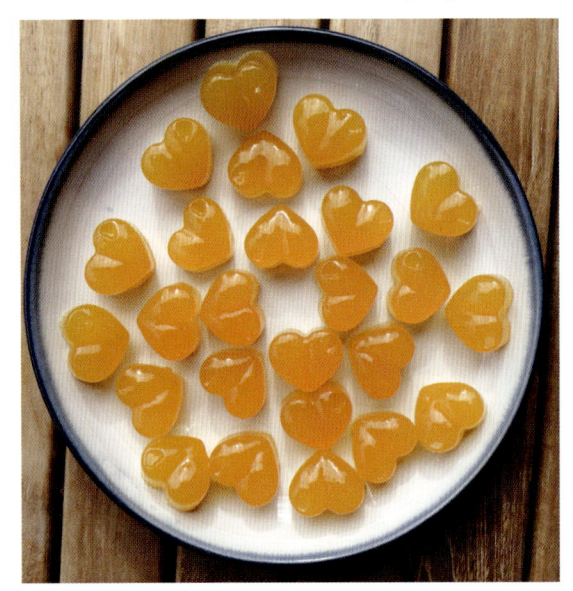

In our family, some of the easiest French recipes have become the favorites, either because my children have been exposed to these so many times or because they really are yummy. If they eat it, we're all happy! Among our favorites, besides bacon, eggs, and hamburgers, are the pork roast, ribs, chops, and shoulder recipes, as well as lamb chops and roasts, pork meatballs, steaks and roasts of beef, and meat stews. These in rotation with chicken, turkey, duck, chili, and fish (usually wild-caught salmon) make for enough of a varied terrain that nobody gets bored. The offal recipes have not yet been accepted by our children, nor has the sauerkraut, I am still working on that!

THE NON-FRENCH FOOD ANGLE

My children admonished me to include more of their favorite non-French originating foods we eat at home, which are numerous:

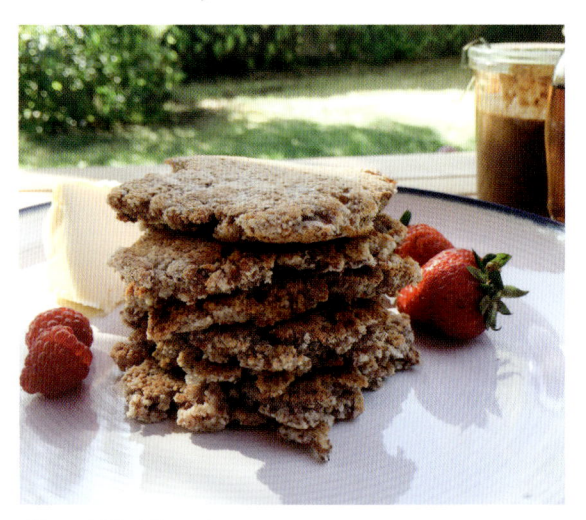

Almond Meal Pancakes

For breakfast, we will occasionally make organic sausages or homemade pork sliders or very rarely, plantain or almond meal "Paleo pancakes" (we slip powdered gelatin into the mix for the extra tummy-soothing, nutrient-dense boost) with grass-fed butter and organic maple syrup. On an even rarer occasion we have "gluten-free" pancakes from a mix, which I do not eat, which is always followed by a behavioral disaster: the sugar high and the withdrawal low that carries on through the day. (A lost weekend day.)

For lunches and dinners, my husband sometimes cooks up a pot of ground beef and kidney bean chili (which I don't eat). I make ground-beef taco meat, served with a few organic corn chips (though we are phasing these out because they are inevitably made with industrial seed oils, even if they are "organic"); we call this "chipped beef," and I always slip a bit of liver powder in there along with fresh chopped herbs, garlic, and extra lard or tallow. Ditto for beef or bison hamburgers, which I fry up in duck fat. There is no comparison to a burger browned in duck fat. I find that in small quantities, the potentially hard-to-digest FODMAP aspect of minced garlic in ground beef is not enough to trouble my stomach, and garlic is incorporated into much of my cooking for flavor and for its antimicrobial properties.

On days when I have forgotten to thaw a larger piece of meat, or I am in need of something mindlessly easy, I thaw some pork, beef, or chicken sausages made by our local organic farmer, beef steaks from the same farmer, or some thin pork cutlets I have sliced ahead of time and frozen. Sometimes the family has bone broth before a meal. I have it with almost every meal, including breakfast. Sometimes we'll have liverwurst, which is actually harder to find in France (because they have so many other liver-based pâtés) than in Germany or German-speaking Switzerland, where we have recently moved, but easy to find in the U.S. at US Wellness Meats. (In fact, US Wellness Meats has three kinds of liverwurst from which to choose.) I grew up on intermittent encounters with liverwurst (*Leberwurst*) during my visits to Germany. It was something I looked forward to eating before every visit. Both our daughters now eat liverwurst, albeit on spelt crackers or else homemade **Seedy Crackers** (page 501) at snack time or sometimes at breakfast or even for dessert! Sometimes we will have a meat-based Russian *borsch*, or I will occasionally make them buckwheat, called *grechnevaya kasha* or just *kasha* in Russian, as a side dish. For vegetables, I sometimes cook up **Oven-Baked French Fries** (page 459) or sweet potato fries with coconut oil (pictured, in a coated pan, before I got rid of it in favor of cast-iron and stainless-steel pans). "As good as McDonald's," says my older daughter, who remembers it from the "good old days." (Gulp.) Another favorite dinner is **Chocolate Pork Chops** (see the recipe on the previous page.) One dessert everybody enjoys is **Chia Coconut Milk Pudding** (on the previous page).

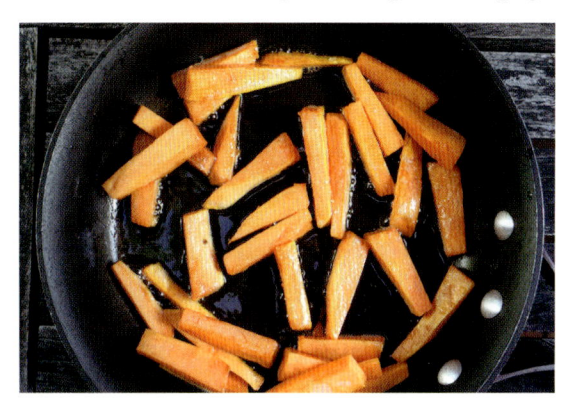

MEAL PLANNING FOR GUESTS

Planning meals for guests is an entirely different beast than planning for your everyday family meals. Here are some tips based on the French style of entertaining.

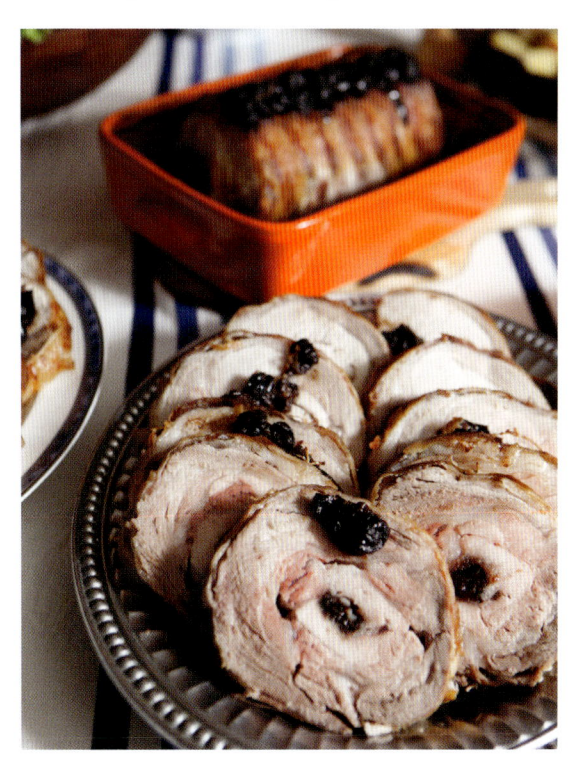

CHAPTER 8

579

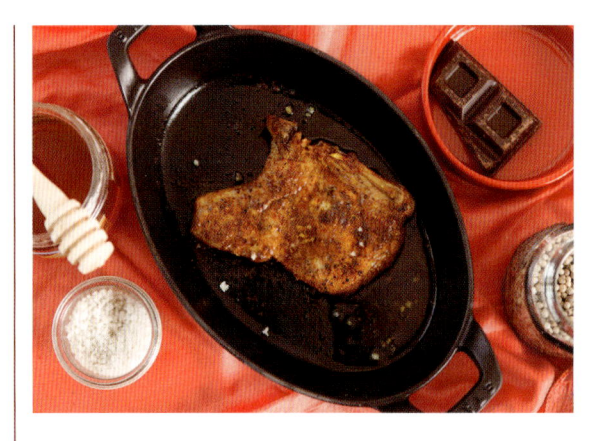

Chocolate Pork Chops Recipe

In an attempt to make pork chops more interesting to my children, I experimented by making a marinade of spices, honey, olive oil, and cocoa powder and place the emphasis on the "chocolate" by calling them **Chocolate Pork Chops**. Not a French dish, but one that sells well in our family and goes well with most vegetables or potatoes, in fried or purée form.

For the meat, use pork chops (with or without the bone) or pork shoulder steaks. For the marinade, combine one teaspoon cocoa powder, one teaspoon honey, two tablespoons olive oil, and dashes of ground ginger, turmeric, cloves, coriander, black pepper, and cinnamon and a pinch of fine sea salt in a bowl and massage the marinade onto both sides of the pork chops. Allow to marinate overnight, for several hours, or not at all if you have no time (which is usually the case for me with this dish). Melt one tablespoon of lard or duck fat in a pan and sear the chops/steaks over medium-high heat briefly then turn down the heat, allowing them to cook through on both sides. You can also finish the cooking by placing them in a hot oven (365°F or 185°C) for 10 minutes.

Serve them with roasted pumpkin (see first half of **Pumpkin Soup** recipe on page 464), plus a side of **Sautéed Swiss Chard** (page 474) or steamed broccoli, and rice or **Sarlat Sautéed Potatoes** (page 468). Pair with a fruity, medium-bodied Bergerac from the Southwest or a floral and fruity rosé from Provence. Yum!

Chia Coconut Milk Pudding Recipe

What is chia coconut milk pudding? It is not a French dessert necessarily, but it is an easy primal/paleo and kid-approved dessert, but something those sensitive to coconut flesh should probably skip. I first saw this recipe on Dr. Alan Christianson's website (www.drchristianson.com) as a part of his *Adrenal Reset Diet* and adapted it slightly.

One can of coconut milk, three tablespoons chia seeds, several drops of almond extract, ½ teaspoon vanilla extract, a few pinches of coconut sugar, and several dashes of powdered cardamom and cinnamon. A teaspoon of cacao powder is optional, but usually requested! Mix and chill overnight in small ramekins. Garnish with in-season berries.

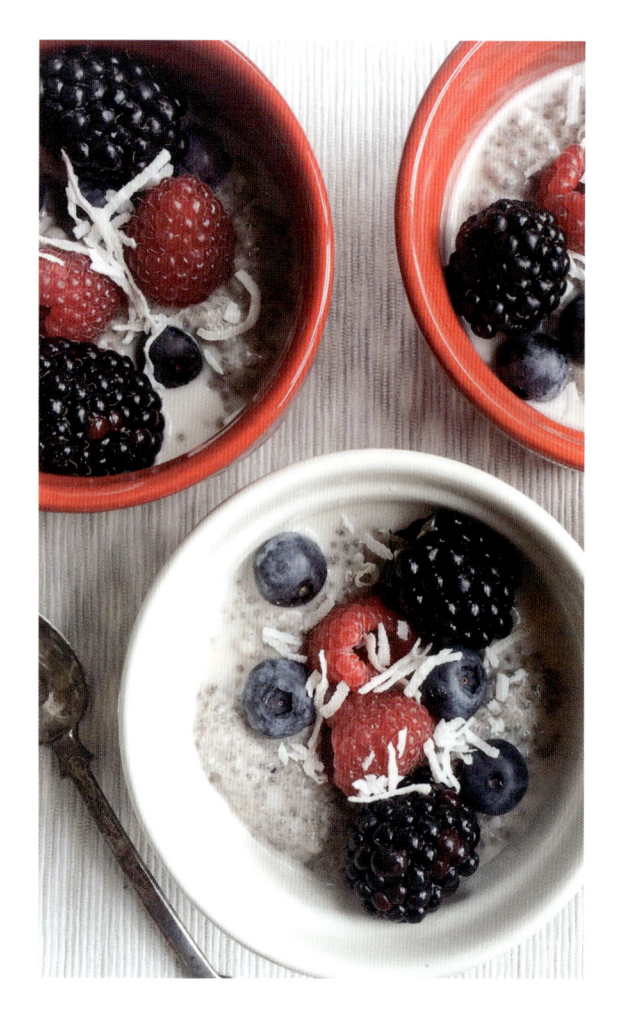

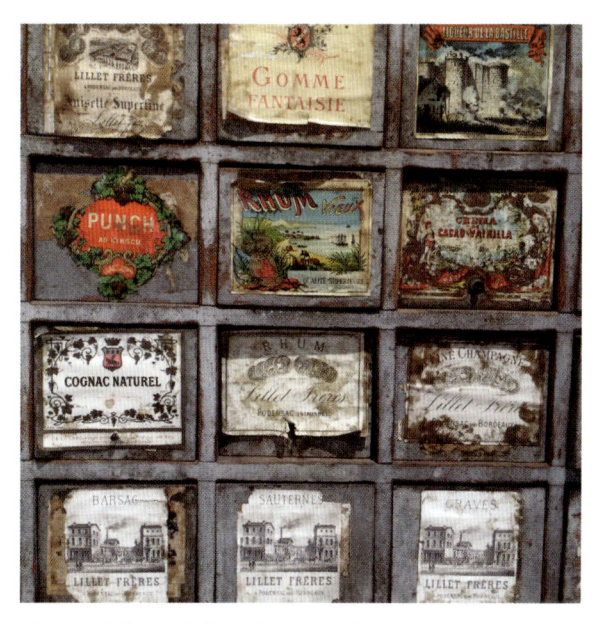

Antique Labels at Lillet Museum, Podensac, Bordeaux

THE APERITIF – *L'APÉRITIF*

When guests arrive at your home, remember to offer them something to drink. (In France, this is invariably alcohol, but sparkling or mineral water is acceptable these days, too.) As I mentioned in the Wine chapter, this first drink offering (*l'apéritif*, sometimes shortened to *l'apéro*) might be champagne, wine, or a drink like *Lillet* (a blend of Bordeaux wines combined with citrus liqueur that comes in *blanc, rouge,* or *rosé*) and usually some *hors d'oeuvre*s (literally "outside of the main work or masterpiece") such as *charcuterie*, raw vegetables (*crudités*) and dip, or even a paste of fish, pork, or poultry (*rillettes*). (See **Pork Meat Pâté** on page 312 and **Spreadable Fish Paste** on page 186.) *Rillettes* can be served with some sort of grain-free cracker, **Seedy Crackers** (page 501) or vegetable chip, such as baked sweet potato or **Beet Chips** (page 457), as can *foie gras* (fatty liver of duck). In France, foie gras is usually served in the winter on spiced bread (*pain d'épices*) or regular bread, often along with sweet wine, especially in the French Southwest. (Though in the U.S. we tend to serve cheese and crackers before dinner, in France, cheese is usually saved for the course between the main dish and dessert or else it is the dessert itself.) Sometimes, if you are only having people over for an *apéritif*, rather than a meal but want to make it a bit more "filling" an event, you can call it *un apéro dinatoire*, in which case you may have some more "finger foods," or *amuse-bouches* (literally, "fun for the mouth"), probably a few of which are warmed. For an *amuse-bouche*, I recommend **Bacon-Wrapped Prunes** (page 287).

THE THREE-COURSE MEAL: ENTRÉE – PLAT – DESSERT

Many recipes in this book could serve as an appetizer, just serve it in a small quantity in a small or medium-sized dish rather than a large plate if you are going for a French style three-course meal. I have indicated in a few recipes where they actually are appetizers or particularly well-suited to serve as such. For the main course, I would serve a meat or fish along with two or more vegetable side dishes (*accompagnements*), including a starchy vegetable such as potato, sweet potato, or other tuber or root vegetable, depending on the guests and their preferences, if you know them. Depending on your guests and your own preferences, you may also wish to serve a cheese course. Find three or four cheeses that you really like, including at least one that is goat (*chèvre*) or sheep (*brebis*), and serve those after dinner, on a separate plate, perhaps, either as an *entremets* (literally "between servings") or as dessert itself. Serve them all on a large platter that you can offer to each guest for them to choose the one(s) they would like. Or else serve the cheeses in courses, from mildest and youngest to most flavorful and/or oldest. For dessert, plan ahead and either make the dessert the day before or have the right fruit or materials on hand, put together, or ready to be put together easily, to serve after dinner or the cheese course. One cheese-related summer appetizer that is fun for kids to both eat *and* prepare is mozzarella, cherry tomato, and basil on a stick. (See photo on the next page.)

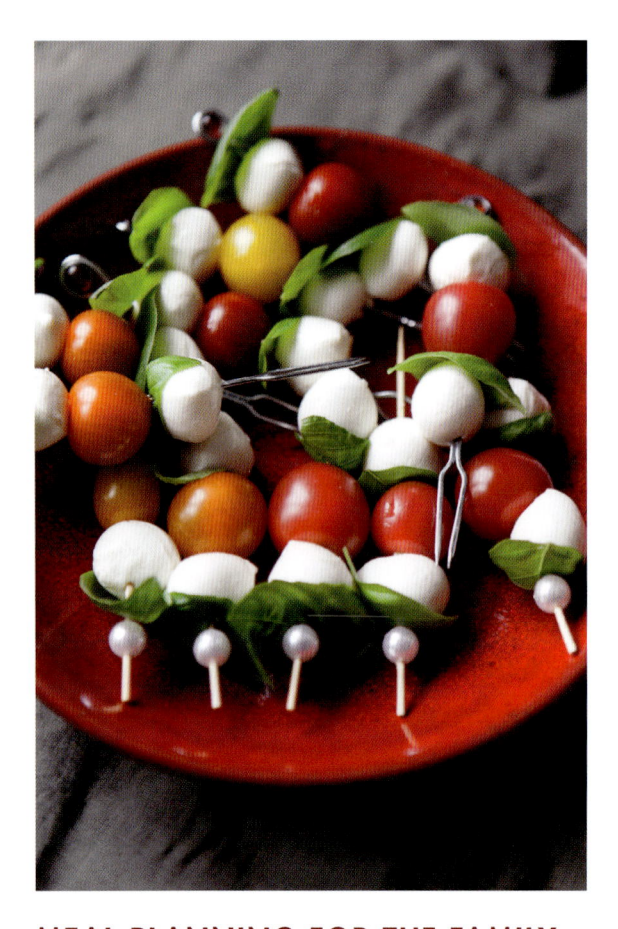

MEAL PLANNING FOR THE FAMILY

For my family, I build my meals in a less formal fashion. Rather than make "starters" for family dinners, I place raw vegetables into nice little bowls and ramekins, in a kind of bento style of small portions with lots of colors, such as the usual suspects of carrots, cherry tomatoes, sliced bell peppers, celery sticks, and cucumber slices, which the children sometimes help to prepare. They choose what they would like along with their meal. Sometimes they receive a mini cup of bone broth or a leaf of something green they say they don't like, just to have them try it now and again. Almost any dish can be served on a small plate as a starter, and if we have company, sometimes we will do this. But most of the time, for family meals, everything is on the table at once, except dessert, so that we can maximize family and eating time and minimize the logistics of running to and from the kitchen.

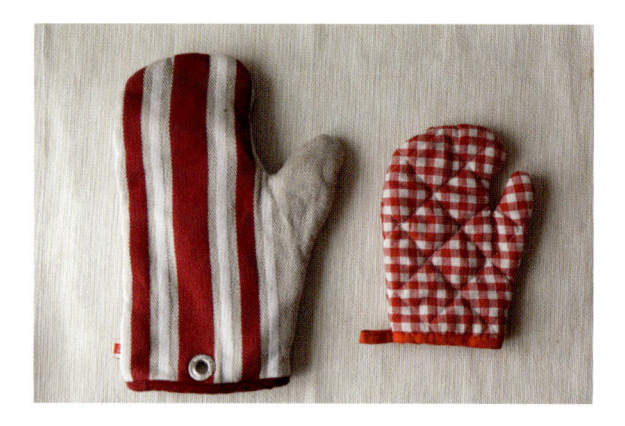

HELPING HANDS

As I have mentioned, I always loved to mix as a child. Mixing potions, colors, rocks and sand, powders, crayon shavings, and melted ice cream. They say you should go back to what you loved as a child. I loved colors and art. And mixing. Cooking and painting are the ultimate in mixing, and I love both! I think most children love to mix. They love to help. (Especially if it's pumpkin pie with homemade nut crust.) My older daughter now makes the white rice or heats up peas and carrots or occasional corn or helps with the hand mixer in making mashed potatoes. I do not eat these things, but I also do not keep them 100% off the table for my children. To all of these we add many spoonfuls of organic, grass-fed, unpasteurized butter.

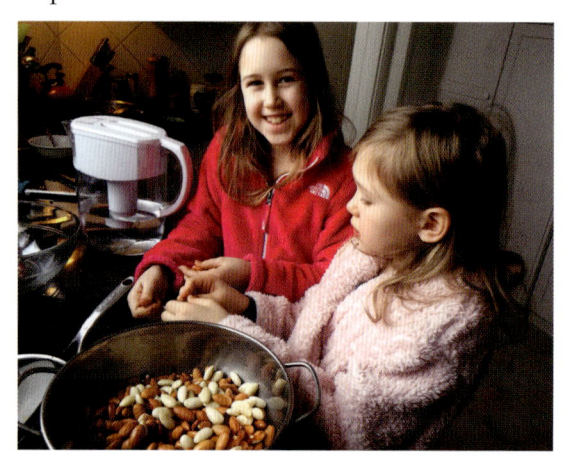

Kids like to help in the kitchen when they get to do something that seems fun to them. Pouring, mixing, even chopping are all tasks that are often more fun than setting the table.

Having them learn to cut their own meat by practicing a little at each dinner with a special knife of their own gives them some ownership over their meal. (We use French Opinel camping knives with a rounded tip, specially made for kids, that are nonetheless sharp.) Helping in the kitchen gives children an understanding of what they are eating and how their food is made and makes them feel like important and useful members of the family. The biggest challenge in nourishing and nurturing a family is keeping things on the fun and positive side, which, when a parent is not feeling well or is tired and frazzled, is extra challenging.

EATING WHILE TRAVELING OR DAY TRIPPING

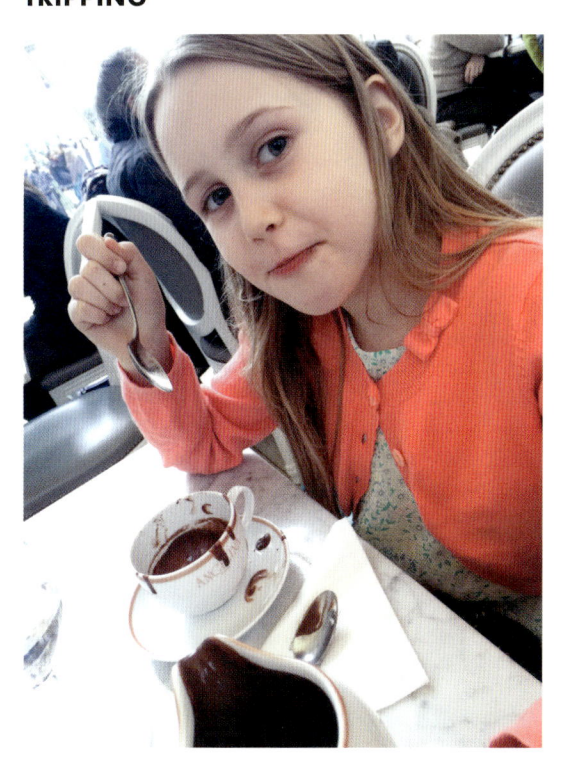

Before I was indoctrinated into good French cooking, we survived road trips by visiting fast food restaurants. They are ubiquitous, and practically anti-social to avoid. But now we try much harder now by traveling with our own food. For treats or snacks, I give my children homemade grain-free zucchini muffins or chocolate-nut date bars, or sometimes we will have an ice cream out or a hot chocolate in a café. Raw veggies travel well (so do olives, which I eat), and it has taken a transition of two years, but we keep the skins on carrots and cucumbers now for freshness, nutrients, and good bacteria.

When we take a road trip nowadays, our children also vote for a home-cooked, take-along thermos lunch, rather than going to a roadside restaurant, even in France! The best meal for this is beef burgers, mixed with minced garlic and rosemary and seared in duck fat. Two patties fit in each lunch thermos. We pack three or four thermoses, so everyone has more than one patty if they need it. It's the most filling meal on the road, served with sides of raw vegetables. I cannot emphasize enough how much it really beats roadside food.

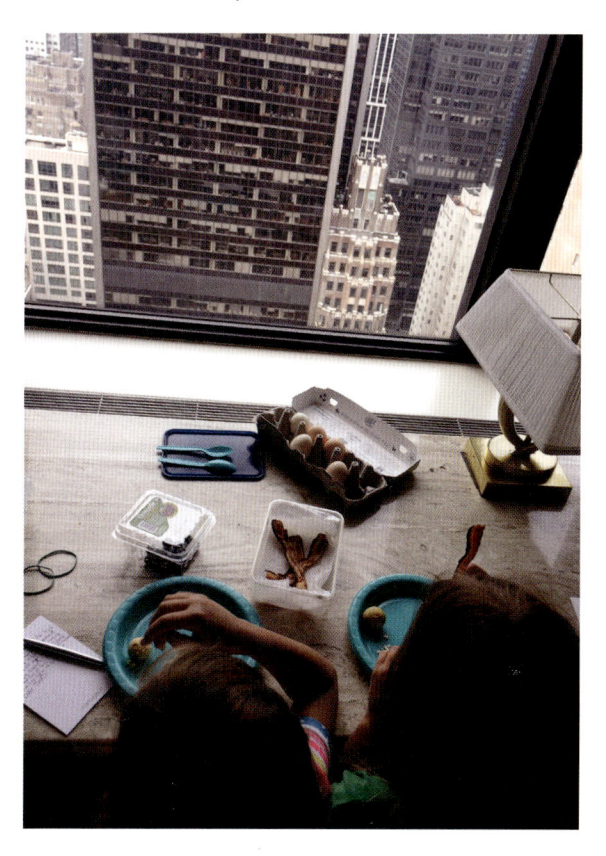

Whenever we are traveling, I try to keep up the same principles by which we live at home: regular mealtimes, nutritious food, no outside distractions. Even visiting New York City from Washington, DC for 48 hours, we packed a lunch for the train, dinner for the first night, and breakfast for the hotel room

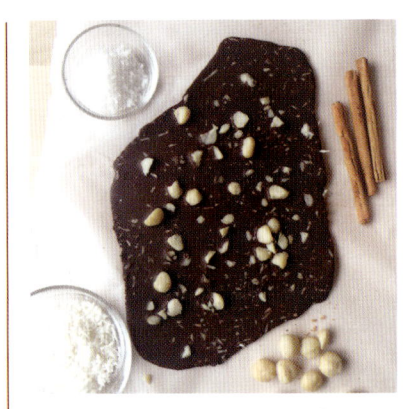

Paleo Chocolate Bark

Melt a bar of dark chocolate in a thick saucepan or double boiler. Stir in one tablespoon coconut oil. Pour the mixture onto a piece of parchment paper on a flat baking sheet. Sprinkle on desired ingredients, such as coconut flakes, chopped macadamia nuts, coconut sugar, cinnamon, *fleur de sel*, as shown here, where I used 100% chocolate. For kids, a lower cocoa percentage (meaning more sugar content) will be more appealing to them. Get them used to this, and they will be less likely to beg for cheap, store-bought, junk chocolate.

consisting of boiled eggs, cold bacon, blueberries, and sea salt. I pack everything in stainless-steel or glass containers, plastic if necessary, depending on how willing I am to carry the heavier containers, along with napkins and cutlery (plastic for planes, metal for car and trains). *Warning:* Bone broth gets confiscated at airport security, sadly. It has happened to us when I forgot it in one of our carry-on bags before a flight across the U.S.

WHEN IN ROME

While it takes more time, planning, and organization to travel with our own food, it gives us a sense of choice and control, rather than be subject to whatever half-baked item is on a fast "food" menu or roadside restaurant. Plus, we save money, we feel good about ourselves, and our stomachs feel much better. Before you travel, prepare and pack yourself real food and snacks, as it is easy while travelling to fall for the non-authentic, über-sugary vices and the pandemic, carbo-loaded "treats" that are at every street corner, rest area, or airport of the modern world. If you travel internationally, consider the ancestral traditions of the local culture you are visiting. Find the local, non-sugary delicacies. Try the charcuterie, cheeses, honeys, pâtés, wines, and regional specialties. This is particularly easy to do in Europe where regional specialties are often legally protected from being counterfeited and are part of the excitement of discovery. If you are buying fresh, local produce, meat, or fish (including oysters) sourced locally from a farmer, butcher, or fishmonger in France, you are sure to get the real thing anyway!

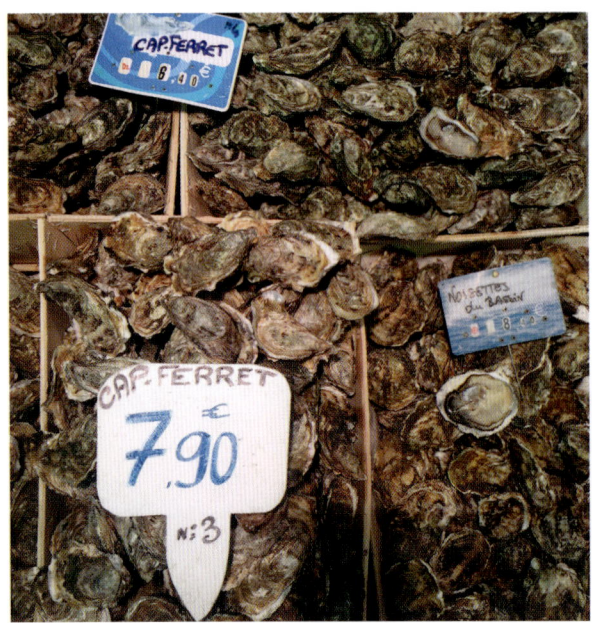

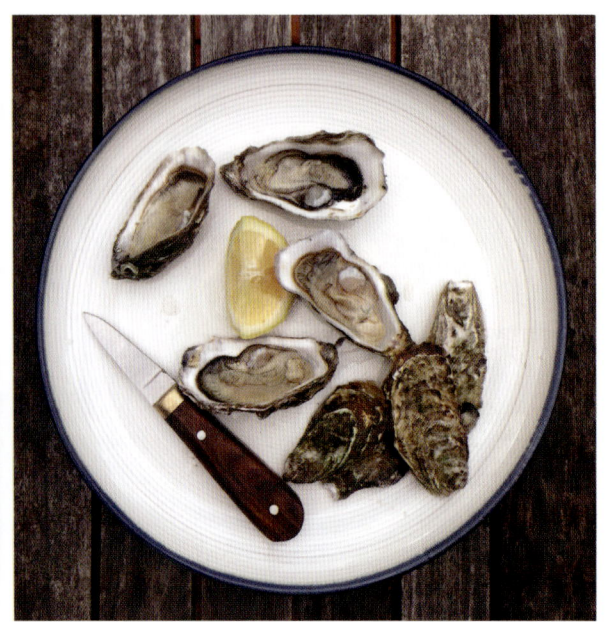

Cap Ferret Oysters, Bay of Arcachon, Bordeaux

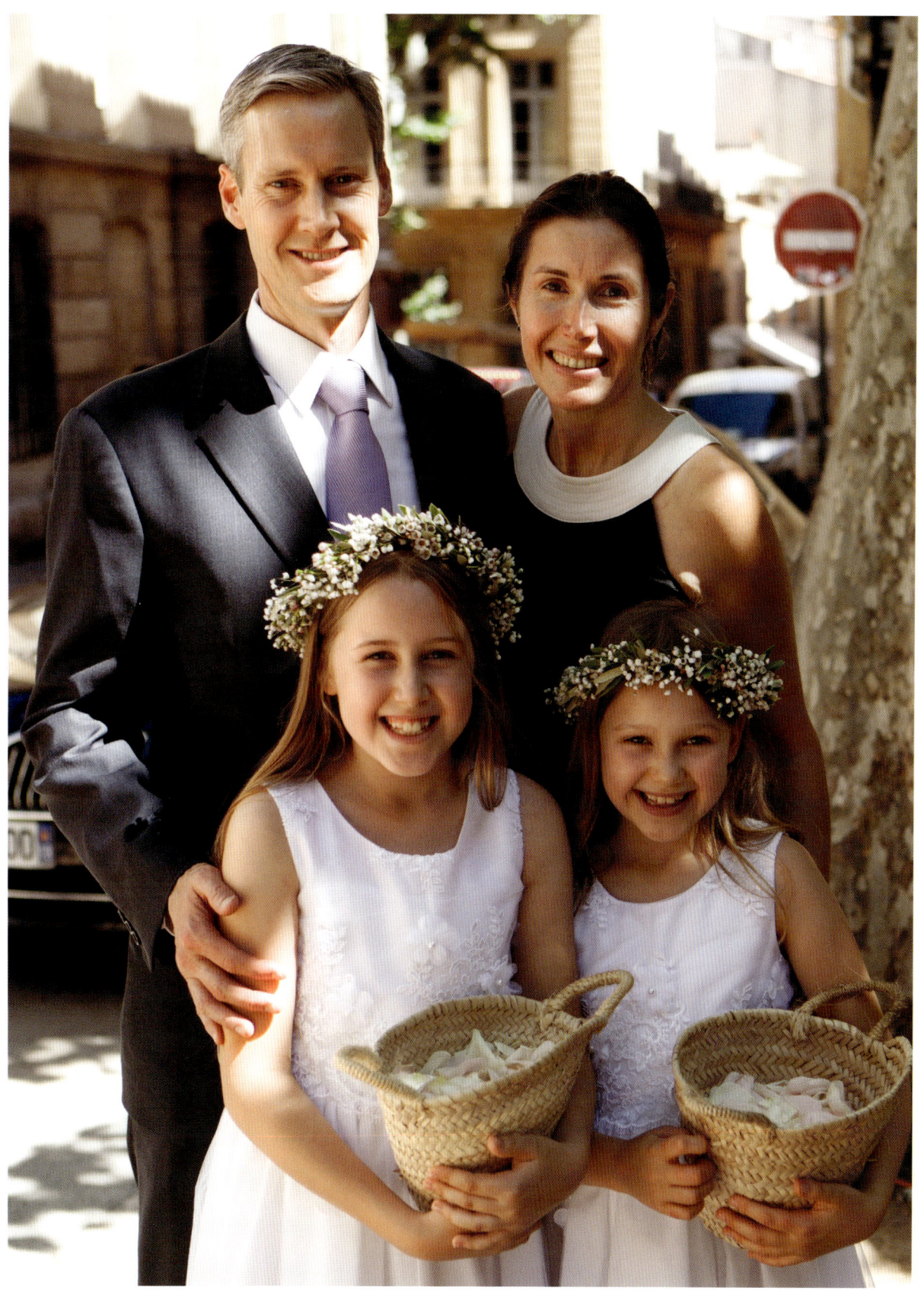

Family Portrait in Aix-en-Provence

APPENDIXES

My Roots	587
Epilogue	591
A Note on the Photography	592
Acknowledgments	593
Cooking Glossary	597
Resources and Further Reading	603
Endnotes	614
Selected Bibliography	623
Index	627

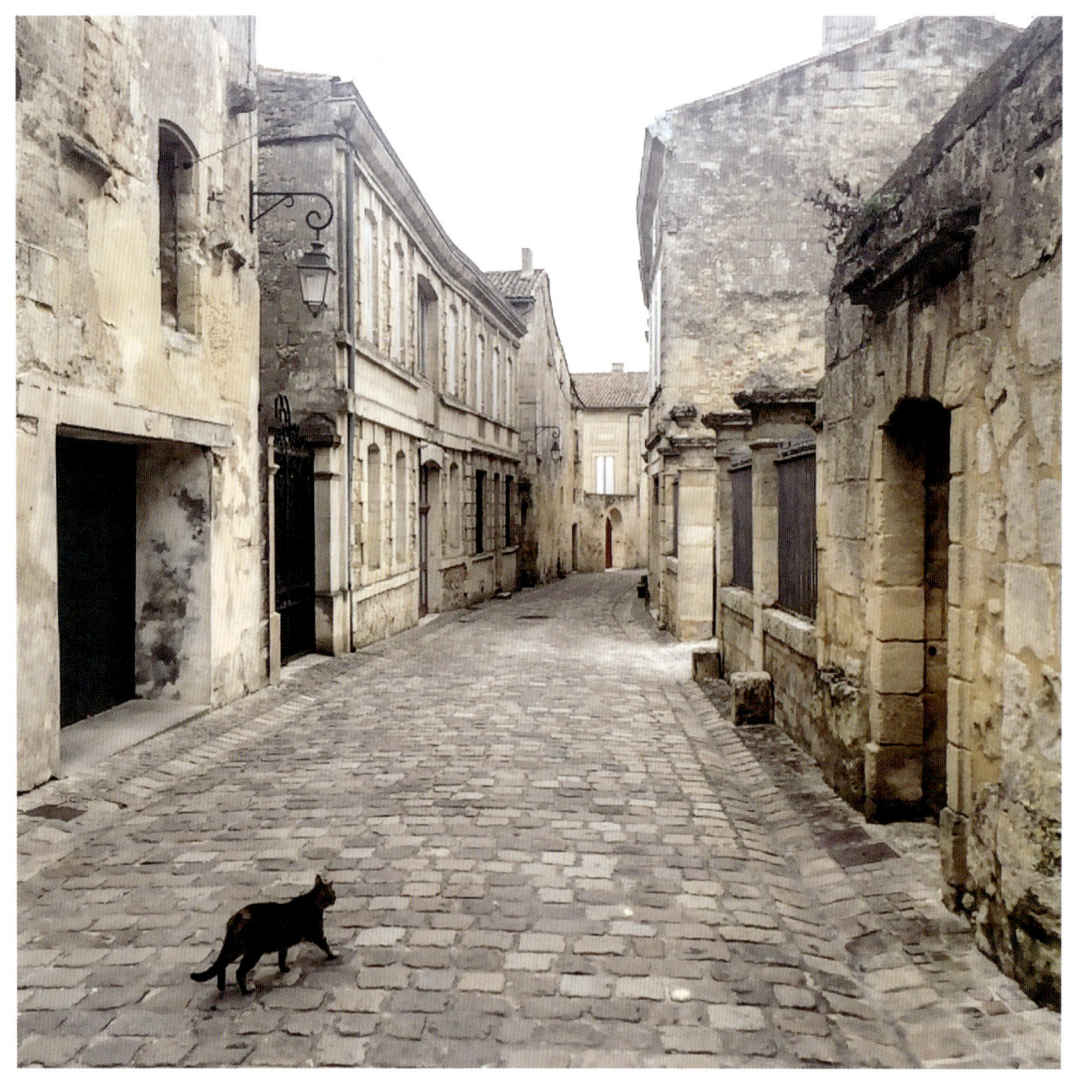

Saint Emilion

MY ROOTS

"Tell me what you eat and I will tell you what you are."
—Gastronome Jean Anthelme Brillat-Savarin (1755-1826)[1]

Born in the U.S. to German immigrant parents, I grew up in Northern California in the 1970s, but my family made frequent trips back to a small German town near Frankfurt to visit (and eat with) my mother's relatives. This was my earliest exposure to natural, unprocessed, and nutrient-dense foods, as well as to a more timeless, family-centered, and sustainable way of living. Liverwurst, butter, and chives were among my earliest food staples on these visits, as were pork sausage (*Bratwurst*), pork patties (*Frikadellen*), and home-cured salami-style pork sausage (*Rote Wurst*) from our relatives' farm. Unfortunately, however, store-bought strawberry popsicles, sugary "children's" chocolate, and chocolate spread smeared on white rolls (*Brötchen*) were also staples for me, as well as the occasional hard candy ("*Bonbon*") from the purse of my loving maternal grandmother, Oma Katharina.

I have a vivid memory of gathering blueberries in the forest with Oma Katharina. Actually, she collected them in her metal milk jug, and instead of filling up my little pail, I ate the blueberries along the way. There were many afternoons of coffee and cake (*Kaffee und Kuchen*), grilling sausages and meat outdoors, and picking black, red, and white currants in my grandmother's vegetable garden just outside of town. Among my fondest memories is one of sitting up high in the cherry tree, picking (and eating) dark cherries in that garden, fenced in by an old gate with peeling green paint and rusting metal locks. Everyone in small-town Germany had a vegetable garden back then, which made for a lot of extra work for the busy relatives like mine who helped my grandmother maintain it on the weekends. But in return there were always fruits and vegetables which were canned and pickled to last everyone through the winter, (though very few of the cherries that *I* picked ever made it into jars or cakes).

One of my earliest memories is of my uncle and aunt, Onkel Hans and Tante Doris, roasting an entire pig on a spit in their garden to serve the relatives and friends who had come to lay the foundation for their new house. It was 1974, and in a true communal effort, one uncle did the brick laying, another did the tile work, and yet another butchered the pig we would feast on. My aunts and mother supplied salads and desserts. My cousin Martina watched over me like an older sister as we sat in the grass with the neighbors eating pieces of barbecued pork.

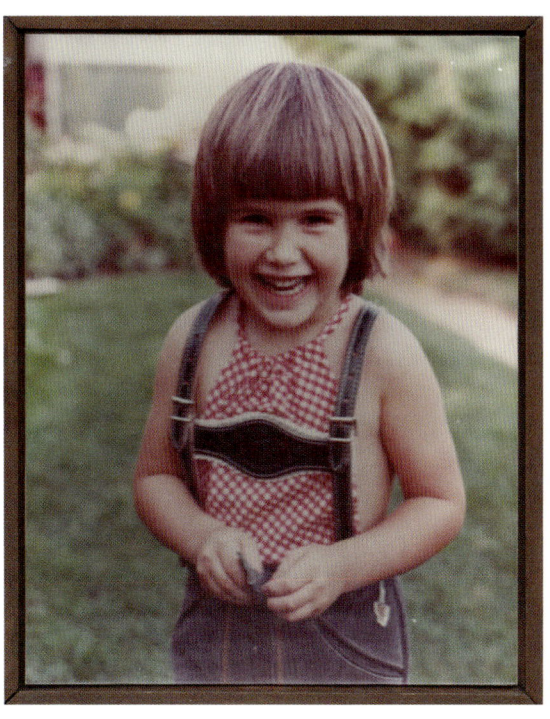

Here I am in my Lederhosen and bowl haircut in Germany in the mid-1970s

Along with home building and communal cooking, my extended German family was both environmentally and economically conscious, especially regarding the conservation of water and electricity and the utility bills that accompany them. Tante Doris in particular encouraged me to take short showers; she saved rainwater in large barrels, and she collected snips of paper or cloth and other bits for later use. But she let me pilfer her vegetable and fruit garden with abandon in the summer. Over the year, when my parents, my younger brother, and I visited our family in Germany, we were treated to all the home cooking and high-fat foods (particularly liverwurst and sausage, which we loved and missed in the U.S.) while seated around the family table, communing at every mealtime. I am forever grateful for the care my relatives took of me and for the cultural and environmentally conscious foundation they helped to form in me, though I did not fully appreciate this gift until years later.

On my father's side, food served as cultural continuity for a family life disrupted by war and immigration. My grandmother, *Oma Herta*, was studying to be a cook in Königsberg (then part of Germany—East Prussia—now Kaliningrad, Russia) when World War II broke out. She and my father, aged two, fled to central Germany by train. Along the way, charitable train passengers offered Oma Herta a few hundred grams (less than a pound) of life-saving butter for her young son, my father. Once reunited after the war, my grandparents learned to adapt as outsiders: first as "Prussian" refugees in central Germany, then as "German" immigrants in Venezuela, and finally settling in Northern California. I remember my Oma Herta's cooking: her roasts, salads, *Rouladen* (meat and pickles dish), and stews, but especially her raspberry blintzes. Everybody loved "Herta's Cooking." It was an institution amidst the group of Germans who lived near each other in California from the 1960s through the early 2000s. How fortunate I was to have grown up exposed to the traditional dishes of my family members, both in California and in Germany, rather than only the highly processed, low-fat, sugary grocery store fare of the 1970s and '80s. Unfortunately for Germany and the rest of Europe, who took clues from America's (as we now know flawed) dietary advice to its own citizens, margarine and vegetable oil and the fear of saturated fat began to creep its way into Europe's kitchens. *The Bordeaux Kitchen* is my way of passing along to you and to future generations an old-world culinary philosophy (prior to the fat-phobias and the modern chronic diseases epidemic) that represents a renewed value for our modern lives and that might otherwise be lost with my grandparents' generation if we do not reclaim and honor it.

After my parents' divorce when I was seven, I split my time between two households. In both households we had breakfasts of cereal, pancakes, and toast, but luckily also bacon, eggs and real butter, and home-cooked and grilled meats and vegetables. It turned out that my grandmothers' generation had influenced both households enough to keep the traditions of home-cooked goodness and gathering alive in our families. Little did I know how these lessons and experiences would later guide me.

When I was twelve, we moved to the East Coast. After high school I left home a young adult, focused on field hockey, lacrosse, Ultimate Frisbee, and my liberal arts studies at my university. I dabbled unsuccessfully in vegetarianism, mostly adopted because I did not really know how to cook meat, nor was I interested in learning. As I have learned and as research shows, being a vegetarian is not a free pass to health and longevity.[2]

Looking back, I am surprised I did not take an interest in cooking more than just vegetables and pasta for myself. My awareness about health and the environment grew while in college, and many of those around me considered vegetarianism a healthy, morally responsible way to live. Sometimes I went off-campus looking for organic (mostly vegetarian) products from the grocery store. I stopped using aluminum-laced deodorants.

And I of course tried not to waste paper, water or electricity. I spent a year studying abroad in Germany, Russia, and France, forcing myself to adapt to the austerities and excesses of each country and culture. But I was still unaware of how to properly nourish myself. With my lack of understanding of the biological need for nutrient-dense foods for healthy brain and hormonal function combined with so many late college nights of sugary ice cream, pizza, and very little sleep, it is no wonder my health began to crumble after college.

I had mostly studied foreign languages in college, and my first "real job" after graduation took me overseas again, this time to the newly independent country of Kazakhstan. Its then capital, Almaty, was a fascinating place to work in the mid-1990s, a real frontier and a relic in many ways of austere Soviet times, and where "new" shops and kiosks were popping up, selling imported ("dumped") bottles of condiments and vegetable oils (nearing or past their expiration dates). I chose not to buy the meats hanging in the local market stalls, opting for the local bread, the imported vegetable oils (try getting your hands on real olive oil in Kazakhstan in 1994!), the fruits and vegetables brought in from the "countryside" but of unclear origin and agricultural treatment. (Chernobyl? Pesticides?) I began to show symptoms of Irritable Bowel Syndrome (IBS), which I now realize was, among other things, due to the severe malnutrition resulting from my lack of understanding of nutrient density or of how to properly nourish myself. After two years in Kazakhstan, my ignorance ultimately resulted in a medical evacuation to a small German hospital, thankfully near my relatives, where I stayed for six weeks, turned 25, and had two major abdominal surgeries for near-fatal peritonitis and related abdominal infections and abscesses. After several weeks in the hospital, three blood transfusions and a narrowly escaping a colostomy bag implantation, I arrived at a moment of unparalleled gratitude to the universe for giving me a second chance.

Moving back home to Connecticut to recover, it became clear to me that I needed to make a change. During the early months of my recovery, I asked an alternative medicine doctor and his wife what they ate for breakfast. That was when I first heard of *Enter the Zone* by Dr. Barry Sears. From then on, I began trying to "balance" my diet in terms of carbohydrates, proteins, and fats, but I mostly just focused on eating meat again to increase my iron levels. I still did not understand the biochemistry of the body and how food plays its role in nourishing us. But I took up Hatha yoga, learned how to move again, and began swimming after my last abdominal scar was cauterized. An older woman, seeing me in the showers at the YWCA pool one day, noticed my large, fresh scar and kindly remarked, "We're glad to have you with us." I was grateful to be there.

Twenty years, 13 moves, and two children later, I am still learning, grateful, and humbled by the ruptured appendix experience. My husband and I have lived, worked, or studied together in many places, including Boston, Washington D.C., New York, Croatia, Germany, France, Russia, Japan, and Switzerland, while always focusing on fitness and eating well. One constant has been preparing eggs for breakfast. From our first summer together, while working in Split, Croatia, we started a daily habit of the "morning hen," or eating an egg with bacon on an English muffin. Wherever we have lived, we have tried to keep up this breakfast ritual (now minus the bread).

Even with the changes I made following my abdominal operations, I still experienced fatigue, anxiety, and brain fog for many years. In the fall of 2013, however, I developed a renewed sense of curiosity and hope. My supportive and resourceful husband, Toby, came across an interview on the *Underground Wellness* podcast (hosted by Sean Croxton, with Dr. David Perlmutter speaking about his then-new bestselling book *Grain Brain*). I became a podcast junkie, burning through every episode of *Underground Wellness*, then Jimmy Moore's podcast *Livin' La Vida Low-Carb Show*, then Robb Wolf's *Paleo Solution Podcast*, then Mark Sisson's *Primal Blueprint Podcast*, and on and on. I listened (and still do) while I cooked, cleaned, drove, or walked, gleaning all manner of knowledge and inspiration.

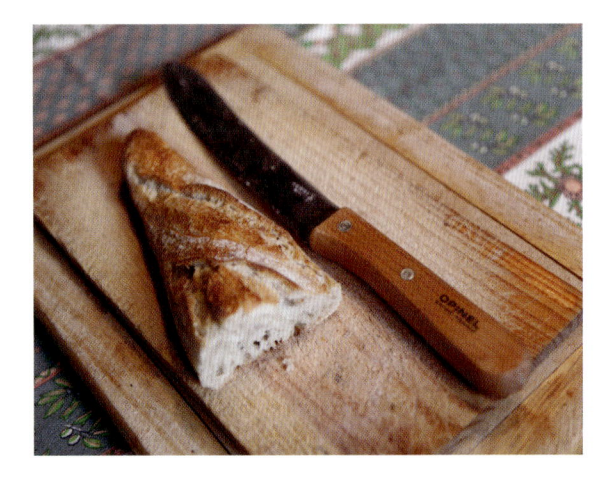

I had one last love affair with gluten and sugar for a few days in April 2014 at an all-you-can-eat resort that brought out the worst in everyone in the cafeteria during mealtimes. After the debauchery of multiple croissants at every breakfast and two desserts at every dinner, I stopped eating breads, pastas, and most desserts and began my long ascent toward a healthier, lower-carbohydrate style of eating.

In the summer of 2014, I poured out my last bottle of "organic" canola oil (I cringe at how long it took me to finally do that), and began eating gluten-free, foregoing the *baguettes*, *croissants*, and *pains au chocolat*, despite their wafting scents at every other street corner in France. In the fall of 2014, despite recurring migraines and fatigue, I forced my brain into action by taking a year-long, science-laden, Bordeaux University wine tasting course, while slowly transitioning to a primal/paleo diet and more ancestral lifestyle. I finally began to grasp the intimate connection between my physical and emotional suffering and fatigue by recognizing my lifelong addiction to high-carbohydrate foods that caused insulin resistance, blood sugar spikes, mood swings and gut discomfort. Realizing I had been unmindfully eating too much, too fast, and too frequently, I tried slowing down and experimenting more with primal- and paleo-friendly recipes and integrating them with traditional French dishes. It was not easy to override the years of carb-glorifying and fat-fearing brainwashing that had been so pervasive for many years. Discovering I also had parasites helped me understand some of my poor digestion, fatigue, and other ills. It has been a cathartic process getting over the "gross factor" of eating organ meats and raw oysters and learning how to butcher a whole carcass down to pieces recognizable in a recipe. My personal dietary choices became less about what I "felt like" eating and more about what would help me heal and give me and my family the most nutrient-dense boost day after day by generally observing the limitations of seasonal, local, and organic foods available, while minding a high-fat, satiating regime of nutrient-dense meats, offal, fish, and vegetables doused in animal fats and olive oil. The two worlds of French ancestral cooking traditions and the primal/paleo/ancestral way of life began to merge in front of me, revealing a new path that I had needed and sought for decades. My friends in both worlds encouraged me on my path despite all my health complexities, helping me to learn and comprehend my role in this new paradigm. I continue to learn, grateful to have the opportunity with *The Bordeaux Kitchen* to pass on knowledge that others may be searching for as well.

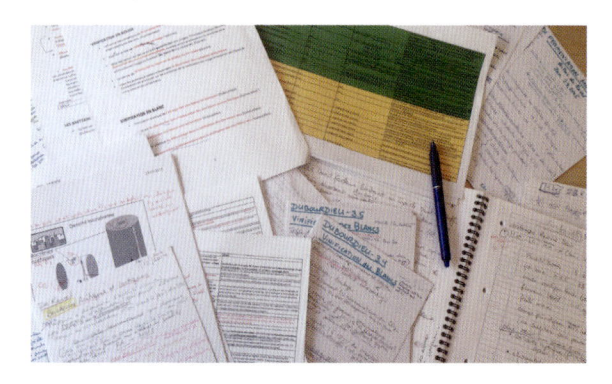

EPILOGUE

Ancestral French cooking has worked well for my family and my health and resonates with my heritage and my life experiences. However, it is by no means the only ancestral cuisine to preserve and integrate into our modern repertoire. Many cultures across the globe do remain and should remain true to their ancestral cuisines. The culinary traditions of Africa, Asia, and the Americas, and the ancestral foods of other European, Jewish, and Middle Eastern cultures are well worth exploring. The longer each of us respects our ancestral heritage, the better chance we have of reclaiming and passing on our renewed good health and the shared joys in life.

I will admit it was a tough sell at first, reversing the brainwashing I had received about fats being unhealthy. But eventually, I reintroduced traditional fats back into my family's diet, just as the French had done for generations (before even they, unfortunately, began succumbing to low-fat dietary fads). I am encouraged by the results of how my family and I feel, as well as by the scientific literature that continues to emerge, including two recent studies showing no greater risk of heart disease mortality from diets high in saturated fats.[1,2]

My hope is that my readers will welcome new ways of looking at their health by taking ownership of it, rather than relying on faulty, conventional food systems and convenience or processed "foods." We all deserve to enjoy healthy, energetic, productive lives as free of disease as possible. I hope the lessons I have learned in my own journey toward better health will encourage others to take control of their nutritional health and to find satisfying and meaningful paths to their own wellness.

The recipes in *The Bordeaux Kitchen* include healthier and tastier alternatives to our current culture of non-fat, starch- and chemical-laden, industrially refined "foods." *The Bordeaux Kitchen* embraces the lessons of our ancestors and invites all of us to move toward a more sustainable, nurturing future for the current and coming generations.

Thank you for sharing in this journey.

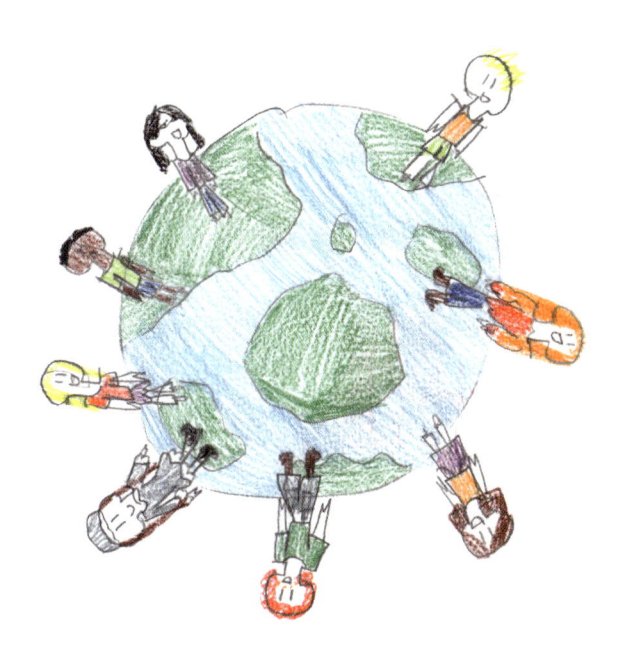

A NOTE ON THE PHOTOGRAPHY FOR THE PHOTO ENTHUSIASTS

I captured all these images using my trusty Canon EOS 5D Mark II using the L Series EF 24-70mm 1:2.8 Zoom lens at 70mm but sometimes at 50mm and occasionally at 35mm, almost always handheld, except when shooting meat-tying demonstrations using the self-timer. Some photos come from my trusty iPhone 5s, because that is what I had on hand in the moment. I used Adobe Lightroom 4 for all my photo editing on a 2013 iMac, while all my writing I have either scribbled on scraps and in notebooks and transferred to my trusty 2011 MacBook Pro, which is just barely hanging in there, thank goodness! I used Photoshop very little, because I'm no good at it. Put me in a real dark room and I can make a mean black and white print, but in Photoshop, I'm a "dummy." My first love was black and white 35mm film (I have a Voigtländer Bessa-R), and I have a medium format (Hasselblad 500 C/M), but for the purpose of surviving the making of this book, digital photography was necessary! In the late 1990s I had a brief internship with *National Geographic* photographer Steve McCurry. I have shot family portraits and a few weddings, Russian and American industrial landscapes, Russian model test shots, European travel and lifestyle, French vineyards and winemaking, and now, food! I have had some of my photography published in magazines in Paris and Tokyo, I have exhibited in Moscow, Paris, and Tokyo, and I have self-published several books and journals, which can be found at www.blurb.com. My personal photography projects can be viewed at www.taniateschke.com. I can be found at Instagram as @TaniaTeschke and Twitter as @BordeauxKitchen. All offers to travel to and shoot in exotic locations with ancestral food or great wine will be considered!

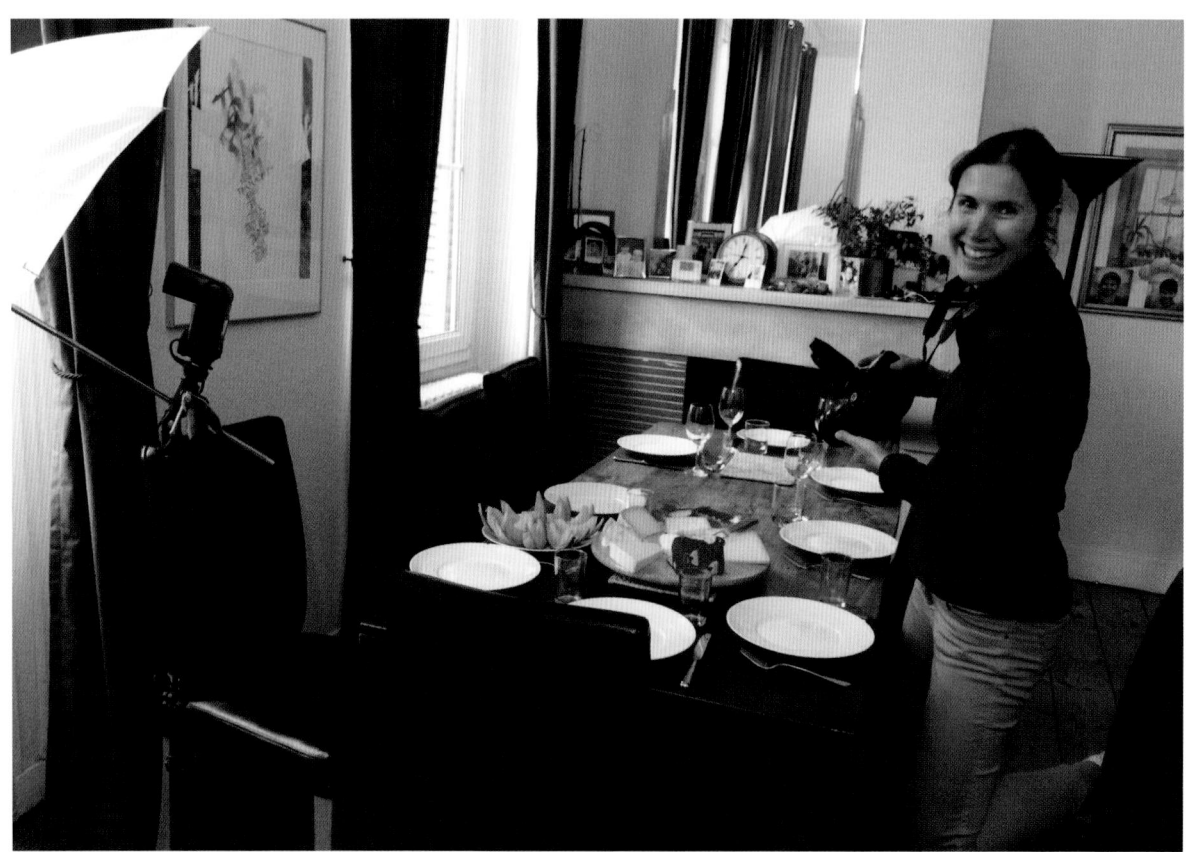

Photo credit: Pascale Davis

ACKNOWLEDGMENTS

The journey of making this book has been a collaborative effort and cathartic experience. It is thanks to those who have forged the path before me who have taught me so much. These include Mark Sisson and Dr. David Perlmutter in the health sphere, Julia Child, Alice Waters, and Paula Wolfert in the cooking world, and the many others whose books, websites and podcasts I have listed in my Resources and Further Reading list.

This book represents the time-honored and life-changing concepts and skills I have learned along this journey. It is the best way I know of sharing what I have learned, knowing others will benefit. It is a great pleasure and privilege to acknowledge the many individuals who have generously helped me in the process of creating this body of work. I am grateful to each person, mentioned here or not, for their moral support, meaningful collaboration, time, and friendship. This book is the beautiful result of their donated time and effort, combined with my stubborn motivation to pull it together on a modest household budget.

I would like to express my sincere gratitude to my generous family, friends, colleagues, and all those who have encouraged and helped me directly and indirectly in the creation of this work:

To my publisher, Brad Kearns, for taking on this project in the first place despite its large scope and long timeline; to Tracy Dunigan, my patient, articulate and supportive editor, who helped tame a monstrous manuscript into a more graceful written work, and whose attention to detail as well as the big picture have made all the difference; to Caroline De Vita for her dedication, patience, and gorgeous design work on the cover and interior, breathing life into the book's visual format; to Tim Tate for his painstaking copyediting efforts, detailed referencing, and endless patience; to Janee Meadows for her cover design magic; to Dr. Catherine Shanahan for her encouragement, generosity, and unique contribution to the Foreword of the book; to Elle Russ for her enthusiasm; to Brian McAndrew, TJ Quillin, Liz Mostaedi, Annie Martin, and the rest of the team at Primal Blueprint and Primal Kitchen for their support; to the team at Sterling Lord Literary for enthusiastically taking on my book; to my helpful distributors Melanie Warren and Justin Bailey and their teams at Gazelle Book Services in the U.K., and to Annette Hughes and the team at Midpoint Trade Books for all of their guidance, enthusiasm, and support. To Christophe Château at the CIVB/Bordeaux Wine Council and to University of California at Davis Professor Emeritus Ann Noble for allowing their diagrams in the book; to Bordeaux native Arnaud Faugas for his lovely animal illustrations; to the Ancestral Health Symposium for being the venue for me to meet so many dedicated health seekers; to Aaron Alexander, Sarah Ballantyne, Aaron Blaisdell, Kevin Boyd, Georges Dagher, Alvin Danenberg, Anne Dann, Romy Dollé, Darryl Edwards, Tony Federico, Nora Gedgaudas, Hilda Labrada Gore, Ben Greenfield, Stephan Guyenet, Tara Grant, Benjamin Kuo, Grace Liu, Marisa Moon, Naomi Norwood, Gina Rieg, Angeles Rios, Ellen Seeley, Scott Solomons, Dr. Terry Wahls, and Marty Wilson for their "ancestral" support; to Michael Dilandro for putting me in touch with Brad initially; and to Mark Sisson for giving the project his blessing and allowing it in to the esteemed Primal Blueprint family.

I extend unending gratitude to my unique and dear collaborative friends who are cooks, chefs, butchers, winemakers, wine advisors, and editors, without whose generosity of time, ideas, and encouragement there would have been no recipes, wine pairings, or stories: Jane Anson, Océanne Auffret, Aline Baly, Philippe Baly, Jean-Luc Beaufils, Bouchra Z., Florent Carriquiry, Stephen Davis, Craig Dennis, Delphine Dentraygues, Malika Faytout, Célia Girard, Ilona Guitz, Lilou and Daniel Leonard, Catherine and Guy-Pétrus Lignac, Vincent Lignac, Joelle Luson, Axel Marchal, Dewey Markam, Jr., Caroline Matthews, Kelley Mouiex, Suzanne Mustacich, Annabelle

Nicolle-Beaufils, Vy Nguyen, Laeticia Ouspointour, Anne Perez, Rébecca Pinsolle, Béatrice Pontallier, Ellen Reeves, Edouard Remont, Véronique Sanders, Frédéric Schueller, and Natalia Youreva. My gratitude goes also to Atelier des Chefs in Bordeaux for their informative hands-on cooking classes and online resources. And to those not already mentioned here, who, among others, kindly allowed me to take photos at their establishments or on their estates: Le Poulailler d'Augustin, Christine Nadalié, Château Rieussec, Château Jean Faure, Château Carbonnieux, Château d'Yquem, Château Palmer, Château La Clémence, Château Coutet, Château Haut-Bailly, Château Guadet, Château Biac, Château La Fleur-Pétrus, and Château Mouton Rothschild.

A big thanks to my friends at Biocoop Cauderan for putting up with me and my many questions during my several months of apprenticing at the butcher counter with Florent Carriquiry; to Romain Camart, Damien Denis, and Nico for their recipe suggestions and butchery lessons; to Florent for his continued butchery support and enthusiasm; to Guillerme for his organic wine insights; to the rest of the staff for their support and enthusiasm; and to Frédérique and Jérôme Mazurier for trusting in me and allowing me to apprentice at their shop.

I am grateful for having had the opportunity to participate in the year-long wine course known as the "DUAD" at the University of Bordeaux, Institute of the Vine and Wine; thanks to my highly esteemed Professors Gilles de Revel, Axel Marchal, and the late Denis Dubourdieu for having accepted me into the program and encouraging me along the way. I am grateful to my DUAD professors including Jean-Claude Berrouet, Philippe Darriet, Sandrine Garbay, and many others who helped teach me the arts of wine making and wine tasting; to my friends Thomas Deroux, Carlyn Whitehouse, the Lignac Family, Sylvie Cazes, Kelly Mouiex, Jane Anson, Wendy Holohan, and Caroline Matthews for encouraging me to apply for the DUAD program, and to Margaret Calvet for her assistance with my application. To the DUAD's Club for providing more opportunities to learn from alumni gatherings. With deepest respect I thank my wine course classmates for their encouraging support throughout the year-long course and beyond: Alexandra, Annabelle G., Annabelle N-B., Anne, Barbara, Bénédicte, Delphine, Elsa, Hubert, Isabelle, Laeticia, Malika, Natalia, Rakusa, Stéphane, and Vy. To the amazing sommelier Annabelle Nicolle-Beaufils, for whose knowledge and efforts to pair my list of recipes with wine I am so very grateful and proud to showcase in this book. An extra word of gratitude to Caroline, Dewey, Ellen, Jane, Stephen, and my husband, Toby, for their tireless review of certain chapters of the book.

To our lovely Bordeaux neighbors, friends, and teachers from the Bordeaux International School, and to the gracious people of Bordeaux (and beyond) not already mentioned who made our experience there all the richer, including the Asseily family, JB and Isabelle Auzely, Sara Babin, Philippe Baly, Violaine Bargues, Stephen Bolger and Lisa La Plant, Olivier Bernard, Sylvain Boivert, Alain Bost, Pascale Bourdessoulles, Anne-Sophie Brieux, Janice Brooks, Audrey and Benoît Cristou, Emmanuel Cruse, Christine Cussac, Philippe Delmas, Philippe Dhalluin, the Davis family, the Decelles, Stéphane and Brigitte Delaux, Noémie Demel, Patrice and Di Dubourdieu, Bernadette and Michel Duclos, the Dugrips, Sophie Emery-Roy, Jennifer Faugere, France Etats-Unis Biarritz Côte Basque, the Forder family, B & JP Frankenhuis, Coach David Garcia, the Garofanos, Antonia Giraud, Ambassador Jane Hartley, Véronique Herpe, Elizabeth Jaubert, Valérie Lavigne, Sophie Lion-Poulain, Pierre Lurton, Virginie Macabet, Solenne Masse, David Maurat, Tamara McIntosh, Sevrine Miailhe, the Mouiex family, Karim Nasser, Pierre de Gaétan Njikam, the Oubru family, Julien Parrou, Daina Paulin, Jean-Charles Perreux, the Perrin family, D & D Pinault, Petra Reineke-Lagarde, the Rides, Pompon and Georges Schell, Jan Schÿler, our wonderful babysitter Sophie Séguin, the Sters, the Swann family, the Teulé family, Oddur and Mimi Thorisson, Bénédicte Trocard, Patrick Viau, the late Bob Wilmers and his wife

Elisabeth, and Mayor Alain Juppé and his wife Isabelle for their encouragement and support along the way. I love Bordeaux!

A big thanks to the shop keepers at Märitladen, the organic farm Biohof Blaser, the Schweizer Fleisch-Fachverband, the head butcher Bislip Mema at Coop Wabern, and organic butcher René Wegmüller at Au Cochon Rose in Bern, for their help with terminology and patience in providing the odd cuts of meat I still needed for several recipes and photos once we had moved to Switzerland after Bordeaux. Also thank you to Richard Cole, Karen Christie, Kathrin Keller, David Lindsay, Rolf Marti, Scott Jackson, Irene Sahli, Ursula Schindler, Nina Schläfli, and the Geiser family and colleagues at Embassy Bern for their help, friendship, and moral support.

A heartfelt thanks to Tressa Johnston at US Wellness Meats for her early support of my work and for giving me the chance to be the August 2016 Chef of the Month and to Benjamin Nutt at PaleoFx for featuring my work ahead of PFX2017. To Ariane Daguin and her team at D'Artagnan, to Sandrine Butteau and her team at the French Cultural Services bookstore Albertine, and to Laura Baddish and the team at the French Cheese Board for all of their dynamism and support. Special thanks also to the members of the International Association of Culinary Professionals who have been so supportive of my work. To my longtime friend and poetry guru Susan Watson, who began teaching me about conscious living, nutrients, and the craft of writing when I was in high school. To Jenn Bloch, Susan Buckley, Nina Furstenau, Professor Patricia Herlihy, Suzanne Mustacich, Ellen Reeves, Hugh Roome, Andrea Suerbaum, and Susan Wolf for their writer's advice and moral and editorial support. To all my dear friends, old and new, in France, Germany, Japan, Kazakhstan, Russia, the U.S., and around the world, I thank you for your support and loyal friendship! To our friends in the State Department and across American Embassies worldwide for their enthusiasm, friendship, and support.

To our extended family around the world, our cousins and their families, and in particular Tante Doris, Tante Lilli, and Martina for always staying close despite the distance. To David and Régine Whittlesey for their wisdom and foresight in giving us the *Larousse de la Cuisine* book and a market basket at our French-themed wedding just before we moved to Paris for my husband's first posting with the Foreign Service.

To Dr. Dan Kalish and his support staff for helping me to begin to unravel my health mysteries and encouraging me to write this book. To Dr. Tim Gerstmar and his assistant Loralei for their ongoing support, compassion and encouragement, as well as Dr. G's elucidations to my many health questions for the book. And to Robin Matthews, who helped to helped me restore calm and reminded me that everything would be okay.

My gratitude goes also to Robin, Pat, Hannah, and Sandra, healing colleagues and friends of my mom's who regularly treated my mom during the last months of my writing this book, helping alleviate the terrible effects of chemo and radiation "treatment" for cancer by using aromatherapy, Emotional Freedom Technique (EFT), Healing Touch, Jin Shin Shiatsu, reflexology, and sound therapy. They, together with my devoted stepfather Sujit and my visiting aunts helped my mom through the weeks and months when I could not help her. I am profoundly thankful.

To my loving parents, Anita and Sujit, Dieter and Jeannie, and my husband's parents, our siblings, siblings-in-law, and their families, I thank you from the bottom of my heart for your sincere and unconditional love and support all these years. And in particular to my brother Clifton: thank you for always being there.

To Toby Wolf, my best friend and husband, who still surprises me with his never-ending patience, and to our daughters, Julia and Annika, who have suffered through my pain and slow recovery and have rejoiced in my small victories along the way. I am humbled by your love and devotion. Thank you for believing in me when I couldn't. You are my inspiration!

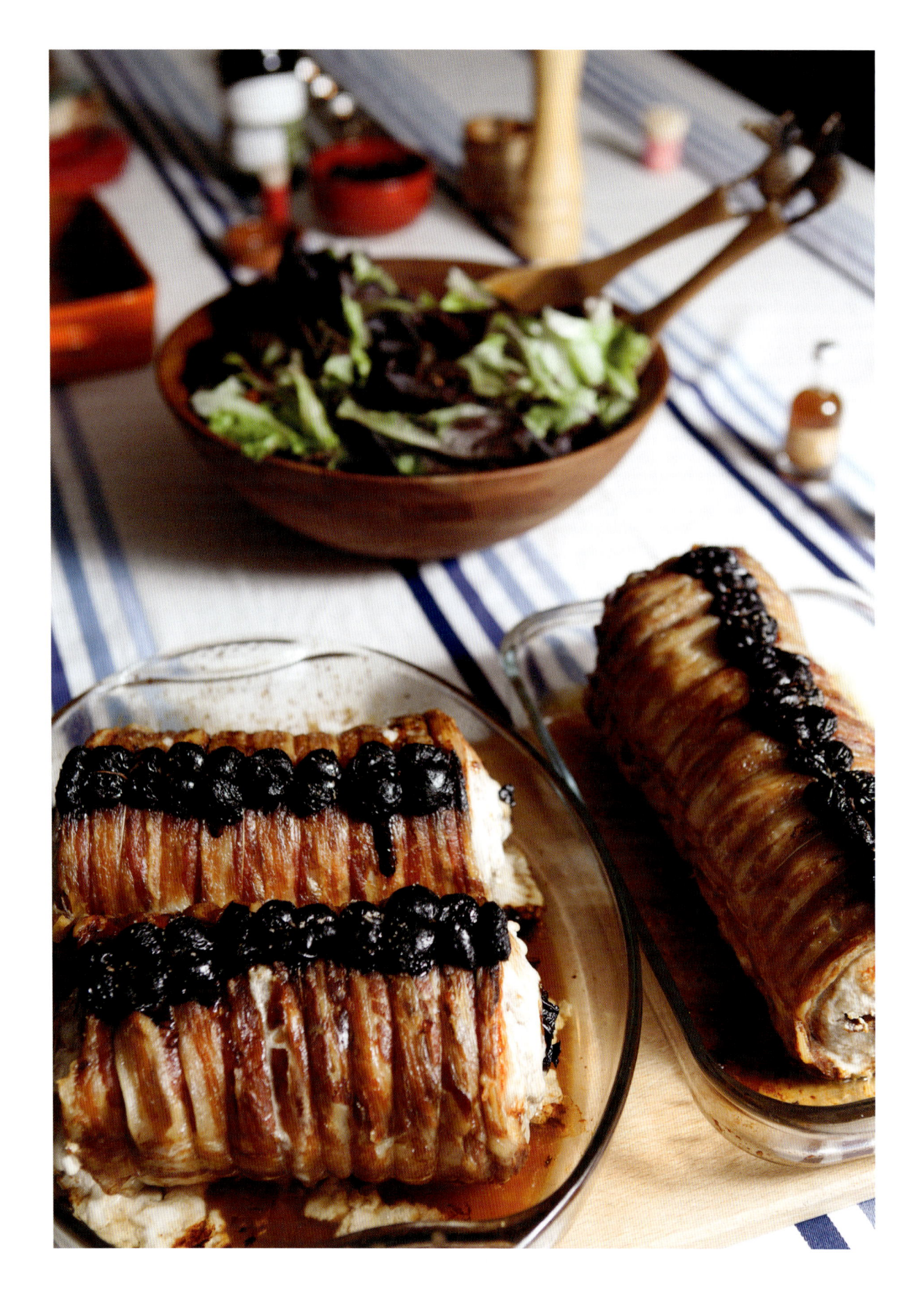

COOKING GLOSSARY

BAIN-MARIE (WATER BATH)
There are two methods for this way of cooking. The first method is to use a double boiler on a *stove* for the purpose of making sauces, or a heavy duty professional saucepan (thick enough to make sauces without using a double boiler). The second method involves pouring water into a tray in the *oven* and placing the food, which is in an oven-safe container such as a ramekin or pâté dish (*terrine*), into the water-filled tray and allowing the water to gently heat the food in the dish. This second "water bath" technique is used to cook foods such as pâté, foie gras, or sometimes *crème brûlée*. The terrines or ramekins containing the pâté are placed into a larger tray that is filled with room temperature, hot, or boiling water (every cook has his or her preference). When the internal temperature of the pâté reaches a certain degree, the terrines are carefully removed from the oven. Cooking something in this manner lowers the risk of burning the food and prevents the food from becoming too hot too quickly.

BAKING IN THE OVEN — *CUIRE AU FOUR*
"Baking" is a term in English used primarily for desserts, whereas in French *cuire* also means "to cook," as does *cuisiner*.

BARDING — *BARDER*
To wrap thin strips of fat (unrendered fatback lard, suet, or bacon strips) around a roast to protect the roast from drying out, to add flavor, and to keep juices in. Barding usually requires the use of butcher's twine or string (*la ficelle*) to hold the strips of fat or bacon in place.

BASIC COOKING METHODS
According to Eugen Pauli, the basic cooking methods include: Blanching, Poaching, Boiling, Steaming, Deep-Fat Frying, Sautéing, Grilling (or Broiling), Gratinating, Baking, Roasting, Braising, Glazing, *Poêler* (steaming in the oven in a covered pot), and Stewing.[1]

BLANCHING — *BLANCHIR*
Placing a vegetable or meat in hot water for one to two minutes, just long enough to apply heat to the surface without wilting or thoroughly boiling the vegetable or meat. Vegetables may be placed in a bowl of ice water which arrests the heating and helps the vegetable retain its color.

BOILING — *BOUILLIR*
Water boils at 212°F (100°C), but it begins showing bubbles (*à ebullition*) at 194°F (90°C), the moment at which you can poach something like an egg or fish. Boiling can last several minutes or several hours, depending on the recipe, but the meat or vegetable is entirely submerged in the boiling liquid. Boiling can be at a very heavy, steady bubble or at a low gurgling boil or simmer. Boiling meats and vegetables fades their color and makes them softer in texture. Some meats, such as those from the front end of animals and the legs or shanks, require several hours of gentle boiling to become tender.

BRAISING — *BRAISER*
Browning meat on all sides (this adds to the flavor of the dish), and then cooking it slowly for several hours (this creates tender meat, breaking down the collagenous fascia and muscle), partially covered with water, broth, wine, or fat in a covered iron pot. The result is a remarkably tender and flavorful meat. I would consider this cooking method to be one of the great secrets to French traditional cooking. Some of my favorite recipes are made by braising meat.

CARPACCIO
Of Italian origin, meaning raw, thinly sliced meat or fish.

CAUL (PORK CAUL) — *LA CRÉPINE*
A kind of web-like fat that is used to hold meatballs or patés together.

COOKING — *CUIRE*
The cooking process begins at 140°F (60°C). Most bacteria, good or bad, are killed between 140°F and 150°F (60°C and 65°C), though an egg yolk, for example, is not "set" until 158°F (70°C) and the white does not coagulate until 176°F (80°C). We cook for certain lengths of time to achieve certain levels of thoroughness of cooking or "doneness," called *la cuisson* in French.

DEGLAZING — *DÉGLACER*
Deglazing is done by pouring cold or room temperature liquid into a pan in which vegetables or meat have been caramelized to remove the remaining caramelized sugars stuck to the pan. The mix of liquid and sugars can be incorporated into a sauce or can augment the flavor of another dish prepared in the pan. For example, I will deglaze a pan of sautéed potatoes with a bit of broth and then throw in some Swiss chard. This has the effect of deglazing the pan while also creating a little warm sauce and flavor for the chard. This can be done with any leafy greens that you might cook. During a January 1994 PBS cooking session with Julia Child, French chef Jacques Pépin defined the glaze as "the solidified or crystallized juices (*les sucs*) glued to bottom of the pan and the process of deglazing (*déglacer*) is to add liquid to those solidified juices and create a sauce." Julia Child adds to this, saying, "One of the great secrets of French cooking is all the care that is taken in deglazing and saving every possible bit of juice."[2] (Of course, the pan requires diffusion of heat throughout the metal—another reason to have high-quality, thick-bottomed equipment.)

Degrees of Doneness – Températures de Cuisson à Coeur or Stades de Cuisson

For Beef — *Pour le Boeuf*

Raw – *Cru*: Uncooked

Bloody or Extra Rare – *Bleu* (briefly seared on the outside, raw on the inside): 113°F to 122°F (45°C to 50°C)

Rare – *Saignant* (cool red center): 122°F to 131°F (50°C to 55°C)

Medium Rare (warm red center): 135°F (57°C)

Medium – *À point* (warm pink center): 140°F to 144°F (60°C to 63°C)

Medium Well (slightly pink center): 144°F to 150°F (63°C to 66°C)

Well Done – *Bien Cuit* (little or no pink, cooked through): 151°F to 160°F (66°C to 71°C)

Note: Americans' "well done" is often considered already "overcooked" (trop cuit).

Very Well Done – *Tres Bien Cuit*: 167°F (75°C). Bordering on overdone. Watch out!

Overdone – *Trop Cuit*: 185°F (85°C). Leathery, over-browned on the inside, no juices left. Because it is the raw juices of the meat that lend it its flavor, once these are cooked off, the meat becomes tougher and less flavorful.

Burned – *Brûlé*: No good. Try it again!

For Lamb — *Pour l'Agneau*

Bloody or Extra Rare – *Bleu*: 131°F to 135°F (55°C to 57°C)

Rare – *Saignant*: 140°F (60°C)

Medium Rare: 140°F to 149°F (60°C to 65°C)

Medium – *À point*: 149°F to 158°F (65°C to 70°C)

Medium Well: 158°F (70°C)

Well Done – *Bien Cuit*: 158°F to 167°F (70°C to 75°C)

Note: Americans' "well done" is often considered already "overcooked" (trop cuit).

For Pork — *Pour le Porc*

Medium Rare: 145°F to 148°F (63°C to 64°C)

Medium – *À point*: 149°F to 160°F (65°C to 71°C)

Well Done – *Bien Cuit*: 170°F to 176°F (77°C to 80°C).

DICING
Cutting into little cubes.

FLEUR DE SEL
Literally, "flower of the salt" (meaning "cream of the crop"), *fleur de sel* is the fine layer of salt that forms on the surface of sea water that has been sequestered in clay beds by the sea. This kind of salt harvesting is a French tradition dating back at least to the Middle Ages. *Fleur de sel* is the most prized of sea salts with its delicate crunch, small crystal size, and pure whiteness. It is skimmed off the top of the water with a special long-handled sieve at the end of each day for several weeks during the summer. Coarse sea salt (*gros sel*) is formed beneath the water's surface. These larger, heavier salt crystals are raked into pyramids and can have shades of grey and pink color. Finely ground sea salt (*sel fin de mer*) is often used for seasoning during cooking, as is course sea salt, while *fleur de sel* is often used as a garnish on both sweet and savory dishes.

"FOUR SPICES" — QUATRE ÉPICES
A blend of spices often used in French cuisine, consisting of ground clove, ginger, nutmeg, and pepper (white, black, or both).

FRENCH PARADOX
University of Bordeaux Professor and renowned French scientist Serge Renaud (1927-2012), considered the father of the term "French Paradox," published a study in the British medical journal *The Lancet* in 1992 explaining the contradictory nature of the consumption of French cuisine—particularly that of the Southwest, which utilizes high amounts of saturated animal fats—and low mortality rates in France (particularly in the French Southwest) from cardiovascular disease. Renaud also proposed in this study that the platelet-inhibiting effects of alcohol (primarily red wine) *consumed slowly and with a high-fat meal* could account for the French, and particularly the French Southwest, populations' protection from coronary heart disease.[3]

FRYING — FRITURE
Cooking over high heat with a large amount of fat for a longer duration than a short sear or a sauté.

GARNISHED BOUQUET — BOUQUET GARNI
A *bouquet garni* is a small bundle of aromatic herbs in a combination which may be comprised of laurel (bay) leaves, thyme, leek, and rosemary, parsley, or savory tied together in a small bundle with string or in cheese cloth.

GLAZING — GLACER
A savory or sweet glaze on top of a food applied by dipping, drizzling, or with a brush.

GOURMAND
A person who enjoys eating and/or often eats too much. The terms "glutton" or "gourmandizer" have negative connotations, connoting someone who overeats and enjoys doing so, whereas a "*bon vivant*," denotes someone who enjoys the luxurious pleasure of food and drink, but is not necessarily concerned with the benefits of the food. In this book, we are concerned more with epicures, foodies, and gourmets: people who care more for quality than quantity, connoisseurs of taking pleasure in good food and drink with a discerning palate, whom I would also call *gastronomes*. "Gourmet" can also be used as an adjective to describe a meal (or a restaurant) using fresh, high-quality ingredients.

GRATINATING — GRATINER
To bake a vegetable or other dish in the oven with the effect of cooking the inside of the dish while browning the outside and turning it a bit crispy on top.

GRILLING — GRILLER
Grilling is a kind of dry cooking of meat or fish by searing it at a high temperature without additional fat (*la matière grasse*). However, when I am grilling in a pan, I usually utilize a fat, either olive oil for fish or tallow for beef, etc., to add flavor to the meat or fish and to aid in cooking. Moisture from the steaks may accumulate in the pan. This can be poured

off in between batches of steaks or cutlets if there is too much, otherwise, the meat will be steamed instead of grilled. As for the fat that drips into the fire, indigenous peoples catch and consume the drippings of fat falling from these tissues. One historical example is herdsmen from South Australia in the 1800s, who "roasted the fattest parts (of their fattest sheep) against a fire with a dripping pan underneath, later dipping the meat into the drippings as they ate."[4]

HERBES DE PROVENCE
A traditional combination of four herbs: savory (a kind of wild basil), oregano, thyme, and rosemary.

LARD (FAT BACK OR BACK FAT)
When pork lard is rendered (heated, separating solid proteins and liquid fat), the end result is a fluffy, creamy, and essentially tasteless lard, (*saindoux*) suitable for cooking and baking.

LARDING — LARDER
The technique of stuffing extra fat into one or more holes in a piece of meat for flavor and enhanced juiciness. Traditionally, strips of lard were "threaded" into meat using a "trussing" needle (*aiguille* à *brider*).

LARDONS
Bacon pieces that are either cut into small cubes or small strips of about a half-inch to one inch (1.25 cm to 2.5 cm) in length.

LEAF LARD AND LARD — SAINDOUX
Visceral pork fat and pork "fat back" (or "back fat") rendered into lard suitable for cooking and baking.

MAILLARD REACTION — LA RÉACTION MAILLARD
Named after French chemist Louis-Camille Maillard who observed in 1912 that amino acids in food become colored or brown when heated, adding to the complexity of aromas and flavors, in what is called non-enzymatic glycation. *Caramelization*, the browning of sugars in food through the application of heat, also adds to the sweetness and complexity of flavor. This browning technique is one of the secrets to flavor in French cuisine. Similarly, our cells undergo a "browning" glycation process as well. There is indeed a tradeoff between cooking and caramelizing food and eating food raw or only steamed without much flavor. Browning food may seem an unnecessary health risk to some because of the glycation of sugars, but browning meats and vegetables is, as I have noted before, one of the keys to flavor in French cooking.

MINCE
Even smaller, and more irregular, than dicing. This may be done by hand or in a mini-chopper.

MIREPOIX
The combination of carrots, onion, and celery (or celery root), often in a 1:2:1 ratio respectively; it is the basis for many stocks, broths, and soups.

NOUVELLE CUISINE
Most famously used by French food critics Gault and Millaut, nouvelle cuisine referred to food prepared by the top chefs of the late 1960s, in particular Paul Bocuse, who published the "*10 Commandments of Nouvelle Cuisine.*" These included using the freshest ingredients and the newest techniques and technology (while not being too modern), shortening menus, outing heavy sauces in favor of butter and herbs, reducing complication by using fewer marinades, shortening cooking times, and steaming. It was an era of inventive combinations and pairings and of chefs paying attention to their clients' dietary needs.[5]

OFFAL — LES ABATS
Also known as variety meats, they are the trimmings, head, feet, and internal organs, used as food. In my definition of offal, I include the skin and bones.

PAN FRYING — POÊLER
Searing a meat with fat over high heat and then continuing to cook the meat in fat over high or medium-high heat.[6]

PINCH — *UNE PINCÉE*
A pinch means using three fingers to grip salt, pepper, herbs, or spices.

POACHING — *POCHER*
Plunging a food (like an egg or a piece of fish) into water that is beginning to show bubbles (at 195°F or 90°C), for a duration of one to several minutes.

PRESERVING — *CONFIRE*
To preserve *meats* by saturating them in fat in a process that includes squeezing out the water content through slow cooking (and sometimes cool storage over weeks or months with the goal of tenderizing, such as with duck legs); to preserve or candy *fruits* by replacing their water content and saturating them in sugar, also in a slow cooking process. The resulting preserves are called "*confit*" such as preserved duck (*confit de canard*) or *confiture* for a marmalade or jam. To *confire* meats means to cook slowly in fat (saturate in one product), which has the effect of squeezing out water in the meat. To c*onfire* fruits means to saturate in sugar, as in making marmalades (*marmalades*). Jams (*confitures*) and jellies (*gelées*) traditionally use sugar or fruit juices as preserving agents but may also be made without added sugar, which however, shortens their shelf life.

RENDERING — *FONDRE LA GRAISSE*
To render fat is to melt raw fat that is finely chopped (usually by a food processor or sausage grinding machine, if not by hand). The liquid fat is run through a sieve and stored in jars. This process is most easily done with beef, pork, and lamb fat. The cracklings (*grattons*), or solids, left over are used like bacon bits.

ROASTING — *RÔTIR*
Cooking something at temperatures between about 355°F and 465°F (180°C and 240°C) to form a crust on the outside while keeping the meat tender and juicy on the inside.[7] Roasting can be done with little or no additional fat. For my beef, lamb, and pork roasts, I often add olive oil for flavor and additional fat. Butter is also often used for certain roasts in traditional French recipes. The practices of barding or larding are also used to add fat to a roast.

SAUTÉING — *SAUTER* (OR *FRICASSER*)
Sauter is the verb meaning "to jump" in French. In cooking, it can mean to fry, cook, or brown in fat, depending on the context. I use this term frequently in my recipes to describe cooking through the meat or vegetables, uncovered, on a medium to medium-high heat, often after having first seared the meat. This process slightly browns the meat or vegetables, adding to both flavor and texture. Sautéing also leaves a crusty brown residue (*fond*) at the bottom of the pan which can be deglazed using liquid or even more fat to dislodge the caramelized pieces of food stuck to the pan, adding flavor to the food.

SEARING — *SAISIR*
To sear meat on the outside creating a light, brown-colored (not blackened) crust while holding the juices inside and keeping the inner meat tender. Meats can be seared (not charred) and then continue to cook or fry in a pan (*poêler*) until the desired "doneness" (*cuisson*) has been reached, such as medium rare. The pan needs to be heated at medium-high to high heat to sear or brown a meat or vegetable. Flicking a drop of water onto the pan to see if it sizzles is the way chefs see whether their pan is hot enough to begin searing. For searing I generally use saturated fats like tallow or lard, as the searing process can oxidize or burn more fragile oils like olive oil. However, there is always a personal call on preference in terms of taste and availability. Olive oil makes things taste good and is often preferred by many cooks for this reason. A combination of butter and olive oil may be used to increase the smoke point of the oil and to enhance flavor.

SIMMER — *MIJOTER*
Heating a pot of liquid over low or medium-low heat to obtain the effect of a gurgling or gentle bubbling; indicates that the liquid is cooking just at or below the boiling point, but not at a rapid, rolling boil.

STEAMING — *CUIRE À LA VAPEUR*
Heating (usually vegetables or fish) in steam from boiling water. This is a "fat-free" way of cooking a vegetable, keeping much of the integrity of the flavor of the vegetable, but it usually requires bathing the steamed vegetable in butter, olive oil, or other fat to bring out more flavor, as well as for the body to be able to absorb the vegetable's fat-soluble nutrients. This method of cooking became popular with the "nouvelle cuisine" of the late 1960s.

STEWING OR SIMMERING — *MIJOTER*
Slow-cooking meat submerged in water, broth, or wine, usually over several hours.

STIR-FRY OR STEAM-FRY — *ÉTUVER*
To cook slowly or soften in a pan, covered, over medium or low heat. This is usually a technique reserved for vegetables and/or thin strips of meat.

SUET — *SUIF*
Hard, protective fat around the kidneys of beef, lamb, and pork.

TALLOW — *SUIF*
Rendered beef or lamb fat. Tallow is the body fat of beef, bison, or lamb that can be rendered into a useable fat for cooking and even for making homemade moisturizing salves.

TRUSSING — *TROUSSER (BRIDER)*
To tie poultry using a special trussing needle (*aiguille* à *brider*).

VACUUM-PACKAGED COOKING — *CUIRE À SOUS-VIDE*
Sous-vide cooking uses soft plastic bags at temperatures just below 212°F (100°C) in a hermetically sealed, humid packaging. The chemical agents in plastic such as Antimony (Sb), Bisphenol A (BPA), and BPS,[8] are known hormone-disrupting and carcinogenic substances and are used to harden and soften plastics. The concern is that these chemicals may leach into the food at higher temperatures around 158°F (70°C), much like a plastic water bottle will leach chemicals into the water if left in the car on a hot summer day. To me, *sous-vide* cooking is neither traditional nor advisable, given the potential risks from heated plastics. It is an example of using new, untested methods to cook for the supposed reasons of economical food preparation, food tenderness, and flavor, when the tried-and-true methods of traditional cooking work just as well without the added dangers from plastics.

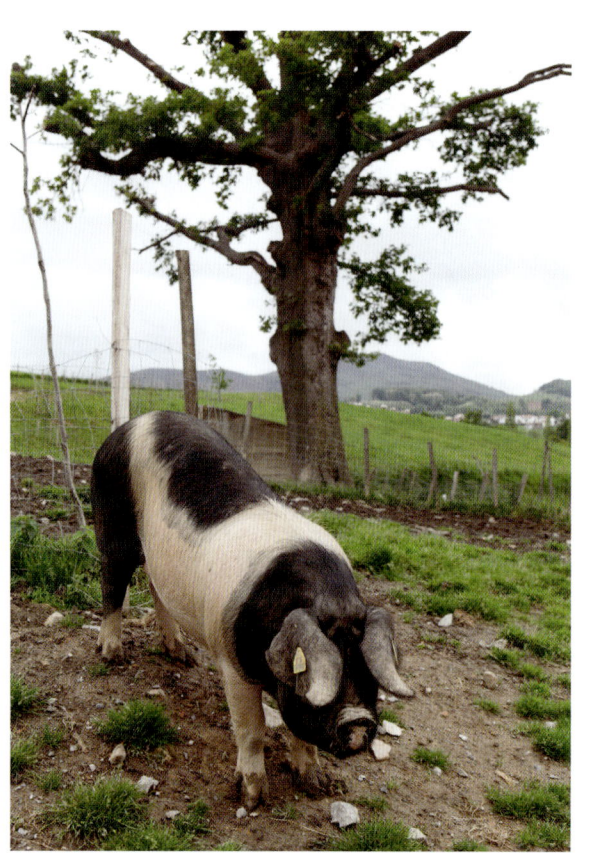

Basque Pig, Agerria Farm

RESOURCES AND FURTHER READING

*"The further a society drifts from truth,
the more it will hate those who speak it."*
—George Orwell

This is my curated selection of primal-paleo-ancestral-related publications, books, podcasts, and websites. This section also includes a few lists of resources and places in France relevant to this book, such as books, shops, and products of interest. Many of these resources fall into multiple categories, but for the sake of brevity, I have chosen one category for each. As research and information evolves and develops, it is advisable to sign up for newsletters or blogs of your favorite sources to get the most up-to-date information. Please refer to my website www.BordeauxKitchen.com where you will find updated resources on food and health-related topics and links to relevant books, practitioners, events, and documentaries, as well as an extensive presentation of the latest research in ancestral health (conveniently organized into an "A to Z of the Primal/Paleo/Ancestral Lifestyle" format).

ADDICTION TO "FOOD" AND MISLEADING "FOOD" LABELING

Always Hungry?, 2016, Dr. David Ludwig

Big Fat Food Fraud: Confessions of a Health-Food Hustler, 2016, Jeff Scot Philips

The Craving Mind: From Cigarettes to Smartphones to Love – Why We Get Hooked and How We Can Break Bad Habits, 2017, Judson Brewer

Death by Food Pyramid, 2014, Denise Minger

The Dorito Effect, 2016, Mark Schatzker,

Food Junkies: The Truth About Food Addiction, 2014, Vera Tarman

The Hungry Brain: Outsmarting the Instincts That Make Us Overeat, 2017, Stephan Guyenet

Real Food/Fake Food: Why You Don't Know What You're Eating and What You Can Do About It, 2016, Larry Olmstead

Salt Sugar Fat: How the Food Giants Hooked Us, Michael Moss

Wired to Eat, 2017, Robb Wolf

ANTIBIOTICS

Beyond Antibiotics, 2009, Michael A. Schmidt

Herbal Antibiotics: Natural Alternatives for Treating Drug-resistant Bacteria, 2nd Edition, 2012 Stephen Harrod Buhner

ANXIETY AND MOOD

The Anti-Anxiety Food Solution, 2011, Trudy Scott

The Diet Cure, 2012, Julia Ross

The Hormone Cure, 2013, Dr. Sara Gottfried

The Mood Cure, 2003, Julia Ross

AUTISM

Biological Treatments for Autism and PDD, 2008, Dr. William Shaw

AutismOne www.autismone.org

Bedrok www.bedrokcommunity.org

Epidemic Answers epidemicanswers.org

Nourishing Hope nourishinghope.com

The Power of Poop thepowerofpoop.com

AUTOIMMUNITY

The Alternative Autoimmune Cookbook, 2014, Angie Alt

The Autoimmune Fix, 2016, Dr. Tom O'Bryan

The Autoimmune Solution, 2017, Dr. Amy Myers

The Autoimmune Wellness Handbook, 2016, Mickey Trescott, and Angie Alt

Gluten Freedom, 2014, Alessio Fasano

The Paleo Approach, 2014, Dr. Sarah Ballantyne

Plague: One Scientist's Intrepid Search for the Truth about Human Retroviruses and Chronic Fatigue Syndrome (ME/CFS), Autism, and Other Diseases, Reprint Edition, 2014, Kent Heckenlively and Judy Mikovits

A Simple Guide to the Paleo Autoimmune Protocol, 2015, Eileen Laird

BORDEAUX AND CHÂTEAUX

The Bordeaux Kitchen (my blog listing my favorite addresses, châteaux, and resources in Bordeaux and France) www.BordeauxKitchen.com

BRAIN HEALTH, ALZHEIMER'S DISEASE, AND NEURODEGENERATIVE DISEASE

The Alzheimer's Antidote: Using a Low-Carb, High-Fat Diet to Fight Alzheimer's Disease, Memory Loss, and Cognitive Decline, 2017, Amy Berger

The Anti-Alzheimer's Prescription: The Science-Proven Prevention Plan to Start at Any Age, 2009, Dr. Vincent Fortanasce

The Better Brain Solution: How to Start Now—at Any Age—to Reverse and Prevent Insulin Resistance of the Brain, Sharpen Cognitive Function, and Avoid Memory Loss, January 2, 2018, Dr. Steven Masley

Brain Building Nutrition, 2006, Michael A. Schmidt

The End of Alzheimer's: The First Program to Prevent and Reverse Cognitive Decline, 2017, Dale Bredesen

The Edge Effect: Achieve Total Health and Longevity with the Balanced Brain Advantage, 2005, Dr. Eric Braverman

Genius Foods: Become Smarter, Happier, and More Productive, While Protecting Your Brain Health for Life, 2018, Max Lugavere and Dr. Paul Gewal

Grain Brain, 2013, Dr. David Perlmutter

Move Into Life: NeuroMovement for Lifelong Vitality, 2016, Ana Baniel

Why Isn't My Brain Working?, 2016, Datis Kharrazian

BUTCHERY, MEAT, CHARCUTERIE, AND KNIVES
The Art of Beef Cutting: A Meat Professional's Guide to Butchering and Merchandising, 2011, Kari Underly

Charcuterie: The Craft of Salting, Smoking and Curing, 2013, Michael Ruhlman

Charcuterie and French Pork Cookery, 2001 (Reprint 2012), Jane Grigson

Sausage Making, 2014, Ryan Farr

Whole Beast Butchery, 2011, Ryan Farr

The Butcher's Guild www.thebutchersguild.org

Fleishers Craft Butchery (butcher shops, butchery education and training) www.fleishers.com

WÜSTHOF knife care and sharpening www.wusthof.com/care-and-sharpening

WÜSTHOF knife skills www.wusthof.com/knife-skills

CANCER
Cancer as a Metabolic Disease, 2012, Thomas Seyfried

Conquering Cancer: Volume One - 50 Pancreatic and Breast Cancer Patients on The Gonzalez Nutritional Protocol, 2016, Dr. Nicholas Gonzalez

Fight Cancer with a Ketogenic Diet, Third Edition: Using a Low-Carb, Fat-Burning Diet as Metabolic Therapy, 2017, Ellen Davis

The Metabolic Approach to Cancer: Integrating Deep Nutrition, the Ketogenic Diet, and Nontoxic Bio-Individualized Therapies, 2017, Dr. Nasha Winters and Jess Higgins Kelley

Tripping Over the Truth, 2017, Travis Christofferson

The Truth About Cancer, 2016, Ty Bollinger

Allison Gannet (a brain cancer conqueror) www.alisongannett.com

Charlie Foundation for Ketogenic Therapies www.charliefoundation.org and ketoconnect.org

Foundation for Metabolic Cancer Therapies www.singlecausesinglecure.org

Integrative cancer therapies search engine www.a4m.com/directory.html#

Quest to Cure Cancer www.questtocurecancer.com

CHILDREN AND PREGNANCY
Nourish Without Nagging, 2016, Dr. Brett Hill

A Compromised Generation: The Epidemic of Chronic Illness in America's Children, 2010, Beth Lambert

Digestive Wellness for Children: How to Strengthen the Immune System & Prevent Disease through Healthy Digestion, 2006, Elizabeth Lipski

Ending the Food Fight, 2008, Dr. David Ludwig

Super Food for Super Children, 2016, Tim Noakes

Real Food Recovery: The Busy Mom's Guide to Health and Healing, 2016, Mandy Blume

Paleo Girl, 2014, Leslie Klenke (for tweens and teens)

The Mama Natural Week-by-Week Guide to Pregnancy and Childbirth, 2017, Genevieve Howland

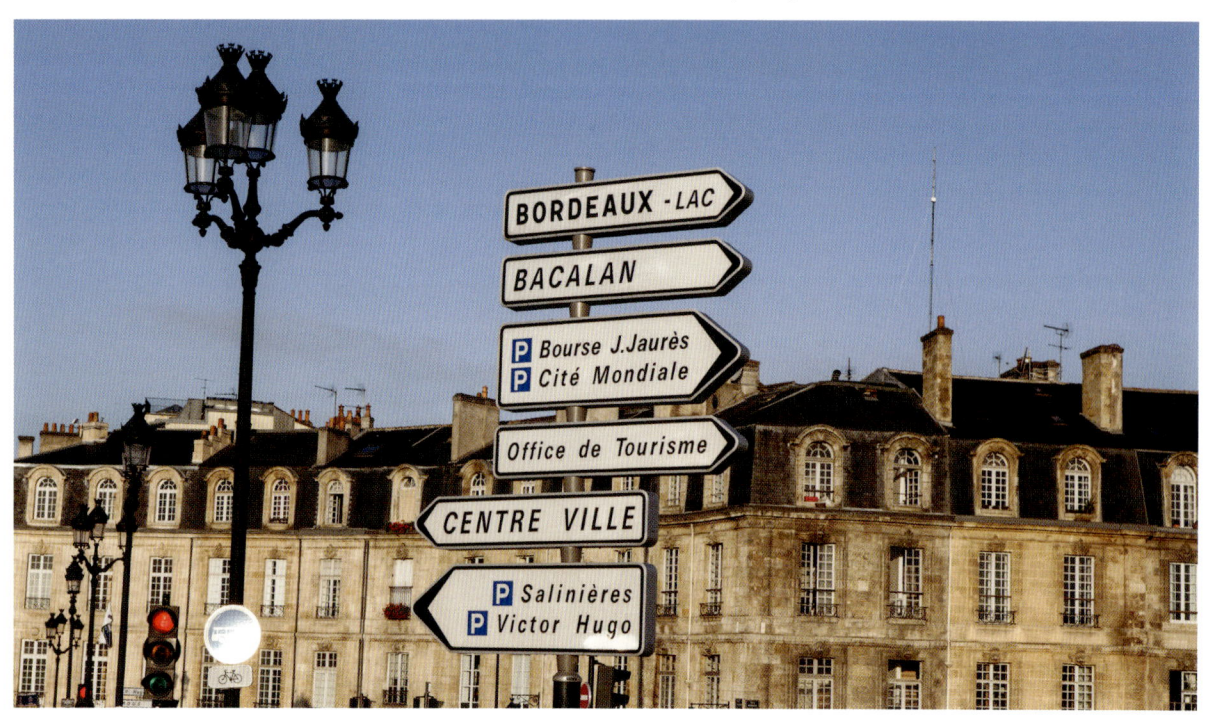

A Compromised Generation: The Epidemic of Chronic Illness in America's Children, 2010, Beth Lambert and Victoria Kobliner

Fat Head Kids: Stuff About Diet and Health I Wish I Knew When I Was Your Age, 2017, Tom Naughton

Eat Like A Dinosaur, 2012, Paleo Parents (recipes kids like and can help with)

Real Food for Rookies: Healthy Cooking – Traditional Food – Vibrant Health, 2015, Kelly Moeggenborg

The N.D.D. Book: How Nutrition Deficit Disorder Affects Your Child's Learning, Behavior, and Health, and What You Can Do About It—Without Drugs (Sears Parenting Library), 2009, Dr. William Sears

Your Healthy Pregnancy with Thyroid Disease: A Guide to Fertility, Pregnancy, and Postpartum Wellness, 2016, Dana Trentini and Mary Shomon

Healthy Kids Happy Kids healthykidshappykids.com

Kids Cook Real Food kidscookrealfood.com

Kitchen Stewardship www.kitchenstewardship.com

Pete Evans: Kids School Lunches peteevans.com/initiatives/kids-school-lunches

CHOLESTEROL, HEART HEALTH, AND STATINS

The 30-Day Heart Tuneup: A Breakthrough Medical Plan to Prevent and Reverse Heart Disease, 2014, Dr. Steven Masley

Cholesterol and Saturated Fat Prevent Heart Disease: Evidence from 101 Scientific Papers, 2012, David Evans

Cholesterol Clarity, 2013, Jimmy Moore and Dr. Eric Westman

The Cholesterol Myths: Exposing the Fallacy that Saturated Fat and Cholesterol Cause Heart Disease, 2000, Dr. Uffe Ravnskov

The Great Cholesterol Myth: Why Lowering Your Cholesterol Won't Prevent Heart Disease—and the Statin-Free Plan that Will, 2012, Johnny Bowden, PhD and Dr. Stephen Sinatra

Human Heart, Cosmic Heart: A Doctor's Quest to Understand, Treat, and Prevent Cardiovascular Disease, 2016, Dr. Thomas Cowan

Low Cholesterol Leads to an Early Death: Evidence from 101 Scientific Papers, 2012, David Evans

Smart Fat, 2017, Dr. Steven Masley and Dr. Johnny Bowden

Statins Toxic Side Effects: Evidence from 500 Scientific Papers, 2015, David Evans

Heart Attack New Approaches (Dr. Knut Sroka) heartattacknew.com

COOKBOOKS AND FOOD BLOGS (PRIMAL-PALEO-ANCESTRAL)

The Ancestral Table, 2014, Russ Crandall

The Autoimmune Paleo Cookbook, 2014, Mickey Trescott

The Bulletproof Diet, 2014, Dave Asprey

Danielle Walker's Against All Grain Celebrations: A Year of Gluten-Free, Dairy-Free, and Paleo Recipes for Every Occasion, 2016, Danielle Walker

Eating on the Wild Side, 2014, Jo Robinson

The Elimination Diet: Discover the Foods That Are Making You Sick and Tired and Feel Better Fast, 2016, Tom Malterre and Alissa Segerston

Food: What the Heck Should I Eat?, 2018, Dr. Mark Hyman

Gather, The Art of Paleo Entertaining, 2013, Bill Staley and Hayley Mason

The Grain Brain Whole Life Plan, 2016, Dr. David Perlmutter

The Homegrown Paleo Cookbook, 2015, Diana Rodgers

It Starts with Food, 2014, and *The Whole 30*, 2015, Dallas and Melissa Hartwig

The Ketogenic Cookbook: Nutritious Low-Carb, High-Fat Paleo Meals to Heal Your Body, 2015, Jimmy Moore and Maria Emmerich

The Ketogenic Kitchen, 2016, Domini Kemp and Patricia Daly

Nourishing Broth: An Old-Fashioned Remedy for the Modern World, 2014, Sally Fallon Morell and Kaayla T. Daniel

Nourishing Traditions: The Cookbook That Challenges Politically Correct Nutrition and Diet Dictocrats, 2001, Sally Fallon Morell and Kaayla T. Daniel

Paleo by Season, 2014, Pete Servold

The Paleo Chef, 2014, Pete Evans

Paleo Grilling: A Modern Caveman's Guide to Cooking with Fire, 2014, Tony Federico and James William Phelan

Practical Paleo, 2016, Diane Sanfilippo

The Primal Kitchen Cookbook: Eat Like Your Life Depends On It!, 2017, Mark Sisson

Raw Paleo: The Extreme Advantages of Eating Paleo Foods in the Raw, 2016, Melissa Henig and Alfredo Urso

Super Food for Super Children, 2016, Tim Noakes

The Wahls Protocol Cooking for Life: The Revolutionary Modern Paleo Plan to Treat All Chronic Autoimmune Conditions, 2017, Dr. Terry Wahls

Weeknight Paleo: 100+ Easy and Delicious Family-Friendly Meals, 2017, Charles and Julie Mayfield

Well Fed, 2011, Melissa Joulwan

The Wellness Mama Cookbook, 2016, Katie Wells

Carrie Brown (keto chef) www.carriebrown.com

Civilized Caveman (George Bryant) www.civilizedcavemancooking.com

Diet Doctor (Dr. Andreas Eenfeldt on low-carb eating) www.dietdoctor.com

Eat REAL (initiative by pediatrician Dr. Robert Lustig) www.eatreal.org

Eat the Butter (vintage eating, Jenni Calihan) www.eatthebutter.org

Elana's Pantry (cookbook author Elana Amsterdam) www.elanaspantry.com

Healing Histamine (non-GMO project) www.healinghistamine.com

Maria Mind Body Health (Maria Emmerich, ketogenic diet and exercise physiology) www.mariamindbodyhealth.com

Non-GMO Project www.nongmoproject.org/about

Non-GMO Project Shopping Guide www.nongmoshoppingguide.com

Nourishing Plot (blog by Becky Plotner, ND) www.nourishingplot.com

Paleo Leap (paleo recipes and articles) www.paleoleap.com

PaleoHacks (blog focusing on health advice, recipes, and natural-movement exercises) www.paleohacks.com

Primal Chef (www.theprimalchef.com)

Tasty Yummies (grain-free recipes and how to make nut butters) www.tasty-yummies.com

The Whole Journey (food as medicine video blog) www.thewholejourney.com/blog

COOKBOOKS AND FOOD BLOGS (NON-PRIMAL-PALEO-ANCESTRAL)

Around My French Table: More than 300 Recipes from My Home to Yours, 2010, Dorrie Greenspan

The Cooking of Southwest France, 2nd ed. 2005, Paula Wolfert

Food and Friends: Recipes and Memories from Simca's Cuisine, 1991, Simone Beck and Suzanne Patterson

Fromages, 2016, Dominique Bouchait

Le Grand Cours de Cuisine de l'Atelier des Chefs, 2013, Hachette Cuisine

I Know How to Cook, 2009 (first published in French in 1932), Geneviève "Ginette" Mathiot

A Kitchen in France: A Year of Cooking in My Farmhouse, 2014, Mimi Thorisson

Mastering the Art of French Cooking, 1961 (Volume 1) and 1970 (Volume 2), Julia Child

Memories of Gascony, 1990, Pierre Koffmann

Morceaux Choisis, 2015, Hugo Desnoyer

My Paris Kitchen, 2014, David Lebovitz

The Nourished Kitchen: Farm-to-Table Recipes for the Traditional Foods Lifestyle, 2014, Jennifer McGruther

Odd Bits: How to Cook the Rest of the Animal, 2011, Jennifer McLagan

Viandes: Encyclopédie des Produits & des Métiers de Bouche, 2013, Jean-François Mallet, Hachette Cuisine

The World Authority Larousse Gastronimique: The Encyclopedia of Food, Wine and Cookery, First American Edition, 1961, Prosper Montagné

La Viande (French website on everything to know about meats) www.la-viande.fr

DIET, DISEASE, AND NUTRITION

5-HTP: The Natural Way to Overcome Depression, Obesity, and Insomnia, 1999, Michael Murray

Big Fat Food Fraud: Confessions of a Health-Food Hustler, 2016, Jeff Scot Philips

The Body Ecology Diet: Recovering Your Health and Rebuilding Your Immunity, 2011, Donna Gates

The Case Against Sugar, 2017, Gary Taubes

The Complete Guide to Fasting: Heal Your Body Through Intermittent, Alternate-Day, and Extended Fasting, 2016, Jimmy Moore and Dr. Jason Fung

Death by Food Pyramid, 2014, Denise Minger

Deep Nutrition, 2017, Dr. Catherine Shanahan

Diabetes Unpacked: Just Science and Sense. No Sugar Coating, 2017, Professor Tim Noakes, Dr. Jason Fung, and Nina Teicholz

The Fibro Fix, 2016, Dr. David Brady

Food and Western Disease: Health and Nutrition from an Evolutionary Perspective, 2010, Staffan Lindeberg

Good Calories, Bad Calories: Fats, Carbs and the Controversial Science of Diet and Health, 2008, Gary Taubes

The Grain Brain Whole Life Plan: Boost Brain Performance, Lose Weight, and Achieve Optimal Health, 2016, Dr. David Perlmutter

Gut and Psychology Syndrome, 2010, Natasha Campbell-McBride

Head Strong, 2017, Dave Asprey

Heal Your Leaky Gut: Secrets to Treating this Dangerous and Hidden Cause of Chronic Diseases, 2017, Dr. David Brownstein

Heal Your Pain Now: The Revolutionary Program to Reset Your Brain and Body for a Pain-Free Life, 2017, Joe Tatta

Honest Medicine: Effective, Time-Tested, Inexpensive Treatments for Life-Threatening Diseases, 2013, Julia E. Schopick

JJ Virgin's Sugar Impact Diet: Drop 7 Hidden Sugars, Lose Up to 10 Pounds in Just 2 Weeks, 2016, J.J. Virgin

The Kalish Method: Healing the Body, Mapping the Mind, 2012, Dr. Daniel Kalish

Lore of Nutrition: Challenging conventional dietary beliefs, 2018, Professor Tim Noakes and Marika Sboros

A Mind of Your Own, 2016, Dr. Kelly Brogan

Never Bet Against Occam: Mast Cell Activation Disease and the Modern Epidemics of Chronic Illness and Medical Complexity, 2016, Dr. Lawrence Afrin

No Grain, No Pain, 2016, Dr. Peter Osborne

Nutrition and Physical Degeneration, 2009, Dr. Weston A. Price

The Primal Prescription, Dr. Doug McGuff and Robert Murphy

Paleo Principles, 2017, Sarah Ballantyne

The Plant Paradox: The Hidden Dangers in "Healthy" Foods That Cause Disease and Weight Gain, 2017, Dr. Steven Gundry

Rich Food Poor Food: The Ultimate Grocery Purchasing System (GPS), 2013, Mira and Jayson Calton

The Salt Fix: Why the Experts Got It All Wrong—and How Eating More Might Save Your Life, 2017, Dr. James DiNicolantonio

Sexy Brain: Sizzling Intimacy & Balanced Hormones Prevent Alzheimer's, Cancer, Depression & Divorce, 2017, Dr. Devaki Lindsey Berkson

Vegetarianism Explained: Making an Informed Decision, 2017, Dr. Natasha Campbell-McBride

The Vitamin D Solution: A 3-Step Strategy to Cure Our Most Common Health Problems, 2011, Dr. Michael Holick

The Wahls Protocol, 2014, Dr. Tery Wahls

Wheat Belly, 2014, Dr. William Davis

Why Stomach Acid Is Good for You: Natural Relief from Heartburn, Indigestion, Reflux and GERD, 2001, Dr. Jonathan Wright

Why We Get Fat, 2011, Gary Taubes

The Wild Diet, 2016, Abel James

Ask Dr. Sears www.askdrsears.com

Aspire Natural Health aspirenaturalhealth.com

Chris Kresser www.chriskresser.com

Healing Histamine (low histamine chef Yasmina Ykelenstam) healinghistamine.com

Kaayla T. Daniel PhD drkaayladaniel.com

Mama Natural www.mamanatural.com

Natural Health 365 www.naturalhealth365.com

Price-Pottenger Nutrition Foundation price-pottenger.org

The Unconventional Traditional (freedom from fibromyalgia) unconventionaltraditional.com

Weston A. Price Foundation www.westonaprice.org [1]

ELECTROMAGNETIC FIELDS (EMFS)
Dirty Electricity, 2012, Samuel Milham

Overpowered, 2015, Martin Blank

Radiation Nation: Fallout of Modern Technology, 2017, Daniel T. & Ryan DeBaun

Sans Mobile, 2015, Marine Richard (French)

Zapped, 2011, Ann Louise Gittleman

The BabySafe Project www.babysafeproject.org

ElectricSense (Lloyd Burrell) www.electricsense.com

EMF Analysis (Jeromy Johnson) www.emfanalysis.com

Environmental Health Trust ehtrust.org

GEOVITAL en.geovital.com

National Association for Children and Safe Technology www.nacst.org

Optimal Health (Dr. Jack Kruse's website) www.jackkruse.com

Show Us the Fine Print showthefineprint.org

ENVIRONMENT, HEALTH, AND FOOD SYSTEM TRANSPARENCY
The Art is Long: Big Health and the New Warrior Activist, 2017, Frank Forencich

Cod: A Biography of a Fish that Changed the World, 1998, Mark Kurlansky

Our Stolen Future, 1997, Theo Colborn

Silent Spring, 1962, Rachel Carson

Earthjustice earthjustice.org

Environmental Working Group www.ewg.org

Feed the Truth www.feedthetruth.org

Moms Across America www.momsacrossamerica.com

The Nature Conservancy www.nature.org

Natural Resources Defense Council www.nrdc.org

Pesticide Action Network North America www.panna.org

Slow Food USA www.slowfoodusa.org

EXERCISE AND MOVEMENT
Beyond Training, 2014, Ben Greenfield

Deskbound: Standing Up to a Sitting World, 2016, Dr. Kelly Starrett

Dynamic Aging: Simple Exercises for Whole-Body Mobility, 2017, Katy Bowman

Eat Well, Move Well, Live Well: 52 Ways to Feel Better in a Week, 2016, Roland and Galina Denzel

The Great Cardio Myth: Why Cardio Exercise Won't Get You Slim, Strong, or Healthy - and the New High-Intensity Strength Training Program that Will, 2017, Craig Ballantyne

How to Eat, Move and Be Healthy, 2004, Paul Chek

Move Your DNA: Restore Your Health Through Natural Movement, Expanded Edition, 2017, Katy Bowman

The Practice of Natural Movement: Reclaim Power, Health and Freedom, 2018, Erwan Le Corre

Primal Endurance, 2016, Mark Sisson and Brad Kearns

The Roll Model: A Step-By-Step Guide to Erase Pain, Improve Mobility, and Live Better in Your Body, 2014, Jill Miller

Weight Training Without Injury: Over 350 Step-by-Step Pictures Including What Not to Do!, 2016, Fred Stellabotte and Rachel Straub

Dagher Strength dagherstrength.com

Primal Play www.primalplay.com

FARMING, ECOLOGY, AND SUSTAINABILITY
Gaining Ground: A Story of Farmers' Markets, Local Food, and Saving the Family Farm, 2013, Forrest Pritchard

Growing Tomorrow: A Farm-to-Table Journey in Photos and Recipes: Behind the Scenes with 18 Extraordinary Sustainable Farmers Who Are Changing the Way We Eat, 2015, Forrest Pritchard

Folks, This Ain't Normal, 2012, Joel Salatin

The Unsettling of America: Culture & Agriculture, 2015, Wendell Barry

The Vegetarian Myth, Lierre Keith

The Cornucopia Institute (third-party information for consumers and farmers on organic food industry and regulatory breaches into the food supply) www.cornucopia.org

Forest Stewardship Council www.fsc.org/en

Grass Based Health grassbasedhealth.blogspot.com

Homestead Honey homestead-honey.com

Hunt Gather Grow Foundation www.huntgathergrowfoundation.com

Marine Stewardship Council www.msc.org

Savory Institute (holistic management) savory.global

Sustainable Table www.sustainabletable.org/1117/welcome-to-sustainable-table

FERMENTATION

Fermented: A Four Season Approach to Paleo Probiotic Foods, 2013, Jill Ciciarelli

Nourishing Traditions, 2001, Sally Fallon

Wild Fermentation: The Flavor, Nutrition, and Craft of Live-Culture Foods, 2nd Edition, 2016, Sandor Ellix Katz

Cultures for Health CulturesForHealth.com

The Kitchn (homemade sauerkraut and cooking techniques) www.thekitchn.com

FAT

Eat Fat, Lose Fat, 2006, Mary Enig and Sally Fallon

Eat the Yolks, 2014, Liz Wolfe

Fat: An Appreciation of a Misunderstood Ingredient, 2008, Jennifer McLagan

The Fat Fallacy: The French Diet Secrets to Permanent Weight Loss, 2003, Will Clower

Fat for Fuel: A Revolutionary Diet to Combat Cancer, Boost Brain Power, and Increase Your Energy, 2017, Dr. Joseph Mercola

Good Fat, Bad Fat, 2016, Romy Dollé

Nourishing Fats: Why We Need Animal Fats for Health and Happiness, 2017, Sally Fallon Morell

The Secret Life of Fat: The Science Behind the Body's Least Understood Organ and What It Means for You, 2016, Sylvia Tara

FRANCE

Bébé Day by Day: 100 Keys to French Parenting, 2013, Pamela Druckerman

French Women Don't Get Fat: The Secret of Eating for Pleasure, 2007, Mireille Guiliano

The Food of France, 1958, Waverley Root,

France à Votre Table: The Gastronomic Routes of France, 1997, Sopexa

Me Talk Pretty One Day, 2001, David Sedaris

My Life in France, 2007, Julia Child and Francis Prud'homme

Questions? Réponses! French non-fiction children's book series by Nathan

Le Tour de France de la Famille Oukilé, 2015, Béatrice Veillon

A Year in Provence and *French Lessons*, Peter Mayle

FRENCH FOODS, SPECIALIZED COOKWARE, AND KITCHEN TOOLS

Amazon (Duralex glassware, Le Creuset mini cocottes, Opinel knives, *piment d'Espelette*, Revol ceramic cookware, Terafeu Basque pottery, Villeroy & Boch wine glasses) www.amazon.com

Artiga (Basque canvas and linens, pillows, kitchen towels, Terafeu Basque pottery) www.artiga.us

Bona Fide Green Goods (Life Factory glass water bottles) www.bonafidegreengoods.com

Chef's Resource (Demeyere Proline pots and pans, Laguiole knives) www.chefsresource.com

Cowgirl Creamery (French-style artisanal cheeses) www.cowgirlcreamery.com

Crate and Barrel (Le Creuset, Staub and Revol cookware, Wüsthof knives) www.crateandbarrel.com/kitchen-and-food/wusthof-classic-cutlery/1

D'Artagnan (Southwest French specialties like charcuterie, chestnuts, duck confit and rillettes, duck fat, foie gras, jambon de Bayonne, quail, truffles, but also grass-fed beef and lamb as well as bison, rabbit and wild boar. Committed to natural, sustainable and humane production.) www.dartagnan.com

Dean & DeLuca (French cheeses, spices, salts, olive oil, olives) *www.deananddeluca.com*

Didriks (Pillivuyt porcelain individual pieces) www.didriks.com

Food52 (Pillivuyt porcelain sets, beautiful photography) www.food52.com

French Brand (Euskal Linge and Jean-Vier kitchen towels and linens) www.french-brand.com

Gracious Style (Le Jacquard Français table linens) www.graciousstyle.com

Healthy Human (Stainless steel hot/cold water bottles) healthyhumanlife.com

Joie de Vivre (Thieffry Frères table linens, "ready-cooked" chestnuts) www.frenchselections.com

Knife Merchant (Demeyere pans, Matfer Bourgeat specialty kitchen tool, Excellent knife selection) www.knifemerchant.com

Laguiole (French knives, corkscrews, and cutlery) www.laguiole.com/index.php?language=en

Le District (Pommery mustards and vinegar, French cheeses, foie gras) www.ledistrict.com – online grocery www.mercato.com/shop/le-district

Revol (porcelain) www.revol1768.com

Sur La Table (Le Creuset cast-iron pots and mini cocottes) *www.surlatable.com*

Williams-Sonoma (Staub, Le Creuset, and Emile Henry cookware) www.williamssonoma.com

ZWILLING J.A. Henckels (Staub cast-iron pots) www.zwillingonline.com

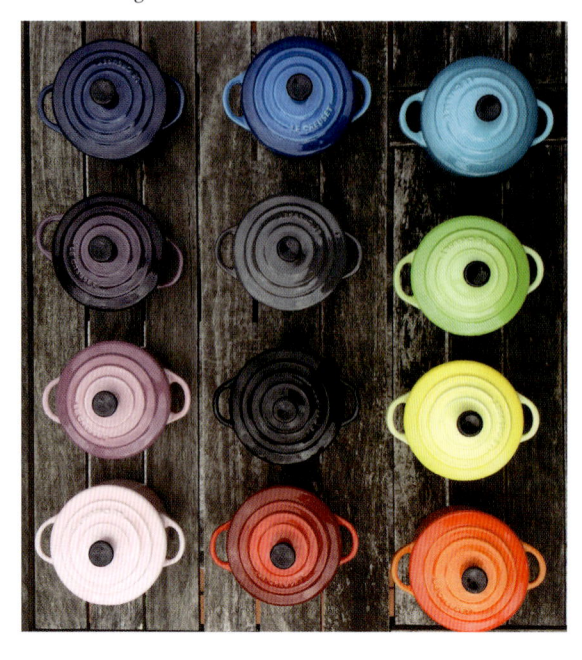

GENETICS AND EPIGENETICS

Dirty Genes: A Breakthrough Program to Treat the Root Cause of Illness and Optimize Your Health, 2018, Dr. Ben Lynch

Pottenger's Prophecy: How Food Resets Genes for Wellness or Illness, 2011, Gray Graham and Deborah Kesten

The Selfish Gene, 1990, Richard Dawkins

Younger: A Breakthrough Program to Reset Your Genes, Reverse Aging, and Turn Back the Clock 10 Years, 2017, Sara Gottfried

GMOS AND GLYPHOSATE

Food Fight: GMOs and the Future of the American Diet, 2017, Mckay Jenkins

Global GMO Free Commission www.gmofreeglobal.org

GMO Free USA (food transparency and food justice) gmofreeusa.org

Mothers Across the World www.momsacrosstheworld.com

Stephanie Seneff people.csail.mit.edu/seneff

U.S. Right to Know (transparency in America's food system) usrtk.org

GRASS-FED MEAT, HIGH-FAT, GRAIN-FREE, AND OTHER PRIMAL/PALEO AND FRENCH FOOD PRODUCTS

2XL Premium Angus (Iowa grass-fed beef) 2xlpremiumangus.com

Anthony's Goods (erythritol, organic coconut flour) www.anthonysgoods.com

Barefoot Provisions barefootprovisions.com

Bulletproof (MCT oil and supplements) www.bulletproofexec.com

ButcherBox www.butcherbox.com

The CowShare www.thecowshare.com

Eatwild (list of grass-fed farms and how to find grass-fed and organic products locally) www.eatwild.com

Edens Garden (essential oils) www.edensgarden.com

EPIC www.epicbar.com

Fatworks (duck fat! goose fat! lard! tallow!) fatworksfoods.com

Four Sigmatic (mushroom superfoods) us.foursigmatic.com

Gourmet Food World (fromage blanc) www.gourmetfoodworld.com/mitica-miticrema-fromage-blanc-11519

Grass-Fed Traditions www.grassfedtraditions.com

Grasspunk Farm (grass-fed beef farm in Southwest France) grasspunk.com

Great Lakes Gelatin Powder greatlakesgelatin.com/storefront

Jilz Crackerz (gluten-free crackers) jilzglutenfree.com

Julian Bakery (grain-free products) www.julianbakery.com

Kerrygold (grass-fed Irish butter and cheese) www.kerrygoldusa.com

Le District (Pommery mustards and vinegar, French cheeses, foie gras) www.ledistrict.com online grocery www.mercato.com/shop/le-district

LocalHarvest (lists local CSAs, farmers' markets and farms around the U.S.) www.localharvest.org

Meatme (grass-fed meats and animal "shares" for Canadian residents) www.meatme.co

Niman Ranch (pork, beef, lamb) www.nimanranch.com

One Stop Paleo Shop (paleo, AIP, and keto foods) www.onestoppaleoshop.com

Otto's Naturals (cassava flour) www.ottosnaturals.com

Over the Grass Farm (grass-fed meat, dairy, poultry, eggs, honey, and vegetables) www.overthegrassfarm.net/

Pete's Paleo (chef-prepared meals) www.petespaleo.com

Pili Hunters (sprouted pili nuts and pili nut butter) www.eatpilinuts.com

Paleo By Maileo (paleo foods, products, and snacks) paleobymaileo.com

Polyface Farms (Joel Salatin's farm) www.polyfacefarms.com

Primal Blueprint / Primal Kitchen (Primal Kitchen foods and supplements) www.primalblueprint.com/shop

Primal Pastures (pasture-raised meats) primalpastures.com

Pure Indian Foods (ghee) www.pureindianfoods.com

Radiant Life (liver powder, herbs) www.radiantlife.com

Real Salt (ancient sea salts from Utah) realsalt.com

Rocky Mountain Naturals (organic and non-GMO products) rockymountainnaturals.greenpolkadotbox.com

Seafood Watch (sustainable seafood) www.seafoodwatch.org

Smith Meadows (sustainable farming) smithmeadows.com

Tendergrass Farms (sustainable organic, NAE, and clean label meat products) tendergrass.com

Thrive Market (socially conscious, online discounted natural foods, vetted for quality) thrivemarket.com

U.S. Wellness Meats (wide selection of grass-fed offal, meats, poultry, rabbit; very supportive of paleo and AIP communities) grasslandbeef.com

Vermont Creamery (fromage blanc) www.vermontcreamery.com/fromage-blanc-1

White Oak Pastures www.whiteoakpastures.com

Wild Mountain Paleo Market www.wildmountainpaleo.com

Vital Choice Seafood www.vitalchoice.com

Vital Proteins (collagen powders) www.vitalproteins.com

HEART HEALTH AND HEALTH CARE

The Paleo Cardiologist: The Natural Way to Heart Health, 2015, Jack Wolfson

Unconventional Medicine: Join the Revolution to Reinvent Healthcare, Reverse Chronic Disease, and Create a Practice You Love, 2017, Chris Kresser

Undoctored: Why Health Care Has Failed You and How You Can Become Smarter Than Your Doctor, 2017, Dr. William Davis

HISTORY OF FOOD IN AMERICA
The Big Fat Surprise, 2014, Nina Teicholz

Eating in America, 1995 ed., Waverley Root and Richard de Rochemont

Ten Restaurants That Changed America, audio book, 2016, Paul Freedman

HOME REMEDIES
Healthy at Home: Get Well and Stay Well Without Prescriptions, Dr. Tieraona Low Dog

Edens Garden (cleaning products using essential oils) www.edensgarden.com

Wellness Mama www.wellnessmama.com

MICROBIOME
Brain Maker, 2015, Dr David Perlmutter

Enlightenweight: Cultivate the Garden Within, 2015, Andrew Miles and Xuelan Qui

Gut: The Inside Story of Our Body's Most Underrated Organ, 2015, Giulia Enders

The Microbiome Diet: The Scientifically Proven Way to Restore Your Gut Health and Achieve Permanent Weight Loss, 2015, Raphael Kellman

Missing Microbes, 2014, Martin J. Blaser

NUTRITIONAL KETOSIS
The Art and Science of Low Carbohydrate Performance, 2012, Jeff S. Volek and Stephen D. Phinney

Conquer Type 2 Diabetes with a Ketogenic Diet: A Practical Guide for Reducing Your HBA1c and Avoiding Diabetic Complications, 2017, Ellen Davis and Dr. Keith Runyan

Eat Rich, Live Long: Mastering the Low-Carb & Keto Spectrum for Weight Loss and Longevity, 2018, Ivor Cummins and Dr. Jeffrey Gerber

Keto: The Complete Guide to Success on The Ketogenic Diet, including Simplified Science and No-cook Meal Plans, 2018, Maria Emmerich and Craig Emmerich

Keto Clarity, 2014, Jimmy Moore and Dr. Eric Westman

The Keto Cure: A Low Carb High Fat Dietary Solution to Heal Your Body and Optimize Your Health, 2017, Jimmy Moore and Dr. Adam Nally

The Keto Diet: The Complete Guide to a High-Fat Diet, 2017, Leanne Vogel

Ketogenic Diet and Metabolic Therapies: Expanded Roles in Health and Disease, 2017, Susan A. Masino, ed.

The Charlie Foundation (ketogenic therapies) www.charliefoundation.org

Ketogenic Diet Resources www.ketogenic-diet-resource.com

KetoNutrition www.ketonutrition.org/resources

ORAL HEALTH
Crazy Good Living, 2017, Dr. Alvin Danenberg

Cure Tooth Decay: Heal and Prevent Cavities with Nutrition, 2nd Edition, 2010, Ramiel Nagel

The Mouth-Body Connection: The 28-Day Program to Create a Healthy Mouth, Reduce Inflammation and Prevent Disease Throughout the Body, 2017, Dr. Gerald P. Curatola

OraWellness www.orawellness.com

PARASITES
Guess What Came to Dinner? Parasites and Your Health, 2001, Ann Louise Gittleman

Lyme Solutions: A Biological Approach to Lyme Disease, 2018, Dr. Dietrich Klinghardt

This Is Your Brain on Parasites: How Tiny Creatures Manipulate Our Behavior and Shape Society, 2017, Kathleen McAuliffe

PODCASTS RELATED TO ANCESTRAL HEALTH AND NUTRITION
2 Keto Dudes, hosted by Carl Franklin and Richard Morris

Align Podcast, hosted by Aaron Alexander

The Ancestral RDs Podcast, hosted by Laura Schoenfeld and Kelsey Marksteiner

Aspire Natural Health Podcast, hosted by Dr. Tim Gerstmar

The Autoimmune Wellness Podcast, hosted by Mickey Trescott and Angie Alt

Balanced Bites: Modern Paleo Living, hosted by Diane Sanfilippo and Liz Wolfe

Ben Greenfield Fitness, hosted by Ben Greenfield

Best Health Radio, hosted by Dr. Devaki Lindsey Berkson

Better Everyday, hosted by Sarah Fragoso and Dr. Brooke Kalanick

Beyond Wellness Radio, hosted by Justin Marchegiani

Bulletproof Radio, hosted by Dave Asprey

The Daily Lipid, hosted by Chris Masterjohn

Daily Meditation Podcast, hosted by Mary Meckley

The Detox and Nutrition Coach Podcast, hosted by Dr. Jay Davidson

Elevate Your Energy, hosted by Evelyne Lambrecht

The Evan Brand Show (formaly *Not Just Paleo*), hosted by Evan Brand

Farm to Table Talk, hosted by Rodger Wasson

Fasting Talk, hosted by Jimmy Moore

Fat Burning Man Podcast, hosted by Abel James

Gut Guardians Podcast, hosted by Grace Liu

The Healing Pain Podcast, hosted by Dr. Joe Tatta

Health, Nutrition and Functional Medicine, hosted by Dr. Michael Ruscio

The Healthy Moms Podcast, hosted by Katie Wells

High Intensity Health Radio, hosted by Mike Mutzel

Hunt Gather Talk, hosted by Hank Shaw

Keto Diet Podcast, hosted by Leanne Vogel

Keto Hacking MD Podcast, hosted by Jimmy Moore, Dr. John Limansky

Keto Talk with Jimmy Moore & The Doc, hosted by Jimmy Moore and Dr. Adam Nally

Ketovangelist Kitchen, hosted by Brian Williamson and Carrie Brown

The Ketovangelist Podcast, hosted by Brian Williamson

Live to 110, hosted by Wendy Myers

The Livin' La Vida Low Carb Show, hosted by Jimmy Moore

MeatCast, hosted by EPIC provisions

The Model Health Show, hosted by Shawn Stevenson

NomNom Paleo, hosted by Michelle Tam

Nourish Balance Thrive, hosted by Chris Kelly

Paleo Magazine Radio, formerly hosted by Tony Federico, now hosted by Ashleigh Van Houten

The Paleo Solution Podcast, hosted by Robb Wolf

The Paleo View, hosted by Sarah Ballantyne and Stacy Toth

The Paleo Women Podcast: Health, Nutrition, Fitness, Hormones, hosted by Noelle Tarr and Stefani Ruper

Phoenix Helix: Reversing Autoimmune Disease Through the Paleo Diet and Lifestyle, hosted by Eileen Laird

Primal Blueprint Podcast, hosted by Brad Kearns, Elle Russ, and Mark Sisson

Primal Body Primal Mind, hosted by Nora Gedgaudas

Primal Diet – Modern Health, hosted by Beverly Meyers

Primal Endurance Podcast, hosted by Brad Kearns

Reset Me with Dr. C, hosted by Dr. Alan Christianson

Revolution Health Radio, hosted by Chris Kresser

Rewild Yourself, hosted by Daniel Vitalis

SuperCharged Health, hosted by Harry Massey and Wendy Myers

Sustainable Dish Podcast, hosted by Diana Rodgers

The SCD Lifestyle Solution, hosted by Jordan Reasoner and Steve Wright

The Spa Dr., hosted by Dr. Trevor Cates

The Ultimate Health Podcast, hosted by Dr. Jesse Chappus and Marni Wasserman

Underground Wellness, hosted by Sean Croxton

Wellness Force Radio, hosted by Josh Trent

Wise Traditions, hosted by Hilda Labrada-Gore of The Weston A. Price Foundation

Women's Wellness Radio, hosted by Bridget Danner

PRIMAL/PALEO/ANCESTRAL HEALTH-RELATED WEBSITES

Brain and Gut Health (Dr. David Perlmutter) www.drperlmutter.com, Expert video interviews, extensive database of relevant scientific studies www.drperlmutter.com/learn/studies

Craig Dennis craigdennismassage.com

Dr. Georgia Ede www.diagnosisdiet.com

Dr. Joseph Mercola www.mercola.com

Gluten Free (Dr. Tom O'Bryen) www.thedr.com

GreenMedInfo www.greenmedinfo.com, GreenMedInfo Research Dashboard www.greenmedinfo.com/research-dashboard

Healthy Digestion (Andrea Nakayama) www.replenishpdx.com

MS/Paleo Protocol (Terry Wahls) terrywahls.com

Naturopathic Doctor (Dr. Tim Gerstmar) aspirenaturalhealth.com

Paleo Health & Lifestyle (Chris Kresser) chriskresser.com

The Paleo Mom (Sarah Ballantyne) www.thepaleomom.com

PaleoFoundation (certification of Paleo products within four certification rubrics) www.PaleoFoundation.com

Dr. Peter Attia eatingacademy.com

Thyroid (Suzy Cohen) www.dearpharmacist.com

Thyroid & Total Health (Reed Davis) bonesandhormones.com/fdn

PRIMAL/PALEO/ANCESTRAL HISTORY AND DIET

Catching Fire – How Cooking Made Us Human, 2009, Richard Rangan

The Diet for Human Beings (DVD), 2012, Beverly Meyer

Health Secrets from the Stone Age, 2005, Philip Goscienski

The Hunter-Gatherer Within: Health and the Natural Human Diet, 2013, Kerry G. Brock and George M. Diggs

Neanderthin, 1995, Ray Audette

The New Evolution Diet, 2011, Arthur DeVany

The New Primal Blueprint, 2016, Mark Sisson

Paleo from A to Z, 2015, Darryl Edwards

The Paleo Cure, 2014, Chris Kresser

The Paleo Diet, 2010, Loren Cordain

The Paleo Manifesto, 2014, John Durant

The Paleo Solution, 2010, Robb Wolf

The Paleolithic Prescription, 1988, Boyd Eaton

Perfect Health Diet, 2013, Paul Jaminet

Primal Body, Primal Mind, 2011, and *Primal Fat Burner*, 2017, Nora Gedgaudas

Primal Connection, 2013, Mark Sisson

Wired to Eat, 2017, Robb Wolf

SLEEP

Better Than Before: What I Learned About Making and Breaking Habits–to Sleep More, Quit Sugar, Procrastinate Less, and Generally Build a Happier Life, 2015, Gretchen Rubin

Go To Bed (eBook), Dr. Sarah Ballantyne www.thepaleomom.com/gotobed

Healing with Essential Oils: How to Use Them to Enhance Sleep, Digestion and Detoxification while Reducing Stress and Inflammation, 2017, Dr. Dietrich Klinghardt

Lights Out, 2001, T.S. Wiley and Bent Formby

Rethinking Fatigue (eBook), 2014, Nora Gedgaudas, (www.primalbody-primalmind.com/rethinking-fatigue)

The Sleep Doctor's Diet Plan, 2011, Michael Breus

Swanwick Sleep blue light-blocking glasses https://www.swanwicksleep.com/

TrueDark™ Twilight blue light-blocking glasses biohacked.com/product/truedarktwilight

SPINE HEALTH
Foundation Training / The Founder by Eric Goodman www.foundationtraining.com

Gokhale Method by Esther Gokhale gokhalemethod.com

THYROID
5 Steps to Restoring Health Protocol: Helping those who haven't been helped with Lyme Disease, Thyroid Problems, Adrenal Fatigue, Heavy Metal Toxicity, Digestive Issues, and More!, 2015, Jay Davidson

The Adrenal Thyroid Revolution: A Proven 4-Week Program to Rescue Your Metabolism, Hormones, Mind & Mood, 2017, Aviva Romm

Hashimoto's Protocol: A 90-Day Plan for Reversing Thyroid Symptoms and Getting Your Life Back, 2017, Izabella Wentz

The Paleo Thyroid Solution, 2016, Elle Russ

The Thyroid Connection: Why You Feel Tired, Brain-Fogged, and Overweight – and How to Get Your Life Back, 2016, Dr. Amy Myers

Why Do I Still Have Thyroid Symptoms, 2010, Datis Kharrazian

Hypothyroid Mom hypothyroidmom.com

Stop the Thyroid Madness™ stopthethyroidmadness.com

Thyroid Pharmacist (Dr. Izabella Wentz) thyroidpharmacist.com

TOXINS
Food Forensics: The Hidden Toxins Lurking in Your Food and How You Can Avoid Them for Lifelong Health, 2016, Mike Adams

Limitless Energy: How to Detox Toxic Metals to End Exhaustion and Chronic Fatigue, 2017, Wendy Myers

The Toxin Solution: How Hidden Poisons in the Air, Water, Food, and Products We Use Are Destroying Our Health—And What We Can Do to Fix It, 2017, Dr. Joseph Pizzorno

VACCINES
Inoculated, 2016, Ken Heckenlively

Vaxxed: From Cover-Up To Catastrophe vaxxedthemovie.com

Cochrane Collaboration swiss.cochrane.org

Erin Elizabeth's Health Nut News www.healthnutnews.com

Physicians for Informed Consent physiciansforinformedconsent.org

ThinkTwice Global Vaccine Institute www.thinktwice.com

World Mercury Project worldmercuryproject.org

Worldwide Choice worldwidechoice.org

WINE
The Bordeaux Wine Guide, Laure Lamendin, ed. L'Ecole du Vin de Bordeaux, Editions de la Martinière, 2015

Cheese & Wine: A Guide to Selecting, Pairing and Enjoying, 2017, Janet Fletcher

The Complete Bordeaux, 2017, Stephen Brook

Dictionnaire des Vins, Bières et Spiritueux du Monde, Claude Chapus and Peter Dunn, Édition Bilingue, Francais/Anglais, Anglais/Francais, BMS Univers Poche & Déclinaisons, 2005.

The Dirty Guide to Wine: Following Flavor from Ground to Glass, 2017, Alice Feiring

The Finest Wines of Bordeaux: A Regional Guide to the Best Chateaux and Their Wines, Richard Lawther, 2010 (ed. 2016)

The Food Lover's Guide to Wine, 2011, K. Page and A. Dornenburg

How to Taste: A Guide to Enjoying Wine, 2008, Jancis Robinson

Le Nez du Vin, 54 wine aromas collection, 2013, Jean Lenoir (available on Amazon)

The Longevity Factor: How Resveratrol and Red Wine Activate Genes for a Longer and Healthier Life, 2009, Dr. Joseph Maroon

The Oxford Companion to Wine, 2015, Jancis Robinson

Oz Clarke's Bordeaux: The Wines, The Vineyards, The Winemakers, 2006, Oz Clarke

Secrets of the Sommeliers, 2010, Rajat Parr

The Taste of Wine: The Art and Science of Wine Appreciation, 1997, Émile Peynaud

What to Drink with What You Eat, 2006, Andrew Dornenburg and Karen Page

What's So Special about Biodynamic Wine? 35 Questions and Answers for Wine Lovers, 2013, Antoine Lepetit de la Bigne

Wine: A Tasting Course, 2013, Marnie Old

Wine Basics: A Quick and Easy Guide, 1993, Dewey Markham, Jr.

Wine Production and Quality, 2nd Edition, 2016, Keith Grainger

Wine Quality: Tasting and Selection, 2009, Keith Grainger

The Wine Bible, 2015, Karen MacNeil

Wine Revolution: The World's Best Organic, Biodynamic and Natural Wines, 2017, Jane Anson

The World Atlas of Wine, 7th Edition, 2013, Hugh Johnson and Jancis Robinson

Guild of Sommeliers Wine Podcasts guildpodcast.com

I'll Drink to That, Talking Wine with Levi Dalton podcast

Wine Enthusiasts Podcast, Wine Enthusiast Magazine

Wine for Normal People podcast, hosted by Elizabeth Schneider and M.C. Ice

Winecast podcast, hosted by Tim Elliott

Anivin de France (French wines resource in English and French) www.vindefrance-cepages.org

Bordeaux Saveurs (Custom wine tourism and events around France) www.bordeauxsaveurs.com/en

Conseil Interprofessionnel du Vin de Bordeaux (CIVB or Bordeaux Wine Council) www.bordeaux.com/us

CellarTracker www.cellartracker.com/default.asp

Dry Farm Wines (biodynamic, natural and organic wines purveyor in the U.S. www.dryfarmwines.com

DMjWineworks (wine tours with Dewey Markham, Jr., along with information on articles, books, classes, and speaking) dmjwineworks.com

Le Figaro Vin (appellations, grape varieties, wine dictionary) avis-vin.lefigaro.fr/connaitre-deguster/tout-savoir-sur-le-vin/guide-des-regions-et-des-appellations

Matching Food & Wine (by UK Food and Wine author Fiona Beckett) www.matchingfoodandwine.com

Taste of Wine (grape varieties, wine tasting 101) www.wine-tasting-reviews.com

Uncorked Wine Tours (wine tours in France, Porto, and Tuscany with Caroline Matthews) www.uncorkedwinetours.com

VINIV (create your own custom blend of Bordeaux wine with Stephen Bolger and his team) www.jmcazes.com/en/viniv

Vin-Vigne (French online guide to French and other wines) www.vin-vigne.com/vin

Vivino (wine app for photographs of labels of wines users have tasted and rated) www.vivino.com/users/taniateschke

Voyages autour du vin (Sommelière and Cellar Master Annabelle Nicolle-Beaufils' wine tours website) voyagesautourduvin.fr

Wine & Spirit Education Trust www.wsetglobal.com

Wine Aroma Wheel (why and how to use the aroma wheel) winearomawheel.com

Wine Folly www.winefolly.com

Wine Spectator (online wine glossary) www.winespectator.com/glossary

Winegeeks (appellations, grapes, vintage wine charts by region) www.winegeeks.com

Winegeeks (wine basics) www.winegeeks.com/articles/18

Wine-Searcher (grape varieties) www.wine-searcher.com/grape-varieties.lml

WINEMAKERS OF FRENCH ORGANIC AND BIODYNAMIC WINES

L'Agence BIO (The BIO Agency) annuaire.agencebio.org/resultats?categorie=2&nom=&product=147&activite=17

Ardoneo Organic Wine www.vin-bio-ardoneo.com

Bio Bourgogne www.biobourgogne-vitrine.org/vins-bio_q11.php

BIODYVIN www.biodyvin.com/en/our-members.html

Demeter www.demeter.fr/type_operateur/viticulteur/ and www.demeter.fr/pres-de-chez-vous

Les Logiques Bio www.eco-bacchus.com/index.php?cPath=1

Pages Vins Bio www.pages-vinsbio.fr/LIENS/Vignerons-Vins-Provence.htm and www.pages-vinsbio.fr/Bordeaux/vins_bordeaux.html

Vignerons Bio d'Aquitaine (organic wine producers in the Aquitaine region of Southwest France) www.vigneronsbio-aquitaine.org

Vinup.com www.vinup.com/producteurs.lasso?&recherche=producteur

WINE PURVEYORS OF FRENCH ORGANIC WINES IN FRANCE

Biocoop www.biocoop.fr/

Petites Caves www.petitescaves.com

Wine et Vin Shop www.wine-et-vin.com/types-de-vins#

WINE PURVEYORS OF FRENCH (AND INTERNATIONAL) ORGANIC, BIODYNAMIC, AND NATURAL WINES IN THE U.S. & U.K.

Buon Vino Natural Wines (U.K.) www.buonvino.co.uk

De Maison Selections (importer located in North Carolina) www.demaisonselections.com/info.html

Dry Farm Wines (organic and biodynamic wine purveyors in U.S., special attention to paleo and ketogenic diets, lab testing for mycotoxins and mold, gluten-free, low alcohol) www.dryfarmwines.com

EcoVine Wine Club (organic and biodynamic wine purveyors in U.S.) www.ecovinewineclub.com

Flatiron Wines & Spirits (NY and SF) flatiron-wines.com

Good Wine Online (U.K.) www.goodwineonline.co.uk/natural-wines

K&L Wine Merchants (limited selection of organic French wines at very reasonable prices) www.klwines.com

Les Caves de Pyrene (U.K.) shop.lescaves.co.uk/lescaves-shopfront

Millésima USA (Manhattan-based fine wine sales specialist) www.millesima-usa.com

Natural Wine Company (based in Colorado) naturalwineco.com

The Organic Wine Company (organic and biodynamic wine purveyor in U.S., selections curated by a French woman living in California) theorganicwinecompany.com

Raw Wine (U.S., Europe & U.K.) www.rawwine.com

Whole Foods (online and local stores in U.S.) www.wholefoodsmarket.com

The Wine Society (U.K.) www.thewinesociety.com

Wine Fellas (organic wine club based in California) winefellas.com

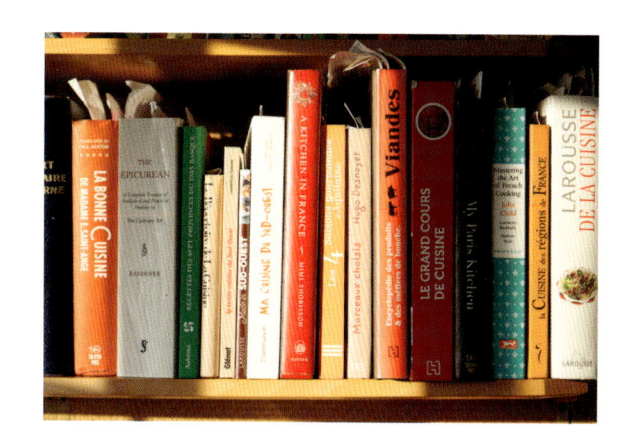

RESOURCES AND FURTHER READING

ENDNOTES

1. INTRODUCTION

1. Waverley Root, *The Food of France* (1958), 9. Historian Jean-Jacques Hémardinquer proposed a similar geographic division of fats used by region in France, based on responses to the usage of fats around France from surveys conducted in 1914, 1936 and 1952 in *L'encycopédie francaise*, by Lucien Febvre, and from surveys conducted between 1942 and 1962, by the Musée des Arts et Traditions in his works, "Essai des cartes des graisses de cuisine en France." *Annales: Economies, Sociétés, Civilisations* 16(1970); and "Pour Une Histoire de l'Alimentation." *Cahiers des Annales*, vol. 28 (Paris: Armand Colin, 1970).
2. www.worldlifeexpectancy.com/cause-of-death/coronary-heart-disease/by-country/ and who.int/nmh/countries/fra_en.pdf?ua=1
3. www.ehnheart.org/cvd-statistics.html

2. DISCOVERING FRENCH ANCESTRAL LIFESTYLE

1. "Salute*m est maxima fortitude.*" – Publius Vergilius Maro (70BC-19BC), Roman philosopher and author of *The Aeneid*.

3. THE FRENCH ART AND TRADITION OF FOOD AND WINE

1. Barbara Ketcham Wheaton, *Savoring the Past: The French Kitchen and Table from 1300 to 1789* (New York: Simon & Shuster, 1983), xix.
2. www.unesco.org/culture/ich/en/RL/gastronomic-meal-of-the-french-00437
3. Representative List of the Intangible Cultural Heritage of Humanity by UNESCO in 2010.
4. Louis Douët d'Arcq, *Treatise on Cooking* (1860), 217. and Wheaton, *Savoring the Past*, 9.
5. Jérôme Pichon and Georges Vicaire, eds. *Le Viandier de Guillaume Tirel, dit Taillevent* (Paris, 1892). H. Leclerc and P. Cornuau. (Reproduced by Kessinger Legacy Reprints.)
6. *Le Ménagier de Paris*, ("*The Goodman of Paris: A Treatise on Moral and Domestic Economy by a Citizen of Paris, c. 1393.*"), translated by Eileen Power. Boydell Press, 2008. (Based on three existing fifteenth-century manuscripts of the *Ménagier*, edited by Jérôme Pichon for the Société des Bibliophile François, Paris, 1846.)
7. Wheaton, *Savoring the Past*, xxi.
8. Ibid., Page 10.
9. Ibid., Page xxi.
10. Nicolas de Bonnefons, on Fruits in *Le Jardinier francois, Epistre aux dames* (1683), 270-276, and on Seasons, 78-79; and on Meats and Fats and Bouillon for Health in *Les Délices de la Campagne, Epistre aux dames* (1679), 170-175.
11. Wheaton, *Savoring the Past*, xxi.
12. www.britannica.com/topic/grande-cuisine
13. Stephane Guyenet, *U.S. Sugar Consumption in the U.S. Diet between 1822 and 2005*, wholehealthsource.blogspot.ch/2012/02/by-2606-us-diet-will-be-100-percent.html
14. Dr. Chris Knobbe, "Food Choices and Vision Loss". presented at the Ancestral Health Symposium, Boulder, Colorado [August 2016]. YouTube video, 40:40. Posted August 2016. www.youtube.com/watch?v=SmrncwpaZ-RM&list=PLbhWKPDKXIEBBybYcY_jUQGE7S0KL-gH5S&index=31.
15. pioneerthinking.com/history-of-white-flour
16. Knobbe, "Food Choices and Vision Loss". YouTube video.
17. www.ashers.com/blog/2013/05/history-of-a-truffle
18. Knobbe, "Food Choices and Vision Loss". YouTube video.
19. Ibid.
20. articles.mercola.com/sites/articles/archive/2014/08/31/trans-fat-saturated-fat.aspx
21. Wheaton, *Savoring the Past*, xx, referencing Jean-Jacques Hémardinquer *Les Graisses de Cuisine en France*, 271.
22. Sally Fallon Morell, *Nourishing Fats: Why We Need Animal Fats for Health and Happiness* (New York: Grand Central Life & Style, 2017), 3-9.
23. Washington Post online: www.washingtonpost.com/wp-srv/special/health/food-pyramid/
24. This intricate story in history is best documented by Nina Teicholz in her book, *The Big Fat Surprise: Why Butter, Meat and Cheese Belong in a Healthy Diet* (New York: Simon & Schuster, 2015).
25. Adele Hite, "2015 Dietary Guidelines for Americans". Presented at Ancestral Health Symposium, Boulder, Colorado [August 2016]. YouTube video, 40:08. Posted August 2016. www.youtube.com/watch?v=nKl1xakEmU-w&list=PLbhWKPDKXIEBBybYcY_jUQGE7S0KL-gH5S&index=28
26. choosemyplate-prod.azureedge.net/sites/default/files/printablematerials/ABriefHistoryOfUSDAFoodGuides.pdf
27. Nina Teicholz interviewed by Jimmy Moore on the *Livin' La Vida Low-Carb Podcast* #1200, December 28, 2016.
28. USDA "Corn sweeteners (notably high-fructose corn syrup, or HFCS)—increased 43 pounds, or 39 percent, between 1950-59 and 2000 (table 2-6)". *Agricultural Fact Book 2001-2002* (Washington, DC: U.S. Government Printing Office, 2003), 20.
29. USDA "Profiling Food Consumption in America," *Agricultural Fact Book 2001-2002* (Washington, DC: U.S. Government Printing Office, 2003), 20.
30. Knobbe, "Food Choices and Vision Loss". YouTube video.
31. EASO easo.org/education-portal/obesity-facts-figures
32. WHO www.who.int/mediacentre/factsheets/fs312/en
33. WHO www.who.int/mediacentre/factsheets/fs317/en
34. Knobbe, "Food Choices and Vision Loss". YouTube video.
35. Sally Schneider, *The Improvisational Cook* (New York: William Morrow Cookbooks, 2011), 19.
36. Paula Wolfert, *The Cooking of Southwest France* (Boston: Houghton Mifflin Harcourt, 2005), 2 and xviii.
37. Washington Post online: www.washingtonpost.com/wp-srv/special/health/food-pyramid
38. www.healthy-eating-politics.com/usda-food-pyramid.html
39. ChooseMyPlate.gov www.choosemyplate.gov
40. Root, *The Food of France*, p. 9.
41. *Le Ménagier de Paris* (*The Goodman of Paris: A Treatise on Moral and Domestic Economy by a Citizen of Paris*, c. 1393).
42. University of Bordeaux II Professor and renowned French scientist, Serge Renaud (1927-2012), considered the father of the French Paradox, published a study in the British medical journal The Lancet in 1992, explaining the contradictory

nature of the consumption of French cuisine, particularly that of the Southwest, which utilizes high amounts of saturated animal fats, and low mortality rates in France (particularly in the Southwest) from cardiovascular disease. Renaud also proposed in this study that the platelet-inhibiting effects of alcohol (primarily red wine) consumed slowly and with a high fat meal could account for the French, and particularly the French Southwest, populations' protection from coronary heart disease. Citation: Wine, alcohol, platelets, and the French paradox for coronary heart disease. Renaud S, de Lorgeril M. INSERM, Nutrition and Vascular Physiopathology Research Unit, (Unit 63), France. Lancet (London, England) [1992, Vol. 339(8808):1523-1526] www.thelancet.com/journals/lancet/article/PII0140-6736(92)91277-F/abstract.

43. Kate Rhéaume-Bleue, *Vitamin K2 and the Calcium Paradox: How a Little-Known Vitamin Could Save Your Life* (Toronto: Wiley, 2012), 68.

44. Dr. Catherine Shanahan, *Deep Nutrition: Why Your Genes Need Traditional Food* (New York: Flatiron Books, 2017), 238-241.

45. Shanahan goes into detail about vegetable oils damaging and toxic effects on the brain and body, particularly in chapters 7 and 8 of her book, *Deep Nutrition: Why Your Genes Need Traditional Foods.*

46. www.unforgettablepaula.com/about-paula and NY Times online: www.nytimes.com/2017/03/21/dining/paula-wolfert-alzheimers.html?_r=1

47. www.lefigaro.fr/conso/2016/09/06/20010-20160906ARTFIG00022-les-francais-depensent-en-moyenne-182-euros-par-mois-en-produits-frais.php

48. www.joe.org/joe/2002february/rb6.php

49. My main source for the lists of fruits, vegetables, and their seasons came out of Béatrice Montevi's *Savoir faire & Recettes de nos Mamies* (Anagramme, 2012).

4. THE THREE SECRETS TO FRENCH COOKING: FARM FATS, FRESH INGREDIENTS, AND CAST-IRON POTS

1. Those individuals with the APOE4 gene mutation may be an exception, potentially faring better on a diet heavily weighted toward consumption of less saturated fat and more monounsaturated fat, such as olive oil. See Dr. Steven Gundry's talk on "Dietary Management of the ApoE4" presented at the Ancestral Health Symposium, Boulder, Colorado [August 2016]. YouTube video, 38:46. Posted August 2016. www.youtube.com/watch?v=Bfr9RPq0HFg&list=PLbhWK-PDKXIEBBybYcY_jUQGE7S0KLgH5S&index=15.

2. Nora Gedgaudas, *Primal Fat Burner* (New York: Atria Books, 2017), 16.

3. Joel Salatin, *Folks, This Ain't Normal* (New York: Center Street, 2012).

4. Gedgaudas, *Primal Fat Burner*, xx.

5. Ibid., xx-xxi.

6. Ibid., xxii-xxiii.

7. Please refer to ketogenic researcher Dr. Jeff Volek's excellent lecture on insulin resistance, carbohydrate over-consumption as the main disease driver in the US, and the history and application of ketogenic diets at Low Carb USA 2016, aired on *The Livin' La Vida Low-Carb Podcast* # 1281 on July 5, 2017. livinlavidalowcarb.com/blog/the-llvlc-show-episode-1281-dr-jeff-volek-2016-low-carb-usa/27981.

8. www.primalbody-primalmind.com/how-much-dietary-fat

9. Howard BV, et al. JAMA. 2006 Feb 8;295(6):655-66. Low-fat dietary pattern and risk of cardiovascular disease: the Women's Health Initiative Randomized Controlled Dietary Modification Trial. www.ncbi.nlm.nih.gov/pubmed/16467234.

10. Women's Health Initiative Clinical Trial and Observational Study dbGaP Study Accession: phs000200.v10. p3. www.ncbi.nlm.nih.gov/projects/gap/cgi-bin/study.cgi?study_id=phs000200.v10.p3.

11. Russell J de Souza et al. BMJ 2015;351:h3978. "Intake of saturated and trans unsaturated fatty acids and risk of all cause mortality, cardiovascular disease, and type 2 diabetes: systematic review and meta-analysis of observational studies". www.bmj.com/content/351/bmj.h3978 and Rajiv Chowdhury, et al. Ann Intern Med. 2014;160(6):398-406. "Association of Dietary, Circulating, and Supplement Fatty Acids with Coronary Risk: A Systematic Review and Meta-analysis". annals.org/aim/article/1846638/association-dietary-circulating-supplement-fatty-acids-coronary-risk-systematic-review?resultClick=3.

12. Marianne U. Jakobsen, et al. Am J Clin Nutr May 2009, vol. 89 no. 5 1425-1432. "Major types of dietary fat and risk of coronary heart disease: a pooled analysis of 11 cohort studies". ajcn.nutrition.org/content/89/5/1425?ijkey=37ccf64f9a226aed8013ee71eb94c63720c9336c&keytype2=tf_ipsecsha#fn-1

13. James J DiNicolantonio, et al. 2014. "The cardiometabolic consequences of replacing saturated fats with carbohydrates or Ω-6 polyunsaturated fats: Do the dietary guidelines have it wrong?" openheart.bmj.com/content/1/1/e000032.full

14. articles.mercola.com/sites/articles/archive/2015/08/31/saturated-fats-heart-disease.aspx#_edn13

15. health.gov/dietaryguidelines/2015/default.asp

16. Saturated fat is not the major issue" BMJ 2013;347:f6340. Published 22 October 2013. www.bmj.com/content/347/bmj.f6340.

17. Paul N. Hopkins, "Effects of Dietary Cholesterol on Serum Cholesterol: A Meta-Analysis and Review," *American Journal of Clinical Nutrition* 55, no. 6 (1992): 1060–1070. 24

18. Gedgaudas, *Primal Fat Burner*, 17.

19. S Kotani et al. Neurosci Res 56 (2), 159-164. 2006 Aug 14. "Dietary Supplementation of Arachidonic and Docosahexaenoic Acids Improves Cognitive Dysfunction". www.ncbi.nlm.nih.gov/labs/articles/16905216

20. www.primalbody-primalmind.com/animal-fat-new-superfood/#_ftn1

21. EC Westman, WS Yancy, et al., *Nutrition & Metabolism*, 2008 Dec 19;5:36. The effect of a low-carbohydrate, ketogenic diet versus a low-glycemic index diet on glycemic control in type 2 diabetes mellitus. www.ncbi.nlm.nih.gov/pubmed/19099589 and livinlavidalowcarb.com/blog/does-butter-raise-insulin-and-make-you-fat-the-low-carb-experts-respond-to-this-claim/7573.

22. Dr. Cate Shanahan in an interview with host Brad Kearns for the *Primal Blueprint Podcast* #152: "Dr. Cate Shanahan, Part II," upon the re-release of her book, *Deep Nutrition*.

23. academic.oup.com/jcem/article/89/6/2548/2870285/Adipose-Tissue-as-an-Endocrine-Organ

24. www.ncbi.nlm.nih.gov/pmc/articles/PMC3648822

25. Dr. Sylvia Tara, author of *The Secret Life of Fat: Behind the Body's Least Understood Organ and What It Means for You* (2016), in an interview on "Understanding Fat to Help You Lose Weight" on the *Bulletproof Radio* podcast, February 21, 2017.

26. www.foodrenegade.com/on-deep-nutrition-genetic-expression
27. Shanahan, *Deep Nutrition*, 207-212.
28. Ibid., p. 154.
29. Ibid., p.219.
30. Ibid., p. 227.
31. Dr. William Davis in an interview with host Jimmy Moore on the *Livin' La Vida Low-Carb Podcast*, 2013.
32. www.westonaprice.org/health-topics/abcs-of-nutrition/nutritional-adjuncts-to-the-fat-soluble-vitamins
33. Tara, *Bulletproof Radio* podcast, February 21, 2017.
34. www.westonaprice.org/health-topics/abcs-of-nutrition/saturated-fat-body-good
35. chriskresser.com/nutrition-for-healthy-skin-part-2
36. AP Simopoulos, "Essential Fatty Acids in Health and Chronic Disease" Am J Clinical Nutrition 1999 Sep;70(3 Suppl):560S-569S. www.ncbi.nlm.nih.gov/pubmed/10479232.
37. Use of omega-6 oils dangerous to health studies: Omega-6s are related to depression: Joseph R. Hibbeln and Norman Salem Jr., "Dietary Polyunsaturated Fatty Acids and Depression: When Cholesterol Does Not Satisfy," *American Journal of Clinical Nutrition* 62, no. 1 (1995): 1–9; J. R. Hibbeln et al., "Do Plasma Polyunsaturates Predict Hostility and Violence?" in *Nutrition and Fitness: Metabolic and Behavior Aspects in Health and Disease, World Review of Nutrition and Diatetics* 82, eds., A. P. Simopoulos and K. N. Pavlou (Basel, Switzerland: Karger, 1996): 175–186. 276; William S. Harris et al., "Omega-6 Fatty Acids and Risk for Cardiovascular Disease. A Scientific Advisory from the American Heart Association Nutrition Subcommittee of the Council of Nutrition, Physical Activity, and Metabolism.
38. M. Kratz, "Atherosclerosis: Diet and Drugs", Volume 170 of the series *Handbook of Experimental Pharmacology*, 195-213 "Dietary Cholesterol, Atherosclerosis and Coronary Heart Disease".
39 Gedgaudas, *Primal Fat Burner*, 15.
40. RA Emken, et al. "Comparison of linolenic and linoleic acid metabolism in man: influence of dietary linoleic acid." www.researchgate.net/publication/43277235_Comparison_of_linolenic_and_linoleic_acid_metabolism_in_man_influence_of_dietary_linoleic_acid
41. For an excellent primer on the issues related to vegetarianism, agriculture, environmental degradation, and sustainability, please refer to former vegan Lierre Keith's 2009 book, *The Vegetarian Myth* (Oakland: PM Press, 2009).
42. Anthony Samsel and Stephanie Seneff, "Glyphosate, pathways to modern diseases II: Celiac sprue and gluten intolerance." *Interdisciplinary Toxicology*, 2013 Dec; 6(4): 159–184. www.ncbi.nlm.nih.gov/pmc/articles/PMC3945755.
43. articles.mercola.com/sites/articles/archive/2016/02/02/how-roundup-damages-mitochondria.aspx
44. James E. Beecham and Stephanie Seneff, "Is there a link between autism and glyphosate-formulated herbicides?" *Journal of Autism*. www.hoajonline.com/autism/2054-992X/3/1.
45. people.csail.mit.edu/seneff
46. R. Mesnage, et al., "Transcriptome profile analysis reflects rat liver and kidney damage following chronic ultra-low dose Roundup exposure." *Environmental Health* (2015) 14:70. www.i-sis.org.uk/pdf/Glyphosate_research_papers_compiled_by_Dr_Alex_Vasquez_and_Dr_Eva_Sirinathsinghji.pdf.
47. Dr. William Shaw on "Most Toxic Chemicals and GPL/Organic Acids Testing" on the *Not Just Paleo* podcast, April 13, 2017. www.evanbrand.com/blog/229-dr-william-shaw-phd-organic-acids-testing-gpl-tox-chemical-profile-testing.
48. A few of my sources include: www.cookingforengineers.com/article/50/Smoke-Points-of-Various-Fats; draxe.com/ghee-benefits; Chris Kresser's list on page 116 in his 2013 edition of *The Paleo Cure*; www.seriouseats.com/2014/05/cooking-fats-101-whats-a-smoke-point-and-why-does-it-matter.html; www.nutriting.com/conseils-sante/quelles-matieres-grasses-pour-la-cuisson; and fr.wikipedia.org/wiki/Point_de_fum%C3%A9e.
49. www.pbs.org/video/cooking-concert-julia-child-and-jacques-pepin-create-classic-holiday-meal
50. chrismasterjohnphd.com/2016/12/29/updates-ultimate-vitamin-k2-resource
51. www.primalbody-primalmind.com/animal-fat-new-superfood/#_ftn6
52. CA Daley, Abbott A, Doyle PS, et al., "A review of fatty acid profiles and antioxidant content in grass-fed and grain-fed beef." Nutr J. 2010; 9: 10. www.ncbi.nlm.nih.gov/pubmed/20219103
53. grasslandbeef.com/your-health#cla.
54. More on ghee, butter, and fats in general at Dr. Axe's website draxe.com/ghee-benefits.
55. Penny M. Kris-Etherton, et al., "High-mono-unsaturated fatty acid diets lower both plasma cholesterol and tracylglycerol concentrations". *American Journal of Clinical Nutrition*, December 1999, vol.70. no.6 1009-1015. ajcn.nutrition.org/content/70/6/1009.full.
56. Seek out the best, organic brands you can afford to ensure you are getting real olive oil drchristianson.com/how-do-you-know-if-your-olive-oil-is-real.
57. In response to the need for a butter substitute for Emperor Napoleon III's army and for the lower classes of French society, Frenchman Hippolyte Mège-Mouriès created in 1869 what was later to be called "margarine."
58. www.marksdailyapple.com/whats-so-healthy-about-avocado-oil
59. Dr. Cate Shanahan, lecture on "Bad Diet, Bad DNA?" Ancestral Health Symposium [August 2016]. YouTube video, 40:40. Posted August 2016. www.youtube.com/watch?v=o8byeJGaOMM&list=PLbhWKPDKXIEBBybY-cY_jUQGE7S0KLgH5S&index=19, and three studies cited: 4HNE Derived from PUFA and Causes Cancer: "Role of Lipid Peroxidation derived 4-hydroxynonenol (4HNE) in Cancer: Focusing on mitochondria" *Redox Biology*, Volume 4, April 2015, 193-199; "4HHE derived from PUFA (omega-3) and Causes Cancer: 4-Hydroxyhexanal- and 4-Hydroxynonenal-Modified Proteins in Pterygia" *Oxidative Medicine and Cellular Longevity*, Volume 2013 (2013); "MDA Derived from PUFA (omega-3 and omega-6) and Causes Cancer: Role of polyunsaturated fatty acids and lipid peroxidation on colorectal cancer risks and treatments". *Current Opinions in Clinical Nutrition Metabolic Care*. 2012 March: 15(2):99-106.
60 *Primal Blueprint Podcast* #151: "Dr. Cate Shanahan, Part I," January 11, 2017.
61. Ibid.
62. Shanahan, Ancestral Health Symposium, August 2016.
63. Ibid.
64. For another informative interview with Dr, Cate Shanahan on "Vegetable Oil – The Silent Killer with Dr. Cate Shanahan," refer to *Bulletproof Radio* podcast #376, January 3, 2017 at blog.bulletproof.com/dr-cate-shanahan-376.
65. Shanahan, Ancestral Health Symposium, August 2016.
66. Shanahan, *Bulletproof Radio* podcast #376, January 3, 2017.

67. José Del Campo, et al., "Antimicrobial effect of rosemary extracts". *Journal of Food Protection*, 2000 Oct;63(10):1359-68. jfoodprotection.org/doi/pdf/10.4315/0362-028X-63.10.1359?code=fopr-site.

68. For more research on rosemary: www.greenmedinfo.com/substance/rosemary

69. Dr. Terry Wahls, MD, on "How to Defy Your Diagnosis and Reverse Autoimmune Disease" on the *Fat-Burning Man* podcast, April 14, 2017. fatburningman.com/dr-terry-wahls-how-to-defy-your-diagnosis-and-reverse-autoimmune-disease.

70. FODMAP is an acronym for "Fermentable, Oligo-, Di-, Mono-saccharides and Polyols," a grouping of carbohydrate compounds that are often poorly digested or can be particularly difficult for some people to digest.

71. EM Sarrell, A. Mandelberg, and HA Cohen, "Efficacy of naturopathic extracts in the management of ear pain associated with acute otitis media". *Archives of Pediatric and Adolescent Medicine*, 2001 Jul;155(7):796-9. www.ncbi.nlm.nih.gov/pubmed/11434846.

72. www.davidlebovitz.com/should-you-remove-the-green-germ-from-garlic

73. Chris Kresser discusses the benefits of eating garlic and other nutrient-dense foods with Jo Robinson, author of *Eating on the Wild Side*, in the *Revolution Health Radio* podcast entitled "Could 'Eating Wild' Be the Missing Link to Optimum Health?" July 17, 2013: chriskresser.com/could-eating-wild-be-the-missing-link-to-optimum-health.

74. deliciousliving.com/blog/new-study-salt-depletes-calcium-what-about-magnesium.

75. More on Celtic and Himalayan salts at draxe.com/10-benefits-celtic-sea-salt-himalayan-salt and www.waterbenefitshealth.com/celtic-sea-salt.html.

76. Sea salt for adrenal fatigue: draxe.com/3-steps-to-heal-adrenal-fatigue. For more on the benefits of sea salt and Himalayan salts: draxe.com/10-benefits-celtic-sea-salt-himalayan-salt and www.waterbenefitshealth.com/celtic-sea-salt.html.

77. www.livestrong.com/article/379070-drinking-salt-water-for-adrenal-fatigue

78. draxe.com/what-is-choline

79. www.healthy-eating-politics.com/organic-eggs.html

80. Shanahan, Ancestral Health Symposium, August 2016.

81. www.causses-cevennes.com/histoire-du-chataignier-en-cevennes

82. SH Ahmed, et al., "Sugar addiction: pushing the drug-sugar analogy to the limit", *Current Opinions in Clinical Nutrition and Metabolic Care*. 2013 Jul;16(4):434-9. www.ncbi.nlm.nih.gov/pubmed/23719144.

83. www.ancient-minerals.com/magnesium-deficiency/need-more

84. articles.mercola.com/sites/articles/archive/2015/01/19/magnesium-deficiency.aspx

85. www.westonaprice.org/health-topics/abcs-of-nutrition/magnificent-magnesium

86. wellnessmama.com/3610/low-magnesium

87. The various health benefits and properties of monk fruit and other sweeteners can be found at Dr. Josh Axe's website: draxe.com/monk-fruit

88. www.greenmedinfo.com/toxic-ingredient/sucralose-aka-splenda

89. Metin Basaranoglu, et al. "Carbohydrate intake and nonalcoholic fatty liver disease: fructose as a weapon of mass destruction". *Hepatobiliary Surgical Nutrition*, 2015 Apr; 4(2): 109–116. www.ncbi.nlm.nih.gov/pmc/articles/PMC4405421.

90. Wheaton, *Savoring the Past*, 87.

91. Ibid., 90-91.

92. For more on the benefits of full-fat and raw, unpasteurized cheese and dairy: blog.grasslandbeef.com/the-many-benefits-of-full-fat-cheese?utm_source=Newsletter+2017-04-02&utm_campaign=20170402&utm_medium=email

93. Dominique Bouchait, *Fromages* (Paris: Hachette Livre: Éditions du Chêne, 2016), 60.

94. Ibid., 140.

95. Ibid., 168.

96. wholehealthsource.blogspot.ch/2008/06/vitamin-k2-menatetrenone-mk-4.html

97. chrismasterjohnphd.com/2016/12/09/the-ultimate-vitamin-k2-resource

98. www.ondietandhealth.com/primal-blueprint-podcast-interview-vitamin-k2

99. draxe.com/is-your-cookware-poisoning-you

100. La-or Chailurkit and Wichai Aekplakorn. "The Association of Serum Bisphenol A with Thyroid Autoimmunity". *Int'l Journal of Environmental Research and Public Health*, 2016, 13(11), 1153. www.mdpi.com/1660-4601/13/11/1153.

101. J Appl Toxicol. 2016 Sep 9. [Epub ahead of print] "Correlation between antibodies to bisphenol A, its target enzyme protein disulfide isomerase and antibodies to neuron-specific antigens". Kharrazian D., Vojdani A. www.ncbi.nlm.nih.gov/pubmed/27610592.

102. www.greenmedinfo.com/blog/scientists-prove-link-between-aluminum-and-early-onset-alzheimer-s-disease

103. Jean de la Fontaine (1621-1625) was one of France's most widely read poets of the 17th century, with his most famous work of rhyming poems, *Fables*, was first published in 1688 and is still recited by children today.

5. BUTCHERY BASICS: KNOW YOUR CUTS AND HONE YOUR KNIVES

1. JF Mallet, with text by Emmanuel Jary, *Viandes: Encyclopédie des Produits & des Métiers de Bouche* (French meat encyclopedia), (Paris: Hachette Livre/Hachette Cuisine, 2013), 9.

2. Paul Freedman, *10 Restaurants that Changed America*, audio book (Ashland, OR: Blackstone Audio, Inc., 2016).

3. Video demonstration: www.seriouseats.com/2010/04/knife-skills-how-to-hone-a-dull-knife.html.

4. Video demonstration: www.wusthof.com/care-and-sharpening/using-a-steel.

5. Video demonstration: www.seriouseats.com/2010/04/knife-skills-how-to-sharpen-a-knife.html.

6. J.F. Mallet, *Viandes: Encyclopédie des Produits & des Métiers de Bouche*.

7. Salatin, *Folks, This Ain't Normal*.

8. www.grass-fed-solutions.com/beef-fat.html

9. Nora Gedgaudas on 100% pasture-fed animal fats: www.primalbody-primalmind.com/animal-fat-new-superfood

10. Dr. Mercola goes into detail about the differences between grass-fed and grain-fed beef at www.mercola.com/beef/cla.htm

11. Dr. Axe describes some of the benefits of CLAs in detail at draxe.com/conjugated-linoleic-acid.

6. RECIPES, STORIES, COOKING TIPS, AND WINE PAIRINGS

1. Diana Rodgers, lecture on "The Global Sustainability -Nutrition Disconnect," Ancestral Health Symposium, [August 2016]. YouTube video, 37:20. Posted September 2016. www.youtube.com/watch?v=_MgaJAu9qJ0&list=PLbhWKPD-KXIEBBybYcY_jUQGE7S0KLgH5S&index=43.
2. For USDA information on food safety: www.fsis.usda.gov/wps/wcm/connect/c33b69fe-7041-4f50-9dd0-d098f11d1f13/Beef_from_Farm_to_Table.pdf?MOD=AJPERES.
3. This cyclical dietary approach is covered in many texts on fasting and nutritional ketosis for its health benefits, such as in Joseph Mercola's 2017 book, *Fat for Fuel* (Carlsbad: Hay House, 2017).
4. See Joseph Mercola's discussion on this topic on "The Empowering Neurologist – David Perlmutter, MD and Dr. Joseph Mercola". YouTube video, 46:37. Posted April 2017. www.youtube.com/watch?v=kvRq50ZFFTU.
5. Franziska Spritzler, registered dietician, speaking at the 2016 Low Carb USA™ conference, aired on *The Livin' La Vida Low-Carb Show*, June 26, 2017.
6. Jean-Louis Flandrin, "Le goût et la nécessité : sur l'usage des graisses dans les cuisines d'Europe occidentale (XIVe-XVIIIe siècle)", in *Annales. Économies, Sociétés, Civilisations*, 38 année, N. 2, 1983, 369-401.
7. Ibid., 369-372.
8. Simone Campos Cavalher-Machado, et al., "The Anti-Allergic Activity of the Acetate Fraction of Schinus Terebinthifolius leaves in IGE induced Mice Paw Edema and Pleurisy". *International Immunopharmacol*, 2008 Nov 29;8(11):1552-60. Epub 2008 Jul 29. www.pubpdf.com/pub/18672096/The-anti-allergic-activity-of-the-acetate-fraction-of-Schinus-terebinthifolius-leaves-in-IgE-induced.
9. Faculté d'Oenologie de Bordeaux – ISVV. Bordeaux School of Oenology, DUAD (Diplôme Universitaire d'Aptitude à la Dégustation) Diploma in Viticulture, Oenology and Professional Tasting, 2014–2015.

BEEF
1. www.la-viande.fr/cuisine-achat/cuisiner-viande/cuisiner-boeuf/morceaux/basses-cotes
2. Ibid.
3. www.certifiedangusbeef.com/kitchen/doneness.php and Atelier des Chefs, Bordeaux. (See photo of their recommended cooked meat temperatures on page 119.)
4. Julia Child, *Mastering the Art of French Cooking*, 9th Printing, 2010, 306.
5. Ibid., 307.
6. Antoine-Augustin Parmentier, *Traité sur la Culture et les Usages des Pommes de Terre, de la Patate, et du Topinambour*, 1789.
7. For a fun glimpse of how Roquefort is made, view "How Do They Do It? - Roquefort cheese". YouTube video, 7:12. Posted Sept 2013. www.youtube.com/watch?v=gWM_R2tDOfA.
8. Wolfert, *The Cooking of Southwest France*, 259.
9. www.winemag.com/2012/11/28/a-wine-lovers-guide-to-herbs
10. www.la-viande.fr/cuisine-achat/cuisiner-viande/cuisiner-boeuf/morceaux/basses-cotes

FISH AND SEAFOOD
1. www.marksdailyapple.com/are-you-eating-these-important-supplemental-foods/#axzz3mMoP1dvW
2. "Oyster Knife - How to Open an Oyster". YouTube video, 2:15. Posted Jan 2010. www.youtube.com/watch?v=97T1Pp4-zyE.
3. www.greatbritishchefs.com/how-to-cook/how-to-open-an-oyster
4. www.ncbi.nlm.nih.gov/pubmed/2614472 and theconversation.com/why-you-shouldnt-wrap-your-food-in-aluminium-foil-before-cooking-it-57220

LAMB
1. Temperature ranges according to www.atelierdeschefs.fr/fr/techniques-de-cuisine/432-tableau-de-temperature-de-cuisson-des-viandes.php and www.beefandlamb.com.au/How_to/Cooking_beef_and_lamb/Preparation_tips/How_to_use_a_meat_thermometer.
2. www.marksdailyapple.com/the-definitive-guide-to-nuts

OFFAL AND FATS
1. www.thepaleomom.com/why-everyone-should-be-eating-organ
2. Nora Gedgaudas' interview on the *Livin' La Vida Low-Carb Show*, #1263: "Nora Gedgaudas on How Fat Can Help You Live Longer," May 24, 2017.
3. www.supertoinette.com/fiche-cuisine/11/abats.html#url://131/28/459
4. documents-dds-ny.un.org/doc/UNDOC/GEN/G08/251/14/PDF/G0825114.pdf?OpenElement
5. Please refer to Mat Lalonde's lecture on "Nutrient Density: Sticking to the Essentials AHS12," presented at the Ancestral Health Symposium 2012, Harvard University [2012]. YouTube video, 51:58. Posted Feb 2013. www.youtube.com/watch?v=HwbY12qZcF4.
6. Chris Kresser, *The Paleo Cure* (New York: Little, Brown and Company, 2013), 68-78.
7. Dr. Terry Wahls speaking on "How to Fuel Your Mitochondria, Organ Meats for Beginners, MCT Oil, and Exogenous Ketones," on *The Ultimate Health Podcast*, #120, September 27, 2016. ultimatehealthpodcast.com/dr-terry-wahls/#.
8. www.wine-searcher.com/regions-pineau+des+charentes

PORK
1. For detailed information on phytic acids, see www.westonaprice.org/health-topics/living-with-phytic-acid. For numerous links on soaking grains, see www.kitchenstewardship.com/seriescarnivals/soaking-grains-an-exploration.

POULTRY, EGGS, AND RABBIT
1. www.marksdailyapple.com/lectins
2. www.marksdailyapple.com/why-grains-are-unhealthy
3. For more on beans and legumes in general, see www.marksdailyapple.com/where-do-legumes-belong-in-the-primal-eating-plan.
4. On cooking duck breast: www.finecooking.com/articles/cooking-duck-brest-medium-rare.aspx.
5. According to the US Department of Health and Human Services, a duck or goose is considered "cooked" at 165°F (74°C). www.foodsafety.gov/keep/charts/mintemp.html.
6. Andrew Dornenburg and Karen Page. *What to Drink with What You Eat* (New York: Bullfinch Press, 2006), 116.
7. This photo tutorial (with captions in French) shows you how to properly debone a rabbit saddle: chefsimon.lemonde.fr/gourmets/chef-simon/recettes/desosser-un-rable-de-lapin.

8. A good resource for cooking chicken can be found at www.recipetips.com/kitchen-tips/t--911/chicken-cooking-times.asp.
9. www.foodsafety.gov/keep/charts/mintemp.html

STOCKS AND SAUCES

1. H.J. Teuteberg, "The General Relationship between Diet and Industrialization," in *Euopean Diet from Pre-Industrial to Modern Times*, Elborg and Robert Forster, eds., (New York: Harper Torchbooks, 1975), 91-92.
2. An interesting discussion of these fears is given by Nick Mailer in his talk "Chemophobia, Appeal to Nature" at the Ancestral Health Symposium in [August 2016]. YouTube video, 38:28. Posted August 2016. www.youtube.com/watch?v=UWxYQMoUJzU.
3. Montagné Prosper, *Larousse Gastronomique*, First American Edition, 1961 (New York: Crown Publishers, Inc.), 851-852.
4. As with the crêpes in the Dessert section (page 503), I have used only Otto's Naturals Cassava Flour in this and the other sauces and cannot vouch for how these sauces might turn out using other brands of cassava flour or other types of flours.
5. Child, *Mastering the Art of French Cooking*, 2010 printing, 60-61.
6. Sarah, T. Peterson, *Acquired Taste: The French Origins of Modern Cooking* (Ithica: Cornell University Press, 1994), 138.
7. Pierre François La Varenne, *Le cuisinier françois enseignant la manière de bien apprester et assaisonner viandes, legumes*, 1651. (Reprint: Paris: Hachette Livre), 214.
8. www.organicfacts.net/health-benefits/animal-product/health-benefits-of-anchovies.html
9. www.epicurious.com/expert-advice/how-to-turn-wine-into-vinegar-article
10. www.saucecuisine.com/Histoires-des-sauces/his-toires-des-sauces.html
11. La Varenne, *Le cuisinier françois enseignant la manière de bien apprester et assaisonner viandes, legumes*, 117.
12. Child, *Mastering the Art of French Cooking*, 2010 printing, 57.
13. Chris Kresser on "What Nutrients Do Kids Need to Thrive?", May 5, 2017, and "CoQ10, Vaccination, and Natural Treatment for Migraines," May 2, 2012, on the *Revolution Health Radio* podcast.
14. www.pbs.org/video/cooking-concert-julia-child-and-jacques-pepin-create-classic-holiday-meal
15. Child, *Mastering the Art of French Cooking*, 2010 printing, 58.
16. Anne Willen, *Great Cooks and Their Recipes: From Taillevent to Escoffier* (New York: McGraw-Hill. 1977), 47.
17. La Varenne, *Le cuisinier françois enseignant la manière de bien apprester et assaisonner viandes, legumes*, 117.
18. Dr. Natasha Campbell McBride, *Gut and Psychology Syndrome: Natural Treatment for Autism, Dyspraxia, A.D.D., Dyslexia, A.D.H.D., Depression, Schizophrenia*, (revised edition, Cambridge: Medinform Publishing, 2010).

VEAL

1. lacuisinedantandepapyjacques.over-blog.com/2015/01/l-histoire-des-paupiettes.html
2. *Le Cuisinier Gascon, ou Traité simplifié des substances alimentaires, revu et aumenté d'un grand nombre de recettes*, ed. Marcel Herbert. 11th Edition, 1864. Editor's Preface pp. 3 and 11-12. (The first edition of *Le Cuisinier Gascon* was published in 1740 in Amsterdam by Louis Auguste de Bourbon, prince de Dombes.)

3. www.gardeningknowhow.com/edible/herbs/cilantro/how-to-grow-cilantro-indoors.htm

VEGETABLES

1. Dr. Steven Gundry discusses lectins at length in his 2017 book *The Plant Paradox* (New York: Harper Way, 2017).
2. Here is a brief sound bite from Dr. Perlmutter's website: www.drperlmutter.com/feeding-good-bacteria-prebiotics.
3. Sarah Fragoso has a great recipe for Paleo Pumpkin Pie in her book *Everyday Paleo* (Las Vegas: Victory Belt Publishing, 2011).
4. espritdepays.com/comprendre/introduction/les-quatre-couleurs-du-perigord#note1

DESSERTS

1. Dr. Joseph Maroon, *The Longevity Factor: How Resveratrol and Red Wine Activate Genes for a Longer and Healthier Life* (New York: Atria Books, 2009), 282.
2. wellnessmama.com/1888/elderberry-syrup
3. wellnessmama.com/4599/flu-busting-gummy-bears
4. Please note: As with the sauces in the Stocks and Sauces section, I have used only Otto's Naturals Cassava Flour to make these crêpes and cannot vouch for how these sauces might turn out using other brands of cassava flour or other types of flours.

7. KNOW YOUR FRENCH WINES, HOW TO TASTE THEM, AND HOW TO PAIR THEM WITH FOOD

1. "Seule, dans le regne végétal, la vigne nous rend intelligible ce qu'est la véritable saveur de la terre." Colette.
2. More from Vincent Lignac in my interview with him for an article of mine published in *The Drinks Business* online edition in October 2014: www.thedrinksbusiness.com/2014/10/st-emilion-balancing-modernity-and-tradition.
3. "On produit un vin à consommer à table et pour avoir une emotion." Eric Boisssenot, Oenologist, Agence Fleurie, Bordeaux, Visiting Professor, University of Bordeaux, ISVV, DUAD Wine Tasting, January 23, 2015. ISVV stands for Institut des Sciences de la Vigne et du Vin, translated as Institute for the Vine and Wine. DUAD stands for *Diplôme Universitaire d'Aptitude à la Dégustation*, translated as "University Diploma in Winetasting."
4. A quote from an article I wrote for *The Drinks Business* online edition in October 2014: www.thedrinksbusiness.com/2014/10/wine-the-kevin-bacon-of-industries.
5. Emile Peynaud, *Connaissance et Travail du Vin* (Paris: Dunod. 1984), 32.
6. S. Renaud, "Wine, Alcohol, Platelets, and the French Paradox for Coronary Heart Disease". *The Lancet* June 20, 1992; 339: 1523–1526.
7. M.S. Ferná dez-Pachón, et al. "Antioxidant activity of wines and relation with their polyphenolic composition." Analytica Chimica Acta, Vol. 513, Issue 1, 18 June 2004, 113-118. www.sciencedirect.com/science/article/pii/S0003267004002181.
8. R. Corder, et al., "Oenology: Red wine procyanidins and vascular health." *Nature* 444. 566, November 30, 2006. www.ncbi.nlm.nih.gov/pubmed/17136085 or www.nature.com/nature/journal/v444/n7119/full/444566a.html#B1 or www.researchgate.net/publication/6662838_Oenology_Red_wine_procyanidins_and_vascular_health

9. Maroon, *The Longevity Factor: How Resveratrol and Red Wine Activate Genes for a Longer and Healthier Life*, 49.
10. M. Lagouge, et al. "Resveratrol improves mitochondrial function and protects against metabolic disease by activating SIRT1 and PGC-1α," Cell 127 (6) (December 15, 2006): 1091-1093. www.ncbi.nlm.nih.gov/pubmed/17112576.
11. Maroon, *The Longevity Factor: How Resveratrol and Red Wine Activate Genes for a Longer and Healthier Life*.
12. Dr. Robert Lustig on "Sugar: The Bitter Truth". YouTube video, 1:29:36. Posted July 2009. www.youtube.com/watch?v=dBnniua6-oM and www.uctv.tv/shows/The-Skinny-on-Obesity-Ep-1-An-Epidemic-for-Every-Body-23305.
13. Olivier Bernard and Thierry Dussard write about this in their 2013 French publication of *The Magic of the 45th Parallel*, French, (Bordeaux: Féret, 2013).
14. *"Très souvent, les expressions les plus originales et singulières d'un cépage se trouvent à la limite Nord de sa zone de maturité, c'est-à-dire dans des endroits où il peut mûrir mais seulement grâce à des efforts importants consentis par les viticulteurs, avec une incidence significative du millésime. C'est le cas par exemple de Sancerre pour le Sauvignon blanc, du Piémont pour le Nebbiolo, de la côte de Nuits pour le Pinot noir ou bien encore du médoc pour le Cabernet-Sauvignon. Comme le disait Denis Dubourdieu, dans les endroits où la vigne est toujours facile à cultiver, le vin est souvent ennuyeux à déguster."*
15. Cornelis Van Leeuwen, Denis Dubourdieu, et al., "Influence of Climate, Soil and Cultivar on Terroir". *American Journal of Enology and Viticulture*, September 2004. www.ajevonline.org/content/55/3/207.
16. Cornelis Van Leeuwen and Gerard Seguin. "The Concept of Terroir in Vitivulture", *Journal of Wine Research*, 2006, Vol. 17, No. 1, 1.
17. The intricate chemical and metabolic intricacies of yeast cells in the fermentation process is explained in detail at winemakermag.com/1078-understanding-yeasts,
18. My personal interview with Dr. Tim Gerstmar on cholesterol, statins, caloric abundance, and sugar addiction, January 27, 2017.
19. Dr. Gary Foresman on the *Primal Blueprint Podcast #155:* Breast Health Part III, February 8, 2017.
20. Miceli, Antonio et al. "Polyphenols, resveratrol, antioxidant activity and ochratoxin a contamination in red table wines, controlled denomination of origin (DOC) wines and wines obtained from organic farming". *Journal of Wine Research*, Vol. 14, Numbers 2-3, August/December 2003, pp. 115-120(6). www.ingentaconnect.com/content/routledg/cjwr/2003/00000014/F0020002/art00004.
21. *L'Ecole du Vin de Bordeaux*, the Bordeaux Wine School, is part of the CIVB, *Conseil Interprofessionnel du Vin de Bordeaux* (The Inter-Professional Council of Bordeaux Wine).
22. www.gardeningknowhow.com/garden-how-to/soil-fertilizers/iron-for-plants.htm and www.ncbi.nlm.nih.gov/pmc/articles/PMC549987/pdf/plntphys00422-0012.pdf
23. I. Gülçin, OI Küfrevioglu, M. Oktay, ME Büyükokuroglu, "Antioxidant, antimicrobial, antiulcer and analgesic activities of nettle (Urtica dioica L.)". Journal of Ethnopharmacol, 2004 Feb;90(2-3):205-15. www.ncbi.nlm.nih.gov/pubmed/15013182.
24. Most of the French *vitis vinifera* vines were ravaged by the the *phylloxera* (a sap-sucking microscopic insect native to North America) infestation during the mid-1800s. Now all vines are grafted with American hybrid rootstocks that are resistant to this "disease."
25. Adapted from *The 2014 Vintage in Bordeaux*, by Professor Denis Dubourdieu and Dr. Laurence Geny, et al., Institute of Vine and Wine Sciences of Bordeaux University, Oenological Research Unit, 2014 and lectures by Professor Dubourdieu during the DUAD wine course 2014-2015. www.bordeauxraisins.fr/images/millesimes/millesime_2014_english.pdf.
26. World renown French oenologist Emile Peynaud, *The Taste of Wine: The Art and Science of Wine Appreciation*. English translation, 28.
27. Axel Marchal, Associate Professor of Oenology, University of Bordeaux: "Il est nécessaire de distinguer la dégustation de la découverte. On ne déguste en effet réellement que les vins que l'on connaît : déguster, c'est revivre une émotion, avec des attentes plus ou moins fortes suscitées par les expériences précédentes vécues avec des vins du même type. Dans l'apprentissage de la dégustation, il est ainsi primordial de mémoriser la sensation globale ressentie lors de la rencontre avec des modèles d'une catégorie donnée de vins. Or, on doit être guidé pour rencontrer ces modèles, par des amis ou des relations connaissant bien la catégorie en question. Trop souvent, le modèle ne représente pas la catégorie, il en constitue l'idéal esthétique, rarement rencontré mais toujours à l'origine d'une émotion singulière."
28. *The Bordeaux Wine Guide, L'École du Vin de Bordeaux*. Translated by Sophie Brissaud. Edited by Laure Lamendin. Paris: Éditions de la Martinière. 2014, 53.
29. Peynaud, *The Taste of Wine: The Art and Science of Wine Appreciation*, 190.
30. A summary of brain signaling as described by Dr. Gilles Sicard, lecture on "The Physiology of Wine Tasting," (*La Physiologie de la Dégustation*), DUAD Wine Course, October 27, 2014, Institute of the Sciences of the Vine and Wine, Bordeaux, France.
31. Peynaud, *The Taste of Wine: The Art and Science of Wine Appreciation*, 190-191. It is worth noting an example of the difference in groupings that the Bordeaux Wine School (L'École du Vin de Bordeaux, part of the CIVB – Conseil Interprofessionnel du Vin de Bordeaux) names an eleventh group, that of "Mineral," (flint, quartz, schist, limestone), which according to Peynaud's list is rolled into the Empyreumatic group, and adds bay leaf, juniper berry and rosemary to the "Spice" category, Havana cigar to the "Animal" category, and green apple to the "Ethers" group.
32. To this list I would add blackcurrant blossom (*bourgeon de cassis*), and boxwood (*buis*), as they are commonly found in Sauvignon blanc wines.
33. I would add to this list dark berries, mashed berries, stewed berries, and stewed fruits (*fruits compotés*), as these come up in Bordeaux wines of vintages that have had a lot of sun, and often these wines are among the "grands vins," such as the Pomerols from 1982, 1985, 1989, 2000, 2003. (Since then, also 2005, and 2009.) Pierre Casamayor, *L'École de la Dégustation: Le Vin en 100 Leçons*, (Paris: Hachette, 2000), 69.
34. Richard Pfister, *Les Parfums du Vin: Sentir et Comprendre le Vin*, (Paris: Delachaux et Niestlé SA, 2013), 42-43.
35. www.guildsomm.com/stay_current/features/b/guest_blog/posts/winetasting-terminology-the-poetry-and-the-prose#pi5772=2
36. For red wines, there were initially only four properties ranked at Premier Cru: Château Haut-Brion, Château Lafite Rothschild, Château Latour, and Château Margaux. Château Mouton Rothschild was added in 1973.

37. "How does our sense of taste work?" www.ncbi.nlm.nih.gov/pubmedhealth/PMH0072592
38. Associate professor of Oenology, University of Bordeaux, *Maître de conférences en œnologie à l'Université de Bordeaux*.
39. "L'équilibre des saveurs contribue notablement à la qualité sensorielle des vins. Comme l'a défini Emile Peynaud, il s'articule autour des saveurs sucrées et acides dans les vins blancs et des saveurs sucrées, acides et amères dans les vins rouges."
40. Data adapted from Jean-Claude Buffin's book, *Educvin: Votre Talent de la Dégustation* and website: www.educvin.com/pages/regions_extrait_chapitre_17.htm.
41. Data adapted from Jean-Claude Buffin's book, *Educ Vin: Votre Talent de la Dégustation* and website: www.educvin.com/pages/regions_extrait_chapitre_36.htm.
42. Carline Matthews is a Level 4 WSET diploma holder and teaches at the Bordeaux Wine School. She gives customized wine tours in France and Italy. www.uncorkedwinetours.com.
43. Robb Wolf, *Wired to Eat: Turn Off Cravings, Rewire Your Appetite for Weight Loss, and Determine the Foods That Work for You* (New York: Harmony Books, 2017).
44. *The Bordeaux Wine Guide*, 147.
45. *The Oxford Companion to Wine*, 4th Edition, Edited by Jancis Robinson and Julia Harding (Oxford: Oxford University Press, 2015), 16.
46. *The Bordeaux Wine Guide*, 15.
47. *The Bordeaux Wine Guide*, 43.
48. www.bourgogne-wines.com/our-wines-our-terroir/our-grape-varietals-our-colors/aligote/aligote-a-100-bourgogne-varietal,2799,10609.html
49. www.vin-vigne.com/vignoble/vin-languedoc-roussillon.html#ixzz4YYmOvLq3
50. *The Oxford Companion to Wine*, 4th Edition, 445.
51. lescepages.free.fr/mollard.html
52. Marnie Old, *Wine: A Tasting Course* (London: Dorling Kindersley, 2013), 203.
53. The Full title of Brillat-Savarin's book is: *Physiologie du Goût, ou Méditations de Gastronomie Transcendante; ouvrage théorique, historique et à l'ordre du jour, dédié aux Gastronomes parisiens, par un Professeur, membre de plusieurs sociétés littéraires et savantes*.
54. espritdepays.com/gastronomie-terroirs-viticulture/specialites-regionales/chabrol-et-tradition-perigourdine#note4

8. FAMILY FOOD ORGANIZATION AND MEAL PLANNING

1. For a serious reality check on the "I'll sleep when I'm dead" mentality and the health benefits of prioritizing sleep, please see Sarah Ballantyne's talk on "Ancestral Sleep in the Modern Age," presented at the Ancestral Health Symposium [August 2016]. YouTube video, 39:41. Posted August 2016. www.youtube.com/watch?v=xb6eI8IBV0M&index-=29&list=PLbhWKPDKXIEBBybYcY_jUQGE7S0KLgH5S.
2. Anne-Marie Chang, et al., "Evening use of light-emitting eReaders negatively affects sleep, circadian timing, and next-morning alertness". Proceedings of the National Academy of Sciences January 27, 2015, 112 (4). 1232–1237. www.pnas.org/content/112/4/1232.
3. www.scientificamerican.com/article/out-of-sync-how-modern-lifestyles-scramble-the-body-s-rhythms
4. Recently, I have discovered two new blue light blocking glasses; they are more expensive, but they are more fitted and stylish: www.swanwicksleep.com and biohacked.com/product/truedarktwilight.
5. www.emfresearch.com/tag/mitochondria
6. www.albany.edu/ihe/assets/Exhibit_G-Mitochondrial_Electrophys_docx.pdf
7. ehtrust.org/france-new-national-law-bans-wifi-nursery-school (The law in French: www.assemblee-nationale.fr/14/ta/ta0468.asp.)
8. alisonmain.me/2017/01/21/the-kids-are-not-all-right
9. www.healthychildren.org/English/safety-prevention/all-around/Pages/Cell-Phone-Radiation-Childrens-Health.aspx
10. See Dr. Kruse's extensive research on EMF exposure: www.jackkruse.com/emf-5-what-are-the-biologic-effects-of-emf.
11. Evan Brand's *Not Just Paleo* podcast interview "Lloyd Burrell: Restoring Health form EMF Sensitivity". January 7, 2017. www.evanbrand.com/blog/216-lloyd-burrell-electric-sensitivity-emf-mitigation. More on EMF protection at: www.electricsense.com/category/electromagnetic-protection.
12. See Lloyd Burrell's extensive list of studies linking cell phones and damage to the brain and DNA: www.electricsense.com/8822/cell-phones-cause-cancer-fact and how to reduce exposure to computer radiation: www.electricsense.com/1138/my-9-tips-to-cut-down-on-exposure-to-computer-radiation.
13. *Ultimate Health Podcast* #120: Interview with Dr. Terry Wahls on "How to Fuel Your Mitochondria, Organ Meats for Beginners, MCT Oil, and Exogenous Ketones." ultimatehealthpodcast.com/dr-terry-wahls/#.
14. Shanahan, *Deep Nutrition*, 227.
15. Dr Robert Lustig, May 2, 2017 in his interview "The Bitter Truth About Sugar" on *The 6th Annual Food Revolution Summit*, hosted by John Robbins and Ocean Robbins, April 29 – May 7, 2017. Dr. Lustig goes on to say, "Sugar is controlling children because it is an addictive substance," which leads to temper tantrums. Dr. Lustig discusses how stress drives visceral fat (which itself driven by our cortisol hormone), and the way to fix it is with stress reduction. "Sugar drives liver fat. Liver fat drives hyper-insulinemia, which drives all the chronic metabolic diseases."
16. J. Bruce German, et al., "A Reappraisal of the Impact of Dairy Foods and Milk Fat on Cardiovascular Disease Risk". *European Journal of Nutrition* 48, no. 4 (2009): 194. www.ncbi.nlm.nih.gov/pubmed/19259609.
17. Frank B. Hu, et al., "Dietary Fat Intake and the Risk of Coronary Heart Disease in Women". *New England Journal of Medicine*, November 20, 1997, 337:1491-1499. www.nejm.org/doi/full/10.1056/NEJM199711203372102%A0%A0#t=article.
18. Enid Blyton, *The Famous Five: Five Run Away Together*, originally published in Great Britain in 1942. ("tongue" p. 192 and "canned salmon" p. 241 in 2001 edition published by Hodder and Stoughton.)
19. Gedgaudas, *Primal Fat Burner*, 20.
20. *Wise Traditions Podcast* #66: "Fibro Hope", March 6, 2017.
21. www.edensgarden.com/blogs/news/5-chemicals-to-avoid-in-cleaning-products?mc_cid=0cf18ed8cd&mc_eid=90fc649ef6
22. www.edensgarden.com/blogs/news/5-chemicals-to-avoid-in-beauty-products?mc_cid=a6f5888dad&mc_eid=90fc649ef6
23. S.M. Vanderhout, et al. "Relation between milk fat percentage, vitamin D and BMI score in early childhood. *The American Journal of Clinical Nutrition*. Nov. 2016. ajcn.nutrition.org/content/early/2016/11/15/ajcn.116.139675.abstract

24. K.P. Kell, et al. Added sugars in the diet are positively associated with diastolic blood pressure and triglycerides in children. *The American Journal of Clinical Nutrition*. April 2014. ajcn.nutrition.org/content/early/2014/04/09/ajcn.113.076505
25. One such interview is on "The Role of the Microbiome in Neurological Health" from Dr. Perlmutter on the *Autism, ADHD and SPD Summit* in June 2017, but there are many other interviews, podcasts as well as his books and website to which to refer. www.autismadhdandsensoryprocessingdisordersummit.com/david-perlmutter-2
26. Natasha Campbell McBride on "GAPS Nutritional Protocol and How It Can Heal Your Child" on the *Autism, ADHD and SPD Summit* in June 2017, but there are many other interviews and podcasts as well as her book, *Gut and Psychology Syndrome*, to which to refer. www.autismadhdandsensoryprocessingdisordersummit.com/natasha-campbell-mcbride
27. Elmer Verner McCollum, *The Newer Knowledge of Nutrition* (New York: MacMillan, 1921), 58.
28. Teicholz, *The Big Fat Surprise*, Ch 6, audio book (Ashland, OR: Blackstone Audio, Inc., 2014).
29. wellnessmama.com/6357/chewable-vitamins

APPENDIXES
MY ROOTS
1. Brillat-Savarin was one of the first if not the first to promote a low-carbohydrate diet, noting that all animals, including humans, grow obese on sugar and white flour in his 1825 book *The Physiology of Taste*.
2. S. Mihrshahi, et al. "Vegetarian diet and all-cause mortality: Evidence from a large population-based Australian cohort – the 45 and Up Study." 2017. PubMed. www.ncbi.nlm.nih.gov/pubmed/28040519

EPILOGUE
1. The April 2016 "Minnesota Coronary Experiment" (www.bmj.com/content/353/bmj.i1246)
2. The international Prospective Urban Rural Epidemiology (PURE) study (www.thelancet.com/journals/lancet/article/PIIS0140-6736(17)32252-3/fulltext)

COOKING GLOSSARY
1. Eugene Pauli. *Classical Cooking the Modern Way* (1979), 219.
2. www.pbs.org/video/1333042208
3. *Wine, alcohol, platelets, and the French paradox for coronary heart disease*. Renaud S, de Lorgeril M. INSERM, Nutrition and Vascular Physiopathology Research Unit, (Unit 63), France. Lancet (London, England) [1992, Vol. 339(8808):1523-1526] www.thelancet.com/journals/lancet/article/PII0140-6736(92)91277-F/abstract
4. Vihjalmur Stefansson, *The Fat of the Land*, English. ed. of *Not by Bread Alone* (1946, reprint, New York: Macmillan, 1956), 128. highsteaks.com/the-fat-of-the-land-not-by-bread-alone-vilhjalmur-stefansson.pdf
5. fr.gaultmillau.com/pages/notre-histoire-gault-millau
6. www.carnivor.fr/termes-de-cuisson-boucher-charcuterie-fromagerie-carnivor
7. gourmandisesansfrontieres.fr/2012/11/je-cuis-tu-cuis-il-cuit-zoom-sur-les-modes-de-cuisson-en-cuisine
8. drgeo.com/plastic-water-bottles-exposed-to-heat-can-be-toxic

RESOURCES AND FURTHER READING
1. The Weston A Price Foundation website, a foundation based on the research of dentist Weston A Price, and functions on the premise of nutrient-dense foods, the way traditional, ancestral societies nourished themselves. For some educational video watching, try The Weston A. Price Foundation's President Sally Fallon-Morell's talk on *Nourishing Traditional Diets: The Key to Vibrant Health*. If you want more, check out her video on *The Oiling of America*. Skip the usual TV series and listen to or watch these videos while you are in the kitchen, which is what I do, but beware, each one is two hours long.

SELECTED BIBLIOGRAPHY

Audinet, Eric, ed. *Les 4 Saisons Gourmandes d'Aquitaine*. Bordeaux: Éditions Confluences, 2008.

Bernard, Olivier and Thierry Dussard. *The Magic of the 45th Parallel* (French). Bordeaux: Féret, 2013.

Blyton, Enid. *The Famous Five: Five Run Away Together*, originally published in Great Britain in 1942. London: Hodder and Stoughton, 2001 reprint.

Bonnefons, Nicolas de. *Les Délices de la campagne*. Paris, 1654.

Bonnefons, Nicolas de. *Le Jardinier François*. Paris, 1651.

The Bordeaux Wine Guide, L'Ecole du Vin de Bordeaux. Translated by Sophie Brissaud. Edited by Laure Lamendin. Paris: Éditions de la Martinière. 2014

Brillat-Savarin, Jean Anthelme. *The Physiology of Taste, Or Meditations on Transcendental Gastronomy*. trans. M.F.K. Fisher. New York: Random House, 2009.

Campbell-McBride, Natasha. *Gut and Psychology Syndrome: Natural Treatment for Autism, Dyspraxia, A.D.D., Dyslexia, A.D.H.D., Depression, Schizophrenia*. Revised edition, Cambridge: Medinform Publishing, 2010.

Carson, Rachel. *Silent Spring*. 1962, 40th Anniversary Edition, New York: Mariner Books, 2002.

Child, Julia. *Mastering the Art of French Cooking*, 9th Printing. New York: Alfred A. Knopf, 2010, 306.

Christianson, Alan. *The Adrenal Reset Diet*. New York: Harmony Books, 2014.

La Cuisine des Régions de France. Rennes: Éditions Ouest-France, 2002.

Le Cuisinier Gascon, ou Traité Simplifié des Substances Alimentaires. Editor anonymous. 1864.

Dawkins, Richard. *The Selfish Gene*. Oxford: Oxford University Press, 1978.

Derue, Alain. *La découpe des viandes de boucherie*. Paris: Éditions J. Lanore, 2004.

Dolle, Romy. *Fruit Belly: A 4-Day Quick Fix To Relieve Bloating Caused By High Carb, High Fruit Diets*. Malibu: Primal Nutrition, Inc., 2015.

Dornenburg, Andrew and Karen Page. *What to Drink with What You Eat*. New York: Bullfinch Press, 2006, 116.

Douet D'arcq, Louis. "Un petit traité de cuisine écrit en français au commencement du XIVe siècle" (original manuscript dates from 1306), *Bibliothèque de l'école des chartes* (1860), tome 21: 209-227.

L'École du Vin de Bordeaux. *The Bordeaux Wine Guide*. Conseil Interprofessionnel du Vin de Bordeaux (CIVB). Translated by Sophie Brissaud. Edited by Laure Lamendin. Bordeaux: Éditions de la Matinière. 2014.

Escoffier, Auguste. *Le Guide Culinaire*. (Originally published in 1902.) Paris: Éditions J'ai Lu, 2015.

Essig, Mark. *Lesser Beasts: A Snout to Tail History of the Humble Pig*. Philadelphia: Basic Books, 2015.

European Diet from Pre-Industrial to Modern Times, Edited by Elborg and Robert Forster. New York: Harper Torchbooks. 1975.

Flandrin, Jean-Louis. "Le Goût et la nécessité: sur l'usage des graisses dans les cuisines d'Europe occidentale (XIVe-XVIIIe siècle)". *Annales. Économies, Sociétés, Civilisations*, 38e Année, no. 2, (1983): 369-401.

Food and Drink in History. Selections from the Annales Economis, Sociétés Civilisation, Volume 5. Edited by Robert Forster and Orest Ranum. Translated by Elborg Forster and Patricia M. Ranum. Baltimore: The Johns Hopkins University Press. 1979.

Fragoso, Sarah. *Everyday Paleo*. Las Vegas: Victory Belt Publishing, 2011.

Frankreich/France Strassenkarte/Carte routière (map). 1990s. Bern: Hallwag AG.

Freedman, Paul. *Ten Restaurants That Changed America*. Audio book. Ashland, OR: Blackstone Audio, Inc., 2016.

Fung, Jason. *The Obesity Code: Unlocking the Secrets of Weight Loss*. Vancouver: Greystone Books Ltd., 2016

Garcia, Stéphane, *Mes Recettes Incontournables Pays Basque*. Toulouse: SG Gastronomie SASU. 2015

Gedgaudas, Nora. *Primal Fat Burner*. New York: Atria Books, 2017, 16.

Gottschall, Elaine. *Breaking the Vicious Cycle: Intestinal Health Through Diet*. Baltimore, ON: The Kirkton Press, 1994.

Le Grand Dictionnaire De L'Académie Françoise, Dédié Au Roy: A-L, Volume 1. Amsterdam: Coignard. 1696, 103.

Green, Aliza. *Field Guide to Meat*. Quirk Books. Philadelphia: 2005.

Guégan, Bertrand. *La Fleur de la Cuisine Française, où l'on trouves les meilleures recettes des meilleurs cuisiniers, pâtissiers et limonadiers de France*, Paris: Éditions de la Sirène, 1920.

Gundry, Steven. *The Plant Paradox*. New York: Harper Way, 2017.

Hémardinquer, Jean-Jacques. "Essai des cartes des graisses de cuisine en France." *Annales: Economies, Sociétés, Civilisations* 16(1970); and "Pour Une Histoire de l'Alimentation." *Cahiiers des Annales*, vol. 28. Paris: Armand Colin, 1970.

Jausserand, Corinne. *Made in Sud-Ouest*. Pairs: Larousse, 2015

Johnson, Hugh and Jancis Robinson. *The World Atlas of Wine*. 7th Edition. London: Octopus Publishing Group Ltd., 2013.

Konner, M., and S.B. Eaton. "Paleolithic nutrition: twenty-five years later." *Nutrition in Clinical Practice*; 25(6) (2010): 594-602.

Kresser, Chris. *The Paleo Cure*. New York: Little, Brown and Company, 2013, 68-78.

Landrieu, François and Fabrice Laroche, *Le Metzger*. Saint-Thibault-Les-Vignes: Autres Voix. 2013.

La Varenne, Pierre François. *Le cuisinier françois enseignant la manière de bien appréster et assaisonner viandes, legumes*. Originally published in 1651. Paris: Hachette Livre, 2012.

Lindeberg, Stefan, PhD. *Food and Western Disease: Health and Nutrition from an Evolutionary Perspective*. Oxford: Wiley-Blackwell, 2010.

Lipski, Elizabeth. *Digestive Wellness: Strengthen the Immune System and Prevent Disease Through Healthy Digestion, 4th Edition*. New York: McGraw-Hill Education, 2011.

Mallet, JF, with text by Emmanuel Jary. *Viandes: Encyclopédie des Produits & des Métiers de Bouche* (French meat encyclopedia). Paris: Hachette Livre/Hachette Cuisine, 2013, 9.

Maroon, Joseph. *The Longevity Factor: How Resveratrol and Red Wine Activate Genes for a Longer and Healthier Life*. New York: Atria Books, 2009.

Massialot, François. *Le Cuisinier Roial et Bourgeois*. (Originally published in 1705.) Paris: Hachette Livre, 2017. (On-demand printing from Amazon, Lavergne, TN, 2017.)

McBride, Natasha Campbell. *Gut and Psychology Syndrome: Natural Treatment for Autism, Dyspraxia, A.D.D., Dyslexia, A.D.H.D., Depression, Schizophrenia*, revised edition. Cambridge: Medinform Publishing, 2010.

McCollum, Elmer Verner. *The Newer Knowledge of Nutrition*. New York: MacMillan, 1921, 58.

McLagan, Jennifer. *Bitter: A Taste of the World's Most Dangerous Flavor, with Recipes*. Berkeley: Ten Speed Press, 2014.

Le Ménagier de Paris ("The Goodman of Paris: A Treatise on Moral and Domestic Economy by a Citizen of Paris, c. 1393."). Edited by Jérome Pichon, Translated by Eileen Power. Woodbridge (U.K.): Boydell Press: 2008. (Based on three existing fifteenth-century manuscripts of the *Ménagier*, Edited by Jérome Pichon for the Société des Bibliophile François, Paris, 1846.)

Mendia, Juan-José Lapitz and Jeanine Pouget. *Recettes des Sept Provinces du Pays Basque*. Aicitrits: Aubéron, 2006.

Mercola, Joseph. *Fat for Fuel*. Carlsbad: Hay House, 2017.

Montevi, Béatrice. *Savoir Faire de Nos Mamies*. Croissy Sur Seine: Anagramme, 2012.

Moore, Jimmy and Jason Fung. *The Complete Guide to Fasting: Heal Your Body Through Intermittent, Alternate-Day, and Extended Fasting*. Las Vegas: Victory Belt Publishing, Inc., 2016.

Moreno, Juan and Rafael Peinado. *Enological Chemistry*. London: Elsevier, 2012, 138.

Morell, Sally Fallon. *Nourishing Fats: Why We Need Animal Fats for Health and Happiness*. New York: Grand Central Life & Style, 2017, 3-9.

Newport, Mary T. *Alzheimer's Disease: What If There Was a Cure?: The Story of Ketones*. Laguna Beach: Basic Health Publications, 2011.

Old, Marnie. *Wine: A Tasting Course*. London: Dorling Kindersley, 2013.

The Oxford Companion to Wine, 4th Edition, Edited by Jancis Robinson and Julia Harding. Oxford: Oxford University Press, 2015.

Pauli, Eugen. *Classical Cooking the Modern Way*, 2nd Edition. Hoboken: John Wiley & Sons, 1989.

Pellaprat, Henri-Paul. *L'Art Culinaire Moderne: La Bonne Table Française et Etrangère*. Paris: Comptoir Français du Livre, 1936.

Peterson, Sarah, T. *Acquired Taste: The French Origins of Modern Cooking*. Ithaca: Cornell University Press. 1994.

Peynaud, Emile. *Connaissance et Travail du Vin*. Paris: Dunod, 1984.

Peynaud, Emile, *The Taste of Wine: The Art and Science of Wine Appreciation*. San Francisco: Wine Appreciation Guild, 1997.

Pfister, Richard. *Les Parfums du Vin: Sentir et Comprendre le Vin*. Paris: Delachaux et Niestlé SA, 2013, 42-43.

Pichon, Jérôme, and Georges Vicaire. *Le Viandier de Guillaume Tirel, dit Taillevent*. Originally published in 1891. Paris: H. Leclerc and P. Cornuau. Reprinted by Kessinger Legacy Reprints, Breinigsville, PA, 2015.

Pomeroy, Elizabeth. *La Cuisine Facile*. (Translated into by Christine Colinet), Paris: Gründ. 1978.

Price, Weston A. *Nutrition and Physical Degeneration*, 8th Edition. Lemon Grove, CA: Price Pottenger, 2016.

Prosper, Montagné. *Larousse Gastronomique*, First American Edition. New York: Crown Publishers, Inc., 1961, 851-852.

Puymirat, Penelope and Kristel Riethmuller. *La Bonne Cuisine du Sud-Ouest*. Grenoble: Glénat, 2014.

Questions? Réponses! Series of nonfiction children's books. Paris: Nathan.

Ranhofer, Charles, *The Epicurean: A Complete Treatise of Analytical and Practical Studies on The Culinary Art*. (Delmonicos Restaurant. First published in 1920.) Mansfield Centre, CT: Martino Publishing, 2011.

Reader's Digest. *Die Reader's Digest Weinschule: Schritt fur Schritt zum Weinkenner*. Stansstad: List Medien AG, 2008.

Rhéaume-Bleue, Kate. *Vitamin K2 and the Calcium Paradox: How a Little-Known Vitamin Could Save Your Life*. Toronto: Wiley, 2012, 68.

Root, Waverley, *The Food of France*. 1958. New York: Alfred A. Knopf, 1958.

Root, Waverley and Richard De Rochemont, *Eating in America: A History*. Hopewell, NJ: The Ecco Presss, 1976.

Saint-Ange, Evelyn. *La Bonne Cuisine de Madame E. Saint-Ange*. First published (in French) in 1927. Translated by Paul Aratow. Las Vegas: Ten Speed Press, 2005 edition.

Salatin, Joel. *Folks, This Ain't Normal*. Audio book. Hachette Audio, 2011.

Saulnier, Louis. *Le Répertoire de la Cuisine, The World Famous Directory of the Culinary Art*. Originally published in 1914. Hauppauge, NY: Barron's Educational Series, 1976 reprint.

Sears, Barry. *Enter The Zone: A Dietary Road map*. New York: Harper Collins, 1995.

Schneider, Sally. *The Improvisational Cook*. New York: William Morrow Cookbooks, 2011, 19.

Shanahan, Catherine, *Deep Nutrition: Why Your Genes Need Traditional Food*. New York: Flatiron Books, 2017, 238-241.

Sopexa. *La France à Votre Table – The Gastronomic Routes of France*, Paris: Le Carrousel, 1974.

Stefansson, Vihjalmur. *The Fat of the Land*, English. ed. of *Not by Bread Alone*, 1946. New York: Macmillan, 1956 reprint, 128.

Suess, Dr. (Theodor Seuss Geisel). *The Lorax*. New York: Random House, 1971.

Teicholz, Nina. *The Big Fat Surprise: Why Butter, Meat and Cheese Belong in a Healthy Diet*. New York: Simon & Schuster, 2015. Audio book: Ashland, OR: Blackstone Audio, Inc., 2014.

Valette-Pariente, Christine, *Ma Cuisine du Sud-Ouest: Des Vignes aux Fourneaux*, Paris: Flammarion, 2015.

Veillon, Béatrice. *Le Tour de France de la Famille Oukilé*. Montrouge:Bayard Jeunesse, 2015.

Westman, Eric, Stephen Phinney, and Jeff Volek. *New Atkins for a New You: The Ultimate Diet for Shedding Weight and Feeling Great*. New York: Fireside, 2010

Wheaton, Barbara Ketcham. *Savoring the Past: The French Kitchen and Table from 1300 to 1789*. New York: Simon & Shuster, 1983.

Willen, Anne. *Great Cooks and Their Recipes: From Taillevent to Escoffier*. New York: McGraw-Hill. 1977.

Wolf, Robb. *Wired to Eat: Turn Off Cravings, Rewire Your Appetite for Weight Loss, and Determine the Foods That Work for You*. New York: Harmony Books, 2017.

Wolfert, Paula, *The Cooking of Southwest France*, revised edition. New York: Houghton Mifflin Harcourt, 2005.

WEBSITES

Adam Liaw, Kitchen Myths: Flambé adamliaw.com/article/kitchen-myths1

Allrecipes.com allrecipes.fr

L'Atelier des Chefs www.atelierdeschefs.fr

Beef Board, Cuts Charts www.beeffoodservice.com/cutsposterbooklet.aspx

Bio Bourgogne www.biobourgogne-vitrine.org/vins-bio_q11.php

BIODYVIN www.biodyvin.com/en/our-members.html

Blaye Côtes de Bordeaux en.vin-blaye.com/our-wines-blaye-cotes-de-bordeaux/our-appellations

Boucheries Nivernaises www.boucheries-nivernaises.com/index.php

Bourgogne Wine Board (BIVB) www.bourgogne-wines.com

Cavacave www.cavacave.com/fr/info/lexique-vin

Certified Angus Beef www.certifiedangusbeef.com/kitchen/doneness.php

Chef Simon, Deboning a Rabbit Saddle chefsimon.lemonde.fr/gourmets/chef-simon/recettes/desosser-un-rable-de-lapin

Chef Simon, Sheep and Lamb (criteria and different pieces) chefsimon.lemonde.fr/produits/morceaux-agneau.html

Chestnut History in the Cevennes www.causses-cevennes.com/histoire-du-chataignier-en-cevennes

Convert Units – Measurement Unit Converter www.convertunits.com

Cooking For Engineers, Smoke Points of Various Fats www.cookingforengineers.com/article/50/Smoke-Points-of-Various-Fats

Crème de Languedoc, Wine Regions and Domains of Languedoc Roussillon, South France www.creme-de-languedoc.com/Languedoc/wine/regions-domains.php

Cuisine a la Francaise www.cuisinealafrancaise.com/fr

Cuisine Bourgeoise web.archive.org/web/20050402231640/www.nicks.com.au/gasthist/page15.html

La Cuisine D'Antan Papyjacques (The Cuisine of Antan Papyjacques Culinary Blog): lacuisinedantandepapyjacques.over-blog.com/2015/01/l-histoire-des-paupiettes.html

La Cuisine du 19 Siecle (Cooking in the 19th Century) lacuisinedu19siecle.wordpress.com/2013/03/14/la-sauce-mornay-la-gloire-du-grand-vefour/

Despi le boucher www.despi-le-boucher.com

Dico-du-Vin www.dico-du-vin.com

Dr. Axe draxe.com

Eater, Fromage Blanc www.eater.com/2016/7/21/12243334/fromage-blanc-dessert-france

Ecocert, Vinification en Agriculture Biologique www.ecocert.fr/sites/www.ecocert.fr/files/FDSVinif.pdf

ElectricSense www.electricsense.com

ElectricSense, Health Risks of Cell Phones and Towers www.electricsense.com/wp-content/uploads/2013/06/emfposter.pdf

Encyclo-ecolo.com www.encyclo-ecolo.com/Calendrier_des_poissons

Esprit de Pays espritdepays.com/comprendre/introduction/les-quatre-couleurs-du-perigord#note1

Le Figaro Vin avis-vin.lefigaro.fr/connaitre-deguster/tout-savoir-sur-le-vin/guide-des-regions-et-des-appellations

Foodsafety.gov www.foodsafety.gov/keep/charts/mintemp.html

FranceAgriMer www.franceagrimer.fr

French Cheese Appellations of Protected Origin www.fromages-aop.com

French Calendar of Seasonal Fruits and Vegetables www.fruits-legumes.org

Grass Fed Solutions www.grass-fed-solutions.com/beef-fat.html

Grasspunk Farm www.grasspunk.com

Guide Hachette des Vins www.hachette-vins.com

GuildSomm www.guildsomm.com

Harvest to Table www.harvesttotable.com

L'Inter-Profession Nationale Porcine (French National Pork Association) www.leporc.com/tout-est-bon-dans-le-cochon/morceaux.html

Jancis Robinson www.jancisrobinson.com

Journal des Femmes, Cuisine cuisine.journaldesfemmes.com

Kitchen Stewardship www.kitchenstewardship.com

The Kitchn www.thekitchn.com

la-Viande.fr www.la-viande.fr/cuisine-achat/cuisiner-viande/cuisiner-boeuf/morceaux/collier-boeuf

Linguee www.linguee.com

Loire Valley Wine Bureau loirevalleywine.com

Madeira Live www.madeira-live.com/fr/wine.html

Marie Claire, Cuisine and Wines of France www.cuisineetvinsdefrance.com

Meilleur du Chef www.meilleurduchef.com/cgi/mdc/l/fr/index.html

Mercola www.mercola.com

Millesimes www.millesimes.fr

Le Monde.fr www.lemonde.fr/m-gastronomie/visuel/2015/11/10/le-retour-de-la-cuisine-bourgeoise_4806422_4497540.html#

Nature et Régions www.nature-regions.com/Bavette-d-aloyau-Lexique-de-la-viande-Informations/p/4/572/95

Nos Petits Mangeurs (French Canadian Website for Childhood Nutrition) www.nospetitsmangeurs.org/fond-bouillon-et-consomme-quelle-est-la-difference

Pages Vins Bio Bordeaux (Organic Wine Growers of Bordeaux Listing) www.pages-vinsbio.fr/Bordeaux/vins_bordeaux.html

Paleo Leap, FODMAPs and Paleo paleoleap.com/fodmaps-and-paleo

Pioneer Thinking, History of White Flour pioneerthinking.com/history-of-white-flour

PlatsNetVins www.platsnetvins.com

Provence Wine Council (Conseil Interprofessionnel des Vins de Provence) www.provencewineusa.com/site

PubMed www.ncbi.nlm.nih.gov/pubmed

Regions of France www.regions-of-france.com

Rosetto, Wine Pairing Guide www.rosetto.com/wine_pairing.php

S.A.I.N.S. Wines vins-sains.org/category/La-charte/English

Savor Each Glass www.savoreachglass.com

Serious Eats www.seriouseats.com

Sommelier Emmanuel Delmas' Blog (Le Blog du Sommelier Emmanuel Delmas) www.sommelier-vins.com

Stanislas Urbi et Orbi, French gastronomic history www.stanislasurbietorbi.com/stanislas/stanislas_gastronomie.htm

Stephan J. Guyenet., PhD www.stephanguyenet.com

A Taste of Wine www.wine-tasting-reviews.com

Terroir France, English Language French Wine Guide www.terroir-france.com

The Truth About Cancer thetruthaboutcancer.com

Tom Cannavan's Wine Pages wine-pages.com

Traditional Over, Concrete Weight Calculator www.traditionaloven.com/conversions_of_measures/concrete-weight.html

United Nations Economic and Social Council (UNECE Standard for Edible Meat Co-Products, 2008) www.unece.org/fileadmin/DAM/trade/agr/standard/meat/e/CoProducts_2008_e_Master.pdf

Urbina Vinos Blog, Desuckering Grape Vines – Viticultural Practice urbinavinos.blogspot.ch/2014/05/desuckering-grape-vines-viticultural.html

Vedura, Seasonal Vegetables in France www.vedura.fr/guide/legumes

Vin de France www.vindefrance-cepages.org/en/

VinePair vinepair.com

Vin-Vigne (Guide to Wine and Vines in France) www.vin-vigne.com/

Vitis, French Viticultural Regions vitis.free.fr/accueil.html

Vitis, Grape Varieties www.lescepages.fr/cepmc.html

WHO Mortality Database apps.who.int/healthinfo/statistics/mortality/whodpms

Wikipedia www.wikipedia.org

The Wine Cellar Insider www.thewinecellarinsider.com

The Wine Cellar Insider, Cote Rotie www.thewinecellarinsider.com/rhone-wines-cote-rotie-hermitage-chateauneuf-du-pape/rhone-wine-cote-rotie-producer-profiles

Wine Enthusiast Magazine (guide to herbs) www.winemag.com/2012/11/28/a-wine-lovers-guide-to-herbs

Wine Folly www.winefolly.com

Wine School of Philadelphia, Wine Terminology & Vocabulary www.vinology.com/wine-terms

The Wine Society, Wine Region List www.thewinesociety.com/wine-region-list

Wine Spectator www.winespectator.com

Winegeeks www.winegeeks.com

WineMaker Magazine winemakermag.com

Wine-Searcher, Grape Varieties www.wine-searcher.com/grape-varieties.lml

Wine-Searcher, Regions of France https://www.wine-searcher.com/regions-france

Wines of Alsace, Taste and Colors www.vinsalsace.com/fr/gouts-et-couleurs/cepages

Wines of Beaujolais, Les Appellations vins-du-beaujolais.com/les-appellations

Wines of Burgundy www.bourgogne-wines.com

Wines of Burgundy www.vins-bourgogne.fr/nos-vins-nos-terroirs/nos-aoc-decodees/vins-de-bourgogne-decodez-les-aoc,2384,9180.html?

Wines of Gaillac www.vins-gaillac.com/en?connect=ok

Wines of Jura www.jura-vins.com/cepages.htm

Wines of Languedoc, Languedoc AOCs www.languedoc-wines.com/en/languedoc-decouverte/les-aoc-du-languedoc

Wine of the Loire Valley loirevalleywine.com

Wines of Luberon www.vins-luberon.fr/en/

Wines of Provence www.vinsdeprovence.com/en

Wines of the Rhône Valley www.rhone-wines.com

INDEX

Italic page numbers indicate images.

A

Abricot Rôti au Lavendre, 486
acidity, wine
  balance, 536–537
  high acidity, 544
Adrenal Reset Diet (Christianson), 580
aerating wine, 540–541
agave, 54
Agneau à l'Ail et au Romarin, 191–192
Agneau Mijoté, 211
Aligoté grapes, 550
Allemande Sauce, 384–385
allspice, 43
almond meal, 49
  Almond Meal Pancakes, *578*
almond milk, making, 48, *48*
almonds
  Coconut Almond Crumble with Seasonal Fruit, 493–494
  grilling, 254, *255*
Alsace region of France/grape varieties, 546
Alsatian Pig's Snout and Ears, 220–221
Altesse grapes, 555
aluminum foil, 66
Ancenis (Malvoisie) grapes, 553
ancestral context of wine, 514
ancestral diets
  perspective of *The Bordeaux Kitchen*, 9–10
  The Bordeaux Kitchen food chart, 68
  versus primal/paleo, 1
ancestral lifestyle, 7–8
ancestral recipes, 3
ancestral secrets to eating, 24
Anchovy Sauce, 386–387
animal aromas, wine, 532
Anson, Jane, 560
aperitif
  meal planning for guests, 581
  wine pairing, 557
appellations of protected origin (AOP)
  cheese, 57, 60
  wine, 517
apples
  Caramelized Apples, 489
  Pork Knuckle with Sauerkraut, 297
apricots
  Baked Apricot with Lavender, 486
  Slow-Cooked Pork Cheeks with Apricots, 272–273
aprons, 66
Araignée de Boeuf à l'Orange, 148–149
Arbois grapes, 552
Armagnac, 555
  Foie Gras with Figs and Armagnac, 247
Armagnac region of France/grape varieties, 555
aroma, wine, 513–533
  balancing with meals, 559
  Aroma Wheel, 532, *533*

asparagus
  Green Asparagus with Bacon and Hazelnuts, 453
  removing toough ends, 453
  Sautéed White Asparagus Slices, 475
Asperges aux Lardons et Noisettes, 453
Asprey, Dave, 46
au gratin, 439
Aubin Vert (Vert Blanc) grapes, 553
Auffret, Oceanne, 167
Aunt Lucie's Millas, 484–485
Auxerrois grapes, 553
avocado oil, 40
Axoa, 420–421

B

bacon
  Bacon-Wrapped Prunes, 287
  barding, 81, 83, 141, *83*
  Canadian bacon, 293
  Chicken Livers with Bacon, 236–237
  elongating for veal cutlets, 429
  fat, 36–37
  Green Asparagus with Bacon and Hazelnuts, 453
  lardons, 109–111, 118, *111*, *118*
  Oven Bacon Strips, 292
  salt-curing, 85–87, *86*, *87*
  Sauerkraut and Bacon, 471
  Sautéed Leeks and Bacon, 472–473
bain-marie, 157, 235
Baked Apricot with Lavender, 486
Baked Whole Mackerel, 175–176
baking with non-grain flours, 49–50
balance, wine, 543
  balancing wine with meals, 559
  red wine, 537, *537*
  white wine, 536, *536*
Ballantyne, Sarah, 575
balsamic aromas, wine, 532
Baly, Aline, 247, 537
Baly, Philippe, 537
Barbaroux grapes, 553
Barbeque Sauce, 389
barding, 81, 83, 141, *83*
Basque, *161*
  piment d'Espelette, 160
Basque Chicken, 334–335
Basque Grandmother's Pâté, 288–289
Basque Grilled Squid, 160–161
Basque Veal with Peppers, 420–421
Bavette à l'Echalotte, 133–134
bay leaves, 43
Bayeux Tapestry, 129
Béarnaise Garbure Soup, 338–339
Béarnaise Sauce, 391
Beaufils, Chef Jean-Luc, 259, 415, 443
Beaujolais region of France/grape varieties, 546–547
"Beauois" (Chardonnay) grapes, 550
Bechameil, Louis de, 392

627

Béchamel Sauce, 392–393, *382*
beef
  cuts, 70, *70*
  degrees of doneness, 119
  grain-finished, 72
  grass-fed/pastured animals, 87–89
  heart, 415
  tallow. *See* tallow
Beef Heart Jerky, 223
beef recipes, 107
  Beef Burgundy, 109–111
  Beef Roast, 113–115
  Beef Stew with Carrots, 116–118
  Beef Tagine Stew, 121–122
  Beef Tongue, 224–225
  Boiled Beef Stew "Pot-Au-Feu," 123–124
  Bone-In Prime Rib, 125
  Braised Oxtail, 127
  Flambéed Sirloin Steak with Cream Sauce, 129–130
  Flambéed Sirloin Steak with Sautéed Vegetables, 131–132
  Flank Steak with Shallots, 133–134
  Grilled Rosemary Beef Skirt Steak, 135
  Ground Beef Parmentier, 137–139
  offal
    Beef Heart Jerky, 223
    Beef Tongue, 224–225
    Roasted Marrow Bones, 269
    Slow-Cooked Beef Cheeks, 271
  Peppered Roast Beef, 141–142
  Roquefort Sirloin Steak, 143
  Sage Butter Sirloin Steak, 145
  Simple Braised Beef Stew with Orange, 153
  Slow-Cooked Beef Shank, 146–147
  Spider Steak with Orange, 148–149
  Wine Trader's Rib Eye Steak, 155–157
  Wine-Braised Beef Stew with Orange, 151–152
beef recipes – French titles
  abats
    Coeur de Boeuf Seché, 223
    Joues de Boeuf, 271
    Langue de Boeuf, 224–225
    Os à Moelle, 269
  Araignée de Boeuf à l'Orange, 148–149
  Bavette à l'Echalotte, 133–134
  Boeuf Bourguignon, 109–111
  Boeuf Carottes, 116–118
  Côte de Boeuf, 125
  Daube de Boeuf à l'Orange, 151–152
  Daube de Boeuf à l'Orange Simple, 153
  Entrecôte Marchand de Vin, 155–157
  Hachis Parmentier, 137–139
  Hampe de Boeuf au Romarin, 135
  Jarret (Gîte) de Boeuf, 146–147
  Pavé de Rumsteck au Beurre à la Sauge, 145
  Pavé de Rumsteck au Roquefort, 143
  Pavé de Rumsteck Flambé avec Garniture de Légumes à la Poêle, 131–132
  Pavés de Rumsteck Flambés, Sauce à la Crème, 129–130
  Pot-au-Feu, 123–124
  Queue de Boeuf, 127
  Rosbif au Poivre, 141–142
  Rôti de Boeuf, 113–115
  Tajine de Boeuf, 121–122

beets
  Beet Salad with Blood Orange, Walnut, and Goat Cheese, 438
  Oven-Baked Beet Chips, 457
Bergerac region of France/grape varieties, 555
berries
  Berry Tart, 487
  Coconut Almond Crumble with Seasonal Fruit, 493–494
  Custard with Seasonal Fruits, 495
Beurre Clarifié, 405
The Big Fat Surprise (Teicholz), 21, 32, 33, 34, 218, 575
biodynamic and organic wines, 520–522
black pepper, 43, 100
Blanc de Seiche Mariné, 178–179
blanching tomatoes, 335
Blanquette de Veau, 422–423, *12*
Blettes Sautées, 474
blind wine tasting, 542
blue light, 568–569
body of wine, 538
Boeuf Bourguignon, 109–111
Boeuf Carottes, 116–118
Boiled Beef Stew "Pot-Au-Feu," 123–124
Boissenot, Eric, 514
bold wine, 543
Bone Broth, 394–396
Bone-In Lamb Shoulder Roast, 195
Bone-In Prime Rib, 125
bones
  marrow, Roasted Marrow Bones, 269
  skin and bones at a butcher's shop, 78
Bonnefons, Nicolas de, 14
Bordeaux. *See also* French Southwest
  conditions necessary to make great wine, 526
  markets, *16*, *23*
  grape varieties, 547–550
  pairing Bordeaux wines, 557
  Saint Seurin Market (pic), 8
  vintages, 527
The Bordeaux Kitchen
  motivation for, 4–5
  perspective on ancestral diets, 9–10
  tenets of, 8–9
Bordeaux Oysters with Pork and Shallot Meatballs, 163–166
Bordeaux wine sauce, 155–157
Bouchait, Dominique, 58, 60
bouillon, 382
  stock/soup vocabulary, 396
Le Bouillon, 394–396
Bouillon de Volaille, 417
Boulettes au Porc, 301–303
bouquet garni, 14, 43, 111, 175, 392, 472, *43*, *111*
Bourboulenc grapes, 554
BPA in plastic containers/utensils, 65
brains, Poached and Sautéed Lamb Brains, 262–264
Brain Building Nutrition and Beyond Antibiotics (Schmidt), 33
brain function/health
  aluminum, 66
  fatty acid ratios, 33
  medium-chain triglycerides (MCTs), 39
braising
  Braised Oxtail, 127
  Braised Veal Shanks, 425–426
  Braised Veal Stew, 422–423

Simple Braised Beef Stew with Orange, 153
Wine-Braised Beef Stew with Orange, 151–152
Brand, Evan, 568
Brazil nut butter, 49
Breaded Veal Sweetbreads "Meunière," 227–229
breakfast, 576
  breaking ceral habit, 575
  non-French food, 578
Bresse chicken, 16, *16*
brightness of wine, 531
Brillat-Savarin, Jean Anthelme, 555, 587
Brittany butter (*beurre de Breton*), 35
broth, 382
  long-cooked in cast-iron pots, 105
  Bone Broth, 394–396
brown butter (*noisette*), 36
Brown Roux, 397
Brown Stock, 398
Bugey region of France/grape varieties, 555
Burgundy region of France/grape varieties, 550
Burrell, Lloyd, 568
butcher's paper, 84
butcher's string, 81–84, *82, 83, 84*
butchery, 71
  butchering a chicken, 336–337
  choosing knives, 81
  cured meats/charcuterie, 84–87, *84–87*
  cuts of meat, 70–72, 78, *70, 72*
  flavors/taste, 71–72
  honing and sharpening knives, 79–80, *79–80*
  learning about meats, 73
  precision, 74–76, *75–76*
  safety, 81
  sausage making, 78–79, *78–79*
  seasonal economics, 72–73
  skin and bones, 78
  symmetry, 76–77, *77*
  vacuum sealing meat, 84
butter, 2, 18, 35–36, 56–57
  Butter-Fried Scallops, 167–169
  ghee, 36
  making clarified butter, 405
  une noisette, 422
butternut squash, *465*
Buzet region of France/grape varieties, 555

C

cabbage
  sauerkraut, 52, *52*
  Stuffed Cabbage Leaves, 326–327
  Stuffed Whole Cabbage, 328–330
Cabernet Franc grapes, 547
Cabernet Sauvignon grapes, 549
cacao, 56
Cahors region of France/grape varieties, 555
Cailles Farcies, 366–367
calf's foot, *415*
Calitor grapes, 553
Camart, Romain, *89, 196,* 594
Canadian bacon, 293
Canard Entier Farci, 375–376
cane sugar, 53–54

canola (rapeseed) oil, 41
Cap Ferret Oysters, *584*
Capucins Market, Bordeaux, *23*
carafing wine, 540–541
Caramelized Apples, 489
Carignan grapes, 551
Carmenère grapes, 549
Carottes Fermentées, 446
Carré d'Agneau aux Herbes, 199–201
Carre d'Agneau Cotes de Filet (or *Carre de Cotes Premieres*), 194
Carre d'Agneau Cotes de Filet Roule, 195
Carre d'Agneau Decouvertes, 194
Carré de Cochon en Croûte de Sel, Gingimbre et à l'Ail, 317–318
Carriquiry, Florent, 75, 76, 85, 146, 196, 202, 209, 213, 288, 428, *74, 75, 89, 196, 289*
carrots
  Beef Stew with Carrots, 116–118
  Fermented Carrots, 446
  pickled, 52
Carson, Rachel, 15
cassava flour
  Cream Sauce (Supreme Sauce), 402
  roux, 392, 397
  Seedy Crackers, 501–502
  Sweet and Savory Crêpes, 503–504
cassoulet vs. *garbure*, 340
cast-iron pots, 64, *64,* 103
  long-cooked stock or broth, 105
  use when making recipes, 103–104
cast-iron skillets, 104
Catch of the Day, 170–171
caul, 37, 164–165, 314, 316, 429, *165, 316*
  Pyrénées Country Pâté, 316
cauliflower
  Cauliflower Gratin, 439–440
  Cauliflower "Rice," 441
Célerisotto, 442
celery root (celeriac), 51
  Celery Root Risotto, 442
Celtic sea salt, 99–100
Cervelles d'Agneau Pochées et Sautées, 262–264
Champagne, 537
Champagne region of France/grape varieties, 550–551
chard, Sautéed Swiss Chard, 474
Chardonnay grapes, 550–551
Chasselas grapes, 546
Chateau Haut-Bailly, 521, *521*
Chateau Jean Faure, 519–520, *520*
Chateau La Fleur Petrus, 560, *560*
Château Palmer, *528*
Château Rieussec, *558*
cheeks
  Slow-Cooked Beef Cheeks, 271
  Slow-Cooked Pork Cheeks with Apricots, 272–273
cheese, 56–62, *57, 58, 60, 62, 69*
  faiselle, 62
  fromage blanc, 495
  goat. *See* goat cheese
  map of French cheese AOPs, 60
  meal planning for guests, 581
  Mornay Cheese Sauce, 407–408

pairing with wine, 61
Roquefort, 61
vitamin K2, 62
Chef Andre Daguin, 143, 244, 351
Chef Auguste Escoffier, 384, 463
Chef Celia Girard, 53, 62, 233, 400, 434, 442, 475, *233*
Chef Craig Dennis, *166, 178, 179*
Chef Edouard Remont, 366, 428, 429, *367, 429*
Chef Frédéric Schueller, 22, 89, 94, 514, *166, 339, 364*
   cast-iron pots, 103
   Chicken Cordon Bleu, 341
   chopping herbs, 350
   Crème Brûlée, 506
   flambe, 131
   foie gras, 244
   food truck, 282, 343
   French Green Peas, 450
   garbure, 340
   Omelet with Herbs, 349–350
   Orange Duck Breast, 351
   oysters, 163
   pinches, 99
   poultry stock, 417
   precise measurements, 97
   Rabbit Stew with Onions and Duck Fat Potatoes, 363
   Veal Liver, 282
Chef Jacques Pepin, 35, 396, 426
Chef Jean-Luc Beaufils, 129, 259, 396, 415, 443, *129*
Chef Nicolas Magie, 53, 233
chemical aromas, wine, 532
chemical toxins in the home, 574
Chenin Blanc grapes, 553
chestnut flour, 49
chestnuts, Kabocha Squash and Chestnut Soup, 454–455
chevre. See goat cheese
Chia Coconut Milk Pudding, 580
chicken
   Bresse chicken, 16, *16*
   butchering, 336–337
   eggs, 47
   fat, 37
chicken recipes
   Basque Chicken, 334–335
   Chicken Cordon Bleu, 341–343
   Chicken in Wine Sauce, 345–348
   offal
      Chicken Hearts with Garlic and Parsley, 230–231
      Chicken Liver Cake with Crab Sauce, 233–235
      Chicken Liver Dip, 238–239
      Chicken Livers with Bacon, 236–237
chicken recipes – French titles
   abats
      Coeurs de Volaille en Persillade, 230–231
      Foies de Volaille aux Lardons, 236–237
      Gâteau de Foies de Volailles Sauce aux Crabes, 233–235
      Sauce aux Foies de Volaille, 238–239
   Cordon Bleu au Poulet, 341–343
   Coq au Vin, 345–348
   Poulet Basquaise, 334–335
Child, Julia, 35, 101, 124, 345, 348, 353, 393, 396, 407, 426
children. *See also* family
   digestive issue, 572–573
   disease prevention, 573

helping with meal preparation, 582–583
picky eaters, 572
snacking, 573–574, 576–577
chipirons, 160
Chipirons à la Plancha, 160–161
Chips de Betterave au Four, 457
chocolate, 55–56
   Chocolate Mousse, 490–491
   Chocolate Pork Chops, 580
   Paleo Chocolate Bark, 584
cholesterol, 31, 34
chopping
   garlic, 44–45, *44*
   herbs, 66, 350
chops
   Chocolate Pork Chops, 580
   Shoulder Chops (lamb), 194
   T-Bone Lamb Chops or Loin Chops, 194
Chou Farci Entier, 328–330
Choucroute aux Lardons, 471
Christianson, Dr. Alan, 580
chutney, Lamb Liver with Onion Chutney, 254–255
cinq epices (five spices), 43
Cinsault grapes, 553–554
circadian rhythms, 568–569
Citeaux, Thomas and Marie-Marie, 46, 178, *46, 179*
CLA (conjugated linoleic acid), 36
   grass-fed beef, 88
Clafoutis aux Légumes, 479
clairet wines, color spectrum, 529–530
Clairette grapes, 554
clarified butter, 36
   making, 405
clarity of wine, 530
clementines, 26
   Orange Plum Sauce, 412
cockles, Catch of the Day, 170–171
coconut milk
   Chia Coconut Milk Pudding, 580
   Vanilla, 508
   Walnuts in Milk, 510
coconut oil, 39–40
cod, 185
Coeur d'Agneau à la Sauge, 248–249
Coeur de Boeuf Seché, 223
Coeurs de Volaille en Persillade, 230–231
coffee, 56
Cognac region of France, 545
Comté cheese, 60, *60*
Confit de Porc Échine, 311–313
Confiture d'Oignons, 411
conjugated linoleic acids (CLAs), 36
   grass-fed beef, 88
The Cooking of Southwest France (Wolfert), 17, 143, 454
cooking time, 95–96
cookware, 64, 65
   oven-safe, 104
   use when making recipes, 103–104
Coq au Vin, 345–348
Coquilles Saint Jacques au Beurre, 167–169
Cordon Bleu au Poulet, 341–343
corn oil, 41
Corsica region of France/grape varieties, 551

Cot (Malbec) grape variety, 549
Côte de Boeuf, 125
Cotelettes de Filet or Cotes Filet, 194
Cotes Decouvertes, 194
cottonseed oil, 41
Courgettes au Four, 461
Courgettes aux Noix et au Fromage de Chèvre, 481
Coustellous au Romarin, 319–320
cows
   grass-fed/pastured, 87–89, *88*
   milk/dairy products, 56, 57
Crab Sauce, 400–401
crackers, Seedy Crackers, 501–502
Craquelins au Graines, 501–502
cream, Vanilla "Burned" Cream, 505–508
Cream of Green Peas, 443, *11*
cream sauce
   Cream Sauce (Supreme Sauce), 402
   Flambéed Sirloin Steak with Cream Sauce, 129–130
Crème Brûlée à la Vanille, 505–508
Crème de Petits Pois, 443
crêpes, Sweet and Savory Crêpes, 503–504
Le Creuset cast-iron pots, 103
Crispy Pork Rinds, 240–241
Croque Madame, 349
Croque Monsieur, 349
Croxton, Sean, 589
Le Crumble au Noix de Coco et aux Fruits de Saison, 493–494
Le Cuisinier Francois (La Varenne), 14, 392
Le Cuisinier Roial et Bourgeois, (Massialot), 403
Cuisses de Canard au Four, 355–356
Cuisses de Canard Confites, 357–358
cured meats/charcuterie, 84–87, *84, 86, 87*
Curnonsky, 557
cuts of meat, 70–72, *70, 72*
   lamb, 188
   Parisian-style cuts, 78
   pork, 284
   poultry, 332
   veal, 418
cuttlefish, Marinated Cuttlefish, 178–179

D

Daguin, Andre, 143, 244, 351
Daguin, Ariane, 244, 351
dairy products, 68
   butter, 35–36
   cheese, 57–62, *57, 58, 60, 62*
   ghee, 36
   raw milk, 36
   tolerance, 56–57
Daly, Patricia, 501
dates, 53, *54*
Daube de Boeuf à l'Orange, 151–152
Daube de Boeuf à l'Orange Simple, 153
Davis, Dr. William, 33
Davis, Stephen, 116, *117*
   Homemade Mayonnaise, 406
   Old-Fashioned Mustard, 410
   Tangy Seafood and Salad Dressing (Tartar Sauce), 414
Death by Food Pyramid (Minger), 34
Deboned Lamb Shoulder Roast, 196

decanting wine, 540–541
Decelle, Olivier, 519
Deep Nutrition (Shanahan), 34, 575
defects in wine, 538
deglazing, 130, 156, 161, 364
degrees of doneness
   beef, 119
   lamb, 193
   pork, 307
dehydrating
   Beef Heart Jerky, 223
   plums, 63
delicate wine, 543
Demeyere saucepans, 65, 104, *64*
demi-glace, 396
Dennis, Craig and Frederique, *166, 178, 179*
Dentraygues, Delphine, 318
Desnoyer, Hugo, 137, 151, 213, 224, 272, 280, 317, 321
dessert recipes, 483
   Aunt Lucie's Millas, 484–485
   Baked Apricot with Lavender, 486
   Berry Tart, 487
   Caramelized Apples, 489
   Chia Coconut Milk Pudding, 580
   Chocolate Mousse, 490–491
   Coconut Almond Crumble with Seasonal Fruit, 493–494
   Custard with Seasonal Fruits, 495
   Paleo Chocolate Bark, 584
   Pears in Butter and Cinnamon, 497
   Raspberry Verbena Syrup and Gelatin, 499–500
   Seedy Crackers, 501–502
   Sweet and Savory Crêpes, 503–504
   Vanilla "Burned" Cream, 505–508
   Walnuts in Milk, 509–510
dessert recipes – French titles
   Abricot Rôti au Lavendre, 486
   Craquelins au Graines, 501–502
   Crème Brûlée à la Vanille, 505–508
   Fromage Blanc aux Fruits de Saison, 495
   Intxaursalsa (Noix au Lait), 509–510
   Le Crumble au Noix de Coco et aux Fruits de Saison, 493–494
   Le Millas de Tante Lucie, 484–485
   Les Crêpes et les Galettes, 503–504
   Mousse au Chocolat, 490–491
   Poires au Beurre Cannelle, 497
   Pommes Caramélisées, 489
   Sirop et Gelée de Verveine à la Framboise, 499–500
   Tarte aux Fruits des Bois, 487
dessert/sweet wine, 544, 560
Diet for a Small Planet (Lappe), 15
digestive issues, 572–573
   gut flora, 575
   FODMAPs, 44, 394, 472
Dijon mustard, 410
dinner, 577
   non-French food, 579
dips
   Chicken Liver Dip, 238–239
   Shallot and Vinegar Dip for Oysters, 413
disease prevention for children, 573
Dolle, Romy, 34, 55
The Dorito Effect (Schatzker), 575
Dornenburg, Andrew, 173

dry wine, 543
DUAD wine course, 101, *102, 103, 235, 559*
Dubourdieu, Denis, 320, 513, 517, 518, 526, 527, 549
duck eggs, 47
duck and goose fat, 2–3, 18, 37, *37*
   Rabbit Stew with Onions and Duck Fat Potatoes, 363–365
   rendering, 266
   smoke point, 37
duck recipes
   Béarnaise Garbure Soup, 338–339
   offal
      Duck Liver Pâté, 242–243
      Duck Rinds, 359
      Foie Gras with Figs and Armagnac, 244–247
   Orange Duck Breast, 351–353
   Oven Roasted Duck Legs, 355–356
   Preserved Duck Legs, 357–358
   Whole Stuffed Duck, 375–376
duck recipes – French titles
   abats
      Grattons de Canard, 359
      Pâté de Foie de Canard, 242–243
      Terrine de Foie Gras aux Figues et à l'Armagnac, 244–247
   Canard Entier Farci, 375
   Cuisses de Canard au Four, 355
   Cuisses de Canard Confites, 357
   La Garbure Béarnaise, 338
   Magret de Canard à l'Orange, 351
Dutch oven, 64, *64*

E

egg recipes
   Omelet with Herbs, 349–350
   Pyrénées Farm Scrambled Eggs, 360
   Traditional Salad from Nice, 476–477
egg recipes – French titles
   Oeufs Brouillés des Pyrénées, 360
   Omelette aux Fines Herbes, 349–350
   Salade Niçoise, 476–477
eggs, 47
elderberry gummies, 500
EMFs (Electro-Magnetic Fields/Frequencies), 568
Enter the Zone (Sears), 589
Entrecôte Marchand de Vin, 155–157
Epaule d'Agneau Entier Roti, 195
Epaule d'Agneau Entier Roti Desossee, 196
erythritol, 54
Escoffier, Chef Auguste, 384, 463
Essig, Mark, 163
establishing healthy habits, 572–575
ether aromas, wine, 532
exotic fruits and year-round eating, 26
experimenting, 104–105

F

Fair Trade products, 55
faire chabrol, 339, 560
faiselle, 62
Fallon, Sally, 34, 52

family
   challenges of establishing healthy habits, 572–575
   living with intention, 563, 564
   market and farm visits, 564–566, *565, 566*
   meal time, 569–571
   reducing chemical toxins in the home, 574
   shifting parents' food paradigm, 574
   sleep and routines, 567–569
family food organization and planning, 575–584
   breakfast, 576, 578
   dinner, 577, 579, 582
   having children help, 582–583
   lunch, 576, 579
   meal planning for guests, 579, 581
   non-French food, 578–579
   simple, quick meals, 579
   snacks, 576–577
   three-course meal, 581
   transitioning to healthier meals, 577–578
   travelling, 583–584
farm and market visits, 564–566, *565, 566*
farm fats, 7–8, 18, 29–39
   bacon fat, 36–37
   butter, 35–36
   cholesterol, 34
   debunking fear of fats, 34
   fatty acid ratios and brain function, 33
   fowl fats, 37
   ghee, 36
   lard, 37
   low-fat diets and heart disease, 32–33
   nutrient density, 33
   olive oil, 38–39
   regional fats in France, 34
   rendering, 265–268
   saturated fat, 30–35
   tallow, 37–38
   use in recipes, 98–99
Farr, Ryan, 220
fat-adapted, 97
fats, 218–219
   avocado oil, 40
   bacon fat, 36–37
   butter, 35–36
   cholesterol, 31, 34
   coconut oil, 39–40
   debunking fear of fats, 34
   dietary fat vs. body fat, 32
   farm fats. *See* farm fats
   fatty acid ratios and brain function, 33
   four fat regions of France, 2–3, *2*
   fowl fats, 37
   ghee, 36
   grapeseed oil, 40
   industrial seed oils, 41
   industrially-refined oils, 19
   lard, 37
   low-fat, 24, 32–33
   macadamia nut oil, 40
   nutrient density, 33
   olive oil, 38–39

palm oil, 39–40
polyunsaturated fatty acids (PUFAs). *See* PUFAs
pork caul (lace fat), 37, 164–165, 314, 316, 429, *165, 316*
regional fats in France, 34
rendering, 265–268
saturated fat, 30–35
sesame seed oil, 40
smoke point, 35
tallow, 37–38
trans fats, 15
use in recipes, 98–99
vitamin K2, 20
walnut oil, 40
fat-soluble vitamins, 30, 33, 35, 38, 47
fatty acid ratios and brain function, 33
Faytout, Malika, 21, 199, 238, 328, 438, 449, 484, *235, 330, 559*
Federico, Tony, 125
Fennel with Red Onion, 445
Fenouil et Onion Rouge, 445
fermentation odors, wine, 532
fermentation of wine, 519
fermented foods
  Fermented Carrots, 446
  Fermented Radishes, 447
  pickling, 52
  sauerkraut, 52
    making, 52, *52*
    Pork Knuckle with Sauerkraut, 297–298
    Sauerkraut and Bacon, 471
Feuilles de Chou Farcies, 326–327
Field Potatoes, 449
figs
  Foie Gras with Figs and Armagnac, 244–247
  Turkey Liver Pâté with Figs, 274
Filet Mignon au Jambon de Pays, 299–300
Filets de Daurade aux Pignons de Pin Grillés, 184–185
filleting fish, 182–183, *182, 183*
fish and seafood
  cod, 185
  cuttlefish, 179
  filleting fish, 182–183, *182, 183*
  haddock, 185
  oysters, 163–166
  sardines, 173
  sea bass, 184
  sea bream, 182–184, *182, 183*
  trout, 184
fish and seafood recipes, 159
  Anchovy Sauce, 387
  Baked Whole Mackerel, 175–176
  Basque Grilled Squid, 160–161
  Bordeaux Oysters with Pork and Shallot Meatballs, 163–166
  Butter-Fried Scallops, 167–169
  Catch of the Day, 170–171
  Fish Stock, 403
  Grilled Mackerel Fillets, 176–177
  Grilled Sardines with Garlic and Parsley, 173
  Mackerel with Garlic and Shallots, 175–177
  Marinated Cuttlefish, 178–179
  Salmon Tartare, 180–181
  Sea Bream Fillets with Grilled Pine Nuts, 184–185
  Spreadable Fish Paste, 186–187

fish and seafood recipes – French titles
  Blanc de Seiche Mariné, 178–179
  Chipirons à la Plancha, 160–161
  Coquilles Saint Jacques au Beurre, 167–169
  Filets de Daurade aux Pignons de Pin Grillés, 184–185
  Huitres à la Bordelaise, Crépinette de Porc à l'Échalote, 163–166
  Maquereau à l'Ail et à l'Échalote, 175–177
  Marmite de Poisson, 170–171
  Rillettes de Poisson, 186–187
  Sardines Grillées à l'Ail et au Persil, 173
  Sauce aux Anchois, 387
  Tartare de Saumon, 180–181
Flambéed Sirloin Steak with Cream Sauce, 129–130
Flambéed Sirloin Steak with Sautéed Vegetables, 131–132
Flank Steak with Shallots, 133–134
flavor (wine), balancing with meals, 559
fleshy/full-flavored Wine, 543
fleur de sel, 47, 99
  harvesting, 46–47, 178, *46, 179*
  using in recipes, 100
floral aromas, wine, 532
flour, 68
  non-grain flours, 49–50
FODMAPs (fermentable oligo-, di-, mono-saccharides, and polyols)
  broths, 394
  garlic, 44
  leeks, 472
Foie d'Agneau à l'Orange, 257
Foie d'Agneau, Chutney d'Onions, 254–255
Foie de Veau, 282–283
Foies de Volaille aux Lardons, 236–237
Folks, This Ain't Normal (Salatin), 18, 85
fond, 396
Fond Blanc de Volaille, 417
Fond Brun et Fond Blanc, 398–399
Fond de Veau, 415–416
Fondre la Graisse de Canard (ou de l'Oie), 266
Fondre le Saindoux, 267
Fondre le Suif, 268
food as medicine, 22
The Food of France (Root), 2, 18, 21, 34
Food Plate, 18
Food Pyramid, 15, 18, 34
four fat regions of France, 2–3
Fragoso, Sarah, 575
France
  AOP (appellations of protected origin)
    cheese, 57, 60
    wine, 517
  butchers
    Parisian-style cuts, 78
    precision, 74–76, *75, 76*
    sausage making, 78–79, *78, 79*
    seasonal economics, 72–73
    skin and bones, 78
    symmetry, 76–77, *77*
    understanding of flavors and cuts, 71–72
  cultural connection with food, 18–24
    ancestral secrets to eating, 24
    culinary diversity, 19–20
    exotic fruits and year-round eating, 26

learning from the past, 21
  markets, 22–24
  school lunches, 21–22
  seasonal eating, 25–26
cultural pride and heritage, 16–18
four fat regions, 2–3
meat processing, 89
mushrooms, 50
regional use of fats, 34
Southwest, 1–2
wine in French culture. *See* wine in French culture
winegrowing regions. *See* winegrowing regions of France
freezing leftovers, 96, 396
French cuisine, 1–3
  ancestral recipes, 3
  fats, 18. *See also* fats
  four fat regions, 2–3
  French Southwest, 1–2
  la nouvelle cuisine, 13
  lack of waste, 118
  nutrient-dense recipes, 4
  preservation of tradition, 13
  preserving tradition, 3
  regional pairing of food and wine, 16-17
  school lunches, 21–22
  taste and *terroir*, 17
  timeline of food culture, 13–15
  wine, 4
French Fries, 459
French Green Peas, 450
French Onion Soup, 451–452
French Paradox, 1, 19–20, 62
French Southwest, 1–2
  Limousine cows, *1, 31*, 88
  regions and grape varieties, 555–556
"Frenched" Rack of Lamb or Bone-In Loin Roast, 194
fresh ingredients, 42
  aromatic herbs, 42
  butter and dairy, 56–57
  cheese, 57–62, *57, 58, 60, 62*
    map of French cheese AOPs, 60
  chocolate, 55, 56
  coffee and tea, 56
  eggs, 47
  Fair Trade products, 55
  fruit/juices, 54–55
  garlic, 44–45, *44*
  legumes, 50
  mushrooms, 50–51, *51*
  natural sugars, 53–54
  nightshade vegetables, 51
  nuts and seeds, 47–50
  pickled vegetables, 52
  preserved lemons, 53
  root vegetables, 51–52, *51*
  salt, 45–47, *46*
  shallots, 45
  spices, 43
  vinegar, 53
fromage blanc, 495
  Fromage Blanc aux Fruits de Saison, 495
Fromages (Bouchait), 60

frozen foods, thawing, 104
fruit, 54–55
  apples
    Caramelized Apples, 489
    Pork Knuckle with Sauerkraut, 297
  apricots
    Baked Apricot with Lavender, 486
    Slow-Cooked Pork Cheeks with Apricots, 272–273
  Berry Tart, 487
  Coconut Almond Crumble with Seasonal Fruit, 493–494
  Custard with Seasonal Fruits, 495
  figs
    Foie Gras with Figs and Armagnac, 244–247
    Turkey Liver Pâté with Figs, 274
  orange. *See* orange
  pears
    Pears in Butter and Cinnamon, 497
    Veal Kidneys with Pickled Pears, 280–281
  plums/prunes, 63
    Bacon-Wrapped Prunes, 287
    Orange Plum Sauce, 412
    Pork Roast Stuffed with Prunes and Tied, 308–309
    Sautéed Pork with Prunes, 324–325
  preserved lemons, 53
  seasonal eating in France, 25
fruit aromas, wine, 532
Fruit Belly (Dolle), 55
full-bodied wine, 543
Fumet de Poisson, 403

G

Gaillac region of France/grape varieties, 555–556
Galettes de Pieds de Cochon, 259–261
Gamay grapes, 547, 550
garbure
  Béarnaise Garbure Soup, 338–339
  vs. *cassoulet*, 340
garlic, 42, 44–45
  crushing, chopping, *44*
  Garlic and Rosemary Lamb, 191–192
  Grilled Sardines with Garlic and Parsley, 173
  Mackerel with Garlic and Shallots, 175–177
  pre-chopped garlic in olive oil, 45
  Rack of Pork in Crusted Salt, Ginger, and Garlic, 317–318
  roasting, 410
  rolling in salt and pepper, 209
garnished bouquet (*bouquet garni*), 14, 43, 111, 175, 392, 472, *43*
garnishing with *fleur de sel*, 100
Gâteau de Foies de Volailles Sauce aux Crabes, 233–235
Gedgaudas, Nora, 30, 218
gelatin, Raspberry Verbena Syrup and Gelatin, 499–500
geography of wine, 516–519
Gewürztraminer grapes, 546
ghee, 36
Gigot D'Agneau des Pyrénées Cuisson Sept Heures, 209–210
ginger, 51
  Rack of Pork in Crusted Salt, Ginger, and Garlic, 317–318
Girard, Chef Celia, 53, 62, 233, 400, 434, 442, 475, *233*
glace, 396
glass, oven cookware, 104
glasses, wine, 540, *540*

gluten-free pancakes, 578
goat cheese, 62, 58, 62
   Beet Salad with Blood Orange, Walnut, and Goat Cheese, 438
   faiselle, 62
   Teulé Goat Farm Market, 566, *566*
   Zucchini with Walnuts and Goat Cheese, 481
Good Calories, Bad Calories (Taubes), 34
Good Fat, Bad Fat (Dolle), 34
goose and duck fat, 2–3, 18, 37
  rendering, 266
goose recipes
   Whole Roast Chicken with *Herbes de Provence*, 373–374
   Whole Stuffed Holiday Goose, 377–378
Grain Brain (Perlmutter), 589
grain-finished beef, 72
grain-free flours, 49–50
grape varieties, 546–556
   Aligoté, 550
   Altesse, 555
   Arbois, 552
   Aubin Vert (Vert Blanc), 553
   Auxerrois, 553
   Barbaroux, 553
   Bourboulenc, 554
   Cabernet Franc, 547
   Cabernet Sauvignon, 549
   Calitor, 553
   Carignan, 551
   Carmenère, 549
   Chardonnay, 551
   Chardonnay ("Beauois"), 550
   Chasselas, 546
   Chenin Blanc, 553
   Cinsault, 553, 554
   Clairette, 554
   Gamay, 547, 550
   Gewürztraminer, 546
   Grenache Blanc, 552, 554
   Grenache Noir, 552, 554
   Grolleau, 552
   Jacquère, 555
   Macabeu, 552
   Malbec (Cot), 549
   Malvoisie, 552
   Malvoisie, 553
   Marsanne, 552, 555
   Melon de Bourgogne, 550, 553
   Merlot, 549
   Mollard, 553
   Mondeuse, 555
   Mourvèdre, 552, 554
   Muscadelle, 549
   Muscat, 546
   Nielluccio, 551
   Petit Verdot, 549
   Picpoul/Picpoul de Pinet, 552
   Pineau d'Aunis, 552
   Pinot Blanc, 546, 550, 553
   Pinot Gris, 546, 553
   Pinot Meunier, 551
   Pinot Noir, 546, 550, 551
   Poulsard, 551, 555
   Riesling, 546
   Rolle (Vermentino), 554
   Romorantin, 553
   Roussanne, 555
   Sauvignon Blanc, 549, 550
   Savagnin, 551
   Sciaccarello, 551
   Sémillon, 549
   Sylvaner, 546
   Syrah, 554
   Téoulier, 554
   Tibouren, 554
   Tressalier, 553
   Tressot, 550
   Trousseau, 551
   Ugni Blanc, 552
   Vermentino, 551
   Viognier, 555
grapeseed oil, 40
grass-fed/pastured animals, 87–89, *88*
  butter, 36
  vs. grass-finished, 88–89
Gratin Dauphinois, 463
Gratin de Choufleur, 439–440
Grattons de Canard, 359
Grattons de Porc Croustillants, 240–241
Green Asparagus with Bacon and Hazelnuts, 453
green peas
  Cream of Green Peas, 443, *11*
  French Green Peas, 450
Grenache Blanc grapes, 552, 554
Grenache Noir grapes, 552, 554
grilling
  almonds, 254, *255*
  Basque Grilled Squid, 160–161
  Grilled Mackerel Fillets, 176–177
  Grilled Rosemary Beef Skirt Steak, 135
  Grilled Sardines with Garlic and Parsley, 173
  pine nuts, 50, *50*
  Sea Bream Fillets with Grilled Pine Nuts, 184–185
Grolleau grapes, 552
gros sel, 47
Ground Beef Parmentier, 137–139
Ground Lamb Parmentier, 197–198
Le Guide Culinaire (Escoffier), 463
Guitz, Ilona, 561
gut flora, 575
Guyenet, Stephan, 62

H

habits, healthy, 572–575
Hachis Parmentier, 137–139
haddock, 185
ham. *See also* pork
  jambon de Bayonne, 85
  Pork Loin Wrapped in Country Ham, 299–300
Hampe de Boeuf au Romarin, 135
hazelnuts,
  Green Asparagus with Bacon and Hazelnuts, 453
  nut butter, 49
health risks of alcohol consumption, 515, 516

The Healthy Moms Podcast (Wells), 575
heart
  beef heart, *415*
  Beef Heart Jerky, 223
  Chicken Hearts with Garlic and Parsley, 230–231
  Lamb Heart with Sage, 248–249
heart disease
  French Paradox, 1, 19–20, 62
  low-fat diets, 32, 33
herbaceous or vegetal aromas, wine, 532
Herbed Rack of Lamb, 199–201
herbes de Provence, 42, 305, 356
  Pork Roast with *Herbes de Provence*, 305–306
  Whole Roast Chicken with *Herbes de Provence*, 373–374
herbs, 42, *100*
  chopping, 66, 350
  fresh vs. dried, 100–101
  garnished bouquet (*bouquet garni*), 14, 43, 111, 175, 392, 472, *43*
  lavender, Baked Apricot with Lavender, 486
  Omelet with Herbs, 349–350
  Roasted Summer Tomatoes with Herbs, 467
  sage, *371*
high acidity wine, 544
Himalayan salt, 46
histamines, leftovers, 96
Hollandaise Sauce, 404–405
Homemade Mayonnaise, 406
honey, 53–54, *53, 54*
Honey-Glazed Pork Belly, 290–291
honing knives, 79–80, *80*
horizontal wine tasting, 542
Huitres à la Bordelaise, Crépinette de Porc à l'Échalote, 163–166
Hure et Oreilles de Cochon à la Façon Alsacienne, 220–221

I

The Improvisational Cook (Schneider), 17
industrial seed oils, 41
ingredients
  freshness. *See* fresh ingredients
  measurements, 97
"instant messaging" of wine, 531
intoxicating/potent wine, 543
Intxaursalsa (Noix au Lait), 509–510
Irouléguy region of France/grape varieties, 556

J

Jacquère grapes, 555
Jallon, Augustin, 16
jambon de Bayonne, 85
Jarret (Gîte) de Boeuf, 146–147
Jarret de Porc à la Choucroute, 297–298
Jarret de Veau (Osso Bucco), 425–426
Jefferson, Thomas, 134
jerky, Beef Heart Jerky, 223
Jerusalem artichokes, 51
  mashed, 456
joie de vivre, 10, 24
Joues de Boeuf, 271
Joues de Porc aux Abricots, 272–273

juice (fruit), 54–55
Jura region of France/grape varieties, 551
Jurançon region of France/grape varieties, 556

K

Kabocha Squash and Chestnut Soup, 454–455
Kefta d'Agneau, 202–203
Kellogg, Will Keith, 21
Kemp, Domini, 501
keto-adapted, 97
ketogenic diet, 96
The *Ketogenic Kitchen* (Daly and Kemp), 501
Keys, Ancel, 15
kidneys
  Lamb Kidneys with Butter and Garlic, 250–251
  Lamb Kidneys with Old-Fashioned Mustard, 252–253
  Lamb Liver with Onion Chutney, 254–255
kitchen, and health, 68
kitchen equipment, 64–66
knives
  care, 81
  choosing, 81
  honing and sharpening, 79, 80, *79, 80*
  mezzaluna knives, 66
  safety, 81
Knobbe, Dr. Chris, 15
knuckle
  Pork Knuckle with Sauerkraut, 297–298
  Pork Loin Wrapped in Country Ham, 299–300
kohlrabi, 52
Kresser, Chris, 575
Kruse, Dr. Jack, 568

L

La Garbure Béarnaise, 338–339
la nouvelle cuisine, 13
La Varenne, Pierre François, 14, 392
lace fat (pork caul), 37, 164, 165. 314, 316, 429, *165, 316*
lamb
  cuts, 70, 188, *70, 188*
  degrees of doneness, 193
  grass-fed, 89
  milk-fed, 89
  tallow. *See* tallow
lamb recipes, 189
  Bone-In Lamb Shoulder Roast, 195
  Deboned Lamb Shoulder Roast, 196
  "Frenched" Rack of Lamb or Bone-In Loin Roast, 194
  Garlic and Rosemary Lamb, 191–192
  Ground Lamb Parmentier, 197–198
  Herbed Rack of Lamb, 199–201
  Lamb Meatballs, 202–203
  Milk-Fed Lamb Roast, 205
  Nut-Encrusted Lamb Shank, 207
  offal
    Lamb Heart with Sage, 248–249
    Lamb Kidneys with Butter and Garlic, 250–251
    Lamb Kidneys with Old-Fashioned Mustard, 252–253
    Lamb Liver with Onion Chutney, 254–255
    Lamb Liver with Orange, 257
    Poached and Sautéed Lamb Brains, 262–264

Pyrénées Seven-Hour Slow-Cooked Leg of Lamb, 209–210
Rack of Lamb, 194
Rolled Lamb Saddle, 195
Rolled Rack of Lamb or Deboned Loin Roast, 195
Shoulder Chops, 194
Simple Lamb Stew, 211
Springtime Lamb Stew, 213–214
T-Bone Lamb Chops or Loin Chops, 194
Topside Roast, 195
lamb recipes – French titles
  abats
    Cervelles d'Agneau Pochées et Sautées, 262–264
    Coeur d'Agneau à la Sauge, 248–249
    Foie d'Agneau à l'Orange, 257
    Foie d'Agneau, Chutney d'Onions, 254–255
    Rognons d'Agneau à la Moutarde à l'Ancienne, 252–253
    Rognons d'Agneau au Beurre et à l'Ail, 250–251
  Agneau à l'Ail et au Romarin, 191–192
  Agneau Mijoté, 211
  Carré d'Agneau aux Herbes, 199–201
  Carre d'Agneau Cotes de Filet (or Carre de Cotes Premieres), 194
  Carre d'Agneau Cotes de Filet Roule, 195
  Carre d'Agneau Decouvertes, 194
  Cotelettes de Filet or Cotes Filet, 194
  Cotes Decouvertes, 194
  Epaule d'Agneau Entier Roti, 195
  Epaule d'Agneau Entier Roti Desossee, 196
  Gigot D'Agneau des Pyrénées Cuisson Sept Heures, 209–210
  Kefta d'Agneau, 202–203
  Navarin Printanier, 213–214
  Noix d'Agneau, 195
  Parmentier Hachis à l'Agneau, 197–198
  Rôti d'Agneau de Lait, 205
  Selle d'Agneau (or Quasi d'Agneau) Roulee, 195
  Souris d'Agneau en Croûte de Noix, 207
Langue de Boeuf, 224–225
Languedoc-Roussillon region of France/grape varieties, 551, 552
Lapin aux Oignons et Pommes de Terre à la Graisse de Canard, 363–365
Lappe, Francis Moore, 15
lard, 2, 18, 37, 29
  rendering, 267
lardons, 109–111, 118, *111, 118*
Lascaux caves, 17, 468
lavender, Baked Apricot with Lavender, 486
Lebovitz, David, 45
LEDs (Light-Emitting Diodes), 568
leeks
  Sautéed Leeks and Bacon, 472–473
  washing, 473
leftovers
  cooling before refrigerating/freezing, 104
  freezing, 96, 396
  French great-grandmothers, 67
  lunch, 576
legs
  calf's foot, 415
  Oven Roasted Duck Legs, 355–356
  Preserved Duck Legs, 357–358
  Pyrénées Seven-Hour Slow-Cooked Leg of Lamb, 209–210
legumes
  peanuts, 49
  soaking, 50

Légumes Racines Rôtis, 466
lemons, preserved, 53
lentils, Salted Pork with Lentils, 321–323
Leonard, Lilou, 205
Les Crêpes et les Galettes, 503–504
Lesser Beasts: A Snout-to-Tail History of the Humble Pig (Essig), 163
Light (or White) Stock, 398–399
light-bodied wine, 543
Lignac, Guy-Petrus and Catherine, 287, 422, 523, 422
Lignac, Vincent, 513, 521, 523
Limousine cows, *1, 31, 88*
liver
  Chicken Liver Dip, 238–239
  Chicken Livers with Bacon, 236–237
  Duck Liver Pâté, 242–243
  Foie Gras with Figs and Armagnac, 244–247
  Lamb Liver with Orange, 257
  pâté. *See* pâté, 274
  pork, Bordeaux Oysters with Pork and Shallot Meatballs, 163–166
  sauteing, 289
  Veal Liver, 282–283
liverwurst, 579
Livin' La Vida Low-Carb Show podcast, 590
living with intention, 563–566, *565, 566*
  challenges of establishing healthy habits, 572–575
  meal time, 569–571
  sleep and routines, 567–569
Loire Valley region of France/grape varieties, 552–553
London Broil, Flank Steak with Shallots, 133–134
long/lengthy finish, 544
Lorraine region of France/grape varieties, 553
low-fat diets, and heart disease, 32–33
lunch, 576
  non-French food, 579
Luson, Joelle, 213, *109*
Lustig, Dr. Robert, 572

M

Macabeu grapes, 552
macadamia nut oil, 40
macadamia nuts, Nut-Encrusted Lamb Shank, 207
mackerel
  Catch of the Day, 170–171
  Mackerel with Garlic and Shallots, 175–177
  Spreadable Fish Paste, 186–187
Madeira, 277
Madiran region of France/grape varieties, 556
Magie, Chef Nicolas, 53, 233
Magret de Canard à l'Orange, 351–353
Maillard reaction, 365
  bacon, 37
  butter, 36
  deglazing a pan, 156
Maillard, Louis-Camille, 365
Malbec (Cot) grapes, 549
Mallet, Jean-Francois, 71, 87, 155, 213, 290, 297, 299
maltitol, 54
Malvoisie grapes, 552, 553
Maquereau à l'Ail et à l'Échalote, 175–177
Marchal, Axel, 517, 534
margarine, 14

Marinated Cuttlefish, 178–179
Marine Stewardship Council (MSC), 167
marjoram, 42
Mark's Daily Apple, 396
market and farm visits, 564–566, *565–566*
markets in France, 22–24, *16*
Markham, Dewey, Jr., 39, 97, 101, 102, 104, 155, 198, 357–358, 359, 513, 541, 558, *198*
marmalade, Onion Marmalade, 411
Marmite de Poisson, 170–171
Maroon, Dr. Joseph, 516
marrow, Roasted Marrow Bones, 269
Marsanne grapes, 552, 555
Mashed Jerusalem Artichokes, 456
Masley, Dr. Stephen, 42
Massialot, Francois, 403
Mastering the Art of French Cooking (Child), 101, 345, 348, 353, 393, 407
Masterjohn, Chris, 62
Matthews, Caroline, 515, 534, 538, 559
mayonnaise
  making, 186, *186*
  Homemade Mayonnaise, 406
  Primal Kitchen Mayo, 40, 186
Mayonnaise Fait Maison, 406
MCTs (medium-chain triglycerides), 39
meal planning
  breakfast, 575–578
  dinner, 577, 579, 582
  guests, 579, 581
  having children help, 582–583
  homemade, 574
  lunch, 576, 579
  non-French food, 578–579
  simple, quick meals, 579
  snacks, 573, 576–577
  three-course meal, 581
  transitioning to healthier meals, 577–578
  travelling, 583–584
meal time, 569–571
measurements, 97
meat. *See also* butchery
  cured meats/charcuterie, 84–87, *84, 86, 87*
  cuts, 70–72, *70, 72*
    lamb, 188, *188*
    Parisian-style cuts, 78
    pork, 284, *284*
    poultry, 332, *332*
    veal, 418, *418*
  pastured animals, 87–89, *88*
  processing, 89
  sausage making, 78–79, *78, 79*
meatballs
  Bordeaux Oysters with Pork and Shallot Meatballs, 163–166
  Lamb Meatballs, 202–203
  Pork Meatballs, 301–303
medium-bodied wine, 543
medium-chain triglycerides (MCTs), 39
Melon de Bourgogne grapes, 550, 553
Merlot grapes, 549
Meyer, Beverly, 62
mezzaluna knives, 66

milk
  almond milk, 48, *48*
  cow's milk, 56–57
  nut milks, 48
  raw milk, 36
  Walnuts in Milk, 509–510
milk-fed lambs, 89
  Milk-Fed Lamb Roast, 205
Le Millas de Tante Lucie, 484–485
Minger, Denise, 34
mirepoix, 43, *43*
molasses, 53, 54
Mollard grapes, 553
Mondeuse grapes, 555
monk fruit sweetener, 54
monounsaturated fatty acids (MUFAs)
  duck and goose fats, 37
  olive oil, 38
Moore, Jimmy, 590
Morceaux Choisis (Desnoyer), 151, 213, 224, 280, 317, 321
Mornay Cheese Sauce, 407–408
Morning Sausage Patties, 327
Morrel, Sally Fallon, 20
Moutard de Meaux Pommery, 199
Moueix, Kelley, 560
Mourvèdre grapes, 552, 554
Mousse au Chocolat, 490–491
mousse, Chocolate Mousse, 490–491
mousseline, 368–369, 405
Moutarde à l'Ancienne, 410
MUFAs (monounsaturated fatty acids)
  duck and goose fats, 37
  olive oil, 38
Muscadelle grapes, 549
Muscat grapes, 546
mushrooms, 50–51, 345–346, *51*
muslin sauce, 405
mussels, Catch of the Day, 170–171
mustard
  Old-Fashioned Mustard, 410
  Moutard de Meaux Pommery, 199
  Veal Kidneys in Old-Fashioned Mustard Sauce, 277–279

N

Navarin Printanier, 213–214
Le Nez Du Vin an aroma kit, 515
Nguyen, Vy, 123, 520, *103, 124, 559*
Niçoise Vinaigrette, 409
Nicolle-Beaufils, Annabelle, 102, 103, 129, 196, 543, 559, *103, 129, 235, 559*
Nielluccio grapes, 551
nightshade vegetables, 51
Noble, Ann, 532, 533
Noix au Lait (Intxaursalsa), 509–510
Noix d'Agneau, 195
Nom Nom Paleo, 575
Not Just Paleo podcast, 568
Nourishing Broths, Nourishing Fats (Morrel), 20
Nourishing Fats (Fallon), 34
Nourishing Traditions (Morrel), 20
Nut-Encrusted Lamb Shank, 207

nutrient density, animal fats, 33
nuts, 47–50
  nut butters, 49
  nut flours, 49–50
  nut milks, 48
  pine nuts, 50, *50*
    Sea Bream Fillets with Grilled Pine Nuts, 184–185

O

oaking wine, 534
Oeufs Brouillés des Pyrénées, 360
offal, 216–219
offal recipes, 217
  Alsatian Pig's Snout and Ears, 220–221
  Basque Grandmother's Pâté, 288–289
  Beef Heart Jerky, 223
  Beef Tongue, 224–225
  Breaded Veal Sweetbreads "Meunière," 227–229
  Chicken Hearts with Garlic and Parsley, 230–231
  Chicken Liver Cake with Crab Sauce, 233–235
  Chicken Liver Dip, 238–239
  Chicken Livers with Bacon, 236–237
  Crispy Pork Rinds, 240–241
  Duck Liver Pâté, 242–243
  Duck Rinds, 359
  Foie Gras with Figs and Armagnac, 244–247
  Lamb Heart with Sage, 248–249
  Lamb Kidneys with Butter and Garlic, 250–251
  Lamb Kidneys with Old-Fashioned Mustard, 252–253
  Lamb Liver with Onion Chutney, 254–255
  Lamb Liver with Orange, 257
  Pig's Feet Sliders, 259–261
  Poached and Sautéed Lamb Brains, 262–264
  Pork Belly Pâté, 294–295
  Pork Meat Pâté, 312
  Pyrénées Country Pâté, 314–316
  Roasted Marrow Bones, 269
  Slow-Cooked Beef Cheeks, 271
  Slow-Cooked Pork Cheeks with Apricots, 272–273
  Turkey Liver Pâté with Figs, 274
  Veal Kidneys in Old-Fashioned Mustard Sauce, 277–279
  Veal Kidneys with Pickled Pears, 280–281
  Veal Liver, 282–283
offal recipes – French titles
  Cervelles d'Agneau Pochées et Sautées, 262–264
  Coeur d'Agneau à la Sauge, 248–249
  Coeur de Boeuf Seché, 223
  Coeurs de Volaille en Persillade, 230–231
  Foie d'Agneau à l'Orange, 257
  Foie d'Agneau, Chutney d'Onions, 254–255
  Foie de Veau, 282–283
  Foies de Volaille aux Lardons, 236–237
  Galettes de Pieds de Cochon, 259–261
  Gâteau de Foies de Volailles Sauce aux Crabes, 233–235
  Grattons de Canard, 359
  Grattons de Porc Croustillants, 240–241
  Hure et Oreilles de Cochon à la Façon Alsacienne, 220–221
  Joues de Boeuf, 271
  Joues de Porc aux Abricots, 272–273
  Langue de Boeuf, 224–225
  Os à Moelle, 269
  Pâté d'Amatxi, 288–289

  Pâté de Foie de Canard, 242–243
  Pâté de Foie de Dinde aux Figues, 274
  Pâté de la Carbonnade de Porc, 294–295
  Rillettes de Porc, 312
  Ris de Veau Meunière, 227–229
  Rognons d'Agneau à la Moutarde à l'Ancienne, 252–253
  Rognons d'Agneau au Beurre et à l'Ail, 250–251
  Rognons de Veau à la Moutarde à l'Ancienne, 277–279
  Rognons de Veau, Pickles de Poires, 280–281
  Sauce aux Foies de Volaille, 238–239
  Terrine de Campagne des Pyrénées, 314–316
  Terrine de Foie Gras aux Figues et à l'Armagnac, 244–247
Oie Farcie pour les Fêtes, 377–378
Oignons Sautés, 474
oils, 38–40
  avocado oil, 40
  coconut oil, 39–40
  grapeseed oil, 40
  industrial seed oils, 41
  macadamia nut oil, 40
  olive oil. *See* olive oil
  palm oil, 39–40
  sesame seed oil, 40
  smoke point, 35
  walnut oil, 40
Old-Fashioned Mustard, 410
  Lamb Kidneys with Old-Fashioned Mustard, 252–253
olive oil, 2, 18, 38, 39
  cooking with, 98–99
  pre-chopped garlic in olive oil, 45
  vs. animal fats, 39
omega-3 fatty acids, 33
Omelet with Herbs, 349–350
Omelette aux Fines Herbes, 349–350
onions
  Rabbit Stew with Onions and Duck Fat Potatoes, 363
  Fennel with Red Onion, 445
  French Onion Soup, 451–452
  Lamb Liver with Onion Chutney, 254–255
  Onion Marmalade, 411
  Sautéed Onions, 474
orange
  Beet Salad with Blood Orange, Walnut, and Goat Cheese, 438
  Lamb Liver with Orange, 257
  Orange Duck Breast, 351–353
  Orange Plum Sauce, 412
  Simple Braised Beef Stew with Orange, 153
  Spider Steak with Orange, 148–149
  Wine-Braised Beef Stew with Orange, 151–152
organic and biodynamic wines, 520–522
Os à Moelle, 269
Osso Bucco (*Jarret de Veau*), 425–426
Ouspointour, Laeticia, 318, *103*
oven
  cookware, 104
  preheating, 104
Oven Bacon Strips, 292
Oven Roasted Duck Legs, 355–356
Oven-Baked Beet Chips, 457
Oven-Baked French Fries, 459
Oven-Baked Sweet Potatoes, 460
oxtail, Braised Oxtail, 127
oysters, 163–164

Bordeaux Oysters with Pork and Shallot Meatballs, 163–166
Cap Ferret Oysters, *584*
opening, 166
Shallot and Vinegar Dip for Oysters, 413

P

Page, Karen, 173
pairing wine. *See* wine pairing
Paleo Chocolate Bark, 584
The Paleo Cure (Kresser), 575
Paleo Grilling (Federico and Phelan), 125
Paleo Pumpkin Pie, 464, *464*
paleo/primal diets
  and moderation, 94
  versus ancestral diets, 1
palm oil, 39, 40
pancakes, 578
Pan-Fried Smoked Pork, 293
pantry, stocking, 67
parents' food paradigm, shifting, 574
Parmentier Hachis à l'Agneau, 197–198
Parmentier, Antoine-Augustin, 137, 197, 382
parsley, Grilled Sardines with Garlic and Parsley, 173
parsnips, 52, 97
pastured meat, 87–89, *88*
Patates Douces au Four, 460
pâté
  Basque Grandmother's Pâté, 288–289
  Duck Liver Pâté, 242–243, *6*
  Pork Belly Pâté, 294–295
  Pork Meat Pâté, 312
  Pyrénées Country Pâté, 314–316
  Turkey Liver Pâté with Figs, 274
Pâté d'Amatxi, 288–289
Pâté de Foie de Canard, 242–243
Pâté de Foie de Dinde aux Figues, 274
Pâté de la Carbonnade de Porc, 294–295
Paupiettes de Veau, 427–429
Pavé de Rumsteck au Beurre à la Sauge, 145
Pavé de Rumsteck au Roquefort, 143
Pavé de Rumsteck Flambé avec Garniture de Légumes à la Poêle, 131–132
Pavés de Rumsteck Flambés, Sauce à la Crème, 129–130
peanuts, 49, 576–577
pears
  Pears in Butter and Cinnamon, 497
  Veal Kidneys with Pickled Pears, 280–281
peas
  Cream of Green Peas, 443, *11*
  French Green Peas, 450
Pepin, Jacques, 35, 396, 426
pepper
  black pepper, 43, 100, *100*
  pinch, 114
  use in recipes, 99, 100
  white, 100
Peppered Roast Beef, 141–142
peppers, Basque Veal with Peppers, 420–421
Perez, Anne, 233
Perlmutter, Dr. David, 575, 589
Petit Pineau (Arbois) grapes, 552
Petit Salé aux Lentilles, 321–323

Petit Verdot grapes, 549
Petits Pois à la Française, 450
Peynaud, Emile, 515, 527, 531, 532, 534
Pfister, Richard, 532
Phelan, James, 125
La Physiologie du Goût (Brillat-Savarin), 555
pickling, 52, 53
picky eaters, 572
Picpoul/Picpoul de Pinet grapes, 552
Pig's Feet Sliders, 259–261, 465
piment d'Espelette, 160, 420, 278
pinch, 114
pine nuts, *50*
  grilling, 50
  Sea Bream Fillets with Grilled Pine Nuts, 184–185
Pineau d'Aunis grapes, 552
Pinot Blanc grapes, 546, 550, 553
pinot grigio, 546
Pinot Gris grapes, 546, 553
Pinot Meunier grapes, 551
Pinot Noir grapes, 546, 550, 551
Pinsolle, Rébecca, 227, 230, 252, 262, 277, 280, 227, 231, 264
plastic
  food containers and utensils, 65
  vacuum sealing meat, 84
play, 513
plums, 63, *63*
  Homemade Plum Preserves, 63
  Orange Plum Sauce, 412
podcasts, 589–590
Poires au Beurre Cannelle, 497
Poitrine de Porc Laquée, 290–291
Poivrons Sautés aux Lardons, 472–473
Polyface Farm, 564, *565*
polyunsaturated fatty-acids (PUFAs), 32
  industrial seed oils, 41
  history of, 14–15
Pommes Caramélisées, 489
Pommes de Terre des Champs, 449
Pommes de Terre Sarladaises, 468–469
Pommes Frites au Four, 459
pork
  bacon fat, 36–37
  Bordeaux Oysters with Pork and Shallot Meatballs, 163–166
  caul, 37, 164–165, 314, 316, 429, *165, 316*
  cuts, 70, 284, *70*
  degrees of doneness, 307
  jambon de Bayonne, 85
  lard. *See* lard
  lardons (pork belly), 109–111, 118, *111, 118*
  Pork Shoulder Confit, *10*
  rendering fat/lard, 267
  rinds, 78
  salt-curing bacon (pork belly), 85–87, *86, 87*
  sausage making, 78–79, 327, *78, 79*
pork recipes, 285
  Bacon-Wrapped Prunes, 287
  Chocolate Pork Chops, 580
  Honey-Glazed Pork Belly, 290–291
  Morning Sausage Patties, 327
  offal
    Alsatian Pig's Snout and Ears, 220–221
    Basque Grandmother's Pâté, 288–289

    Crispy Pork Rinds, 240–241
    Pig's Feet Sliders, 259–261
    Pork Belly Pâté, 294–295
    Pork Meat Pâté, 312
    Pyrénées Country Pâté, 314–316
    Slow-Cooked Pork Cheeks with Apricots, 272–273
  Oven Bacon Strips, 292
  Pan-Fried Smoked Pork, 293
  Pork Knuckle with Sauerkraut, 297–298
  Pork Loin Wrapped in Country Ham, 299–300
  Pork Meatballs, 301–303
  Pork Roast Stuffed with Prunes and Tied, 308–309
  Pork Roast with *Herbes de Provence*, 305–306
  Pork Shoulder Cooked in Fat, 311–313
  Rack of Pork in Crusted Salt, Ginger, and Garlic, 317–318
  Rosemary Pork Ribs, 319–320
  Salted Pork with Lentils, 321–323
  Sautéed Pork with Prunes, 324–325
  Stuffed Cabbage Leaves, 326–327
  Stuffed Whole Cabbage, 328–330
 pork recipes – French titles
  abats
    Galettes de Pieds de Cochon, 259–261
    Grattons de Porc Croustillants, 240–241
    Hure et Oreilles de Cochon à la Façon Alsacienne, 220–221
    Joues de Porc aux Abricots, 272–273
    Pâté d'Amatxi, 288–289
    Pâté de la Carbonnade de Porc, 294–295
    Rillettes de Porc, 312
    Terrine de Campagne des Pyrénées, 314–316
  Bacon Fumé à la Poêle, 293
  Boulettes au Porc, 301–303
  Carré de Cochon en Croûte de Sel, Gingimbre et à l'Ail, 317–318
  Chou Farci Entier, 328–330
  Confit de Porc Échine, 311–313
  Coustellous au Romarin, 319–320
  Feuilles de Chou Farcies, 326–327
  Filet Mignon au Jambon de Pays, 299–300
  Jarret de Porc à la Choucroute, 297–298
  Petit Salé aux Lentilles, 321–323
  Poitrine de Porc Laquée, 290–291
  Pruneaux au Lard Fumé, 287
  Rôti de Porc aux Herbes de Provence, 305–306
  Rôti de Porc aux Pruneaux à la Ficelle, 308–309
  Sauté de Porc aux Pruneaux, 324–325
  Tranches de Poitrine Fumée au Four, 292
 potatoes
  Field Potatoes, 449
  Ground Beef Parmentier, 137–139
  Ground Lamb Parmentier, 197–198
  Oven-Baked French Fries, 459
  Peppered Roast Beef, 141–142
  Potato Gratin, 463
  Rabbit Stew with Onions and Duck Fat Potatoes, 363–365
  Sarlat Sautéed Potatoes, 468–469
 Pot-au-Feu, 123–124
 potent/intoxicating wine, 543
 pots and pans, 64–65, 64
 Poulet Basquaise, 334–335
 Poulet Rôti aux Herbes de Provence, 373–374
 Poulsard grapes, 551, 555
 poultry fats, 37. See also duck and goose fat

 poultry recipes, 333
  Basque Chicken, 334–335
  Béarnaise Garbure Soup, 338–339
  Chicken Cordon Bleu, 341–343
  Chicken in Wine Sauce, 345–348
  offal
    Chicken Hearts with Garlic and Parsley, 230–231
    Chicken Liver Cake with Crab Sauce, 233–235
    Chicken Liver Dip, 238–239
    Chicken Livers with Bacon, 236–237
    Duck Liver Pâté, 242–243
    Duck Rinds, 359
    Foie Gras with Figs and Armagnac, 244–247
    Turkey Liver Pâté with Figs, 274
  Orange Duck Breast, 351–353
  Oven Roasted Duck Legs, 355–356
  Preserved Duck Legs, 357–358
  Stuffed Quail, 366–367
  Turkey Ragout, 370–371
  White Poultry Stock, 417
  Whole Roast Chicken with *Herbes de Provence*, 373–374
  Whole Stuffed Duck, 375–376
  Whole Stuffed Holiday Goose, 377–378
 poultry recipes – French titles
  abats
    Coeurs de Volaille en Persillade, 230–231
    Gateau de Foies de Volailles Sauce aux Crabes, 233–235
    Grattons de Canard, 359
    Foies de Volaille aux Lardons, 236–237
    Pate de Foie de Canard, 242–243
    Pâté de Foie de Dinde aux Figues, 274
    Sauce aux Foies de Volaille, 238–239
    Terrine de Foie Gras aux Figues et a l'Armagnac, 244–247
  Cailles Farcies, 366–367
  Canard Entier Farci, 375–376
  Coq au Vin, 345–348
  Cordon Bleu au Poulet, 341–343
  Cuisses de Canard au Four, 355–356
  Cuisses de Canard Confites, 357–358
  La Garbure Béarnaise, 338–339
  Magret de Canard à l'Orange, 351–353
  Oie Farcie pour les Fêtes, 377–378
  Poulet Basquaise, 334–335
  Poulet Rôti aux Herbes de Provence, 373–374
  Ragoût de Dinde, 370–371
 preheating the oven, 104
 preparation time, 94–95
 preservation of French tradition, 13
 Preserved Duck Legs, 357–358
 preserved lemons, 53
 Primal Blueprint, 513, 516
 Primal Blueprint Podcast, 590
 Primal Fat Burner (Gedgaudas), 30, 218
 Primal Kitchen Mayo, 40, 186
 primal/paleo diets
  and moderation, 94
  versus ancestral diets, 1
 Prime Rib (Bone-In), 125
 processed foods, 21–22
 processing meat in France, 89
 proportions, 94
 Proust, Joseph Louis, 382

Provence region of France/grape varieties, 553–554
Pruneaux au Lard Fumé, 287
prunes, 63
    Bacon-Wrapped Prunes, 287
    Pork Roast Stuffed with Prunes and Tied, 308–309
    Sautéed Pork with Prunes, 324–325
PUFAs (polyunsaturated fatty-acids), 32
    industrial seed oils, 41
    history of, 14–15
Pumpkin Soup, 464–465
Purée de Potiron, 464–465
Purée de Topinambour, 456
Pyrénées Country Pâté, 314–316
Pyrénées Farm Scrambled Eggs, 360
Pyrénées Seven-Hour Slow-Cooked Leg of Lamb, 209–210
Pyrex bowls, 65

Q

quail, Stuffed Quail, 366–367
Quasi d'Agneau (Selle d'Agneau) Roulee, 195
quatre epices (four spices), 43
Questions? Reponses!, 17
Queue de Boeuf, 127

R

rabbit, *332, 368, 369*
    Rabbit Stew with Onions and Duck Fat Potatoes, 363–365
    Stuffed Rabbit Saddle, 368–369
rabbit recipes – French titles
    Lapin aux Oignons et Pommes de Terre à la Graisse de Canard, 363–365
    Râble de Lapin Farci, 368–369
    Râble de Lapin Farci, 368–369
rack of lamb
    "Frenched" Rack of Lamb or Bone-In Loin Roast, 194
    Herbed Rack of Lamb, 199–201
    Rack of Lamb, 194
Rack of Pork in Crusted Salt, Ginger, and Garlic, 317–318
Radis Fermentés, 447
radishes, Fermented Radishes, 447
ragout, Turkey Ragout, 370–371
Ragoût de Dinde, 370–371
Raspberry Verbena Syrup and Gelatin, 499–500
raw milk, 36
Real Salt, 99
recipes
    appropriate seasons, 94
    beef. *See* beef recipes
    cooking time, 95–96
    desserts. *See* dessert recipes
    experimenting, 104–105
    fish and seafood. *See* fish and seafood recipes
    lamb. *See* lamb recipes
    measurements, 97
    moderation, 94
    offal. *See* offal recipes
    organization of, 93
    oven cookware, 104
    preheating the oven, 104
    preparation time, 94–95
    proportions, 94
    serving suggestions, 101
    servings and serving sizes, 96–97
    slow cooking, 105
    thawing frozen foods, 104
    use of fats, 98–99
    use of herbs, fresh vs. dried, 100–101
    use of salt and pepper, 99–100
    utensils and equipment, 103–104
    variations, 101
    veal. *See* veal recipes
    wine pairing tips, 101–103
red wines
    balance, 537, *537*
    color spectrum, 530
réduction, 396
regional wine tasting, 542
Remont, Chef Edouard, 366, 428, 429, *367, 429*
rémoulade
    Spreadable Fish Paste, 186
    Tangy Seafood and Salad Dressing (Tartar Sauce), 414
Renaud, Dr. Serge, 19
rendering farm fats, 265, 266, 267, 268
Le Repertoire de la Cuisine (Saulnier), 227
resveratrol, 516
Rhéaume-Bleue, Dr. Kate, 20, 62
Rhone Valley region of France/grape varieties, 554–555
rib eye steak
    Bone-In Prime Rib, 125
    Wine Trader's Rib Eye Steak, 155–157
ribs, Rosemary Pork Ribs, 319–320
rice bran oil, 41
Riesling grapes, 546
rillettes, 186–187
    Rillettes de Poisson, 186–187
    Rillettes de Porc, 312
rinds
    Crispy Pork Rinds, 240–241
    Duck Rinds, 359
    skin and bones at a butcher's shop, 78
Ris de Veau Meunière, 227–229
risotto, Celery Root Risotto, 442
Riz au Chou-Fleur, 441
roast beef, Peppered Roast Beef, 141–142
Roasted Marrow Bones, 269
Roasted Summer Tomatoes with Herbs, 467
roasting garlic, 410
roasts
    barding, 81, 83, *83*
    beef, 114
    lamb, 192
        Bone-In Lamb Shoulder Roast, 195
        Deboned Lamb Shoulder Roast, 196
        "Frenched" Rack of Lamb or Bone-In Loin Roast, 194
        Milk-Fed Lamb Roast, 205
        Rolled Rack of Lamb or Deboned Loin Roast, 195
        Topside Roast, 195
    pork, 307
    Pork Roast Stuffed with Prunes and Tied, 308–309
    Pork Roast with *Herbes de Provence*, 305–306
    tying, 82–83, *82, 83, 84*
Rodgers, Diana, 94

Rognons d'Agneau à la Moutarde à l'Ancienne, 252–253
Rognons d'Agneau au Beurre et à l'Ail, 250–251
Rognons de Veau à la Moutarde à l'Ancienne, 277–279
Rognons de Veau, Pickles de Poires, 280–281
Rolle (Vermentino) grapes, 554
Rolled Lamb Saddle, 195
Rolled Rack of Lamb or Deboned Loin Roast, 195
Romorantin grapes, 553
root vegetables, 51–52, *51*
   Roasted Root Vegetables, 466
Root, Waverley, 2, 3, 18, 19, 21, 34, 98
Roquefort, 61
   Roquefort Sirloin Steak, 143
Rosbif au Poivre, 141–142
rosé wines, color spectrum, 529
rosemary, 42
   chopping, 66
   fresh vs. dried, 100
   Garlic and Rosemary Lamb, 191–192
   Grilled Rosemary Beef Skirt Steak, 135
   Rosemary Pork Ribs, 319–320
   Salted Pork with Lentils, 321–323
Rôti d'Agneau de Lait, 205
Rôti de Boeuf, 113–115
Rôti de Porc aux Herbes de Provence, 305–306
Rôti de Porc aux Pruneaux à la Ficelle, 308–309
Roussanne grapes, 555
routines
   bedtime, 567
   family mealtime, 570
   French great-grandmothers, 67
   value of, 567–569
roux, 397
   Béchamel Sauce, 392
   Brown Roux and White Roux, 397
Roux Brun et Roux Blanc, 397
rutabaga, 52

S

SAD diet (Standard American Diet), 32
saddle
   lamb, 195
   rabbit, 368–369, *332, 368, 369*
safflower oil, 41
sage, 100, *371*
Sage Butter Sirloin Steak, 145
Sailland, Maurice Edmond, 557
salad
   Beet Salad with Blood Orange, Walnut, and Goat Cheese, 438
   Traditional Salad from Nice, 476–477
Salade de Betteraves aux Oranges Sanguines, Noix et Chèvre, 438
Salade Niçoise, 476–477
Salatin, Joel, 18, 85, 87, 564, *565*
salmon
   Catch of the Day, 170–171
   Salmon Tartare, 180–181
salsify, 52
salt, 45–47, 67, 99
   Celtic sea salt, 99–100
   fleur de sel, 47, 100, *99*
   harvesting sea salt, 46–47, 178, *46, 179*

Himalayan salt, 46
pinch, 114
Rack of Pork in Crusted Salt, Ginger, and Garlic, 317–318
sea salt, 178–179
use in recipes, 99–100
salt-curing bacon, 85–87, *86, 87*
Salted Pork with Lentils, 321–323
Sanders, Veronique, 521, 557
Sardenne, Joel and Josiane, 123–124, *124*
sardines, Grilled Sardines with Garlic and Parsley, 173
Sardines Grillées à l'Ail et au Persil, 173
Sarlat Sautéed Potatoes, 468–469
saturated fat, 30–35
Sauce à Barbeque, 389
Sauce Allemande, 384–385
Sauce aux Anchois, 386–387
Sauce aux Crabes, 400–401
Sauce aux Foies de Volaille, 238–239
Sauce aux Prunes à l'Orange, 412
Sauce Béarnaise, 391
Sauce Béchamel, 392–393
Sauce Chantilly, 405
Sauce Hollandaise, 404–405
Sauce Mornay, 407–408
Sauce Mousseline, 368–369, 405
Sauce Rémoulade, 414
Sauce Suprême (Sauce Velouté à la Crème), 402
Sauce Velouté à la Crème (Sauce Suprême), 402
sauces, 381–382
   Allemande Sauce, 384–385
   Anchovy Sauce, 386–387
   Barbeque Sauce, 389
   Béarnaise Sauce, 391
   Béchamel Sauce, 392–393, *382*
   Coq au Vin, 345–348
   Crab Sauce, 400–401
   cream sauce, 129–130
   Cream Sauce (Supreme Sauce), 402
   deglazing, 156
   Fish Stock, 403
   Hollandaise Sauce, 404–405
   Homemade Mayonnaise, 406
   Mornay Cheese Sauce, 407–408
   mousseline, 368–369, 405
   orange sauce, 148
   tartar sauce (*rémoulade*)
   Spreadable Fish Paste, 186
   Tartar Sauce, 414
   wine sauce, 155–157
saucepans, 64–65, *64*
   use when making recipes, 103–104
sauerkraut, 52
   making, 52, *52*
   Pork Knuckle with Sauerkraut, 297–298
   Sauerkraut and Bacon, 471
Saulnier, Louis, 227
sausage
   making, 78–79, *78, 79*
   Morning Sausage Patties, 327
Sauté de Porc aux Pruneaux, 324–325
Sautéed Leeks and Bacon, 472–473
Sautéed Onions, 474

Sautéed Pork with Prunes, 324–325
Sautéed Swiss Chard, 474
Sautéed White Asparagus Slices, 475
Sauvignon Blanc grapes, 549, 550
Savagnin grapes, 551
Savoie-Bugey region of France/grape varieties, 555
scallops, Butter-Fried Scallops, 167–169
Schatzker, Mark, 575
Schmidt, Michael A., 33
Schmit, Alexandre, 515
Schneider, Sally, 17
school lunches in France, 21, 22
Schueller, Chef Frédéric. *See* Chef Frédéric Schueller
Sciaccarello grapes, 551
scoring
  cuttlefish, 179
  steaks, 155
scrambled eggs, Pyrénées Farm Scrambled Eggs, 360
sea bass, 184
sea bream, 182–183, *182, 183*
  filleting, 182–183, *182, 183*
  Sea Bream Fillets with Grilled Pine Nuts, 184–185
sea salt. *See* salt

seafood
  cod, 185
  Crab Sauce, 400–401
  cuttlefish, 179
  filleting fish, 182–183, *182, 183*
  haddock, 185
  oysters, 163–166
  sardines, 173
  sea bass, 184
  sea bream, 182–185, *182, 183*
  Tangy Seafood and Salad Dressing (Tartar Sauce), 414
  trout, 184
Sears, Dr. Barry, 589
seasonal butcher economics, 72–73
seasonal eating in France, 25–26
  appropriate seasons for recipes, 94
seeds, 47–49
  nut butters, 49
Seedy Crackers, 501–502
sel de mer fin, 47
Selle d'Agneau (or Quasi d'Agneau) Roulee, 195
Sémillon grapes, 549
servings and serving sizes, 96–97
sesame seed oil, 40
shallots, 45
  Bordeaux Oysters with Pork and Shallot Meatballs, 163–166
  Flank Steak with Shallots, 133–134
  Mackerel with Garlic and Shallots, 175–177
  Shallot and Vinegar Dip for Oysters, 413
Shanahan, Dr. Catherine (Cate), 20, 34, 41, 572, 575
shank, Slow-Cooked Beef Shank, 146–147
sharpening knives, 79–80, *79*
sheep. *See* lamb
Shiraz (Syrah) grapes, 554
Shoulder Chops (lamb), 194
Silent Spring (Carson), 15
silky tannins, 543
Simple Braised Beef Stew with Orange, 153

Simple Lamb Stew, 211
Simple Vinaigrette, 413
simple wine, 544
sirloin steak
  Flambéed Sirloin Steak with Cream Sauce, 129–130
  Flambéed Sirloin Steak with Sautéed Vegetables, 131–132
  Roquefort Sirloin Steak, 143
  Sage Butter Sirloin Steak, 145
Sirop et Gelée de Verveine à la Framboise, 499–500
Sisson, Mark, 40, 396, 513, 516, 590
skin
  Crispy Pork Rinds, 240–241
  Duck Rinds, 359
  skin and bones at a butcher's shop, 78
skirt steak, Grilled Rosemary Beef Skirt Steak, 135
sleep, 567–569
sliders, Pig's Feet Sliders, 259–261, *11*
slow cooking, 105
  Slow-Cooked Beef Cheeks, 271
  Slow-Cooked Beef Shank, 146–147
  Slow-Cooked Pork Cheeks with Apricots, 272–273
smoke point of fat/oil, 35
  avocado oil, 40
  duck, goose, and chicken fat, 37
  macadamia nut oil, 40
  olive oil, 38
  sesame seed oil, 40
  tallow, 37
snacks, 573–577
soaking
  legumes, 50
  nuts and seeds, 48
sommeliers, 102
soup. *See also* stocks
  Béarnaise Garbure Soup, 338–339
  faire chabrol, 339, 560
  French Onion Soup, 451–452
  stock/soup vocabulary, 396
Soupe à l'Oignon, 451–452
Souris d'Agneau en Croûte de Noix, 207
Southwest, 1–2
sovereignty of French wine, 514
soybean oil, 41
sparkling wines, 529
  balance, 536–537
spices, 43
  pinch, 114
spicy aromas, wine, 532
Spider Steak with Orange, 148–149
spitting out wine (*cracher*), 516
Spreadable Fish Paste, 186–187
Springtime Lamb Stew, 213–214
sprouting nuts and seeds, 48
squash
  butternut squash, *465*
  Kabocha Squash and Chestnut Soup, 454–455
squid, Basque Grilled Squid, 160–161
stainless-steel pans
  saucepans, 64–65, *64*
  using when making recipes, 103–104
Standard American Diet (SAD diet), 32

Staub cast-iron pots, 103
steak
　Bone-In Prime Rib, 125
　Flambéed Sirloin Steak with Cream Sauce, 129–130
　Flambéed Sirloin Steak with Sautéed Vegetables, 131–132
　Flank Steak with Shallots, 133–134
　Grilled Rosemary Beef Skirt Steak, 135
　Roquefort Sirloin Steak, 143
　Sage Butter Sirloin Steak, 145
　Slow-Cooked Beef Shank, 146–147
　Spider Steak with Orange, 148–149
　T-Bone Lamb Chops, 194
　Wine Trader's Rib Eye Steak, 155–157
stevia, 54
stew
　Braised Veal Stew, 422–423
　Simple Braised Beef Stew with Orange, 153
　Simple Lamb Stew, 211
　Springtime Lamb Stew, 213–214
　Veal Tagine Stew, 431–432
　Wine-Braised Beef Stew with Orange, 151–152
stocking your pantry, 67
stocks, 382
　Brown and White (or Light) Stock, 398–399
　freezing vegetable leftovers for use in stock, 396
　long-cooked in cast-iron pots, 105
　Veal Stock, 415–416
　White Poultry Stock, 417
stocks and sauces recipes, 381
　Allemande Sauce, 384–385
　Anchovy Sauce, 386–387
　Barbeque Sauce, 389
　Béarnaise Sauce, 391
　Béchamel Sauce, 392–393
　Bone Broth, 394–396
　Brown and White (or Light) Stock, 398–399
　Brown Roux and White Roux, 397
　Crab Sauce, 400–401
　Cream Sauce (Supreme Sauce), 402
　Fish Stock, 403
　Hollandaise Sauce, 404–405
　Homemade Mayonnaise, 406
　Mornay Cheese Sauce, 407–408
　Niçoise Vinaigrette, 409
　Old-Fashioned Mustard, 410
　Onion Marmalade, 411
　Orange Plum Sauce, 412
　Shallot and Vinegar Dip for Oysters, 413
　Simple Vinaigrette, 413
　Tangy Seafood and Salad Dressing (Tartar Sauce), 414
　Veal Stock, 415–416
　White Poultry Stock, 417
stocks and sauces recipes – French titles
　Bouillon de Volaille or *Fond Blanc de Volaille*, 417
　Confiture d'Oignons, 411
　Fond Brun et Fond Blanc, 398–399
　Fond de Veau, 415–416
　Fumet de Poisson, 403
　Le Bouillon, 394–396
　Mayonnaise Fait Maison, 406
　Moutarde à l'Ancienne, 410
　Roux Brun et Roux Blanc, 397
　Sauce à Barbeque, 389

Sauce Allemande, 384–385
Sauce aux Anchois, 386–387
Sauce aux Crabes, 400–401
Sauce aux Prunes à l'Orange, 412
Sauce Béarnaise, 391
Sauce Béchamel, 392–393
Sauce Hollandaise, 404–405
Sauce Mornay, 407–408
Sauce Rémoulade, 414
Sauce Velouté à la Crème (Sauce Suprême), 402
Une Vinaigrette Simple, 413
Vinaigre aux Echalotes pour les Huîtres, 413
Vinaigrette Niçoise, 409
string. *See* butcher's string
structured/tannic wine, 544
Stuffed Cabbage Leaves, 326–327
Stuffed Quail, 366–367
Stuffed Rabbit Saddle, 368–369
Stuffed Veal Cutlets, 427–429
Stuffed Whole Cabbage, 328–330
suet, 268
sugar, 53–54, 68
　health risks, 515–516
sugar alcohols, 54
sunflower oil, 41
sunflower seeds, 48
supple wine, 544
Supreme Sauce (Cream Sauce), 402
Sweet and Savory Crêpes, 503–504
sweet potatoes, Oven-Baked Sweet Potatoes, 460
sweet wines, 544
　balance, 537
　color, 529
sweetbreads, 227–229
Swiss chard, Sautéed Swiss Chard, 474
Sylvaner grapes, 546
Syrah grapes, 554

T

tagines (*tajines*), 53
　Beef Tagine Stew, 121–122
　Veal Tagine Stew, 431–432
Tajine de Boeuf, 121–122
Tajine de Veau, 431–432
tallow, 3, 37–38
　rendering, 268
Tan, Michelle, 575
Tangy Seafood and Salad Dressing (Tartar Sauce), 414
tannins
　tannic/structured wine, 544
　well-blended tannins, 544
Tante Lucie, 21
Tapestry of Bayeux, 129
tart, Berry Tart, 487
tartar sauce
　Spreadable Fish Paste, 186
　Tangy Seafood and Salad Dressing (Tartar Sauce), 414
tartare
　Salmon Tartare, 180–181
　Veal Tartare, 433–434
Tartare de Saumon, 180–181
Tartare de Veau, 433–434

Tarte aux Fruits des Bois, 487
The Taste of Wine (Peynaud), 531
tasting notes, wine, 538–540
tasting parties, 542
Taubes, Gary, 34
T-Bone Lamb Chops or Loin Chops, 194
tea, 56
Teflon-coated pans, 65
Teicholz, Nina, 21, 32, 33, 34, 218, 575
temperatures for wine storing/serving, 541
tenets of The Bordeaux Kitchen, 8–9
Téoulier grapes, 554
Terafeu cookware, 65, *65*
Terrine de Campagne des Pyrénées, 314–316
Terrine de Foie Gras aux Figues et à l'Armagnac, 244–247
terroir
   dairy and cheese, 58
   organic and biodynamic wines, 522
   and taste, 17
   wine growing, 517–518, 521–522
Teschke, Tania
   background/roots, 587–590
   illness and recovery, 7, 589–590
   motivation for *The Bordeaux Kitchen*, 4–5
   pictures
     butcher apprenticeship, *76, 89*
     Catherine and Guy-Pétrus Lignac, *422*
     DUAD wine course, *102, 103, 235, 559*
     Germany as a child, *587*
     Polyface Farm visit, *565*
     Saint Seurin Market in Bordeaux, *8*
     setting table, *592*
     Stephen Davis, *117*
     Teschke family portrait, *565, 585*
Teulé Goat Farm Market, 566, *566*
Teule's goat cheese farm, Bouliac, 62
thawing frozen foods, 104
The Thirty-Day Heart Tune-Up (Masley), 42
thyme, 42
Tibouren grapes, 554
timeline of food culture in France and the U.S., 13–15
Tomates d'Été Rôties au Herbes, 467
tomatoes
   blanching, 335
   Roasted Summer Tomatoes with Herbs, 467
tongue, 224–225
Topside Roast, 195
Toth, Stacy, 575
Le Tour de France de la Famille Oukile (Veillon), 17
towels, kitchen, 66
Traditional Salad from Nice, 476–477
Tranches Bacon Fumé à la Poêle, 293
Tranches de Poitrine Fumée au Four, 292
Tranches Fines d'Asperges Blanches Pôelées, 475
trans fats, 15
travelling, meal planning, 583–584
Tressalier grapes, 553
Tressot grapes, 550
Trousseau grapes, 551
trout, 184
truffles, 50–51
   Omelet with Herbs, 350

turkey recipes
   Turkey Cordon Bleu, 343
   Turkey Liver Pâté with Figs, 274
   Turkey Ragout, 370–371
turmeric, 52
turnip cabbage (kohlrabi), 52
turnips, 52, 97
tying with butcher's string, 81–84, *82, 83, 84*
   Pork Roast Stuffed with Prunes and Tied, 308–309

U

Ugni Blanc grapes, 552
Underground Wellness podcast, 589
Une Vinaigrette Simple, 413
US Wellness Meats, 579
USDA dietary guidelines, 15, 18
   cholesterol, 31
   food pyramid, 34
utensils, 65, 103–104

V

vacuum sealing meat, 84
vanilla, 505
   Vanilla "Burned" Cream, 505–508
varietal wine tasting, 542
veal cuts, 418
veal recipes, 419
   Basque Veal with Peppers, 420–421
   Braised Veal Shanks, 425–426
   Braised Veal Stew, 422–423
   offal
     Breaded Veal Sweetbreads "Meunière," 227–229
     Veal Kidneys in Old-Fashioned Mustard Sauce, 277–279
     Veal Kidneys with Pickled Pears, 280–281
     Veal Liver, 282–283
   Stuffed Veal Cutlets, 427–429
   Veal Cordon Bleu, 343
   Veal Stock, 416
   Veal Tagine Stew, 431–432
   Veal Tartare, 433–434
veal recipes – French titles
   abats
     Foie de Veau, 282–283
     Ris de Veau Meunière, 227–229
     Rognons de Veau à la Moutarde à l'Ancienne, 277–279
     Rognons de Veau, Pickles de Poires, 280–281
   Axoa, 420–421
   Blanquette de Veau, 422–423
   Fond de Veau, 415
   Osso Bucco (Jarret de Veau), 425–426
   Paupiettes de Veau, 427–429
   Tajine de Veau, 431–432
   Tartare de Veau, 433–434
"vegetable" oil, 41
vegetable recipes
   Beet Salad with Blood Orange, Walnut, and Goat Cheese, 438
   Cauliflower Gratin, 439–440
   Cauliflower "Rice," 441
   Celery Root Risotto, 442
   Cream of Green Peas, 443, *11*

Fennel with Red Onion, 445
Fermented Carrots, 446
Fermented Radishes, 447
Field Potatoes, 449
French Green Peas, 450
French Onion Soup, 451–452
Green Asparagus with Bacon and Hazelnuts, 453
Kabocha Squash and Chestnut Soup, 454–455
Mashed Jerusalem Artichokes, 456
Oven-Baked Beet Chips, 457
Oven-Baked French Fries, 459
Oven-Baked Sweet Potatoes, 460
Oven-Baked Zucchini, 461
Potato Gratin, 463
Pumpkin Soup, 464–465
Roasted Root Vegetables, 466
Roasted Summer Tomatoes with Herbs, 467
Sarlat Sautéed Potatoes, 468–469
Sauerkraut and Bacon, 471
Sautéed Leeks and Bacon, 472–473
Sautéed Onions, 474
Sautéed Swiss Chard, 474
Sautéed White Asparagus Slices, 475
Traditional Salad from Nice, 476–477
Vegetable "Clafoutis," 479
Zucchini with Walnuts and Goat Cheese, 481
vegetable recipes – French titles
Asperges aux Lardons et Noisettes, 453
Blettes Sautées, 474
Carottes Fermentées, 446
Célerisotto, 442
Chips de Betterave au Four, 457
Choucroute aux Lardons, 471
Clafoutis aux Légumes, 479
Courgettes au Four, 461
Courgettes aux Noix et au Fromage de Chèvre, 481
Crème de Petits Pois, 443
Fenouil et Onion Rouge, 445
Gratin Dauphinois, 463
Gratin de Choufleur, 439–440
Légumes Racines Rôtis, 466
Oignons Sautés, 474
Patates Douces au Four, 460
Petits Pois à la Française, 450
Poivrons Sautés aux Lardons, 472–473
Pommes de Terre des Champs, 449
Pommes de Terre Sarladaises, 468–469
Pommes Frites au Four, 459
Purée de Potiron, 464–465
Purée de Topinambour, 456
Radis Fermentés, 447
Riz au Chou-Fleur, 441
Salade de Betteraves aux Oranges Sanguines, Noix et Chèvre, 438
Salade Niçoise, 476–477
Soupe à l'Oignon, 451–452
Tomates d'Été Rôties au Herbes, 467
Tranches Fines d'Asperges Blanches Pôelées, 475
Velouté de Potimarron aux Chataignes, 454–455
vegetables
blanching tomatoes, 335
FODMAPs, 44, 394, 472

nightshades, 51
pickled, 52
roots, 51–52, *51*
seasonal eating in France, 26
vegetal or herbaceous aromas, wine, 532
vegetarian diet, 35
Veillon, Beatrice, 17
Velouté de Potimarron aux Chataignes, 454–455
Vermentino grapes, 551
  Malvoisie, 552
  Rolle, 554
Vert Blanc (Aubin Vert) grapes, 553
vertical wine tasting, 542
Viandes (Mallet), 87, 155, 213, 290, 297, 299
Vinaigre aux Echalotes pour les Huîtres, 413
vinaigrettes
  Niçoise Vinaigrette, 409
  Simple Vinaigrette, 413
vinegar, 53
  deglazing pans, 161
  Shallot and Vinegar Dip for Oysters, 413
vineyards
  tasks throughout the year, 523–525
  winegrowing regions of France. *See* winegrowing regions of France
vintages of wine, 527
Viognier grapes, 555
vitamins
  fat-soluble, 30, 33, 35, 38, 47
  vitamin D, and animal fats, 35, 37
  vitamin K2, 20, 36, 62

W

walnut oil, 40
walnuts
  Beet Salad with Blood Orange, Walnut, and Goat Cheese, 438
  Walnuts in Milk, 509–510
  Zucchini with Walnuts and Goat Cheese, 481
warm wine, 544
well-blended tannins, 544
Wellness Mama, 575
The Wellness Mama Cookbook (Wells), 575
Wells, Katie, 575
Weston A. Price Foundation, 20, 34, 36, 49
What to Drink with What You Eat (Dornenburg and Page), 173
Wheat Belly (Davis), 33
Wheaton, Barbara Ketcham, 13
White (or Light) Stock, 398–399
white asparagus, Sautéed White Asparagus Slices, 475
white pepper, 100, 137, 479, *100*
White Poultry Stock, 417
White Roux, 397
white wine
  balance, 536, *536*
  color spectrum, 529
Whole Beast Butchery (Farr), 220
Whole Roast Chicken with *Herbes de Provence*, 373–374
Whole Stuffed Duck, 375–376
Whole Stuffed Holiday Goose, 377–378
Why We Get Fat (Taubes), 34
Wi-Fi routers, 568

wine, 4
  aerating, carafing, decanting, 540–541
  aroma, 513–515, 531, 533–534
    balancing with meals, 559
  balance, 536–537, 543, *536, 537*
  barrels, 534, *535*
  body, 538
  bouquet, 533
  color, 528–531
  cooking wines, 155
  defects, 538
  faire chabrol, 339, 560
  fermentation process, 519
  flavor, 513–514, 534
    balancing with meals, 559
  geography, 516–519
  glasses, 540, *540*
  oaking, 534
  regional pairing of food and wine, 16–17
  tasting. *See* wine tasting
  temperatures for storing/serving, 541
  terminology, 543–544
  vintages, 527
wine bars, 542
wine cellars, building, 561
wine in French culture, 513
  ancestral context, 514
  geography of wine, 516–519
  growing up with wine, 514–515
  health risks of alcohol consumption, 515–516
  nature's cycles, 519–520
  organic and biodynamic wines, 520–522
  sensory experience, 513–514
  sovereignty of French wine, 514
  spitting out wine (*cracher*), 516
  training sense of smell, 515
wine pairing, 101–103, 557–560. *See also* individual recipes
  aperitif (before dinner), 557
  Bordeaux wines, 557
  cheese, 61
  main dish, 559
  questions to ask, 557–559
  rules of thumb, 559
  sweet wines, 560
wine sauce, 155–157
wine tasting, 527
  aerating, carafing, decanting wine, 540–541
  aroma, 531, 533–534
  balance, 536–537, *536, 537*
  body, 538
  bouquet, 533
  descriptors/language, 528–531
  detecting defects, 538
  discovery, 527
  flavors, 534
  glasses, 540, *540*
  "instant messaging" of wine, 531
  model/archetypical wines, 527–528
  protocol, 539–540
  serving temperatures, 541
  tasting notes, 538–540
  tasting parties, 542
Wine Trader's Rib Eye Steak, 155–157
Wine-Braised Beef Stew with Orange, 151–152
winegrowers
  fermentation of wine, 519
  following nature's cycles, 519–520
  organic and biodynamic wines, 520–521
  soil type, 518–519
  terroir, 517–518, 521–522
  water, 518
winegrowing regions of France, 545–556
  Alsace, 546
  Beaujolais, 546–547
  Bordeaux, 547–550
  Burgundy, 550
  Champagne, 550–551
  Corsica, 551
  Jura, 551
  Languedoc-Roussillon, 551–552
  Loire Valley, 552–553
  Lorraine, 553
  map, *512, 548*
  Provence, 553–554
  Rhone Valley, 554–555
  Savoie-Bugey, 555
  Southwest, 555–556
winemakers
  conditions necessary to make great wine, 526
  tasks throughout the seasons, 523–525
Wired to Eat (Wolf), 539, 575
Wolf, Robb, 539, 575
Wolfert, Paula, 17, 22, 143, 454
wood aromas, wine, 532

X

xylitol, 54

Z

zucchini
  Oven-Baked Zucchini, 461
  Vegetable "Clafoutis," 479
  Zucchini with Walnuts and Goat Cheese, 481